Prevention and Management of Cardiovascular and Metabolic Disease

Prevention and Management of Cardiovascular and Metabolic Disease

Diet, Physical Activity and Healthy Aging

Christina N. Katsagoni
Agia Sofia Children's Hospital, Thivon 1 & Papadiamantopoulou Str, Athens, GR, 11527

Peter Kokkinos
Rutgers University, 295 Halsey road, Annapolis, MD, US, 21401

Labros S. Sidossis
Rutgers University, 70 Lipman Drive, New Brunswick, NJ, US, 08901-8525

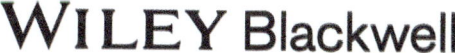

This edition first published 2023
© 2023 John Wiley & Sons Ltd

All rights reserved. No part of this publication may be reproduced, stored in a retrieval system, or transmitted, in any form or by any means, electronic, mechanical, photocopying, recording or otherwise, except as permitted by law. Advice on how to obtain permission to reuse material from this title is available at http://www.wiley.com/go/permissions.

The right of Christina N. Katsagoni, Peter Kokkinos, and Labros S. Sidossis to be identified as the authors of this work has been asserted in accordance with law.

Registered Office
John Wiley & Sons Ltd, The Atrium, Southern Gate, Chichester, West Sussex, PO19 8SQ, UK

For details of our global editorial offices, customer services, and more information about Wiley products visit us at www.wiley.com.

Wiley also publishes its books in a variety of electronic formats and by print-on-demand. Some content that appears in standard print versions of this book may not be available in other formats.

Trademarks: Wiley and the Wiley logo are trademarks or registered trademarks of John Wiley & Sons, Inc. and/or its affiliates in the United States and other countries and may not be used without written permission. All other trademarks are the property of their respective owners. John Wiley & Sons, Inc. is not associated with any product or vendor mentioned in this book.

Limit of Liability/Disclaimer of Warranty
The contents of this work are intended to further general scientific research, understanding, and discussion only and are not intended and should not be relied upon as recommending or promoting scientific method, diagnosis, or treatment by physicians for any particular patient. In view of ongoing research, equipment modifications, changes in governmental regulations, and the constant flow of information relating to the use of medicines, equipment, and devices, the reader is urged to review and evaluate the information provided in the package insert or instructions for each medicine, equipment, or device for, among other things, any changes in the instructions or indication of usage and for added warnings and precautions. While the publisher and authors have used their best efforts in preparing this work, they make no representations or warranties with respect to the accuracy or completeness of the contents of this work and specifically disclaim all warranties, including without limitation any implied warranties of merchantability or fitness for a particular purpose. No warranty may be created or extended by sales representatives, written sales materials or promotional statements for this work. The fact that an organization, website, or product is referred to in this work as a citation and/or potential source of further information does not mean that the publisher and authors endorse the information or services the organization, website, or product may provide or recommendations it may make. This work is sold with the understanding that the publisher is not engaged in rendering professional services. The advice and strategies contained herein may not be suitable for your situation. You should consult with a specialist where appropriate. Further, readers should be aware that websites listed in this work may have changed or disappeared between when this work was written and when it is read. Neither the publisher nor authors shall be liable for any loss of profit or any other commercial damages, including but not limited to special, incidental, consequential, or other damages.

Library of Congress Cataloging-in-Publication Data

Names: Katsagoni, Christina, N., author. | Kokkinos, Peter, author.| Sidossis, Labros S., author.
Title: Prevention and management of cardiovascular and metabolic disease : diet, physical activity and healthy aging / Christina N. Katsagoni, Peter Kokkinos, Labros S. Sidossis.
Description: First edition. | Chichester, West Sussex, UK ; [Hoboken] : Wiley-Blackwell, 2023. | Includes bibliographical references and index.
Identifiers: LCCN 2023013406 (print) | LCCN 2023013407 (ebook) | ISBN 9781119833444 (cloth) | ISBN 9781119833451 (adobe pdf) | ISBN 9781119833468 (epub)
Subjects: MESH: Cardiovascular Diseases–prevention & control | Metabolic Diseases–prevention & control | Exercise | Healthy Aging
Classification: LCC RC684.D5 (print) | LCC RC684.D5 (ebook) | NLM WG 120 | DDC 616.1/0654–dc23/eng/20230323
LC record available at https://lccn.loc.gov/2023013406
LC ebook record available at https://lccn.loc.gov/2023013407

Cover Design: Wiley
Cover Image: © Science Photo Library/Alamy Stock Photo,Simone van den Berg/Adobe Stock Photos, Explode/Shutterstock

Set in 9.5/12pts of STIXTwoText by Straive, Pondicherry, India

Contents

Preface — vii
List of Contributors — ix

UNIT 1
DIET AND PHYSICAL ACTIVITY AS DETERMINANTS OF HUMAN HEALTH

1. The Link between Sub-optimal Diet and Physical Inactivity with Non-communicable Diseases — 3
2. Lifestyle and Epigenetics — 19
3. Healthy/Prudent Diets and Health Benefits in Adults — 35

UNIT 2
BASIC CONCEPTS OF PHYSICAL ACTIVITY AND FITNESS

4. Definition of Fitness and Its Components — 63
5. Defining Physical Activity and Exercise — 69
6. Implications and Health Benefits of Physical Activity in Adults — 79

UNIT 3
DETERMINANTS OF HEALTHY AGING

7. Healthy Aging: Definition and Scope — 93
8. The Interface Between Healthy Aging, Longevity, and Disease — 105
9. Physiological Changes in Multiple Organ Systems Through Aging: Measuring and Monitoring Aging — 117
10. The Role of Plant-based Diets on Healthy Aging — 133
11. Physical Activity as a Determinant of Healthy Aging — 159

UNIT 4
CARDIOVASCULAR HEALTH, DIET, AND PHYSICAL ACTIVITY

12. Heart Failure — 171
13. Atrial/Flutter Fibrillation — 191
14. Endothelial Function — 205

UNIT 5
CARDIO-METABOLIC HEALTH, DIET, AND PHYSICAL ACTIVITY

15. Diabetes Mellitus — 223
16. Hypertension — 241

17 Dyslipidemia	259	**21** Cancer	347
18 Obesity and Metabolic Syndrome	275	**Appendix** Answers to Self-assessment Questions	367
19 Obstructive Sleep Apnea	299	Abbreviations	381
		Glossary	385
20 Chronic Kidney Disease	327	Index	393

Preface

Approximately 2500 years ago, the Greek physician and father of medicine Hippocrates wrote: *"If we could give every individual the right amount of nourishment and exercise, not too little and not too much, we would have found the safest way to health."* In more recent years, a plethora of scientific evidence supports this concept.

In this book, we present strong scientific evidence that supports the important role of proper diet and physical activity on the prevention and management of cardio-metabolic diseases and mortality. Our focus is on older adults and healthy aging, as the aging population is increasing globally and is expected to nearly double by 2050. Millions of deaths worldwide are attributed to some of today's most common diseases such as cardiovascular disease, obesity, type 2 diabetes mellitus, and others.

It is now well-accepted that individuals who follow a healthy lifestyle live longer and are in better health. Key health behaviors such as physical activity and healthy diet are among the factors that contribute to reducing the risk of chronic diseases, improving quality of life, and promoting healthy aging.

The main aim of this book is to provide health professionals, clinicians, and students in medical and health-related disciplines with the most recent scientific evidence on the impact of diet and physical activity in the prevention and management of several chronic diseases that are prevalent in aging populations. Our goal is to provide accurate and well-established knowledge and to identify gaps in our knowledge as well as new challenges for current and future health professionals in our quest to find the safest way to healthy aging via proper diet and physical activity.

This book can serve as a primer for all health-care professionals involved in the prevention and management of cardiovascular and metabolic conditions with a special focus on older adults, or in a research lab that studies some aspects of lifestyle in relation to healthy aging.

The book is divided into five units. In every chapter, readers are provided with the latest, in-depth scientific evidence in specific areas.

Unit 1: Diet and Physical Activity as Determinants of Human Health. In Unit 1, we discuss the dual role of lifestyle, e.g., the negative (unhealthy lifestyle) or positive (healthy lifestyle) effects on health. We first describe the link between a suboptimal diet and physical inactivity with non-communicable diseases. Next, we discuss the concept and mechanisms of epigenetics, presenting how lifestyle stimuli can change our gene expression. We finish this unit by describing the beneficial role of healthy/prudent diets on health.

Unit 2: Basic Concepts of Physical Activity and Fitness. Unit 2 begins with an introduction to the fundamental knowledge needed for both basic and more complex definitions of physical activity, exercise, and fitness. We then describe the implications and health benefits of physical activity in adults.

Unit 3: Determinants of Healthy Aging. In Unit 3, we begin with a discussion on aging and age-related disease (e.g., the definition of healthy aging, the interface between healthy aging, longevity, and disease, the physiological changes in multiple organ systems through aging, measuring and monitoring tools). Next, we emphasize the role of nutrients, foods, and healthy dietary patterns on aging. For example, we discuss in detail the Mediterranean dietary pattern, the Nordic diet, the Dietary Approaches to Stop Hypertension (DASH) diet, the vegetarian diet, and the Okinawan diet by presenting the latest evidence-based data on this topic. We finish this unit by including the applicability of metrics used in physical activity for older adults as well as mechanisms to reduce sarcopenia and frailty, common health issues in older adults. We hope that this section will be a useful guide in the hands of health professionals and clinicians who manage older-adult patients by acknowledging the instrumental role of diet and physical activity as determinants of healthy aging.

Unit 4: Cardiovascular Health, Diet, and Physical Activity. Unit 4 is devoted to specific cardiovascular diseases common in older adults, e.g., heart failure and atrial/flutter fibrillation as well as the loss of normal endothelial function as a hallmark of vascular diseases. We discuss the challenges faced in the assessment and management of these diseases in adults and older adults. We also present specific exercise training and dietary interventions for these populations.

Unit 5: Cardio-metabolic Health, Diet, and Physical Activity. In Unit 5, we describe the most common metabolic diseases, which include diabetes mellitus, hypertension, dyslipidemia, obesity, metabolic syndrome, obstructive sleep apnea, chronic kidney disease, and obesity-induced cancers. Most of these conditions require a weight-loss intervention as part of the strategy to prevent and manage the disease. We provide evidence on the impact of diet- or exercise-alone interventions on muscle physiology in these patients and older adults. We also discuss the synergistic effects of diet and physical activity in achieving optimal health.

Some of the distinctive features of the book are:

1. Well-established knowledge related to cardiovascular and metabolic diseases that affect human health.

2. Applicability to those interested in studying or working with older-adult patients.
3. An easy-to-use and read format that can be used for undergraduate and graduate teaching.
4. The latest evidence-based data to describe some of the healthiest dietary patterns according to the 2015 Dietary Guidelines for Americans: the Mediterranean-style eating pattern, the DASH diet, the Nordic dietary pattern, and the vegetarian-type dietary pattern.
5. Highlighted main messages (key points) at the end of each chapter.
6. Over 200 "Self-assessment Questions" and answers that offer readers the most comprehensive, and up-to-date coverage in relation to the material presented in the book.
7. Useful links and related bibliographies at the end of each chapter with patent-related information and services.
8. A collection of clinical "Case scenarios" at the end of each chapter in Units 4 and 5, for students and health professionals to enhance their knowledge and practice skills relevant to each clinical condition.

We hope that this book can serve as a valuable tool to students in medical and health-related disciplines and to health professionals, including dietitians and nutritionists, exercise physiologists, athletic trainers, nurses, physicians, geriatricians, and other health professionals. We hope that the information included in this book will advance the implementation of non-pharmacological strategies that include proper dietary and exercise interventions to better manage cardiovascular and metabolic diseases in adults and older adults, ultimately leading to healthy aging.

We are grateful to Ioanna Katsaroli MSc, Mara Alepoudea cMMedSci, Athanasia Kyrkili MSc, Alexandros Tsigkas MSc, Michael Georgoulis PhD, Natasha Kolomvotsou PhD, Eleftheria Papachristou MSc, Despoina Chaloutsi, and Alexandra Foskolou PhD. These passionate young scientists contributed tremendously to completing this book with thorough literature reviews, drafting and editing chapters, and helping during the final stages of book editing. Last, but not least we would like to thank the Wiley team for their dedication and professionalism; Mandy Collison, Tom Marriott, Ranjith Kumar Thanigasalam, Anitha Jasmine Stanley, and Ada Hagan, PhD.

We would like also to thank our families for their continuous love and support.

Christina N. Katsagoni, PhD
Athens, Greece

Peter Kokkinos, PhD
Annapolis, Maryland, USA

Labros S. Sidossis, PhD
Princeton, New Jersey, USA

AUTHORS

Christina N. Katsagoni, PhD is a Clinical Dietitian at Agia Sofia Children's Hospital; Research Associate at the Department of Nutrition and Dietetics, School of Health Sciences and Education, Harokopio University of Athens, Greece; and post-doctoral researcher at the Department of Kinesiology and Health at Rutgers University, NJ, USA

Peter Kokkinos, PhD, FACSM, FAHA is a Professor in the Department of Kinesiology and Health at Rutgers University, New Brunswick, NJ, USA; Professor of Medicine at George Washington University School of Medicine and Health Sciences; and Physiologist in the Cardiology Department at the Veterans Affairs Medical Center, Washington DC, USA.

Labros S. Sidossis, PhD is a Distinguished Professor at the Department of Kinesiology and Health at Rutgers University, NJ, USA; Professor of Medicine at Robert Wood Johnson Medical School; and President of the Mediterranean Lifestyle Medicine Institute.

List of Contributors

Alepoudea Maria, cMMedSci
Nutritionist-Dietitian, Sfantos and Partners
cMMedSci in General Pediatrics and Pediatric Subspecialties, National and Kapodistrian University of Athens
Research Associate, Department of Nutrition and Dietetics, School of Health Sciences and Education, Harokopio University of Athens, Greece

Foscolou Alexandra, PhD
Dietitian-Nutritionist, Epidemiologist
PhD in Nutritional Epidemiology, Department of Nutrition and Dietetics, School of Health Sciences and Education, Harokopio University of Athens, Greece

Katsaroli Ioanna, MSc
Clinical Dietitian-Nutritionist,
MSc in Sport Science, Department of Nutrition and Dietetics, School of Health Sciences and Education, Harokopio University of Athens, Greece

Kolomvotsou Natasha, PhD
Chief Clinical Dietitian, Polyclinic of Olympic Village, Athens, Greece
PhD in the Department of Food Science & Human Nutrition at the Agricultural University of Athens-Greece

Kyrkili Athanasia, MSc
Dietitian-Nutritionist,
MSc in Clinical Nutrition, Research Associate, Department of Nutrition and Dietetics, School of Health Sciences and Education, Harokopio University of Athens, Greece

Georgoulis Michael, PhD
Dietitian-Nutritionist
Post Doctoral Researcher, Department of Nutrition and Dietetics, School of Health Sciences and Education, Harokopio University of Athens, Greece

Pantelis-Tsigkas Alexandros, MSc
Dietitian-Nutritionist,
MSc in Clinical Nutrition, Research Associate, Department of Nutrition and Dietetics, School of Health Sciences and Education, Harokopio University of Athens, Greece

Papachristou Eleftheria, MSc
Clinical Dietitian-Nutritionist,
MSc in Clinical Nutrition, Department of Nutrition and Dietetics, School of Health Sciences and Education, Harokopio University of Athens, Greece

Diet and Physical Activity as Determinants of Human Health

UNIT 1

The Link between Sub-optimal Diet and Physical Inactivity with Non-communicable Diseases

CHAPTER 1

Introduction	3
Sub-optimal Diet in Terms of Nutrients	5
Low Dietary Fiber Intake	5
High Dietary Sodium Intake	5
High Saturated Fatty Acid Intake	7
High Trans Fatty Acids Intake	7
Sub-optimal Diet in Terms of Foods and Food Groups	7
Low Consumption of Fruits and Vegetables	7
Low Consumption of Whole-grain Products	8
High Intake of Added/Free Sugar and Sweetened Beverages	8
Foods and Food Groups Rich in Saturated Fatty Acids	9
High Processed-meat Consumption	10
Sub-optimal Diet in Terms of Dietary Patterns	11
The Western Dietary Pattern	11
Physical Inactivity	11
Key Points	13
Self-assessment Questions	14
References	14
Further Reading	16
Bibliography	16
Links	17

INTRODUCTION

Non-communicable diseases (NCDs), also known as chronic diseases, are medical conditions linked with genetic, physiological, behavioral, and environmental factors among others. NCDs are the leading cause of death worldwide, equivalent to 71% of all deaths globally (WHO, 2021). The NCDs with the highest numbers of deaths globally are cardiovascular diseases (CVDs) followed by cancers, respiratory diseases, and diabetes mellitus (DM). Other health problems included under the umbrella of NCDs are obesity, hypertension, gastrointestinal diseases, liver, and renal disorders. Although nothing can be done about non-modifiable risk factors such as age, gender, genetic factors, race, and ethnicity, most of these disorders could be prevented if behavioral and metabolic changes are achieved (Budreviciute et al., 2020). Key metabolic changes that increase the risk of NCDs include hypertension, overweight/obesity, hyperglycemia, and hyperlipidemia (WHO, 2021). The main modifiable behavioral risk factors involve unhealthy diets (i.e., specific nutrients, foods, and food groups as well as dietary patterns) physical inactivity, tobacco use, and alcohol abuse. In 2017, a sub-optimal diet was responsible for more deaths than any other risks globally, including tobacco smoking: 11 million deaths and 255 million disability-adjusted life-years (DALYs; 22% of all deaths and 15% of all DALYs in adults aged 25 years or older) (**Figure 1.1**) (Murray et al., 2020).

With regards to nutrients, high sodium intake (defined by WHO [World Health Organization] as >2 g/day, equivalent to 5 g salt/day) ranks first for mortality worldwide (Murray et al., 2020). High sodium intake contributes to high blood pressure and increases the overall risk for stroke and heart disease. Moreover, the low intake of whole grains and fruit along with high sodium intake constitute more than half of all diet-related deaths and two-thirds of diet-related DALYs (Forouhi & Unwin, 2019). Sub-optimal intake of fruits and vegetables increases the risk for ischemic heart disease, stroke, and gastrointestinal cancers. Also, a high consumption of processed meat is associated with increased all-cause mortality as well as several types of cancer, DM and CVD mortality.

Prevention and Management of Cardiovascular and Metabolic Disease: Diet, Physical Activity and Healthy Aging,
First Edition. Christina N. Katsagoni, Peter Kokkinos, and Labros S. Sidossis.
© 2023 John Wiley & Sons Ltd. Published 2023 by John Wiley & Sons Ltd.

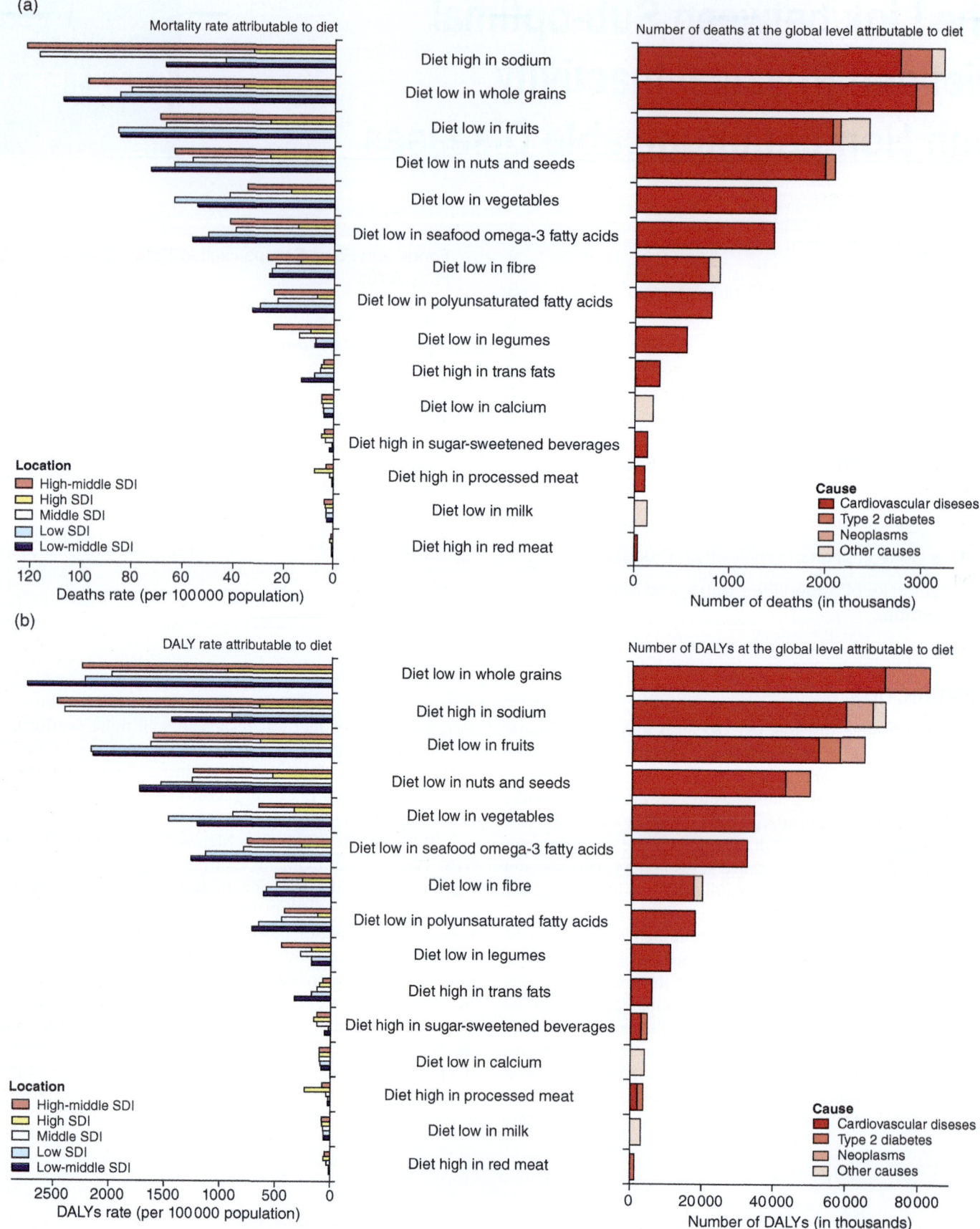

FIGURE 1.1 (a) Number of deaths and DALYs and (b) age-standardized mortality rate and DALY rate (per 100 000 population) attributable to individual dietary risks at the global and SDI level in 2017. DALY = disability-adjusted life-year. SDI = Socio-demographic Index. Source: Adapted from (Afshin et al., 2019).

Along with sub-optimal diet, according to a 2010 WHO report (WHO, 2010), insufficient physical activity was the fourth leading risk factor for mortality, leading to 3.2 million deaths and 32.1 million DALYs (about 2.1% of global DALYs) annually. In 2016, 27.5% of adults globally were insufficiently physically active.

In the following paragraphs, we will focus on the link between a sub-optimal diet and physical inactivity with NCDs.

SUB-OPTIMAL DIET IN TERMS OF NUTRIENTS

LOW DIETARY FIBER INTAKE

Based on a 2017 Global Burden of Disease (GBD) report, in the European Union (EU), the deaths and DALYs attributable to a diet low in fiber (defined as an average daily consumption of <23.5 g/day) account for approximately 97 000 deaths and more than 1 440 000 DALYs, mainly ischemic heart disease as well as colon and rectal cancer (European Commission. Health Promotion and Disease Prevention Knowledge Gateway; Stanaway et al., 2018).

Fiber, according to the US Food and Drug Administration (FDA), is the edible part(s) of plants that are resistant to digestion and absorption in the human small intestine. Good fiber sources are whole grains, vegetables, pulses, and some fruits. Based on their physicochemical characteristics, namely their solubility in water (i.e., they dissolve in water), their viscosity (i.e., the degree of resistance to flow), and their fermentation in the colon, they are categorized as soluble (fermentable)—like pectin, gum, mucilage, β-glucan and polydextrose—and insoluble (non-fermentable)—like cellulose, resistance starches, chitosan, hemicellulose, and lignin—fibers (**Figure 1.2**) (Gill, Rossi, Bajka, & Whelan, 2021). Fiber, like carbohydrates, fats, and proteins, is a source of metabolic energy for the human body and provides, on average, 2 kcal/g (European Commission. Health Promotion and Disease Prevention Knowledge Gateway).

Dietary fiber is considered a protective nutrient against the risk of NCDs, namely type 2 diabetes (T2D), CVDs, and colorectal cancer as well as a reduced risk of gaining weight. This is because high fiber intake improves gut microbiome diversity while increasing the production of short-chain fatty acids (SCFAs) and reduces the risk of obesity and other diseases such as DM and inflammation.

In an umbrella review of systematic reviews with 18 meta-analyses (that included 298 prospective observational studies), the highest versus the lowest quantile of dietary fiber intake was associated with a lower risk of CVD (i.e., coronary artery disease and CVD-related death). Evidence also associate the highest category of dietary fiber intake compared to the lowest with a lower risk of several cancers (e.g., pancreatic, gastric, esophageal adenocarcinoma, colon, endometrial, breast, and renal), stroke, and T2D (Veronese et al., 2018).

According to the Dietary Reference Intakes (DRIs) recommended by the United States Department of Agriculture (USDA), the adequate daily intake of fiber from all sources including fruits, vegetables, grains, legumes, and pulses is 14 g per 1,000 kcal, which is approximately 25 g/day for women and 38 g/day for men (European Commission. Health Promotion and Disease Prevention Knowledge Gateway).

HIGH DIETARY SODIUM INTAKE

Although the global age-standardized rates of deaths and DALYs attributable to high sodium intake decreased for both sexes between 1990 and 2019, the total absolute number of deaths and

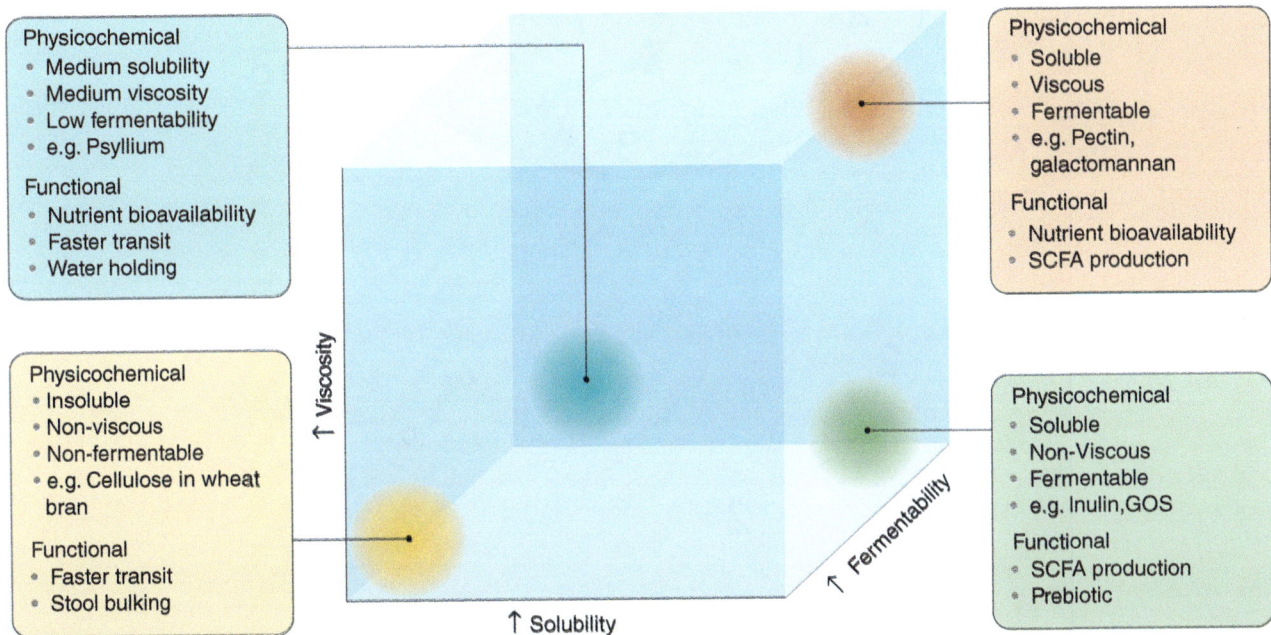

FIGURE 1.2 Spectrum of the physicochemical characteristics of dietary fiber. The physicochemical characteristics of fiber (solubility, viscosity, and fermentability) form a continuum and work in concert to determine its functional properties in the gastrointestinal tract. The combination of these three physicochemical characteristics determines the functional effects of fiber in the gut. Source: (Gill et al., 2020).

DALYs have increased due to population growth and aging (Chen, Du, Wu, Cao, & Sun, 2021). As most of the diseases associated with high sodium intake are age-related, the burden is expected to increase. Indeed, there is a long-standing association between high dietary sodium intake and hypertension as well as CVD (Rhee, 2015). This is related to water retention, systemic peripheral resistance increase, changes in the endothelial function, changes within the structure and function of large elastic arteries, altered activity of the sympathetic system, and altered autonomic neuronal modulation of the cardiovascular system (Grillo, Salvi, Coruzzi, Salvi, & Parati, 2019). High sodium intake is also associated with an increased risk of kidney disease and stomach cancer (Chen et al., 2021).

Numerous meta-analyses have indicated the positive association, either linear or U-shaped, between CVD risk and high sodium intake. In a 2020 meta-analysis of 36 cohort studies that included 616 905 participants, researchers identified a linear relationship between dietary sodium intake and CVD risk, with an increase in risk up to 6% for every 1 g increase in sodium intake per day (Y.-J. Wang, Yeh, Shih, Tu, & Chien, 2020). The U-shaped association was supported in another meta-analysis of cohort studies in which participants with both low (<115 mmol) and high (>215 mmol) sodium intakes had higher mortality compared to participants with a recommended dietary sodium intake (115–215 mmol) (Graudal, Jürgens, Baslund, & Alderman, 2014).

Salt (a combination of sodium and chloride) is the major source of sodium in the diet. Classic sources of salt are processed foods, ready-to-eat meals, salt added during food preparation and cooking as well as table salt (Y.-J. Wang et al., 2020) (**Figure 1.3**). The WHO recommends an overall sodium intake of less than 2 000 mg/day of sodium (<5 g of salt/day)

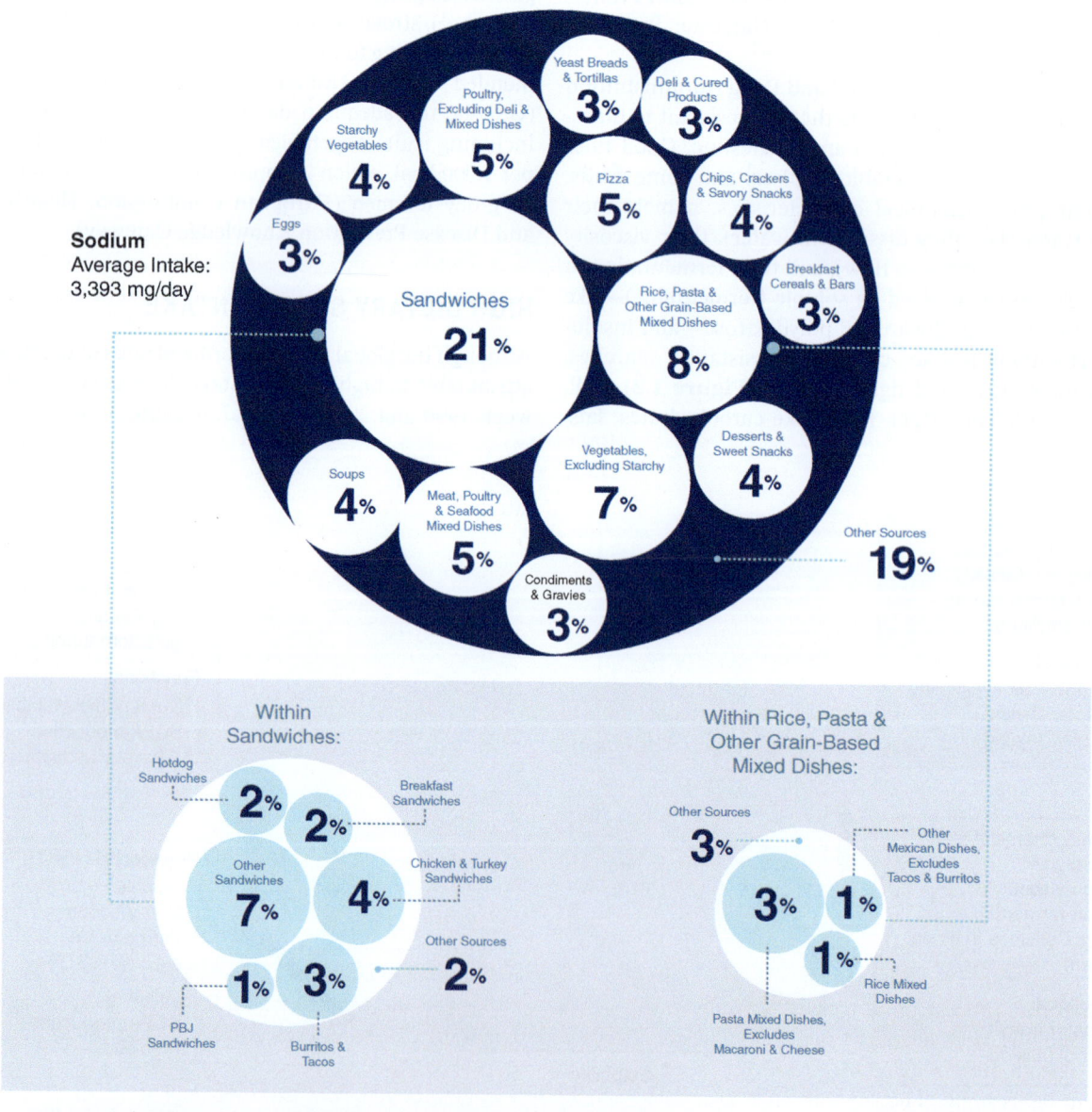

FIGURE 1.3 Source and average intake of sodium for US populations ages 1 and older. Source: (US Department of Agriculture and US Department of Health and Human Services. Dietary Guidelines for Americans, 2020-2025).

(WHO, 2012), whereas the 2020–2025 US Dietary Guidelines for adults recommend limiting sodium intake to 2 300 mg/day (US Department of Agriculture and US Department of Health and Human Services. Dietary Guidelines for Americans, 2020–2025). However, the average sodium intake across the US exceeds these recommendations at 3 393 mg/day (range 2000–5000mg/day) for those ages 1 and older (US Department of Agriculture and US Department of Health and Human Services. Dietary Guidelines for Americans, 2020–2025).

A reduction in dietary sodium can reduce blood pressure in both hypertensive and normotensive individuals, regardless of sex and ethnic group, as well as the incidence of hypertension; it was also linked to a reduction in morbidity and mortality from CVDs (Grillo et al., 2019). More details will be discussed in **Chapter 16**.

HIGH SATURATED FATTY ACID INTAKE

Over the last decade, numerous studies have investigated the role of saturated fats on several cardiovascular outcomes, but they fail to demonstrate rigorous evidence that supports continued recommendations to either limit saturated fatty acid (SFA) consumption or replace them with poly-unsaturated fatty acids (PUFAs) like omega-3 (Astrup et al., 2021). However, the 2020–2025 Dietary Guidelines for Americans continued the recommendation to limit SFAs to 10% or less of total energy intake, based on insufficient and inconsistent evidence (Dietary Guidelines Advisory Committee, 2020).

Indeed, results from clinical trials data are inconclusive. Although researchers concluded that reducing dietary saturated fat for at least 2 years could reduce the risk of combined cardiovascular events by 21%, a systematic review of 15 randomized controlled trials (RCTs) with about 59 000 participants, found little or no effect of reducing saturated fat on all-cause mortality or cardiovascular mortality, including non-fatal myocardial infarction, stroke, and coronary heart disease (CHD) events. Little or no effect was also found for cancer diagnoses, DM diagnosis, HDL cholesterol, serum triglycerides, or blood pressure. There were small reductions in weight, serum total cholesterol, LDL cholesterol, and BMI (Hooper et al., 2020).

Similarly, the epidemiological data from several meta-analyses of prospective observational studies have shown no significant associations between SFA consumption and CHD or CVD (Heileson, 2020).

HIGH TRANS FATTY ACIDS INTAKE

Trans fatty acids (TFAs) are unsaturated fatty acids with one or more unconjugated double bonds in the trans configuration. They are present in foods from ruminant animals (i.e., cattle, sheep, goats, and camels), although most are generated during the manufacturing processing of partially hydrogenated vegetable and marine oils, such as margarines, confectionery fats, and fat spreads. The amount of TFAs in partially hydrogenated vegetable oils can be as high as 60%. Foods that commonly contain margarine, such as deep-fried foods, baked goods, and snacks are therefore high in TFAs. Compared to animal fats, hydrogenated vegetable oils are more stable and less likely to become rancid during repeated deep-frying processes. Thus, they are widely used commercially (Oteng & Kersten, 2019).

Collectively, evidence strongly suggests that industrial TFA consumption is associated with increased risk of CHD-related mortality and CVD. Therefore, several countries have passed laws that either restrict or completely ban food companies from incorporating TFAs into their food products. However, there is an ongoing debate as to whether industrially or naturally produced ruminant TFAs exert the same effects on cardiovascular health (Pipoyan et al., 2021).

A meta-analysis of RCTs that explored naturally occurring or industrially produced TFAs and plasma LDL-to-HDL ratios revealed that, independent of their source, all TFAs could lead to an increase in the LDL-to-HDL ratio. However, a systematic review and meta-analysis of prospective studies found that industrially produced, but not naturally occurring TFAs, are associated with an increased risk of CHD. Interestingly, new evidence supports that specific animal-derived TFAs do not have detrimental health effects but may be beneficial for human health (Pipoyan et al., 2021). In a 2016 systematic review and meta-analysis authorized by the WHO, replacing total or industrial TFAs with either cis-MUFA or cis-PUFA improved lipid and lipoprotein profiles, which further lead to a reduction of CVD risk.

According to a 2020 review, mechanistically, in vivo and in vitro studies show that industrial TFAs might promote inflammation, endoplasmic reticulum (ER) stress, and fat storage in the liver instead of adipose tissue, compared with cis-unsaturated fatty acids and SFAs (Oteng & Kersten, 2020).

Therefore, in 2018, the WHO published an action package to reduce the TFA use in the global food supply called the 'REPLACE action package' (**Figure 1.4**). Based on a six-step strategy, each country should implement actions to eliminate industrially produced TFAs.

SUB-OPTIMAL DIET IN TERMS OF FOODS AND FOOD GROUPS

LOW CONSUMPTION OF FRUITS AND VEGETABLES

The low consumption of fruit and vegetables is associated with an increased risk of CVD, T2D, and cancer. The WHO recommends eating five portions of fruit and vegetables per day (equivalent to 400 g).

According to a meta-analysis of 27 prospective cohort studies as well as the results from the Nurses' Health Study (1984–2014, 66 719 women) and the Health Professionals Follow-up Study (1986–2014, 42 016 men), fruit and vegetable intake was inversely associated with with total mortality and cause-specific mortality attributable to cancer, CVD, and respiratory disease. Interestingly, consuming about 5 servings/day of fruit and vegetables, or two fruit servings and three vegetable servings, was associated with the lowest mortality, without additional risk reduction at higher intakes (D. D. Wang et al., 2021).

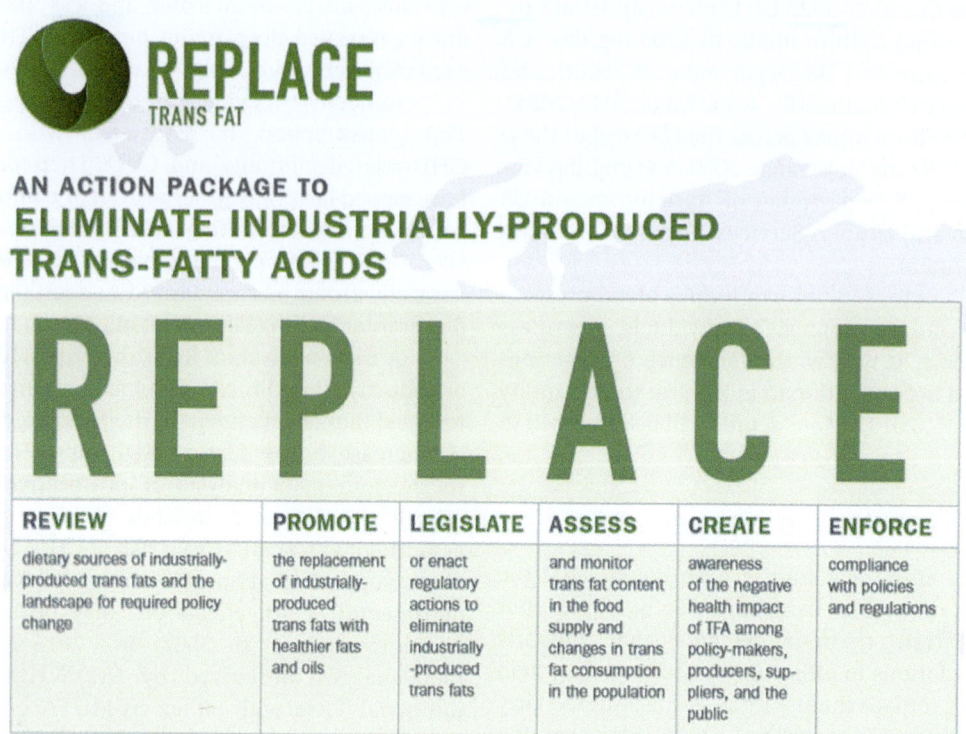

FIGURE 1.4 The 'REPLACE' action package developed by the WHO to reduce trans fatty acids from the global food supply. Source: [https://www.who.int/teams/nutrition-and-food-safety/replace-trans-fat (accessed 3 May 2022)].

LOW CONSUMPTION OF WHOLE-GRAIN PRODUCTS

In 2017, the Healthy Grain Forum (Ross et al., 2017) in accordance with the International Carbohydrate Quality Consortium (ICQC) Scientific Consensus on Whole Grains, published a definition for whole-grain foods. According to this definition, a food might be labeled as whole grain "if it contains at least 30% whole-grain ingredients in the overall product and more whole grain than refined grain ingredients, both on a dry-weight basis" (Ross et al., 2017).

A low consumption of whole-grain food products usually leads to a low fiber intake (especially insoluble fractions) as well as B vitamins, minerals, and phytochemicals with antioxidant properties, all of which are linked to many health benefits.

Epidemiological data support that the high intake of whole grains is correlated with decreased mortality from CVD as well as the prevention and management of T2D (Tieri et al., 2020). Moreover, whole grains are considered an important factor for maintaining a healthy body weight and reducing the risk of obesity (Tieri et al., 2020).

Despite the health benefits from high consumption, the intake of whole grains globally is lower than general recommendations, which increases the risk for mortality associated with chronic disease (Tieri et al., 2020). With regards to morbidity, low whole-grain intake is associated with the highest number of DALYs (Murray et al., 2020).

There are several recommendations for the daily consumption of whole grains; in the USA, it is recommended to consume at least 85 g/day (Arnold, Harding, & Conley, 2021), while in European countries, such as Denmark, it is 75 g or 10 megajoules (MJ, 2 388 kcal) per day (Frølich, Åman, & Tetens, 2013).

HIGH INTAKE OF ADDED/FREE SUGAR AND SWEETENED BEVERAGES

The WHO defines added/free sugar as "monosaccharides and disaccharides added to foods and beverages by the manufacturer, cook, or consumer, and sugars naturally present in honey, syrups, fruit juices, and fruit juice concentrates" (WHO, 2015).

In many high-income countries, sugar-sweetened beverages and added/free sugars are consumed above the recommended daily limits (**Table 1.1**), while it is on the rise in low- and middle-income countries.

This is a major problem for public health, as there is a strong association between a high sugar diet and obesity, which was stated in 2015 reports from both the WHO (WHO, 2015) and the UK's Scientific Advisory Committee on Nutrition (SACN) (Carbohydrates and Health Report, 2015). Added/free sugars, particularly those coming from sugar-sweetened beverages (SSBs), increase overall energy intake while lowering the intake of nutritional foods, leading to an unhealthy diet, weight gain, and increased risk of NCDs (WHO, 2015). A major concern is also the positive association between free sugar intake and dental caries. Similarly, results from prospective cohort studies have linked SSBs to an increased risk of T2D (Moore & Fielding, 2016). Both obesity and T2D are important risk factors for cardio-metabolic diseases, which supports the evidence that a very high sugar diet could also be associated with CVD mortality (Moore & Fielding, 2016).

Table 1.1 Recently published recommendations on the consumption of dietary sugars.

Organization (year)	Recommendations
2020–2025 Dietary Guidelines for Americans (US Department of Agriculture and US Department of Health and Human Services. Dietary Guidelines for Americans, 2020)	Consume less than 10% of calories per day from added sugars.
World Health Organization (2015) (WHO, 2015)	The intake of free sugars should be reduced to less than 10% of total energy intake in both adults and children.
UK Scientific Advisory Committee on Nutrition (SACN) (2015) (Carbohydrates and Health Report, 2015)	The average population intake of free sugars should not exceed 5% of the total dietary energy for age groups from 2 years onward.
2015–2020 Dietary Guidelines for Americans (2015) (US Department of Health and Human Services and US Department of Agriculture, 2015)	Consume less than 10% of calories per day from added sugars.
Australian National Health and Medical Research Council (2013) (Australian Guidelines, 2013)	Limit intake of foods and drinks containing added sugars such as confectionery; sugar-sweetened soft drinks and cordials; fruit drinks; vitamin waters; energy and sport drinks.
European Food Safety Authority (2010) (EFSA Panel on Dietetic Products & Allergies, 2010)	The available evidence is insufficient to set an upper limit for the intake of (added) sugars based on their effects on body weight or a risk reduction of dental caries.

Source: (Moore and Fielding, 2016).

The harmful association between SSBs and several health outcomes may reflect a general unhealthy lifestyle whereby individuals with greater SSB intake are more likely to have a poorer diet quality, higher caloric intake, and a sedentary lifestyle (Semnani-Azad et al., 2020). The pathophysiology behind the high amounts of sugar consumption via SSBs and ultra-processed foods is that the latter may lead to the production of high reactive oxygen-carbons (ROCs), which further increases the possibility of atherosclerosis, hypertension, peripheral vascular disease, coronary artery disease, cardiomyopathy, heart failure, and cardiac arrhythmia (Haque et al., 2020).

Based on the aforementioned evidence, most scientific organizations, in order to limit the rising trends of obesity and related metabolic diseases, suggest reducing total dietary intake of added/free sugars to 5% to 10% of total energy intake (**Table 1.1**).

Nevertheless, the effect of specific dietary sugars, e.g., glucose, fructose and others, on metabolism and human health is less clear (Moore & Fielding, 2016). Especially when considering that the postprandial glucose response, commonly known as the glycemic index used to measure the blood glucose-raising potential of foods, varies between people, as it is affected by several factors such as the gut microbiome, anthropometric data, physical activity, and blood lipids (Zeevi et al., 2015).

However, it seems that the effects of total sugars, added sugars or specific dietary sugars in human health depends on the consumed amount. In a systematic review and dose-response meta-analysis of 10 prospective cohort studies, including 624 128 individuals with 11 856 cases of CVD incidence and 12 224 cases of CVD mortality (Khan et al., 2019), authors investigated the relation of total and added fructose-containing sugars with CVD risk. A harmful association of total sugars, fructose, and added sugars with CVD mortality was found for intakes above 133 g (26% energy) of total sugars, 58 g (11% energy) of fructose, and 65 g (13% energy) of added sugars. No harmful association was found with lower intake of these sugars or at any dose for sucrose (Khan et al., 2019).

Attention should be given to other major food sources of fructose-containing sugars such as yogurt, fruit, 100% fruit juice, and mixed-fruit juice, as the latest data support the notion of a possible, even protective role, of those foods with cardio-metabolic conditions such as metabolic syndrome. In a systematic review and meta-analysis of 13 prospective cohort studies (including 49 591 participants and 14 205 metabolic syndrome cases), although a positive association was found between SSBs and the risk of metabolic syndrome incidence, an L-shaped protective dose-response association was observed for yogurt and fruit with metabolic syndrome (Semnani-Azad et al., 2020). Regarding fruit juices (mixed and 100%), a U-shaped dose-response association was found, suggesting a protective association between 75 and 150 mL/d but an adverse association for more than 175 to 200 mL/d. Yogurt, fruit, and 100% fruit juices are highly nutritious food groups.

FOODS AND FOOD GROUPS RICH IN SATURATED FATTY ACIDS

Whole-fat dairy products, unprocessed meat, eggs, and dark chocolate were thought to increase the risk of CVD due to their high SFA content. However, it is now apparent that the relationship or effect of any food cannot be predicted by its nutrient content without considering the overall macronutrient distribution (**Figure 1.5**) (Astrup et al., 2020).

Robust evidence from prospective and clinical trial studies show no increase, or even a small benefit, in CVD risk from full-fat dairy consumption (Giosuè, Calabrese, Vitale, Riccardi, & Vaccaro, 2022). Based on an umbrella review of observational studies, there is also convincing and probable evidence of a decreased risk of colorectal cancer, hypertension, elevated blood pressure, and fatal stroke as well as a possible decreased risk of breast cancer, metabolic syndrome, stroke, and T2D (Godos et al., 2020). The potential mechanisms of the attenuating effects of dairy foods remain to be fully elaborated, but seem to involve food matrix effects on fat bioavailability and changes in the gut microbiome as well as glucose, insulin, and other hormonal responses (Giosuè et al., 2022).

Eggs are rich in SFAs. However, they provide important nutrients such as high-quality protein, iron, other minerals, vitamins, and carotenoids. Several meta-analyses of prospective studies have concluded that higher egg consumption is not associated with CHD risk and may be associated with a lower

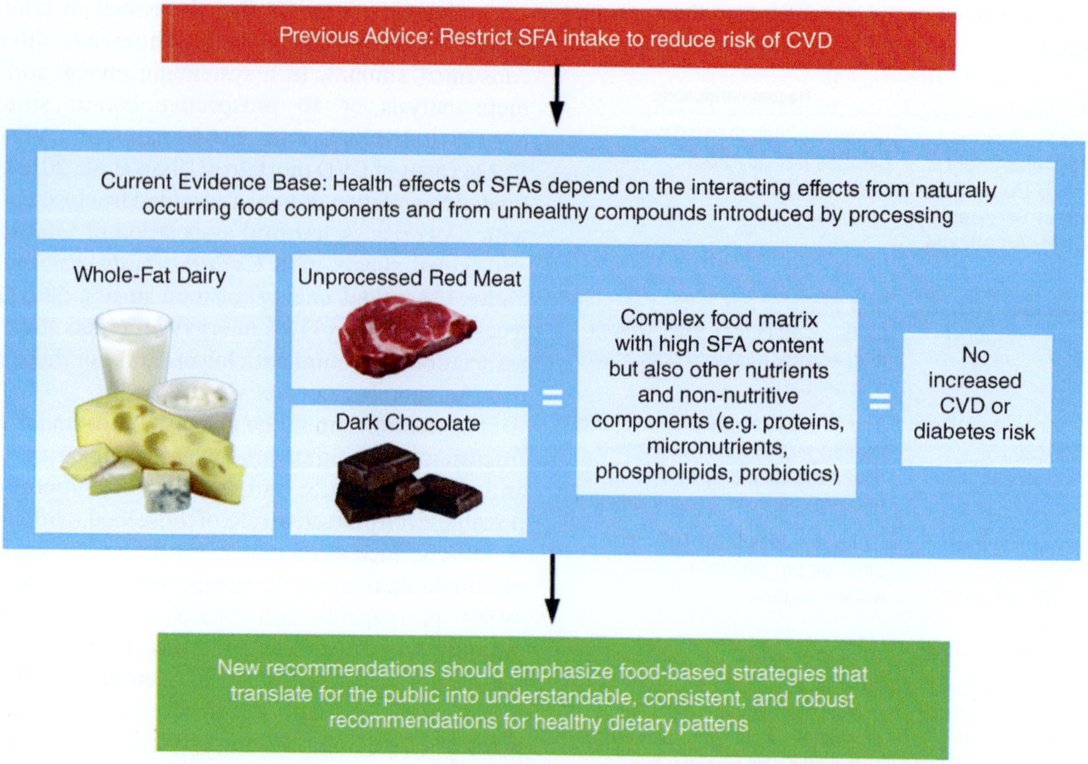

FIGURE 1.5 Previous and current evidence regarding the health effects of high SFA content foods (e.g., whole-fat dairy, unprocessed red meat, and dark chocolate) and CVD risk. Source: (Astrup et al., 2020 / with permission of Elsevier).

risk of stroke (Drouin-Chartier et al., 2020; Geiker, Larsen, Dyerberg, Stender, & Astrup, 2018). Moreover, results from RCTs show neutral or beneficial effects on cardio-metabolic risk markers in people with prediabetes and T2D (Fuller et al., 2018).

Dark chocolate has a high SFA content but also contains stearic acid, which is considered of neutral effect on CVD risk. Moreover, epidemiological and experimental data suggest that dark chocolate has anti-oxidative, antihypertensive, anti-inflammatory, anti-atherogenic, and anti-thrombotic properties, which have preventive effects against CVD and T2D (Astrup et al., 2020).

Likewise, evidence regarding the association of unprocessed meat with all-cause mortality, CVD, CHD, and T2D risk is low to very low compared to processed meat that shows increased risks. The results from a meta-analysis of RCTs found no differences in blood lipids, lipoproteins, or blood pressure between groups of individuals consuming more, or fewer, than 0.5 daily servings of meat (O'Connor, Kim, & Campbell, 2017). In the same meta-analysis, processed meat raised the risk of T2D to 19%, but red-meat consumption was not significantly associated with DM (O'Connor et al., 2017).

In a meta-analysis of RCTs that compared diets with red meat with diets that replaced red meat with a high-quality plant protein sources, animal sources (i.e., chicken/poultry/fish; fish only; poultry only), mixed-animal protein sources (including dairy); and carbohydrates found no significant differences between red meat and all the comparison diets combined in the blood concentrations of total, low-density lipoprotein, high-density lipoprotein cholesterol, apolipoproteins A1 and B, or blood pressure. However, relative to the combined comparison diets, red-meat intake resulted in lower decreases in triglyceride levels (Guasch-Ferré et al., 2019).

Although the evidence regarding red-meat consumption is inconclusive regarding cardio-metabolic diseases, there is strong evidence that consuming either red or processed meat is positively associated with colorectal cancer (Huang et al., 2021), as it will be further discussed in **Chapter 21**.

HIGH PROCESSED-MEAT CONSUMPTION

As mentioned in the previous section, a high consumption of processed meat like bacon, sausages, salami, or other cold cuts, may increase the risk for chronic diseases, namely T2D (Yang et al., 2020) and certain cancers, e.g., colorectal and esophageal cancer.

Indeed, in an umbrella review including 72 meta-analysis of both cohort and case-control studies, 100g/day increments of red meat and 50 g/day increments of processed meat were associated with 11% to 51% and 8% to 72% increased risk of multiple cancers, respectively (Huang et al., 2021). During the high-temperature cooking process of red meat, several potential carcinogens, such as polycyclic aromatic hydrocarbons and heterocyclic amines are formed, which increases the possibility of cancer risk.

Also, the high sodium content of processed meat increases the risk of developing hypertension and vascular stiffness. However, the magnitude of association of processed meat consumption with adverse cardio-metabolic outcomes is very small and the evidence is low (Zeraatkar et al., 2020).

SUB-OPTIMAL DIET IN TERMS OF DIETARY PATTERNS

Beyond single nutrients, foods, and food groups, in the last decades there is a shift in nutrition research to more holistic dietary patterns. The assessment of whole dietary patterns either *a priori* or *a posteriori* is likely to provide a better explanation of diet–health interactions as it takes into consideration combinations of different foods and beverages. To this context, sub-optimal, unhealthy or Western dietary patterns increase the risk of CVD, obesity, metabolic syndrome, T2D (Fung, Schulze, Manson, Willett, & Hu, 2004; Walsh, Jacka, Butterworth, Anstey, & Cherbuin, 2017), and cancer. However, according to a 2020 umbrella systematic review (Jayedi, Soltani, Abdolshahi, & Shab-Bidar, 2020) that evaluated the evidence obtained by published meta-analyses of prospective cohort studies on the association between empirically derived unhealthy dietary patterns and the risk of NCDs, found a very low to moderate quality of evidence. Notably, positive associations between unhealthy dietary patterns and the risk of NCDs were confirmed only for all-cause mortality, colorectal adenoma, T2D, and metabolic syndrome but not CVD or CHD mortality (Jayedi et al., 2020).

THE WESTERN DIETARY PATTERN

The Western pattern is characterized by a high intake of processed meat, red meat, butter, eggs, refined grains, fast food, SSBs, sweets, and desserts while it is low in fruit and vegetables. Therefore, Western-type diets are enriched in total fat, animal proteins, n-6 PUFAs, and added sugars, while they are low in fiber (Hu, 2002).

Numerous cohort (Oikonomou et al., 2018), such as the ATTICA study (Panagiotakos et al., 2009), and case-control studies, such as the INTERHEART study (Iqbal et al., 2008), have shown statistically significant associations between unhealthy dietary patterns and increased odds or risk for developing CVD. However, the pooled estimation from several meta-analyses assessing the associations of unhealthy dietary patterns with CVD has not always revealed statistical results (Li et al., 2015; Rodríguez-Monforte, Flores-Mateo, & Sánchez, 2015). This is because an unhealthy pattern is not always synonymous with developing CVD as those patterns do not necessarily represent food choices that pose the highest CVD risk rather than a mix of food choices including those with a protective role.

Regarding metabolic syndrome and T2D, evidence is more constant and clearer. Data from observational cohort studies show that the adherence to the highest compared to the lowest category of Western diet is associated with an increased risk of metabolic syndrome, general and central obesity, higher BMI, and waist circumference in several countries (Rodríguez-Monforte, Sánchez, Barrio, Costa, & Flores-Mateo, 2017). Also, a large body of evidence from meta-analyses of prospective cohort studies (Alhazmi, Stojanovski, McEvoy, & Garg, 2014; Jannasch, Kröger, & Schulze, 2017) suggest that an unhealthy dietary pattern characterized by red and processed meats, high-fat dairy, and refined grains may also increase the risk of T2D incidence by almost 30% (Maghsoudi, Ghiasvand, & Salehi-Abargouei, 2016) through exacerbated insulin secretion and insulin resistance.

The proposed mechanisms behind the harmful associations between Western-type diets and health include the increased production of reactive-oxygen species, low-grade inflammation, abnormal activation of the sympathetic nervous and renin-angiotensin-systems (Kopp, 2019). There is also evidence that as well as alterations in the structure and diversity of gut microbiome affect both systemic and mucosal immune responses (Statovci, Aguilera, MacSharry, & Melgar, 2017), all of which play a pivotal role in the development of NCDs.

PHYSICAL INACTIVITY

Physical activity is a widely accepted global public health issue. Data regarding physical inactivity worldwide is disappointing. More than a quarter of all adults globally (27.5%) were physically inactive in 2016, putting more than 1.4 billion adults at risk for developing diseases associated with physical inactivity such as CVD (Guthold, Stevens, Riley, & Bull, 2018). Women were less active than men (31.7% woman versus 23.4% men) (**Figure 1.6**), as were older adults compared to younger adults. High-income countries showed almost a double prevalence of inactivity (36.8%) compared with low-income countries (16%) (Guthold et al., 2018).

Globally, in 2022, physical inactivity was deemed responsible for 7.2% and 7.6% of all cause and CVD deaths, respectively (Katzmarzyk, Friedenreich, Shiroma, & Lee, 2022). Regarding the proportions of all NCDs attributable to physical inactivity, these varied from 5% for CHD, 4.5% for T2D, 7.2% of renal cancer, and 8.1% for dementia (Katzmarzyk et al., 2022). Moreover, despite the high prevalence-based population attributable risks in high-income countries, 69% of total deaths and 74% of CVD deaths associated with physical inactivity occurred in middle-income countries due to the greater populations of these countries (Katzmarzyk et al., 2022). The high levels of physical inactivity in wealthier countries might be attributed to more sedentary occupations and personal motorized transportation, while more activity is undertaken at work and for transport in low-income countries (Guthold et al., 2018).

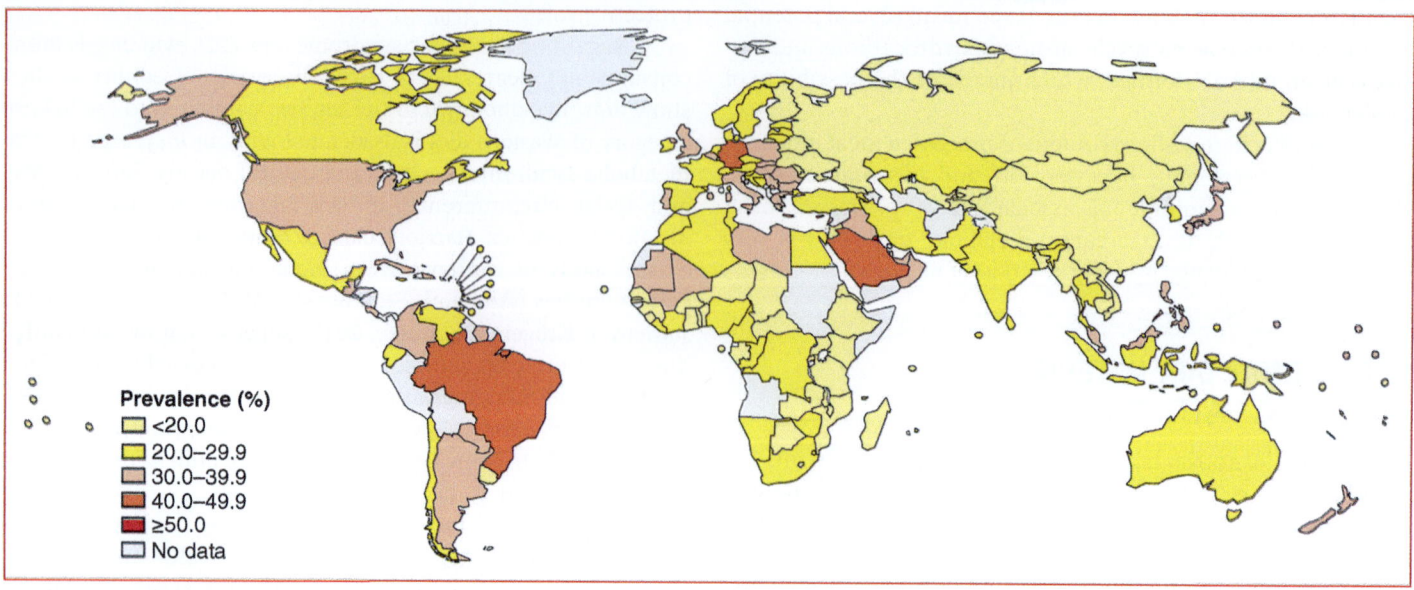

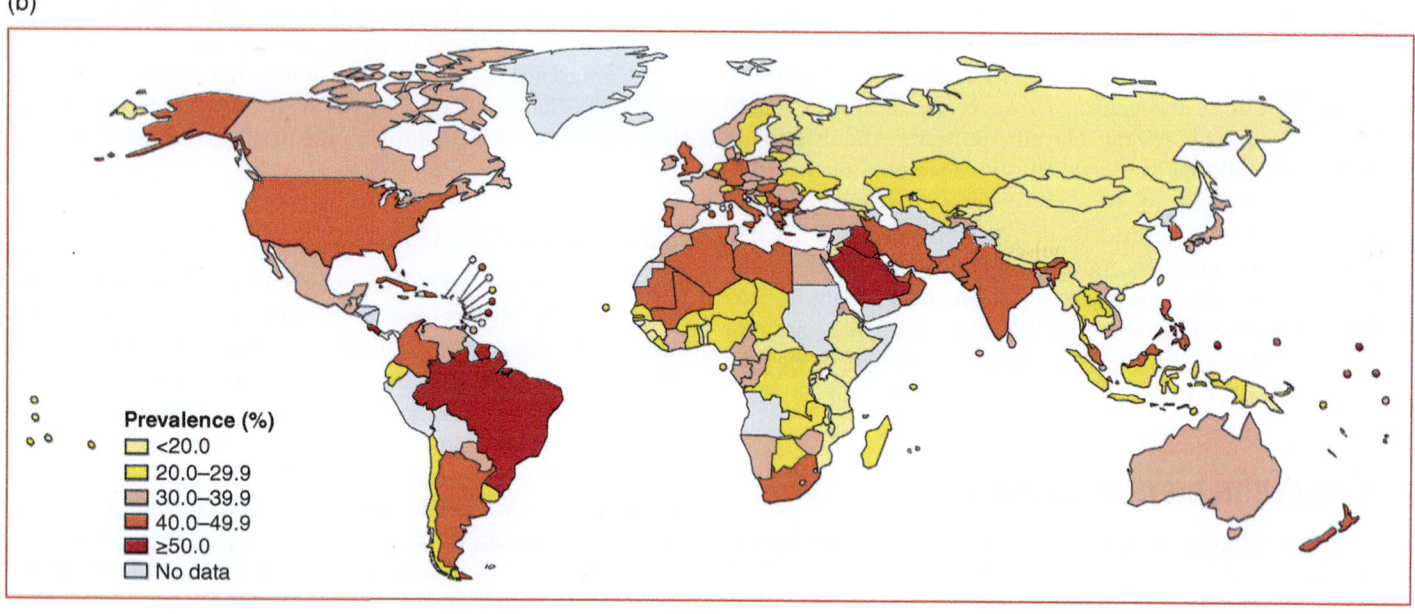

FIGURE 1.6 Country prevalence of insufficient physical activity in (a) men and (b) women in 2016. Women were less active than men (31.7% versus 23.4%). Source: (Guthold et al., 2018 / Elsevier / CC BY 3.0 IGO).

Globally, reasons for insufficient participation in physical activity include the increased use of technology, alterations in transportation patterns, and economic development in many countries (Kohl et al., 2012). According to the US Centers for Disease Control and Protection (CDC), people report lack of time and safety issues as common barriers, while other reasons cited are a lack of self-motivation; confidence in the capability to be physically active; encouragement, support, or companionship during exercise; feeling inconvenienced by exercise; or feeling bored during or not enjoying, exercise. Moreover, several environmental factors may influence individuals' participation in physical activity in all domains, such as an increase in violence, high-density traffic, and air pollution as well as a lack of parks, sidewalks, and sports/recreation facilities. In both middle aged (50 to 64) and older (65 to 70 years old) adults, environmental factors, and resources as well as social influences and beliefs about being capable of exercising seem to be among the most frequently identified barriers (Spiteri et al., 2019).

According to 2020 WHO guidelines on physical activity and sedentary behavior (WHO, 2020), physical inactivity is defined as individuals' inability to follow their current age group recommendations regarding weekly levels of physical activity.

More information will be given in **Unit 2**. Briefly, for children and youth aged 5 to 17, guidelines recommend at least 60 minutes of moderate- to vigorous-intensity physical activity daily, preferably aerobic and performed as play. For adults, recommendations suggest at least 150 minutes of moderate-intensity aerobic physical activity per week or at least 75 minutes of vigorous-intensity aerobic physical activity throughout the week, or an equivalent combination of moderate- and vigorous-intensity activity (WHO, 2020).

KEY POINTS

- Non-communicable diseases (NCDs), also known as chronic diseases, are medical conditions linked with several factors such as genetic, physiological, behavioral, and environmental factors.
- The NCDs with the highest numbers of deaths globally are cardiovascular diseases (CVDs) followed by cancers, respiratory diseases, and DM. Other health problems included under the umbrella of NCDs are obesity, hypertension, gastrointestinal diseases, and liver and renal disorders.
- A diet low in fiber is defined as an average daily consumption of less than 23.5 g of fiber per day.
- The adequate daily intake of fiber from all sources including fruits, vegetables, grains, legumes, and pulses is 14 g per 1 000 kcal, which is approximately 25 g/day for women and 38 g/day for men.
- High sodium intake (defined by WHO as >2 g /day, equivalent to 5 g salt/day) ranks first for mortality worldwide.
- Salt (a combination of sodium and chloride) is the major source of sodium in the diet. Classic sources of salt are processed foods, ready-to-eat meals, salt added during food preparation and cooking as well as table salt.
- The WHO recommends an overall sodium intake of less than 2 000 mg/day of sodium (<5 g salt/day), whereas the 2020–2025 US Dietary Guidelines for adults recommend limiting sodium intake to 2 300 mg/day.
- Numerous studies have failed to demonstrate rigorous evidence supporting continued recommendations either to limit the consumption of saturated fatty acids (SFAs) or replace them with poly-unsaturated fatty acids (PUFAs) like omega-3.
- The 2020–2025 Dietary Guidelines for Americans continues the recommendation to limit SFAs to 10% or less of total energy intake, based on insufficient and inconsistent evidence.
- Evidence strongly suggest that industrial trans fatty acid (TFA) consumption is associated with an increased risk of CHD, related mortality, and CVD.
- The WHO published an action package to reduce TFA using the global food supply called the 'REPLACE action package'.
- The low consumption of fruit and vegetables has been associated with increased risk of CVD, T2D and cancer. WHO recommends eating five portions of fruit and vegetables per day (equivalent to 400 g).
- A low consumption of whole-grain food products leads to a low fiber intake (especially insoluble fractions) in addition to B vitamins, minerals, and phytochemicals with antioxidant properties, all of which are components linked to many health benefits.
- There are several recommendations for the daily consumption of whole grains; in the USA, at least 85 g/day is recommended, while in European countries, such as Denmark, the recommendation is 75 g/10 megajoules (MJ, 2 388 kcal) per day.
- Added/free sugars, particularly those from sugar-sweetened beverages (SSBs) increase overall energy intake and lowers the intake of nutritional foods, which leads to an unhealthy diet, weight gain, and increased risk of NCDs.
- The postprandial glucose response, commonly known as the glycemic index used to measure the blood glucose-raising potential of foods, varies between people, as it is affected by several factors such as the gut microbiome, anthropometric data, physical activity, and blood lipids.
- It seems that the effects of total sugars, added sugars, or specific dietary sugars on human health depends on the consumed amount.
- Attention should be given to other major food sources of fructose-containing sugars such as yogurt, fruit, 100% fruit juice, and mixed-fruit juice, as the latest data support a potentially protective role of those foods against cardio-metabolic conditions such as metabolic syndrome.
- Whole-fat dairy products, unprocessed meat, eggs, and dark chocolate were thought to increase the risk of CVD due to their high SFA content. However, it is now apparent that the relationship or effect of any food cannot be predicted by its nutrient content without considering the overall macronutrient distribution.
- During the high-temperature cooking process of red meat, several potential carcinogens, such as polycyclic aromatic hydrocarbons and heterocyclic amines are formed, increasing cancer risk.
- The assessment of whole dietary patterns either *a priori or a posteriori* is likely to provide a better explanation of diet–health interactions as it considers the combination of different foods and beverages.
- The proposed mechanisms behind the harmful associations between Western-type diets and health include (i) the increased production of reactive-oxygen species, (ii) low-grade inflammation, (iii) abnormal activation of the sympathetic nervous and renin-angiotensin systems as well as (iv) alterations in the structure and diversity of the gut microbiome, which affects both systemic and mucosal immune responses, all of whom have a pivotal role in the development of NCDs.
- Data regarding physical inactivity worldwide is disappointing. More than a quarter of all adults globally (27.5%) were physically inactive in 2016, putting more than 1.4 billion adults at risk for developing diseases associated with physical inactivity.
- The high levels of physical inactivity in wealthier countries might be attributed to more sedentary occupations and personal motorized transportation, while more activity is undertaken at work and for transport in low-income countries

SELF-ASSESSMENT QUESTIONS

1. Indicate whether the following statements are true or false:

   (a) A low in fiber diet is defined as an average daily fiber consumption of less than 23.5 g per day.

   (b) A low in fiber diet is defined as an average daily fiber consumption of less than 25 g per day.

   (c) A low in fiber diet is defined as an average daily fiber consumption of less than 15.0 g per day.

   (d) All the above answers are incorrect.

2. Fill in the blanks:

   (a) A high sodium intake is considered as and equivalent to according to WHO.

   (b) The physicochemical characteristics of fibers include their _____, _____, and _____ in the gut.

   (c) The 2020–2025 Dietary Guidelines for Americans recommend limiting saturated fatty acids to of total energy intake.

   (d) WHO recommends eating of fruit and vegetables per day (equivalent to_____).

   (e) Most scientific organizations, to limit the rising trends of obesity and the related metabolic diseases, suggest reducing total dietary intake of added/free sugars to.

   (f) The Western type diets are enriched in _____, _____, n-6 poly-unsaturated fatty acids and, while they are low in.

3. Through what mechanisms do trans fatty acids act to affect human health?

4. Provide the WHO definition for added/free sugars.

5. Provide the WHO definition for physical inactivity.

6. Children should perform:

   (a) 30 minutes or more per day of moderate- to vigorous-intensity physical activity.

   (b) 60 minutes or more per day of moderate- to vigorous-intensity physical activity.

   (c) 90 minutes or more per day of moderate- to vigorous-intensity physical activity.

   (d) 150 minutes or more per day of moderate- to vigorous-intensity physical activity.

7. What is the physical activity recommendation for adults?

8. Are unhealthy dietary patterns always synonymous with developing CVD?

9. What is the pathophysiology of high amounts of sugar via sugar-sweetened beverages?

10. Fill in the blanks:

    (a) There is a long-standing association between high dietary sodium intake and _____ as well as _____.

    (b) The 2020–2025 US Dietary Guidelines for adults recommend limiting sodium intake to_____.

    (c) _____ is the major source of sodium in the diet.

    (d) Classic sources of salt are_____, _____, _____, and_____ as well as _____.

    (e) A reduction in dietary sodium reduces regardless of sex and ethnic group.

REFERENCES

Alhazmi, A., Stojanovski, E., McEvoy, M., & Garg, M. (2014). The association between dietary patterns and type 2 diabetes: a systematic review and meta-analysis of cohort studies. *Journal of Human Nutrition and Dietetics*, 27(3), 251–260.

Arnold, M. J., Harding, M. C., & Conley, A. T. (2021). Dietary Guidelines for Americans 2020–2025: Recommendations from the US Departments of Agriculture and Health and Human Services. *American Family Physician*, 104(5), 533–536.

Astrup, A., Magkos, F., Bier, D. M., Brenna, J. T., de Oliveira Otto, M. C., Hill, J. O., ... Volek, J. S. (2020). Saturated fats and health: a reassessment and proposal for food-based recommendations: JACC state-of-the-art review. *Journal of the American College of Cardiology*, 76(7), 844–857.

Astrup, A., Teicholz, N., Magkos, F., Bier, D. M., Brenna, J. T., King, J. C., ... Krauss, R. M. (2021). Dietary Saturated Fats and Health: Are the US Guidelines Evidence-Based? *Nutrients*, 13(10), 3305. Retrieved from https://www.mdpi.com/2072-6643/13/10/3305

Budreviciute, A., Damiati, S., Sabir, D. K., Onder, K., Schuller-Goetzburg, P., Plakys, G., ... Kodzius, R. (2020). Management and Prevention Strategies for Non-communicable Diseases (NCDs) and Their Risk Factors. *Frontiers in Public Health*, 8. doi:10.3389/fpubh.2020.574111

Carbohydrates and Health Report, S. (2015). Scientific Advisory Committee on Nutrition. In. London: TSO (The Stationery Office).

Chen, X., Du, J., Wu, X., Cao, W., & Sun, S. (2021). Global burden attributable to high sodium intake from 1990 to 2019. *Nutr Metab Cardiovasc Dis*, 31(12), 3314–3321. doi:10.1016/j.numecd.2021.08.033

European Commission. Health Promotion and Disease Prevention Knowledge Gateway. Retrieved from https://knowledge4policy.ec.europa.eu/health-promotion-knowledge-gateway/dietary-fibre_en#references (assessed May 22, 2022)

Dietary Guidelines Advisory Committee. (2020). Scientific report of the 2020 Dietary Guidelines Advisory Committee: advisory report to the Secretary of Agriculture and the Secretary of Health and Human Services. *Agricultural Research Service*, 2020–2007.

National Health and Medical Research Council (2013) Australian Dietary Guidelines. Canberra: National Health and Medical Research Council. Retrieved from https://www.health.gov.au/sites/default/files/australian-dietary-guidelines.pdf

Drouin-Chartier, J.-P., Chen, S., Li, Y., Schwab, A. L., Stampfer, M. J., Sacks, F. M., ... Bhupathiraju, S. N. (2020). Egg consumption and risk of cardiovascular disease: three large prospective US cohort studies, systematic review, and updated meta-analysis. *BMJ, 368*.

EFSA Panel on Dietetic Products, N., & Allergies. (2010). Scientific opinion on dietary reference values for carbohydrates and dietary fibre. *EFSA Journal, 8*(3), 1462.

Forouhi, N. G., & Unwin, N. (2019). Global diet and health: old questions, fresh evidence, and new horizons. *The Lancet, 393*(10184), 1916–1918.

Frølich, W., Åman, P., & Tetens, I. (2013). Whole grain foods and health–a Scandinavian perspective. *Food & nutrition research, 57*(1), 18503.

Fuller, N. R., Sainsbury, A., Caterson, I. D., Denyer, G., Fong, M., Gerofi, J., . . . Januszewski, A. S. (2018). Effect of a high-egg diet on cardiometabolic risk factors in people with type 2 diabetes: the Diabetes and Egg (DIABEGG) Study—randomized weight-loss and follow-up phase. *Am J Clin Nutr, 107*(6), 921-931.

Fung, T. T., Schulze, M., Manson, J. E., Willett, W. C., & Hu, F. B. (2004). Dietary Patterns, Meat Intake, and the Risk of Type 2 Diabetes in Women. *Arch Intern Med, 164*(20), 2235-2240. doi:10.1001/archinte.164.20.2235

Geiker, N., Larsen, M. L., Dyerberg, J., Stender, S., & Astrup, A. (2018). Egg consumption, cardiovascular diseases and type 2 diabetes. *European journal of clinical nutrition, 72*(1), 44–56.

Gill, S. K., Rossi, M., Bajka, B., & Whelan, K. (2021). Dietary fibre in gastrointestinal health and disease. *Nature Reviews Gastroenterology & Hepatology, 18*(2), 101–116.

Giosuè, A., Calabrese, I., Vitale, M., Riccardi, G., & Vaccaro, O. (2022). Consumption of Dairy Foods and Cardiovascular Disease: A Systematic Review. *Nutrients, 14*(4), 831. Retrieved from https://www.mdpi.com/2072-6643/14/4/831

Godos, J., Tieri, M., Ghelfi, F., Titta, L., Marventano, S., Lafranconi, A., . . . Grosso, G. (2020). Dairy foods and health: an umbrella review of observational studies. *International Journal of Food Sciences and Nutrition, 71*(2), 138–151. doi:10.1080/09637486.2019.1625035

Graudal, N., Jürgens, G., Baslund, B., & Alderman, M. H. (2014). Compared With Usual Sodium Intake, Low- and Excessive-Sodium Diets Are Associated With Increased Mortality: A Meta-Analysis. *American Journal of Hypertension, 27*(9), 1129–1137. doi:10.1093/ajh/hpu028

Grillo, A., Salvi, L., Coruzzi, P., Salvi, P., & Parati, G. (2019). Sodium Intake and Hypertension. *Nutrients, 11*(9), 1970. Retrieved from https://www.mdpi.com/2072-6643/11/9/1970

Guasch-Ferré, M., Satija, A., Blondin, S. A., Janiszewski, M., Emlen, E., O'Connor, L. E., . . . Stampfer, M. J. (2019). Meta-Analysis of Randomized Controlled Trials of Red Meat Consumption in Comparison With Various Comparison Diets on Cardiovascular Risk Factors. *Circulation, 139*(15), 1828–1845. doi:doi:10.1161/CIRCULATIONAHA.118.035225

Guthold, R., Stevens, G. A., Riley, L. M., & Bull, F. C. (2018). Worldwide trends in insufficient physical activity from 2001 to 2016: a pooled analysis of 358 population-based surveys with 1·9 million participants. *The lancet global health, 6*(10), e1077–e1086.

Haque, M., McKimm, J., Sartelli, M., Samad, N., Haque, S. Z., & Bakar, M. A. (2020). A narrative review of the effects of sugar-sweetened beverages on human health: A key global health issue. *J Popul Ther Clin Pharmacol, 27*(1), e76–e103. doi:10.15586/jptcp.v27i1.666

Heileson, J. L. (2020). Dietary saturated fat and heart disease: a narrative review. *Nutrition reviews, 78*(6), 474–485.

Hooper, L., Martin, N., Jimoh, O. F., Kirk, C., Foster, E., & Abdelhamid, A. S. (2020). Reduction in saturated fat intake for cardiovascular disease. *Cochrane Database of Systematic Reviews*(5). doi:10.1002/14651858.CD011737.pub2

Hu, F. B. (2002). Dietary pattern analysis: a new direction in nutritional epidemiology. *Current opinion in lipidology, 13*(1), 3–9.

Huang, Y., Cao, D., Chen, Z., Chen, B., Li, J., Guo, J., . . . Wei, Q. (2021). Red and processed meat consumption and cancer outcomes: Umbrella review. *Food Chemistry, 356*, 129697. doi:https://doi.org/10.1016/j.foodchem.2021.129697

Iqbal, R., Anand, S., Ounpuu, S., Islam, S., Zhang, X., Rangarajan, S., . . . Yusuf, S. (2008). Dietary patterns and the risk of acute myocardial infarction in 52 countries: results of the INTERHEART study. *Circulation, 118*(19), 1929–1937. doi:10.1161/circulationaha.107.738716

Jannasch, F., Kröger, J., & Schulze, M. B. (2017). Dietary Patterns and Type 2 Diabetes: A Systematic Literature Review and Meta-Analysis of Prospective Studies. *The Journal of Nutrition, 147*(6), 1174–1182. doi:10.3945/jn.116.242552

Jayedi, A., Soltani, S., Abdolshahi, A., & Shab-Bidar, S. (2020). Healthy and unhealthy dietary patterns and the risk of chronic disease: an umbrella review of meta-analyses of prospective cohort studies. *British Journal of Nutrition, 124*(11), 1133–1144. doi:10.1017/S0007114520002330

Katzmarzyk, P. T., Friedenreich, C., Shiroma, E. J., & Lee, I. M. (2022). Physical inactivity and non-communicable disease burden in low-income, middle-income and high-income countries. *British Journal of Sports Medicine, 56*(2), 101. doi:10.1136/bjsports-2020-103640

Khan, T. A., Tayyiba, M., Agarwal, A., Mejia, S. B., de Souza, R. J., Wolever, T. M. S., . . . Sievenpiper, J. L. (2019). Relation of Total Sugars, Sucrose, Fructose, and Added Sugars With the Risk of Cardiovascular Disease: A Systematic Review and Dose-Response Meta-analysis of Prospective Cohort Studies. *Mayo Clinic Proceedings, 94*(12), 2399–2414. doi:https://doi.org/10.1016/j.mayocp.2019.05.034

Kohl, H. W., 3rd, Craig, C. L., Lambert, E. V., Inoue, S., Alkandari, J. R., Leetongin, G., . . . Lancet Physical Activity Series Working, G. (2012). The pandemic of physical inactivity: global action for public health. *Lancet, 380*(9838), 294–305. doi:10.1016/S0140-6736(12)60898-8

Kopp, W. (2019). How Western Diet And Lifestyle Drive The Pandemic Of Obesity And Civilization Diseases. *Diabetes, metabolic syndrome and obesity: targets and therapy, 12*, 2221–2236. doi:10.2147/DMSO.S216791

Li, F., Hou, L.-n., Chen, W., Chen, P.-l., Lei, C.-y., Wei, Q., . . . Zheng, S.-b. (2015). Associations of dietary patterns with the risk of all-cause, CVD and stroke mortality: a meta-analysis of prospective cohort studies. *British Journal of Nutrition, 113*(1), 16–24. doi:10.1017/S000711451400289X

Maghsoudi, Z., Ghiasvand, R., & Salehi-Abargouei, A. (2016). Empirically derived dietary patterns and incident type 2 diabetes mellitus: a systematic review and meta-analysis on prospective observational studies. *Public Health Nutrition, 19*(2), 230–241. doi:10.1017/S1368980015001251

Moore, J. B., & Fielding, B. A. (2016). Sugar and metabolic health: is there still a debate? *Current opinion in clinical nutrition and metabolic care, 19*(4), 303–309.

Murray, C. J. L., Aravkin, A. Y., Zheng, P., Abbafati, C., Abbas, K. M., Abbasi-Kangevari, M., . . . Lim, S. S. (2020). Global burden of 87 risk factors in 204 countries and territories, 1990–2019: a systematic analysis for the Global Burden of Disease Study 2019. *The Lancet, 396*(10258), 1223–1249. doi:10.1016/S0140-6736(20)30752-2

O'Connor, L. E., Kim, J. E., & Campbell, W. W. (2017). Total red meat intake of ≥ 0.5 servings/d does not negatively influence cardiovascular disease risk factors: a systemically searched meta-analysis of randomized controlled trials. *Am J Clin Nutr, 105*(1), 57–69.

Oikonomou, E., Psaltopoulou, T., Georgiopoulos, G., Siasos, G., Kokkou, E., Antonopoulos, A., . . . Tousoulis, D. (2018). Western Dietary Pattern

Is Associated With Severe Coronary Artery Disease. *Angiology, 69*(4), 339–346. doi:10.1177/0003319717721603

Oteng, A.-B., & Kersten, S. (2019). Mechanisms of Action of trans Fatty Acids. *Advances in Nutrition, 11*(3), 697–708. doi:10.1093/advances/nmz125

Oteng, A.-B., & Kersten, S. (2020). Mechanisms of action of trans fatty acids. *Advances in Nutrition, 11*(3), 697–708.

Panagiotakos, D., Pitsavos, C., Chrysohoou, C., Palliou, K., Lentzas, I., Skoumas, I., & Stefanadis, C. (2009). Dietary patterns and 5-year incidence of cardiovascular disease: a multivariate analysis of the ATTICA study. *Nutr Metab Cardiovasc Dis, 19*(4), 253–263. doi:10.1016/j.numecd.2008.06.005

Pipoyan, D., Stepanyan, S., Stepanyan, S., Beglaryan, M., Costantini, L., Molinari, R., & Merendino, N. (2021). The Effect of Trans Fatty Acids on Human Health: Regulation and Consumption Patterns. *Foods (Basel, Switzerland), 10*(10), 2452. doi:10.3390/foods10102452

Rhee, M.-Y. (2015). High sodium intake: review of recent issues on its association with cardiovascular events and measurement methods. *Korean circulation journal, 45*(3), 175–183. doi:10.4070/kcj.2015.45.3.175

Rodríguez-Monforte, M., Flores-Mateo, G., & Sánchez, E. (2015). Dietary patterns and CVD: a systematic review and meta-analysis of observational studies. *British Journal of Nutrition, 114*(9), 1341–1359. doi:10.1017/S0007114515003177

Rodríguez-Monforte, M., Sánchez, E., Barrio, F., Costa, B., & Flores-Mateo, G. (2017). Metabolic syndrome and dietary patterns: a systematic review and meta-analysis of observational studies. *European Journal of Nutrition, 56*(3), 925–947. doi:10.1007/s00394-016-1305-y

Ross, A. B., van der Kamp, J.-W., King, R., Lê K.-A., Mejborn, H., Seal, C. J., & Thielecke, F., on behalf of the Healthgrain Forum (2017). Perspective: A Definition for Whole-Grain Food Products—Recommendations from the Healthgrain Forum. *Advances in Nutrition, 8*(4), 525–531. doi:10.3945/an.116.014001

Semnani-Azad, Z., Khan, T. A., Blanco Mejia, S., de Souza, R. J., Leiter, L. A., Kendall, C. W. C., . . . Sievenpiper, J. L. (2020). Association of Major Food Sources of Fructose-Containing Sugars With Incident Metabolic Syndrome: A Systematic Review and Meta-analysis. *JAMA Network Open, 3*(7), e209993-e209993. doi:10.1001/jamanetworkopen.2020.9993

US Department of Health and Human Services and US Department of Agriculture. 2015–2020 Dietary Guidelines for Americans. 8th Edition. December 2015. Available at https://health.gov/our-work/food-nutrition/previous-dietary-guidelines/2015.

US Department of Agriculture and US Department of Health and Human Services. Dietary Guidelines for Americans, 2020-2025. 9th Edition. December 2020. Available at DietaryGuidelines.gov (assessed 18 April 2022).

Spiteri, K., Broom, D., Bekhet, A. H., de Caro, J. X., Laventure, B., & Grafton, K. (2019). Barriers and Motivators of Physical Activity Participation in Middle-aged and Older-adults - A Systematic Review. *J Aging Phys Act, 27*(4), 929–944. doi:10.1123/japa.2018-0343

Stanaway, J. D., Afshin, A., Gakidou, E., Lim, S. S., Abate, D., Abate, K. H., . . . Murray, C. J. L. (2018). Global, regional, and national comparative risk assessment of 84 behavioural, environmental and occupational, and metabolic risks or clusters of risks for 195 countries and territories, 1990–2017: a systematic analysis for the Global Burden of Disease Study 2017. *The Lancet, 392*(10159), 1923–1994. doi:10.1016/S0140-6736(18)32225-6

Statovci, D., Aguilera, M., MacSharry, J., & Melgar, S. (2017). The Impact of Western Diet and Nutrients on the Microbiota and Immune Response at Mucosal Interfaces. *Frontiers in immunology, 8*, 838–838. doi:10.3389/fimmu.2017.00838

Tieri, M., Ghelfi, F., Vitale, M., Vetrani, C., Marventano, S., Lafranconi, A., . . . Grosso, G. (2020). Whole grain consumption and human health: an umbrella review of observational studies. *International Journal of Food Sciences and Nutrition, 71*(6), 668–677. doi:10.1080/09637486.2020.1715354

Veronese, N., Solmi, M., Caruso, M. G., Giannelli, G., Osella, A. R., Evangelou, E., . . . Tzoulaki, I. (2018). Dietary fiber and health outcomes: an umbrella review of systematic reviews and meta-analyses. *Am J Clin Nutr, 107*(3), 436–444. doi:10.1093/ajcn/nqx082

Walsh, E. I., Jacka, F. N., Butterworth, P., Anstey, K. J., & Cherbuin, N. (2017). The association between Western and Prudent dietary patterns and fasting blood glucose levels in type 2 diabetes and normal glucose metabolism in older Australian adults. *Heliyon, 3*(6), e00315. doi:https://doi.org/10.1016/j.heliyon.2017.e00315

Wang, D. D., Li, Y., Bhupathiraju, S. N., Rosner, B. A., Sun, Q., Giovannucci, E. L., . . . Hu, F. B. (2021). Fruit and Vegetable Intake and Mortality. *Circulation, 143*(17), 1642–1654. doi:doi:10.1161/CIRCULATIONAHA.120.048996

Wang, Y.-J., Yeh, T.-L., Shih, M.-C., Tu, Y.-K., & Chien, K.-L. (2020). Dietary Sodium Intake and Risk of Cardiovascular Disease: A Systematic Review and Dose-Response Meta-Analysis. *Nutrients, 12*(10), 2934. doi:10.3390/nu12102934

WHO. (2010). *Global recommendations on physical activity for health*: World Health Organization.

WHO. (2012). *Guideline: sodium intake for adults and children*: World Health Organization.

WHO. (2015). *Guideline: sugars intake for adults and children*: World Health Organization.

WHO. (2020). World Health Organization guidelines on physical activity and sedentary behaviour: at a glance.

WHO. (2021). Noncommunicable Diseases (NCD). Retrieved from https://www.who.int/news-room/fact-sheets/detail/noncommunicable-diseases

Yang, X., Li, Y., Wang, C., Mao, Z., Zhou, W., Zhang, L., . . . Li, L. (2020). Meat and fish intake and type 2 diabetes: Dose–response meta-analysis of prospective cohort studies. *Diabetes & Metabolism, 46*(5), 345–352. doi:https://doi.org/10.1016/j.diabet.2020.03.004

Zeevi, D., Korem, T., Zmora, N., Israeli, D., Rothschild, D., Weinberger, A., . . . Lotan-Pompan, M. (2015). Personalized nutrition by prediction of glycemic responses. *Cell, 163*(5), 1079–1094.

Zeraatkar, D., Guyatt, G. H., Alonso-Coello, P., Bala, M. M., Rabassa, M., Han, M. A., . . . Johnston, B. C. (2020). Red and Processed Meat Consumption and Risk for All-Cause Mortality and Cardiometabolic Outcomes. *Ann Intern Med, 172*(7), 511–512. doi:10.7326/L20-0070

FURTHER READING

Bibliography

Afshin, A., Sur, P. J., Fay, K. A., Cornaby, L., Ferrara, G., Salama, J. S., . . . & Murray, C. J. (2019). Health effects of dietary risks in 195 countries, 1990–2017: a systematic analysis for the Global Burden of Disease Study 2017. *The Lancet, 393*(10184), 1958–1972.

Althoff, T., Sosič, R., Hicks, J. L., King, A. C., Delp, S. L., & Leskovec, J. (2017). Large-scale physical activity data reveal worldwide activity inequality. *Nature, 547*(7663), 336–339. doi: 10.1038/nature23018.

Gill, S. K., Rossi, M., Bajka, B., et al. (2020). Dietary fibre in gastrointestinal health and disease. *Nature Reviews Gastroenterology & Hepatology* doi:10.1038/s41575-020-00375-4.

Grillo, A., Salvi, L., Coruzzi, P., Salvi, P., & Parati, G. (2019). Sodium intake and hypertension. Nutrients, *11*(9), 1970. doi: 10.3390/nu11091970.

Oteng, A. B., & Kersten, S. (2020). Mechanisms of action of trans fatty acids. Advances in Nutrition, *11*(3), 697–708.

Scientific Advisory Committee on Nutrition (2015). Carbohydrates and health. https://www.gov.uk/government/publications/sacn-carbohydrates-and-health-report (accessed 30 June 2022).

World Health Organization (2018), REPLACE trans fat: an action package to eliminate industrially produced trans-fatty acids. ISBN 978-92-4-002110-5

Zeevi, D., Korem, T., Zmora, N., Israeli, D., Rothschild, D., Weinberger, A., . . . & Segal, E. (2015). Personalized nutrition by prediction of glycemic responses. *Cell*, *163*(5), 1079–1094.

Links

- https://www.who.int/news-room/fact-sheets/detail/noncommunicable-diseases
- www.fda.gov/nutritioneducation
- https://www.gov.uk/government/groups/scientific-advisory-committee-on-nutrition
- https://www.cdc.gov/chronicdisease/resources/publications/factsheets/physical-activity.htm
- wholegrainscouncil.org
- carbquality.org
- https://www1.nyc.gov/site/doh/health/health-topics/national-salt-sugar-reduction-initiative.page
- sweeteners.org
- nutrition.gov
- dietaryguidelines.gov
- https://www.fao.org/home/en
- https://www.who.int/teams/nutrition-and-food-safety/replace-trans-fat

Lifestyle and Epigenetics

CHAPTER 2

Introduction	19	Psychological Stress	28
Epigenetics Overview	19	Cigarette Smoking	28
Epigenetics Definition	19	Alcohol Consumption	29
Epigenetic Mechanisms	20	Endocrine Disruptors	29
Epigenetics and Disease Epidemiology	21	Physical Activity and Epigenetic Alterations	29
The Barker Hypothesis	22	Key Points	30
Epigenetics *in utero* and Maternal Lifestyle	23	Self-assessment Questions	30
Maternal Undernutrition	23	References	30
Maternal Overnutrition	24	Further Reading	33
Dietary Pattern as an Epigenetic Mark	25	Bibliography	33
Epigenetics and Stress	27		

INTRODUCTION

Our genetic background and way of life as well as environmental factors are closely related and synergistically control our physiology and health status. Though we are the imprint of our genes, a plethora of scientific evidence confirms that lifestyle stimuli such as diet, physical activity, stress, smoking, alcohol consumption, and pollutants, among others, can influence the genome by triggering epigenetic mechanisms that potentially can cause changes in gene expression (Alegría-Torres, Baccarelli, & Bollati, 2011; Ramsay, 2015). Epigenetic alterations occur during the entire lifespan, from conception to adulthood. In the broad sense of the term, epigenetics, which literally means "above the genes", are the bridge between genotype and phenotype and modify genome function by offering a way to control the expression of genes (Dupont, Armant, & Brenner, 2009). Admittedly, internal and external cues influence the epigenetic landscape, disrupt genetic programming, and eventually modify DNA, mainly through regulating which genes are turned on or off (Peral-Sanchez, Hojeij, Ojeda, Steegers-Theunissen, & Willaime-Morawek, 2021).

EPIGENETICS OVERVIEW

EPIGENETICS DEFINITION

The term "epigenetics" was first introduced by Conrad Waddington in 1942 (Waddington, 1956) who referred to the study of epigenesis, namely how phenotypes derive from genotypes during development (Casadesús & Noyer-Weidner, 2013; Dupont et al., 2009). He defined epigenetics as "the branch of biology that studies the causal interactions between genes and their products which bring the phenotype into being" (Noble, 2015; Waddington, 1956). With the rapid growth of genetics, the meaning of the term has undergone several transitions and is now used to describe the study of changes in gene function that are heritable and are not attributed to alterations in the DNA sequence (Deans & Maggert, 2015). While the sequence of DNA remains constant, the epigenetic state of the genome (i.e., epigenome) changes dynamically in the cells of different tissues and, by using many coordinating enzymes, regulates the expression of genes to alter the phenotypes in different cell types (Lacal & Ventura, 2018). Epigenetic mechanisms can influence genes at

Prevention and Management of Cardiovascular and Metabolic Disease: Diet, Physical Activity and Healthy Aging,
First Edition. Christina N. Katsagoni, Peter Kokkinos, and Labros S. Sidossis.
© 2023 John Wiley & Sons Ltd. Published 2023 by John Wiley & Sons Ltd.

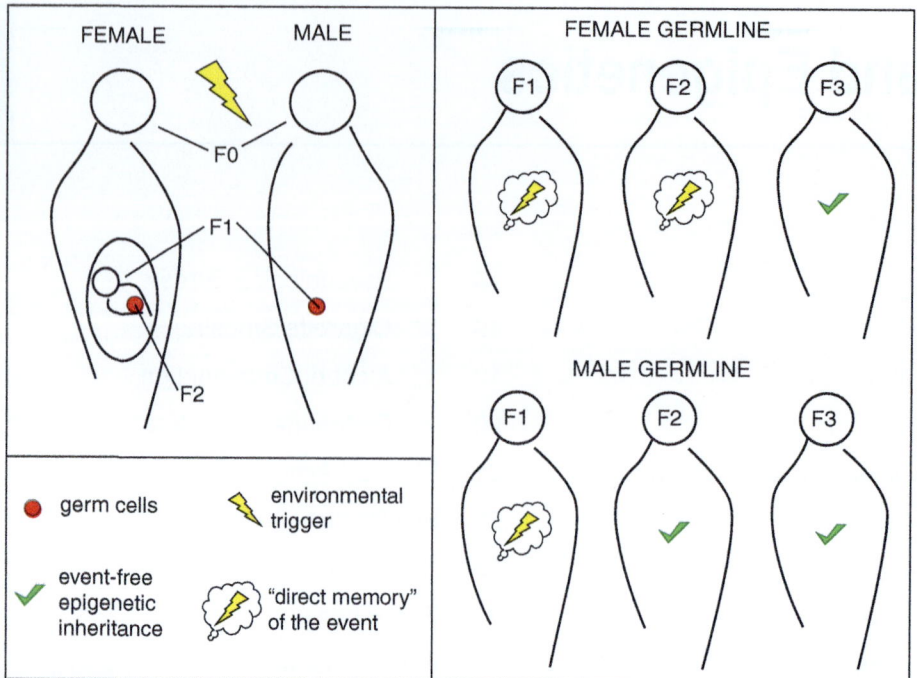

FIGURE 2.1   Transgenerational epigenetic inheritance. Source: (Lacal & Ventura, 2018 / Frontiers Media S.A / CC BY-4.0).

the transcriptional and post-transcriptional levels and/or at the translational and post-translational level (Gibney & Nolan, 2010).

Epigenetic and genetic information are both inherited, but contrary to genetic information, epigenetic data are reversible (called epigenetic plasticity) and may be affected by various stimuli or environmental factors (Bohacek & Mansuy, 2013). These changes may persist through multiple cell divisions, even for all of a cell's life, and may also be transferred to the offspring, lasting for multiple generations via trans-generational epigenetic inheritance (Wei, Huang, Yang, & Kang, 2017). The knowledge of the mechanism by which epigenetic information is transmitted is poor, but it is known to be transferred differently between sexes. More specifically, an exposure to an environmental factor, such as a toxicant, to a gestating F0 female individual promotes an epigenetic alteration in the germ cell programming of the F1 generation fetus (**Figure 2.1**). The altered germ cell epigenetics is then transmitted in the second (2) and the third (3) generations (Lacal & Ventura, 2018; Nilsson, Ben Maamar & Skinner, 2022), and consequently, only the fourth generation can be considered as "event free". An exposure to an environmental factor in the father, it can only modify his sperm, producing an epigenetic change in the F1 generation, effecting a reliable non-genetic inheritance in the third generation (Donkin & Barrès, 2018; Lacal & Ventura, 2018).

EPIGENETIC MECHANISMS

The fundamental molecular mechanisms that mediate epigenetic modulation are DNA methylation, histone posttranslational modification, and non-coding RNA regulation (Dupont et al., 2009) (**Figure 2.2**). The above-mentioned epigenetic mechanisms are controlled by several enzymes, the writers that add chemical residues to DNA and histones, the erasers that remove them, and the readers, specialized domain-containing proteins that identify and interpret those modifications (Biswas & Rao, 2018).

The most-studied epigenetic mechanism is DNA methylation, which includes the addition of a methyl group (CH_3) at the nucleotide cytosine (Dupont et al., 2009). The most common DNA methylation process is the covalent addition of the methyl group at the 5-carbon of the cytosine ring resulting in 5-methylcytosine (5-mC). In mammals, DNA methylation occurs at cytosines in any context of the genome; in somatic cells methylation occurs almost exclusively in a cytosine–guanine site (CpGs), while in embryonic stem cells (ESCs) as much as a quarter of all methylation appears in a non-CpG context. When methyl groups are present on a gene, that gene is turned off or silenced, and a protein is not produced from that gene.

Furthermore, histone modifications are key epigenetic regulators that control chromatin structure and gene transcription, thereby affecting various cellular phenotypes (Molina-Serrano, Kyriakou, & Kirmizis, 2019). Histone modification includes multiple, mostly reversible, chemical alterations (e.g., acetylation, methylation, and phosphorylation) of nucleosome core histones, particularly at their N-terminal sequences, and of the linker histone H1. Due to this characteristic, epigenetic modifications are reversible and thus able to dynamically modulate chromatin structure to activate or silence gene expression (Bannister & Kouzarides, 2011).

Novel insights have highlighted the important role of non-coding RNA transcripts in epigenetic gene regulation (Mattick & Makunin, 2006; Wei et al., 2017). The term

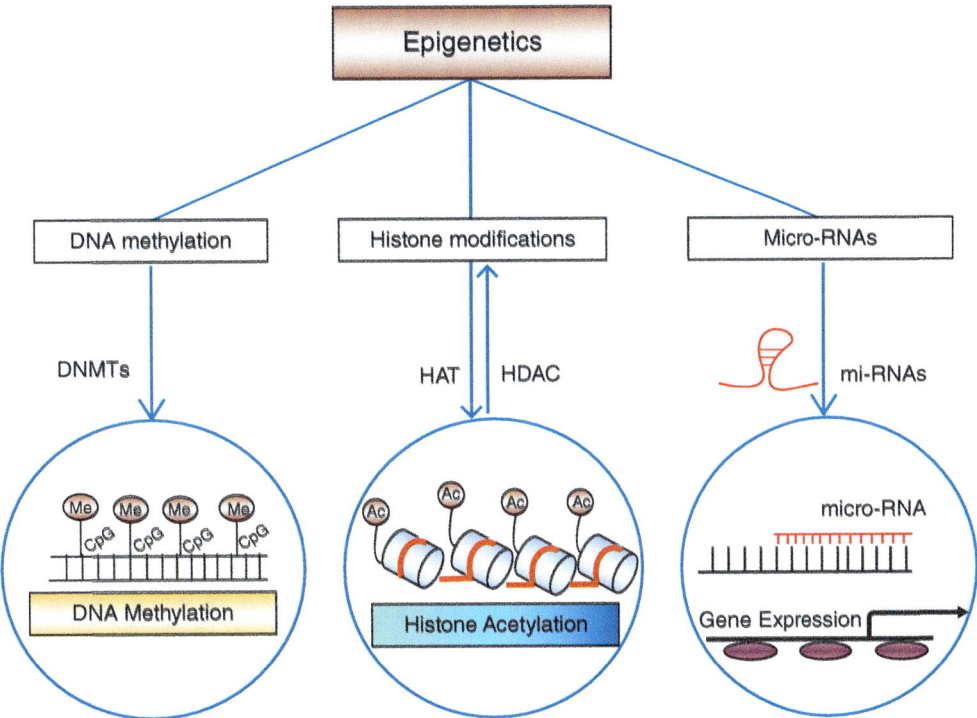

FIGURE 2.2 Overview of epigenetic modifications. Source: (Chaturvedi and Tyagi, 2014 / with permission of Elsevier).

non-coding RNA (ncRNA) is commonly used for RNA that does not encode a protein, however, many of these RNAs do contain information and are functional. Non-coding RNA helps control gene expression by attaching to coding RNA, along proteins that break down the coding RNA and prevent it from making proteins. Non-coding RNA may also recruit proteins that modify histones to turn genes on or off by making them more or less accessible, respectively, to RNA-making machinery.

EPIGENETICS AND DISEASE EPIDEMIOLOGY

Alterations in epigenetic marks such as modification of the wrong gene or the failure to add a chemical group to a particular gene or histone, could lead to abnormal gene activity or inactivity (Casadesús & Noyer-Weidner, 2013). Such epigenetic mechanisms could result in a vast spectrum of cell differentiations, morphogenesis, variability, and adaptability. Epigenetic modifications can directly cause disease, such as Beckwith Weidemann syndrome (BWS), an imprinting disorder caused by abnormal DNA methylation (Bakulski & Fallin, 2014). Epigenetics can also be the mechanism linking environmental exposures and disease, and classic example of this interaction is oxidative DNA damage caused by toxicants. Epigenetics may also influence the relationships between exposure and disease or genotype and disease via effect modification (i.e., exposure to air pollution and increased risk of cardiovascular disease). When targeting treatment, epigenetic factors can serve as useful biomarkers of disease status or disease subtype.

Incorrect epigenetic marks can result in birth defects, childhood diseases, or diseases during a person's lifespan. In this regard, epigenetic errors are associated with multiple NCDs, including cancer, cardiovascular, respiratory, and neurodegenerative diseases (Romani, Pistillo, & Banelli, 2015). Indeed, epigenetic modifications may be behind middle to late life functional declines. Early studies on epigenetic functions mainly focused on fetal development, aging, and cancer. As epigenetic research has progressed and epigenetic mechanisms have become better understood, possible epigenetic pathways have been implicated in complex diseases etiology, such as autoimmune diseases, inflammation, allergy, obesity, insulin resistance, type 2 diabetes (T2D), neurodegenerative diseases, autism spectrum disorders, bipolar disorder, and schizophrenia (Dupont et al., 2009; Ramsay, 2015).

Epigenetic errors are also implicated in imprinting disorders, such as Silver–Russell syndrome (SRS) and Beckwith–Weidemann syndrome (BWS), for individuals conceived by assisted reproductive technologies (ART) (Peral-Sanchez et al., 2021). ART conception is associated with an approximately two-fold increased risk of preterm birth, low birth weight, being small for gestational age or perinatal mortality, some of which may be attributable to epigenetic variation induced in the periconceptional period. Genome-wide DNA methylation profiling in cord blood and placenta revealed differences in the methylation status between ART and spontaneous conceiving populations (Novakovic et al., 2019).

Across epigenomic sites, particular regions show change in methylation within the same person over time (Bakulski & Fallin, 2014). Furthermore, it was recently demonstrated that some epigenetic marks can be reversible, a trait that it is as challenging as it is promising (Bohacek & Mansuy, 2013; Foley et al., 2008). This characteristic makes the genome flexible to respond and adapt to external stimuli, such as nutrition, stress, exercise, pollutants, and drugs, since epigenetic modifications are dynamic and intertwined with environmental and lifestyle cues.

THE BARKER HYPOTHESIS

What is beyond any doubt is that we are not born *tabula rasa*, as blank slates. Utero is the first environment that we are exposed to, and maternal stimuli can epigenetically modify the expression of our genes. It is well established that the environmental stimuli experienced during the first 1000 days of life, as early as pre-conception, the nine months of pregnancy and the first two years of life, are transmitted to offspring and subsequent generations (Gabbianelli & Damiani, 2018) (**Figure 2.3**). Contrary to the common notion that the interaction between genes and the environment starts right after the birth, the fetal origins hypothesis was a scientific breakthrough in the late 1980s (Barker, 1995). Up until then, scientific research mainly focused on childhood environmental exposures and how these affected

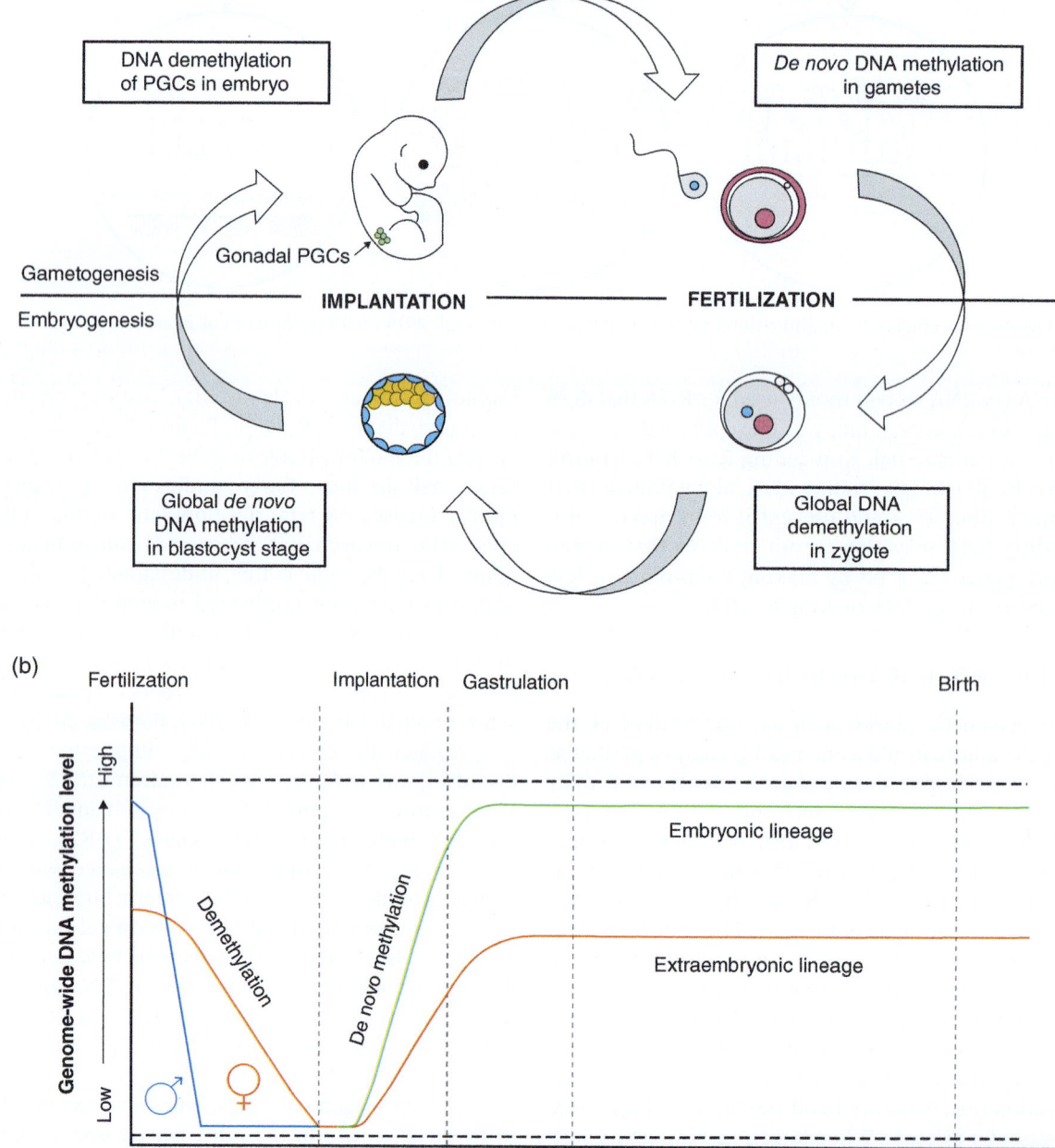

FIGURE 2.3 (a) Epigenetic reprogramming in the germ line and somatic cells. (b) Epigenetic reprogramming in embryos. Source: (Wallén et al., 2021 / MDPI / CC BY-4.0).

the risk of developing chronic diseases and mortality. On the other hand, Professor Barker, an innovating researcher, observed that a higher incidence of cardiovascular and infant mortality in regions of England and Wales was related to low birth weight, which was in turn associated with poor maternal nutrition and higher maternal mortality rates. These observations, along with the fact that offspring who weighed more at birth and were still breastfed 1 year later had lower death rates, led to Barker's hypothesis of "the fetal and infant origins of adult disease". According to this hypothesis, fetal undernutrition in middle to late gestation leads to disproportionate fetal growth, which predisposes them to certain diseases in adulthood. Hales and Barker later published the thrifty phenotype hypothesis, proposing that "the epidemiological associations between poor fetal and infant growth and the subsequent development of T2D and the metabolic syndrome result from the effects of poor nutrition in early life, which produces permanent changes in glucose-insulin metabolism" (Hales & Barker, 2001).

This influential theory aroused a great deal of research interest and activity in the field of developmental plasticity, and over the years, vast scientific data were documented that closely linked maternal obesity and gestational diabetes with several metabolic implications in offspring (Gabbianelli & Damiani, 2018). In addition, the Barker hypothesis set the basis for the developmental origins of health and disease hypothesis that "recognizes the broader scope of developmental cues, extending from the oocyte to the infant and beyond, and captures the concept that the early life environment has widespread consequences for later life" (Gillman, 2005; Koemel & Skilton, 2022). In fact, environmental exposures and lifestyle behaviors, from the prenatal period and on, seem to be the origin of diseases such as diabetes, cardiovascular diseases, obesity, and cancer. While one's lifestyle clearly affects an individual's health, vast epidemiological data emphasize that maternal and paternal lifestyle(s) can modify the risk of chronic diseases in subsequent generations (Donkin & Barrès, 2018).

EPIGENETICS *IN UTERO* AND MATERNAL LIFESTYLE

The ability of a given genotype to produce different phenotypes in response to different environments is plasticity and is part of the organism's adaptability to environmental factors to provide the best chances to survive and reproduce (Bateson, Barker, et al., 2004). Our nature is designed to use placental, nutritional, and endocrine cues to set long-term biological, mental, and behavioral alterations in response to internal and external stimuli (Kuzawa, 2005) (**Figure 2.4**). The window of developmental plasticity extends from conception to early childhood and adolescence and could be epigenetically transmitted to next generations. The epigenome, *in utero* and early in life, presents a high degree of plasticity. A wide spectrum of gestational cues, including diet, stress, toxins, and maternal lifestyle overall, significantly impacts fetal growth and epigenetically modulates the offspring's phenotype and health (Koemel & Skilton, 2022). Maternal nutrition is an important genetic regulator, since nutritional exposures mediate fetal epigenetic modifications.

MATERNAL UNDERNUTRITION

Very interesting scientific data concerning the effect of nutrition during gestation arose from a classic epidemiological study during the Dutch famine of 1944–1945 (World War II), which demonstrated that individuals conceived during the famine were at a greater risk of CVD and metabolic disorders, such as obesity, diabetes, impaired glucose tolerance, and hyperlipidemia in adulthood (Lumey, 1992). Decades later, a significant reduction in DNA methylation in famine-exposed offspring was observed at the promoter of the insulin-like growth factor 2 (IGF2) gene, which regulates fetal development and growth. Most importantly, the Dutch famine data highlight that nutritional deprivation can have adverse effects on health beyond a person's lifespan and leave a lasting epigenetic imprint on offspring. Similarly,

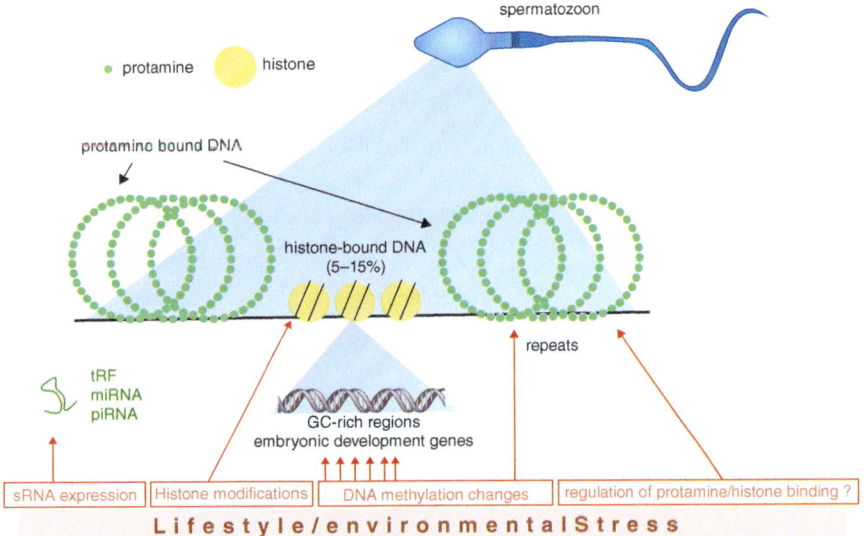

FIGURE 2.4 Overview of epigenetic marks susceptible to remodeling with environmental stimuli. Source: (Donkin & Barrès, 2018 / with permission of Elsevier).

epidemiological data from other famine studies (Hult et al., 2010; Li et al., 2010) demonstrate that adults exposed *in utero* or early in life to energy deficits had an increased risk for developing hypertension, glucose intolerance, and obesity compared to individuals conceived after the famine.

Additionally, maternal malnutrition along with low-protein diets from the pre-implantation period to late lactation, is associated with the onset of metabolic diseases in adult offspring, which are mediated by epigenetic modifications (Koemel and Skilton, 2022; Peral-Sanchez et al., 2021). Undernutrition during pregnancy may alter the fetal epigenome through reduced intake and bioavailability of protein, amino acids, and key micro-nutrients involved in one-carbon metabolism, such as folate, methionine, choline, betaine, vitamin B12, vitamin B6, antioxidants, and other bioactive compounds (Cai et al., 2021; Jankovic-Karasoulos et al., 2021). The above-mentioned nutrients are involved in one carbon metabolism and subsequently in DNA-methylation process as co-factors or methyl donors. More specifically, methionine, choline, and folate are substrates needed for the methylation process (methyl-donor nutrients); the vitamins B2, B6, and B12 are co-factors needed for methyl-transferases, the enzymes involved in the methylation process (Kohil, Al-Asmakh, Al-Shafai, & Terranegra, 2021). Vitamin B6 serves as a coenzyme to serine hydroxymethyltransferase, the key enzyme in the folate cycle converting tetrahydrofolate (THF) to 5,10-methyleneTHF. Riboflavin (vitamin B2) is a precursor for flavin adenine dinucleotides, which is a cofactor to methylenetetrahydrofolate reductase (MTHFR) in the conversion of 5,10-methylene THF to 5-methyl THF. Vitamin B12 is the coenzyme of methionine synthase, which catalyzes the reaction of homocysteine involved in the production of methionine from homocysteine and betaine (**Figure 2.5**) (Anderson, Sant, & Dolinoy, 2012).

Folate-mediated one-carbon metabolism refers to a complex network of interconnected metabolic pathways, which ultimately result in a supply of methyl groups for DNA, RNA, or protein methylation. Folate, in particular, is a key source of the methyl group required for DNA and histone methylation, and sub-optimal intake during gestation may alter methylation patterns that are vital for fetal development and the offspring's health (Lintas, 2019). Most importantly, folate deficiency is correlated with methylation changes in brain tissue and may alter epigenetic marks implicated in neural tube defects, thus neurocognitive and neurobehavioral deficits (Joubert et al., 2016).

Interestingly, there is little evidence that nutritional interventions during early or mid-pregnancy, like providing undernourished mothers with protein, energy, and micronutrient supplements, reduces the cardio-metabolic disease risk in offspring. Data from animal studies suggest that it may be more crucial to intervene earlier in the pregnancy, when the developmental window is more critical, or even pre-conception, to modify placentation and organogenesis (which occur mainly in the first trimester) as well as peri-conceptional epigenetic changes (Fall & Kumaran, 2019).

MATERNAL OVERNUTRITION

Excess fat and caloric consumption during gestation as well as a mother's pre-pregnancy obesity are also linked to epigenetic changes (**Figure 2.6**). Maternal metabolic disorders (e.g., poor glycemic control, hypertension) are associated with epigenetic alterations of the offspring too. Notably, genes that regulate energy and glucose metabolism as well as adipogenesis, leptin encoding, and transcription factors are controlled by epigenetic mechanisms (Elshenawy & Simmons, 2016). Maternal overnutrition may modify the expression of hypothalamic genes that can increase fetal and neonatal energy intake (Şanlı & Kabaran, 2019). Moreover, considering that lipids act as both transcriptional activators and signaling molecules, excess lipid exposure may regulate genes involved in lipid sensing and metabolism. It was suggested that the prevalence of an obese phenotype is closely related to epigenetic marks, originating from *in utero* stimuli and passing on through trans-generational transmission (Heerwagen, Miller, Barbour, & Friedman, 2010).

More specifically, leptin and insulin signals modify the development of eating behaviors by affecting the neuronal circuits in the hypothalamus. According to these neuroendocrine factors, increased fetal appetite, energy intake, and adiposity

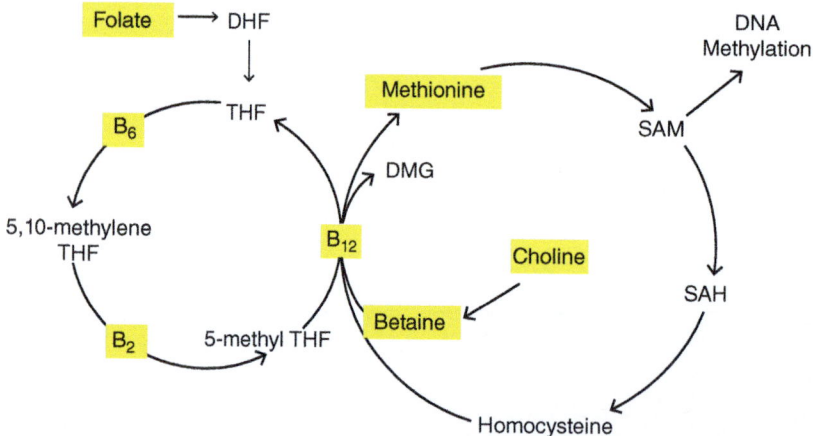

FIGURE 2.5 Dietary methyl donors and one carbon metabolism. Source: (Anderson et al., 2012 / with permission of Elsevier).

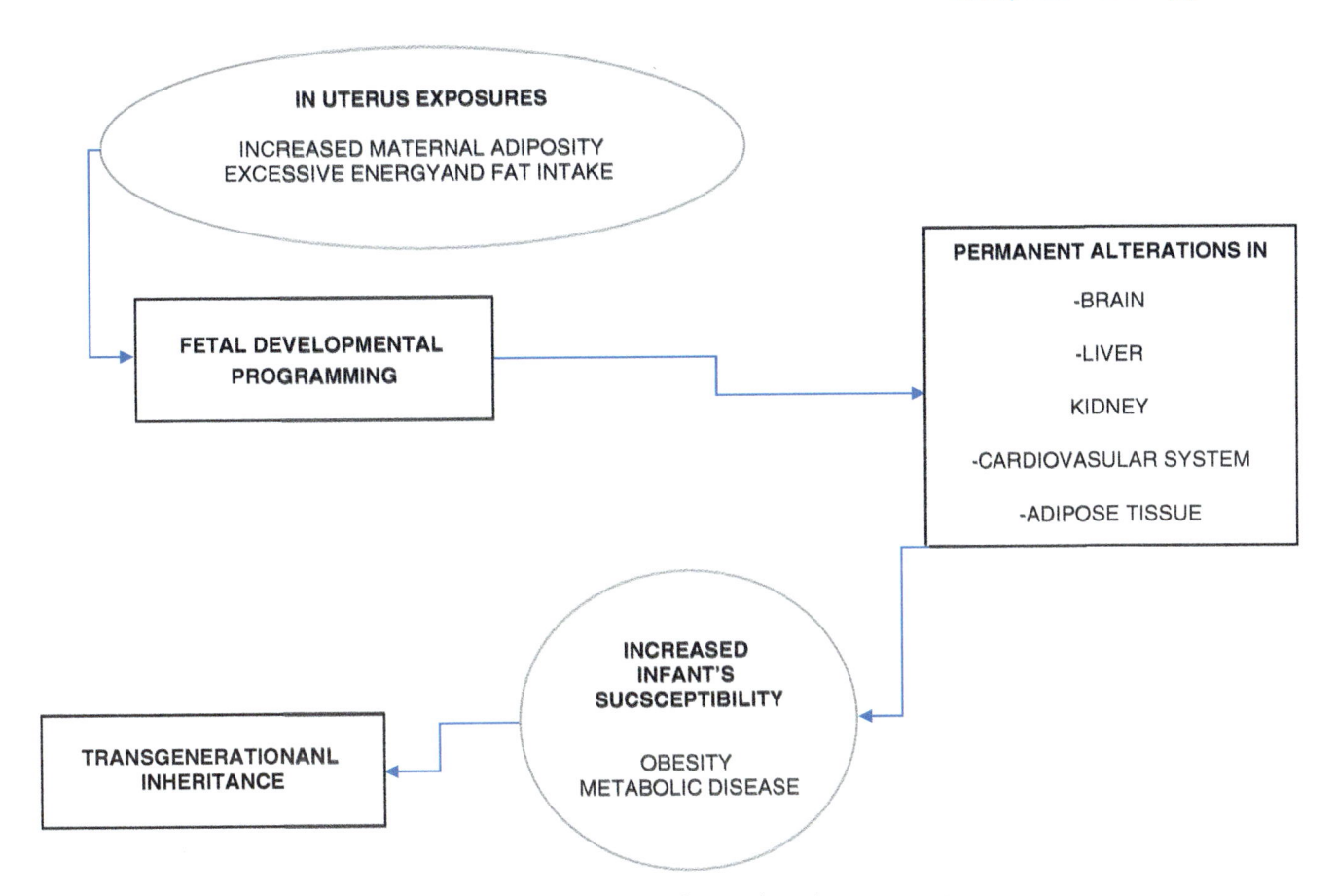

FIGURE 2.6 Consequences of an early-life exposure in an intrauterine obesogenic environment.

alter the food preferences and body composition after birth (Lawlor et al., 2006). Overall, maternal obesity and overnutrition can lead to permanent changes in metabolic and epigenetic mechanisms, and their offspring are predisposed to be overweight or with obesity themselves. Siblings born to mothers with obesity before and after the mother's bariatric surgery had different obesity risks; the children born after weight loss had a lower risk of being overweight or with obesity (Şanlı & Kabaran, 2019). Therefore, considering the public health burden of obesity and metabolic diseases across generations, perinatal weight control interventions including lifestyle modifications through a healthy and balanced dietary pattern and exercise in mothers with obesity should be considered (**Figure 2.7**).

DIETARY PATTERN AS AN EPIGENETIC MARK

It is well documented that increased energy and nutrient supply during gestation, especially a high fat and sugar diet, leads to rapid weight gain of the fetus, which induces permanent epigenetic changes within the central energy balance and appetite regulatory pathways (Şanlı & Kabaran, 2019). A typical example of this dietary pattern is the Western diet, which tends to be high in saturated fats, red meats, and sugar but low in fresh fruits and vegetables, whole grains, seafood, and poultry. The Western diet is linked to many diseases (hypertension, heart disease, diabetes, and obesity), and it is speculated that these physiological dysfunctions might be mediated via epigenetic changes from intrauterine life till adulthood (Kopp, 2019). So, it is reasonable to assume that there is a dynamic interplay between dietary patterns and genes, which suggests that diet composition may result in epigenetic signatures during lifespan. One of the best examples of a profound and seemingly direct diet-mediated epigenetic effect in nature occurs in honeybee colonies, where the behavior, function, lifespan, and morphology of genetically identical bees can be changed in response to a specific food (Ideraabdullah & Zeisel, 2018).

There is growing interest that dietary compounds can epigenetically reprogram gene expression, and these nutrition-induced health properties may have important implications for cancer prevention and chronic disease (Tiffon, 2018). Emerging data suggest that bioactive compounds and, most importantly, dietary phytochemicals have epigenetic targets, especially in the cancer prevention field: dietary polyphenols present in fruits and vegetables; catechins in tea; resveratrol in peanuts, mulberries, cranberries, and blueberries, but most abundant in grape skin; curcumin in turmeric; isoflavones and genistein in soybeans (the most studied); and isothiocyanates in cruciferous vegetables including broccoli, cabbage, and kale (Hardy & Tollefsbol, 2011) (**Table 2.1**). Nevertheless, the exact mechanism that mediates the relationship between dietary components and the epigenome, and mostly how this interaction impacts human health, is not fully understood since data from

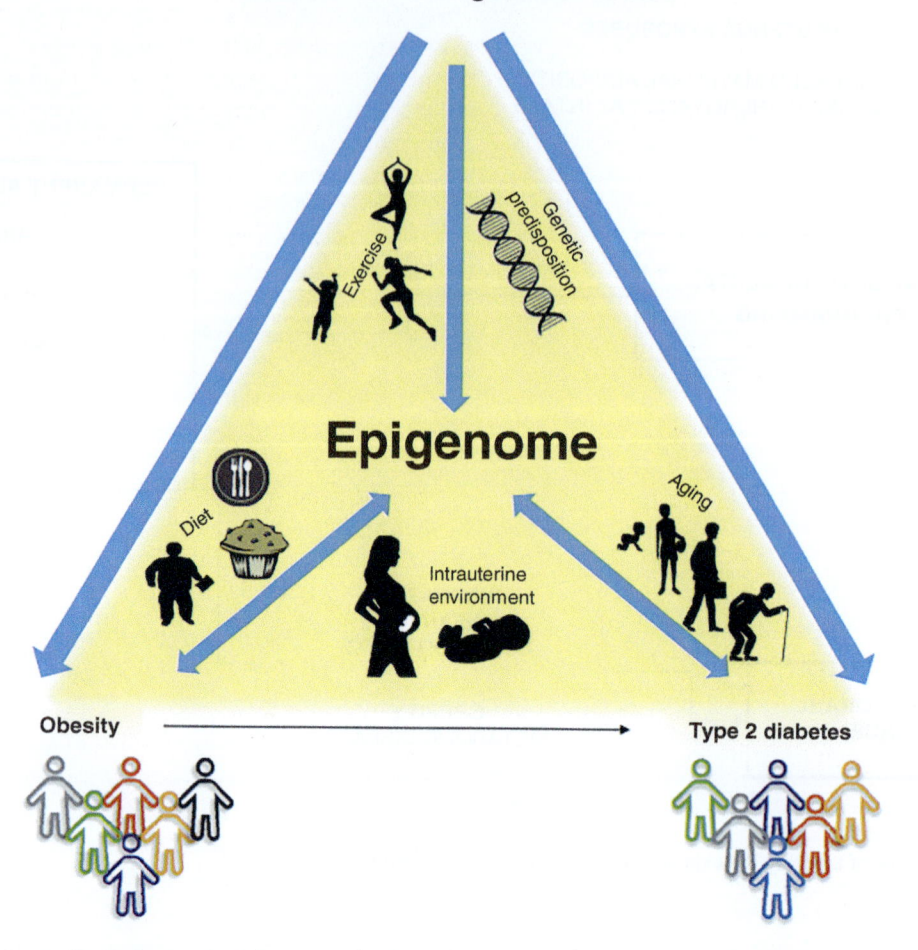

FIGURE 2.7 Interactions between the environment, epigenome, obesity, and type 2 diabetes. Source: (Ling & Rönn, 2019 / with permission of Elsevier).

Table 2.1 A summary of some dietary components considered to be protective against cancer.

Nutrient	Food origin	Epigenetic role
Methionine	Sesame seeds, brazil nuts, fish, peppers, spinach	SAM synthesis
Folic acid	Leafy vegetables, sunflower seeds, baker's yeast, liver	Methionine synthesis
Vitamin B12	Meat, liver, shellfish, milk	Methionine synthesis
Vitamin B6	Meats, whole grain products, vegetables, nuts	Methionine synthesis
SAM-e (SAM)	Popular dietary supplement pill; unstable in food	Enzymes transfer methyl groups from SAM directly to the DNA
Choline	Egg yolks, liver, soy, cooked beef, chicken, veal, and turkey	Methyl donor to SAM
Betaine	Wheat, spinach, shellfish, and sugar beets	Break down the toxic byproducts of SAM synthesis
Resveratrol	Red wine	Removes acetyl groups from histones, improving health (shown in lab mice)
Genistein	Soy, soy products	Increased methylation, cancer prevention, unknown mechanism
Sulforaphane	Broccoli	Increased histone acetylation, upregulates anti-cancer genes
Butyrate	Fermented dietary fiber in the GI tract	Increased histone acetylation, upregulates 'protective' genes, increased lifespan (shown in the lab in flies)
Diallyl sulphide (DADS)	Garlic	Increased histone acetylation, upregulates anti-cancer genes

Source: (Tiffon, 2018 / MDPI / CC BY-4.0).

studies in humans are limited. These nutrients may either supply the molecules that comprise the epigenetic mark (e.g., methyl groups for DNA methylation) or interact directly to induce or repress the activity of epigenetic regulatory enzymes; thus, they might act as intermediate signaling molecules for the dietary regulation of cell metabolism (Ideraabdullah & Zeisel, 2018).

Nevertheless, nutritional components interact with each other, and it would be sounder to consider a holistic diet approach. In this regard, epigenetic diets are a dietary pattern that provides bioactive nutritional factors that can influence epigenetic mechanisms capable of protecting against cancer, aging, and metabolic diseases (Kontogiorgis, Bompou, Ntella, & Berghe, 2010; Tiffon, 2018). Also termed nutrigenomics, the interaction of nutrient intake and individual genetic differences on genetic expression represents an opportunity for personalized medicine to prevent and manage chronic diseases and cancer (Ideraabdullah & Zeisel, 2018).

The Mediterranean diet (MD) is an excellent model of an epigenetic diet, since it is characterized by a high consumption of whole grains, vegetables, fruit, and legumes, the use of olive oil, a regular consumption of fresh fish and moderate red-meat consumption. Numerous studies provide strong evidence that adhering to the MD is inversely associated with total mortality, CVD, cancer, and metabolic diseases. Undoubtably, the MD is a lifestyle pattern that can improve health status and favorably contribute to a better quality of life, thus increasing lifespan both directly and through its own epigenetic mechanisms (Carlos-Reyes et al., 2019). Key MD foods, such as olive oil, oily fish, nuts, yogurt, fruits, spices, and herbs, are considered functional foods due to their nutraceutical content (Chrysohoou & Stefanadis, 2013) (**Figure 2.8**). Bioactive compounds and nutraceuticals found in abundance in the MD, interact with gene polymorphisms that play a role in aging and atherosclerosis, but also interfere with carcinogenesis mechanisms, by restoring the inflammatory balance through preserving the intestinal microbiota and epigenetically altering oncogenic and oncosuppressive factors (Divella, Daniele, Savino, & Paradiso, 2020). The MD as a dietary pattern presents a high antioxidant and nutrigenomic modulation power with all the characteristics of an example of the environment-livings-environment relationship (Caradonna, Consiglio, Luparello, & Gentile, 2020).

EPIGENETICS AND STRESS

Emerging scientific data advocate that maternal exposures to stress, such as psychological stress, mother's depression, smoking, alcohol, and environmental pollutants, can alter epigenetic gene programming related to neurodevelopmental and behavioral deficits in the offspring that persist throughout childhood and adulthood (Gheorghe, Goyal, Mittal, & Longo, 2010) (**Figure 2.9**). The main pathway that stress stimuli mediate epigenetic changes in fetal programming is through exposure to maternal cortisol. More specifically, prenatal maternal stress may activate the pituitary-adrenal (HPA) axis, triggering glucocorticoid secretion that reaches the fetus; relatively small increases in maternal cortisol can double fetal concentrations. Glucocorticoid receptors bind to cortisol and other glucocorticoids to create a negative feedback within the HPA axis and regulate the body's response to stress. The effects of maternal stress on fetal development include a wide range of physiological implications in immune function, brain development, and behavior outcomes (Cao-Lei, Laplante, & King, 2016). Of special

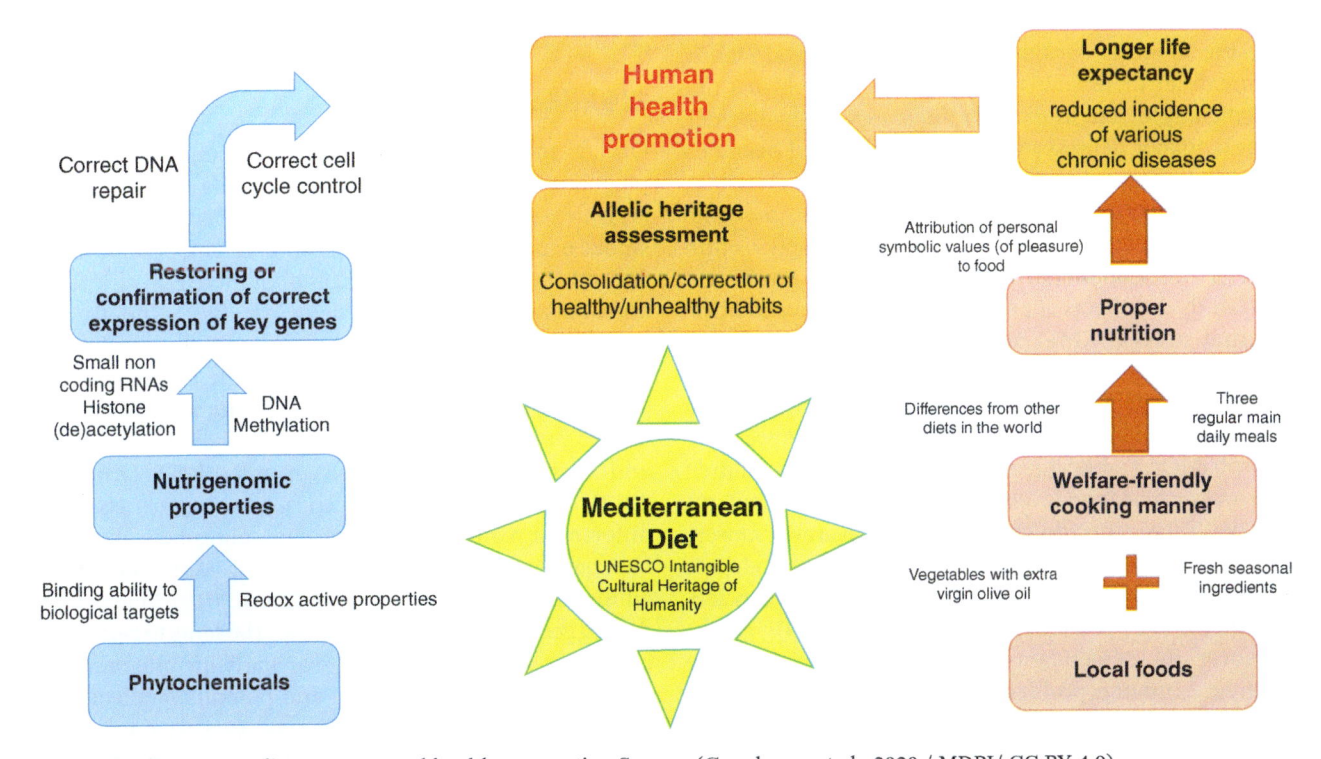

FIGURE 2.8 Mediterranean diet concepts and healthy properties. Source: (Caradonna et al., 2020 / MDPI/ CC BY-4.0).

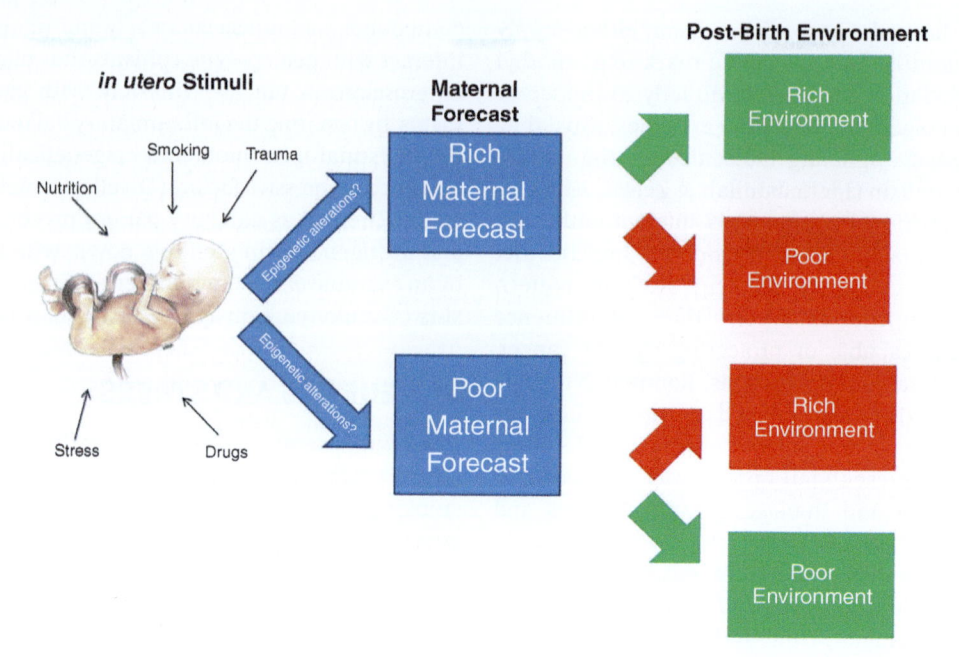

FIGURE 2.9 *In utero* stimuli-associated epigenetic alterations and maternal forecasts. Source: (Knopik et al., 2012 / with permission of Cambridge University Press).

concern is the role of epigenetics in synaptic plasticity, memory and cognitive processes, and shaping stress-vulnerable phenotypes and behavioral adaptations to chronic stress (Stankiewicz, Swiergiel, & Lisowski, 2013).

PSYCHOLOGICAL STRESS

Psychological stress during pregnancy, like maternal depression and anxiety disorders, are closely associated with long-term epigenome alterations in offspring (Monk, Spicer, & Champagne, 2012; Serpeloni et al., 2019). Numerous studies suggest that *in utero* exposure to stress cues affect the child's mental health, mainly through an increased risk of psychiatric problems like attention-deficit hyperactivity disorder, autism spectrum disorder, schizophrenia, major depression, and anxiety-related disorders (Lupien, McEwen, Gunnar, & Heim, 2009; O'Connor et al., 2005; Serpeloni et al., 2019). The most interesting data come from studies that examine the gene-by-environment interactions during the *in utero* developmental window. Project Ice Storm was designed to study the effects of exposure to varying levels of prenatal maternal stress (PNMS), resulting from an independent stressor, on childrens' development from birth through childhood (Laplante, Brunet, Schmitz, Ciampi, & King, 2008). Children exposed *in utero* to high levels of objective stress had lower full-scale IQs, verbal IQs, and language abilities compared to children exposed to low or moderate levels of objective PNMS. Similarly, data from the Tutsi genocide study (Musanabaganwa, Jansen, Fatumo, et al., 2020), demonstrated that the terror of genocide was associated with chemical modifications to the DNA of genocide-exposed women and their offspring (Perroud et al., 2014).

Moreover, the descendants of Holocaust survivors have different stress hormone profiles than their peers, which perhaps predisposes them to anxiety disorders (Kellermann, 2013). Despite previous research that assumed that such transmission was caused by environmental factors, such as the parents' behavior, new research indicates that these trans-generational effects may also be epigenetically transmitted to their children. Many of these modifications occur in genes previously implicated with a risk for mental disorders such as post-traumatic stress disorders and depression, suggesting that, unlike gene mutations, these chemical epigenetic modifications can retain a rapid response to trauma across generations (Stankiewicz et al., 2013). The stress regulatory system prepares us for the fight, flight, or freeze reflex, and epigenetic changes may train offspring to fight harder, flee faster, or freeze faster when facing stressful stimuli.

CIGARETTE SMOKING

One of the most hazardous environmental exposures during pregnancy with long-lasting effects on the offspring's epigenome is cigarette smoking. Numerous studies have associated prenatal smoke exposure with reduced birth weight, poor developmental and psychological outcomes, and an increased risk for diseases and behavioral disorders later in life (Knopik, Maccani, Francazio, & McGeary, 2012). Many of the mechanisms that underlie fetal growth and development defects are epigenetically modified. More specifically maternal cigarette smoking during pregnancy is associated with altered DNA methylation and dysregulated expression of microRNA (Knopik et al., 2012). Furthermore, smoke exposure *in utero* is associated with differential methylation of cytosine–phosphate–guanine (CpG) base pairs in newborns, children, young adults, and middle-aged adults (Zong, Liu, Li, Ouyang, & Chen, 2019). Maternal smoking during gestation potentially exposes the fetus to cigarette-related chemicals and toxins leading to an early life programming effect that persists into adolescence and potentially affects long-term health. These epigenetic changes are suggested to be associated with increased body mass index, blood pressure, and blood lipids levels in adulthood, which increase the risk for diabetes, heart disease, and stroke later in life (Rauschert, Melton, Burdge, et al., 2019). Overall, cigarette smoking affects global epigenetic regulation of transcription across tissue types and is associated with genome instability (Kaur, Begum, Thota, & Batra, 2019). A growing body of evidence supports the importance of epigenetic alterations in the initiation and development of smoking-induced diseases, such as CVDs, chronic obstructive pulmonary disease, and cancers (Zong et al., 2019).

ALCOHOL CONSUMPTION

Prenatal alcohol exposure is one of the most significant causes of developmental disability termed alcohol spectrum disorders (Oei, 2020). Alcohol consumption during pregnancy leads to an increased risk of neurological deficits and developmental abnormalities in the fetus. Apparently, early pregnancy is a sensitive period for environmentally induced epigenetic changes and is, therefore, prone to molecular changes caused by alcohol exposure. Undoubtedly, alcohol alters epigenetic marks, including DNA methylation, histone modifications, and non-coding RNAs, though the exact molecular mechanisms are not fully understood. One suggested mechanism is the alcohol-induced reduction in folate, B6, or B12 vitamins in the methionine cycle, which decreases both DNA and histone methylation (Wallén, Auvinen, & Kaminen-Ahola, 2021). This, in turn, influences several genes associated with brain development, oxidative stress, and proinflammatory cytokine production. Consequently, physical and cognitive abnormalities known as fetal alcohol spectrum disorder (FASD) are observed in children exposed to alcohol in utero.

Notably, both genetic and epigenetic factors affect alcohol consumption and interfere with the transition from use to abuse, to addiction via neuroadaptations (Krishnan, Sakharkar, Teppen, Berkel, & Pandey, 2014). Ethanol usually dysregulates neuronal functions via epigenetic modifiers and could lead to positive and negative affective states of addiction (Ciafrè et al., 2019). In particular, the enzymes responsible for chromatin remodeling (e.g., histone deacetylases and methyltransferases, DNA methyltransferases, or DNMT enzymes) were identified as common molecular mechanisms for the interaction of stress and alcohol (Palmisano & Pandey, 2017). Noticeably, alcohol intake can modulate the amygdala epigenome, thus acute and chronic alcohol consumption can lead to a reduction in the alcohol-induced anxiety state. After alcohol cessation, the chromatin returns to its initial state, and this leads to the development of the anxiety and drinking behaviors usually found in alcoholism. A deeper knowledge of alcoholism mechanisms, which are under complex epigenetic regulation, may inform addiction management and lead to promising therapeutic interventions to treat alcoholism.

ENDOCRINE DISRUPTORS

Endocrine-disrupting chemicals (EDCs) are chemicals such as drugs, pesticides, plastic softeners, and flame retardants that mimic, block, or interfere with hormones in the body's endocrine system and are associated with various health issues (la Merrill et al., 2020). Dioxin and dioxin-like compounds, heavy metals, inhaled pollutants, plastic components such as bisphenol A (BPA) and phthalates, parabens, and various flame retardants are examples of EDCs. The best-studied mechanism by which ECDs mediate their negative impact on human health is through the interaction of EDCs with hormone receptors of the nuclear receptor family, such as estrogen, androgen, and thyroid hormone receptors (Nettore, Franchini, Palatucci, Macchia, & Ungaro, 2021).

Numerous data strongly demonstrate that early exposure during the critical developmental window of fetus life can increase the risk of reproductive defects, metabolic diseases, cognitive dysfunctions, and cancers, among other diseases (Alavian-Ghavanini & Rüegg, 2018). Though the exact mechanism that mediates these abnormalities later in life is not fully understood, novel insights emphasize that epigenetic alterations might be responsible since endocrine disruptors act on the epigenome in several ways, mainly through global and gene-specific action (Alavian-Ghavanini & Rüegg, 2018).

PHYSICAL ACTIVITY AND EPIGENETIC ALTERATIONS

Physical inactivity and sedentary behavior are leading risk factors closely related to the pathogenesis of metabolic diseases such as insulin resistance, T2D, inflammation, cardiovascular risk, obesity, cancer, and dyslipidemias. Cumulative evidence suggests that regular physical exercise can improve the negative consequences of physical inactivity via epigenetic alterations in several tissues, including adipose, liver, brain, and blood cells (Sellami, Bragazzi, Prince, Denham, & Elrayess, 2021). Complex molecular mechanisms are activated in the skeletal muscle and several metabolites may be substrates for epigenetic modifications, enabling transcriptional changes to key pathways and leading to muscle adaptation and remodeling. Skeletal muscle initiates cross talk with other tissues, especially the central nervous system, by releasing protein hormones and myokines, which can exert autocrine, paracrine, and long-distance endocrine effects.

Recent data suggest that physical fitness might exceed its beneficial effect beyond the individual and impact its offspring health through trans-generational epigenetic regulation. While scientific data are limited, those existing support the hypothesis that parental exercise induces epigenetic changes in offspring by modifying both global DNA methylation and promoter-region methylation of specific genes (Barrón-Cabrera et al., 2019). Interestingly, exercise also attenuates or reverses some high-fat diet–associated methylation patterns. Many of the physical activity–mediated epigenetic marks are implicated in metabolic functions, such as the regulation of oxidative metabolism and glucose transportation, alterations that are clinically significant for offspring (Barrón-Cabrera et al., 2019). Moreover, exercise improves cognitive development, as hippocampal DNA methylation is lower in exercise-exposed offspring (Mega et al., 2018). More specifically, adults whose mothers had exercised on a treadmill during pregnancy had a better learning curve and offspring of mothers who had practiced strength training showed slightly better results in terms of memorization and learning tasks.

KEY POINTS

- Epigenetics literally means "above the genes", and is the study of changes in gene function that are heritable and not attributed to alterations of the DNA sequence. Epigenetic alterations occur during the entire lifespan, from conception to adulthood, and are reversible.
- Epigenetic errors are associated with a variety of human disorders, including cancer, cardiovascular, respiratory, and neurodegenerative diseases, among others.
- Our genes are flexible to respond and adapt to external stimuli, such as nutrition, stress, exercise, pollutants, and drugs; epigenetic modifications are dynamic and intertwined with environmental and lifestyle cues.
- Environmental exposures and lifestyle behaviors, from the prenatal period onward, seem to be the origin of NCDs such as diabetes, CVD, obesity, and cancer.
- Maternal over- and undernutrition is closely related to fetal development and the risk of metabolic abnormalities in the offspring.
- The prevalence of an obese phenotype is closely related to epigenetic marks that originate from *in utero* stimuli and pass on through transgenerational transmission.
- Diet is a strong epigenetic modulator and nutrigenomics represents an opportunity for personalized medicine to prevent and manage chronic diseases and preventable cancers.
- Maternal exposure to stress (psychological, smoking, alcohol) activates the pituitary-adrenal (HPA) axis and is related to neurodevelopmental and behavioral deficits in the offspring.
- Prenatal alcohol exposure is one of the most significant causes of developmental disability termed alcohol spectrum disorders. Moreover, alcohol addiction might be mediated by epigenetic mechanisms.

SELF-ASSESSMENT QUESTIONS

1. True or False: Can epigenetic changes be inherited to the next generations?

2. Which of the following diet compounds have epigenetic effects?
   (a) Mercury
   (b) Curcumin
   (c) Genistein
   (d) All the above are correct.

3. How can excessive gain weight during pregnancy affect the health status of the offspring?

4. In what ways does our environment predispose us to be obese?

5. Maternal anxiety:
   (a) Is related to the offspring's depression.
   (b) Can lead to offspring metabolic abnormalities.
   (c) Can be epigenetically transmitted to the offspring.
   (d) All the above are correct.

6. True or False: Epigenetic alterations are mainly inherited from the mother. Why?

7. How can air pollutants and living in the city lead to epigenetic alterations?

8. How can epigenetics lead the way for a personalized healthcare approach?

9. What is an epigenetic diet?

10. Physical activity can modulate gene expression through epigenetic alterations.
    (a) The exact type and dose need to be determined.
    (b) Mainly aerobic activities activate epigenetic alterations.
    (c) By decreasing basal levels of inflammation.
    (d) All the above are correct.

REFERENCES

Alavian-Ghavanini, A., & Rüegg, J. (2018). Understanding epigenetic effects of endocrine disrupting chemicals: From mechanisms to novel test methods. *Basic & Clinical Pharmacology & Toxicology*, 122 (1): 38–45. doi: 10.1111/bcpt.12878.

Alegría-Torres, J. A., Baccarelli, A., & Bollati, V. (2011). Epigenetics and lifestyle. *Epigenomics* 3 (3): 267–277. doi: 10.2217/epi.11.22.

Anderson, O. S., Sant, K. E., & Dolinoy, D. C. (2012). Nutrition and epigenetics: an interplay of dietary methyl donors, one-carbon metabolism and DNA methylation. The Journal of nutritional biochemistry, 23(8), 853–859. https://doi.org/10.1016/j.jnutbio.2012.03.003.

Bakulski, K. M., & Fallin, M. D. (2014). Epigenetic epidemiology: promises for public health research. *Environmental and molecular mutagenesis*, 55(3), 171–183. https://doi.org/10.1002/em.21850

Bannister, A. J., & Kouzarides, T. (2011). Regulation of chromatin by histone modifications. *Cell Research* 21 (3): 381–395. doi: 10.1038/cr.2011.22.

Barker, D. J. P. (1995). Fetal origins of coronary heart disease. *BMJ* 311 (6998): 171–174. doi: 10.1136/bmj.311.6998.171.

Barrón-Cabrera, E., Ramos-Lopez, O., González-Becerra, K., Riezu-Boj, J. I., Milagro, F. I., Martínez-López, E., & Martínez, J. A. (2019). Epigenetic modifications as outcomes of exercise interventions related to specific metabolic alterations: A systematic review. *Lifestyle Genomics* 12 (1–6): 25–44. doi: 10.1159/000503289.

Bateson, P., Barker, D., Clutton-Brock, T., Deb, D., D'Udine, B., Foley, R. A., ... Sultan, S. E. (2004). Developmental plasticity and human health. *Nature* 430 (6998): 419–421. doi: 10.1038/nature02725.

Biswas, S., & Rao, C. M. (2018). Epigenetic tools (the writers, the readers, and the erasers) and their implications in cancer therapy. *European Journal of Pharmacology 837*: 8–24. doi: 10.1016/j.ejphar.2018.08.021.

Bohacek, J., & Mansuy, I. M. (2013). Epigenetic inheritance of disease and disease risk. *Neuropsychopharmacology 38* (1): 220–236. doi: 10.1038/npp.2012.110.

Cai, S., Quan, S., Yang, G., Ye, Q., Chen, M., Yu, H., . . . Qiao, S. (2021). One carbon metabolism and mammalian pregnancy outcomes. *Molecular Nutrition & Food Research 65* (2): 2000734. doi: 10.1002/mnfr.202000734.

Cao-Lei, L., Laplante, D. P., & King, S. (2016). Prenatal maternal stress and epigenetics: Review of the human research. *Current Molecular Biology Reports 2* (1): 16–25. doi: 10.1007/s40610-016-0030-x.

Caradonna, F., Consiglio, O., Luparello, C., and Gentile, C. (2020). Science and healthy meals in the world: Nutritional epigenomics and nutrigenetics of the Mediterranean diet. *Nutrients 12* (6): 1748. doi: 10.3390/nu12061748.

Carlos-Reyes, Á., López-González, J. S., Meneses-Flores, M., Gallardo-Rincón, D., Ruíz-García, E., Marchat, L. A., . . . López-Camarillo, C. (2019). Dietary compounds as epigenetic modulating agents in cancer. *Frontiers in Genetics*. doi: 10.3389/fgene.2019.00079.

Casadesús, J., & Noyer-Weidner, M. (2013). Epigenetics. In: *Brenner's Encyclopedia of Genetics*, 2e (ed. S. Maloy and K. Hughes), 500–503. Cambridge, MA: Academic Press. doi: 10.1016/B978-0-12-374984-0.00480-0.

Chaturvedi, P., & Tyagi, S. C. (2014). Epigenetic mechanisms underlying cardiac degeneration and regeneration. *International Journal of Cardiology 173* (1): 1–11. doi: 10.1016/j.ijcard.2014.02.008.

Chrysohoou, C., & Stefanadis, C. (2013). Longevity and diet. Myth or pragmatism? *Maturitas 76* (4): 303–307. doi: 10.1016/j.maturitas.2013.09.014.

Ciafrè, S., Carito, V., Ferraguti, G., Greco, A., Chaldakov, G. N., Fiore, M., & Ceccanti, M. (2019). How alcohol drinking affects our genes: An epigenetic point of view. *Biochemistry and Cell Biology 97* (4): 345–356. doi: 10.1139/bcb-2018-0248.

Deans, C., & Maggert, K. A. (2015). What do you mean, "epigenetic"? *Genetics 199* (4): 887–896. doi: 10.1534/genetics.114.173492.

Divella, R., Daniele, A., Savino, E., & Paradiso, A. (2020). Anticancer effects of nutraceuticals in the Mediterranean diet: An epigenetic diet model. *Cancer Genomics & Proteomics 17* (4): 335–350. doi: 10.21873/cgp.20193.

Donkin, I., & Barrès, R. (2018). Sperm epigenetics and influence of environmental factors. *Molecular Metabolism 14*: 1–11. doi: 10.1016/j.molmet.2018.02.006.

Dupont, C., Armant, D., & Brenner, C. (2009). Epigenetics: Definition, mechanisms and clinical perspective. *Seminars in Reproductive Medicine 27* (05): 351–357. doi: 10.1055/s-0029-1237423.

Elshenawy, S., & Simmons, R. (2016). Maternal obesity and prenatal programming. *Molecular and Cellular Endocrinology 435*: 2–6. doi: 10.1016/j.mce.2016.07.002.

Fall, C. H. D., & Kumaran, K. (2019). Metabolic programming in early life in humans. *Philosophical Transactions of the Royal Society B: Biological Sciences 374* (1770): 20180123. doi: 10.1098/rstb.2018.0123.

Foley, D. L., Craig, J. M., Morley, R., Olsson, C. J., Dwyer, T., Smith, K., & Saffery, R. (2008). Prospects for epigenetic epidemiology. *American Journal of Epidemiology 169* (4): 389–400. doi: 10.1093/aje/kwn380.

Gabbianelli, R., & Damiani, E. (2018). Epigenetics and neurodegeneration: Role of early-life nutrition. *The Journal of Nutritional Biochemistry 57*: 1–13. doi: 10.1016/j.jnutbio.2018.01.014.

Gheorghe, C. P., Goyal, R., Mittal, A., & Longo, L. D. (2010). Gene expression in the placenta: Maternal stress and epigenetic responses. *The International Journal of Developmental Biology 54* (2–3): 507–523. doi: 10.1387/ijdb.082770cg.

Gibney, E. R., & Nolan, C. M. (2010). Epigenetics and gene expression. *Heredity 105* (1): 4–13. doi: 10.1038/hdy.2010.54.

Gillman, M. W. (2005). Developmental origins of health and disease. *New England Journal of Medicine 353* (17): 1848–1850. doi: 10.1056/NEJMe058187.

Hales, C. N., & Barker, D. J. P. (2001). The thrifty phenotype hypothesis. *British Medical Bulletin 60* (1): 5–20. doi: 10.1093/bmb/60.1.5.

Hardy, T. M., & Tollefsbol, T. O. (2011). Epigenetic diet: impact on the epigenome and cancer. *Epigenomics 3* (4): 503–518. doi: 10.2217/epi.11.71.

Heerwagen, M. J. R., Miller, M. R., Barbour, L. A., & Friedman, J. E. (2010). Maternal obesity and fetal metabolic programming: A fertile epigenetic soil. *American Journal of Physiology-Regulatory, Integrative and Comparative Physiology 299* (3): R711–R722. doi: 10.1152/ajpregu.00310.2010.

Hult, M., Tornhammar, P., Ueda, P., Chima, C., Edstedt Bonamy, A.-K., Ozumba, B., & Norman, M. (2010). Hypertension, diabetes and overweight: Looming legacies of the Biafran famine. *PLoS ONE 5* (10): e13582. doi: 10.1371/journal.pone.0013582.

Ideraabdullah, F. Y., & Zeisel, S. H. (2018). Dietary modulation of the epigenome. *Physiological Reviews 98* (2): 667–695. doi: 10.1152/physrev.00010.2017.

Jankovic-Karasoulos, T., Furness, D. L., Leemaqz, S. Y., Dekker, G. A., Grzeskowiak, L. E., Grieger, J. A., ... Roberts, C. T. (2021). Maternal folate, one-carbon metabolism and pregnancy outcomes. *Maternal & Child Nutrition 17*(1). doi: 10.1111/mcn.13064.

Joubert, B. R., den Dekker, H. T., Felix, J. F., Bohlin, J., Ligthart, S., Beckett, E., ... London, S. J. (2016). Maternal plasma folate impacts differential DNA methylation in an epigenome-wide meta-analysis of newborns. *Nature Communications 7* (1): 10577. doi: 10.1038/ncomms10577.

Kaur, G., Begum, R., Thota, S., and Batra, S. (2019). A systematic review of smoking-related epigenetic alterations. *Archives of Toxicology 93* (10): 2715–2740. doi: 10.1007/s00204-019-02562-y.

Kellermann, N. P. (2013). Epigenetic transmission of Holocaust trauma: Can nightmares be inherited? *The Israel Journal of Psychiatry and Related Sciences 50* (1): 33–39.

Knopik, V. S., Maccani, M. A., Francazio, S., & McGeary, J. E. (2012). The epigenetics of maternal cigarette smoking during pregnancy and effects on child development. *Development and Psychopathology 24* (4): 1377–1390. doi: 10.1017/S0954579412000776

Koemel, N. A., & Skilton, M. R. (2022). Epigenetic aging in early life: Role of maternal and early childhood nutrition. *Current Nutrition Reports*. doi: 10.1007/s13668-022-00402-7

Kohil, A., Al-Asmakh, M., Al-Shafai, M., & Terranegra, A. (2021). The interplay between diet and the epigenome in the pathogenesis of type-1 diabetes. *Frontiers in Nutrition*. doi: 10.3389/fnut.2020.612115

Kontogiorgis, C. A., Bompou, E.-M., Ntella, M., & Berghe, W. vanden. (2010). Natural products from Mediterranean diet: From anti-inflammatory agents to dietary epigenetic modulators. *Anti-Inflammatory & Anti-Allergy Agents in Medicinal Chemistry 9* (2): 101–124. doi: 10.2174/187152310791110652

Kopp, W. (2019). How Western Diet And Lifestyle Drive The Pandemic Of Obesity And Civilization Diseases. *Diabetes, Metabolic Syndrome and Obesity: Targets and Therapy, Volume 12*, 2221–2236. doi: 10.2147/DMSO.S216791

Krishnan, H. R., Sakharkar, A. J., Teppen, T. L., Berkel, T. D. M., & Pandey, S. C. (2014). *The Epigenetic Landscape of Alcoholism*. doi: 10.1016/B978-0-12-801311-3.00003-2

Kuzawa, C. W. (2005). Fetal origins of developmental plasticity: Are fetal cues reliable predictors of future nutritional environments? *American Journal of Human Biology 17* (1): 5–21. doi: 10.1002/ajhb.20091

la Merrill, M. A., Vandenberg, L. N., Smith, M. T., Goodson, W., Browne, P., Patisaul, H. B., ... Zoeller, R. T. (2020). Consensus on the key characteristics of endocrine-disrupting chemicals as a basis for hazard identification. *Nature Reviews Endocrinology 16* (1): 45–57. doi: 10.1038/s41574-019-0273-8

Lacal, I., & Ventura, R. (2018). Epigenetic inheritance: Concepts, mechanisms, and perspectives. *Frontiers in Molecular Neuroscience*. doi: 10.3389/fnmol.2018.00292

Laplante, D. P., Brunet, A., Schmitz, N., Ciampi, A., & King, S. (2008). Project Ice Storm: Prenatal maternal stress affects cognitive and linguistic functioning in 5½-year-old children. *Journal of the American Academy of Child & Adolescent Psychiatry 47* (9): 1063–1072. doi: 10.1097/CHI.0b013e31817eec80

Lawlor, D. A., Smith, G. D., O'Callaghan, M., Alati, R., Mamun, A. A., Williams, G. M., & Najman, J. M. (2006). Epidemiologic evidence for the fetal overnutrition hypothesis: Findings from the Mater-University study of pregnancy and its outcomes. *American Journal of Epidemiology 165* (4): 418–424. doi: 10.1093/aje/kwk030

Li, Y., He, Y., Qi, L., Jaddoe, V. W., Feskens, E. J. M., Yang, X., ... Hu, F. B. (2010). Exposure to the Chinese famine in early life and the risk of hyperglycemia and type 2 diabetes in adulthood. *Diabetes 59* (10): 2400–2406. doi: 10.2337/db10-0385

Ling, C., & Rönn, T. (2019). Epigenetics in human obesity and type 2 diabetes. *Cell Metabolism, 29*(5), 1028–1044. doi: 10.1016/j.cmet.2019.03.009

Lintas, C. (2019). Linking genetics to epigenetics: The role of folate and folate-related pathways in neurodevelopmental disorders. *Clinical Genetics 95* (2): 241–252. doi: 10.1111/cge.13421

Lumey, L. H. (1992). Decreased birthweights in infants after maternal in utero exposure to the Dutch famine of 1944–1945. *Paediatric and Perinatal Epidemiology 6* (2): 240–253. doi: 10.1111/j.1365-3016.1992.tb00764.x

Lupien, S. J., McEwen, B. S., Gunnar, M. R., & Heim, C. (2009). Effects of stress throughout the lifespan on the brain, behaviour and cognition. *Nature Reviews Neuroscience 10* (6): 434–445. doi: 10.1038/nrn2639

Mattick, J. S., & Makunin, I. v. (2006). Non-coding RNA. *Human Molecular Genetics 15* (suppl_1): R17–R29. doi: 10.1093/hmg/ddl046

Mega, F., de Meireles, A., Piazza, F. V., Spindler, C., Segabinazi, E., Dos Santos Salvalaggio, G., Achaval, M., & Marcuzzo, S. (2018). Paternal physical exercise demethylates the hippocampal DNA of male pups without modifying the cognitive and physical development. *Behavioural brain research, 348*, 1–8. https://doi.org/10.1016/j.bbr.2018.03.040

Molina-Serrano, D., Kyriakou, D., & Kirmizis, A. (2019). Histone modifications as an intersection between diet and longevity. *Frontiers in Genetics*. doi: 10.3389/fgene.2019.00192

Monk, C., Spicer, J., & Champagne, F. A. (2012). Linking prenatal maternal adversity to developmental outcomes in infants: The role of epigenetic pathways. *Development and Psychopathology 24* (4): 1361–1376. doi: 10.1017/S0954579412000764

Musanabaganwa, C., Jansen, S., Fatumo, S., Rutembesa, E., Mutabaruka, J., Gishoma, D., ... Mutesa, L. (2020). Burden of post-traumatic stress disorder in postgenocide Rwandan population following exposure to 1994 genocide against the Tutsi: A meta-analysis. *Journal of Affective Disorders 275*: 7–13. doi: 10.1016/j.jad.2020.06.017

Nettore, I. C., Franchini, F., Palatucci, G., Macchia, P. E., & Ungaro, P. (2021). Epigenetic mechanisms of endocrine-disrupting chemicals in obesity. *Biomedicines 9* (11): 1716. doi: 10.3390/biomedicines9111716

Nilsson, E. E., Ben Maamar, M., & Skinner, M. K. (2022). Role of epigenetic transgenerational inheritance in generational toxicology. *Environmental epigenetics, 8*(1), dvac001. doi.org/10.1093/eep/dvac001

Noble, D. (2015). Conrad Waddington and the origin of epigenetics. *Journal of Experimental Biology 218* (6): 816–818. doi: 10.1242/jeb.120071

Novakovic, B., Lewis, S., Halliday, J., Kennedy, J., Burgner, D. P., Czajko, A., Kim, B., Sexton-Oates, A., Juonala, M., Hammarberg, K., Amor, D. J., Doyle, L. W., Ranganathan, S., Welsh, L., Cheung, M., McBain, J., McLachlan, R., & Saffery, R. (2019). Assisted reproductive technologies are associated with limited epigenetic variation at birth that largely resolves by adulthood. *Nature communications, 10*(1), 3922. https://doi.org/10.1038/s41467-019-11929-9

O'Connor, T. G., Ben-Shlomo, Y., Heron, J., Golding, J., Adams, D., & Glover, V. (2005). Prenatal anxiety predicts individual differences in cortisol in pre-adolescent children. *Biological Psychiatry 58* (3): 211–217. doi: 10.1016/j.biopsych.2005.03.032

Oei, J. L. (2020). Alcohol use in pregnancy and its impact on the mother and child. *Addiction 115* (11): 2148–2163. doi: 10.1111/add.15036

Palmisano, M., & Pandey, S. C. (2017). Epigenetic mechanisms of alcoholism and stress-related disorders. *Alcohol 60*: 7–18. doi: 10.1016/j.alcohol.2017.01.001

Peral-Sanchez, I., Hojeij, B., Ojeda, D. A., Steegers-Theunissen, R. P. M., & Willaime-Morawek, S. (2021). Epigenetics in the uterine environment: How maternal diet and ART may influence the epigenome in the offspring with long-term health consequences. *Genes 13* (1): 31. doi: 10.3390/genes13010031

Perroud, N., Rutembesa, E., Paoloni-Giacobino, A., Mutabaruka, J., Mutesa, L., Stenz, L., ... Karege, F. (2014). The Tutsi genocide and transgenerational transmission of maternal stress: epigenetics and biology of the HPA axis. *The World Journal of Biological Psychiatry 15* (4): 334–345. doi: 10.3109/15622975.2013.866693

Ramsay, M. (2015). Epigenetic epidemiology: is there cause for optimism? *Epigenomics, 7* (5): 683–685. doi: 10.2217/epi.15.48

Rauschert, S., Melton, P. E., Burdge, G., Craig, J. M., Godfrey, K. M., Holbrook, J. D., ... Huang, R.-C. (2019). Maternal smoking during pregnancy induces persistent epigenetic changes Into adolescence, independent of postnatal smoke exposure and is associated with cardiometabolic risk. *Frontiers in Genetics*. doi: 10.3389/fgene.2019.00770

Romani, M., Pistillo, M. P., & Banelli, B. (2015). Environmental epigenetics: Crossroad between public health, lifestyle, and cancer prevention. *BioMed Research International*. doi: 10.1155/2015/587983

Şanlı, E., & Kabaran, S. (2019). Maternal obesity, maternal overnutrition and fetal programming: Effects of epigenetic mechanisms on the development of metabolic disorders. *Current Genomics 20*(6): 419–427. doi: 10.2174/1389202920666191030092225

Sellami, M., Bragazzi, N., Prince, M. S., Denham, J., & Elrayess, M. (2021). Regular, intense exercise training as a healthy aging lifestyle strategy: Preventing DNA damage, telomere shortening and adverse DNA methylation changes over a lifetime. *Frontiers in Genetics*. doi: 10.3389/fgene.2021.652497

Serpeloni, F., Radtke, K. M., Hecker, T., Sill, J., Vukojevic, V., Assis, S. G. de, ... Nätt, D. (2019). Does prenatal stress shape postnatal resilience? – An epigenome-wide study on violence and mental health in humans. *Frontiers in Genetics*. doi: 10.3389/fgene.2019.00269

Stankiewicz, A. M., Swiergiel, A. H., & Lisowski, P. (2013). Epigenetics of stress adaptations in the brain. *Brain Research Bulletin 98*: 76–92. doi: 10.1016/j.brainresbull.2013.07.003

Tiffon, C. (2018). The impact of nutrition and environmental epigenetics on human health and disease. *International Journal of Molecular Sciences 19* (11): 3425. doi: 10.3390/ijms19113425

Waddington, C. H. (1956). Genetic Assimilation of the Bithorax Phenotype. *Evolution 10* (1): 1. doi: 10.2307/2406091

Wallén, E., Auvinen, P., & Kaminen-Ahola, N. (2021). The effects of early prenatal alcohol exposure on epigenome and embryonic development. *Genes 12* (7): 1095. doi: genes12071095

Wei, J.-W., Huang, K., Yang, C., and Kang, C.-S. (2017). Non-coding RNAs as regulators in epigenetics. *Oncology Reports 37* (1): 3–9. doi: 10.3892/or.2016.5236

Zong, D., Liu, X., Li, J., Ouyang, R., & Chen, P. (2019). The role of cigarette smoke-induced epigenetic alterations in inflammation. *Epigenetics & Chromatin 12* (1): 65. doi: 10.1186/s13072-019-0311-8

FURTHER READING

Bibliography

Bošković, A. & Rando, O. J. (2018) Transgenerational epigenetic inheritance. *Annual Review of Genetics*. doi: 10.1146/annurev-genet-120417-031404.

Cavalli, G. & Heard, E. (2019). Advances in epigenetics link genetics to the environment and disease. *Nature*. doi: 10.1038/s41586-019-1411-0.

Franzago, M., Santurbano, D., Vitacolonna, E., & Stuppia, L. (2020). Genes and diet in the prevention of chronic diseases in future generations. *International Journal of Molecular Sciences*. doi: 10.3390/ijms21072633.

Gayon, J. (2016) From Mendel to epigenetics: History of genetics. *Comptes Rendus Biologies*. doi: 10.1016/j.crvi.2016.05.009.

Moore, D.S. (2017). Behavioral epigenetics. *Wiley Interdisciplinary Reviews: Systems Biology and Medicine*. doi: 10.1002/wsbm.1333.

Medline Plus. What is epigenetics; 2021 update. [cited 2022 September 30]. Available from: https://medlineplus.gov/genetics/understanding/howgeneswork/epigenome/

Centers for Disease Control and Prevention. What is epigenetics; 2022 review. [cited 2022 September 30]. Available from: https://www.cdc.gov/genomics/disease/epigenetics.htm

National Human Genome Research Institute (NIH). Epigenomics Fact Sheet; 2020 update. [cited 2022 September 30]. Available from: https://www.genome.gov/about-genomics/fact-sheets/Epigenomics-Fact-Sheet

Genetics Science Learning Center. Epigenetics. [cited 2022 September 30]. Available from: https://learn.genetics.utah.edu/content/epigenetics/

Healthy/Prudent Diets and Health Benefits in Adults

CHAPTER 3

Introduction	35
A Healthy/Prudent Diet Definition	36
Dietary Patterns that are Considered Healthy	37
The Mediterranean-type Dietary Pattern	37
Health Effects of the Mediterranean Diet	39
All-cause and Disease-specific Mortality	39
Cardiovascular Diseases	40
Hypertension	41
Type 2 Diabetes Mellitus	41
Dyslipidemia	42
Obesity/Metabolic syndrome	42
Cancer	42
Healthy Aging	42
The Dietary Approaches to Stop Hypertension (DASH) Dietary Pattern	44
Initial Dietary Approaches to Stop Hypertension (DASH) Trials	44
The Dietary Approaches to Stop Hypertension (DASH) Diet Characteristics	44
The Dietary Approaches to Stop Hypertension (DASH) Diet Health Effects	44
All-cause and Specific-cause Mortality	45
Cardiovascular Diseases	45
Obesity/Metabolic Syndrome	45
Type 2 Diabetes Mellitus/Hyperglycemia	46
Hyperlipidemia	46
Cancer	46
Chronic Kidney Disease	46
The Healthy Nordic Dietary Pattern	46
Health Effects of the Nordic Diet	47
Chronic Disease Risk	47
All-cause and Specific-cause Mortality	48
Inflammation	48
Physical Performance and Cognitive Health in Older Adults	48
The Healthy Vegetarian-type Dietary Pattern	48
Health Effects of the Healthy Vegetarian–type Dietary Pattern	50
CVD Risk and Mortality	50
Blood Pressure/Hypertension	50
Type 2 Diabetes	50
Metabolic Syndrome	50
Cancer	51
Considerations in Implementing a Healthy Vegetarian-type Dietary Pattern	51
The Healthy US-style Dietary Pattern	51
Effectiveness of Healthy/Prudent Dietary Patterns	52
Key Points	52
Self-assessment Questions	54
References	54
Further Reading	59
Bibliography	59
Links	59

INTRODUCTION

Historically, nutrition research has focused on the relationship between specific nutrients, foods, and food groups with numerous health conditions. However, current research shows that various nutrients or foods have a cumulative effect in the context of a whole dietary pattern, which might differ from the effects of a single nutrient or food item in health (Hu, 2002). Due to the multiple combinations of nutrients that may correlate and interact with each other as we eat through food synergy (Jacobs & Tapsell, 2013), as well as the different

Prevention and Management of Cardiovascular and Metabolic Disease: Diet, Physical Activity and Healthy Aging,
First Edition. Christina N. Katsagoni, Peter Kokkinos, and Labros S. Sidossis.
© 2023 John Wiley & Sons Ltd. Published 2023 by John Wiley & Sons Ltd.

food and food groups that can be consumed in a meal, dietary patterns have been examined in the literature in relation to chronic diseases and non-communicable diseases (NCDs) (Jacobs, Tapsell, & Temple, 2011). Different approaches to assess adherence to several dietary patterns, including *a priori* and *a posteriori* scores, have been proposed.

Chapter 1 outlined the link between the Western dietary pattern and NCDs. This chapter will describe the health benefits associated with adherence to healthy/prudent dietary patterns.

A HEALTHY/PRUDENT DIET DEFINITION

Four principles were used to characterize and define a dietary pattern as a healthy or prudent: the avoidance of excess energy intake, increased dietary fiber intake, reduced total fat intake to approximately 30% of energy intake, and an increase in polyunsaturated fat consumption (Mann, 1979). More recently, according to a 2020 World Health Organization (WHO) report, a healthy diet should protect against all types of malnutrition (e.g., undernutrition, overnutrition, micronutrient abnormalities, sarcopenia, frailty, and re-feeding syndrome (Cederholm et al., 2017)) and NCD development; limiting added/free sugars and salt are also included in the key facts that characterize healthy diets (WHO, 2020). Based on the 2020–2025 Dietary Guidelines for Americans, a healthy dietary pattern should represent all foods and beverages consumed, including foods and beverages across all food groups in nutrient-dense forms, in the recommended amounts and within calorie limits, while individuals should have more than one way to achieve a healthy dietary pattern (US Department of Agriculture and US Department of Health and Human Services. Dietary Guidelines for Americans, 2020–2025). Unfortunately, more than 80% of Americans follow dietary patterns that are low in vegetables, fruits, and dairy, while more than half of the population is meeting or exceeding total grain and total protein recommendations, but are not meeting the recommendations for the subgroups within each of these food groups (**Figure 3.1**) (US Department of Agriculture and US Department of Health and Human Services. Dietary Guidelines for Americans, 2020–2025).

A healthy diet starts from infancy through breastfeeding. Healthy practices throughout childhood and adolescence helps to foster a healthy growth and cognitive development (WHO, 2020). However, it is important to understand that apart from some key elements, a healthy diet varies across populations as it depends on personal characteristics, age, gender, physical activity habits, dietary preferences, and cultural habits, but also on food availability and accessibility.

Nevertheless, to ensure good health, physical activity should also be considered among the essential components of everyday life. Physical activity may include planned exercise (e.g., sports), occupational (e.g., at work), domestic (e.g., household chores), transportation/utilitarian, and leisure time physical activities (e.g., physically active hobbies like bicycling) (Strath, Smith, & Swartz, 2013). Combining aerobic and muscle-strengthening exercises seems to provide an additive health benefit (Walker, Tullar, Diamond, Kohl, & Amick, 2017). The basic concepts of physical activity and

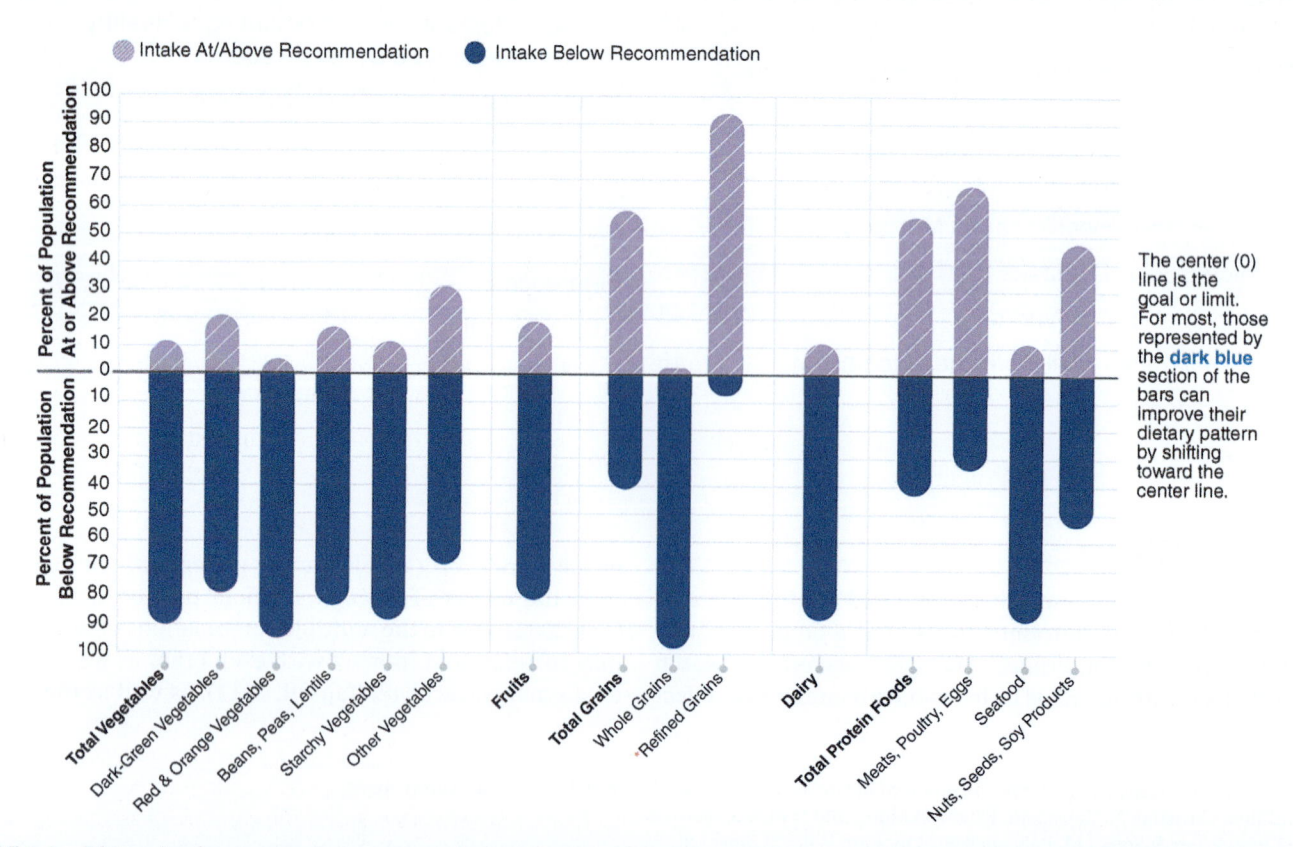

FIGURE 3.1 Dietary intake compared to recommendations: Percent of the US population ages 1 and older who are below and at or above each dietary goal. Source: (US Department of Agriculture and US Department of Health and Human Services. Dietary Guidelines for Americans, 2020–2025).

fitness as well as its implications and health benefits in adults will be discussed in **Unit 2**.

This chapter will focus on dietary patterns that are considered healthy based on long-standing literature.

DIETARY PATTERNS THAT ARE CONSIDERED HEALTHY

The Mediterranean-type dietary pattern, the Dietary Approaches to Stop Hypertension (DASH) diet, the US-style dietary patterns, and vegetarian eating patterns are all highlighted as healthy dietary patterns in the 2020–2025 Dietary Guidelines for Americans.

THE MEDITERRANEAN-TYPE DIETARY PATTERN

The healthy Mediterranean-type dietary pattern (MD) is the result of several interactions between multiple civilizations, cultures, religions, and environments of populations living around the Mediterranean basin. Therefore, more than one version of this dietary pattern exists. Consequently, the MD reflects a way of living that incorporates an assortment of knowledge, expertise, customs, and rituals from different populations around the Mediterranean region that can be conveyed from previous generations to the next (Davis, Bryan, Hodgson, & Murphy, 2015).

A large body of evidence has led to the MD's recognition as the gold standard dietary pattern of healthy nutrition and one of the best studied dietary patterns (Sepideh Soltani, Jayedi, Shab-Bidar, Becerra-Tomás, & Salas-Salvadó, 2019). November 16, 2020, was the tenth anniversary since the MD was included on the UNESCO Representative List of the Intangible Cultural Heritage of Humanity. UNESCO acknowledged several characteristics (Bonaccio, Iacoviello, Donati, & de Gaetano, 2022) of the MD including:

- The MD promotes social exchange and community events, as shared meals are the cornerstone of social customs in the context of traditional festivities.
- Eating together is a fundamental aspect of the MD's cultural identity.
- Local markets play a key role in cultivating and transmitting the MD during the daily practice of exchanging traditional products.

The MD has evolved over the centuries. Despite the many versions and depending on local conditions, the MD essentials have remained the same. It is a diet with a semi-vegetarian character high in olive oil (particularly cold-pressed extra-virgin olive oil) and it is based in the daily consumption of seasonal fruit and vegetables (including leafy green vegetables); whole-grain cereals, nuts, and pulses/legumes; the moderate intake of fish and other meat, dairy products, and red wine; and a low intake of eggs and sweets (Davis et al., 2015; Hidalgo-Mora et al., 2020). It is important to note that the MD is not a low fat dietary pattern as the main sources include olive oil and nuts (**Table 3.1**). Frugality is an important feature of MD due to the scarcity of food during winter or periods of financial constraints.

The recommended number of servings for the aforementioned food groups are usually depicted in a pyramid. A significant number of MD pyramids exist in the literature as each depends on the population and their national organizations' policies (Davis et al., 2015). The latest MD pyramid was published in 2011 by the Mediterranean Diet Foundation (**Figure 3.2**) (Bach-Faig et al., 2011). In this pyramid, sugary foods were moved to the vertex of the pyramid, shifting the consumption of red meat one place lower than in previous versions of the MD. Apart from the general principles of the MD that regard the frequency and approximate quantities of the MD food groups, other aspects of the Mediterranean lifestyle (MedLife), such as the healthy lifestyle and cultural elements were also added. Socialization, cooking, and sharing meals with friends and family as well as seasonality, biodiversity, and the eco-friendly characteristics of the MD are included at the bottom of the pyramid to highlight aspects such as relaxation, community, and sustainability that constitute the MedLife.

Regular physical activity (such as walking, using the stairs instead of the lift, housework for at least 30 min throughout the day) is also represented in the pyramid for balancing energy intake, weight maintenance, and other health benefits (Bach-Faig et al., 2011). Moreover, a reference to adequate water intake was added to highlight the essential role of water to human function and hydration, as regions around the Mediterranean Sea have climates that are hot and dry for several months of the year. Herbal infusions, such as herbal teas, low-fat broths, and other non-alcoholic beverages also contribute to adequate daily hydration.

Another significant aspect of the MedLife that is described in the 2011 MD pyramid is the conviviality of meals, i.e., the practice of eating a friendly, lively meal together in a pleasant environment. Indeed, people in Mediterranean countries seems to spend more time eating with others than people anywhere else in the world, which demonstrates the social character of meals in southern European countries. Moreover, although the culinary practices of human health have not been thoroughly studied, they are thought to contribute to individuals' nutritional status, which is why they were incorporated into the 2011 MD pyramid. Many studies suggest that home cooking is positively correlated with better diet quality, while homemade meals are associated with increased consumption of fruits, vegetables, and whole grains. Improved cooking skills are linked to reduced fast-food consumption, more shared meals, and cooking with low-cost basic ingredients. Homemade meals are considered less energy-dense, containing lower concentrations of total fat and saturated fatty acids, dietary cholesterol and sodium, but more nutrient-dense, having greater fiber, calcium and iron content.

Sleep, an important aspect of the MedLife, is also highlighted in the latest version of the MD pyramid (Bach-Faig et al., 2011). Indeed, adequate rest, both at night and during the day in the form of short naps or siestas is recommended. Siestas usually last 20 to 40 min. Mid-day naps can be helpful for memory consolidation, subsequent learning, executive functioning enhancement, and emotional stability. As sleep deprivation narrows cognitive abilities, mid-day naps can recover these abilities. However, more frequent and longer naps are linked to numerous negative outcomes such as hypertension and T2D, particularly in older adults.

The MD dietary pattern has many similarities and unique features with the US-style and DASH dietary patterns, which

Table 3.1 Healthy Mediterranean-style dietary pattern for ages 2 and older, with daily or weekly amounts from food groups, subgroups, and components.

Calorie level of pattern	1,000	1,200	1,400	1,600	1,800	2,000	2,200	2,400	2,600	2,800	3,000	3,200
Food group or subgroup	\multicolumn{12}{c}{Daily amount of food from each group (Vegetable and protein foods subgroup amounts are per week.)}											
Vegetables (cup eq/day)	1	1 ½	1 ½	2	2 ½	2 ½	3	3	3 ½	3 ½	4	4
Vegetable subgroups in weekly amounts												
Dark-green vegetables (cup eq/wk)	½	1	1	1 ½	1 ½	1 ½	2	2	2 ½	2 ½	2 ½	2 ½
Red and orange vegetables (cup eq/wk)	2 ½	3	3	4	5 ½	5 ½	6	6	7	7	7 ½	7 ½
Beans, peas, lentils (cup eq/wk)	½	½	½	1	1 ½	1 ½	2	2	2 ½	2 ½	3	3
Starchy vegetables (cup eq/wk)	2	3 ½	3 ½	4	5	5	6	6	7	7	8	8
Other vegetables (cup eq/wk)	1 ½	2 ½	2 ½	3 ½	4	4	5	5	5 ½	5 ½	7	7
Fruits (cup eq/day)	1	1	1 ½	2	2	2 ½	2 ½	2 ½	2 ½	3	3	3
Grains (ounce eq/day)	3	4	5	5	6	6	7	8	9	10	10	10
Whole grains (ounce eq/day)	1 ½	2	2 ½	3	3	3	3 ½	4	4 ½	5	5	5
Refined grains (ounce eq/day)	1 ½	2	2 ½	2	3	3	3 ½	4	4 ½	5	5	5
Dairy (cup eq/day)	2	2 ½	2 ½	2	2	2	2	2 ½	2 ½	2 ½	2 ½	2 ½
Protein foods (ounce eq/day)	2	3	4	5 ½	6	6 ½	7	7 ½	7 ½	8	8	8
Protein foods subgroups in weekly amounts												
Meats, poultry, eggs (ounce eq/wk)	10	14	19	23	23	26	28	31	31	33	33	33
Seafood (ounce eq/wk)	3	4	6	11	15	15	16	16	17	17	17	17
Nuts, seeds, soy products (ounce eq/wk)	2	2	3	4	4	5	5	5	5	6	6	6
Oils (grams/day)	15	17	17	22	24	27	29	31	34	36	44	51
Limit on calories for other uses (kcal/day)	130	80	90	120	140	240	250	280	300	330	400	540
Limit on calories for other uses (%/day)	13%	7%	6%	8%	8%	12%	11%	12%	12%	12%	13%	17%

[1] Amounts of dairy recommended for children and adolescents, regardless of the calorie level: for age 2 years, 2 cup-eq per day; for ages 3 to 8 years, 2 ½ cup-eq per day; for ages 9 to 18 years, 3 cup-eq per day.

[2] The US Food and Drug Administration (FDA) and the US Environmental Protection Agency (EPA) provide joint advice regarding seafood consumption to limit methylmercury exposure for women who might become or are pregnant or lactating, and children. Depending on body weight, some women and children should choose seafood lowest in methylmercury or eat less seafood than the amounts in the healthy US-style dietary pattern. Source: FDA.gov/fishadvice; EPA.gov/fishadvice.

[3] Foods are assumed to be in nutrient-dense forms; lean or low-fat; and prepared with minimal added sugars, refined starches (a calorie source with few or no nutrients), saturated fat, or sodium. If all food choices to meet food group recommendations are in nutrient-dense forms, a small number of calories remain within the overall limit (i.e., limit on calories for other uses). The amount of calories depends on the total calorie level of the pattern and the amounts of food from each food group required to meet nutritional goals. Calories up to the specified limit can be used for added sugars, saturated fat, and/or alcohol (for nonpregnant adults of legal drinking age only) or to eat more than the recommended amount of food in a food group.

Source: (US Department of Agriculture and US Department of Health and Human Services. Dietary Guidelines for Americans, 2020–2025).

NOTE: The total dietary pattern should not exceed dietary guideline limits for added sugars, saturated fat, and alcohol; be within the acceptable macronutrient distribution ranges for protein, carbohydrate, and total fats; and stay within calorie limits. Values are rounded.

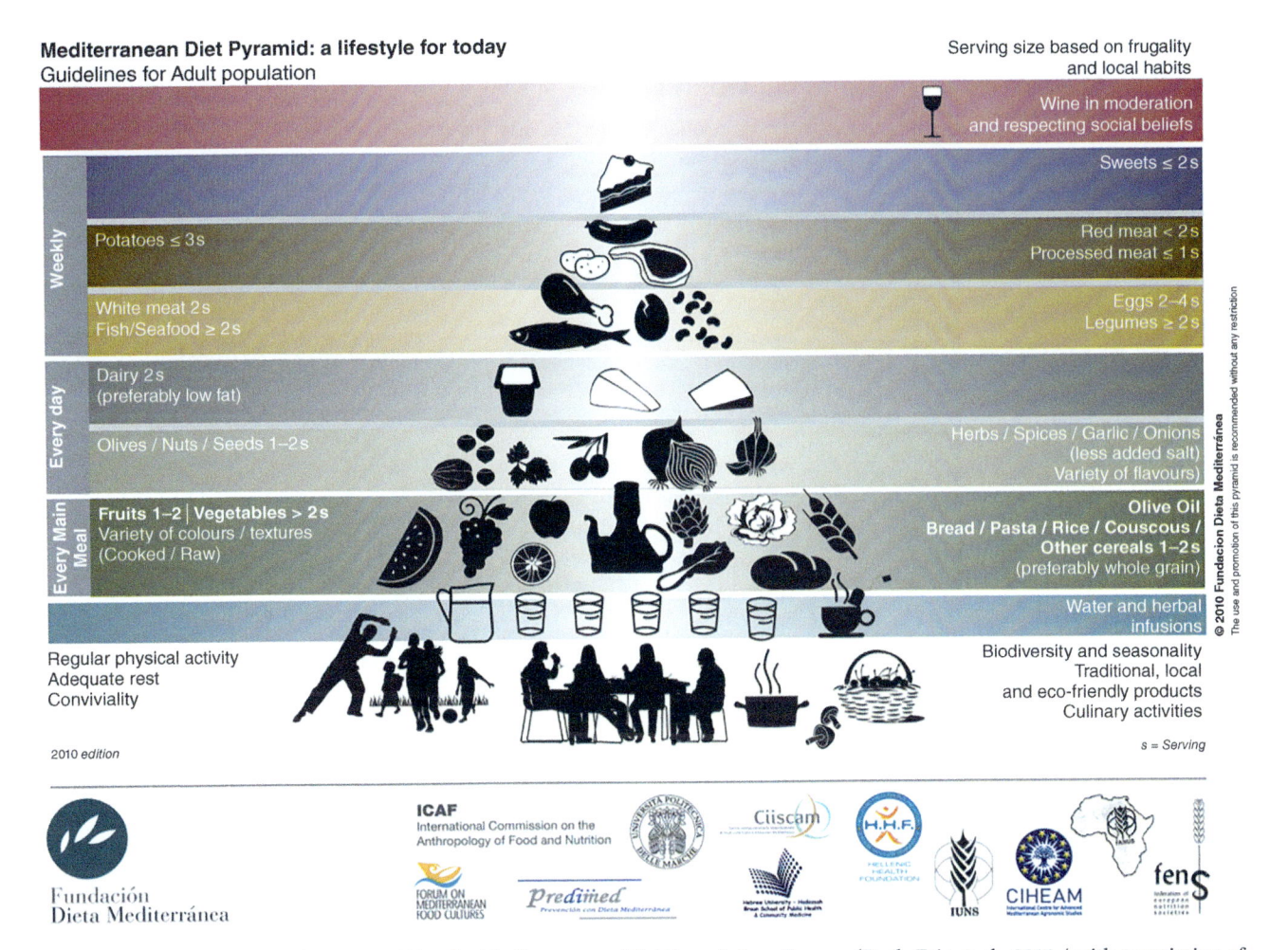

FIGURE 3.2 The Mediterranean-diet pyramid by the Mediterranean Diet Foundation. Source: (Bach-Faig et al., 2011 / with permission of Cambridge University Press).

will be described throughout this chapter (**Figure 3.3**) (Richter, Skulas-Ray, & Kris-Etherton, 2014).

HEALTH EFFECTS OF THE MEDITERRANEAN DIET

Numerous epidemiological and intervention studies have established the effectiveness of the MD in preventing and managing NCDs and other conditions. The beneficial effect of the MD on lifespan was first suggested in 1960s (Sepideh Soltani et al., 2019). In the following paragraphs, we will review the health benefits associated with all-cause mortality, NCDs (namely cardiovascular diseases [CVD], dyslipidemia, metabolic syndrome, hypertension, T2D, and cancer), and healthy aging with the long-term adherence to the MD.

ALL-CAUSE AND DISEASE-SPECIFIC MORTALITY

Since the 1960s, several epidemiological studies have linked the MD to better survival and a protective association against all-cause and disease-specific mortality. In 2014, a meta-analysis by Sofi et al. (Sofi, Macchi, Abbate, Gensini, & Casini, 2014) of 16 prospective cohort studies, including 4 172 412 subjects, revealed that a quite moderate 2-point increase in the MD adherence score could lead to an 8% decrease in all-cause mortality, a 10% decrease in CVD-related mortality, and a 4% decrease in malignancies-associated mortality. Another meta-analysis (Sepideh Soltani et al., 2019) of 29 prospective studies with 1 676 901 participants and 221 603 cases of all-cause mortality concluded similarly. The same meta-analysis supported that the decrease in mortality risk was evident in both Mediterranean and non-Mediterranean regions, although it was stronger in the former. A linear inverse association between adherence to the MD and risk of all-cause mortality was also suggested.

The link between better adherence to MD and reduced all-cause and disease-specific mortality is attributed to the beneficial effects of some individual components. Meta-analytic data support that those consuming more vegetables, fruits/nuts, legumes, cereals, and fish as well as less dairy and meat/poultry have a higher mono-unsaturated to saturated fatty acids (MUFA:SFA) ratio, and those who consume moderate amounts of ethanol have better cardiovascular and cognitive health than those consuming less (Davis et al., 2015). However, the quantity used to define these associations varies across studies, one cutoff point may lead to loosing subtle improvements of specific food groups, e.g., nuts, in health. Nevertheless, the high fruit and vegetable content of the MD correlates with a 10% to 30%

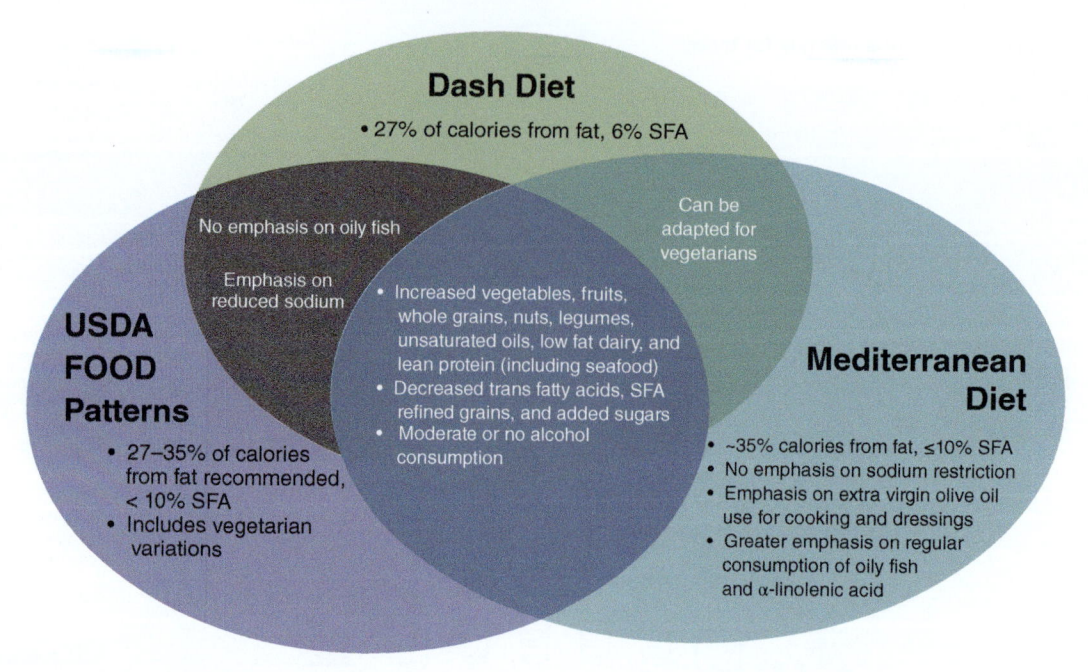

FIGURE 3.3 Common and unique features of the USDA food patterns, DASH diet, and Mediterranean dietary patterns. SFA: saturated fatty acid. Source: (Richter et al., 2014 / with permission of Elsevier).

decrease in overall mortality among CVD patients (Grosso et al., 2017; D. D. Wang et al., 2021), especially when using a threshold of five servings of fruit and vegetables per day (X. Wang et al., 2014). With regard to olive oil, each 10-g increment of olive oil has been associated with decreased CVD and mortality risk by 10% and 7%, respectively (Foscolou, Critselis, & Panagiotakos, 2018; Guasch-Ferré et al., 2014), with the maximum benefit obtained consuming 20 to 30 g/day (Donat-Vargas et al., 2022).

CARDIOVASCULAR DISEASES

CVDs include coronary heart disease (CHD), stroke, heart failure, and other conditions that affect the heart and blood vessels (more on CVD in **Unit 4**).

The bulk of evidence comes mainly from prospective epidemiological studies that investigated the role of the MD on total CVD risk. All have found an inverse association between adherence to the MD and the risk of CVDs (Jordi Salas-Salvadó, Becerra-Tomás, García-Gavilán, Bulló, & Barrubés, 2018). Overall, a 20% to 25% lower risk of total CVDs is suggested when compliance with the MD or Mediterranean-like dietary patterns is high, compared to low (Rosato et al., 2019). The results align with meta-analyses assessing the role of the MD on CVD incidence, comparing the highest versus the lowest categories of MD adherence showing a 25% to 47% lower risk of CVD incidence (Grosso et al., 2017; Rosato et al., 2019). The beneficial effect of the MD on strokes was also assessed by meta-analyses of both observational and interventional studies, which show an approximately 30% lower risk and 35% favorable effect of the MD on stroke risk (Jordi Salas-Salvadó et al., 2018) from high compared to low adherence, but not to moderate (Saulle, Lia, De Giusti, & La Torre, 2019). Furthermore, the beneficial effects of the MD were evaluated in lowering concentrations of inflammatory markers and improving endothelial dysfunction, atherosclerosis, and arterial stiffness, all well-established factors for stroke (Saulle et al., 2019). Regarding heart failure, in a meta-analysis of prospective cohort studies, a higher adherence to the MD, compared to a lower adherence, was associated with 8% lower risk (Liyanage et al., 2016). Moreover, the results from randomized controlled trials (RCTs) show a protective effect of the MD on the incidence of heart failure or worsening of cardiac function parameters for patients with previous cardiovascular disease (Sanches Machado d'Almeida, Ronchi Spillere, Zuchinali, & Corrêa Souza, 2018).

Mechanistically, based on population and RCT data, several components of the MD are associated with beneficial effects on total CVD prevention and risk (Widmer, Flammer, Lerman, & Lerman, 2015). With regard to foods and food groups, whole grains, fruit (especially citrus and deep yellow-orange), and vegetables (especially dark green leafy, cruciferous, and deep yellow-orange), fish, and olive oil, which are shown in **Table 3.2** (Sala-Vila, Estruch, & Ros, 2015; Widmer et al., 2015), as well as their bioactive components namely polyphenols, unsaturated fatty acids, all prevent CVD and ameliorate a host of CVD features.

Olive oil induces cardio-protective effects due to the presence of a plethora of polyphenolic compounds. A number of mechanistic studies have demonstrated that olive-oil polyphenols increase the high-density lipoprotein level; prevent damage from oxidative stress; reduce thrombogenic, endothelial dysfunction, blood pressure (BP), and inflammation; and alter gene expression responsible for atherosclerosis (Mehmood, Usman, Patil, Zhao, & Wang, 2020).

Alcohol, and especially red wine, a typical component of the MD, is thought to play a significant role in CVD prevention due to its high concentration of polyphenols, which decrease

Table 3.2 Effects of foods and food groups of the Mediterranean diet along with its bioactive components on the cardiovascular risk.

Food group	Population-based data	RCT data	Bioactive components	CVD effect	Proposed mechanisms
MedDiet	+++	+++		+++	Improves lipids, reduces ROS, endothelial Function, Platelet function
Fruits/ vegetables	++	+	slow-release carb and fiber	+	Improves lipid profiles, glucemic control and BP; reduces ROS
Unsaturated fats	+	+		+	Improves lipids, reduces ROS, endothelial function, Platelet function
Fish	+/−	++	Long-chain n-3 fatty acids	+	Improves lipid profiles and BP (antiarrhythmic)
Whole grains	++	+	Slow-release carb and fiber	+	improves glucose metabolism, reduced inflammation, ROS, lipid profiles (eg cholesterol), and blood pressure
			beta-glucan (oats)		
			Polyphenols		
Eggs	+/−	+/−	Lecithin; ACE inhibitory peptides	NC	controversial data; seems to imporve BP;
Nuts	++	++	Unsaturated fatty acids	+	+/− ROS and lipid profiles (eg cholesterol); improves BP and endothelial function
			Non-sodium minerals		
			Polyphenols		
Alcohol	++	+	Ethanol	++	Improves lipid profiles, BP, (+/−) ROS, and endothelial function
			Polyphenols		

ACE: angiotensin converting enzyme; BP: blood pressure; Carb: carbohydrates; CVD: cardiovascular disease; NC: no change; RCT: randomized controlled trial; ROS: reactive oxygen species; +: positive effect; - Negative effect.
Sources: Sala-Vila, Estruch, and Ros, 2015; Widmer et al., 2015.

oxidized LDL levels, prevent platelet aggregation, and improve endothelium function (Widmer et al., 2015).

HYPERTENSION

High BP is a common and serious medical condition as it is a well-documented risk factor of CVDs, brain, renal, and other diseases (Bakaloudi, Chrysoula, Leonida, et al., 2021) (more on hypertension in **Unit 5**). A healthful lifestyle is a fundamental strategy for decreasing hypertension, and the MD improves endothelial function by reducing reactive oxygen species (ROS), offering a considerable benefit against the risk of hypertension (De Pergola & D'Alessandro, 2018).

Although different versions of the MD exist, different populations or types of studies with high heterogeneity, multiple ways of monitoring BP (home or office), and/or patients with differing hypertension severity (De Pergola & D'Alessandro, 2018), pooled data from interventional studies (Bakaloudi, Chrysoula, Leonida, et al., 2021; Filippou et al., 2021; Nissensohn, Román-Viñas, Sánchez-Villegas, Piscopo, & Serra-Majem, 2016), show a reduction in both systolic (SBP) and diastolic (DBP) in adults with normal BP or mild hypertension after adopting the MD. However, the magnitude of the effect is small, supporting a low clinical effect. Therefore, more convincing evidence is needed to support the beneficial effect of MD on BP.

Nevertheless, in a dose-response meta-analysis of 19 RCTs with 4137 participants and 16 observational studies on 59 001 participants, authors concluded that interventions based on the MD might reduce SBP and DBP by a mean 1.4 mmHg and 1.5 mmHg, respectively, versus control. In observational studies, the likelihood of developing hypertension was 13% lower with higher versus lower MD adherence (Cowell et al., 2021).

TYPE 2 DIABETES MELLITUS

Diabetes mellitus is a group of metabolic diseases characterized by hyperglycemia resulting from defects in insulin production, insulin action, or both. Diet is considered a pillar for the prevention and progression of type 2 diabetes (T2D). Meta-analytic evidence from observational studies have demonstrated an association between the adherence to the MD pattern and a decrease in T2D risk, showing an approximately 20% reduction of T2D incidence in individuals with the highest, versus the lowest, adherence to the MD (Koloverou, Esposito, Giugliano, & Panagiotakos, 2014; Martín-Peláez, Fito, & Castaner, 2020; Lukas Schwingshackl, Missbach, König, & Hoffmann, 2015).

Concerning data from clinical trials, the large-scale, multi-center, controlled randomized PREDIMED trial (J. Salas-Salvadó et al., 2011; Jordi Salas-Salvadó et al., 2014) enrolled 418 non-diabetic individuals with a high risk of CVD and randomly assigned them to a low-fat diet (control group) or the MD supplemented either with extra-virgin olive oil (1 L/week) or nuts (30 g/day). After approximately 4 years of follow-up, the groups following the MD supplemented with olive oil or nuts exhibited a 50% lower risk of developing T2D, compared to controls. Approximately 5 years after the end of the study, non-diabetic patients who had received the MD supplemented with olive oil had a 40% reduced risk of developing T2DM, whereas those received the nut-enhanced MD had a 20% lower risk, compared with the control group. These beneficial effects were attributed to the overall composition of the dietary pattern, not caloric restriction, increased physical activity, or weight loss (Martín-Peláez et al., 2020).

Some of the mechanisms that contribute to the impaired insulin secretion of β-cells include insulin resistance, lipotoxicity, glucotoxicity, oxidative stress, activation of inflammatory pathways, endoplasmic reticulum stress, and cellular mitochondrial dysfunction. The MD seems to play a role in these T2D-related mechanisms through actions and interactions by different nutrients including anti-inflammatory/antioxidant actions, glucagon-like peptide agonist compounds, and changes in gut microbiota (Martín-Peláez et al., 2020).

DYSLIPIDEMIA

The MD has been found to lower total, medium-small, and very small atherogenic LDL particles, large very-low density lipoprotein (VLDL) fractions and total cholesterol (TC) concentration. Indeed, results from the PREDIMED trial study show that the MD supplemented with olive oil or nuts effectively reduced plasma concentrations of LDL; the MD supplemented with nuts changed the lipoprotein subfractions to a less atherogenic pattern, suggesting a mechanism for the reduction of CVD events noticed in this group (Damasceno et al., 2013). Moreover, pooled data from observational studies support that HDL-cholesterol levels are higher and triglycerides levels lower in individuals with a high adherence also to the MD compared to those with low adherence (Bakaloudi, Chrysoula, Kotzakioulafi, Theodoridis, & Chourdakis, 2021).

A possible mechanism explaining the alterations in lipid profiles of patients with high adherence to the MD is the high content of olive-oil polyphenols and oleic acid as part of the MD, through the amelioration of the antioxidant and inflammatory status of the subjects (Tsartsou, Proutsos, Castanas, & Kampa, 2019). Moreover, phytosterol intakes of 0.6 to 3.3 g/day—including plant sterols and stanols, compounds in vegetable oils, nuts, seeds, grain products, fruits, and vegetables—can also reduce LDL-cholesterol concentrations (Ras, Geleijnse, & Trautwein, 2014).

OBESITY/METABOLIC SYNDROME

There is a long-term (>12 months) effect of the MD on weight loss in individuals with overweight or obesity trying to lose weight (Mancini, Filion, Atallah, & Eisenberg, 2016). This seems to be mediated by decreased hepatic fat content (Gepner et al., 2019) and improvements in several cardio-metabolic risk factors (Gepner et al., 2019; Mancini et al., 2016).

Considering the effects of the MD on metabolic syndrome (MetS), MD is a possible therapy for MetS, as it reduces the excess of adiposity and the obesity-related inflammatory response. Moreover, pooled results from prospective and cross-sectional data (Justyna Godos et al., 2017; Kastorini et al., 2011) support that a higher adherence to the MD is associated with a 19% lower risk of developing MetS, while its components (e.g., waist circumference, BP, hyperlipidemia, and hyperglycemia) can also be improved (Castro-Barquero, Ruiz-León, Sierra-Pérez, Estruch, & Casas, 2020).

CANCER

Cancer is a major public health problem worldwide, accounting for nearly 10 million deaths in 2020 (Sung et al., 2021). Based on 2014 data, an estimated proportion of 42% of all cancers in adults over the age of 30, were attributed to potentially modifiable risk factors (**Figure 3.4**) (Islami et al., 2018). Cigarette smoking had, by far, the highest proportion (19.0% of all cases), followed by excess body weight (7.8% of all cases), alcohol intake (5.6% of all cases), and physical inactivity (2.9% of all cases).

The MD is inversely associated with the development of several cancer types, such as colorectal, epithelial, breast, prostate, pancreas, endometrial, and cancers of the upper aerodigestive tract. Some of MD components, such as whole-grain cereals, fruits, and vegetables, seem to lower the risk of cancers associated with the gastrointestinal, breast, and female genital tracts and epithelium.

In 2018, the World Cancer Research Fund along with the American Institute for Cancer Research (WCRF/AIRC) reported that the MD is "convincingly" associated with a reduced risk of weight gain, and overweight or obesity, suggesting that the MD might indirectly have a huge impact on cancer development. Moreover, the 2018 WCRF/AIRC recommendations suggest specific quantities of some foods and nutrients that are a part of the MD, including at least 30 g of fiber and 400 g of non-starchy vegetables/fruits per day as well as limiting red meat consumption to no more than three portions (350 to 500 g) per week (Rock et al., 2020; WCRF/AICR, 2018).

HEALTHY AGING

Extended longevity is emerging globally and its impending effects on high-income countries are based on whether

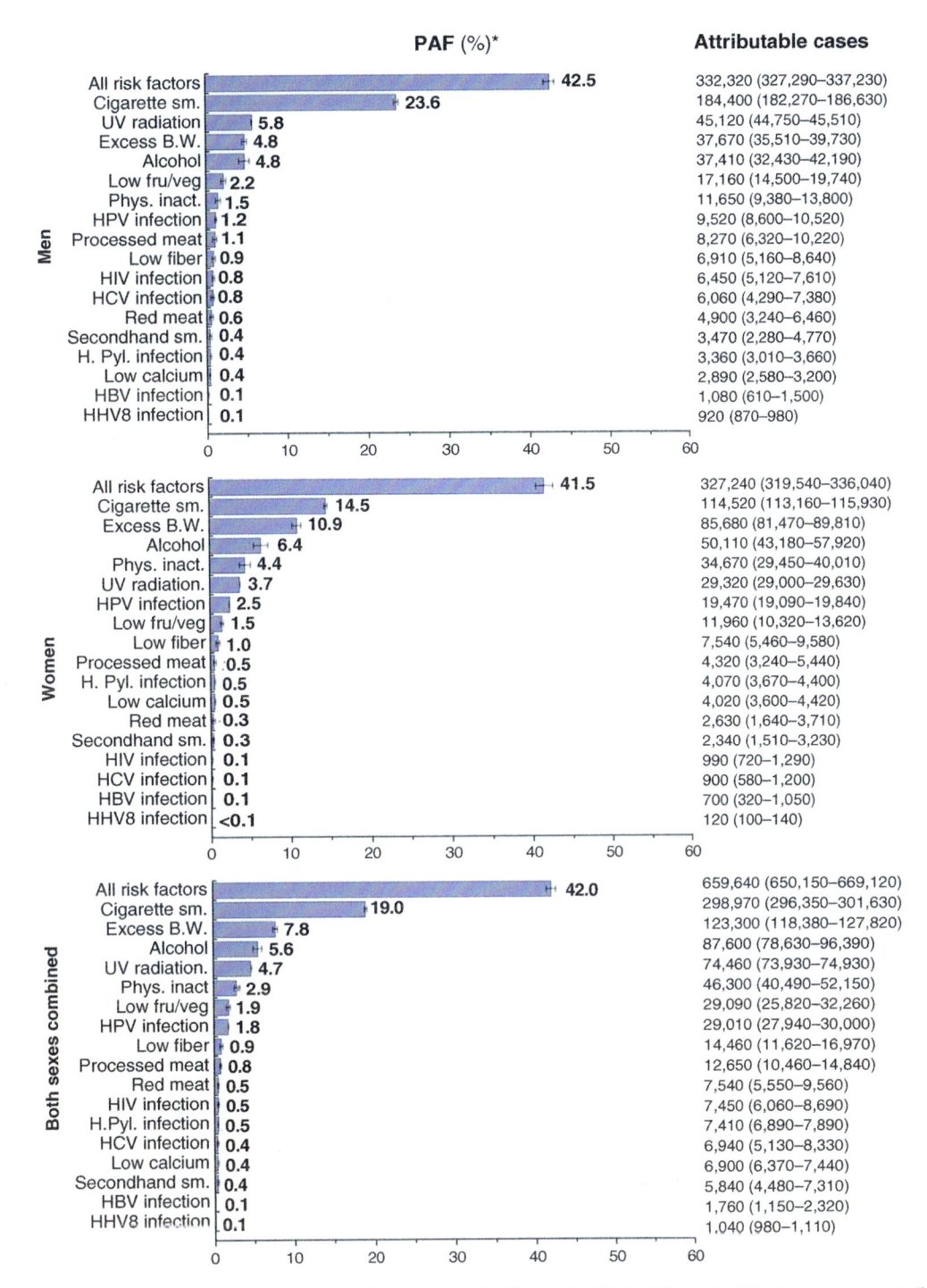

FIGURE 3.4 An estimated 42% of all cancers in adults aged 30 years and older in the United States in 2014 by sex were attributed to potentially modifiable risk factors, e.g., cigarette smoking, excess body weight, alcohol intake, and physical inactivity. PAF: the population-attributable fraction. Source: (Islami et al., 2018 / with permission of John Wiley & Sons).

individuals' extended lifespans are accompanied by the adverse effects of aging. Indeed, aging is accompanied by a progressive loss of physical, mental, and cognitive functions, that if not treated, will ultimately lead to morbidity and mortality (Critselis & Panagiotakos, 2020). Although, specific hallmarks of aging exist (Shannon et al., 2021), there are some modifiable lifestyle factors, namely diet and physical activity, which, if altered via related interventions, can facilitate healthy aging (Critselis & Panagiotakos, 2020).

Of all the dietary patterns linked to healthy aging (e.g. MD, Okinawan and DASH diets), most predominantly, the MD was associated with numerous health benefits and the prevention of a variety of age-related disorders, such as all-cause mortality, CVDs, T2D, MetS, and cancers as well as longevity (L. J. Dominguez,

Di Bella, Veronese, & Barbagallo, 2021) and mental health (Ventriglio et al., 2020).

Of note, olive oil, and in particular virgin olive oil, which is rich in oleic acid and polyphenols (namely secoiridoids), a major component of the MD, impacts the biological pathways implicated in the hallmarks of aging (Critselis & Panagiotakos, 2020; Fernandez del Rio, Gutierrez-Casado, Varela-Lopez, & Villalba, 2016) (more on healthy aging in **Unit 3**).

THE DIETARY APPROACHES TO STOP HYPERTENSION (DASH) DIETARY PATTERN

INITIAL DIETARY APPROACHES TO STOP HYPERTENSION (DASH) TRIALS

The Dietary Approaches to Stop Hypertension (DASH) was first designed to prevent and treat hypertension. In the 1990s, the goals of DASH diet trials (Appel et al., 1997) were to create patterns similar to the BP lowering benefits of vegetarian diets, yet contain enough animal products to make them palatable to non-vegetarians.

The initial trial, DASH (Appel et al., 1997), tested the effects on BP of (1) a diet rich in fruits, vegetables, low-fat dairy foods, and low in total fat, saturated fat and dietary cholesterol (2) a diet high in fruits and vegatables and (3) a control diet similar to what many Americans consume. Daily sodium intake ranged from 2.5 to 4.0 g, depending on the energy level. Two years later, the DASH-Sodium trial (Svetkey et al., 1999) compared the effects on BP of the DASH diet using three dietary sodium levels—low (40–80 mmol or 920–1840 mg), intermediate (80–160 mmol or 1840–3680 mg), and high (120–240 mmol or 2760–5520 mg)—in adults with above-optimal BP or stage 1 hypertension over the typical American diet (control diet). In both trials, reductions in BP were significantly higher for participants eating the DASH dietary patterns either with or without sodium restriction compared to control diets.

Since then, several DASH diet alternatives have been tested including other lifestyle parameters or nutrients that seem to affect BP. The DEW-IT trial (Diet, Exercise, and Weight Loss Intervention Trial) (Miller 3rd et al., 2002) and the PREMIER trial (a Trial of Lifestyle Interventions for Blood Pressure Control) (Funk et al., 2008), showed improvements in BP after implementing the DASH diet, along with weight loss, physical activity, sodium and alcohol restriction, compared to control diets; however, the effect of multiple lifestyle changes on BP were not be fully additive to that of the DASH diet alone on the aforementioned trials. With regard to nutrient content, a high-fat DASH diet (HF-DASH) compared to the original DASH diet had similar reductions in BP, although plasma triglyceride and VLDL levels decreased more in the HF-DASH diet, without differences in LDL-cholesterol levels (S. Chiu et al., 2016). Moreover, a DASH diet where the main protein source (55% of total proteins) was lean pork (DASH-P) instead of chicken and fish (DASH-CF), showed similar results in improving BP, suggesting an alternative DASH-style diet for BP reduction (Sayer, Wright, Chen, & Campbell, 2015).

THE DIETARY APPROACHES TO STOP HYPERTENSION (DASH) DIET CHARACTERISTICS

The DASH diet is a plant-based dietary pattern characterized by a high intake of vegetables, fruits, whole grains, nuts; the addition of some fish, poultry, and low-fat dairy products; and the minimization of processed/red meat, sugar, and processed foods. As a result, it provides low amounts of saturated fat (6% of energy), total fat (27% of daily calorie intake), dietary cholesterol (about 150 mg/day), and reduced sodium content (1500 to 2300 mg/day), while endorsing dietary fiber (>30 g/day), potassium (K), magnesium (Mg), and calcium (Ca) intake (Castro-Barquero et al., 2020; Craddick et al., 2003).

A typical serving guide of the DASH diet (**Figure 3.5**) includes (Akhlaghi, 2020; Challa, Ameer, & Uppaluri, 2021) (University of Arcancas System):

- Fruit: 4–5 servings/day (e.g., low glycemic index fruits)
- Vegetables: 4–5 servings/day (e.g., kale, broccoli, spinach, collards)
- Grain and grain products: 6–8 servings/day, whole grains are 3.8 servings/day (e.g., cracked wheat, millets, oats)
- Low-fat dairy foods: about 2–3 servings/day, with reduced total (25.6 % of energy) and saturated (7% of energy) fat
- Legumes: 0.7 servings/day
- Fish: 0.5 servings/day (e.g., rich in omega-3 fatty acids)
- Red meat: 0.5 servings/day
- Lean meat products: about two or fewer servings/day
- Sweets and sugar-sweetened beverages: 0.7 servings/day, <5 servings/week
- Nuts, seeds: 4–5 servings per week (e.g., avocados, hempseeds, flax seeds)

THE DIETARY APPROACHES TO STOP HYPERTENSION (DASH) DIET HEALTH EFFECTS

Over the last two decades, the DASH has emerged as a healthy-eating guideline. Aside from its positive effects on hypertension, the DASH dietary pattern seems to positively affect the risk of several chronic diseases. It is inversely associated with the risk of CVD (Chiavaroli et al., 2019), MetS (Akhlaghi, 2020), chronic kidney disease (Raphael, 2019), and several types of cancer (Onvani, Haghighatdoost, & Azadbakht, 2015). There is also evidence that it improves lipid profile (Miller, Erlinger, & Appel, 2006), insulin sensitivity, inflammation, and oxidative stress in T2D (Fernandez & Murillo, 2022). Most importantly, even modest adherence to the DASH diet is associated with a lower risk of all-cause mortality, while high versus low adherence seems to strengthen this risk-reducing association (S. Soltani, Arablou, Jayedi, & Salehi-Abargouei, 2020). Its high content in some bioactive compounds (such as fiber, vitamins, minerals, trace elements, and phytochemicals) found in whole grains, fruits, and vegetables, combined with its low content in harmful compounds found in processed meat and sugary beverages explain the above associations. (Akhlaghi, 2020). The

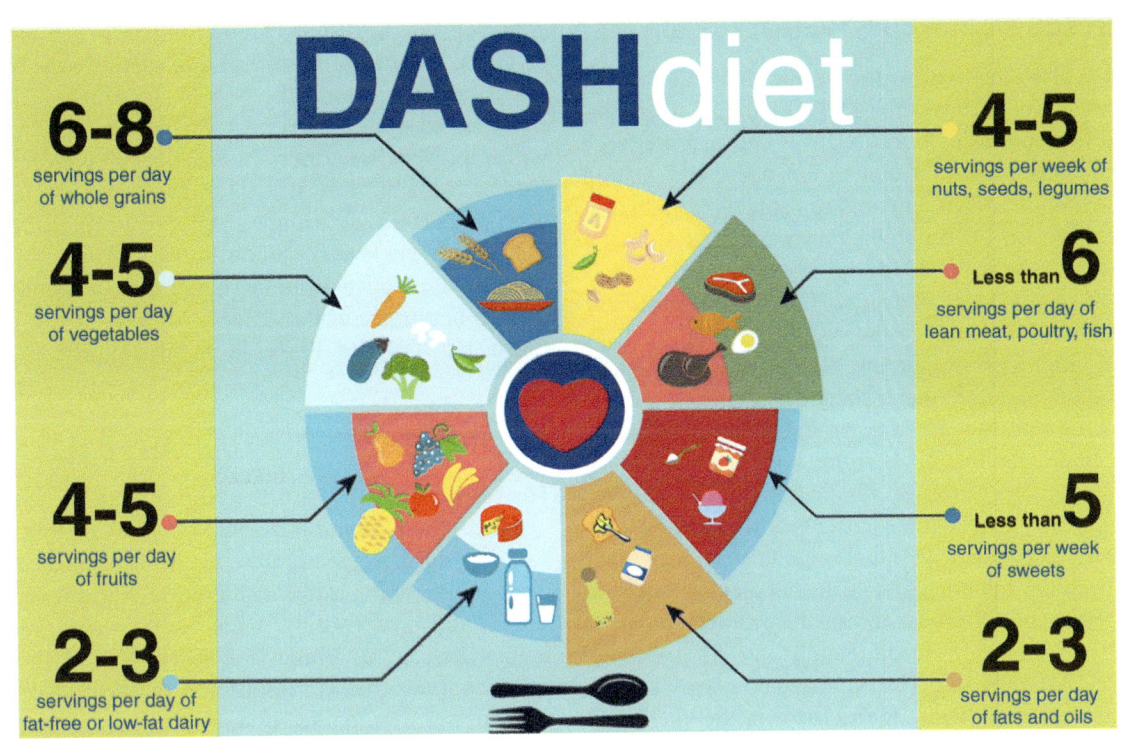

FIGURE 3.5 The DASH dietary pattern. Source: University of Arkancas System, Department of Agriculture. Research & Extension Lowering Your Blood Pressure with the DASH Eating Plan.

DASH diet is also suggested to have antioxidant, anti-atherogenic, anti-inflammatory, antiproliferative, and anti-tumor properties.

The health effects of the DASH diet on the aforementioned chronic conditions will be discussed next.

ALL-CAUSE AND SPECIFIC-CAUSE MORTALITY

The DASH diet has a significant, inverse dose-response association with all-cause, CVD, stroke, and cancer mortality. A meta-analysis and systematic review (S. Soltani et al., 2020) of 17 prospective cohort studies revealed that for each 5-point increment in adherence to the DASH diet, there was a lower of risk 5% for all-causes, 4% for CVD, 3% for stroke, and 3% for cancer mortality. In the same meta-analysis, the non-linear dose-response analysis showed that the DASH-mortality association becomes stronger when the adherence score exceeds 20 points (medium to high adherence) (S. Soltani et al., 2020).

CARDIOVASCULAR DISEASES

Adherence to the DASH diet seems to reduce the incidence of CVDs, stroke, CHD, and heart failure. A meta-analysis of six prospective observational studies (Salehi-Abargouei, Maghsoudi, Shirani, & Azadbakht, 2013) with follow-ups from 7 to 24 years showed that a DASH-like diet was protective against CVDs, CHD, stroke, and heart-failure risk by 20%, 21%, 19%, and 29%, respectively.

Data from interventional studies regarding the DASH diet and heart failure comes from the DASH-Diastolic Heart-failure (DASH-DHF) trial; a non-blinded, non-randomized, and non-controlled pilot study conducted among 13 primarily obese, post-menopausal women with heart failure-preserved ejection fraction results (Hummel et al., 2012; Hummel et al., 2013; Mathew, Seymour, Byun, Pennathur, & Hummel, 2015). The DASH-DHF trial showed improvements in heart-failure biomarkers (e.g. urinary sodium, BNP, and oxidative stress), BP, and cardiac function, along with weight loss. The aforementioned results agreed with another RCT (Rifai, Pisano, Hayden, Sulo, & Silver, 2015), in which DASH was compared to general heart-failure recommendations in 48 patients with mild-moderate heart failure, although weight loss was not observed after 12 weeks (Kerley, 2018).

OBESITY/METABOLIC SYNDROME

As the DASH dietary pattern is limited in fat and high in fiber and Ca content, individuals on this diet are less prone to develop overweight and obesity as well as MetS (Akhlaghi, 2020). A meta-analysis of 13 clinical trials assessed the potential beneficial effects of the DASH diet on body weight and abdominal obesity compared to control diets (western or population's usual diet). Adherence to the DASH diet significantly decreased body weight, body mass index (BMI), and waist circumference (WC) compared to the control diets. The mean weight reduction was about 1.42 kg for study periods 8 to 24 weeks long, for short-term periods it was 1.64 kg, and in participants with overweight and obesity it was 1.63 kg. Of note, a low-calorie DASH diet was even more effective (−2.27 kg) compared with other low-energy diets (S. Soltani, Shirani, Chitsazi, & Salehi-Abargouei, 2016).

Furthermore, epidemiological data assessing the benefits of the DASH diet on MetS show that high adherence to the DASH diet is associated with a lower likelihood of having MetS compared to low adherence (Castro-Barquero et al., 2020).

TYPE 2 DIABETES MELLITUS/HYPERGLYCEMIA

The DASH diet is also effective on glucose and insulin levels. In a randomized crossover clinical trial, 31 T2D patients were randomly assigned to a control diet or the DASH eating pattern for 8 weeks. Participants in DASH diet group decreased fasting blood glucose levels and A1C compared to controls (Azadbakht et al., 2010). Indeed, in an umbrella review of 60 systematic review and meta-analysis of RCTs and observational studies assessing the role of the DASH diet and MD in the prevention of T2D, found that both can reduce the risk of developing T2D, especially in the high-risk population. Some food groups and nutrients that demonstrated the associated beneficial effects were whole-grain foods, low-fat dairy products, cheese, yogurt, olive oil, total fiber, dietary magnesium, and flavonoids (Toi et al., 2020).

Moreover, nearly two of three patients with diabetes have hypertension. Therefore, the DASH diet might also be beneficial for people with both hypertension and diabetes (Campbell, 2017). In a cross-sectional study aiming to evaluate possible associations of the food groups recommended in DASH with BP values in 225 T2D patients, 80 g/1000 kcal and 50 g/1000 kcal of fruits and vegetables, respectively, found to lower the likelihood of having high BP (de Paula et al., 2012).

HYPERLIPIDEMIA

The benefits of DASH diet on lipid profiles are not consistent. The original DASH study was tested on altering plasma lipids with improvements in TC and LDL-cholesterol but modest effects on HDL-cholesterol and no changes in triacylglycerol (TAG) levels (Obarzanek et al., 2001). In a meta-analysis of 20 RCTs including 1917 participants, DASH improved total and LDL-cholesterol but did not change HDL-cholesterol or TAG levels (Siervo et al., 2015). The effects of DASH on total and LDL-cholesterol could be attributed to the decreased intake of saturated fat, while the high Ca content of DASH may explain the total cholesterol–lowering effect of the DASH diet (Akhlaghi, 2020).

CANCER

The DASH dietary pattern has been also associated with lower cancer mortality risk. In a meta-analysis of 27 cohort studies (Milajerdi, Namazi, Larijani, & Azadbakht, 2018), diet quality and cancer mortality was assessed. Nine studies evaluated the DASH diet and risk of mortality from all cancer types. A significant inverse correlation between the DASH diet and total cancer mortality was found, although this association remained significant only between high-quality studies. The association between the DASH diet and cancer mortality was not significant among studies assessing colorectal cancer death (Milajerdi et al., 2018). More will be discussed in **Chapter 21**.

CHRONIC KIDNEY DISEASE

Adherence to a DASH dietary pattern could also help prevent chronic kidney disease (CKD). In a systematic review and meta-analysis of observational studies (Mozaffari, Ajabshir, & Alizadeh, 2020) with 568 213 participants including 16 694 cases of CKD, a significant inverse association was found between DASH adherence and the risk of developing CKD. Notably, a stratified analysis of this relationship remained significant only within prospective cohort studies but not within cross-sectional studies (Mozaffari et al., 2020). Moreover, the DASH diet has been associated with higher glomerular filtration rates (GFRs) as well as lower levels of albuminuria and inflammatory markers such as C-reactive protein (CRP) and e-selectin, which suggests a nephroprotective effect and lower CKD risk (Quintela, Carioca, de Oliveira, Fraser, & da Silva Junior, 2021).

THE HEALTHY NORDIC DIETARY PATTERN

The Nordic diet (ND) shares many similarities with the MD. For instance, the MD and ND share similar nutritional recommendations and there is a preference for seasonal, locally available foods while taking into consideration cultural heredity, sustainability, and preservation of the environment (Krznarić, Karas, Ljubas Kelečić, & Vranešić Bender, 2021). However, the ND includes foods that are traditional to northern European countries such as Denmark, Finland, Iceland, Norway, and Sweden. The ND is considered a plant-based diet that is locally sourced, ensuring an environmentally friendly characteristic in terms of production, especially when consumed in the Baltic region. The Baltic Sea pyramid is addressed to the general healthy population to depict healthier dietary choices based on foods typically grown in Nordic countries. Its most commonly used ingredients and foods can be seen in **Figure 3.6** (Kanerva, Kaartinen, Schwab, Lahti-Koski, & Männistö, 2014; Renzella et al., 2018).

The core statements upon which the ND was developed are: (1) more calories from plant-based foods and less from meat; (2) use of more foods sourced from lakes and the sea (e.g., sea weeds and shellfish); and (3) including more wild local foods from the countryside (plants, berries, mushrooms, and aromatic herbs) (Ligia J. Dominguez et al., 2022).

The pyramid illustrates the relative, recommended amount of foods and food groups. The staple components of ND are berries, apples, pears, and Nordic fruits in general, fatty fish (Baltic herring, mackerel, and salmon), lean fish, vegetables (cabbage, tomatoes, lettuce, cucumbers, legumes, and roots—except for potatoes) and whole-grain cereals (barley, oats, and rye) (Perälä et al., 2016; Renzella et al., 2018). Nordic vegetables and fruits are located at the bottom of the pyramid (**Figure 3.6**) due to their crucial role in health preservation and promotion. Whole-grain products, which are rich in fiber, are found in the intermediate levels of the pyramid before fish, low-fat or fat-free milk products and oils used for cooking (Noora Kanerva et al., 2014). A notable difference between the ND and MD is the use of rapeseed (canola) oil instead of olive oil (Renzella et al., 2018). Canola oil is rich in MUFAs and alpha-linolenic acid, a plant-based n-3 poly-unsaturated fatty acids (PUFAs). Milk and sour milk are the only drinks illustrated in the ND pyramid, because of its important role in Nordic nutrition (Noora Kanerva et al., 2014). Water and tea are preferred to address thirst, while light to moderate alcohol drinks are tolerated (Perälä et al., 2016). Foods like processed meat, butter, sweets,

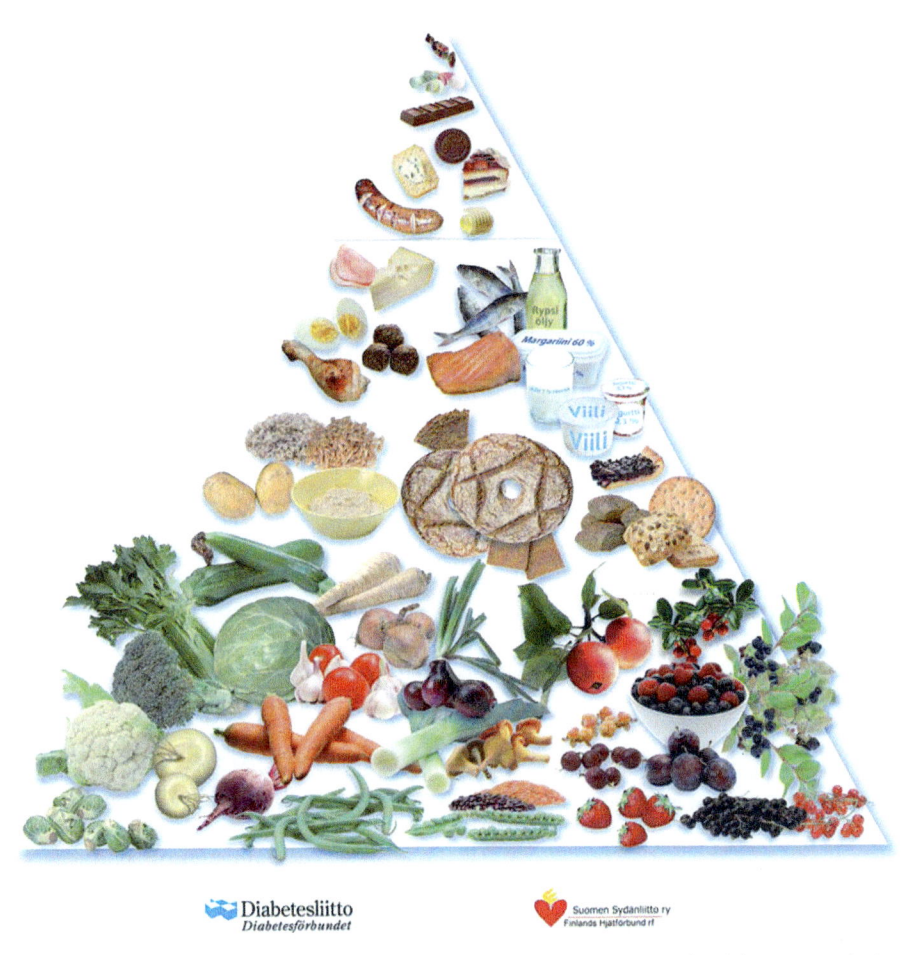

FIGURE 3.6 The Baltic Sea diet pyramid. Created by the Finnish Heart Association, the Finnish Diabetes Association, and the University of Eastern Finland. Source: (Noora Kanerva et al., 2014 / with permission of Cambridge University Press).

chocolate, and sweet baker products are located at the top of the pyramid, implying the need for very considerate consumption (Noora Kanerva et al., 2014).

HEALTH EFFECTS OF THE NORDIC DIET

Although the ND was developed only recently, the literature on this healthy dietary pattern has grown, showing significant associations between the ND and several health outcomes. This includes improvements in several CVD parameters, namely blood-lipid levels, systolic and diastolic BP, glucose metabolism, insulin sensitivity (Berild, Holven, & Ulven, 2017; Ramezani-Jolfaie, Mohammadi, & Salehi-Abargouei, 2019), inflammation (Maria Lankinen, Matti Uusitupa, & Ursula Schwab, 2019), and the risks of all-cause mortality and death due to cancer and CVD (Castro-Espin & Agudo, 2022; Jalilpiran, Jayedi, Djafarian, & Shab-Bidar, 2022) as well as physical performance and cognitive health in older adults (Männikkö et al., 2015; Perälä et al., 2016).

CHRONIC DISEASE RISK

Several epidemiological studies have investigated the association between greater ND adherence and chronic diseases, namely CVD risk (e.g., myocardial infarction [MI], ischemic heart disease [IHD], stroke), T2D, and cancer. However, data are not always consistent.

In the Danish Diet Cancer and Health cohort study (Gunge et al., 2017) that included 57 053 men and women aged 50 to 64 years, 1669 men and 653 women developed MIs during follow-up (median of 13.6 years). The highest adherence to the ND, as assessed using a healthy Nordic food index, was associated with 23% lower MI risk in men and 45% lower MI risk in women compared to those with the lowest adherence. Moreover, in the same cohort (Kyrø et al., 2013), a greater ND compliance, using the same index was related to a lower risk of developing colorectal cancer by 35% among women, with only a tendency found in men. It was further indicated that per point adherence to the healthy Nordic food index, women had a 9% lower risk of colorectal cancer occurrence, but no significant effect was found for men (Kyrø et al., 2013). In the EPIC-Potsdam cohort study (Galbete et al., 2018) that recruited 27 548 participants with chronic diseases (e.g., T2D, MI, stroke, and cancer), the ND showed a possible beneficial effect on MI and T2D in the overall population, but only in men for stroke. Conversely, data from the prospective Swedish Women's Lifestyle and Health cohort (Roswall et al., 2015), which included 43 310 women, 8383 of whom developed CVD, showed no association between ND adherence and CVD risk.

However, pooled data from 13 prospective cohort studies with 930 153 participants (Jalilpiran et al., 2022) showed that the highest category of ND adherence was associated with 12%, 20%, and 10% lower risk for stroke, MI, and T2D, compared to the lowest.

Results from RCTs regarding CVD factors are still inconsistent. A meta-analysis of five RCTs (Ramezani-Jolfaie et al., 2019) investigating the effect of the ND on circulating lipid levels and BP, showed that ND significantly reduces total and LDL-cholesterol, but not HDL-cholesterol and TAG. These results, however, were not in accordance with a previously published meta-analysis of three cohort studies that showed an increased risk of lowered HDL-cholesterol on those with high ND adherence compared to low (N. Kanerva et al., 2014). Nevertheless, the ND was found to beneficially reduce systolic and diastolic BP based on interventional data (Ramezani-Jolfaie et al., 2019).

A lack of significant findings between ND and chronic diseases is most likely due to methodological issues regarding the *a priori* development of dietary indexes that represent the ND diet and not underlying associations per se (Gunge et al., 2017). Indeed, several food items comprising the ND have long-standing associations with reduced risk for chronic diseases, such as the consumption of oily fish, whole grains and oats, and fruits and vegetables (e.g., apples and pears) (Gunge et al., 2017).

ALL-CAUSE AND SPECIFIC-CAUSE MORTALITY

Although evidence regarding the associations between the ND with chronic disease risk is still inconclusive, a dose-response meta-analysis of prospective observational studies (Jalilpiran et al., 2022) investigating all-cause and specific-cause mortality and ND adherence in the general population found promising results. An inverse linear association was found for ND adherence and mortality due to all-cause, CVD, and cancer. Participants with the highest ND adherence compared to lowest showed a 22% lower risk for all-cause and CVD mortality and 14% for cancer mortality. Moreover, a model-based simulation study to find the number of deaths attributable to CVDs that could be prevented or delayed in Nordic countries indicated that the most lives could be saved by increasing fruit and vegetable intake.

INFLAMMATION

Few epidemiological data in the literature exist supporting the effective role of the ND in lowering inflammation levels compared to the MD for which the evidence is more robust (L Schwingshackl & Hoffmann, 2014). Data from interventional studies are needed to confirm the anti-inflammatory effects of the ND. A narrative review of two observational studies and eight intervention trials evaluated the associations of ND with inflammation. Based on observational studies, the authors reported an inverse association between ND adherence and the concentration of high-sensitivity (hs) CRP. The results of two out of four intervention studies showed a significant decrease in hsCRP levels, while other single intervention studies reported beneficial effects on interleukin-1 receptor agonist and cathepsin S (M. Lankinen, M. Uusitupa, & U. Schwab, 2019).

PHYSICAL PERFORMANCE AND COGNITIVE HEALTH IN OLDER ADULTS

The rapid increase in the prevalence of poor physical performance and cognitive impairment associated with aging populations has stimulated interest in identifying modifiable lifestyle factors, such as diet, that could prevent these conditions. Männikkö et al., (Männikkö et al., 2015) evaluated cross-sectional and longitudinal associations of the ND with cognitive function. High adherence to the ND at baseline was positively associated with verbal fluency and word-list learning after 4 years of the diet. Moreover, the Helsinki Birth Cohort study that examined associations between the ND and measures of physical performance 10 years later in older adults found that women with the highest ND compliance had better physical performance, even after controlling for physical activity, compared to the lowest ND compliance. The role of the ND in older adults and healthy aging will discussed further in **Chapter 10**.

THE HEALTHY VEGETARIAN-TYPE DIETARY PATTERN

Healthy vegetarian dietary patterns are an alternative to the healthy US-style dietary pattern and are primarily considered plant-based diets that exclude all kinds of meats, including fowl, poultry, fish, or seafood (**Table 3.3**) (US Department of Agriculture and US Department of Health and Human Services. Dietary Guidelines for Americans, 2020-2025). Healthy vegetarian dietary patterns are high in soy products (mainly tofu and other processed soy products); beans, peas, and lentils; nuts and seeds; and whole grains. All foods in those patterns should be prepared with minimal added sugars, refined starches, or sodium and in nutrient-dense forms. Therefore, no calories for added sugars, saturated fat, or calories for extra food than recommended, are included. Moreover, due to the plant-based origin of foods, those patterns are high in fiber, Mg, K, vitamin C and E, folate, carotenoids, and other phytochemical substances (US Department of Agriculture and US Department of Health and Human Services. Dietary Guidelines for Americans, 2020–2025).

The two most common types of the healthy vegetarian dietary patterns are the vegan diet, in which all animal products are avoided (e.g., meat, poultry, fish, seafood, eggs, and dairy products) and the vegetarian diet, which may include eggs (ovo-vegetarian), dairy products (lacto-vegetarian), eggs and dairy products (lacto-ovo-vegetarian) or eggs, dairy products, and fish and/or shellfish (pescetarian) (**Figure 3.7**) (Kahleova H, 2020; Pieters & Swanepoel, 2021).

The flexitarian or semi-vegetarian diet is considered a non-strict vegetarian diet in which individuals may occasionally eat meat or fish. In all of these occasions, lean or low-fat forms of foods are advised, apart from dairy, for which whole-fat milk, reduced-fat plain yogurt, and reduced-fat cheese are included.

Table 3.3 Healthy vegetarian-type dietary pattern for ages 2 and older, with daily or weekly amounts from food groups, subgroups, and components.

Calorie level of pattern	1,000	1,200	1,400	1,600	1,800	2,000	2,200	2,400	2,600	2,800	3,000	3,200
Food group or subgroup	\multicolumn{12}{c}{Daily amount of food from each group (Vegetable and protein foods subgroup amounts[b] are per week.)}											
Vegetables (cup eq/day)	1	1 ½	1 ½	2	2 ½	2 ½	3	3	3 ½	3 ½	4	4
Vegetable subgroups in weekly amounts												
Dark-green vegetables (cup eq/wk)	½	1	1	1 ½	1 ½	1 ½	2	2	2 ½	2 ½	2 ½	2 ½
Red and orange vegetables (cup eq/wk)	2 ½	3	3	4	5 ½	5 ½	6	6	7	7	7 ½	7 ½
Beans, peas, lentils (cup eq/wk)	½	½	½	1	1 ½	1 ½	2	2	2 ½	2 ½	3	3
Starchy vegetables (cup eq/wk)	2	3 ½	3 ½	4	5	5	6	6	7	7	8	8
Other vegetables (cup eq/wk)	1 ½	2 ½	2 ½	3 ½	4	4	5	5	5 ½	5 ½	7	7
Fruits (cup eq/day)	1	1	1 ½	1 ½	1 ½	2	2	2	2	2 ½	2 ½	2 ½
Grains (ounce eq/day)	3	4	5	5 ½	6 ½	6 ½	7 ½	8 ½	9 ½	10 ½	10 ½	10 ½
Whole grains (ounce eq/day)	1 ½	2	2 ½	3	3 ½	3 ½	4	4 ½	5	5 ½	5 ½	5 ½
Refined grains (ounce eq/day)	1 ½	2	2 ½	2 ½	3	3	3 ½	4	4 ½	5	5	5
Dairy (cup eq/day)	2	2 ½	2 ½	3	3	3	3	3	3	3	3	3
Protein foods (ounce eq/day)	1	1 ½	2	2 ½	3	3 ½	3 ½	4	4 ½	5	5 ½	6
Protein food subgroups in weekly amounts												
Eggs (ounce eq/wk)	2	3	3	3	3	3	3	3	3	4	4	4
Beans, peas, lentils (cup eq/wk)	1	2	4	4	6	6	6	8	9	10	11	12
Soy products (ounce eq/wk)	2	3	4	6	6	8	8	9	10	11	12	13
Nuts, seeds (ounce eq/wk)	2	2	3	5	6	7	7	8	9	10	12	13
Oils (grams/day)	15	17	17	22	24	27	29	31	34	36	44	51
Limit on calories for other uses (kcal/day)	170	140	160	150	150	250	290	350	350	350	390	500
Limit on calories for other uses (%/day)	17%	12%	11%	9%	8%	13%	13%	15%	13%	13%	13%	16%

[1] About half of beans, peas, and lentils are shown as vegetables (cup eq), and half as protein foods (ounce eq). Beans, peas, and lentils (cup eq), is the amount in the vegetable group plus the amount in protein foods group (in ounce eq) divided by four.

Source: (US Department of Agriculture and US Department of Health and Human Services. Dietary Guidelines for Americans, 2020–2025).

NOTE: The total dietary pattern should not exceed dietary guideline limits for added sugars, saturated fat, and alcohol; be within the acceptable macronutrient distribution ranges for protein, carbohydrate, and total fats; and stay within calorie limits. Values are rounded.

Plant-based ↑ / Animal-based ↓

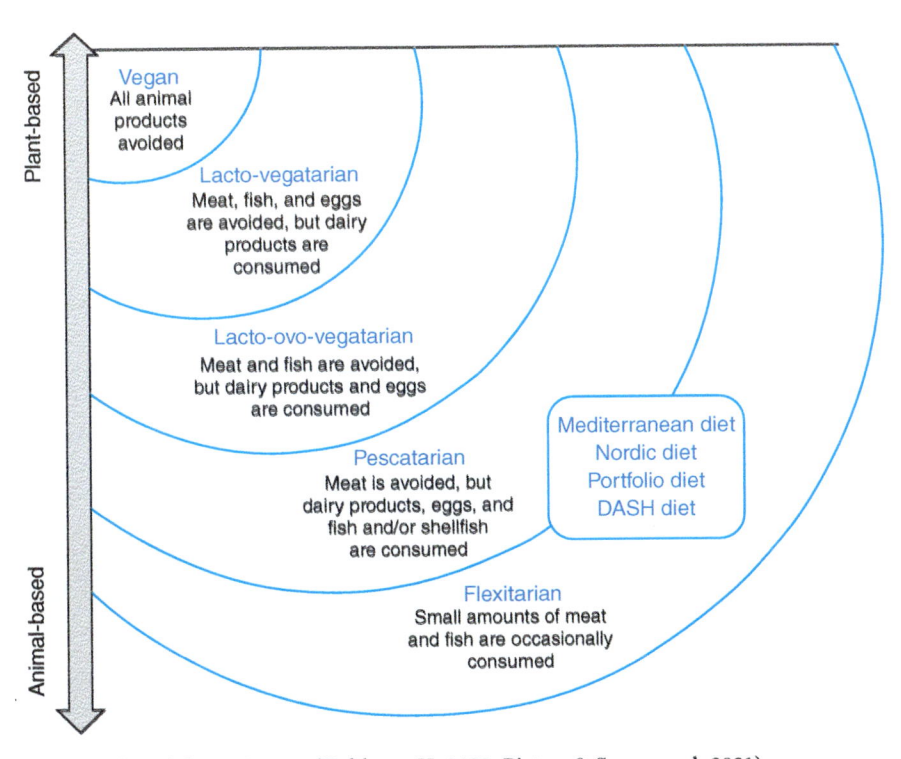

- **Vegan** — All animal products avoided
- **Lacto-vegetarian** — Meat, fish, and eggs are avoided, but dairy products are consumed
- **Lacto-ovo-vegetarian** — Meat and fish are avoided, but dairy products and eggs are consumed
- **Pescatarian** — Meat is avoided, but dairy products, eggs, and fish and/or shellfish are consumed
- **Flexitarian** — Small amounts of meat and fish are occasionally consumed

Mediterranean diet / Nordic diet / Portfolio diet / DASH diet

FIGURE 3.7 The spectrum of plant-based diets. Source: (Kahleova H, 2020; Pieters & Swanepoel, 2021).

HEALTH EFFECTS OF THE HEALTHY VEGETARIAN-TYPE DIETARY PATTERN

Most of the observational data regarding the role of vegetarianism in health and disease come from the Seventh-day Adventist (SDA) population. The studies focused on this population have investigated associations between lifestyle, diet, and disease (Kahn, Phillips, Snowdon, & CHOI, 1984; Snowdon & Phillips, 1985; Tonstad, Butler, Yan, & Fraser, 2009; Wynder, Lemon, & Bross, 1959) among members of the SDA church, a Christian denomination that encourages vegetarian diet patterns while calling for abstinence from alcohol and tobacco.

CVD RISK AND MORTALITY

Vegetarian dietary patterns may reduce CVD mortality and the risk of CHD by 40% (Kahleova, Levin, & Barnard, 2018). Several meta-analyses of cross-sectional and prospective studies (Dinu, Abbate, Gensini, Casini, & Sofi, 2017; Jabri et al., 2021; Kwok, Umar, Myint, Mamas, & Loke, 2014) have concluded that a vegetarian diet, compared with a non-vegetarian diet, may be associated with a reduced risk of IHD mortality, but not cerebrovascular or all-cause mortality, although the evidence remains low, certainty for all CVD outcomes. The protective effect of vegetarian diets on CHD risk and mortality seems to be mediated by the reduced meat consumption and the increased consumption of fruits and vegetables. The findings from systematic reviews and meta-analyses of prospective cohort studies suggesting lowering meat consumption provide further evidence that vegetarian dietary patterns may be beneficial for CVD risk reduction (Glenn et al., 2019). Indeed, according to American Heart Association/American College of Cardiology (AHA/ACC) recommendations, vegetarian diets are dietary patterns that could help meet the AHA/ACC guidelines along with DASH and the MD (Van Horn et al., 2016).

BLOOD PRESSURE/HYPERTENSION

Consistent, robust data from both epidemiological and clinical trial studies show clear benefits of plant-based diets, including vegetarian diets, for BP, suggesting that they may play a fundamental role in the primary prevention and management of hypertension.

In a 2014 meta-analysis (Yokoyama et al., 2014), comparing vegetarian and omnivorous diets, both RCTs and observational studies were found to improve BP levels. The RCTs revealed a reduction in both systolic and diastolic BP by 4.8 mmHg and 2.2 mmHg, respectively. In observational studies, vegetarian diets were associated with a reduction in BP of 6.9 mmHg and 4.7 mmHg for systolic and diastolic BP, respectively.

In a meta-analysis of 15 RCTs with 856 subjects (Lee, Loh, Ching, Devaraj, & Hoo, 2020), the vegan diet reduced systolic and diastolic BP by 3.12 mmHg and 1.92 mmHg, respectively, compared to a lacto-ovo-vegetarian diet, in which the BP reductions were lower (1.75 mmHg for systolic but none for diastolic). Notably, vegan diets seem to provide a greater reduction in BP in patients with a systolic BP above 130 mm Hg. Furthermore, its effects do not seem to be affected by patient medical status, particularly obesity or T2D. Therefore, vegan diets without calorie restriction are suggested to be comparable with diets recommended by medical societies [e.g., AHA-, American Dietetic Association (ADA) -, or DASH-type diets] and portion-controlled diets (Lopez, Cativo, Atlas, & Rosendorff, 2019).

TYPE 2 DIABETES

Research to date has looked at the role of a vegetarian diet at both the prevention and treatment of diabetes.

Previous results from a cohort study (Vang, Singh, Lee, Haddad, & Brinegar, 2008) that examined and followed 8401 SDA adults without diabetes for 17 years, showed that a lifelong adherence to a vegetarian diet was associated with a 74% reduction of the risk to develop diabetes compared to a diet that included weekly meat consumption. Another cohort study (T. H. Chiu, Pan, Lin, & Lin, 2018) including 2918 non-smoking, non-alcohol drinking Buddhists with a mean follow-up of 5 years showed a 35% lower risk of developing diabetes in those adhering to a vegetarian diet compared to non-vegetarian. Most importantly, non-vegetarians that altered their diet to a vegetarian one had a 53% lower risk for developing diabetes than non-vegetarians who kept the same diet.

With regard to diabetes management, results from large clinical trials suggest that vegetarian diets, compared to conventional diets, can improve insulin dosage, HbA1c, insulin and fasting glucose levels, and insulin sensitivity in T2D patients as well as their quality of life (Olfert & Wattick, 2018).

METABOLIC SYNDROME

Pooled data from epidemiological studies, namely cohort, cross-sectional, and case–control studies as well as RCTs show mixed results about the associations of vegetarian diets with the likelihood of developing MetS.

Several, individual studies have shown an inverse association between the consumption of a vegetarian dietary pattern and the prevalence or risk of developing MetS (Sabaté & Wien, 2015). Regarding the MetS criteria, pooled data of cross-sectional studies (Dinu et al., 2017) with more than 56 000 subjects following a plant-based dietary pattern, showed lower BMI, TC, LDL-cholesterol, triglycerides, and blood glucose when vegetarians were compared with non-vegetarians, and lower BMI, TC, and LDL-cholesterol in vegans were compared to non-vegans. The studies that support this notion rely on the beneficial synergistic combination of antioxidants, fiber, K, Mg, and phytochemicals, which may result in decreased

BMI, BP, TAG, oxidative stress, insulin resistance (IR), and systemic inflammation that result in improved MetS risk (Sabaté & Wien, 2015).

Conversely, a meta-analysis of 71 studies (six RCTs, two cohorts, and 63 cross-sectional) (Picasso, Lo-Tayraco, Ramos-Villanueva, Pasupuleti, & Hernandez, 2019), including 103 008 individuals aimed to reveal associations between vegetarian diets and MetS compared to omnivorous diets. The data from cross-sectional studies on vegetarian diets were not associated with a lower risk of MetS, although they were associated with significant lower levels of systolic and diastolic BP, fasting glucose, WC, and HDL-cholesterol. This association did not hold in the meta-analysis of RCTs and cohort studies (Picasso et al., 2019).

Overall, there are studies that favor an improvement in MetS components independently, but not all MetS components together when comparing vegetarian and omnivorous diets. This might be explained by the differing definitions of MetS data and biomarkers used for the MetS diagnosis (Picasso et al., 2019).

CANCER

Previous studies on the association of vegetarian diets and specific cancer-type mortality have partially conflicting results, although vegetarian diets seem to be associated with a lower cancer incidence. Data come mainly from epidemilogical studies.

Pooled data of seven prospective studies (Huang et al., 2012) with a total of 124 706 participants showed that vegetarians had a significantly lower overall cancer incidence by 18% compared to non-vegetarians. The mechanism mediating the effect of vegetarian diets on cancer incidence is not known. Vegetarians may have lower levels of hs-CRP compared to non-vegetarians. Moreover, the antioxidant and anti-inflammatory effects of the food groups, e.g., fruits and vegetables, that constitute this pattern may also result in lower inflammation in the long term. Indeed, a variety of phytochemicals, such as sulforaphane, ferulic acid, genistein, indole-3-carbinol, curcumin, epigallocatechin-3-gallate, diallyl disulfide, resveratrol, lycopene, and quercetin appear in vegetables, legumes, fruits, spices, and whole grains may provide protection against cancer (Melina, Craig, & Levin, 2016).

Another meta-analysis among prospective cohort studies (Dinu et al., 2017) revealed an 8% reduction of total cancer incidence, but not cancer mortality when vegetarians were compared to non-vegetarians. The overall analysis in the cohort studies reported no significant associations with specific cancer types, such as incidence and mortality from breast, lung, colon-rectum, and stomach cancer (Dinu et al., 2017). Moreover, a 2017 meta-analysis of six cohorts studies (Godos, Bella, Sciacca, Galvano, & Grosso, 2017) including 686 629 individuals and 3441, 4062, and 1935 cases of breast, colorectal, and prostate cancer, respectively, found no associations. In particular, there were no associations between the vegetarian diet and the risk of either breast, colorectal, and prostate cancer compared to a non–vegetarian diet.

The aforementioned results, although partly surprising, may be explained by the fact that incidence and mortality are two very different outcomes, as they are greatly influenced by the treatment approaches, while a low number of studies exist that evaluate specific cancer types (Dinu et al., 2017).

CONSIDERATIONS IN IMPLEMENTING A HEALTHY VEGETARIAN-TYPE DIETARY PATTERN

In 2009, the American Dietetic Association (ADA) published a position statement regarding the nutrient adequacy and safety of a vegetarian diet (Craig & Mangels, 2009): "*It is the position of the American Dietetic Association that appropriately planned vegetarian diets, including total vegetarian or vegan diets, are healthful, nutritionally adequate, and may provide health benefits in the prevention and treatment of certain diseases. Well-planned vegetarian diets are appropriate for individuals during all stages of the lifecycle, including pregnancy, lactation, infancy, childhood, and adolescence, and for athletes*".

Years later, in 2016, the Academy of Nutrition and Dietetics also published a position statement about vegetarian diets that was more or less in accordance with the ADA's statement (Melina et al., 2016). It supported that a well-structured vegetarian diet can provide adequate nutrient intake throughout the lifecycle and be helpful as a therapeutic approach to some chronic diseases, e.g., hypertension, T2D, etc. However, it also stated that some vegetarian diets, e.g., vegan diets, may be low in certain nutrients, such as calcium and vitamin B-12 and D, omega-3 fatty acids, iodine, iron, and zinc. Therefore, individuals following such a dietary pattern may need appropriate planning and encouraged them to habitually consume good sources of those micronutrients to avoid becoming deficient. This notion was also supported by the position statement of the working group of the Italian Society of Human Nutrition published in 2017 (Agnoli et al., 2017).

Of all nutrients, vitamin B12 may be the most difficult to get in a vegetarian diet as it is not available from plant foods. Although it is in some fermented foods like nori as well as spirulina, chlorella algae, and unfortified nutritional yeast, this may not be adequate. Therefore, some fortified foods or supplements may be recommended for people adhering to vegetarian diets while showing specific micronutrient depletions or deficiencies (Melina et al., 2016).

THE HEALTHY US-STYLE DIETARY PATTERN

As mentioned earlier in this chapter, the US-style (USDA) dietary patterns (US Department of Agriculture and US Department of Health and Human Services. Dietary Guidelines for Americans, 2020–2025) were highlighted by the 2020–2025 Dietary Guidelines for Americans (DGA) as healthy along with other dietary patterns such as the healthy MD, DASH diet and vegetarian eating patterns.

The USDA dietary patterns were created to help Americans meet their nutrient needs within energy requirements based on the Dietary Reference Intakes (DRIs). These patterns recommend that the included foods and food groups be eaten in nutrient-dense forms, prepared with minimal added sugars, refined starches, and sodium, and consumed in appropriate amounts (US Department of Agriculture and US Department of Health and Human Services. Dietary Guidelines for Americans, 2020–2025). They emphasize fruits, vegetables, whole grains, low- and fat-free dairy, healthy fats (20–25% of total calories), while calories from saturated fats (<10% of calories), added sugars and refined starches are limited. Several plant and animal-based foods, including lean meats, poultry, eggs, seafood, nuts, seeds, and soy products constitute the dietary sources of protein in these patterns that account for nearly 40% of total dietary protein. Dairy foods contribute nearly 30% of total dietary protein (**Table 3.4**).

EFFECTIVENESS OF HEALTHY/PRUDENT DIETARY PATTERNS

The 2021 AHA guidance to improve cardiovascular health (Lichtenstein et al., 2021) emphasizes the important role of the USDA dietary patterns (US Department of Agriculture and US Department of Health and Human Services. Dietary Guidelines for Americans, 2020-2025), the healthy MD, DASH, and vegetarian eating patterns as heart healthy.

According to the Dietary Patterns Methods Project study (Liese et al., 2015), which used data from three large cohorts of US adults, those with high adherence to high-quality dietary patterns were found to have 14% to 28% lower CVD mortality than those with a low adherence. Another study (Cifelli, Fulgoni, Stylianou, & Jolliet, 2022) using a representative sample of 13 331 Americans aged at least 25 years old from the National Health and Nutrition Examination Survey (NHANES) 2011–2016 database aimed to estimate the health burden (DALY) and benefit (in minutes of healthy life) of three DGA-recommended dietary patterns the: USDA, vegetarian, and MD. The USDA diets were correlated with a gain of 32 minutes of healthy life/day, while the vegetarian and MD dietary patterns were associated with gains of 56 and 38 minutes of healthy life/day, respectively. The largest contributors to gaining minutes of healthy life were increases in fruit (15–19 min/day), whole grains (11 min/day), vegetables (6 min/day) and milk (4–6 min/day); the increased fish consumption of the MD provided additional benefits of 10 min/day (Cifelli et al., 2022).

Similar to AHA recommendations, several of the aforementioned eating patterns have been acknowledged and accepted for diabetes management based on ADA guidelines (American Diabetes Association, 2018). With regard to their positive effects on glycemia, evidence is more clear to support the MD and vegetarian eating patterns, although all eating patterns may help T2D patients improve their health, especially when individualized (Benson & Hayes, 2020).

Moreover, overall, both observational and intervention studies show an inverse association between plant-based diets, namely the Mediterranean and DASH diets, and oxidative stress as well as proinflammatory biomarkers; the vegetarian and USDA diets have an inverse association with oxidative stress and inflammation (Aleksandrova, Koelman, & Rodrigues, 2021).

KEY POINTS

- According to the 2020 WHO update, a healthy diet should protect against all types of malnutrition (e.g., undernutrition, overnutrition, micronutrient abnormalities, sarcopenia, frailty, and re-feeding syndrome) and NCDs development.

- A large body of evidence supports the recognition of the MD as the gold standard dietary pattern for healthy nutrition; it is one of the best studied dietary patterns.

- The MD has evolved over the centuries. Despite its different versions and depending on local conditions, the essentials of the diet have remained the same. It is a diet with a semi-vegetarian character, high in olive oil (particularly cold-pressed extra-virgin olive oil) and based in the daily consumption of seasonal fruit and vegetables (including leafy green vegetables), whole-grain cereals, nuts, and pulses/legumes as well as a moderate intake of fish and other meat, dairy products, and red wine with a low intake of eggs and sweets.

- Several epidemiological studies have been published linking the MD to better survival and a protective association against all-cause and disease-specific mortality and the risk for several chronic diseases namely CVD, hypertension, T2D, dyslipidemia, obesity, MetS, and cancer.

- Of all the dietary patterns linked to healthy aging, the MD is most predominantly associated with numerous health benefits and the prevention of a variety of age-related disorders.

- The DASH diet is a plant-based dietary pattern characterized by a high intake of vegetables, fruits, whole grains, nuts, the addition of some fish, poultry, and low-fat dairy products as well as the minimization of processed/red meat, sugar, and processed foods.

- Except for its positive effects on hypertension, the DASH dietary pattern seems to be effective in reducing the risk of all-cause and specific-cause mortality, the incidence of CVDs, stroke, CHD, and heart failure as well as the risk of cancer and CKD.

- Individuals on DASH are less prone to present overweight and obesity or develop MetS. The DASH diet is also effective at maintaining glucose and insulin levels.

- The core statements upon which the Nordic diet (ND) was developed are: (1) more calories from plant-based foods and less from meat; (2) more lake- and sea-sourced foods (e.g., sea weeds and shellfish); and (3) more wild local foods (plants, berries, mushrooms, and aromatic herbs).

Table 3.4 Healthy US-style dietary pattern for ages 2 and older, with daily or weekly amounts from food groups, subgroups, and components.

Calorie level of pattern	1,000	1,200	1,400	1,600	1,800	2,000	2,200	2,400	2,600	2,800	3,000	3,200
Food group or subgroup												
	\multicolumn{12}{c}{Daily amount of food from each group}											
	\multicolumn{12}{c}{(Vegetable and protein foods subgroup amounts are per week.)}											
Vegetables (cup eq/day)	1	1½	1½	2	2½	2½	3	3	3½	3½	4	4
	\multicolumn{12}{c}{Vegetable subgroups in weekly amounts}											
Dark-green vegetables (cup eq/wk)	½	1	1	1½	1½	1½	2	2	2½	2½	2½	2½
Red and orange vegetables (cup eq/wk)	2½	3	3	4	5½	5½	6	6	7	7	7½	7½
Beans, peas, lentils (cup eq/wk)	½	½	½	1	1½	1½	2	2	2½	2½	3	3
Starchy vegetables (cup eq/wk)	2	3½	3½	4	5	5	6	6	7	7	8	8
Other vegetables (cup eq/wk)	1½	2½	2½	3½	4	4	5	5	5½	5½	7	7
Fruits (cup eq/day)	1	1	1½	1½	1½	2	2	2	2	2½	2½	2½
Grains (ounce eq/day)	3	4	5	5	6	6	7	8	9	10	10	10
Whole grains (ounce eq/day)	1½	2	2½	3	3	3	3½	4	4½	5	5	5
Refined grains (ounce eq/day)	1½	2	2½	2	3	3	3½	4	4½	5	5	5
Dairy (cup eq/day)	2	2½	2½	3	3	3	3	3	3	3	3	3
Protein foods (ounce eq/day)	2	3	4	5	5	5½	6	6½	6½	7	7	7
	\multicolumn{12}{c}{Protein food subgroups in weekly amounts}											
Meats, poultry, eggs (ounce eq/wk)	10	14	19	23	23	26	28	31	31	33	33	33
Seafood (ounce eq/wk)	2-3	4	6	8	8	8	9	10	10	10	10	10
Nuts, seeds, soy products (ounce eq/wk)	2	2	3	4	4	5	5	5	5	6	6	6
Oils (grams/day)	15	17	17	22	24	27	29	31	34	36	44	51
Limit on calories for other uses (kcal/day)	130	80	90	100	140	240	250	320	350	370	440	580
Limit on calories for other uses (%/day)	13%	7%	6%	6%	8%	12%	11%	13%	13%	13%	15%	18%

[1] Patterns at 1000, 1200, and 1400 kcal levels are designed to meet the nutritional needs of children ages 2 to 8 years. Patterns from 1600 to 3200 kcal are designed to meet the nutritional needs of children 9 years and older as well as adults. If a child 4 to 8 years of age needs more energy and, therefore, is following a pattern at 1600 calories or more, his/her recommended amount from the dairy group should be 2½ cup eq/day. Dairy for children ages 9 to 18 is 3 cup eq/day regardless of calorie level. The 1000 and 1200 kcal level patterns are not intended for children 9 and older or adults. The 1400 kcal level is not intended for children ages 10 and older or adults.

Source: (US Department of Agriculture and US Department of Health and Human Services. Dietary Guidelines for Americans, 2020–2025).

- Although the ND was recently developed, it is associated with improvements in several CVD parameters, namely blood-lipid levels, systolic and diastolic BP, glucose metabolism, insulin sensitivity, and inflammation; the risk of all-cause mortality and death due to cancer and CVD; and physical performance and cognitive health in older adults.
- The vegetarian diet patterns are an alternative to the USDA dietary pattern. They are primarily considered plant-based diets that exclude all kinds of meats including fowl, poultry, fish, or seafood.
- Vegetarian dietary patterns may reduce CVD mortality and the risk of CHD while they play a fundamental role in the primary prevention and management of hypertension and diabetes; They are linked with mixed results regarding MetS and cancer risk.
- Vitamin B12 may be the most difficult nutrient to get in a vegetarian diet as it is not found in any plant foods.
- The USDA dietary patterns were highlighted by the 2020–2025 DGA as healthy along with other dietary patterns including the MD, DASH diet, and vegetarian eating patterns.
- The USDA dietary patterns were created to help Americans meet their nutrient needs within energy requirements based on the DRIs.

SELF-ASSESSMENT QUESTIONS

1. According to the 2020–2025 Dietary Guidelines for Americans, what should a healthy dietary pattern include?

2. Based on the latest MD pyramid published in 2011 by the Mediterranean Diet Foundation, which food group is at the vertex of the pyramid?
   (a) Red meat
   (b) Sweets
   (c) Eggs
   (d) Full-fat dairies
   (e) None of the above.

3. Which food components of the MD have cardio-protective effects and why?

4. Please complete the phrase:
   (a) The DASH diet provides low amounts of saturated fat (_____), total fat (_____) and dietary cholesterol (_____).
   (b) The sodium content of the DASH diet varies_____.
   (c) The dietary fiber intake of the DASH diet is_____.
   (d) The Dietary Approaches to Stop Hypertension (DASH) was first designed to _____.

5. The ND shares many similarities with MD. However, they have a notable difference. What is this difference?

6. What are the two most common types of healthy vegetarian dietary patterns?

7. The flexitarian or semi-vegetarian diet is considered _____.

8. Are there any considerations when implementing a vegetarian-type dietary pattern?

9. According to 2021 AHA guidance to improve cardiovascular health, which dietary patterns are considered heart healthy?

10. Indicate whether each statement is true or false:
    (a) Vegetarian dietary patterns may reduce CVD mortality and the risk of CHD.
    (b) The staple components of the ND fruit category are watermelon, strawberries, banana, and pineapple.
    (c) The DASH diet is ineffective at managing glucose and insulin levels.
    (d) Alcohol, and especially red wine, a typical component of the MD, is thought to play a significant role in CVD prevention.

REFERENCES

Agnoli, C., Baroni, L., Bertini, I., Ciappellano, S., Fabbri, A., Papa, M., . . . Sieri, S. (2017). Position paper on vegetarian diets from the working group of the Italian Society of Human Nutrition. *Nutr Metab Cardiovasc Dis*, *27*(12), 1037–1052. doi:10.1016/j.numecd.2017.10.020

Akhlaghi, M. (2020). Dietary Approaches to Stop Hypertension (DASH): potential mechanisms of action against risk factors of the metabolic syndrome. *Nutr Res Rev*, *33*(1), 1–18. doi:10.1017/s0954422419000155

Aleksandrova, K., Koelman, L., & Rodrigues, C. E. (2021). Dietary patterns and biomarkers of oxidative stress and inflammation: A systematic review of observational and intervention studies. *Redox Biology*, *42*, 101869. doi:https://doi.org/10.1016/j.redox.2021.101869

Appel, L. J., Moore, T. J., Obarzanek, E., Vollmer, W. M., Svetkey, L. P., Sacks, F. M.,. . . Harsha, D. W. (1997). A Clinical Trial of the Effects of Dietary Patterns on Blood Pressure. *New England Journal of Medicine*, *336*(16), 1117–1124. doi:10.1056/nejm199704173361601

American Diabetes Association, (2018). 5. Lifestyle Management: Standards of Medical Care in Diabetes—2019. *Diabetes Care*, *42*(Supplement_1), S46–S60. doi:10.2337/dc19-S005

Azadbakht, L., Fard, N. R. P., Karimi, M., Baghaei, M. H., Surkan, P. J., Rahimi, M., . . . Willett, W. C. (2010). Effects of the Dietary Approaches to Stop Hypertension (DASH) Eating Plan on Cardiovascular Risks Among Type 2 Diabetic Patients: A randomized crossover clinical trial. *Diabetes Care*, *34*(1), 55–57. doi:10.2337/dc10-0676

Bach-Faig, A., Berry, E. M., Lairon, D., Reguant, J., Trichopoulou, A., Dernini, S., . . . Mediterranean Diet Foundation Expert, G. (2011). Mediterranean diet pyramid today. Science and cultural updates. *Public Health Nutr*, *14*(12A), 2274–2284. doi:10.1017/S1368980011002515

Bakaloudi, D. R., Chrysoula, L., Kotzakioulafi, E., Theodoridis, X., & Chourdakis, M. (2021). Impact of the Level of Adherence to Mediterranean Diet on the Parameters of Metabolic Syndrome: A Systematic Review and Meta-Analysis of Observational Studies. *Nutrients*, *13*(5), 1514. Retrieved from https://www.mdpi.com/2072-6643/13/5/1514

Bakaloudi, D. R., Chrysoula, L., Leonida, I., Kotzakioulafi, E., Theodoridis, X., & Chourdakis, M. (2021). Impact of the level of adherence to the Mediterranean Diet on blood pressure: A systematic review and meta-analysis of observational studies. *Clinical nutrition*, *40*(12), 5771–5780. doi:10.1016/j.clnu.2021.10.002

Benson, G., & Hayes, J. (2020). An Update on the Mediterranean, Vegetarian, and DASH Eating Patterns in People With Type 2 Diabetes. *Diabetes spectrum: a publication of the American Diabetes Association*, *33*(2), 125–132. doi:10.2337/ds19-0073

Berild, A., Holven, K. B., & Ulven, S. M. (2017). Recommended Nordic diet and risk markers for cardiovascular disease. *Tidsskr Nor Laegeforen*, *137*(10), 721–726. doi:10.4045/tidsskr.16.0243

Bonaccio, M., Iacoviello, L., Donati, M. B., & de Gaetano, G. (2022). The tenth anniversary as a UNESCO world cultural heritage: an unmissable opportunity to get back to the cultural roots of the Mediterranean diet. *European journal of clinical nutrition*, *76*(2), 179–183.

Campbell, A. P. (2017). DASH Eating Plan: An Eating Pattern for Diabetes Management. *Diabetes Spectrum*, *30*(2), 76–81. doi:10.2337/ds16-0084

Castro-Barquero, S., Ruiz-León, A. M., Sierra-Pérez, M., Estruch, R., & Casas, R. (2020). Dietary Strategies for Metabolic Syndrome: A Comprehensive Review. *Nutrients*, *12*(10), 2983. Retrieved from https://www.mdpi.com/2072-6643/12/10/2983

Castro-Espin, C., & Agudo, A. (2022). The role of diet in prognosis among cancer survivors: A systematic review and meta-analysis of dietary patterns and diet interventions. *Nutrients*, *14*(2), 348.

Cederholm, T., Barazzoni, R., Austin, P., Ballmer, P., Biolo, G., Bischoff, S. C., . . . Holst, M. (2017). ESPEN guidelines on definitions and terminology of clinical nutrition. *Clinical nutrition*, *36*(1), 49–64.

Challa, H. J., Ameer, M. A., & Uppaluri, K. R. (2021). DASH diet to stop hypertension. In *StatPearls [Internet]*: StatPearls Publishing.

Chiavaroli, L., Viguiliouk, E., Nishi, S. K., Blanco Mejia, S., Rahelić, D., Kahleová, H., . . . Sievenpiper, J. L. (2019). DASH Dietary Pattern and Cardiometabolic Outcomes: An Umbrella Review of Systematic Reviews and Meta-Analyses. *Nutrients*, *11*(2), 338. doi:10.3390/nu11020338

Chiu, S., Bergeron, N., Williams, P. T., Bray, G. A., Sutherland, B., & Krauss, R. M. (2016). Comparison of the DASH (Dietary Approaches to Stop Hypertension) diet and a higher-fat DASH diet on blood pressure and lipids and lipoproteins: a randomized controlled trial. *Am J Clin Nutr*, *103*(2), 341–347. doi:10.3945/ajcn.115.123281

Chiu, T. H., Pan, W.-H., Lin, M.-N., & Lin, C.-L. (2018). Vegetarian diet, change in dietary patterns, and diabetes risk: a prospective study. *Nutrition & diabetes*, *8*(1), 1–9.

Cifelli, C., Fulgoni, V., Stylianou, K., & Jolliet, O. (2022). Dietary Guidelines for Americans Dietary Patterns Are Associated with Significant Improvements in Healthy Life As Assessed by the Health Nutritional Index (HENI). *Current developments in nutrition*, *6*(Suppl 1), 894–894. Retrieved from http://europepmc.org/abstract/PMC/PMC9193600 https://www.ncbi.nlm.nih.gov/pmc/articles/PMC9193600/?tool=EBI https://www.ncbi.nlm.nih.gov/pmc/articles/PMC9193600/pdf/?tool=EBI https://europepmc.org/articles/PMC9193600 https://europepmc.org/articles/PMC9193600?pdf=render

Cowell, O. R., Mistry, N., Deighton, K., Matu, J., Griffiths, A., Minihane, A. M., . . . Siervo, M. (2021). Effects of a Mediterranean diet on blood pressure: a systematic review and meta-analysis of randomized controlled trials and observational studies. *J Hypertens*, *39*(4), 729–739. doi:10.1097/hjh.0000000000002667

Craddick, S. R., Elmer, P. J., Obarzanek, E., Vollmer, W. M., Svetkey, L. P., & Swain, M. C. (2003). The DASH diet and blood pressure. *Current atherosclerosis reports*, *5*(6), 484–491.

Craig, W. J., & Mangels, A. R. (2009). Position of the American Dietetic Association: vegetarian diets. *Journal of the American dietetic association*, *109*(7), 1266.

Critselis, E., & Panagiotakos, D. (2020). Adherence to the Mediterranean diet and healthy ageing: Current evidence, biological pathways, and future directions. *Crit Rev Food Sci Nutr*, *60*(13), 2148–2157. doi:10.1080/10408398.2019.1631752

Damasceno, N. R., Sala-Vila, A., Cofán, M., Pérez-Heras, A. M., Fitó, M., Ruiz-Gutiérrez, V., . . . Ros, E. (2013). Mediterranean diet supplemented with nuts reduces waist circumference and shifts lipoprotein subfractions to a less atherogenic pattern in subjects at high cardiovascular risk. *Atherosclerosis*, *230*(2), 347–353. doi:10.1016/j.atherosclerosis.2013.08.014

Davis, C., Bryan, J., Hodgson, J., & Murphy, K. (2015). Definition of the Mediterranean diet; a literature review. *Nutrients*, *7*(11), 9139–9153.

de Paula, T. P., Steemburgo, T., de Almeida, J. C., Dall'Alba, V., Gross, J. L., & de Azevedo, M. J. (2012). The role of Dietary Approaches to Stop Hypertension (DASH) diet food groups in blood pressure in type 2 diabetes. *British Journal of Nutrition*, *108*(1), 155–162. doi:10.1017/S0007114511005381

De Pergola, G., & D'Alessandro, A. (2018). Influence of Mediterranean Diet on Blood Pressure. *Nutrients*, *10*(11), 1700. doi:10.3390/nu10111700

Dinu, M., Abbate, R., Gensini, G. F., Casini, A., & Sofi, F. (2017). Vegetarian, vegan diets and multiple health outcomes: A systematic review with meta-analysis of observational studies. *Critical Reviews in Food Science and Nutrition*, *57*(17), 3640–3649. doi:10.1080/10408398.2016.1138447

Dominguez, L. J., Di Bella, G., Veronese, N., & Barbagallo, M. (2021). Impact of Mediterranean Diet on Chronic Non-Communicable Diseases and Longevity. *Nutrients*, *13*(6). doi:10.3390/nu13062028

Dominguez, L. J., Veronese, N., Baiamonte, E., Guarrera, M., Parisi, A., Ruffolo, C., . . . Barbagallo, M. (2022). Healthy Aging and Dietary Patterns. *Nutrients*, *14*(4), 889. Retrieved from https://www.mdpi.com/2072-6643/14/4/889

Donat-Vargas, C., Sandoval-Insausti, H., Peñalvo, J. L., Moreno Iribas, M. C., Amiano, P., Bes-Rastrollo, M., . . . Guallar-Castillón, P. (2022). Olive oil consumption is associated with a lower risk of cardiovascular disease and stroke. *Clinical nutrition*, *41*(1), 122–130. doi:10.1016/j.clnu.2021.11.002

Fernandez del Rio, L., Gutierrez-Casado, E., Varela-Lopez, A., & Villalba, J. M. (2016). Olive Oil and the Hallmarks of Aging. *Molecules*, *21*(2), 163. doi:10.3390/molecules21020163

Fernandez, M. L., & Murillo, A. G. (2022). Dietary Treatments to Reduce Insulin Resistance and Inflammation in Type-2 Diabetic Patients. *Medical Research Archives*, *10*(4). doi:10.18103/mra.v10i4.2768

Filippou, C. D., Thomopoulos, C. G., Kouremeti, M. M., Sotiropoulou, L. I., Nihoyannopoulos, P. I., Tousoulis, D. M., & Tsioufis, C. P. (2021). Mediterranean diet and blood pressure reduction in adults with and without hypertension: A systematic review and meta-analysis of randomized controlled trials. *Clinical nutrition*, *40*(5), 3191–3200. doi:10.1016/j.clnu.2021.01.030

Foscolou, A., Critselis, E., & Panagiotakos, D. (2018). Olive oil consumption and human health: A narrative review. *Maturitas*, *118*, 60–66.

Funk, K. L., Elmer, P. J., Stevens, V. J., Harsha, D. W., Craddick, S. R., Lin, P. H.,... Appel, L. J. (2008). PREMIER--a trial of lifestyle interventions for blood pressure control: intervention design and rationale. *Health Promot Pract*, 9(3), 271–280. doi:10.1177/1524839906289035

Galbete, C., Kröger, J., Jannasch, F., Iqbal, K., Schwingshackl, L., Schwedhelm, C., ... Schulze, M. B. (2018). Nordic diet, Mediterranean diet, and the risk of chronic diseases: the EPIC-Potsdam study. *BMC Medicine*, 16(1), 99. doi:10.1186/s12916-018-1082-y

Gepner, Y., Shelef, I., Komy, O., Cohen, N., Schwarzfuchs, D., Bril, N., ... Shai, I. (2019). The beneficial effects of Mediterranean diet over low-fat diet may be mediated by decreasing hepatic fat content. *Journal of Hepatology*, 71(2), 379–388. doi:https://doi.org/10.1016/j.jhep.2019.04.013

Glenn, A. J., Viguiliouk, E., Seider, M., Boucher, B. A., Khan, T. A., Blanco Mejia, S., ... Sievenpiper, J. L. (2019). Relation of Vegetarian Dietary Patterns With Major Cardiovascular Outcomes: A Systematic Review and Meta-Analysis of Prospective Cohort Studies. *Frontiers in Nutrition*, 6. doi:10.3389/fnut.2019.00080

Godos, J., Bella, F., Sciacca, S., Galvano, F., & Grosso, G. (2017). Vegetarianism and breast, colorectal and prostate cancer risk: an overview and meta-analysis of cohort studies. *Journal of Human Nutrition and Dietetics*, 30(3), 349–359.

Godos, J., Zappalà, G., Bernardini, S., Giambini, I., Bes-Rastrollo, M., & Martinez-Gonzalez, M. (2017). Adherence to the Mediterranean diet is inversely associated with metabolic syndrome occurrence: a meta-analysis of observational studies. *International Journal of Food Sciences and Nutrition*, 68(2), 138–148.

Grosso, G., Marventano, S., Yang, J., Micek, A., Pajak, A., Scalfi, L., ... Kales, S. N. (2017). A comprehensive meta-analysis on evidence of Mediterranean diet and cardiovascular disease: Are individual components equal? *Critical Reviews in Food Science and Nutrition*, 57(15), 3218–3232. doi:10.1080/10408398.2015.1107021

Guasch-Ferré, M., Hu, F. B., Martínez-González, M. A., Fitó, M., Bulló, M., Estruch, R., ... Salas-Salvadó, J. (2014). Olive oil intake and risk of cardiovascular disease and mortality in the PREDIMED Study. *BMC Medicine*, 12(1), 78. doi:10.1186/1741-7015-12-78

Gunge, V. B., Andersen, I., Kyrø, C., Hansen, C. P., Dahm, C. C., Christensen, J., ... Olsen, A. (2017). Adherence to a healthy Nordic food index and risk of myocardial infarction in middle-aged Danes: the diet, cancer and health cohort study. *European journal of clinical nutrition*, 71(5), 652–658. doi:10.1038/ejcn.2017.1

Hidalgo-Mora, J. J., García-Vigara, A., Sánchez-Sánchez, M. L., García-Pérez, M.-Á., Tarín, J., & Cano, A. (2020). The Mediterranean diet: A historical perspective on food for health. *Maturitas*, 132, 65–69.

Hu, F. B. (2002). Dietary pattern analysis: a new direction in nutritional epidemiology. *Current opinion in lipidology*, 13(1), 3–9.

Huang, T., Yang, B., Zheng, J., Li, G., Wahlqvist, M. L., & Li, D. (2012). Cardiovascular Disease Mortality and Cancer Incidence in Vegetarians: A Meta-Analysis and Systematic Review. *Annals of Nutrition and Metabolism*, 60(4), 233–240. doi:10.1159/000337301

Hummel, S. L., Seymour, E. M., Brook, R. D., Kolias, T. J., Sheth, S. S., Rosenblum, H. R., ... Weder, A. B. (2012). Low-sodium dietary approaches to stop hypertension diet reduces blood pressure, arterial stiffness, and oxidative stress in hypertensive heart failure with preserved ejection fraction. *Hypertension*, 60(5), 1200–1206.

Hummel, S. L., Seymour, E. M., Brook, R. D., Sheth, S. S., Ghosh, E., Zhu, S., ... Kolias, T. J. (2013). Low-sodium DASH diet improves diastolic function and ventricular–arterial coupling in hypertensive heart failure with preserved ejection fraction. *Circulation: Heart Failure*, 6(6), 1165–1171.

Islami, F., Goding Sauer, A., Miller, K. D., Siegel, R. L., Fedewa, S. A., Jacobs, E. J., ... Jemal, A. (2018). Proportion and number of cancer cases and deaths attributable to potentially modifiable risk factors in the United States. *CA Cancer J Clin*, 68(1), 31–54. doi:10.3322/caac.21440

Jabri, A., Kumar, A., Verghese, E., Alameh, A., Kumar, A., Khan, M. S., ... Kalra, A. (2021). Meta-analysis of effect of vegetarian diet on ischemic heart disease and all-cause mortality. *American Journal of Preventive Cardiology*, 7, 100182. doi:https://doi.org/10.1016/j.ajpc.2021.100182

Jacobs, D. R., & Tapsell, L. C. (2013). Food synergy: the key to a healthy diet. *Proceedings of the Nutrition Society*, 72(2), 200–206. doi:10.1017/S0029665112003011

Jacobs, D. R., Tapsell, L. C., & Temple, N. J. (2011). Food Synergy: The Key to Balancing the Nutrition Research Effort. *Public Health Reviews*, 33(2), 507–529. doi:10.1007/BF03391648

Jalilpiran, Y., Jayedi, A., Djafarian, K., & Shab-Bidar, S. (2022). The Nordic diet and the risk of non-communicable chronic disease and mortality: a systematic review and dose-response meta-analysis of prospective cohort studies. *Critical Reviews in Food Science and Nutrition*, 62(11), 3124–3136. doi:10.1080/10408398.2020.1863906

Kahleova H, B.-T. N., Blanco Mejia S, et al. (2020). Plant-based eating and cardiometabolic health. *Alpro Foundation*.

Kahleova, H., Levin, S., & Barnard, N. D. (2018). Vegetarian Dietary Patterns and Cardiovascular Disease. *Prog Cardiovasc Dis*, 61(1), 54–61. doi:10.1016/j.pcad.2018.05.002

Kahn, H. A., Phillips, R. L., Snowdon, D. A., & CHOI, W. (1984). Association between reported diet and all-cause mortality: twenty-one-year follow-up on 27, 530 adult Seventh-Day Adventists. *American Journal of Epidemiology*, 119(5), 775–787.

Kanerva, N., Kaartinen, N. E., Rissanen, H., Knekt, P., Eriksson, J. G., Sääksjärvi, K., ... Männistö, S. (2014). Associations of the Baltic Sea diet with cardiometabolic risk factors--a meta-analysis of three Finnish studies. *Br J Nutr*, 112(4), 616–626. doi:10.1017/s0007114514001159

Kanerva, N., Kaartinen, N. E., Schwab, U., Lahti-Koski, M., & Männistö, S. (2014). The Baltic Sea Diet Score: a tool for assessing healthy eating in Nordic countries. *Public Health Nutrition*, 17(8), 1697–1705.

Kastorini, C.-M., Milionis, H. J., Esposito, K., Giugliano, D., Goudevenos, J. A., & Panagiotakos, D. B. (2011). The effect of Mediterranean diet on metabolic syndrome and its components: a meta-analysis of 50 studies and 534,906 individuals. *Journal of the American College of Cardiology*, 57(11), 1299–1313.

Kerley, C. P. (2018). Nutritional Interventions in Heart Failure: Challenges and Opportunities. *Curr Heart Fail Rep*, 15(3), 131–140. doi:10.1007/s11897-018-0388-6

Koloverou, E., Esposito, K., Giugliano, D., & Panagiotakos, D. (2014). The effect of Mediterranean diet on the development of type 2 diabetes mellitus: a meta-analysis of 10 prospective studies and 136,846 participants. *Metabolism*, 63(7), 903–911.

Krznarić, Ž., Karas, I., Ljubas Kelečić, D., & Vranešić Bender, D. (2021). The Mediterranean and Nordic Diet: A Review of Differences and Similarities of Two Sustainable, Health-Promoting Dietary Patterns. *Frontiers in Nutrition*, 8. doi:10.3389/fnut.2021.683678

Kwok, C. S., Umar, S., Myint, P. K., Mamas, M. A., & Loke, Y. K. (2014). Vegetarian diet, Seventh Day Adventists and risk of cardiovascular mortality: A systematic review and meta-analysis. *International Journal of Cardiology*, 176(3), 680–686. doi:https://doi.org/10.1016/j.ijcard.2014.07.080

Kyrø, C., Skeie, G., Loft, S., Overvad, K., Christensen, J., Tjønneland, A., & Olsen, A. (2013). Adherence to a healthy Nordic food index is associated with a lower incidence of colorectal cancer in women: the Diet,

Cancer and Health cohort study. *Br J Nutr, 109*(5), 920–927. doi:10.1017/s0007114512002085

Lankinen, M., Uusitupa, M., & Schwab, U. (2019). Nordic Diet and Inflammation-A Review of Observational and Intervention Studies. *Nutrients, 11*(6). doi:10.3390/nu11061369

Lankinen, M., Uusitupa, M., & Schwab, U. (2019). Nordic Diet and Inflammation—A Review of Observational and Intervention Studies. *Nutrients, 11*(6), 1369. Retrieved from https://www.mdpi.com/2072-6643/11/6/1369

Lee, K. W., Loh, H. C., Ching, S. M., Devaraj, N. K., & Hoo, F. K. (2020). Effects of Vegetarian Diets on Blood Pressure Lowering: A Systematic Review with Meta-Analysis and Trial Sequential Analysis. *Nutrients, 12*(6), 1604. Retrieved from https://www.mdpi.com/2072-6643/12/6/1604

Lichtenstein, A. H., Appel, L. J., Vadiveloo, M., Hu, F. B., Kris-Etherton, P. M., Rebholz, C. M., . . . Wylie-Rosett, J. (2021). 2021 dietary guidance to improve cardiovascular health: a scientific statement from the American Heart Association. *Circulation, 144*(23), e472–e487.

Liese, A. D., Krebs-Smith, S. M., Subar, A. F., George, S. M., Harmon, B. E., Neuhouser, M. L., . . . Reedy, J. (2015). The Dietary Patterns Methods Project: synthesis of findings across cohorts and relevance to dietary guidance. *The Journal of Nutrition, 145*(3), 393–402.

Liyanage, T., Ninomiya, T., Wang, A., Neal, B., Jun, M., Wong, M. G., . . . Perkovic, V. (2016). Effects of the Mediterranean Diet on Cardiovascular Outcomes-A Systematic Review and Meta-Analysis. *PLoS One, 11*(8), e0159252. doi:10.1371/journal.pone.0159252

Lopez, P. D., Cativo, E. H., Atlas, S. A., & Rosendorff, C. (2019). The Effect of Vegan Diets on Blood Pressure in Adults: A Meta-Analysis of Randomized Controlled Trials. *The American journal of medicine, 132*(7), 875–883.e877. doi:https://doi.org/10.1016/j.amjmed.2019.01.044

Mancini, J. G., Filion, K. B., Atallah, R., & Eisenberg, M. J. (2016). Systematic review of the Mediterranean diet for long-term weight loss. *The American journal of medicine, 129*(4), 407–415. e404.

Mann, J. I. (1979). A prudent diet for the nation. *J Hum Nutr, 33*(1), 57–63. doi:10.3109/09637487909143350

Männikkö, R., Komulainen, P., Schwab, U., Heikkilä, H. M., Savonen, K., Hassinen, M., . . . Rauramaa, R. (2015). The Nordic diet and cognition – The DR's EXTRA Study. *British Journal of Nutrition, 114*(2), 231–239. doi:10.1017/S0007114515001890

Martín-Peláez, S., Fito, M., & Castaner, O. (2020). Mediterranean Diet Effects on Type 2 Diabetes Prevention, Disease Progression, and Related Mechanisms. A Review. *Nutrients, 12*(8), 2236. doi:10.3390/nu12082236

Mathew, A. V., Seymour, E. M., Byun, J., Pennathur, S., & Hummel, S. L. (2015). Altered metabolic profile with sodium-restricted dietary approaches to stop hypertension diet in hypertensive heart failure with preserved ejection fraction. *Journal of cardiac failure, 21*(12), 963–967.

Mehmood, A., Usman, M., Patil, P., Zhao, L., & Wang, C. (2020). A review on management of cardiovascular diseases by olive polyphenols. *Food Science & Nutrition, 8*(9), 4639–4655.

Melina, V., Craig, W., & Levin, S. (2016). Position of the Academy of Nutrition and Dietetics: vegetarian diets. *J Acad Nutr Diet, 116*(12), 1970–1980.

Milajerdi, A., Namazi, N., Larijani, B., & Azadbakht, L. (2018). The Association of Dietary Quality Indices and Cancer Mortality: A Systematic Review and Meta-analysis of Cohort Studies. *Nutrition and Cancer, 70*(7), 1091–1105. doi:10.1080/01635581.2018.1502331

Miller 3rd, E. R., Erlinger, T. P., Young, D. R., Jehn, M., Charleston, J., Rhodes, D., . . . Appel, L. J. (2002). Results of the Diet, Exercise, and Weight Loss Intervention Trial (DEW-IT). *Hypertension, 40*(5), 612–618.

Miller, E. R., Erlinger, T. P., & Appel, L. J. (2006). The effects of macronutrients on blood pressure and lipids: An overview of the DASH and omniheart trials. *Current atherosclerosis reports, 8*(6), 460–465. doi:10.1007/s11883-006-0020-1

Mozaffari, H., Ajabshir, S., & Alizadeh, S. (2020). Dietary Approaches to Stop Hypertension and risk of chronic kidney disease: A systematic review and meta-analysis of observational studies. *Clin Nutr, 39*(7), 2035–2044. doi:10.1016/j.clnu.2019.10.004

Nissensohn, M., Román-Viñas, B., Sánchez-Villegas, A., Piscopo, S., & Serra-Majem, L. (2016). The Effect of the Mediterranean Diet on Hypertension: A Systematic Review and Meta-Analysis. *J Nutr Educ Behav, 48*(1), 42–53.e41. doi:10.1016/j.jneb.2015.08.023

Obarzanek, E., Sacks, F. M., Vollmer, W. M., Bray, G. A., Miller, E. R., 3rd, Lin, P. H., . . . Proschan, M. A. (2001). Effects on blood lipids of a blood pressure-lowering diet: the Dietary Approaches to Stop Hypertension (DASH) Trial. *Am J Clin Nutr, 74*(1), 80–89. doi:10.1093/ajcn/74.1.80

Olfert, M. D., & Wattick, R. A. (2018). Vegetarian Diets and the Risk of Diabetes. *Current diabetes reports, 18*(11), 101–101. doi:10.1007/s11892-018-1070-9

Onvani, S., Haghighatdoost, F., & Azadbakht, L. (2015). Dietary approach to stop hypertension (DASH): diet components may be related to lower prevalence of different kinds of cancer: A review on the related documents. *Journal of research in medical sciences: the official journal of Isfahan University of Medical Sciences, 20*(7), 707–713. doi:10.4103/1735-1995.166233

Perälä, M. M., von Bonsdorff, M., Männistö, S., Salonen, M. K., Simonen, M., Kanerva, N., . . . Eriksson, J. G. (2016). A healthy Nordic diet and physical performance in old age: findings from the longitudinal Helsinki Birth Cohort Study. *Br J Nutr, 115*(5), 878–886. doi:10.1017/s0007114515005309

Picasso, M. C., Lo-Tayraco, J. A., Ramos-Villanueva, J. M., Pasupuleti, V., & Hernandez, A. V. (2019). Effect of vegetarian diets on the presentation of metabolic syndrome or its components: A systematic review and meta-analysis. *Clinical nutrition, 38*(3), 1117–1132. doi:https://doi.org/10.1016/j.clnu.2018.05.021

Pieters, M., & Swanepoel, A. C. (2021). The effect of plant-based diets on thrombotic risk factors. *Pol Arch Intern Med, 131*(10). doi:10.20452/pamw.16123

Quintela, B., Carioca, A. A. F., de Oliveira, J. G. R., Fraser, S. D. S., & da Silva Junior, G. B. (2021). Dietary patterns and chronic kidney disease outcomes: A systematic review. *Nephrology (Carlton), 26*(7), 603–612. doi:10.1111/nep.13883

Ramezani-Jolfaie, N., Mohammadi, M., & Salehi-Abargouei, A. (2019). The effect of healthy Nordic diet on cardio-metabolic markers: a systematic review and meta-analysis of randomized controlled clinical trials. *European Journal of Nutrition, 58*(6), 2159–2174.

Raphael, K. L. (2019). The Dietary Approaches to Stop Hypertension (DASH) diet in chronic kidney disease: should we embrace it? *Kidney Int, 95*(6), 1296–1298. doi:10.1016/j.kint.2019.01.026

Ras, R. T., Geleijnse, J. M., & Trautwein, E. A. (2014). LDL-cholesterol-lowering effect of plant sterols and stanols across different dose ranges: a meta-analysis of randomised controlled studies. *British Journal of Nutrition, 112*(2), 214–219. doi:10.1017/S0007114514000750

Renzella, J., Townsend, N., Jewell, J., Breda, J., Roberts, N., Rayner, M., & Wickramasinghe, K. (2018). *What national and subnational interventions and policies based on Mediterranean and Nordic diets are recommended or implemented in the WHO European region, and is there evidence of effectiveness in reducing noncommunicable diseases?*: World Health Organization. Regional Office for Europe.

Richter, C. K., Skulas-Ray, A. C., & Kris-Etherton, P. M. (2014). Recent findings of studies on the Mediterranean diet: what are the implications for current dietary recommendations? *Endocrinol Metab Clin North Am, 43*(4), 963–980. doi:10.1016/j.ecl.2014.08.003

Rifai, L., Pisano, C., Hayden, J., Sulo, S., & Silver, M. A. (2015). *Impact of the DASH diet on endothelial function, exercise capacity, and quality of life in patients with heart failure.* Paper presented at the Baylor University Medical Center Proceedings.

Rock, C. L., Thomson, C., Gansler, T., Gapstur, S. M., McCullough, M. L., Patel, A. V., . . . Doyle, C. (2020). American Cancer Society guideline for diet and physical activity for cancer prevention. *CA Cancer J Clin, 70*(4), 245–271. doi:10.3322/caac.21591

Rosato, V., Temple, N. J., La Vecchia, C., Castellan, G., Tavani, A., & Guercio, V. (2019). Mediterranean diet and cardiovascular disease: a systematic review and meta-analysis of observational studies. *European Journal of Nutrition, 58*(1), 173–191. doi:10.1007/s00394-017-1582-0

Roswall, N., Sandin, S., Scragg, R., Löf, M., Skeie, G., Olsen, A., . . . Weiderpass, E. (2015). No association between adherence to the healthy Nordic food index and cardiovascular disease amongst Swedish women: a cohort study. *Journal of Internal Medicine, 278*(5), 531–541. doi:https://doi.org/10.1111/joim.12378

Sabaté, J., & Wien, M. (2015). A perspective on vegetarian dietary patterns and risk of metabolic syndrome. *British Journal of Nutrition, 113*(S2), S136–S143. doi:10.1017/S0007114514004139

Sala-Vila, A., Estruch, R., & Ros, E. (2015). New insights into the role of nutrition in CVD prevention. *Current Cardiology Reports, 17*(5), 1–11.

Salas-Salvadó, J., Becerra-Tomás, N., García-Gavilán, J. F., Bulló, M., & Barrubés, L. (2018). Mediterranean Diet and Cardiovascular Disease Prevention: What Do We Know? *Progress in Cardiovascular Diseases, 61*(1), 62–67. doi:https://doi.org/10.1016/j.pcad.2018.04.006

Salas-Salvadó, J., Bulló, M., Babio, N., Martínez-González, M., Ibarrola-Jurado, N., Basora, J., . . . Ros, E. (2011). Reduction in the incidence of type 2 diabetes with the Mediterranean diet: results of the PREDIMED-Reus nutrition intervention randomized trial. *Diabetes Care, 34*(1), 14–19. doi:10.2337/dc10-1288

Salas-Salvadó, J., Bulló, M., Estruch, R., Ros, E., Covas, M.-I., Ibarrola-Jurado, N., . . . Ruiz-Gutiérrez, V. (2014). Prevention of diabetes with Mediterranean diets: a subgroup analysis of a randomized trial. *Ann Intern Med, 160*(1), 1–10.

Salehi-Abargouei, A., Maghsoudi, Z., Shirani, F., & Azadbakht, L. (2013). Effects of Dietary Approaches to Stop Hypertension (DASH)-style diet on fatal or nonfatal cardiovascular diseases--incidence: a systematic review and meta-analysis on observational prospective studies. *Nutrition, 29*(4), 611–618. doi:10.1016/j.nut.2012.12.018

Sanches Machado d'Almeida, K., Ronchi Spillere, S., Zuchinali, P., & Corrêa Souza, G. (2018). Mediterranean Diet and Other Dietary Patterns in Primary Prevention of Heart Failure and Changes in Cardiac Function Markers: A Systematic Review. *Nutrients, 10*(1), 58. doi:10.3390/nu10010058

Saulle, R., Lia, L., De Giusti, M., & La Torre, G. (2019). A systematic overview of the scientific literature on the association between Mediterranean Diet and the Stroke prevention. *Clin Ter, 170*(5), e396–e408. doi:10.7417/ct.2019.2166

Sayer, R. D., Wright, A. J., Chen, N., & Campbell, W. W. (2015). Dietary Approaches to Stop Hypertension diet retains effectiveness to reduce blood pressure when lean pork is substituted for chicken and fish as the predominant source of protein. *Am J Clin Nutr, 102*(2), 302–308. doi:10.3945/ajcn.115.111757

Schwingshackl, L., & Hoffmann, G. (2014). Mediterranean dietary pattern, inflammation and endothelial function: a systematic review and meta-analysis of intervention trials. *Nutrition, Metabolism and Cardiovascular Diseases, 24*(9), 929–939.

Schwingshackl, L., Missbach, B., König, J., & Hoffmann, G. (2015). Adherence to a Mediterranean diet and risk of diabetes: a systematic review and meta-analysis. *Public Health Nutrition, 18*(7), 1292–1299.

Siervo, M., Lara, J., Chowdhury, S., Ashor, A., Oggioni, C., & Mathers, J. C. (2015). Effects of the Dietary Approach to Stop Hypertension (DASH) diet on cardiovascular risk factors: a systematic review and meta-analysis. *Br J Nutr, 113*(1), 1–15. doi:10.1017/s0007114514003341

Snowdon, D. A., & Phillips, R. L. (1985). Does a vegetarian diet reduce the occurrence of diabetes? *American Journal of Public Health, 75*(5), 507–512. doi:10.2105/ajph.75.5.507

Sofi, F., Macchi, C., Abbate, R., Gensini, G. F., & Casini, A. (2014). Mediterranean diet and health status: an updated meta-analysis and a proposal for a literature-based adherence score. *Public Health Nutrition, 17*(12), 2769–2782. doi:10.1017/S1368980013003169

Soltani, S., Arablou, T., Jayedi, A., & Salehi-Abargouei, A. (2020). Adherence to the dietary approaches to stop hypertension (DASH) diet in relation to all-cause and cause-specific mortality: a systematic review and dose-response meta-analysis of prospective cohort studies. *Nutr J, 19*(1), 37. doi:10.1186/s12937-020-00554-8

Soltani, S., Jayedi, A., Shab-Bidar, S., Becerra-Tomás, N., & Salas-Salvadó, J. (2019). Adherence to the Mediterranean Diet in Relation to All-Cause Mortality: A Systematic Review and Dose-Response Meta-Analysis of Prospective Cohort Studies. *Advances in Nutrition, 10*(6), 1029–1039. doi:10.1093/advances/nmz041

Soltani, S., Shirani, F., Chitsazi, M. J., & Salehi-Abargouei, A. (2016). The effect of dietary approaches to stop hypertension (DASH) diet on weight and body composition in adults: a systematic review and meta-analysis of randomized controlled clinical trials. *Obes Rev, 17*(5), 442–454. doi:10.1111/obr.12391

Strath, S. J., Kaminsky, Leonard A Ainsworth, Barbara E Ekelund, Ulf Freedson, Patty S Gary, Rebecca A Richardson, Caroline R, Smith, D. T., & Swartz, A. M. (2013). Guide to the assessment of physical activity: clinical and research applications: a scientific statement from the American Heart Association. *Circulation, 128*(20), 2259–2279.

Sung, H., Ferlay, J., Siegel, R. L., Laversanne, M., Soerjomataram, I., Jemal, A., & Bray, F. (2021). Global Cancer Statistics 2020: GLOBOCAN Estimates of Incidence and Mortality Worldwide for 36 Cancers in 185 Countries. *CA Cancer J Clin, 71*(3), 209–249. doi:10.3322/caac.21660

Svetkey, L. P., Sacks, F. M., Obarzanek, E., Vollmer, W. M., Appel, L. J., Lin, P. H., . . . Laws, R. L. (1999). The DASH Diet, Sodium Intake and Blood Pressure Trial (DASH-sodium): rationale and design. DASH-Sodium Collaborative Research Group. *J Am Diet Assoc, 99*(8 Suppl), S96-104. doi:10.1016/s0002-8223(99)00423-x

Toi, P. L., Anothaisintawee, T., Chaikledkaew, U., Briones, J. R., Reutrakul, S., & Thakkinstian, A. (2020). Preventive Role of Diet Interventions and Dietary Factors in Type 2 Diabetes Mellitus: An Umbrella Review. *Nutrients, 12*(9), 2722. Retrieved from https://www.mdpi.com/2072-6643/12/9/2722

Tonstad, S., Butler, T., Yan, R., & Fraser, G. E. (2009). Type of Vegetarian Diet, Body Weight, and Prevalence of Type 2 Diabetes. *Diabetes Care, 32*(5), 791–796. doi:10.2337/dc08-1886

Tsartsou, E., Proutsos, N., Castanas, E., & Kampa, M. (2019). Network Meta-Analysis of Metabolic Effects of Olive-Oil in Humans Shows the Importance of Olive Oil Consumption With Moderate Polyphenol Levels as Part of the Mediterranean Diet. *Frontiers in Nutrition*, *6*. doi:10.3389/fnut.2019.00006

University of Arkancas System, Department of Agriculture. Research & Extension Lowering Your Blood Pressure with the DASH Eating Plan. Retrieved from https://www.uaex.uada.edu/counties/miller/news/fcs/meal-prep-healthy-eating/Lowering-Your-Blood-Pressure-with-the-DASH-Eating-Plan.aspx

US Department of Agriculture and US Department of Health and Human Services. Dietary Guidelines for Americans, 2020–2025. 9th Edition. December 2020. Available at DietaryGuidelines.gov.

Van Horn, L., Carson, J. A., Appel, L. J., Burke, L. E., Economos, C., Karmally, W.,. . . Kris-Etherton, P. (2016). Recommended Dietary Pattern to Achieve Adherence to the American Heart Association/American College of Cardiology (AHA/ACC) Guidelines: A Scientific Statement From the American Heart Association. *Circulation*, *134*(22), e505–e529. doi:10.1161/cir.0000000000000462

Vang, A., Singh, P. N., Lee, J. W., Haddad, E. H., & Brinegar, C. H. (2008). Meats, processed meats, obesity, weight gain and occurrence of diabetes among adults: findings from Adventist Health Studies. *Annals of Nutrition and Metabolism*, *52*(2), 96–104.

Ventriglio, A., Sancassiani, F., Contu, M. P., Latorre, M., Di Slavatore, M., Fornaro, M., & Bhugra, D. (2020). Mediterranean Diet and its Benefits on Health and Mental Health: A Literature Review. *Clinical practice and epidemiology in mental health: CP & EMH*, *16*(Suppl-1), 156–164. doi:10.2174/1745017902016010156

Walker, T. J., Tullar, J. M., Diamond, P. M., Kohl, H. W., 3rd, & Amick, B. C., 3rd. (2017). The Relation of Combined Aerobic and Muscle–Strengthening Physical Activities With Presenteeism. *J Phys Act Health*, *14*(11), 893–898. doi:10.1123/jpah.2016-0696

Wang, D. D., Li, Y., Bhupathiraju, S. N., Rosner, B. A., Sun, Q., Giovannucci, E. L., . . . Stampfer, M. J. (2021). Fruit and vegetable intake and mortality: results from 2 prospective cohort studies of US men and women and a meta-analysis of 26 cohort studies. *Circulation*, *143*(17), 1642–1654.

Wang, X., Ouyang, Y., Liu, J., Zhu, M., Zhao, G., Bao, W., & Hu, F. B. (2014). Fruit and vegetable consumption and mortality from all causes, cardiovascular disease, and cancer: systematic review and dose-response meta-analysis of prospective cohort studies. *BMJ: British Medical Journal*, *349*, g4490. doi:10.1136/bmj.g4490

WCRF/AICR. (2018). *Diet, nutrition, physical activity and cancer: a global perspective. Continuous Update Project Expert Report 2018*. Retrieved from https://www.wcrf.org/dietandcancer

WHO. (2020, 29 April 2020). Healthy diet. Retrieved from https://www.who.int/news-room/fact-sheets/detail/healthy-diet

Widmer, R. J., Flammer, A. J., Lerman, L. O., & Lerman, A. (2015). The Mediterranean diet, its components, and cardiovascular disease. *The American journal of medicine*, *128*(3), 229–238.

Wynder, E. L., Lemon, F. R., & Bross, I. J. (1959). Cancer and coronary artery disease among Seventh-Day Adventists. *Cancer*, *12*(5), 1016–1028.

Yokoyama, Y., Nishimura, K., Barnard, N. D., Takegami, M., Watanabe, M., Sekikawa, A.,. . . Miyamoto, Y. (2014). Vegetarian diets and blood pressure: a meta-analysis. *JAMA Intern Med*, *174*(4), 577–587. doi:10.1001/jamainternmed.2013.14547

FURTHER READING

Bibliography

Allen, T. S., Bhatia, H. S., Wood, A. C., Momin, S. R., & Allison, M. A. (2022). State-of-the-art review: Evidence on red meat consumption and hypertension outcomes. American Journal of Hypertension.

Bôto, J. M., Rocha, A., Miguéis, V., Meireles, M., & Neto, B. (2022). Sustainability Dimensions of the Mediterranean Diet: A Systematic Review of the Indicators used and Its Results. Advances in Nutrition.

Briggs, M. A., Fleming, J. A., & Kris-Etherton, P. M. (2016). Food-Based approaches for achieving nutritional adequacy with the Mediterranean, DASH, and USDA food patterns. In Mediterranean Diet (pp. 239–259). Humana Press, Cham.

Calella, P., Gallè, F., Di Onofrio, V., Cerullo, G., Liguori, G., & Valerio, G. (2022). Adherence to Mediterranean diet in athletes: a narrative review. Sport Sciences for Health, 1–8.

Cena, H., & Calder, P. C. (2020). Defining a healthy diet: evidence for the role of contemporary dietary patterns in health and disease. Nutrients, *12*(2), 334.

Gallego-Narbón, A., & Vaquero, M. (2019). Are vegetarian diets nutritionally adequate? A revision of the scientific evidence. Nutricion Hospitalaria, *36*(4), 950–961.

Parker, H. W., & Vadiveloo, M. K. (2019). Diet quality of vegetarian diets compared with nonvegetarian diets: a systematic review. Nutrition reviews, *77*(3), 144–160.

Solch, R. J., Aigbogun, J. O., Voyiadjis, A. G., Talkington, G. M., Darensbourg, R. M., O'Connell, S.,. . . & Maraganore, D. M. (2022). Mediterranean diet adherence, gut microbiota, and Alzheimer's or Parkinson's disease risk: A systematic review. Journal of the Neurological Sciences, *120166*.

Links

- mediterradiet.org
- https://oldwayspt.org/traditional-diets/mediterranean-diet
- https://ich.unesco.org/en/RL/mediterranean-diet-00884
- dashdiet.org/
- eatright.org/
- vndpg.org
- vegetariannutrition.net
- veganhealth.org
- vegweb.com
- usda.gov/
- nal.usda.gov/
- health.gov

Basic Concepts of Physical Activity and Fitness

UNIT 2

UNIT 2

Basic Concepts of Physical Activity and Fitness

Definition of Fitness and Its Components

CHAPTER 4

Definition of Physical Fitness	63	Flexibility	65
Aerobic and Anaerobic Fitness	63	Skill-Related Physical Fitness Components	65
Health-related Physical Fitness Components	64	Speed, Agility, Balance, Reaction Time, Power	65
Cardiovascular or Cardiorespiratory Fitness	64	Key Points	66
Body Composition	64	Self-assessment Questions	66
Muscular Fitness	64	References	66
Muscular Strength	64	Further Reading	67
Muscular Endurance	65	Bibliography	67
Muscular Endurance Versus Aerobic Endurance	65	Links	67

DEFINITION OF PHYSICAL FITNESS

In 2006, the American College of Sports Medicine (ACSM) defined physical fitness as, "a set of physical attributes that people have or achieve that relates to the ability to perform physical activity" (Wilder et al., 2006).

Until then, physical fitness was defined in several ways, but according to 2013 ACSM guidelines (Thompson, Arena, Riebe, Pescatello, & American College of Sports, 2013), the most well-accepted definition for physical fitness was "the ability to carry out daily tasks with vigor and alertness, without undue fatigue, and with ample energy to enjoy leisure-time pursuits and meet unforeseen emergencies".

AEROBIC AND ANAEROBIC FITNESS

To perform any task, energy is needed. Because physical performance involves muscular work, the degree of performance of the task at hand (i.e., the degree of fitness) depends mainly on how the energy is made available and used by the muscles. In specific, it is not energy that is delivered to the muscles but the raw materials for example fat or glycogen. From these materials, the muscle cells extract the energy required for the task at hand. Cells can extract the necessary energy in one of two ways: with the use of oxygen and without oxygen. The use of oxygen to extract energy is referred to as **aerobic** metabolism (from the Greek word "aerobiosis", air-dependent living). Conversely, extracting energy without using oxygen is referred to as **anaerobic** (air-independent living) metabolism.

The derivation of energy aerobically or anaerobically depends exclusively on the intensity of the activity. In high-intensity activities energy is mainly derived without oxygen from components that are already stored in our body and are readily available. In low-intensity activities oxygen is used from the muscles to break down energy sources like fats or glucose to perform the exercise. Thus, activities referred to as **aerobic or anaerobic** accordingly. In general, in aerobic processes more energy is produced from the use of the oxygen than anaerobic processes, but anaerobic processes release energy faster. Aerobic fitness refers to the degree or ability to provide the required energy for a specific task aerobically. Conversely, anaerobic fitness refers to the body's ability to provide the required energy for a specific task anaerobically.

Aerobic exercises or activities consist of repetitive, low resistance movements (walking or cycling) that last over a relatively long period of time (generally 5 minutes or more). Anaerobic exercises or activities, on the other hand, are characterized by bursts of intense activity lasting only a short time. Such activities include lifting a very heavy weight, jumping, sprinting, etc. These activities challenge the body to maximum or near maximum efforts. They require a great deal of energy within a short span of time and can only be sustained for a few seconds to minutes. The energy requirements are met predominately without the use of oxygen. For example, no oxygen is

Prevention and Management of Cardiovascular and Metabolic Disease: Diet, Physical Activity and Healthy Aging,
First Edition. Christina N. Katsagoni, Peter Kokkinos, and Labros S. Sidossis.
© 2023 John Wiley & Sons Ltd. Published 2023 by John Wiley & Sons Ltd.

Table 4.1 Physical fitness categorization into health-related and skill-related components.

Health-related physical fitness components	Skill-related physical fitness components
Cardiorespiratory fitness	Speed
Body composition	Agility
Muscular strength	Coordination
Muscular endurance	Power
Flexibility	Reaction time
	Balance

Source: (Adapted from Thompson et al., 2013).

required to meet the energy necessary to run 100 meters or lift a heavy weight.

These two energy systems (aerobic and anaerobic) almost always work together harmoniously, sharing the responsibility for providing the energy for the entire body. However, one is likely to be the predominant system and provide most of the energy for the particular activity at hand.

As it will be described in the next paragraphs, physical fitness can be further grouped into health- and skill-related components (**Table 4.1**) (Thompson et al., 2013).

HEALTH-RELATED PHYSICAL FITNESS COMPONENTS

Health-related components of physical fitness include five components of physical fitness:

1. cardiorespiratory fitness,
2. body composition,
3. muscular strength,
4. muscular endurance, and
5. flexibility.

CARDIOVASCULAR OR CARDIORESPIRATORY FITNESS

Cardiorespiratory fitness (CRF), also known as cardiovascular fitness, is the ability to perform dynamic exercise using large muscles for prolonged periods, at specific intensities and frequency.

The degree of CRF depends on the coordinated functional state of three systems: (1) the respiratory system (lungs) to provide the necessary oxygen for the muscles, (2) the cardiovascular system (heart and vessels) to deliver the nutrients and oxygen requirements to the working muscles, and (3) the muscular system that uses the oxygen and nutrients delivered to meet the energy demands of the activity at hand. Naturally, the more efficiently these three systems become, the higher the performance will be.

Thus, aerobic fitness can be defined as the ability of the circulatory and the respiratory systems to supply the necessary oxygen for the muscle during prolonged work. Consequently, aerobic fitness is referred to as CRF or endurance. Because cardiovascular, cardiorespiratory, and aerobic fitness or aerobic capacity terms are so closely related, they can be used inter-changeably.

Low CRF is considered as a independent predictor of cardiovascular disease (CVD) and all-cause mortality in adults. Today, it is well-known that being physically active is linked to better health outcomes independent of CRF, a concept that would have been considered unorthodox a few decades ago (Myers, Kokkinos, Arena, & LaMonte, 2021). The role of physical activity in health will be discussed further in **Chapter 6**.

BODY COMPOSITION

With respect to health and fitness, body composition is used to describe both the fat-free mass (FFM), which includes the skeleton, muscles, and body water, and the fat mass (FM) in human bodies. Both FFM and FM are very important for the assessment of health status.

Variations in FFM may expose people at risk of malnutrition, for example undernutrition or sarcopenia, especially in older adults that could lead to disability. Conversely, increased visceral FM in people with obesity is associated with CVD and diabetes (Buffa, Floris, Putzu, & Marini, 2011). More will be discussed in **Units 4** and **5**, meanwhile body composition could explain why two people at the same height and same body weight may have different health issues.

Body composition in athletes is associated with enhancements in CRF and strength. In sports nutrition, body composition is used by experts to develop specific dietary interventions, and strength coaches to create, optimize, and evaluate training programs (Moon, 2013).

MUSCULAR FITNESS

The ACSM defines muscular fitness as the ability of the muscle to perform tasks that require muscular strength or muscular endurance.

MUSCULAR STRENGTH

Muscular strength is defined as the ability of the muscle or muscle groups to exert force during a voluntary contraction (Caspersen, Powell, & Christenson, 1985; Wilder et al., 2006). Traditionally, the maximal force a muscle or group of muscles can exert is assessed by tests that require maximum effort against the greatest resistance one can move through the full range of motion once; this is known as the 1-repetition maximum (1-RM). A percentage of this 1-RM is then used to determine the number of repetitions one should perform to enhance the strength for a specific muscle. Generally, 8 to 12 repetitions at 40% to 60% of the 1-RM are sufficient to enhance muscular strength. However, intensities as much as 80% and higher with relatively few repetitions (3 to 5) can be more effective for rapid strength gains (Wilder et al., 2006).

It is important to mention that the level of intensity for resistance exercises is not easy to determine and the 1-RM does not depict a true intensity. The number of repetitions and the percent of resistance based on the 1-RM differ significantly between individuals and muscle groups. Thus, the 1-RM should only be used as a general guideline (Wilder et al., 2006).

MUSCULAR ENDURANCE

Muscular endurance is defined as the ability of the muscle or muscle groups to perform repetitive contractions over a period of time against a resistance, such as lifting a set amount of weight several times (Wilder et al., 2006). Muscular endurance is assessed by tests requiring more than 12 repetitions. A simple test of muscular endurance is the maximum number of push-ups or sit-ups one can execute without rest (Wilder et al., 2006).

Generally, muscular endurance is best developed with relatively high repetitions (12 to 20) and low resistance. However, more than 25 repetitions appear to have no further contribution to the development of muscular endurance.

MUSCULAR ENDURANCE VERSUS AEROBIC ENDURANCE

Muscular endurance often is confused with aerobic endurance. Some people claim that lifting a relatively light weight several times and quickly, moving from exercise to exercise with no more than a few seconds of rest between sessions or stations, as is the case with circuit weight training, can increase aerobic performance. These claims are based on the substantial increase in heart rate observed during circuit weight training or resistance training in general. Although small gains in aerobic capacity with such training can occur, it is not an efficient way to improve aerobic endurance for several reasons, which involve the following two principles.

Specificity Principle

First, the body's response and adaptation to a specific type of exercise (stimulus) is very specific to that exercise. This is known as the specificity principle. Based on this principle, only exercises that require increased oxygen consumption to meet their energy demand will enhance the aerobic capacity of the individual. The small gains in aerobic endurance reported by some scientists support this concept (Beckham & Earnest, 2000). It is important to remember that almost all physical activities have both an aerobic and anaerobic component, and none are purely aerobic or purely anaerobic. The degree of involvement by each system depends mostly on the intensity of the activity. During circuit weight training, the resistance (intensity) used is relatively light and the number of repetitions high, which allows a certain degree of involvement by the aerobic system. Because this system is challenged, it responds by small improvements in its function.

Oxygen Consumption Link with Heart Rate

Second, there is a linear relationship between oxygen consumption and heart rate during a graded aerobic activity. That is, as the intensity of the exercise increases, the oxygen consumption and heart rate increase in a linear fashion. Oxygen consumption reaches maximal levels when the maximal heart rate is achieved.

Heart rate, thus, can be used as a surrogate for oxygen consumption and as an indicator of aerobic work only if this linear relationship exists. Indeed, exercise intensity is based on a percentage of maximal heart rate when aerobic activity is involved.

In resistance training, however, the increase in heart rate is the result of catecholamine surge and not oxygen demand. Thus, the heart rate increase is disproportionate to the increase in oxygen consumption (Beckham & Earnest, 2000; Wilmore et al., 1978). Because the relationship between heart rate and oxygen consumption is no longer linear, the heart rate cannot be used as an indicator of aerobic work. The terms muscular fitness or muscular endurance therefore should be used to describe the ability of the muscle to perform mostly anaerobic work.

FLEXIBILITY

Body flexibility is often measured in terms of the joint range of motion (RoM).

The RoM generally decreases as age increases, and this is reflected by age-associated functional changes in the musculoskeletal tissues, such as losses in the resilience of cartilage, reduced elasticity of ligaments, and fat redistribution (Jeong, Heo, Lee, & Park, 2018). Pre-obesity and obesity have been associated with reduced RoM for somebody joint motions, which is related to muscle mass changes and excess FM.

Moreover, women compared to men are generally more flexible for most body joint motions. This is linked to differences in sex hormones, such as such as estrogen, progesterone, relaxin, and oxytocin that are reported to increase the laxity of connective tissues. Conversely, testosterone is increases muscle mass, which might reduce joint RoM. This is because affected muscles occupy more space between the adjacent body segments of a joint and therefore reduce the inter-segmental rotation (Jeong et al., 2018).

Physical inactivity may also reduce body flexibility. Prolonged inactivity is known to proliferate fibro-fatty connective tissues and cause fibrous adhesions into joint space (Jeong et al., 2018).

SKILL-RELATED PHYSICAL FITNESS COMPONENTS

Skill-related physical fitness consists of six components: agility, speed, power, balance, coordination, reaction time. These components are movements that an individual needs to successfully demonstrate a variety of motor skills and movement patterns (DeMet & Wahl-Alexander, 2019).

SPEED, AGILITY, BALANCE, REACTION TIME, POWER

Speed is the ability to achieve high movement velocity within a short period of time. Agility is the ability to change the direction of speed and mode of response to a stimulus. It involves perceptual and decision-making components. Speed and agility incorporate strength, neuromuscular coordination, and flexibility by allowing the person to move at a higher rate of speed (Walankar & Shetty, 2020). The ability to use the senses, such as sight and hearing, in conjunction with other body parts to perform tasks efficiently and accurately is known as coordination.

However, power is needed to perform a task, while stationary or in motion and maintaining balance (Thompson et al., 2013). Reaction time is the time elapsed between any stimulus and the initiation of the motor response to the stimulus (Walankar & Shetty, 2020).

Knowledge about the relationship between balance, strength, and power are important for identifying individuals at risk, such as older adults or in populations with other clinical conditions such diabetes. This is because deficits in these neuromuscular components are linked to an increased risk of sustaining injuries and falls (Muehlbauer, Gollhofer, & Granacher, 2015). These will be discussed further in **Chapter 6**, along with the implications and health benefits of physical activity in adults.

KEY POINTS

- According to the 2013 American College of Sports Medicine guidelines, physical fitness is defined by the ability to carry out daily tasks with vigor and alertness, without undue fatigue, and with ample energy to enjoy leisure-time pursuits and meet unforeseen emergencies.
- Physical activities or exercise can be defined as aerobic or anaerobic. The derivation of energy aerobically or anaerobically depends exclusively on the intensity of the activity.
- Aerobic exercises or activities consist of repetitive, low resistance movements (walking or cycling) that last a relatively long period of time (generally 5 minutes or more).
- Anaerobic exercises or activities are characterized by bursts of intense activity lasting only a short time. Their energy requirements are derived predominantly without oxygen (anaerobic metabolism).
- Health-related components of physical fitness include: (1) cardiorespiratory fitness, (2) body composition, (3) muscular strength, (4) muscular endurance, and (5) flexibility.
- Skill-related physical fitness consists of six components: agility, speed, power, balance, coordination, and reaction time.

SELF-ASSESSMENT QUESTIONS

1. Define aerobic and anaerobic metabolism.
2. What is cardiorespiratory fitness?
3. What does body composition refer to?
4. What is the 1-repetition maximum (1-RM)?
5. Which factors affect the joint range of motion (RoM)?

REFERENCES

Beckham, S. G., & Earnest, C. P. (2000). Metabolic cost of free weight circuit weight training. *J Sports Med Phys Fitness*, 40(2), 118–125. Retrieved from https://www.ncbi.nlm.nih.gov/pubmed/11034431

Buffa, R., Floris, G. U., Putzu, P. F., & Marini, E. (2011). Body composition variations in ageing. *Collegium antropologicum*, 35(1), 259–265.

Caspersen, C. J., Powell, K. E., & Christenson, G. M. (1985). Physical activity, exercise, and physical fitness: definitions and distinctions for health-related research. *Public Health Rep*, 100(2), 126–131. Retrieved from https://www.ncbi.nlm.nih.gov/pubmed/3920711

DeMet, T., & Wahl-Alexander, Z. (2019). Integrating skill-related components of fitness into physical education. *Strategies*, 32(5), 10–17.

Jeong, Y., Heo, S., Lee, G., & Park, W. (2018). Pre-obesity and obesity impacts on passive joint range of motion. *Ergonomics*, 61(9), 1223–1231. doi: 10.1080/00140139.2018.1478455

Moon, J. R. (2013). Body composition in athletes and sports nutrition: an examination of the bioimpedance analysis technique. *Eur J Clin Nutr*, 67 Suppl 1, S54–59. doi:10.1038/ejcn.2012.165

Muehlbauer, T., Gollhofer, A., & Granacher, U. (2015). Associations between measures of balance and lower-extremity muscle strength/power in healthy individuals across the lifespan: a systematic review and meta-analysis. *Sports medicine*, 45(12), 1671–1692.

Myers, J., Kokkinos, P., Arena, R., & LaMonte, M. J. (2021). The impact of moving more, physical activity, and cardiorespiratory fitness: Why we should strive to measure and improve fitness. *Prog Cardiovasc Dis*, 64, 77–82. doi:10.1016/j.pcad.2020.11.003

Thompson, P. D., Arena, R., Riebe, D., Pescatello, L. S., & American College of Sports, M. (2013). ACSM's new preparticipation health screening recommendations from ACSM's guidelines for exercise testing and prescription, ninth edition. *Curr Sports Med Rep*, 12(4), 215–217. doi:10.1249/JSR.0b013e31829a68cf

Walankar, P., & Shetty, J. (2020). Speed, agility and quickness training: A review.

Wilder, R. P., Greene, J. A., Winters, K. L., Long, W. B., 3rd, Gubler, K., & Edlich, R. F. (2006). Physical fitness assessment: an update. *J Long Term Eff Med Implants*, 16(2), 193–204. doi:10.1615/jlongtermeffmedimplants.v16.i2.90

Wilmore, J. H., Parr, R. B., Ward, P., Vodak, P. A., Barstow, T. J., Pipes, T. V., . . . Leslie, P. (1978). Energy cost of circuit weight training. *Med Sci Sports*, 10(2), 75–78. Retrieved from https://www.ncbi.nlm.nih.gov/pubmed/692305

FURTHER READING

Bibliography

Myers, J., Kokkinos, P., Arena, R., & LaMonte, M. J. (2021). The impact of moving more, physical activity, and cardiorespiratory fitness: Why we should strive to measure and improve fitness. Progress in cardiovascular diseases, *64*, 77–82.

Toomey, C. M., Cremona, A., Hughes, K., Norton, C., & Jakeman, P. (2015). A review of body composition measurement in the assessment of health. Topics in Clinical Nutrition, *30*(1), 16–32. doi:10.1097/TIN.0000000000000017

Bosy-Westphal, A., & Müller, M. J. (2021). Diagnosis of obesity based on body composition-associated health risks—Time for a change in paradigm. Obesity Reviews, *22*, e13190. doi: 10.1111/obr.13190.

Earnest, C. P., Rothschild, J., Harnish, C. R., & Naderi, A. (2019). Metabolic adaptations to endurance training and nutrition strategies influencing performance. Research in Sports Medicine, *27*(2), 134–146.

Links

- https://www.acsm.org/education-resources/trending-topics-resources/physical-activity-guidelines
- https://www.cdc.gov/physicalactivity/basics/older_adults/index.htm
- https://www.nia.nih.gov/health/exercise-physical-activity
- https://www.cdc.gov/diabetes/managing/active.html

Defining Physical Activity and Exercise

CHAPTER 5

Definition of Physical Activity and Exercise	69	VO_2 Reserve Method	76
Quantifying the Intensity of Physical Activity	69	Exercise Duration	76
Total Energy Expenditure	69	Exercise Frequency	76
Physical Activity Level	71	Exercise Volume	76
Perceived Exertion (Borg Rating of Perceived Exertion Scale)	72	Key Points	77
		Self-assessment Questions	77
Metabolic Equivalents of Task	72	References	77
VO_2max	74	Further Reading	78
Percent of Maximum Heart Rate	75	Bibliography	78
Heart Rate Reserve Method (Karvonen Method)	75	Links	78

DEFINITION OF PHYSICAL ACTIVITY AND EXERCISE

According to the 2020 WHO guidelines, physical activity (PA) is defined as "any bodily movement produced by skeletal muscles that requires energy expenditure" (Bull, 2020). Other alternatives of this definition were proposed in the literature and used; however, all are derived from the same initial definition by Caspersen et al. (Caspersen, 1985).

In terms of mode, there are four PA domains: (i) occupational (i.e., work), (ii) domestic (i.e., household chores), (iii) transportation/utilitarian, and (iv) leisure time (Strath, Smith, & Swartz, 2013). Examples of these physical-activity domains are shown in **Table 5.1**. The assessment of PA should include all four domains as they impact health and should be considered separately. This is evident as an increase in one PA domain (e.g., occupation activity) may lead to decreased activity in another domain (e.g., leisure time) that causes an overall increase in sedentary time. Sedentary time is positively correlated with poor health and premature death as it will be discussed in **Chapter 6**.

PA is further classified as structured or incidental. Structured PA or exercise is a planned, structured program designed to beneficially promote health and physical fitness. Incidental PA is not planned and usually is the result of daily activities at work, at home, or during transport (Strath et al., 2013).

PA and exercise can be quantified based on (Hills, 2014): (i) mode or type of activity, i.e., specific activity performed; (ii) frequency of performing the activity, i.e., number of sessions per day or per week; (iii) duration of performing activity, i.e., time (minutes or hours) of the activity bout during a specified time frame; and (iv) intensity of performing the activity, i.e., rate of energy expenditure (**Table 5.2**) (Strath et al., 2013).

QUANTIFYING THE INTENSITY OF PHYSICAL ACTIVITY

The result of participating in PA or exercise is the expenditure of energy, which is commonly quantified in terms of intensity. There are several methods to quantify PA intensity (Liguori, 2020) : energy expenditure as a result of PA, metabolic equivalents (METs), oxygen consumption (VO_2), heart rate (HR), heart rate reserve (HRR), and specifying a percentage of oxygen uptake reserve (VO_2R). Each of these methods has strengths and limitations (Hills, 2014; Liguori, 2020).

TOTAL ENERGY EXPENDITURE

PA is commonly quantified by determining the energy expended for physical activity. Assessing energy expenditure and estimated PA in free-living individuals is very important in the

Prevention and Management of Cardiovascular and Metabolic Disease: Diet, Physical Activity and Healthy Aging,
First Edition. Christina N. Katsagoni, Peter Kokkinos, and Labros S. Sidossis.
© 2023 John Wiley & Sons Ltd. Published 2023 by John Wiley & Sons Ltd.

Table 5.1 Physical-activity domains.

Occupational	Work-related: involving manual labor tasks, walking, carrying or lifting objects
Domestic	Housework: yard work, child care, chores, self-care, shopping, incidental
Transportation/ utilitarian	Purpose of going somewhere: walking, bicycling, climbing/descending stairs to public transportation, standing while riding transportation
Leisure time	Discretionary or recreational activities: sports, hobbies, exercise, volunteer work

Source: (Strath et al., 2013).

Table 5.2 Physical-activity dimensions: mode, frequency, duration, and intensity.

Dimension	Definition and context
Mode	Specific activity performed (e.g., walking, gardening, cycling). Mode can also be defined in the context of physiological and biomechanical demands/types (e.g., aerobic versus anaerobic activity, resistance or strength training, balance, and stability training).
Frequency	Number of sessions per day or per week. In the context of health-promoting PA, frequency is often qualified as number of sessions (bouts) ≥10 min in duration/length.
Duration	Time (minutes or hours) of the activity bout during a specified time frame (e.g., day, week, year, past month).
Intensity	Rate of energy expenditure. Intensity is an indicator of the metabolic demand of an activity. It can be objectively quantified with physiological measures (e.g., oxygen consumption, heart rate, respiratory exchange ratio), subjectively assessed by perceptual characteristics (e.g., rating of perceived exertion, walk-and-talk test), or quantified by body movement (e.g., stepping rate, 3-dimensional body accelerations).

Source: (Strath et al., 2013).

global context of non-communicable diseases (NCDs), such as malnutrition, obesity, and diabetes.

The gold-standard method by which total energy expenditure (TEE) is assessed in a free-living context is the doubly labeled water technique. However, this method requires sophisticated laboratory-based equipment for sample analysis, which are high cost and time-prohibitive, thus restricting its use to large-scale studies only. The most common approach to assess TEE is by measuring oxygen consumption and/or the production of carbon dioxide via indirect calorimetry or by using prediction equations. Direct calorimetry, in which heat production is measured in a metabolic chamber, is not widely used (Hills, 2014).

TEE represents the total energy that a person expends in a day for processes essential for life (e.g., to digest, absorb, and convert food as well as exercise). It is comprised of three components including: resting energy expenditure, physical-activity energy expenditure, and the thermic effect of food (**Figure 5.1**).

Resting energy expenditure (REE) or the resting metabolic rate (RMR) represents the energy expended at rest by an individual in fasting conditions and a thermo-neutral environment. It accounts for approximately 60% of the TEE. It is the largest proportion of TEE. RMR is typically slightly higher than the basal metabolic rate (BMR), which is measured under stricter conditions.

The thermic effect of food (TEF), also called the specific dynamic action (SDA) or dietary-induced thermogenesis, is the energy expended processing and storing food as well as assimilating nutrients. The TEF accounts for approximately 10% of the TEE (Calcagno, 2019).

The activity energy expenditure (AEE) represents all energy expended above the resting level and includes the exercise energy expenditure (ExEE) as well as non-exercise activity thermogenesis (NEAT) (Hills, 2014). ExEE is required for intentional (e.g., sports-related) PA and accounts for between 0% and 10% of the total daily energy expenditure, although in

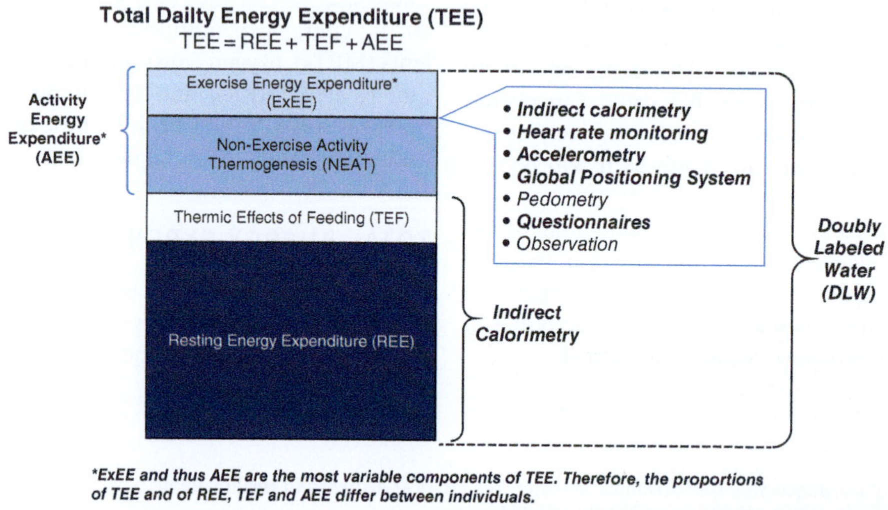

Total Daily Energy Expenditure (TEE)
TEE = REE + TEF + AEE

Activity Energy Expenditure* (AEE):
- Exercise Energy Expenditure* (ExEE)
- Non-Exercise Activity Thermogenesis (NEAT)

Thermic Effects of Feeding (TEF)

Resting Energy Expenditure (REE)

Indirect Calorimetry:
- Indirect calorimetry
- Heart rate monitoring
- Accelerometry
- Global Positioning System
- Pedometry
- Questionnaires
- Observation

Doubly Labeled Water (DLW)

*ExEE and thus AEE are the most variable components of TEE. Therefore, the proportions of TEE and of REE, TEF and AEE differ between individuals.

FIGURE 5.1 Components of total daily energy expenditure and measurement approaches. Source: (Hills, 2014 / Frontiers Media S.A. / CC BY-3.0).

extremely active individuals, it may constitute up to 60% to 70% of TEE. NEAT (e.g., daily living activities, fidgeting, maintenance of posture) accounts for the roughly 20% of remaining TEE (Calcagno, 2019).

If we know the REE and assume that the TEF constitutes 10%, which is relatively stable, we can then calculate the AEE:

$$\text{AEE kcal/day} = 0.9 \times \text{TEE kcal/day} - \text{REE kcal/day}$$
$$(\text{Hills, 2014})$$

PA can be expressed either in kilocalories (kcal) or in metabolic equivalents of task (METs). One kcal is equivalent to the energy required to raise the temperature of 1 kilogram of water by 1 degree Celsius. When 1 L of oxygen is used, approximately 5 kcal of energy are released. Therefore, if a 70 kg individual walks for 60 min at an intensity that requires a 1 L/min rate of oxygen consumption, they would consume 60 L of oxygen. In this case, the TEE (including the REE) for those 60 min would be ~300 kcal (i.e., 60 L x 5 kcal/L). The total daily energy for PA is the sum of all the physical activities performed on a given day.

PHYSICAL ACTIVITY LEVEL

The physical-activity level (PAL) is a way to describe a person's daily physical activity as a number, and it can be estimated using the average 24-hour TEE and BMR.

$$\text{PAL} = \text{TEE} \div \text{BMR}$$

For example, a male with a PAL of 1.68 and a mean BMR of 6.0 MJ/day (1434 kcal/day) has a mean energy requirement of $1.68 \times 6.0 = 10.08$ MJ/day (2409 kcal/day).

The mean PAL per day is derived from multiplying the energy cost of each activity (expressed as multiples of BMR, or physical-activity ratio (PAR) with the time spent in each activity (**Table 5.3**) [Joint Food and Agriculture Organization (FAO) of the United Nations, World Health Organization (WHO) & United Nations University (UNU) (1985)].

There are different levels of activity associated with an individual's lifestyle. The categories are shown in **Table 5.4**. PAL values that can be sustained for a long period of time by

Table 5.3 Factorial calculations of total energy expenditure for a population group.

Main daily activities	Time allocation	Energy cost[1]	Time × energy cost	Mean PAL[2]
	Hours	PAR		Multiple of 24-hour BMR
Sedentary or light activity lifestyle				
Sleeping	8	1	8.0	
Personal care (dressing, showering)	1	2.3	2.3	
Eating	1	1.5	1.5	
Cooking	1	2.1	2.1	
Sitting (office work, selling produce, tending shop)	8	1.5	12.0	
General household work	1	2.8	2.8	
Driving car to/from work	1	2.0	2.0	
Walking at varying paces without a load	1	3.2	3.2	
Light leisure activities (watching TV, chatting)	2	1.4	2.8	
Total	24		36.7	36.7/24 = 1.53
Active or moderately active lifestyle				
Sleeping	8	1	8.0	
Personal care (dressing, showering)	1	2.3	2.3	
Eating	1	1.5	1.5	
Standing, carrying light loads (waiting on tables, arranging merchandise)[3]	8	2.2	17.6	
Commuting to/from work on the bus	1	1.2	1.2	
Walking at varying paces without a load	1	3.2	3.2	
Low-intensity aerobic exercise	1	4.2	4.2	
Light leisure activities (watching TV, chatting)	3	1.4	4.2	
Total	24		42.2	42.2/24 = 1.76
Vigorous or vigorously active lifestyle				
Sleeping	8	1	8.0	
Personal care (dressing, bathing)	1	2.3	2.3	

(Continued)

Table 5.3 (Continued)

Main daily activities	Time allocation	Energy cost[1]	Time × energy cost	Mean PAL[2]
	Hours	PAR		Multiple of 24-hour BMR
Vigorous or vigorously active lifestyle				
Eating	1	1.4	1.4	
Cooking	1	2.1	2.1	
Non-mechanized agricultural work (planting, weeding, gathering)	6	4.1	24.6	
Collecting water/wood	1	4.4	4.4	
Non-mechanized domestic chores (sweeping, washing clothes and dishes by hand)	1	2.3	2.3	
Walking at varying paces without a load	1	3.2	3.2	
Miscellaneous light leisure activities	4	1.4	5.6	
Total	24		53.9	53.9/24 = 2.25

[1] Energy costB16s of activities, expressed as multiples of basal metabolic rate, or physical-activity ratio (PAR).
[2] PAL = physical-activity level, or energy requirement expressed as a multiple of 24-hour BMR.
[3] Composite of the energy cost of standing, walking slowly, and serving meals or carrying a light load.
Source: Joint Food and Agriculture Organization (FAO) of the United Nations, World Health Organization (WHO) & United Nations University (UNU) (1985).

Table 5.4 Classification of lifestyles in relation to the intensity of habitual physical activity, or PAL

Category	PAL value
Sedentary or light activity lifestyle	1.40–1.69
Active or moderately active lifestyle	1.70–1.99
Vigorous or vigorously active lifestyle	2.00–2.40[1]

[1] Physical activity level (PAL) values >2.40 are difficult to maintain over a long period of time.
Source: Joint Food and Agriculture Organization (FAO) of the United Nations, World Health Organization (WHO) & United Nations University (UNU) (1985).

Table 5.5 The Borg scale of perceived exertion.

How you might describe your exertion	Borg rating of your exertion	Examples (for most adults <65 years old)
None	6	Reading a book, watching television
Very, very light	7 to 8	Tying shoes
Very light	9 to 10	Chores like folding clothes that seem to take little effort
Fairly light	11 to 12	Walking through the grocery store or other activities that require some effort but not enough to speed up your breathing
Somewhat hard	13 to 14	Brisk walking or other activities that require moderate effort and speed your HR and breathing but don't make you out of breath
Hard	15 to 16	Bicycling, swimming, or other activities that take vigorous effort and get the heart pounding and make breathing very fast
Very hard	17 to 18	The highest level of activity you can sustain
Very, very hard	19 to 20	A finishing kick in a race or other burst of activity that you can't maintain for long

HR: heart rate.
Source: (Borg, 1982).

free-living adult populations range from about 1.40 to 2.40. Although there is no physiological basis for establishing the duration of that period, it may be defined as one month or longer [Joint Food and Agriculture Organization (FAO) of the United Nations, World Health Organization (WHO) & United Nations University (UNU) (1985)].

PERCEIVED EXERTION (BORG RATING OF PERCEIVED EXERTION SCALE)

Another way for an individual to measure PA intensity is the Borg rating of perceived exertion scale (Borg, 1982).

The scale is based on an individual's experiences during PA, namely HR, breathing rate, sweating, and muscle fatigue. It includes a rating from 6, meaning "no exertion at all" to 20, a "maximal exertion" of effort (**Table 5.5**). It is important to know that this is a subjective measure. However, it may provide a good estimate of someone's HR during PA (Borg, 1982).

METABOLIC EQUIVALENTS OF TASK

One metabolic equivalent (1 MET) represents the amount of oxygen used during resting conditions or sitting quietly, and it is assumed to be 3.5 mL of oxygen per kg of body weight per minute

Table 5.6 Metabolic equivalents (METs) values of common physical activities classified as light, moderate, or vigorous intensity.

Very Light/Light (<3.0 METs)	Moderate (3.0–5.9 METs)	Vigorous (≥6.0 METs)
Walking	**Walking**	**Walking, jogging, and running**
Walking slowly around home, store, or office = 2.0[a]	Walking 3.0 mi · h^{-1} = 3.0[a] Walking at very brist pace 4.0 mi · h^{-1} = 5.0[a]	Walking at very, very brisk pace 4.5 mi · h^{-1} = 6.3[a] Walking/hiking at moderate pace and grade with no or light pack (<10 lb) = 7.0 Hiking at steep grades and pack 10–42 lb = 7.5–9.0 Jogging at 5 mi · h^{-1} = 8.0[a] Jogging at 6 mi · h^{-1} = 10.0[a] Running at 7 mi · h^{-1} = 11.5[a]
Household and occupation	**Household and occupation**	**Household and occupation**
Standing performing light work, such as making bed, washing dishes, ironing, preparing food, or store clerk = 2.0–2.5	Cleaning, heavy — washing windows, car, clean garage = 3.0 Sweeping floors or carpet, vacuuming, mopping — 3.0–3.5 Carpentry — general = 3.6 Carrying and stacking wood = 5.5 Mowing lawn — walk power mower = 5.5	Shoveling sand, coal, etc. = 7.0 Carrying heavy loads, such as bricks = 7.5 Heavy farming, such as bailing hay — 8.0 Shoveling, digging ditches = 8.5
Leisure time and sports	**Leisure time and sports**	**Leisure time and sports**
Arts and crafts, playing cards = 1.5 Billiards = 2.5 Boating — power = 2.5 Croquet = 2.5 Darts — 2.5 Fishing — sitting — 2.5 Playing most musical instruments = 2.0–2.5	Badminton — recreational = 4.5 Basketball — shooting around = 4.5 Dancing — ballroom slow = 3.0; ballroom fast = 4.5 Fishing from riverbank and walking = 4.0 Golf — walking, pulling clubs = 4.3 Sailing boat, wind surfing = 3.0 Table tennis = 4.0 Tennis doubles = 5.0 Volleyball — noncompetitive = 3.0–4.0	Bicycling on flat — light (10 – 12 mi · h^{-1}) = 6.0 Basketball game = 8.0 Bicycling on flat — moderate effort (12 – 14 mi · h^{-1}) = 8.0; fast (14 – 16 mi · h^{-1}) = 10.0 Skiing cross-country — slow (2.5 mi · h^{-1}) = 7.0; fast (5.0 – 7.9 mi · h^{-1}) = 9.0 Soccer — casual = 7.0; competitive = 10.0 Swimming leisurely = 6.0[b]; swimming — moderate/ hard = 8.0 – 11.0[b] Tennis singles — 8.0 Volleyball — competitive at gym or beach = 8.0

[a] On flat, hard surface.
[b] MET values can vary substantially between individuals.
Source: (Liguori, 2020).

(3.5 mL O$_2$/kg/min). Thus, tasks that require twice that amount (7 ml O$_2$/kg/min) require 2 METs and those triple the amount of oxygen require 3 METs, and so on.

A sample of select activities in METs for each of the intensity rates is presented in **Table 5.6** (Liguori, 2020).

METs are an easy, useful, and standardized way to describe the absolute intensity of several physical activities (Liguori, 2020). Absolute intensity is the amount of energy needed for an activity without considering the cardio-respiratory fitness or aerobic capacity of an individual. Absolute intensity is expressed in METs. Conversely, relative intensity is the level of effort based on the individual's level of cardio-respiratory fitness (Piercy et al., 2018), and it is expressed as either the maximal oxygen uptake (VO$_2$max, the maximum amount of oxygen used in 1 minute), or maximal heart rate (HRmax).

Any kind of PA can be performed at a variety of intensities. According to the current Physical Activity Guidelines for Americans, published in 2018 (Piercy et al., 2018), the absolute rates of energy expenditure during PA are considered as light, moderate, or vigorous (high) intensity.

According to the most recent WHO definition of PA, an energy expenditure of 1 MET refers to the REE. Therefore, sedentary behaviors are defined as any waking behaviors characterized by an energy expenditure ≤ 1.5 METs in a sitting, reclining, or lying position (Tremblay et al., 2017a). Indicators of sedentary behaviors are usually screen time and sitting time.

Light intensity activities are defined as activities performed at or under 3 METs, which require the least amount of effort compared to moderate and vigorous activities. Some examples include walking slowly (i.e., shopping, walking around the office), doing household shores (e.g., preparing food, and washing dishes) or activities of daily living (e.g., sitting at your computer, making the bed, eating).

Moderate-intensity activities are activities that require 3.0 to 5.9 METs. Examples include walking briskly, playing doubles tennis, raking the yard, slow dancing, or washing windows.

Vigorous-intensity activities are defined as activities that require 6.0 or more METs. Vigorous activities are performed using the highest amount of oxygen consumption to complete the activity. Examples include running, jogging, playing soccer, swimming, shoveling snow, and carrying heavy loads.

An easy and practical way to determine whether an activity is of moderate or vigorous intensity is the talk test. While performing a moderate-intensity activity, an individual can talk, but not sing. However, during a vigorous-intensity activity, they cannot say more than a few words without taking a breath.

Aerobic capacity decreases with age after peaking in young adulthood. Therefore, relative intensity is a better guide for older adults than absolute intensity.

VO_2MAX

Maximal oxygen uptake (VO_2max) is one of the most widely used measurements in exercise science. The VO_2max measurement applies from elite athletes to individuals with several pathologic conditions. It is considered the gold standard for assessing a person's cardio-respiratory fitness. People who present with a low VO_2max have an increased risk of premature death and developing several NCDs, whereas individuals with a high VO_2max have a lower likelihood of developing NCDs, all-cause mortality, and coronary artery disease (Buttar, Saboo, & Kacker, 2019).

The VO_2max is the maximum amount of oxygen (or true maximum aerobic capacity) that the body can use during work, and the value does not change despite an increase in workload over time. This can be established using direct or indirect methods. VO_2max is expressed as liters per minute (L/min), an absolute value, or in milliliters of oxygen per kilogram (kg) of body weight per minute (ml/kg/min) as the relative VO_2max.

In the direct method, VO_2max is estimated in laboratories by trained personnel using elaborate, expensive equipment. Individuals are submitted to an ergometric test with progressive loads to analyze their pulmonary ventilation by measuring inspired oxygen (O_2) and expired carbon dioxide (CO_2) through breath analysis.

The individual breathes room air via a mouthpiece (with the nose occluded) that is connected by plastic tubes to an automated, computerized system called a metabolic cart. The mouthpiece is designed to allow the expired air (or a sample of it) to enter the metabolic cart where it is analyzed for its O_2 and CO_2 content. After resting samples are taken, the individual is subjected to a standardized exercise protocol on a treadmill or stationary bike (**Figure 5.2**) (Rusdiana, 2020). The exercise begins at a very low workload and increases every 2 to 3 minutes, depending on the exercise protocol. The workload is determined by a standardized and progressive increase in the speed and/or elevation of a treadmill or the increased resistance of a bike. HR and oxygen uptake are continuously monitored and recorded. Blood pressure is measured and recorded every 2 to 3 minutes.

Exercise protocols are designed to fatigue most people within 10 to 12 minutes. When the individual reaches fatigue, the test is terminated. This is the maximal aerobic capacity of the individual. The oxygen used by the body at the point of fatigue is the individual's VO_2max, which is expressed in L/min or ml/kg/min.

The advantage of measuring VO_2max is its high accuracy, since it allows the assessment of an individual's exercise intensity based on a measured—not estimated—aerobic capacity. Its high cost and time requirements make it prohibitive for the population at large, so this method is mostly used in patients with specific needs and for research purposes.

Since the VO_2max is not practical for measuring the exercise intensity during training, indirect methods are used instead. These methods include field tests, estimating a person's aerobic capacity based on their HR (which corresponds to the percentage of oxygen consumption), their distance covered, and/or their time completing a trial.

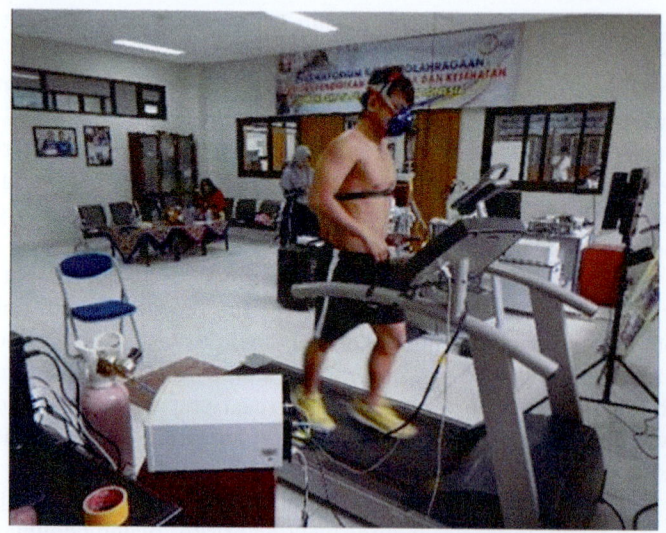

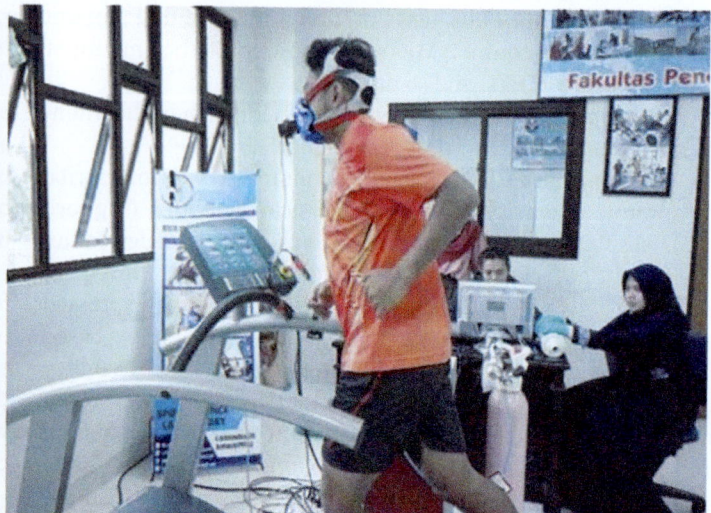

FIGURE 5.2 VO_2max test with direct measurement in badminton. Source: (Rusdiana, 2020).

PERCENT OF MAXIMUM HEART RATE

The easiest and most straightforward method to establish exercise intensity is to measure the percentage of the maximum heart rate (HRmax). This method is based on the concept that the HR increases linearly with an increase in workload and oxygen consumption (**Figure 5.3**).

Theoretically, when the VO_2max is achieved, HRmax is also achieved. Thus, a percentage of the individual's HRmax can be used to establish their desired exercise intensity (**Table 5.7**).

The HRmax of an individual can be easily estimated, with an acceptable degree of accuracy, by subtracting the individual's age from 220.

$$HRmax = 220 - age$$

Table 5.7 Average HRs by age.

Age (years)	Moderate intensity (Target: 50%-70%)	Vigorous intensity (Target: 70%-85%)	Average maximum HR (100%)
20	100–140	140–170	200
30	95–133	133–162	190
35	93–130	130–157	185
40	90–126	126–153	180
45	88–123	123–149	175
50	85–119	119–145	170
55	83–116	116–140	165
60	80–112	112–136	160
65	78–109	109–132	155
70	75–105	105–128	150

HR: heart rate.
Source: Adapted from American Heart Association.

For example, for a 20-year-old individual, the HRmax will be 200 beats per minute (bpm; 220−20), and for a 50-year-old, the HRmax will be 170 bpm (220−50).

Table 5.8 summarizes examples for absolute and relative intensities at different levels of intensity based on METs, % HRmax, the Borg scale score, and the talk test (Visseren et al., 2021).

HEART RATE RESERVE METHOD (KARVONEN METHOD)

Another way to determine the exercise HR is the heart rate reserve (HRR) method, the Karvonen method (Karvonen, 1957). It is more precise because it considers the individual's resting HR. The exercise intensity used for this method is 60% to 80% of the HRmax. There are five steps to determine the exercise intensity using the HRR method:

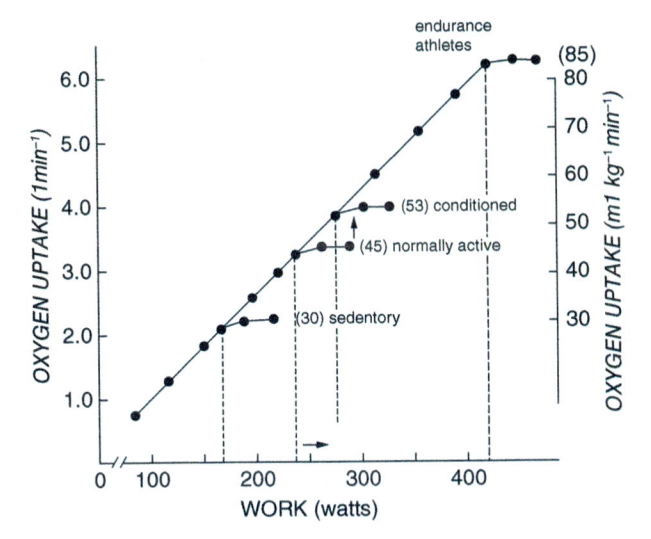

FIGURE 5.3 The relationship between exercise intensity and oxygen uptake is similar in human subjects with different levels of physical conditioning, but their maximal oxygen uptakes are quite different. Values for oxygen consumption are expressed in l/min (left y-axis) and ml × min^{-1} × kg^{-1} (right y-axis). Source: (Adapted from Laughlin, 1999).

Table 5.8 Classification of physical-activity intensity and examples of absolute and relative intensity levels.

	Absolute Intensity		Relative Intensity		
Intensity	MET[1]	Examples	%HRmax	RPE (Borg scale score)	Talk Test
Light	1.1–2.9	Walking <4.7 km/h, light household work.	57–63	10–11	
Moderate	3.0–5.9	Walking at moderate or brisk pace (4.1–6.5 km/h), slow cycling (15 km/h), painting/decorating, vacuuming, gardening (mowing lawn), golf (pulling clubs in trolley), tennis (doubles), ballroom dancing, water aerobics.	64–76	12–13	Breathing is faster but compatible with speaking full sentences.
Vigorous	≥6	Race-walking, jogging or running, bicycling >15 km/h, heavy gardening (continuous digging or hoeing), swimming laps, tennis (singles).	77–95	14–17	Breathing very hard, incompatible with carrying on a conversation comfortably.

[1] MET is estimated as the energy cost of a given activity divided by REE: 1 MET = 3.5 mL oxygen kg^{-1} min^{-1} VO_2. %HRmax = percentage of measured or estimated maximum heart rate (220 - age); MET = metabolic equivalent of task; RPE = rating of perceived exertion (Borg scale 620); VO_2 = oxygen consumption.
Source: (Visseren et al., 2021).

1. Calculate the HRmax of an individual by subtracting their age from 220.
2. Determine the resting HR after resting for 5 minutes.
3. Subtract the resting HR from the HRmax to determine the HRR.
4. Multiply the HRR by 0.6 or 60% and add the resting HR to that number. This is the lower limit of the exercise HR.
5. Multiply the HRR by 0.80 or 80% and add the resting HR to determine the higher limit of the exercise HR.

The 60% to 80% exercise heart rate values derived from the HRR method are associated with the heart rate that corresponds to 60% to 80% of the directly measured VO_2max for most physically fit individuals. However, the method overestimates the intensity for low fit individuals.

Example:

A 50-year-old with a resting HR of 70 bpm.
HRmax = 220 − 50
= 170 bpm

HRR = HRmax − resting HR
= 170 − 70
= 100 bpm

Exercise Heart Rate
Lower Limit = (HRR × 0.60) + resting HR (100 × 0.60)
= 60 + 70
= 130 bpm

Upper Limit = (HRR × 0.80) + resting HR (100 × 0.80)
= 80 + 70
= 150 bpm

VO_2 RESERVE METHOD

To correct for the overestimation of intensity for low-fitness individuals, Swain and Franklin (Swain & Franklin, 2002) proposed using the difference between VO_2max and the resting O_2 uptake (VO_2 reserve) as a more accurate method to estimate exercise intensity.

When the VO_2 reserve method is applied, the association becomes stronger across all fitness levels. That is, 60% of the HRR corresponds very closely to the HR at 60% of VO_2 reserve. For example, let us assume that the VO_2max value of an individual is 40 ml/kg/min. Sixty percent of that value is 24 ml/kg/min. According to the VO_2 reserve method:

VO_2 reserve = VO_2 max − 3.5
= 40 − 3.5 ml/kg/min
= 36.5 ml/kg/min

Thus, 60% of VO_2 reserve = $(36.5 \text{ ml/kg/min} \times 0.60)$
= 21.9 ml/kg/min
+ 3.5 ml/kg/min (at rest)
= 25.4 ml/kg/min

EXERCISE DURATION

Exercise duration is inversely related to intensity of the activity and, therefore, intensity and duration can interact to produce the desired results. It is also possible that a high-intensity, low-duration activity can yield similar results if the intensity for the same activity is reduced, and the duration increased. Accordingly, manipulations in duration and intensity can be applied for different populations to make exercise safe while achieving the desired health benefits.

The 2010 WHO recommendations (World Health Organization, 2010) only specified minimum weekly thresholds, however, current WHO recommendations (Bull, 2020) suggest a weekly range of recommended aerobic activity volume. Moreover, moderate-intensity aerobic exercise is recommended in any duration, which highlights the value of total PA volume, irrespective of bout length, which differs from the 2010 requirement for bouts of at least 10 min.

Longer exercise durations offer added health and physical performance benefits (muscular and cardiovascular endurance). However, the interaction between exercise intensity and duration is also important. Generally speaking, the higher the exercise intensity, the lower the duration will be and *vice versa*. Thus, the cost of any given activity can be similar or identical to a different combination of exercise intensity and duration.

EXERCISE FREQUENCY

The frequency of exercise, i.e., the number of days per week performing a PA is another important exercise component. The Physical Activity Guidelines for Americans (Piercy et al., 2018), the American College of Sports Medicine (Liguori, 2020), and other health organizations (Weggemans et al., 2018) recommend that exercise be spread throughout the week. There is evidence to support that the more frequent the activity occurs, the more health benefits exist, although the relative benefits tend to diminish at higher levels of PA.

Current RCTs use PA programs that repeat exercises more than once a week (Weggemans et al., 2018), suggesting that activity on more than one day produces certain benefits. However, other schemes could also work, especially for specific populations, such as older adults. As it will be discussed in **Unit 3**.

EXERCISE VOLUME

Exercise volume is the byproduct of all exercise components. That is, exercise volume is the outcome of: (i) exercise intensity, (ii) exercise duration, and (iii) frequency.

In general, a long-duration and low-intensity exercise can yield similar benefits as those of a short-duration and high-intensity, if the exercise volumes are similar. Therefore, daily walks can be as effective in yielding health benefits as jogging three times per week. Thus, when conducting exercise-related research, one must be mindful of the total volume of exercise achieved.

KEY POINTS

- According to the 2020 WHO guidelines, physical activity (PA) is defined as "any bodily movement produced by skeletal muscles that requires energy expenditure".
- In terms of mode, there are four domains of physical activity: 1) occupational, 2) domestic, 3) transportation/utilitarian, and 4) leisure time.
- PA is commonly quantified by determining energy expenditure for physical activity.
- Total energy expenditure (TEE) represents the total energy that a person expends in a day for essential for life processes (e.g., to digest, absorb, and convert food as well as exercise).
- Exercise energy expenditure is required for intentional (e.g., sports-related) PA and accounts for between 0% and 10% of total energy expenditure, although in extremely active individuals, it may constitute up to 60 to 70% of TEE.
- Non-exercise activity thermogenesis (NEAT) (e.g., daily living activities, fidgeting, maintenance of posture) accounts for the remaining roughly 20% of TEE.
- Physical activity can be expressed either in kilocalories (kcal) or METs.
- The mean physical-activity level of a day is derived from the multiplication of the energy cost of each activity (expressed as multiples of basal metabolic rate, or physical-activity ratio (PAR) with the time spent in each activity.
- One metabolic equivalent (1 MET) represents the amount of oxygen used during resting conditions or sitting quietly, and it is assumed to be 3.5 mL of oxygen per kg of body weight per minute (3.5 mL O_2/kg/min).
- Absolute intensity is the amount of energy needed for an activity without accounting for the cardio-respiratory fitness or aerobic capacity of an individual, and it is expressed in METs.
- Relative intensity is the level of effort based on an individual's level of cardio-respiratory fitness.
- According to the current Physical Activity Guidelines for Americans, published in 2018, the absolute rates of energy expenditure during PA are considered as light, moderate, or vigorous (high) intensity.
- The talk test is an easy and practical way to determine whether an activity is of moderate or vigorous intensity.
- VO_2max is the maximum amount of oxygen (or true maximum aerobic capacity) the body can use during work, and the value does not change despite an increase in workload over time.
- The easiest and most straightforward method to establish exercise intensity is to measure the percentage of the maximum heart rate (HR_{max}), which is based on a linear increase of the HR with an increase in workload and oxygen consumption.
- According to 2020 WHO recommendations, a weekly range of moderate-intensity aerobic exercise of 150 to 300 minutes or vigorous intensity of 75 to 150 minutes along with 2 or more days of muscle-strengthening activities are recommended for the general population.
- The Physical Activity Guidelines for Americans, the American College of Sports Medicine, and other health organizations recommend that exercise is spread throughout the week.

SELF-ASSESSMENT QUESTIONS

1. Define structured physical activity.
2. Which components do you need to know to quantify physical activity?
3. State three methods to quantify physical-activity intensity.
4. Your resting energy expenditure is 1450 kcal/d and your total energy expenditure is 2380 kcal/day. Estimate your activity energy expenditure per day.
5. Your total energy expenditure is 2220 kcal/d and your basal metabolic rate is 1350 kcal/day. Estimate your average physical-activity level. Do you have a sedentary, active, or vigorous lifestyle?
6. According to the Borg rating of perceived exertion scale, you got a score of 9. How might you describe your exertion? Please give examples of activities under this score.
7. Indicate which activities require between 3.0 and 6.0 METs:
   (a) Walking around the office
   (b) Washing dishes
   (c) Running at 7 mi . h^{-1}
   (d) Playing doubles tennis
   (e) Washing windows
   (f) Jogging at 5 mi . h^{-1}
8. For an individual of 52 years old, calculate their HR_{max}.
9. How much moderate-intensity aerobic exercise duration would you recommended to an individual?
10. Define exercise volume.

REFERENCES

Borg, G. A. (1982). Psychophysical bases of perceived exertion. *Medicine & science in sports & exercise*.

Bull, F. C. A.-A., Salih S Biddle, Stuart Borodulin, Katja Buman, Matthew P Cardon, Greet Carty, Catherine Chaput, Jean Philippe Chastin, Sebastien Chou, Roger. (2020). World Health Organization 2020 guidelines on physical activity and sedentary behaviour. In (Vol. *54*, pp. 1451–1462): BMJ Publishing Group Ltd and British Association of Sport and Exercise Medicine.

Buttar, K. K., Saboo, N., & Kacker, S. (2019). A review: Maximal oxygen uptake (VO₂max) and its estimation methods. *IJPESH, 6*, 24–32.

Calcagno, M. K., Hana Alwarith, Jihad Burgess, Nora N Flores, Rosendo A Busta, Melissa L Barnard, Neal D. (2019). The thermic effect of food: a review. In (Vol. *38*, pp. 547–551): Taylor & Francis.

Caspersen, C. J. P., Kenneth E Christenson, Gregory M. (1985). Physical activity, exercise, and physical fitness: definitions and distinctions for health-related research. In (Vol. *100*, pp. 126): SAGE Publications.

Hills, A. P., Mokhtar, Najat Byrne, Nuala M (2014). Assessment of physical activity and energy expenditure: an overview of objective measures. In (Vol. *1*, pp. 5): Frontiers.

Joint Food and Agriculture Organization (FAO) of the United Nations, World Health Organization (WHO) & United Nations University (UNU) (1985). *Energy and protein requirements: report of a Joint FAO/WHO/UNU Expert Consultation [held in Rome from 5 to 17 October 1981]*: World Health Organization.

Karvonen, M. J. (1957). The effects of training on heart rate: A longitudinal study. *Ann med exp biol fenn, 35*, 307–315.

Laughlin, M. H. (1999). Cardiovascular response to exercise. *Advances in physiology education, 277*(6), S244.

Liguori, G. (2020). ACSM's guidelines for exercise testing and prescription. In: Lippincott Williams & Wilkins.

World Health Organization, (2010). *Global recommendations on physical activity for health*: World Health Organization.

Piercy, K. L., Troiano, R. P., Ballard, R. M., Carlson, S. A., Fulton, J. E., Galuska, D. A., . . . Olson, R. D. (2018). The physical activity guidelines for Americans. *JAMA, 320*(19), 2020–2028.

Rusdiana, A. (2020). Analysis Differences of VO₂max between Direct and Indirect Measurement in Badminton, Cycling and Rowing. *International Journal of Applied Exercise Physiology, 9*(3), 162–170.

Strath, S. J., Kaminsky, Leonard A Ainsworth, Barbara E Ekelund, Ulf Freedson, Patty S Gary, Rebecca A Richardson, Caroline R, Smith, D. T., & Swartz, A. M. (2013). Guide to the assessment of physical activity: clinical and research applications: a scientific statement from the American Heart Association. *Circulation, 128*(20), 2259–2279.

Swain, D. P., & Franklin, B. A. (2002). VO₂ reserve and the minimal intensity for improving cardiorespiratory fitness. *Med Sci Sports Exerc, 34*(1).

Tremblay, M. S., Aubert, S., Barnes, J. D., Saunders, T. J., Carson, V., Latimer-Cheung, A. E., . . . Chinapaw, M. J. (2017a). Sedentary behavior research network (SBRN)–terminology consensus project process and outcome. *International journal of behavioral nutrition and physical activity, 14*(1), 1–17.

Visseren, F. L., Mach, F., Smulders, Y. M., Carballo, D., Koskinas, K. C., Bäck, M., . . . & Williams, B. (2021). 2021 ESC Guidelines on cardiovascular disease prevention in clinical practice: Developed by the Task Force for cardiovascular disease prevention in clinical practice with representatives of the European Society of Cardiology and 12 medical societies With the special contribution of the European Association of Preventive Cardiology (EAPC). *European heart journal, 42*(34), 3227–3337.

Weggemans, R. M., Backx, F. J., Borghouts, L., Chinapaw, M., Hopman, M. T., Koster, A., . . . Mosterd, A. (2018). The 2017 Dutch physical activity guidelines. *International journal of behavioral nutrition and physical activity, 15*(1), 1–12.

FURTHER READING

Bibliography

Lightfoot, J. T., De Geus, E. J., Booth, F. W., Bray, M. S., Den Hoed, M., Kaprio, J., . . . & Bouchard, C. (2018). Biological/genetic regulation of physical activity level: consensus from GenBioPAC. *Medicine and Science in Sports and Exercise, 50*(4), 863. doi: 10.1249/MSS.0000000000001499.

Mendes, M. D. A., Da Silva, I., Ramires, V., Reichert, F., Martins, R., Ferreira, R., & Tomasi, E. (2018). Metabolic equivalent of task (METs) thresholds as an indicator of physical activity intensity. *PLoS one, 13*(7), e0200701.

Rimbach, R., Yamada, Y., Sagayama, H., Ainslie, P. N., Anderson, L. F., Anderson, L. J., . . . & Pontzer, H. (2022). Total energy expenditure is repeatable in adults but not associated with short-term changes in body composition. *Nature Communications, 13*(1), 1–8. doi: 10.1038/s41467-021-27246-z.

Tremblay, M. S., Aubert, S., Barnes, J. D., Saunders, T. J., Carson, V., Latimer-Cheung, A. E., . . . & Chinapaw, M. J. (2017b). Sedentary behavior research network (SBRN)–terminology consensus project process and outcome. *International Journal of Behavioral Nutrition and Physical Activity, 14*(1), 1–17.

Links

- https://www.cdc.gov/nccdphp/dnpa/physical/pdf/pa_intensity_table_2_1.pdf
- https://www.who.int/publications/i/item/9789240015128
- https://www.cdc.gov/physicalactivity/index.html
- https://www.shapeamerica.org/publications/resources/default.aspx?hkey=55103b9c-7979-4a38-a483-c1669fefbc6e
- https://www.fao.org/3/y5686e/y5686e00.htm#Contents
- https://www.who.int/news-room/fact-sheets/detail/physical-activity

Implications and Health Benefits of Physical Activity in Adults

CHAPTER 6

Introduction	79	Interventions to Increase Physical Activity	86
Physical Activity and Inactivity Estimations Worldwide	79	Key Points	88
		Self-assessment Questions	88
Sedentary Behavior	80	References	88
Premature All-cause Mortality	81	Further Reading	90
Health Impact of Physical Activity	81	Bibliography	90
Physical Activity Guidelines	83	Links	90

INTRODUCTION

The literature shows irrefutable evidence that document the health benefits of physical activity (PA). The common message within health promotion settings is to be physically active. Physical inactivity and sedentary behavior correlate with numerous chronic diseases as well as premature all-cause mortality. Several public health organizations as well as the World Health Organization (WHO) provide recommendations for the amount (frequency, intensity, duration) and types of PA for people in all age groups and those living with chronic conditions or disability.

In this chapter, we will discuss the estimations of physical activity/inactivity worldwide, the health effects of PA, and the current PA recommendations.

PHYSICAL ACTIVITY AND INACTIVITY ESTIMATIONS WORLDWIDE

There is increasing evidence of poor PA worldwide.

The estimates on insufficient PA in 2010 using data from 146 countries was 23.3%, with higher levels among women and older age groups. Pooled data from 358 surveys across 168 countries, including 1.9 million participants, showed that in 2016, the global age-standardized prevalence of insufficient PA increased to 27.5%, with a difference between sexes of more than 8 percentage points (i.e., 23.4% in men versus 31.7% in women) (Guthold, Stevens, Riley, & Bull, 2018). This practically means that more than one in four adults globally are physically inactive. This increase in physical inactivity correlates with technology advances including increased television viewing as well as computer, mobile device, and video game use (Anderson & Durstine, 2019).

Physical inactivity prevalence seems to increase with age: 25% of young adults aged 18 to 44 years, 33% of middle-aged adults aged 45 to 64 years, 36% of older adults aged 65 to 74 years, and 53% of the elderly aged ≥75 years are considered inactive (Anderson & Durstine, 2019).

The definition of physical inactivity has changed through the years, from failing to meet the previous recommendations—*30 min of moderate-intensity PA at least 5 days per week, 20 min of vigorous PA at least 3 days per week, or a combination of walking, moderate-intensity, and vigorous-intensity activities to total 600 MET minutes per week* (Pate et al., 1995)—to the current recommendations (US Department of Agriculture and US Department of Health and Human Services 2018; World Health Organization, 2020; World Health Organization, 2010)— *at least 150 min of moderate-to-vigorous-intensity physical activity per week regardless of over how many days activity is accumulated.* This has led to an artificial decline in the global prevalence of physical inactivity, although estimates, as mentioned previously are high (Ding Ding et al., 2020).

According to a 2010 WHO report (World Health Organization, 2010), insufficient PA is considered the fourth leading risk factor for mortality, leading to 3.2 million deaths and 32.1 million disability-adjusted life years (DALYs) (about 2.1% of global DALYs) annually. Individuals that are physically inactive have a 20% to 30% increased risk of all-cause mortality compared to those with at least 30 minutes of moderate-intensity PA most days of the week (World Health Organization, 2010).

Prevention and Management of Cardiovascular and Metabolic Disease: Diet, Physical Activity and Healthy Aging,
First Edition. Christina N. Katsagoni, Peter Kokkinos, and Labros S. Sidossis.
© 2023 John Wiley & Sons Ltd. Published 2023 by John Wiley & Sons Ltd.

There is a strong link between physical inactivity and major non-communicable diseases (NCDs). In high-income countries with a high prevalence of insufficient PA levels, high prevalence rates of NCDs also occur. Physical inactivity is directly responsible for 6% of the global burden of coronary heart disease (CHD), 7% of type 2 diabetes (T2D), and 10% of breast cancer. For instance, if a patient with T2D increases sedentary time by just 60min/day, independently of moderate-to-vigorous PA (MVPA), all-cause mortality will increase by 13% (Loprinzi & Sng, 2016). Similarly, patients with symptomatic chronic heart failure (HF), who are physically inactive have a greater risk of all-cause death and cardiac death (Doukky et al., 2016). Other health problems associated with physical inactivity are impaired circulation, osteoporosis, arthritis and/or other skeletal disabilities, diminished self-concept, a greater dependence on others for daily living, reduced opportunity and ability for normal social interactions, and an overall diminished quality of life (Anderson & Durstine, 2019).

Due to the strong association of physical inactivity with NCDs, member states of the WHO agreed to a 10% relative reduction in the prevalence of insufficient PA by 2025 as one of the nine global goals for the prevention and treatment of NCDs (**Figure 6.1**) (World Health Organization, 2021).

SEDENTARY BEHAVIOR

In 2012, the Sedentary Behavior Research Network proposed (González, Fuentes, & Márquez, 2017) a definition of sedentary behavior as waking behavior with an energy expenditure of ≤1.5 METs. The term 'sedentary' comes from the Latin '*sedere*' (to sit). Sedentary behavior, therefore, typically refers to sitting, lying, and reclining behaviors during waking hours rather than a simple absence of MVPA. The term 'physical inactivity' as already mentioned, describes the insufficient amounts of PA that are performed, that is, failing to meet specified PA guidelines (González et al., 2017).

US adults seem to spent 54.9% of their waking time, or 7.7 hours/day, in sedentary behaviors, while older adults aged ≥60 years spent about 60% of their waking time sedentary (Matthews et al., 2008). Accordingly, in Europe, an average of 40% of leisure time is spent watching TV. However, sufficient levels of MVPA does not automatically mean low levels of sedentary time and *vice versa*. Moreover, the inverse health effects of sedentary behaviors tend to persist, with some attenuation, after considering MVPA (Patterson et al., 2018).

There is strong evidence of a positive relationship between sedentary behavior and all-cause mortality, fatal and non-fatal cardiovascular disease (CVD), T2D (Wilmot et al., 2012), and

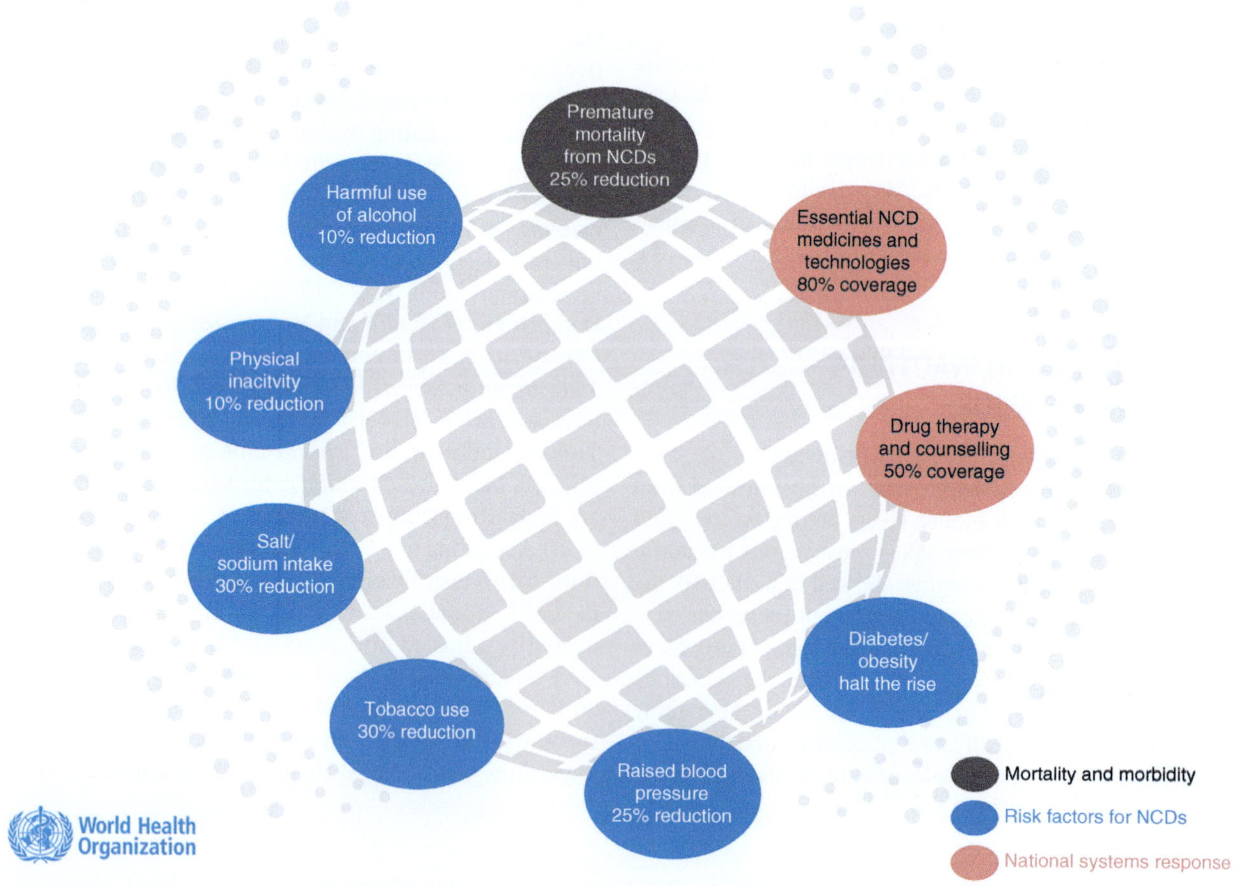

FIGURE 6.1 The set of nine voluntary global NCD targets for 2025; NCD = non-communicable diseases. Source: (World Health Organization, 2021)

metabolic syndrome (MetS). In addition, there is moderate evidence for incidence rates of ovarian, colon, and endometrial cancers with sedentary behavior (i.e., overall sitting time, sitting outside of work, and TV viewing).

PREMATURE ALL-CAUSE MORTALITY

The first epidemiological data that demonstrated a clear dose-response relationship between PA and lower risk for all-cause mortality was from the Harvard alumni study (Paffenbarger Jr, Hyde, Wing, & Hsieh, 1986). The study showed that all-cause mortality was lower among active individuals compared to less active participants; large risk reductions were found with relatively small changes in PA behavior (Paffenbarger Jr et al., 1986).

Since then, numerous meta-analyses and systematic reviews of epidemiological and interventional studies (Ekelund et al., 2016; Kraus et al., 2019; Ramakrishnan et al., 2021) have verified these early data.

More recently, a prospective study by Dohm and colleagues (Dohrn, Kwak, Oja, Sjöström, & Hagströmer, 2018) followed up with 851 women and men for 14.2 years (standard deviation of 1.9) during which time 79 deaths occurred (24 deaths from CVD, 27 from cancer, and 28 from other causes). Researchers showed that replacing 30 minutes/day of sedentary time with light-intensity PA was linked to a significant reduction in all-cause and CVD mortality risk. Replacing only 10 minutes of sedentary time with MVPA was associated with a reduction in CVD mortality risk. These results clearly suggest that replacing sedentary behavior with PA for the same amount of time could also impact all-cause mortality.

Any PA rather than none, is also beneficial for all-cause mortality, which may help those struggling to follow the guidelines to engage more with PA. In a systematic review and harmonized meta-analysis of eight observational studies (n = 36 383; mean age 62.6 years; 72.8% women), with a median follow-up of 5.8 years and 2149 (5.9%) deaths, Ekelund and colleagues (Ekelund et al., 2019) showed that any PA, regardless of intensity, and less time spent sedentary, were associated with a lower risk for premature mortality in a non-linear dose-response.

In conclusion, it seems that PA decreases remarkably the risk for premature all-cause mortality, even with relatively small participation.

HEALTH IMPACT OF PHYSICAL ACTIVITY

Routine PA is an effective method for the primary and secondary prevention of more than 25 chronic medical conditions and premature mortality (D. E. R. Warburton & Bredin, 2017). In particular, there is an inverse relationship between routine PA and CVD/coronary artery disease (CAD), hypertension, stroke, osteoporosis, T2D, MetS, obesity, and 13 types of cancers (breast, bladder, rectal, head and neck, colon, myeloma, myeloid leukemia, endometrial, gastric cardia, kidney, lung, liver, and esophageal adenocarcinoma) (Liguori & Medicine, 2020) (**Figure 6.2**). Data from interventional studies, large-scale population-based, and observational studies show strong evidence of a dose-response inverse relationship between these conditions and PA.

Of note, the greatest health benefits are observed in individuals who are physically inactive and become more physically active (D. E. Warburton, Nicol, & Bredin, 2006; D. E. R. Warburton & Bredin, 2019) (**Figure 6.3**) (D. E. Warburton & Bredin, 2016).

Moreover, the domain of PA seems to positively affect health. In a prospective cohort study including participants from 17 countries (Lear et al., 2017), both leisure-time and non-leisure-time PA were protective of mortality and CVD in low-, middle-, and high-income countries. Furthermore, occupational PA is protective of several NCDs, including some cancers. In an umbrella review of 23 health outcomes across 158 observational studies (Cillekens et al., 2020), those engaging in high versus low occupational PA had better health effects, considering multiple cancer outcomes (i.e., colon and prostate), ischemic stroke, CHD, and mental health (i.e., mental well-being and life satisfaction) (Cillekens et al., 2020). However, high occupational PA was associated with unfavorable health outcomes for all-cause mortality in men, mental ill health (i.e., depression and anxiety), osteoarthritis, and sleep quality and duration, suggesting a potential paradox. This observation received some criticism. The misclassification of occupational activities using simple questionnaires as well as incomplete adjustments for covariates, e.g., cigarette smoking and socio-economic status, may explain the observed paradox (Ding Ding et al., 2020).

In older adults, increased PA is linked to improved functional health, performance capabilities, mental health, sleep, and quality of life (autonomy and vitality) (D. Ding et al., 2020). Moreover, age-related losses of bone mineral density in women as well as hip fracture risk and falls are reduced (Chodzko-Zajko et al., 2009). PA is suggested to both prevent and improve cognitive function in terms of preventing and lowering both age-related cognitive decline and the risk for neurological disorders, such as Alzheimer's disease (Gheysen et al., 2018) (More will be discussed in **Unit 3**).

The mechanisms by which routine PA is thought to be effective in primary and secondary prevention strategies of chronic diseases include (Rhodes, Janssen, Bredin, Warburton, & Bauman, 2017):

- improved cardio-respiratory and health-related physical fitness,
- better exercise toleration and functional status,
- improved body composition (e.g., strategies against obesity, reduced central obesity, weight management),
- improved lipid profiles (e.g., reduced triglycerides, higher high-density lipoprotein (HDL) -cholesterol, lower low density lipoprotein (LDL)-to-HDL ratios, improved glucose parameters (e.g., glucose homeostasis, insulin resistance, insulin sensitivity),
- improved blood pressure,
- improved autonomic tone,

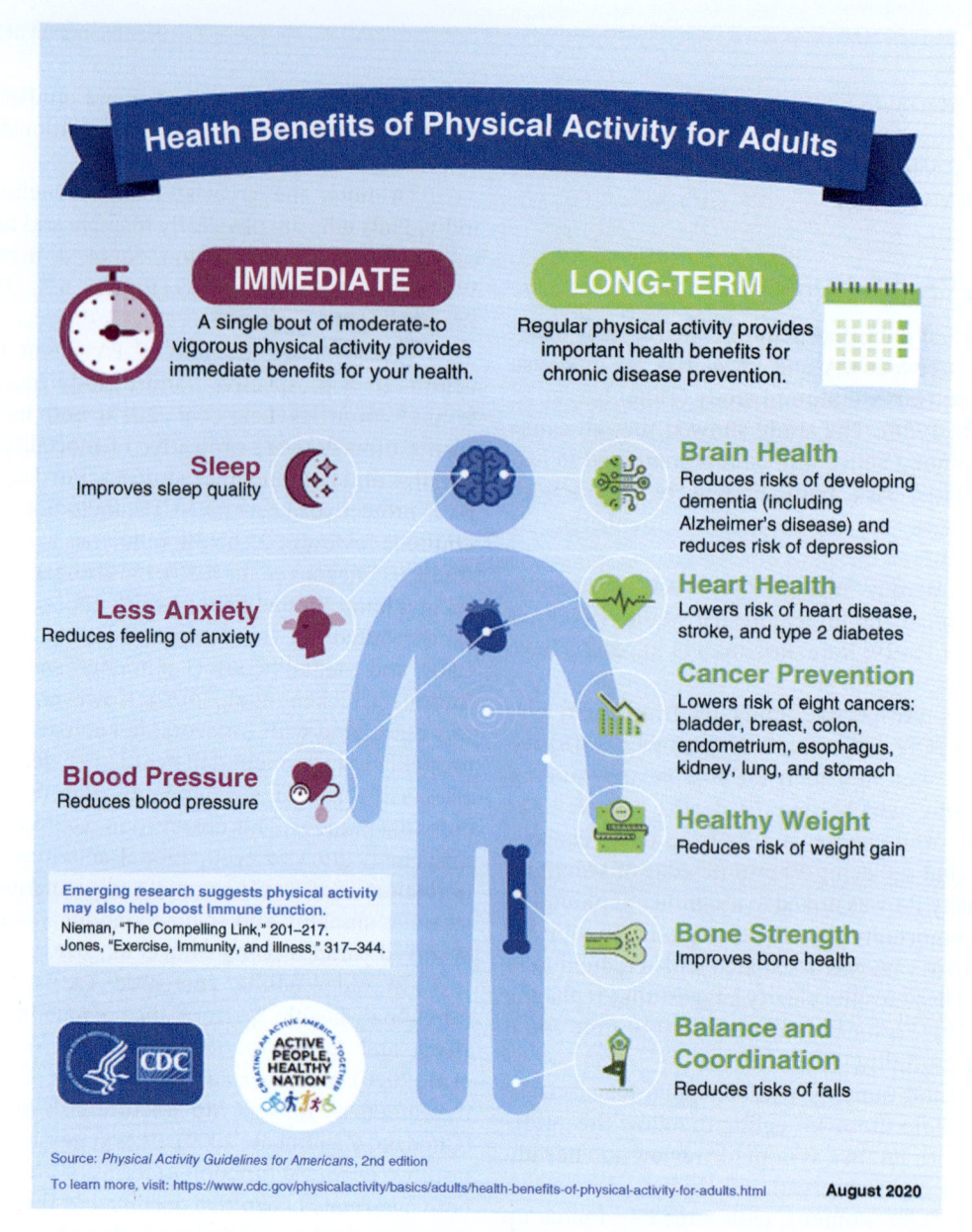

FIGURE 6.2 Health benefits of PA in adults. Source: CDC 2020 / US Department of Health & Human Services / Public domain.

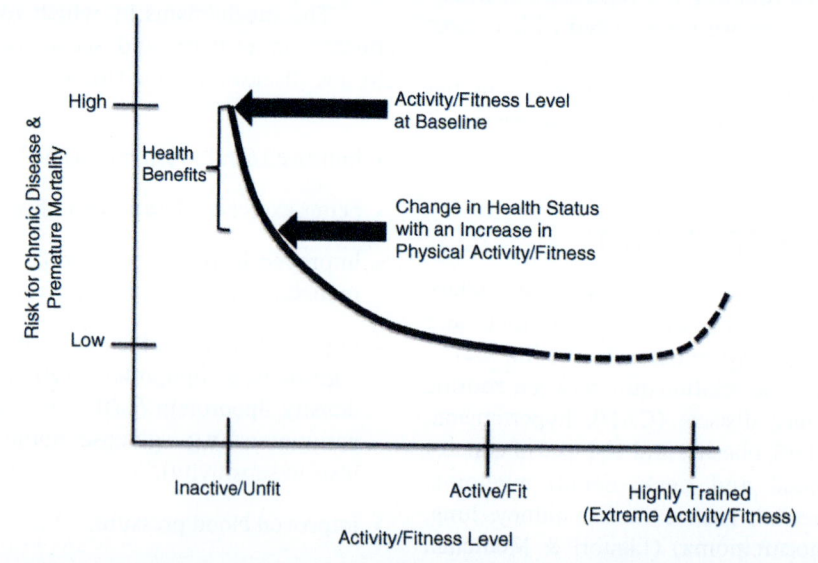

FIGURE 6.3 In individuals who are physically inactive/unfit, a small change in physical activity/fitness will lead to a significant improvement in health status, including a reduction in the risk for chronic disease and premature mortality. The dashed line represents the potential attenuation in health status seen in highly (extremely) trained endurance athletes. Source: (D. E. Warburton & Bredin, 2016 / with permission of Elsevier).

- better blood coagulation,
- improved coronary blood flow,
- augmented cardiac function,
- improved endothelial function,
- less systemic inflammation, and
- improved psychological well-being (e.g., improvements in stress, anxiety, and depression).

PHYSICAL ACTIVITY GUIDELINES

The 2020 WHO Guidelines on Physical Activity and Sedentary Behavior (Bull et al., 2020) provide recommendations on the amount (frequency, intensity, duration) and types of PA for children, adolescents, adults, and older adults as well as pregnant and postpartum women and people living with chronic conditions or disability (**Figure 6.4**) (World Health Organization, 2020).

These guidelines (**Table 6.1**) (Bull et al., 2020) include some major developments compared to previous published guidelines. They address, for the first time, the health impact of sedentary behavior, support the evidence for additional health benefits (e.g., improved cognitive health, health-related quality of life, mental health, and sleep) apart from previously known health effects on specific conditions, provide recommendations for specific groups, i.e., pregnant and postpartum women and people living with chronic conditions or disability, while clearly supporting the notion that "any physical activity is better than none" (D. Ding et al., 2020).

Previously published PA guidelines (**Figure 6.5**) focused mainly on continuous vigorous aerobic exercise to improve performance or cardiac rehabilitation. The American College of Sports Medicine (ACSM) has published guidelines for PA since 1975. Through the years, the PA recommendations of the ACSM were focused on how much exercise someone following the recommendations should do, suggesting that a PA level that does not meet these specific criteria is of limited or no value.

Indeed, most international guidelines recommend MVPA of 150 min/wk. However, many health agencies translated these recommendations to indicate that this is the minimum volume of activity required for health benefits. However, recent data, support that this threshold-centered messaging is not evidence-based and may create an unnecessary barrier to those who could benefit greatly from simply becoming more active (D. E. R. Warburton & Bredin, 2017).

There is increasing evidence for the health benefits of moderate-intensity PA (i.e., walking), while guidelines show a shift from exercise (i.e., planned and structured) to PA, as part of daily living (Bull et al., 2020). Moreover, the benefits of light-intensity PA are now clearly stated, highlighting the value of replacing sedentary time, regardless of the time spent, with any duration of light-intensity PA.

In the prospective cohort study by LaCroix and colleagues (LaCroix et al., 2019), scientists aimed to investigate whether higher levels of light PA were associated with reduced risks of CHD or CVD in older women. According to their findings, the highest quartile of light PA was associated with a 42% reduced risk of myocardial infarction or CHD and a 22% reduced risk of

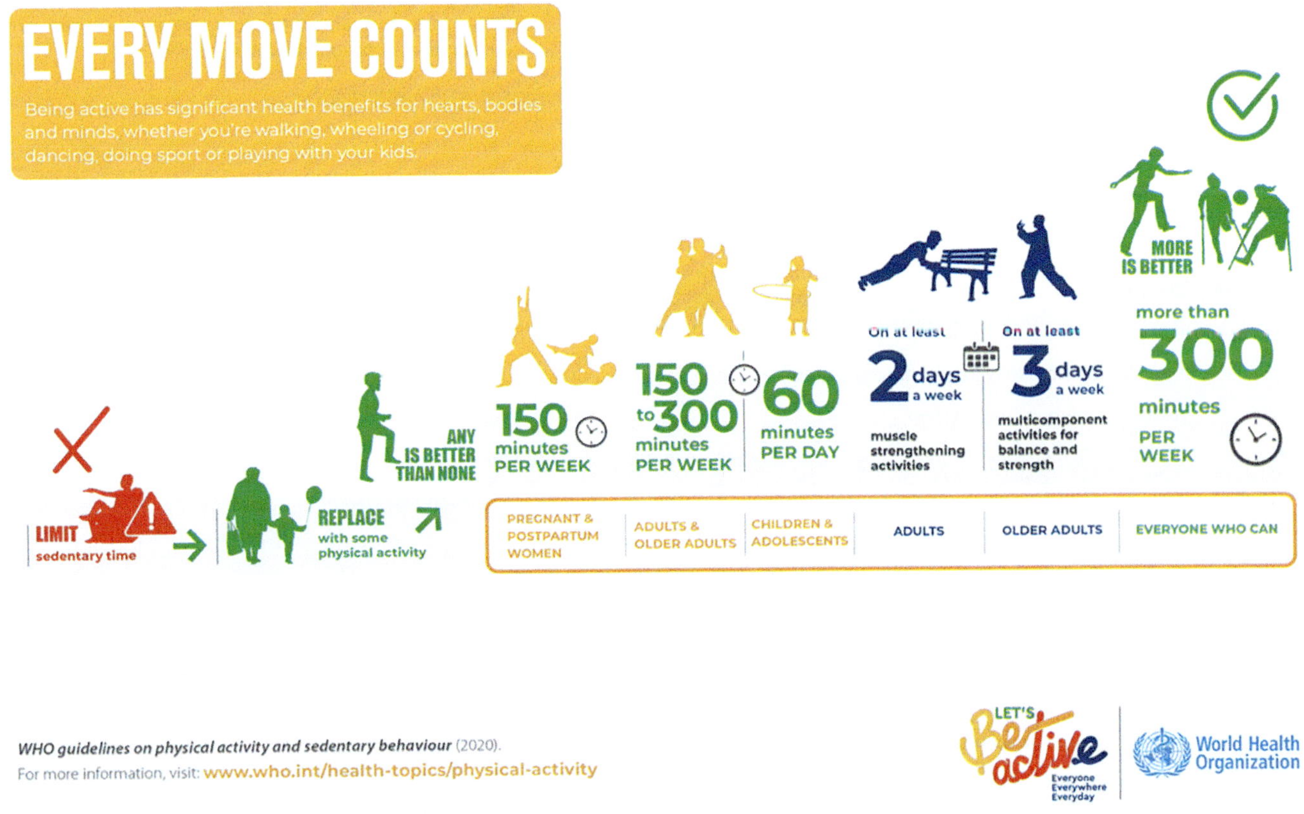

FIGURE 6.4 2020 World Health Organization physical-activity guidelines. Source: (World Health Organization, 2020).

Table 6.1 Summary of WHO guidelines on PA and sedentary behavior.

These public health guidelines are for all populations across the age groups from 5 years of age and above, irrespective of gender, cultural background or should try to meet these recommendations where possible and as able.

	Physical activity	Sedentary behaviour
Children and adolescents *(aged 5–17 years), including those living with disability*	In children and adolescents, physical activity confers benefits for the following health outcomes: physical fitness (cardiorespiratory and muscular fitness), cardiometabolic health (blood pressure, dyslipidaemia, glucose and insulin resistance), bone health, cognitive outcomes (academic performance, executive function) and mental health (reduced symptoms of depression) and reduced adiposity. It is recommended that: • Children and adolescents should do at least an average of 60 min/day of moderate-to-vigorous intensity, mostly aerobic, physical activity, across the week; • Vigorous-intensity aerobic activities, as well as those that strengthen muscle and bone should be incorporated at least 3 days a week. *Strong recommendation*	In children and adolescents, higher amounts of sedentary behaviour are associated with detrimental effects on the following health outcomes: fitness and cardiometabolic health, adiposity, behavioural conduct/pro-social behaviour and sleep duration. It is recommended that: • Children and adolescents should limit the amount of time spent being sedentary, particularly the amount of recreational screen time. *Strong recommendation*
Adults *(aged 18–64 years) including those with chronic conditions and those living with disability*	In adults, physical activity confers benefits for the following health outcomes: all-cause mortality, cardiovascular disease mortality, incident hypertension, incident type 2 diabetes, incident site-specific cancers, mental health (reduced symptoms of anxiety and depression), cognitive health and sleep ; measures of adiposity may also improve. It is recommended that: • All adults should undertake regular physical activity; • Adults should do at least 150-300 min of moderate-intensity aerobic physical activity, or at least 75-150 min of vigorous-intensity aerobic physical activity, or an equivalent combination of moderate-intensity and vigorous-intensity activity throughout the week for substantial health benefits; • Adults should also do muscle-strengthening activities at moderate or greater intensity that involve all major muscle groups on 2 or more days a week, as these provide additional health benefits. *Strong recommendation* • Adults may increase moderate-intensity aerobic physical activity to >300 min, or do >150 min of vigorous-intensity aerobic physical activity, or an equivalent combination of moderate-intensity and vigorous-intensity activity throughout the week for additional health benefits (when not contraindicated for those with chronic conditions). *Conditional recommendation*	In adults, higher amounts of sedentary behaviour are associated with detrimental effects on the following health outcomes: all-cause mortality, cardiovascular disease mortality and cancer mortality and incidence of cardiovascular disease, type 2 diabetes and cancer. It is recommended that: • Adults should limit the amount of time spent being sedentary. Replacing sedentary time with physical activity of any intensity (including light intensity) provides health benefits; • To help reduce the detrimental effects of high levels of sedentary behaviour on health, adults should aim to do more than the recommended levels of moderate-to-vigorous physical activity. *Strong recommendation*
Older adults *(aged 65 years and older) including those with chronic conditions and those living with disability*	In older adults, physical activity also helps prevent falls and falls-related injuries and declines in bone health and functional ability. It is recommended that: As for adults, plus • As part of their weekly physical activity, older adults should do varied multicomponent physical activity that emphasises functional balance and strength training at moderate or greater intensity on 3 or more days a week, to enhance functional capacity and to prevent falls. *Strong recommendation*	As for adults *Strong recommendation*

(Continued)

Table 6.1 (Continued)

These public health guidelines are for all populations across the age groups from 5 years of age and above, irrespective of gender, cultural background or should try to meet these recommendations where possible and as able.

	Physical activity	Sedentary behaviour
Pregnant and postpartum women	In women, physical activity during pregnancy and the postpartum period confers benefits for the following maternal and fetal health outcomes: reduced risk of preeclampsia, gestational hypertension, gestational diabetes, excessive gestational weight gain, delivery complications and postpartum depression and no increase in risk of stillbirth, newborn complications or adverse effects on birth weight. It is recommended that all pregnant and postpartum women without contraindication should: • undertake regular physical activity throughout pregnancy and post partum; • do at least 150 min of moderate-intensity aerobic physical activity throughout the week for substantial health benefits; • incorporate a variety of aerobic and muscle-strengthening activities. Adding gentle stretching may also be beneficial. In addition: Women who, before pregnancy, habitually engaged in vigorous-intensity aerobic activity or who were physically active can continue these activities during pregnancy and the postpartum period. *Strong recommendation*	• Pregnant and postpartum women should limit the amount of time spent being sedentary. Replacing sedentary time with physical activity of any intensity (including light intensity) provides health benefits. *Strong recommendation*

Additional explanatory and practical notes:

Some physical activity is better than none.

If not currently meeting these recommendations, doing some physical activity will bring benefits to health. Start with small amounts of physical activity and gradually increase frequency, intensity and duration over time. Pre-exercise medical clearance is generally unnecessary for individuals without contraindications prior to beginning light-intensity or moderate-intensity physical activity not exceeding the demands of brisk walking or everyday living.

It is important to provide all children and adolescents with safe and equitable opportunities and encouragement to participate in physical activities that are appropriate for their age and ability, that are enjoyable, and that offer variety.

Older adults should be as physically active as their functional ability allows and adjust their level of effort for physical activity relative to their level of fitness.

When not able to meet the recommendations, adults with chronic conditions should aim to engage in physical activity according to their abilities. Adults with chronic conditions may wish to consult with a physical activity specialist or healthcare professional for advice on the types and amounts of activity appropriate for their individual needs, abilities, functional limitations/complications, medications and overall treatment plan.

If pregnant and postpartum women are not currently meeting these recommendations, doing some physical activity will bring benefits to health. They should start with small amounts of physical activity and gradually increase frequency, intensity and duration over time. Pelvic floor muscle training may be performed on a daily basis to reduce the risk of urinary incontinence.

Additional on safety considerations when undertaking physical activity for pregnant women are:

• Avoid physical activity during excessive heat, especially with high humidity;
• Stay hydrated by drinking water before, during and after physical activity;
• Avoid participating in activities which involve physical contact, pose a high risk of falling or might limit oxygenation (such as activities at high altitude, when not normally living at altitude);
• Avoid activities in supine position after the first trimester of pregnancy;
• Pregnant women should be informed by their healthcare provider of the danger signs for when to stop, or limit physical activity and to consult a qualified healthcare provider immediately if they occur.

Return to physical activity gradually after delivery and in consultation with a healthcare provider in the case of delivery by caesarean section.

There are no major risks to people living with disability engaging in physical activity when it is appropriate to an individual's current activity level, health status and physical function and the health benefits accrued outweigh the risks. People living with disability may need to consult a healthcare professional or other physical active specialist to help determine the type and amount of activity appropriate for them.

Source: (Bull et al., 2020).

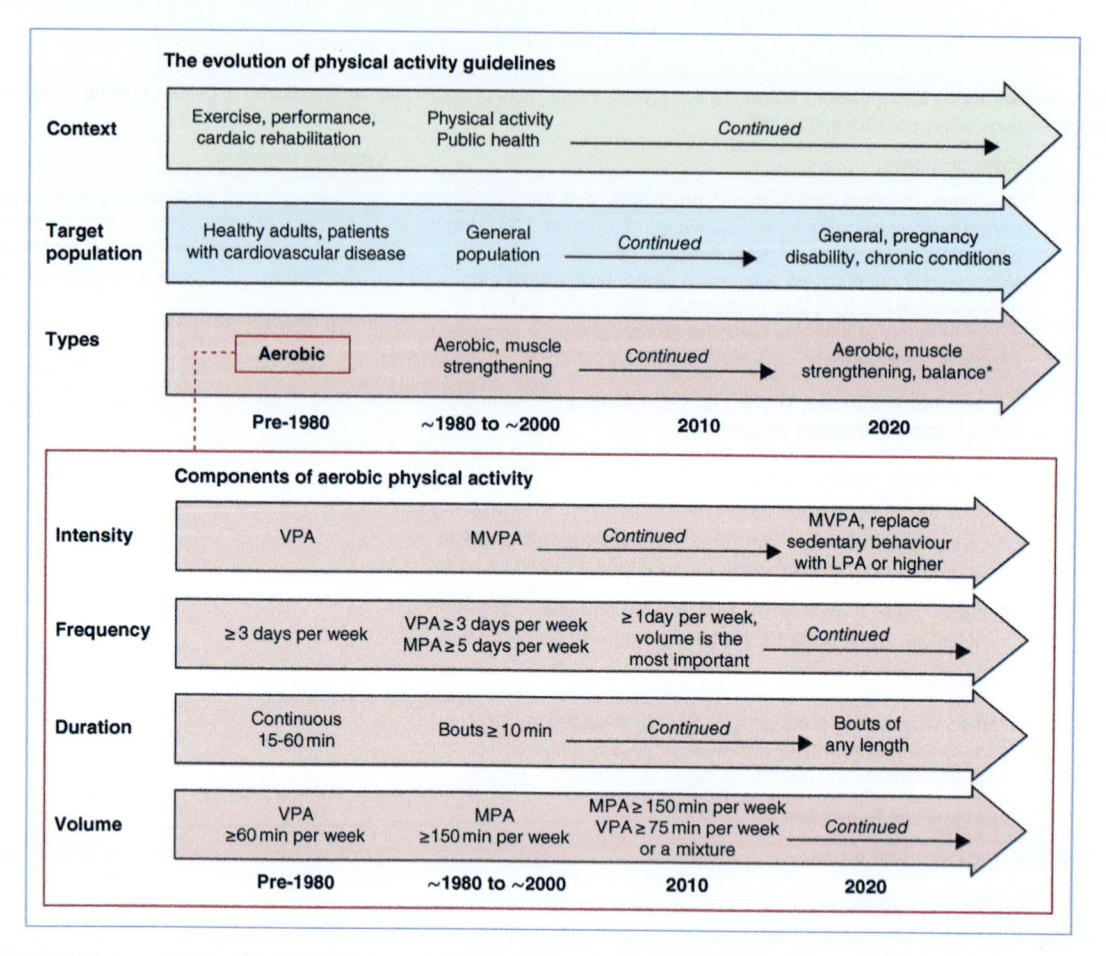

FIGURE 6.5 The evolution of physical-activity guidelines and components of aerobic physical-activity. Source: (D. Ding et al., 2020 / with permission of Elsevier).

CVD events compared with the lowest quartile of light PA (LaCroix et al., 2019).

The aforementioned study aligns very well with the scientific report published by the 2018 Physical Activity Guidelines Advisory Committee as well as the 2018 Physical Activity Guidelines for Americans (Piercy et al., 2018), both of which highlighted the association of low-dose light PA with a reduced risk of CVD incidence and mortality. The previous 2008 Physical Activity Guidelines for Americans (Hootman, 2009) recommended accumulating MVPA in bouts of 10 minutes or more. It is now well-documented that any amount of MVPA counts and could contribute to the health benefits associated with PA.

INTERVENTIONS TO INCREASE PHYSICAL ACTIVITY

To facilitate regular participation in recommended PA levels and/or reduce sedentary time, a multidimensional approach is required. This basically means setting individual, interpersonal, organizational, environmental, and policy targets (Ozemek, Lavie, & Rognmo, 2019).

With regards to personal self-monitoring, many individuals require additional support to follow the PA guidelines. Wearable health and PA devices have garnered attention in recent years as a method by which individuals could become more physically active, especially among populations with chronic diseases. These remote interventions mainly use smartphone-assisted interventions as well as web-, mail-, and/or email-based interventions. These device-based interventions have a strong efficacy in both adult and older adult populations including patients with T2D and musculoskeletal disorders in the short term (Keadle, Bustamante, & Buman, 2021; Muellmann et al., 2018). For instance, meta-analytic findings show that device-based interventions are also effective for increasing PA behaviors among populations with cardio-metabolic conditions (Kirk, Amiri, Pirbaglou, & Ritvo, 2019). However, data are still missing on whether these devices could help individuals adopt PA targets on a long term (≥1 year) basis (Ozemek et al., 2019).

Wearable health and PA devices are also tested in workplace health promotion programs, also known as wellness programs, to promote routine PA. Such interventions improve cardio-respiratory fitness, body-mass index, blood pressure, blood glucose, total cholesterol, and triglycerides (Ozemek et al., 2019). These programs should be implemented in institutions to improve employees' well-being. Therefore, employees could stay more engaged in the long term by avoiding economical losses of unproductivity associated with cardio-metabolic risk factors (Souza, Miyagawa, Melo, & Maciel, 2017).

At the environmental level, several interventions exist in the literature that target changes in PA behaviors to overcome environmental barriers such as a lack of access to gyms and workout facilities, few parks, and green spaces, etc. These interventions have a small but broad impact of behaviors. A classic example is using the stairs instead the elevators to increase activity and stair use. Other interventions include modifying environmental characteristics (e.g., walkability, land-use mix, or destinations) and implementing programs that support active transportation (e.g., walking to school, biking to work) (Keadle et al., 2021).

As already mentioned, the 2018 Physical Activity Guidelines for Americans emphasized the benefits of engaging in any of the PA domains to improve health. For instance, cycling to work is associated with reduced all-cause mortality, CVD mortality, cancer mortality, and cancer incidence (Patterson et al., 2020). Indeed, the WHO created an infographic showing how PA could be part of people's daily life, namely being active at home, at work, at school, and/or in the community (**Figure 6.6**).

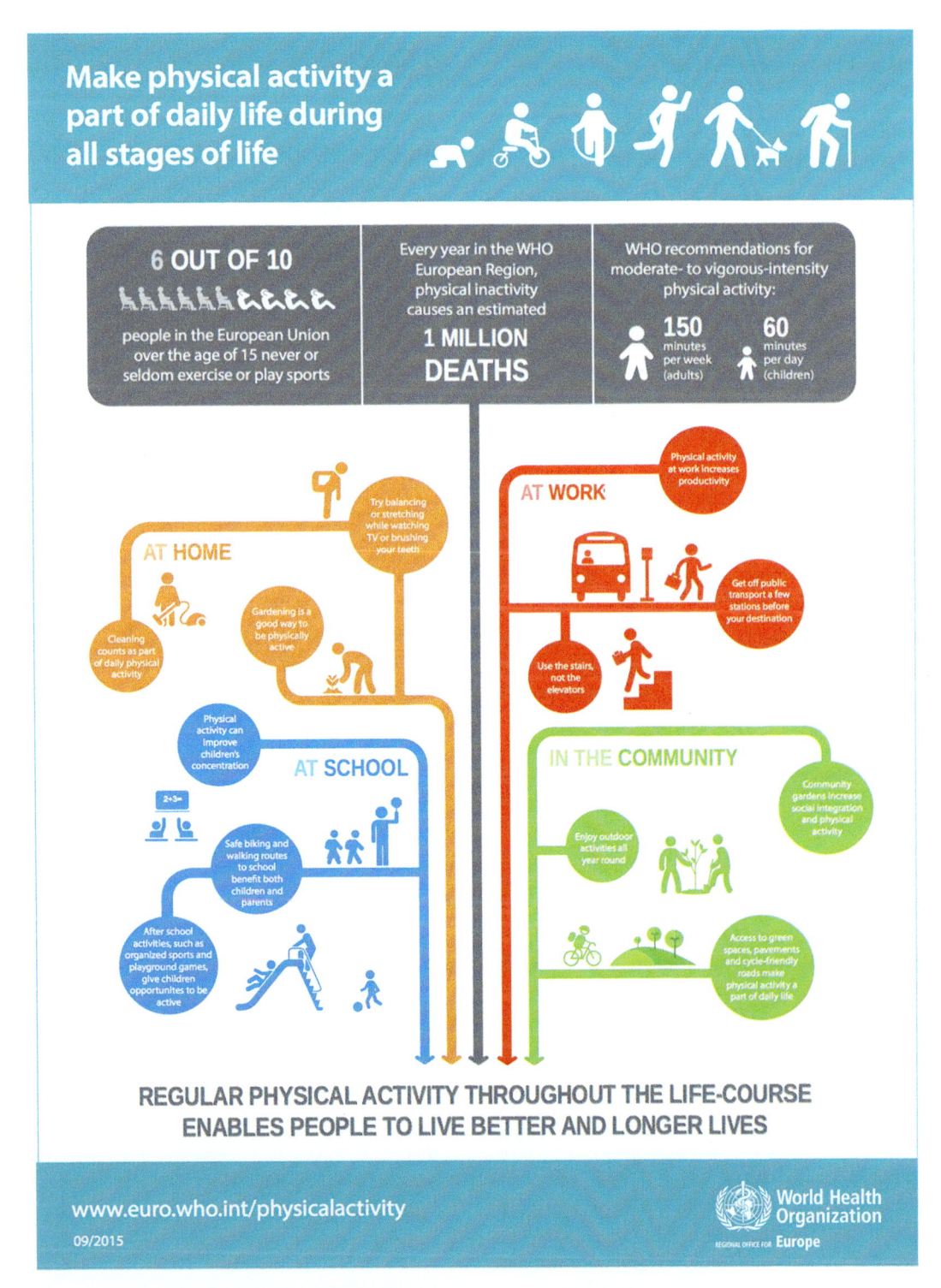

FIGURE 6.6   WHO infographic on integrating physical activity as a part of people's daily life. Source: (World Health Organization, 2015).

KEY POINTS

- More than one in four adults globally are physically inactive. Physical inactivity is correlated with technology advances including increased television viewing as well as computer, mobile device, and video game use.
- According to the WHO, insufficient PA is considered the fourth leading risk factor for mortality.
- There is a strong link between physical inactivity and major NCDs. Physical inactivity is directly responsible for 6% of the global burden of CHD, 7% of T2D, and 10% of breast cancer.
- Member states of the WHO agreed to a 10% relative reduction in the prevalence of insufficient PA by 2025, as one of the nine global goals for the prevention and treatment of NCDs.
- Sedentary behavior typically refers to sitting, lying, and reclining behaviors during waking hours rather than an absence of MVPA.
- There is strong evidence of a positive relationship between sedentary behavior and all-cause mortality, fatal and non-fatal CVD, T2D, and MetS.
- PA remarkably decreases the risk for premature all-cause mortality, even with relatively small participation.
- Routine PA is an effective method for the primary and secondary prevention of more than 25 chronic medical conditions.
- The greatest health benefits of PA are observed in individuals who are physically inactive and become more physically active.
- The domain of PA seems to affect health positively.
- In older adults, increased PA is linked to improved functional health, performance capabilities, mental health, sleep, and quality of life.
- There is increasing evidence for the health benefits of moderate-intensity PA (i.e., walking), while guidelines show a shift from exercise (i.e., planned and structured) to PA.
- The benefits of light-intensity PA are now clearly stated, highlighting the value of replacing sedentary time, regardless of the time spent, with any duration of light-intensity PA.
- A low-dose, light PA is associated with a reduced risk of CVD incidence and mortality.
- To facilitate regular participation at recommended PA levels and/or to reduce sedentary time, a multidimensional approach is required. This means setting individual, interpersonal, organizational, environmental, and policy targets.

SELF-ASSESSMENT QUESTIONS

1. Define physical inactivity based on previous and current recommendations.
2. Complete the sentence: Physical inactivity is directly responsible for _____, _____, and _____.
3. Define sedentary behavior.
4. Could someone who struggles to follow the physical-activity recommendations benefit from any physical activity rather than none?
5. List five clinical conditions that physical activity could be effective at preventing.
6. Indicate whether the following statements are true or false:
   (a) The domain of physical activity does not seem to positively affect health.
   (b) Both leisure-time and non-leisure-time physical activities protect against mortality and cardiovascular disease.
   (c) Those who engage in high versus low occupational physical activity have the same health effects.
   (d) In older adults, increased physical activity is linked to improved functional health.
7. Provide three mechanisms by which physical activity may benefit health.
8. What are the 2020 WHO physical activity recommendations for adults?
9. How could wearable health and physical activity devices could help individuals become more physically active?
10. Provide examples of environmental level interventions to increase physical activity.

REFERENCES

Anderson, E., & Durstine, J. L. (2019). Physical activity, exercise, and chronic diseases: A brief review. *Sports Medicine and Health Science, 1*(1), 3–10. doi:https://doi.org/10.1016/j.smhs.2019.08.006

Bull, F. C., Al-Ansari, S. S., Biddle, S., Borodulin, K., Buman, M. P., Cardon, G., . . . Chou, R. (2020). World Health Organization 2020 guidelines on physical activity and sedentary behaviour. *British journal of sports medicine, 54*(24), 1451–1462.

Chodzko-Zajko, W. J., Proctor, D. N., Singh, M. A. F., Minson, C. T., Nigg, C. R., Salem, G. J., & Skinner, J. S. (2009). Exercise and physical activity for older adults. *Medicine & science in sports & exercise, 41*(7), 1510–1530.

Cillekens, B., Lang, M., van Mechelen, W., Verhagen, E., Huysmans, M. A., Holtermann, A., . . . Coenen, P. (2020). How does occupational physical activity influence health? An umbrella review of 23 health outcomes across 158 observational studies. *Br J Sports Med, 54*(24), 1474–1481. doi:10.1136/bjsports-2020-102587

Ding, D., Mutrie, N., Bauman, A., Pratt, M., Hallal, P. R. C., & Powell, K. E. (2020). Physical activity guidelines 2020: comprehensive and inclusive recommendations to activate populations. *Lancet, 396*(10265), 1780–1782. doi:10.1016/S0140-6736(20)32229-7

Ding, D., Ramirez Varela, A., Bauman, A. E., Ekelund, U., Lee, I. M., Heath, G.,... Pratt, M. (2020). Towards better evidence-informed global action: lessons learnt from the Lancet series and recent developments in physical activity and public health. *British journal of sports medicine, 54*(8), 462. doi:10.1136/bjsports-2019-101001

Dohrn, M., Kwak, L., Oja, P., Sjöström, M., & Hagströmer, M. (2018). Replacing sedentary time with physical activity: a 15-year follow-up of mortality in a national cohort. *Clinical epidemiology, 10*, 179.

Doukky, R., Mangla, A., Ibrahim, Z., Poulin, M.-F., Avery, E., Collado, F. M.,... Powell, L. H. (2016). Impact of Physical Inactivity on Mortality in Patients With Heart Failure. *The American Journal of Cardiology, 117*(7), 1135–1143. doi:https://doi.org/10.1016/j.amjcard.2015.12.060

Ekelund, U., Steene-Johannessen, J., Brown, W. J., Fagerland, M. W., Owen, N., Powell, K. E.,... Group, L. S. B. W. (2016). Does physical activity attenuate, or even eliminate, the detrimental association of sitting time with mortality? A harmonised meta-analysis of data from more than 1 million men and women. *The Lancet, 388*(10051), 1302–1310.

Ekelund, U., Tarp, J., Steene-Johannessen, J., Hansen, B. H., Jefferis, B., Fagerland, M. W.,... Chernofsky, A. (2019). Dose-response associations between accelerometry measured physical activity and sedentary time and all cause mortality: systematic review and harmonised meta-analysis. *bmj, 366*.

Gheysen, F., Poppe, L., DeSmet, A., Swinnen, S., Cardon, G., De Bourdeaudhuij, I.,... Fias, W. (2018). Physical activity to improve cognition in older adults: can physical activity programs enriched with cognitive challenges enhance the effects? A systematic review and meta-analysis. *International Journal of Behavioral Nutrition and Physical Activity, 15*(1), 1–13.

González, K., Fuentes, J., & Márquez, J. L. (2017). Physical Inactivity, Sedentary Behavior and Chronic Diseases. *Korean J Fam Med, 38*(3), 111–115. doi:10.4082/kjfm.2017.38.3.111

Guthold, R., Stevens, G. A., Riley, L. M., & Bull, F. C. (2018). Worldwide trends in insufficient physical activity from 2001 to 2016: a pooled analysis of 358 population-based surveys with 1·9 million participants. *The Lancet Global Health, 6*(10), e1077–e1086. doi:https://doi.org/10.1016/S2214-109X(18)30357-7

US Department of Agriculture and US Department of Health and Human Services (2018). Physical activity guidelines advisory committee. 2018 physical activity guidelines advisory committee scientific report. *Published online*.

Hootman, J. M. (2009). 2008 Physical Activity Guidelines for Americans: an opportunity for athletic trainers. *Journal of athletic training, 44*(1), 5–6.

Keadle, S. K., Bustamante, E. E., & Buman, M. P. (2021). Physical activity and public health: four decades of progress. *Kinesiology Review, 10*(3), 319–330.

Kirk, M. A., Amiri, M., Pirbaglou, M., & Ritvo, P. (2019). Wearable technology and physical activity behavior change in adults with chronic cardiometabolic disease: a systematic review and meta-analysis. *American Journal of Health Promotion, 33*(5), 778–791.

Kraus, W. E., Powell, K. E., Haskell, W. L., Janz, K. F., Campbell, W. W., Jakicic, J. M.,... Piercy, K. L. (2019). Physical activity, all-cause and cardiovascular mortality, and cardiovascular disease. *Medicine and science in sports and exercise, 51*(6), 1270.

LaCroix, A. Z., Bellettiere, J., Rillamas-Sun, E., Di, C., Evenson, K. R., Lewis, C. E.,... Rosenberg, D. E. (2019). Association of light physical activity measured by accelerometry and incidence of coronary heart disease and cardiovascular disease in older women. *JAMA Network Open, 2*(3), e190419-e190419.

Lear, S. A., Hu, W., Rangarajan, S., Gasevic, D., Leong, D., Iqbal, R.,... Yusuf, S. (2017). The effect of physical activity on mortality and cardiovascular disease in 130 000 people from 17 high-income, middle-income, and low-income countries: the PURE study. *Lancet, 390*(10113), 2643–2654. doi:10.1016/s0140-6736(17)31634-3

Liguori, G., & Medicine, A. C. o. S. (2020). *ACSM's guidelines for exercise testing and prescription*: Lippincott Williams & Wilkins.

Loprinzi, P. D., & Sng, E. (2016). The effects of objectively measured sedentary behavior on all-cause mortality in a national sample of adults with diabetes. *Preventive Medicine, 86*, 55–57. doi:https://doi.org/10.1016/j.ypmed.2016.01.023

Matthews, C. E., Chen, K. Y., Freedson, P. S., Buchowski, M. S., Beech, B. M., Pate, R. R., & Troiano, R. P. (2008). Amount of Time Spent in Sedentary Behaviors in the United States, 2003–2004. *American Journal of Epidemiology, 167*(7), 875–881. doi:10.1093/aje/kwm390

Muellmann, S., Forberger, S., Möllers, T., Bröring, E., Zeeb, H., & Pischke, C. R. (2018). Effectiveness of eHealth interventions for the promotion of physical activity in older adults: A systematic review. *Preventive Medicine, 108*, 93–110. doi:https://doi.org/10.1016/j.ypmed.2017.12.026

Ozemek, C., Lavie, C. J., & Rognmo, Ø. (2019). Global physical activity levels - Need for intervention. *Progress in Cardiovascular Diseases, 62*(2), 102–107. doi:https://doi.org/10.1016/j.pcad.2019.02.004

Paffenbarger Jr, R. S., Hyde, R., Wing, A. L., & Hsieh, C.-c. (1986). Physical activity, all-cause mortality, and longevity of college alumni. *New England journal of medicine, 314*(10), 605–613.

Pate, R. R., Pratt, M., Blair, S. N., Haskell, W. L., Macera, C. A., Bouchard, C.,... King, A. C. (1995). Physical activity and public health: a recommendation from the Centers for Disease Control and Prevention and the American College of Sports Medicine. *Jama, 273*(5), 402–407.

Patterson, R., McNamara, E., Tainio, M., de Sá, T. H., Smith, A. D., Sharp, S. J.,... Wijndaele, K. (2018). Sedentary behaviour and risk of all-cause, cardiovascular and cancer mortality, and incident type 2 diabetes: a systematic review and dose response meta-analysis. *European Journal of Epidemiology, 33*(9), 811–829. doi:10.1007/s10654-018-0380-1

Patterson, R., Panter, J., Vamos, E. P., Cummins, S., Millett, C., & Laverty, A. A. (2020). Associations between commute mode and cardiovascular disease, cancer, and all-cause mortality, and cancer incidence, using linked Census data over 25 years in England and Wales: a cohort study. *The Lancet Planetary Health, 4*(5), e186-e194. doi:https://doi.org/10.1016/S2542-5196(20)30079-6

Piercy, K. L., Troiano, R. P., Ballard, R. M., Carlson, S. A., Fulton, J. E., Galuska, D. A.,... Olson, R. D. (2018). The physical activity guidelines for Americans. *Jama, 320*(19), 2020–2028.

Ramakrishnan, R., He, J.-R., Ponsonby, A.-L., Woodward, M., Rahimi, K., Blair, S. N., & Dwyer, T. (2021). Objectively measured physical activity and all cause mortality: a systematic review and meta-analysis. *Preventive Medicine, 143*, 106356.

Rhodes, R. E., Janssen, I., Bredin, S. S., Warburton, D. E., & Bauman, A. (2017). Physical activity: Health impact, prevalence, correlates and interventions. *Psychology & Health, 32*(8), 942–975.

Souza, M., Miyagawa, T., Melo, P., & Maciel, F. (2017, 2017//). *Wellness Programs: Wearable Technologies Supporting Healthy Habits and Corporate*

Costs Reduction. Paper presented at the HCI International 2017 – Posters' Extended Abstracts, Cham.

Warburton, D. E., & Bredin, S. S. (2016). Reflections on Physical Activity and Health: What Should We Recommend? *Can J Cardiol, 32*(4), 495–504. doi:10.1016/j.cjca.2016.01.024

Warburton, D. E., Nicol, C. W., & Bredin, S. S. (2006). Health benefits of physical activity: the evidence. *CMAJ, 174*(6), 801–809. doi:10.1503/cmaj.051351

Warburton, D. E. R., & Bredin, S. S. D. (2017). Health benefits of physical activity: a systematic review of current systematic reviews. *Curr Opin Cardiol, 32*(5), 541–556. doi:10.1097/HCO.0000000000000437

Warburton, D. E. R., & Bredin, S. S. D. (2019). Health Benefits of Physical Activity: A Strengths-Based Approach. *J Clin Med, 8*(12). doi:10.3390/jcm8122044

Wilmot, E. G., Edwardson, C. L., Achana, F. A., Davies, M. J., Gorely, T., Gray, L. J.,. . . Biddle, S. J. H. (2012). Sedentary time in adults and the association with diabetes, cardiovascular disease and death: systematic review and meta-analysis. *Diabetologia, 55*(11), 2895–2905. doi:10.1007/s00125-012-2677-z

World Health Organization. (2010). *Global recommendations on physical activity for health*: World Health Organization.

World Health Organization. (2020). WHO guidelines on physical activity and sedentary behaviour: web annex: evidence profiles.

World Health Organization. (2021). The WHO Global Monitoring Framework on noncommunicable diseases. Retrieved from https://www.who.int/teams/ncds/surveillance/monitoring-capacity/gmf

FURTHER READING

Bibliography

Geidl, W., Schlesinger, S., Mino, E., Miranda, L., & Pfeifer, K. (2020). Dose–response relationship between physical activity and mortality in adults with noncommunicable diseases: a systematic review and meta-analysis of prospective observational studies. International Journal of Behavioral Nutrition and Physical Activity, 17(1), 1–18.

Katsagoni, C. N., Papachristou, E., Sidossis, A., & Sidossis, L. (2020). Effects of dietary and lifestyle interventions on liver, clinical and metabolic parameters in children and adolescents with non-alcoholic fatty liver disease: A systematic review. Nutrients, 12(9), 2864.

Klepac Pogrmilovic, B., O'Sullivan, G., Milton, K., Biddle, S. J., Bauman, A., Bull, F.,. . . & Pedisic, Z. (2018). A global systematic scoping review of studies analysing indicators, development, and content of national-level physical activity and sedentary behaviour policies. International Journal of Behavioral Nutrition and Physical Activity, 15(1), 1–17.

Kokkinos, P., & Myers, J. (2019). Physical activity, cardiorespiratory fitness, and health: A historical perspective. In Cardiorespiratory fitness in cardiometabolic diseases (pp. 1–9). Springer, Cham.

Tambalis, K. D., & Sidossis, L. S. (2019). Physical activity and cardiometabolic health benefits in children. In Cardiorespiratory fitness in cardiometabolic diseases (pp. 405–423). Springer, Cham.

Links

- https://www.cdc.gov/chronicdisease/resources/infographic/physical-activity.htm
- https://www.cdc.gov/chronicdisease/resources/publications/factsheets/physical-activity.htm
- https://www.who.int/health-topics/physical-activity#tab=tab_1
- https://apps.who.int/iris/bitstream/handle/10665/337001/9789240014886-eng.pdf
- www.acsm.org/
- https://www.exerciseismedicine.org/wp-content/uploads/2021/08/ExerciseIsMedicine_v8.pdf

Determinants of Healthy Aging

UNIT 3

Healthy Aging: Definition and Scope

CHAPTER 7

Introduction	93	Special Considerations	101
Overview of the Aging Process	93	Key Points	102
Biology of Aging	93	Self-assessment Questions	102
Early Concepts of Healthy Aging	96	References	103
The Concept of Successful Aging	97	Further Reading	104
Healthy Aging	98	Bibliography	104
Definition	98		
Life-course Approach to Healthy Aging	99		

INTRODUCTION

A new era has begun for human aging (Cosco, Howse & Brayne, 2017). Nowadays, people worldwide are living longer than before, and they are expected to pass their 60s (Beard & Cassels, 2016). The world is experiencing a rapid aging, namely a considerable increase in the older population. By 2050, the number of those over 60-years old will nearly double. In real terms, in 2015, the population of older people was 900 million, and this is expected to increase to about 2 billion by 2050. According to the United Nations definition, when the population over 60-years old surpasses 7% in a country, the country is considered aged (United Nations, 2019). This demographic transition toward aging invokes public action to find ways of improving health and maintaining well-being throughout the life course (Beard & Cassels, 2016).

Yet, living longer does not necessarily mean living healthier, as longevity (typically defined as reaching an age of ≥85 years) does not always entail experiencing better health (Beard & Cassels, 2016). In fact, scarce evidence exists that older people today are experiencing better health than their ancestors at the same age. Indeed, as human life expectancy is prolonged, age-related diseases are common (Carmona, 2016), with three chronic disorders constituting the leading causes of death: ischemic heart disease, stroke, and chronic obstructive pulmonary disease (Beard & Cassels, 2016). Above all, living longer must be congruent with living well, and that is why adding health to years is the key factor for well-being in later life (Beard & Cassels, 2016).

Although 70 does not yet seem to be the new 60, undoubtedly, the extension of life span is extremely valuable, since it provides the chance to reconsider what older age might be and to rethink the endless prospects through which to spend these extra years fruitfully (Beard & Cassels, 2016). Older people can contribute to society in many ways and living these extra years in prosperity provides them with limitless opportunities. To illustrate this point, in high-income countries, people over 60 are very likely to start looking for new career, continue lifelong learning, or a new hobby. Likewise, younger people, knowing that they will live more, might plan to live their lives differently (Green, 2013). However, if these additional years are dominated by decreased physical and mental capacities, they can ultimately lead to higher health and social costs (Goldman, 2016).

Evidently, enabling people to age better and maintain better health, as well as to prolong good function and high levels of well-being in the second half of life, are of major importance. This notion is highlighted by the fact that globally, public health agendas are investing in policies that promote healthy aging (Beard & Cassels, 2016). Nevertheless, there is clearly some difficulty in building a framework aimed at advancing quality aging while confusion as to the nature of the concept itself remains; reaching a consensus on the definition of healthy has proven to be a difficult task (Estebsari et al., 2020).

OVERVIEW OF THE AGING PROCESS

BIOLOGY OF AGING

Aging is the process of gradual physiological deterioration that all living beings experience with time (Carmona, 2016). At the biological level, aging results from the impact of an accumulated

---

Prevention and Management of Cardiovascular and Metabolic Disease: Diet, Physical Activity and Healthy Aging,
First Edition. Christina N. Katsagoni, Peter Kokkinos, and Labros S. Sidossis.
© 2023 John Wiley & Sons Ltd. Published 2023 by John Wiley & Sons Ltd.

variety of molecular and cellular damage over time. This leads to a gradual decrease in physical and mental capacity, a growing risk of disease, and ultimately, death. This deterioration is the primary risk factor for major human pathologies including cancer, diabetes, cardiovascular disorders, and neurodegenerative diseases (Carmona, 2016). Nine hallmarks are generally considered responsible for this macromolecular damage: genomic instability, telomere attrition, epigenetic alterations, loss of proteostasis, deregulated nutrient-sensing, mitochondrial dysfunction, cellular senescence, stem-cell exhaustion, and altered intercellular communication (López-Otín et al., 2013) (**Figure 7.1**).

For example, molecular integrity of the genome, telomere length, epigenetic landscape stability, and protein homeostasis are all features linked to "youthful" states (**Figure 7.2**). Indeed, healthy aging refers to the prevention of this molecular and cellular decline to reach the longest lifespan (López-Otín et al., 2013).

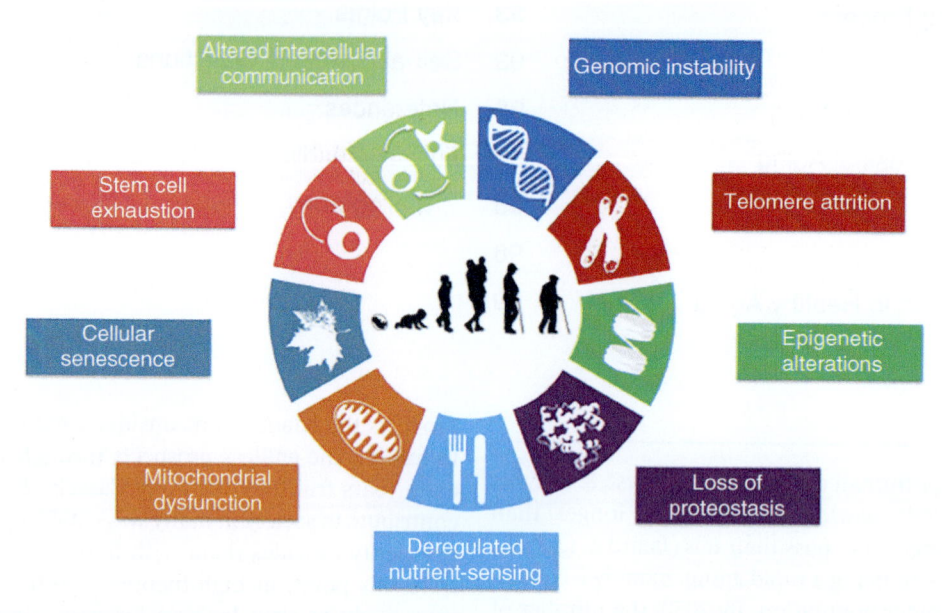

FIGURE 7.1 The hallmarks of aging. The scheme enumerates the nine hallmarks: genomic instability, telomere attrition, epigenetic alterations, loss of proteostasis, deregulated nutrient-sensing, mitochondrial dysfunction, cellular senescence, stem-cell exhaustion, and altered intercellular communication. Source: (López-Otín et al., 2013 / with permission of Elsevier).

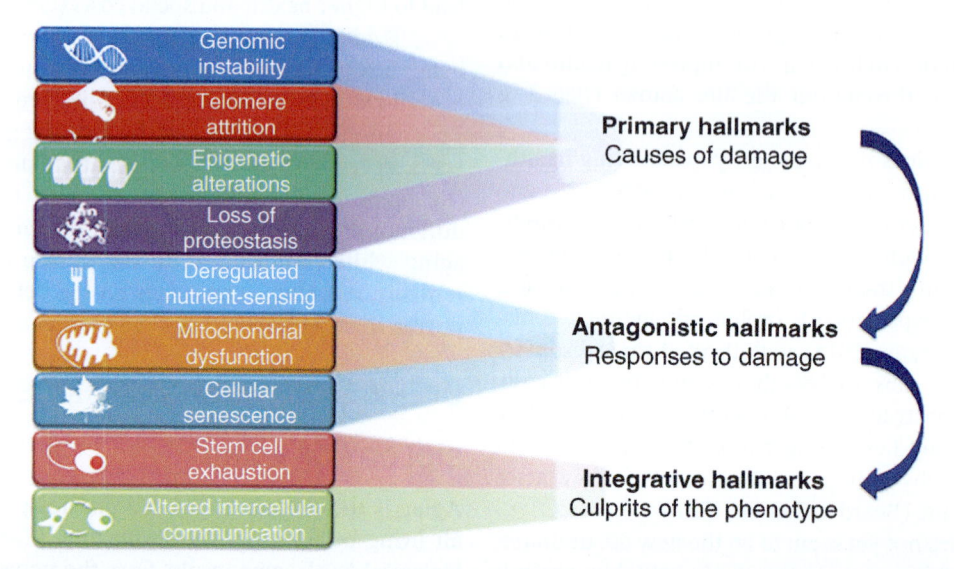

FIGURE 7.2 Functional interconnections between the hallmarks of aging. The nine proposed hallmarks of aging are grouped into three categories. In the top, those hallmarks considered to be the primary causes of cellular damage. In the middle are those considered to be part of compensatory or antagonistic responses to the damage. These responses initially mitigate the damage, but eventually, if chronic or exacerbated, they become deleterious themselves. At the bottom are the integrative hallmarks that are the end result of the previous two groups of hallmarks and are ultimately responsible for the functional decline associated with aging. Source: (López-Otín et al., 2013 / with permission of Elsevier).

A plethora of scientific evidence supports the claim that there is not a single cause of aging and that multiple mechanisms modulate the aging process (Wagner, Cameron-Smith, Wessner & Franzke, 2016). Aging research has experienced remarkable progress over recent years. Specifically, the discovery that the rate of aging is controlled, at least to some extent, by genetic pathways and biochemical processes, was a scientific breakthrough (Wagner et al., 2016). The genome does not solely account for physiological traits or disease risk. Presumably, genetics have a low impact on the age of death (between 12% and 25%) (Passarino, de Rango & Montesanto, 2016). Although many longevity genes have been investigated, only two genes have been widely replicated, *ApoE* and *FOX03A*, as discussed in **Chapter 8**. In the longest-living families, these variants have an impact on the age of death between 1% to 10% of a birth cohort.

It is unclear, however, how these complex molecular signs interrelate with personal lifestyle and the diverse environments to which humans are exposed, especially considering that the dynamic interaction between a living being and its environment defines the rate and fate of aging (Carmona, 2016). Notably, beyond genetic variations and biological factors, aging is strongly associated with the physical and social environment (external factors: race/ethnicity, culture, religion, and security as well as social inequities and scientific/technological advances) as well as personal characteristics, such as sex, ethnicity, or socio-economic status (Eaton et al., 2012) (**Figure 7.3**). The environments that people live in, combined with their personal characteristics, have long-term effects on how they age. Environments have a strong impact on establishing healthy behaviors throughout life (Hernandez & Johnston, 2017), like a balanced diet (Black & Bowman, 2020), engaging in regular physical activity (Daskalopoulou et al., 2017), and refraining from tobacco use, habits that all contribute to reducing the risk of non-communicable diseases and improving physical and mental capacity.

Furthermore, it is well accepted that environmental factors orchestrate epigenetic (which literally means "above the genes", as discussed in **Chapter 2**) and gene transcription changes to affect health and aging process itself (Carmona, 2016). While genes have traditionally been a nonmodifiable factor, there is growing evidence linking epigenetic DNA modification through environmental exposures to a wide range of aging phenotypes (Eaton et al., 2012). The diversity seen in older adults is not random. Aging is an heterogenous and heterochronic process and is only loosely associated with a person's age in years (Carmona, 2016). After all, there is no "typical" older person (Beard & Cassels, 2016). For instance, while some 70-year-olds enjoy extremely good health and functioning, others are frail and require significant help from others.

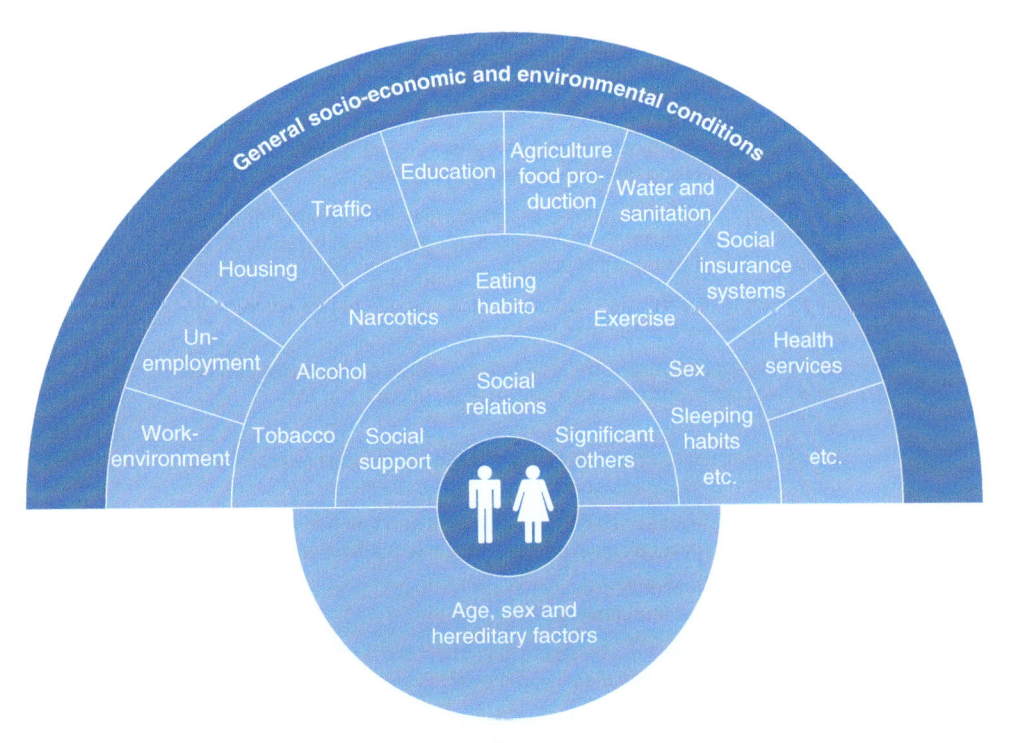

FIGURE 7.3 Health determinants. Source: (Adapted from WHO, 2015).

EARLY CONCEPTS OF HEALTHY AGING

Quality of life in older people has been variously conceptualized as "successful", "active", "productive", "healthy", and "positive" aging, among others (Estebsari et al., 2020). What do people need to age well? For most, the answer seems clear, since many people prioritize good health as an important goal in their lives and consider health and functioning in old age as a prerequisite for healthy aging (Reich et al., 2020). Notably, some might consider the term "healthy aging" an oxymoron, since the healthy usually implies optimal function and absence of disease yet aging is synonymous with co-morbidities, physical or mental (Aronson, 2020). Conversely, many people worldwide experience high levels of well-being despite their body's decline. This "aging well-being paradox" resembles the "disability paradox" in which people with severe physical disabilities rate their own well-being rather positively, which is unexpected to outsiders. It is reasonable, however, that people adapt to their own disabilities (Rowe & Kahn, 1987). Therefore, maintaining good physical health might not be the only prerequisite for aging healthy.

According to this scope, any critical analysis of the definitions of healthy aging should start with a clear understanding of the historical perspective on the concepts of aging (Urtamo, 2019a) (**Table 7.1**). Carl Jung's work on aging during the 1920s and 1930s may be considered the most significant forerunner of modern gerontology, as he identified late life as a process of turning inward. One of the earliest definitions of successful aging found in the gerontology literature is that introduced by Robert Havighurst in 1961 (Neugarten, Havighurst & Tobin, 1961). According to this conceptualization, successful aging should promote maximum satisfaction and happiness with one's present and past lives. This pioneering point of view was published in 1953, in a book titled Older People. This book was a milestone, it introduced a novel aspect of aging well, outside the medical domain, described through

Table 7.1 Historical preview of key concepts in successful/healthy aging.

Concept	Description	Author
Activity theory (1961)	Maintaining middle-aged activities and attitudes into later adulthood	Cumming
Disengagement theory (1961)	Desire and ability of older people to disengage from active life to prepare themselves for death	Cumming
Successful aging (1961)	Conditions promoting a maximum of satisfaction and happiness	Havighurst
Successful aging (1963)	Having feelings of happiness and satisfaction with one's present and past life	Havighurst
Index of activities of daily living (ADL) (1963)	Systematic approach to measuring physical performance in a population of older or chronically ill persons	Katz
Aging successfully (1972)	Coping style, prior ability to adapt, and expectations of life as well as income, health, social interactions, freedoms, and constraints; coalescence of personality, which plays into the enormous complexity of successful aging	Neugarten
Successful aging (1987; 1998)	Interplay between social engagement with life, health, and functioning for a positive aging experience (low probability of disease and disease-related disability)	Rowe
Selective optimization with compensation (1990)	(i) Selective adaptation and transformation of internal and external resources. (ii) Optimization and compensation. (iii) Maintaining function, maximizing gains, and minimizing losses	Baltes
Productive aging (1990)	Any activity by an older individual that contributes to producing goods or services, or develops the capacity to produce them (whether or not the individual is paid for this activity)	Butler
Active aging (2002)	The process of optimizing opportunities for health, participation, and security to enhance quality of life as people age	WHO
Healthy aging (2006)	Optimizing opportunities for good health, so that older people can take an active part in society and enjoy an independent and high quality of life	Swedish National Institute of Public Health
Cultural aspects of "good aging" (2007)	Cultures have different understandings and interactions to promote or detract from a good old age	Fry
Successful aging and diseases (2009)	Successful aging may coexist with diseases and functional limitations if compensatory psychological and/or social mechanisms are used	Young
Healthy and active aging (2011)	The process of optimizing opportunities for health to enhance quality of life as people age and grow old	European Commission
Healthy aging (2015)	More than the absence of disease; it is the process of developing and maintaining the functional ability that enables well-being in older age	WHO
Active and healthy aging (2015)	An ability to perform daily activities, feeling happy, remaining free of cognitive or functional impairments, and free of major chronic diseases	Helsinki Businessmen Study cohort

Source: (Adapted from Martin et al., 2015).

the eyes of older people themselves, the challenges people face daily, as they grow older. At the time, descriptions of old-age problems were based on the perception of younger adults and there were two contrasting theories of aging well: activity theory and disengagement theory (Cumming, 1968). Activity theory stated that older adults are happiest when they stay active and maintain social interactions; gerontologists generally preferred this theory because it was assumed to capture the desire of aging individuals. Disengagement theory, on the other hand, stated that a person aging in success would want, over time, to disengage from an active life.

Moreover, an innovative publication by Katz et al. in 1963 viewed successful aging as a process from the perspective of researchers or clinicians: to be "successful", older persons should maintain their functioning within the bounds predetermined by researchers (Katz, 1963). Following this, the Index of Activities of Daily Living (ADL) (Instrumental ADL, IADL) was introduced as a systematic approach to measure physical performance in a population of older or chronically ill adults. This instrument was proposed as an objective guide to distinguish "usual" and "successful" aging within an older population, and it was used frequently in later studies on successful aging to make this distinction.

A multidimensional approach was introduced by Neugarten, which emphasized personality type as a predictor for successful aging, such as coping style, prior ability to adapt, and life expectations as well as income, health, social interactions, freedoms, and constraints (Neugarten, 1972). The successfully aging individuals not only play an active role in adapting to the biological and social changes with time, but also in creating patterns of life that will give them the greatest ego involvement and life satisfaction. The author also suggested that there might be differences in age norms even among older adults. She identified two major groups of aged adults: the "young-old," aged 55 to 75, and the "old-old," aged 75 or above. A few years later, Suzman and Riley added the "oldest -old" to the Neugarten framework (Suzman, 1985).

THE CONCEPT OF SUCCESSFUL AGING

Probably the most well-known aging model was introduced by Rowe and Kahn in 1987, which advocated for a successful aging model for biomedical research purposes (Stowe & Cooney, 2015). Geriatrician John W. Rowe and social psychologist Robert L. Kahn argued that there is substantial heterogeneity among older persons and added an extra category to the traditional "normal aged" and "diseased aged" categories. "Normal" aging should be divided into two vastly different groups: a large group of people undergoing usual aging and a smaller group undergoing successful aging, differentiated from usual aging by the impact of extrinsic factors. For decades, studies on human aging believed that intrinsic factors such as genetics were the primary determinant of losses commonly seen in older people. The critical role of extrinsic factors such as diet, physical activity, and lifestyle in general was overlooked. It appeared that usual aging could be modified by personal, behavioral, and psychosocial parameters and that there was a causal relationship between extrinsic factors and the process of aging (Stowe & Cooney, 2015).

The Rowe's and Kahn's biomedical model, which is arguably the best known and widely applied model (Estebsari et al., 2020), views "better than average" aging as a combination of three components: (i) being free of disease and disability, (ii) having high cognitive and physical abilities, and (iii) engaging with life (**Figure 7.4**). This model was a hallmark in gerontology and a major turning point in developing programs that view older adults as able, valuable social members. Nevertheless, this conceptualization has a relatively static nature since it emphasizes personal control over one's later-life outcomes and neglects developmental processes and the trajectories of continuity and change in function over time (Rowe & Kahn, 1987). In 2015, Rowe and Kahn suggested adding societal-level principles to evaluations of successful aging: more opportunities for employment, voluntary work, and social activities; trust in older people, due to their knowledge and capacity for problem-solving; and investment in training and education for older adults, rather than exclusion due to their chronological age (Stowe & Cooney, 2015).

Moving beyond Rowe and Kahn's model, psychosocial theories view aging as a lifelong process; the most well-known model of this perspective is the one developed by Baltes and Baltes (Freund & Baltes, 1998). In agreement with lifespan developmental psychology, development and aging are synonyms for behavioral changes across the life span, emphasizing the presence of three components of successful aging (SOC): selection, optimization, and compensation. The lifelong process of selective optimization with compensation allows people to age successfully, i.e., to engage in life tasks that are important to them despite a reduction in energy. Subsequent studies provided evidence that the SOC components were correlated to subjective indicators of well-being such as positive emotions, autonomy, personal growth, and self-acceptance, among others (Urtamo, 2019b).

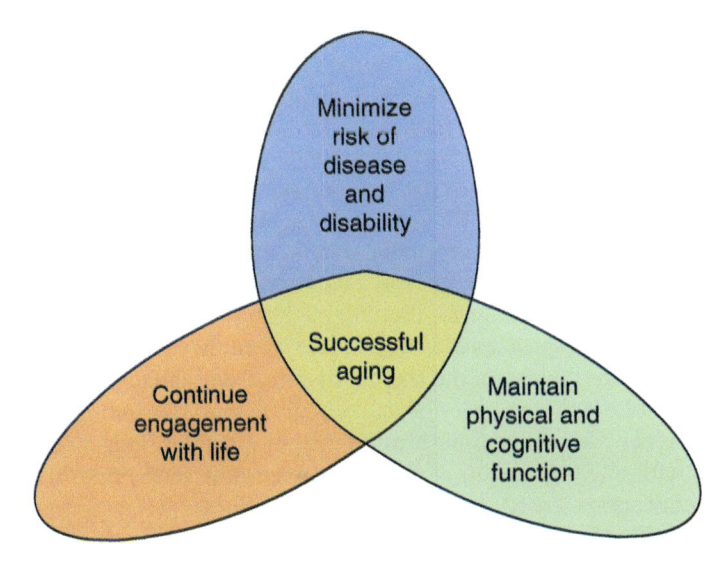

FIGURE 7.4 The Rowe and Kahn's successful aging model in 1997. Source: (Adapted from Stowe & Cooney, 2015).

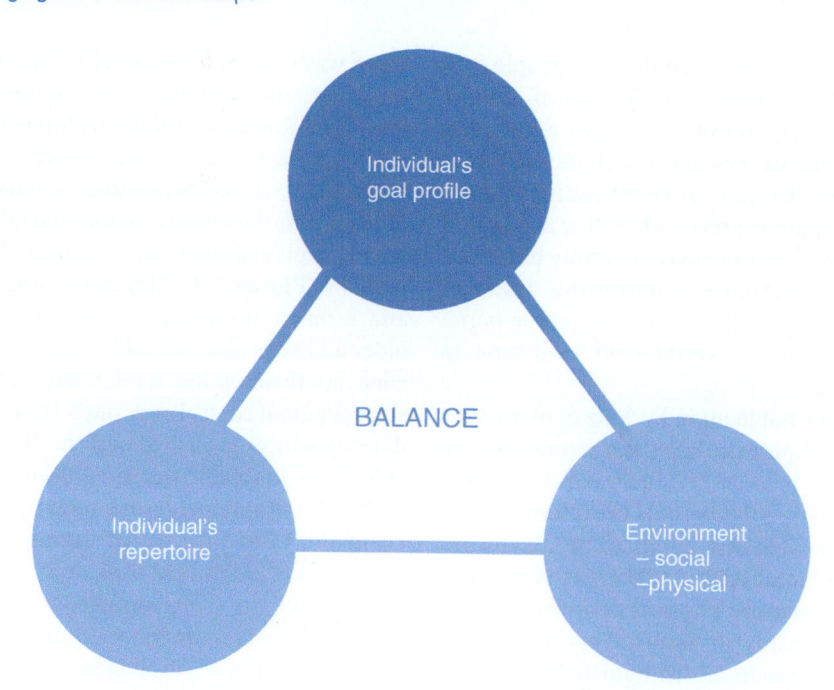

FIGURE 7.5 The balance between capacity, goals, and environments. Source: (Adapted from Beard et al., 2016).

A novel approach argued that, due to aging heterogeneity, there cannot be a single approach to success (Young, Frick & Phelan, 2009). A person can be successful in the absence of diseases and functional impairments (physiologic); in a high-cognition function, emotion vitality, coping, and resilience (psychological); engagement with life, spirituality, and the use of social support (social). One can be successful in three states, with the highest score being achieved in the third condition. Eventually, successful aging occurs whenever a person has a high well-being, quality of life, and personal fulfillment. Unlike others, this model allows for varied degrees and types of success as well as accommodating both physically healthy people and those with age-related limitations (**Figure 7.5**).

An interesting analysis of the literature proposed that the ideal definition should be acceptable to everyone involved: clinicians and older people themselves (Depp & Jeste, 2006). The authors acknowledged that successful aging is described and measured in several ways and highlighted the need to expand those definitions. They argued that there was a gap between operationalized definitions, and the perception of successful aging according to older adults themselves. In accordance, later publications noted that although objective criteria are important components of successful aging, they do not tell the whole story. They pointed out that success is a function of value judgments as well as objective criteria, thus highlighting the importance of adaptive processes that adults undergo when they grow older.

Nevertheless, in the current literature one can distinguish two different concepts of successful aging, depending on whether the individual himself or an outsider judges the situation (Kusumastuti et al., 2016). According to the first, the publications based on the Havighurst's model (Havighurst-cluster), advocate older people's perspectives of aging well, highlighting the possible risk of medical categorization of successful and usual aging. On the other hand, the second group of publications called the "Katz-cluster", tend to analyze successful aging purely from the perspective of researchers or clinicians, using quantitatively physical functioning assessments and predictors. These different points of view are useful to explain the aging paradox, as successful aging lies in the eyes of the beholder (Kusumastuti et al., 2016). Over time, the two clusters seemed to be moving closer to each other on the horizontal axis, suggesting that they started to acknowledge the importance of each other perspectives.

HEALTHY AGING

DEFINITION

Leading health organizations have adopted definitions that incorporate key attributes of biomedical and social sciences, in line with older adult's views. In 2003, the Swedish National Institute of Public Health, with the support of the European Commission and 12 partners including the World Health Organization (WHO), European Older Peoples Platform, EuroHealthNet, and concerned stakeholders initiated the Healthy Aging project under the European Union Public Health Program (The Swedish National Institute of Public Health, 2006). Healthy aging is described as "a lifelong process optimizing opportunities for improving and preserving health and physical, social, and mental wellness, independence, quality of life and enhancing successful life-course transitions." Healthy aging fostered by systematically planned health promotion efforts was mentioned in 1998 as Target 5 in the WHO policy "Health for All in the 21st Century".

The WHO first introduced "active aging" in 2002 as "the process of optimizing opportunities for health, participation, and security in order to enhance the quality of life as people age." Along with this approach, the WHO in 2006 defined healthy aging (World Health Organization, 2015) as "the process of developing and maintaining the functional ability that enables well-being in older age." Furthermore, it is noted that "functional ability" is about having the capabilities that enable all people to be and do what they have reason to value. This includes a person's ability to meet their basic needs; learn, grow, and make decisions; be mobile; build and maintain relationships; and contribute to society. Functional ability consists of the intrinsic capacity of the individual, relevant environmental characteristics, and the interaction between them. Intrinsic capacity comprises all the mental and physical capacities that a person can draw on and includes their ability to walk, think, see, hear, and remember. The level of intrinsic capacity is influenced by several factors such as the presence of diseases, injuries, and age-related changes." Our fixed "personal characteristics (e.g., gender or ethnicity), social norms (e.g., occupation, education, wealth, or social security), and other factors (e.g., smoking, drinking, deprivation, or air pollution) across our life span can affect later health characteristics such as physiological risk factors, diseases, injuries, and broader geriatric syndromes. The cumulative effects of these health characteristics determine one's intrinsic capacity."

Likewise, Health Canada (The Healthy Aging and Wellness Working Group, 2006) describes healthy aging as "a lifelong process of optimizing opportunities for improving and preserving health and physical, social, and mental wellness, independence, quality of life and enhancing successful life-course transitions." Reaching a consensus about defining healthy aging has proven a difficult task, since there is no universally accepted definition. Nonetheless, according to the current literature, the main definitive variables of healthy aging are high physical, cognitive, and social functioning; adjusting to age-related changes; and self-perception of health and well-being.

LIFE-COURSE APPROACH TO HEALTHY AGING

Recently it was proposed that healthy aging may be linked to physical, cognitive, and emotional development in early life as well as to lifetime environmental factors and lifestyles (Kuh, Karunananthan, Bergman & Cooper, 2014). An integrated life-course healthy biological aging (Michel & Ecarnot, 2019) approach might provide insight about how to preserve health-span through the lifespan. Under this scope, it is important first, to evaluate healthy aging through the prism of the WHO's definition of health (WHO, 1948) as a "state of complete physical, mental, and social well-being and not merely the absence of disease or infirmity" and not merely as the opposite of aging, as the absence of disease and impairments. Indeed, health reflects the ability to respond adaptively to environmental challenges and to self-manage, "based on resilience to cope, maintain, and restore one's integrity equilibrium, and sense of well-being in three areas: biologically, in terms of physiological resilience; mentally, in terms of capacity to cope; and socially, in terms of the capacity to fulfill potential and obligations, manage independent living, and social participation" (Kuh, 2007).

Health is dynamic and differentiates across age stages; therefore, a constant assessment of health status is needed throughout a lifespan instead of an evaluation at one point in time (Michel & Ecarnot, 2019). In this facet, healthy aging is a life-course process and early life exposures might be related to changes in health and disease risk in later life (Kuh et al., 2014) Growing evidence suggests that the aging process starts at the beginning of life and that dynamic relationships exist between different aging trajectories. Specifically, "health reserve" is stocked during development, reaches a plateau at maturity (structural or functional reserve), and then declines with age. The "biological capital" acquired during growth and the rate of decline determine how long aging individuals remain above a critical threshold of risk for adverse outcomes associated with loss of function. Thus, where an individual ends up in old age (**Figure 7.6**), depends on both the peak attained and the rate of decline (Kuh et al., 2014).

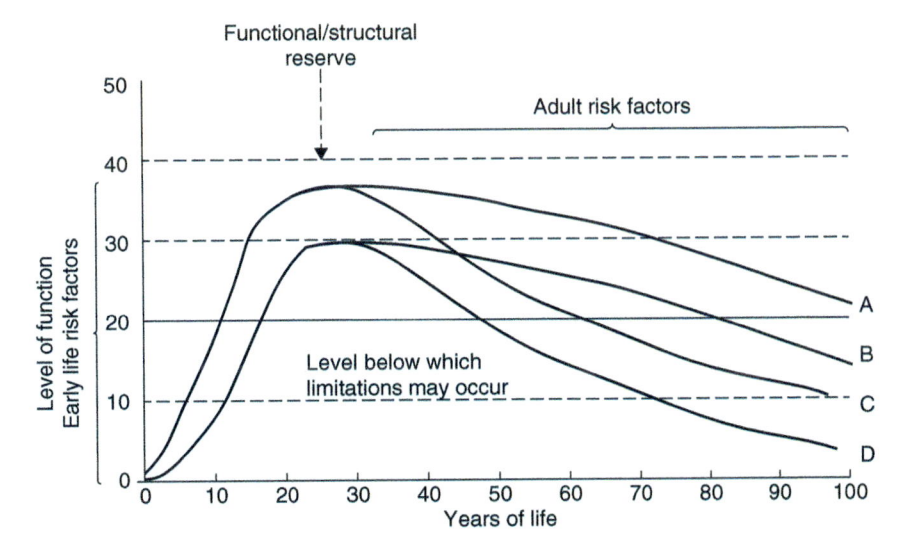

FIGURE 7.6 Life-course functional trajectories. (A) Normal development, and decline; (B) sub-optimal development resulting in reduced functional reserve at maturity; (C) accelerated age-related decline; (D) a combination of trajectories B and C. Source: (Kuh, 2007 / with permission of Oxford University Press).

Physical and social exposures from gestation to adult life can affect health status and disease risk in a lifetime. Exposures in early life, such as nutrition, activity, and chance events act across the lifespan, particularly during a critical developmental window, and may affect the structure or function of body systems, whereas exposures after the developmental period can only affect the timing and rate of decline. This concept is supported by the fact that age-related chronic diseases have their origins in early life and share common risk factors and causative mechanisms (Kuh, 2007).

According to the life-course aging concept, healthy aging is separated into healthy biological aging and well-being (**Figure 7.6**) (Kuh, 2007). Healthy biological aging is defined as "the maintenance, post maturity, of optimal physical and cognitive functioning for as long as possible, delaying the onset and rate of functional decline, and clinical disorders; well-being, on the other hand, represents positive emotional health, and participation in valued social roles, engaging with others, leading meaningful lives, maintaining autonomy, and independence." The healthy biological health theory provides us clear standards to evaluate and measure healthy aging, whereas the WHO concepts establish the framework for public health strategies to achieve healthy aging (Lu, Pikhart & Sacker 2019).

In 2018, the American Geriatrics Society white paper on healthy aging stated that: "Promotion of a realistic, dynamic, multidimensional view of healthy aging is an important goal obtainable through traditional and innovative models of health promotion and prevention" (Friedman et al., 2019). The WHO proposed "a public health framework for healthy aging across the life course, which involved developing strategies for health services, long-term care, and environments (Beard & Cassels, 2016)." This report also suggested that "before shaping policies, a quantitative assessment of healthy aging to help identify older people's health and needs are essential."

Apparently, there is no agreed-upon standard measure, given the complexity of the aging process and the lack of consensus about how to define healthy aging (Estebsari et al., 2020; Urtamo, 2019b). Despite the variety of approaches, the maintenance of functional independence seems to be a key element. Basically, healthy aging is a mix of functions, including physical capability, cognition, metabolic and physiological health, psychological well-being, and social well-being (Aronson, 2020; Friedman et al., 2019; Lu et al., 2019; Michel, 2019; Wagner et al., 2016) (**Figure 7.7; Table 7.2**).

- Physical capability is the degree to which a person can manage the physical tasks of daily living and encompasses a broad range of physical functions (Kuh et al., 2014). ADLs and IADLs are recommended for community-based studies to predict physical capabilities, whereas direct observations of performance such as grip strength, walking speed, balance, and the chair-rise test improve the predictability, especially among men (Lu et al., 2019).

- Cognitive function is an intellectual process by which one becomes aware of, perceives, or comprehends ideas. It is related to knowledge, attention, memory, judgment, and evaluation, among others. The Mini Mental State Examination (MMSE) is not the most appropriate scale to evaluate cognitive functions, but it can provide a brief cognitive screening test, and therefore, its application along with other cognitive tests, especially in memory and executive functions, is recommended (Lu et al., 2019).

- Regarding physiological health evaluation, the self-reported absence of chronic diseases may result in reporting bias, which is why objective tests for cardiovascular and lung functions, glucose metabolism, sleeping problems, vision, audition, and body pain are preferred (Wagner et al., 2016).

- The validity and reliability of psychological scales is well documented, yet it is necessary to clearly distinguish between the concepts behind the measurements.

- Measurements of social well-being are fuzzy; thus, it is preferable to use measurements of specific social roles.

Additionally, the importance of assessing sensorial functions was identified. For instance, olfactory function may be an indicator of the integrity of the aging brain in older people, as smell dysfunction is among the earliest 'preclinical' signs of

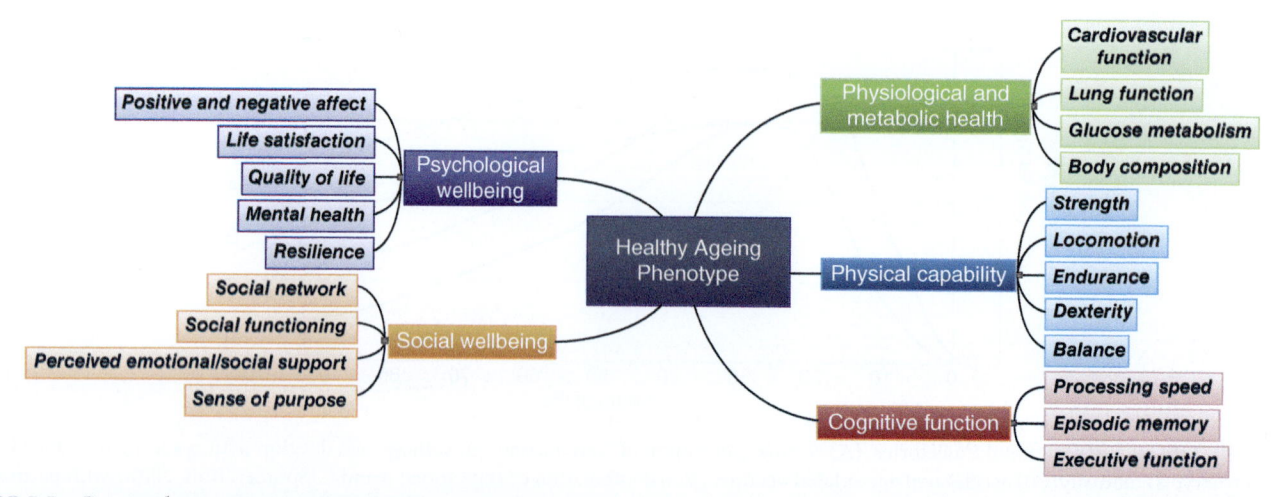

FIGURE 7.7 Proposed measurement domains for the healthy aging phenotype. Source: (Lara et al., 2013 / with permission of Elsevier).

Table 7.2 Tools to measure selected domains and sub-domains of the healthy aging phenotype.

Domain	Sub-domain	Tool/measure
Physiological and metabolic health	Cardiovascular function	Blood pressure
	Lung function	Blood lipids
	Glucose metabolism	Forced expiratory volume (FEC1)
	Body composition	Glycated hemoglobin (HbA1C)
		Blood glucose
		Waist circumference
		Waist-to-hip ratio
		Body-mass index
Physical capability	Strength	Handgrip strength
	Locomotion	Gait speed
	Endurance	Walk endurance test
	Dexterity	Pegboard dexterity test
	Balance	Standing balance test
		IADL
Cognitive function	Processing speed	Speed reaction time
	Episodic memory	Symbol digit modalities test
	Executive function	Story recall
		Word list recall
		Paired associate learning
		Stroop
		Trail making test A and B
Physiological well-being	Positive and negative affect	Positive and negative affect schedule (PANAS)
	Live satisfaction	Satisfaction with life scale (SWLS)
	Quality of life	Control, autonomy, pleasure, and self-realization, quality of life scale (CASP-19)
	Mental health	WHO quality of life -BREF (WHOQOL-BREF)
	Resilience	Center for Epidemiological Studies depression scale (CES-D)
		Warwick–Edinburgh mental well-being scale (WEMWBS)
		Psychological resilience scale

Sources: (Lara et al., 2013; Michel et al., 2019; Mount et al., 2016).

neurodegenerative diseases, such as Alzheimer's disease and sporadic Parkinson's disease (Lara et al., 2013).

SPECIAL CONSIDERATIONS

Undoubtedly, vast differences exist between how healthy aging is scientifically defined and how aging is viewed from the older adult's perspective (Reich et al., 2020). More specifically, in the medical literature, it is often viewed as the absence of disease and physical or cognitive disabilities (Michel, Graf, & Ecarnot, 2019). Social scientists, however, describe it as a state of well-being, socialization, and life satisfaction, highlighting the need to be portrayed by individual criteria. Others emphasize that aging well is aging in health, not merely avoiding a disease, and that it is important to incorporate both objective and subjective dimensions into the definition (Martin et al., 2015).

From the older adult's point of view, healthy aging is not a singular outcome, or the absence of changes compared with younger adults, thus it cannot be evaluated only by traditional health metrics. Older adults indicate that "well-being is produced by having the capability to mobilize resources to achieve goals and respond effectively to circumstances (Reich et al., 2020)." People's perceptions are not static either, as they often change over the life span and vary according to the person's psyche and sociocultural variables. Additionally, different cultures have different understandings and interact differently to promote or detract from a "good old age" (Aronson, 2020).

Many terms are used to describe an ideal aging trajectory, including successful, well, active, optimal, healthy, harmonious, and productive (Depp & Jeste, 2006; Mount, Lara, Schols & Mathers, 2016). "Healthy aging" is particularly current in Australian and European literature but appears also to underlie health policy development in the US (Depp & Jeste, 2006). Currently, healthy and successful aging are the most frequent terminologies, and they are often used interchangeably. Yet, is this identification correct? Following the previous analysis, concerns remain whether, in clinical practice, healthy and successful aging should be used as synonyms.

The term "successful" has been criticized. In high-income countries, "success" is usually associated with economic achievement, employment status, income, and assets (Aronson, 2020). Apart from this materialistic point of view, successful aging encompasses failure and questions whether functional decline is inevitable. Therefore, it is not considered appropriate for describing positive health outcomes, yet after decades of use, it will be difficult to eliminate its use.

Thereby, in accordance with McLaughlin et al., a distinction between successful and healthy aging can be made (McLaughlin, Jette, Connell, 2012). Successful aging requires the absence of disease and signals optimal health and functioning, whereas healthy aging does not. Basically, "healthy aging becomes a goal present across old age, yet successful aging signals human optimal health and functioning." According to the American Geriatrics Society, "By scaling expectations, compensating in creative ways, drawing assistance from others when needed, and both accommodating ourselves to changed circumstances and altering the environment to suit our circumstances, we can optimize chances for a rich and rewarding phase of late life (Friedman et al., 2019)."

What characteristics should a healthy ager have? Which parameters establish a healthy aging phenotype (Lara et al., 2013)? Expanding Rowe and Kahn's concept of "successful aging", healthy agers are the group with a "low probability of disease and disease-related disability, high cognitive and physical function capacity, and active engagement with life." It is important to consider that as people grow older, declining health is likely to occur. Although, for instance, some older adults remain free of chronic illness until late in life, over 80% of older adults have at least one chronic condition (Rowe & Kahn, 1987). Even individuals with healthy lifestyles and habits can usually expect some degree of physical, mental, and/or functional decline in old age. The distinction between "usual" and "successful" classifies many individuals with inconsequential health problems as unhealthy. There is a clear need to clarify the definition of healthy aging and specify its dimensions to identify older adults with reasonably good health from those whose health places them at risk of adverse events.

KEY POINTS

- The world population is aging rapidly, a demographic transition that necessitates a thorough evaluation of the aging process.
- Living longer does not necessarily entail experiencing better health, since age-related diseases are common.
- Aging is a complex process. Genetics, environment, and personal characteristics interrelate in several ways that lead to different aging phenotypes.
- A critical analysis of the historical development of aging theories is extremely important to understand the multidimensional nature of aging well.
- Rowe and Kahn's biomedical model of successful aging is a milestone in gerontology.
- There are two main scientific approaches: advocating for the older adults' aspects of aging and evaluating successful aging from the clinician's perspectives.

- There is not an agreed-upon definition of healthy aging. The WHO's definition is the one most often used.
- Healthy aging is a life-course process, and early life exposures might be related to changes in health and disease risk in later life.
- Healthy aging is a combination of functions, including physical capability, cognition, metabolic and physiological health, psychological well-being, and social well-being.
- The lack of an agreed-upon definition for healthy aging limits the development of tools for its measurement.
- Successful and healthy aging must not be used interchangeably; they represent different parameters. Successful aging requires the absence of disease and signals optimal health and functioning, whereas healthy aging does not. Basically, "healthy aging becomes a goal present across old age, yet successful aging signals human optimal health and functioning."

SELF-ASSESSMENT QUESTIONS

1. Aging is a multi-factorial process. Which variables account the most for the aging phenotype?
2. What factors are associated with successful aging?
3. Successful aging is a well-stated theory:
   (a) Examining life as a life-course procedure
   (b) Advocating older people's view
   (c) Distinguishing older from usual and unusual aging
   (d) Evaluating aging from the psychological point of view
4. In the literature, healthy and successful aging are used synonymously. Is this correct?
5. What are the key components of healthy aging?
6. True or False: Healthy aging is a dynamic life-course process.
7. True or False: A person with disabilities cannot be considered a healthy ager.
8. What is the aging paradox?
9. True or False: Healthy aging interventions are advised to start as soon as pre-conception. Why?
10. True or False: Physiological measures most commonly used to evaluate health status (i.e., glucose, lipid profile) are the most appropriate to assess healthy aging. Why?

REFERENCES

Aronson, L. (2020). Healthy Aging Across the Stages of Old Age. *Clinics in Geriatric Medicine*, *36*(4), 549–558. https://doi.org/10.1016/j.cger.2020.06.001

Beard, J. R., Officer, A., de Carvalho, I. A., Sadana, R., Pot, A. M., Michel, J.-P., Lloyd-Sherlock, P., Epping-Jordan, J. E., Peeters, G. M. E. E. (Geeske), Mahanani, W. R., Thiyagarajan, J. A., & Chatterji, S. (2016). The World report on ageing and health: a policy framework for healthy ageing. *The Lancet*, *387*(10033), 2145–2154. https://doi.org/10.1016/S0140-6736(15)00516-4

Beard, J. R., Officer, A. M., & Cassels, A. K. (2016). The World Report on Ageing and Health. *The Gerontologist*, *56*(Suppl 2), S163–S166. https://doi.org/10.1093/geront/gnw037

Black, M., & Bowman, M. (2020). Nutrition and Healthy Aging. *Clinics in Geriatric Medicine*, *36*(4), 655–669. https://doi.org/10.1016/j.cger.2020.06.008

Carmona JJ, M. S. (2016). Biology of Healthy Aging and Longevity. *Rev Invest Clin.*, *68*(1), 7–16.

Cosco, T. D., Howse, K., & Brayne, C. (2017). Healthy ageing, resilience and wellbeing. *Epidemiology and Psychiatric Sciences*, *26*(6), 579–583. https://doi.org/10.1017/S2045796017000324

Cumming, E. (1968). New thoughts on the theory of disengagement. *International Journal of Psychiatry*, *6*(1), 53–67.

Daskalopoulou, C., Stubbs, B., Kralj, C., Koukounari, A., Prince, M., & Prina, A. M. (2017). Physical activity and healthy ageing: A systematic review and meta-analysis of longitudinal cohort studies. *Ageing Research Reviews*, *38*, 6–17. https://doi.org/10.1016/j.arr.2017.06.003

Depp, C. A., & Jeste, D. v. (2006). Definitions and Predictors of Successful Aging: A Comprehensive Review of Larger Quantitative Studies. *The American Journal of Geriatric Psychiatry*, *14*(1), 6–20. https://doi.org/10.1097/01.JGP.0000192501.03069.bc

Eaton, N. R., Krueger, R. F., South, S. C., Gruenewald, T. L., Seeman, T. E., & Roberts, B. W. (2012). Genes, Environments, Personality, and Successful Aging: Toward a Comprehensive Developmental Model in Later Life. *The Journals of Gerontology Series A: Biological Sciences and Medical Sciences*, *67A*(5), 480–488. https://doi.org/10.1093/gerona/gls090

Estebsari, F., Dastoorpoor, M., Khalifehkandi, Z. R., Nouri, A., Mostafaei, D., Hosseini, M., Esmaeili, R., & Aghababaeian, H. (2020). The Concept of Successful Aging: A Review Article. *Current Aging Science*, *13*(1), 4–10. https://doi.org/10.2174/1874609812666191023130117

Freund, A. M., & Baltes, P. B. (1998). Selection, optimization, and compensation as strategies of life management: Correlations with subjective indicators of successful aging. *Psychology and Aging*, *13*(4), 531–543. https://doi.org/10.1037/0882-7974.13.4.531

Friedman, S. M., Mulhausen, P., Cleveland, M. L., Coll, P. P., Daniel, K. M., Hayward, A. D., Shah, K., Skudlarska, B., & White, H. K. (2019). Healthy Aging: American Geriatrics Society White Paper Executive Summary. *Journal of the American Geriatrics Society*, *67*(1), 17–20. https://doi.org/10.1111/jgs.15644

Goldman, D. (2016). The Economic Promise of Delayed Aging. *Cold Spring Harbor Perspectives in Medicine*, *6*(2), a025072. https://doi.org/10.1101/cshperspect.a025072

Green, G. (2013). Age-Friendly Cities of Europe. *Journal of Urban Health*, *90*(S1), 116–128. https://doi.org/10.1007/s11524-012-9765-8

Healthy Aging and Wellness Working Group of the Federal/Provincial/Territorial (F/P/T) Committee of Officials (Seniors). (2006). *Healthy Aging in Canada: A New Vision, A Vital Investment From Evidence to Action.* Https://Www.Health.Gov.Bc.ca/Library/Publications/Year/2006/Healthy_Aging_A_Vital_latest_copy_October_2006.Pdf.

Hernandez, D. C., & Johnston, C. A. (2017). Individual and Environmental Barriers to Successful Aging. *American Journal of Lifestyle Medicine*, *11*(1), 21–23. https://doi.org/10.1177/1559827616672617

Katz, T. F. A. D. L. (1963). Activities of Daily Living. *Journal of American Medical Association*, *185*, 914–919.

Kuh, D. (2007). A Life Course Approach to Healthy Aging, Frailty, and Capability. *The Journals of Gerontology Series A: Biological Sciences and Medical Sciences*, *62*(7), 717–721. https://doi.org/10.1093/gerona/62.7.717

Kuh, D., Karunananthan, S., Bergman, H., & Cooper, R. (2014). A life-course approach to healthy ageing: maintaining physical capability. *Proceedings of the Nutrition Society*, *73*(2), 237–248. https://doi.org/10.1017/S0029665113003923

Kusumastuti, S., Derks, M. G. M., Tellier, S., di Nucci, E., Lund, R., Mortensen, E. L., & Westendorp, R. G. J. (2016). Successful ageing: A study of the literature using citation network analysis. *Maturitas*, *93*, 4–12. https://doi.org/10.1016/j.maturitas.2016.04.010

Lara, J., Godfrey, A., Evans, E., Heaven, B., Brown, L. J. E., Barron, E., Rochester, L., Meyer, T. D., & Mathers, J. C. (2013). Towards measurement of the Healthy Ageing Phenotype in lifestyle-based intervention studies. *Maturitas*, *76*(2), 189–199. https://doi.org/10.1016/j.maturitas.2013.07.007

López-Otín, C., Blasco, M. A., Partridge, L., Serrano, M., & Kroemer, G. (2013). The Hallmarks of Aging. *Cell*, *153*(6), 1194–1217. https://doi.org/10.1016/j.cell.2013.05.039

Lu, W., Pikhart, H., & Sacker, A. (2019). Domains and Measurements of Healthy Aging in Epidemiological Studies: A Review. *The Gerontologist*, *59*(4), e294–e310. https://doi.org/10.1093/geront/gny029

Martin, P., Kelly, N., Kahana, B., Kahana, E., Willcox, B. J., Willcox, D. C., & Poon, L. W. (2015). Defining Successful Aging: A Tangible or Elusive Concept? *The Gerontologist*, *55*(1), 14–25. https://doi.org/10.1093/geront/gnu044

McLaughlin, S. J., Jette, A. M., & Connell, C. M. (2012). An Examination of Healthy Aging Across a Conceptual Continuum: Prevalence Estimates, Demographic Patterns, and Validity. *The Journals of Gerontology Series A: Biological Sciences and Medical Sciences*, *67*(7), 783–789. https://doi.org/10.1093/gerona/glr234

Michel, J.-P. (2019). Identification of the Best Societal Measurement of Healthy Aging. *Annals of Geriatric Medicine and Research*, *23*(2), 45–49. https://doi.org/10.4235/agmr.19.0017

Michel, J.-P., & Ecarnot, F. (2019). Integrating functional ageing into daily clinical practice. *Journal of Frailty, Sarcopenia and Falls*, *04*(02), 30–35. https://doi.org/10.22540/JFSF-04-030

Michel, J.-P., Graf, C., & Ecarnot, F. (2019). Individual healthy aging indices, measurements and scores. *Aging Clinical and Experimental Research*, *31*(12), 1719–1725. https://doi.org/10.1007/s40520-019-01327-y

Mount, S., Lara, J., Schols, A. M. W. J., & Mathers, J. C. (2016). Towards a multidimensional healthy ageing phenotype. *Current Opinion in Clinical Nutrition & Metabolic Care*, *19*(6), 418–426. https://doi.org/10.1097/MCO.0000000000000318

Neugarten, B. L. (1972). Personality and the Aging Process. *The Gerontologist*, *12*(1 Part 1), 9–15. https://doi.org/10.1093/geront/12.1_Part_1.9

Neugarten, B. L., Havighurst, R. J., & Tobin, S. S. (1961). The Measurement of Life Satisfaction. *Journal of Gerontology*, *16*(2), 134–143. https://doi.org/10.1093/geronj/16.2.134

Passarino, G., de Rango, F., & Montesanto, A. (2016). Human longevity: Genetics or Lifestyle? It takes two to tango. *Immunity & Ageing, 13*(1), 12. https://doi.org/10.1186/s12979-016-0066-z

Reich, A. J., Claunch, K. D., Verdeja, M. A., Dungan, M. T., Anderson, S., Clayton, C. K., Goates, M. C., & Thacker, E. L. (2020). What Does "Successful Aging" Mean to you? — Systematic Review and Cross-Cultural Comparison of Lay Perspectives of Older Adults in 13 Countries, 2010–2020. *Journal of Cross-Cultural Gerontology, 35*(4), 455–478. https://doi.org/10.1007/s10823-020-09416-6

Rowe, J. W., & Kahn, R. L. (1987). Human Aging: Usual and Successful. *Science, 237*(4811), 143–149. https://doi.org/10.1126/science.3299702

Stowe, J. D., & Cooney, T. M. (2015). Examining Rowe and Kahn's Concept of Successful Aging: Importance of Taking a Life Course Perspective. *The Gerontologist, 55*(1), 43–50. https://doi.org/10.1093/geront/gnu055

Suzman, R., & R. M. W. (1985). Introducing the "oldest old"Introducing the "oldest old." *The Milbank Memorial Fund Quarterly. Health and Society, 63*(2), 177–186.

The Swedish National Institute of Public Health. (2006). Healthy Aging. *A challenge for Europe.* Https://Ec.Europa.Eu/Health/Ph_projects/2003/Action1/Docs/2003_1_26_frep_en.Pdf.

United Nations. (2019). *World Population Ageing* 2019. Https://Www.Un.Org/En/Development/Desa/Population/Publications/Pdf/Ageing/WorldPopulationAgeing2019-Highlights.Pdf.

Urtamo, A., J. S. K., & S. T. E. (2019a). Definitions of successful ageing: a brief review of a multidimensional concept. *Acta Bio-Medica : Atenei Parmensis, 90*(2), 359–363.

Urtamo, A., J. S. K., & S. T. E. (2019b). Definitions of successful ageing: a brief review of a multidimensional concept. *Acta Bio-Medica : Atenei Parmensis, 90*(2), 359–363.

Wagner, K.-H., Cameron-Smith, D., Wessner, B., & Franzke, B. (2016). Biomarkers of Aging: From Function to Molecular Biology. *Nutrients, 8*(6), 338. https://doi.org/10.3390/nu8060338

World Health Organization. (1948). *The definition of Health.* Https://Www.Who.Int/about/Who-We-Are/Constitution.

World Health Organization. (2015). *World Report on Healthy Aging.* Https://Apps.Who.Int/Iris/Bitstream/Handle/10665/186468/WHO_FWC_ALC_15.01_eng.Pdf;Jsessionid=80D6ABD990647FDC364B4A95DC6504D0?Sequence=1.

Young, Y., Frick, K. D., & Phelan, E. A. (2009). Can Successful Aging and Chronic Illness Coexist in the Same Individual? A Multidimensional Concept of Successful Aging. *Journal of the American Medical Directors Association, 10*(2), 87–92. https://doi.org/10.1016/j.jamda.2008.11.003

FURTHER READING

Bibliography

Brooks-Wilson A. R. (2013). Genetics of healthy aging and longevity. *Human Genetics 132* (12), 1323–1338. doi: 10.1007/s00439-013-1342-z.

Daniel K. M. (2020). Best practices for promoting healthy aging. *Clinics in Geriatric Medicine 36* (4): 713–718. doi: 10.1016/j.cger.2020.06.012.

Friedman S. M. (2020). Lifestyle (medicine) and healthy aging. *Clinics in Geriatric Medicine 36* (4): 645–653. doi: 10.1016/j.cger.2020.06.007.

Roberts, S. B., Silver, R. E., Das, S. K., Fielding, R. A., Gilhooly, C. H., Jacques, P. F., Kelly, J. M., Mason, J. B., McKeown, N. M., Reardon, M. A., Rowan, S., Saltzman, E., Shukitt-Hale, B., Smith, C. E., Taylor, A. A., Wu, D., Zhang, F. F., Panetta, K., & Booth, S. (2021). Healthy aging-nutrition matters: Start early and screen often. *Advances in Nutrition 12* (4): 1438–1448. doi: 10.1093/advances/nmab032.

Sharda, N., Wong, S., & White, H. (2020). The role of prevention in healthy aging. *Clinics in Geriatric Medicine 36* (4): 697–711. doi: 10.1016/j.cger.2020.06.011.

Age Platform Europe. Healthy Aging. [cited 2022 September 30]. Available from: https://www.age-platform.eu/policy-work/healthy-ageing

European Commission. Active and Healthy Living in the Digital World. [cited 2022 October 30]. Available from: https://ec.europa.eu/eip/ageing/home_en.html

National Institutes of Health. What Do We Know About Healthy Aging; February 23, 2022. [cited 2022 September 30]. Available from: https://www.nia.nih.gov/health/what-do-we-know-about-healthy-aging

United Nations. Ageing, Older Persons and the 2030 Agenda for Sustainable Development. 2017 update. [cited 2022 October 30]. Available from: https://www.un.org/development/desa/ageing/news/2017/07/ageing-older-persons-and-the-2030-agenda-for-sustainable-development/

World Health Organization. Healthy ageing and functional ability; October 20, 2020. [cited 2022 October 30]. Available from: https://www.who.int/philippines/news/q-a-detail/healthy-ageing-and-functional-ability

World Health Organization. What is the UN Decade of Healthy Ageing? [cited 2022 October 30]. Available from: https://www.who.int/initiatives/decade-of-healthy-ageing

The Interface Between Healthy Aging, Longevity, and Disease

CHAPTER 8

Introduction	105	The Heritability of Longevity and Healthy Aging	109
Overview of Longevity	107	Epigenetic Mechanisms and Longevity	110
The Longevity Boom	107	How to Achieve a Healthy and Long Life Span	111
Sex Differences	107	Key Points	113
Geographical Longevity Clusters	108	Self-assessment Questions	113
Overview of the Concepts of Morbidity and Mortality	108	References	113
Longevity as a Healthy Aging Model	109	Further Reading	115
Are the Long Lived, Healthy Lived?	109	Bibliography	115
		Links	115

INTRODUCTION

Over the last 200 years, human life expectancy has nearly doubled. Demographic data confirm that at the beginning of the nineteenth century, a child born could only expect a short life, considering that globally, no country had a life expectancy more than 40 years. In the United Kingdom (UK), for instance, the country with the longest time-series, in 1765, a baby girl was expected to live up to 42 years and a boy to 40. In 2019, life expectancy was 83 and 79 years old for women and men, respectively (Roser, Ortiz-Ospina, Ritchie, 2019). In the 150 years since 1765, some parts of the world experienced great improvements in life expectancy. This shift was mainly related to a significant reduction in early life mortality observed during the first half of the twentieth century, followed by an almost twofold reduction in mortality at ages 70 years and older in the past 50 years (Oeppen & Vaupel, 2002) (**Figure 8.1**).

Worldwide, according to the United Nations (UN), the mean life span over the last few decades, has increased from 52.5 in the 1960s, to 73 years old today (The World Bank group, 2021) (**Figure 8.2**). However, since the 1950s, increases in life expectancy have slowed, demonstrating that human life expectancy might have reached its biological upper limit (Cardona & Bishai, 2018). Similarly, the maximum life span has only modestly increased too. These observations prompted the notion that the human life span might have reached its maximal natural limit of about 115 years (Brooks-Wilson, 2013). The oldest documented person in the world to date, lived to 122 (Robine & Allard, 1998). Others argue that the lack of increase does not exclude the possibility that the maximum human life span might increase in the future. These observations make us wonder: is our life span flexible or fixed by genetics?

Although the human life span is prolonged, there is no evidence to suggest that older people are experiencing better health than their ancestors at the same age (Calder et al., 2018). It is true that the healthy life expectancy has increased around the world in recent decades, though it is also a fact that improved healthcare increased the number of years experiencing disease or disability; as people age, they have an increased risk for disease and disability (**Figure 8.3**). Aging was described as an accumulation of the impact of time, environmental factors, and disease (Bussee, 1969). Notably, older people have a higher incidence of cerebrovascular and ischemic heart disease, chronic obstructive lung disease, dementia, vision disorders, and cancer (Byles, 2007). These conditions apparently contribute to a great loss of years and significantly affect quality of life. Considering that increases in lifespan exceed increases in health span, an important question arises about how people can live longer and healthier lives.

Modern medical research focuses mostly on learning the causes of disease pathology, noting that disease is the major challenge to tackle. For some this pathology-oriented approach

---

Prevention and Management of Cardiovascular and Metabolic Disease: Diet, Physical Activity and Healthy Aging,
First Edition. Christina N. Katsagoni, Peter Kokkinos, and Labros S. Sidossis.
© 2023 John Wiley & Sons Ltd. Published 2023 by John Wiley & Sons Ltd.

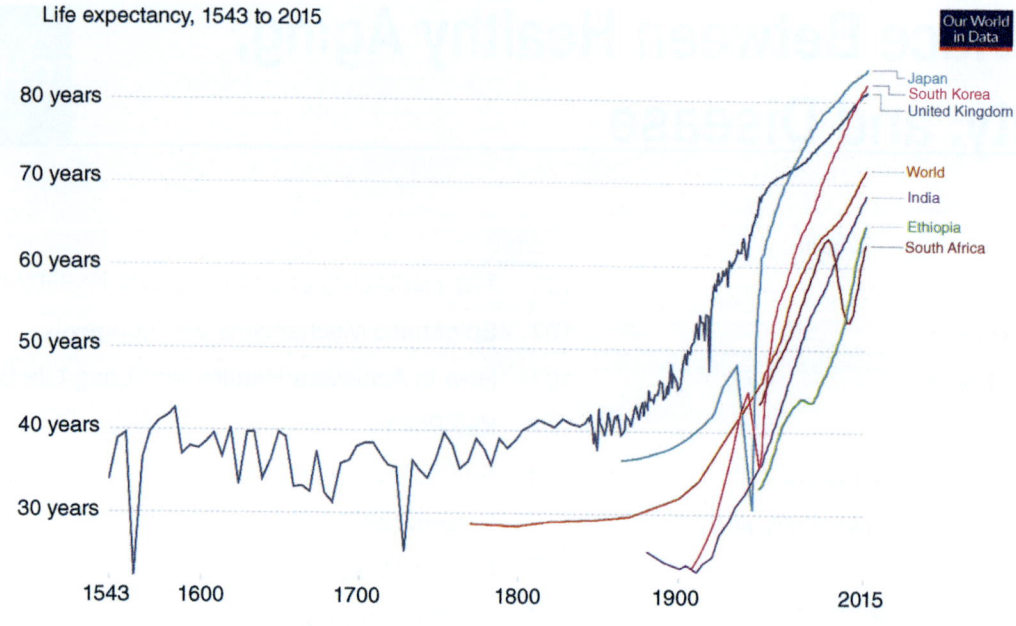

FIGURE 8.1 Life expectancy, 1543 to 2015. Source: (Riley, 2005).

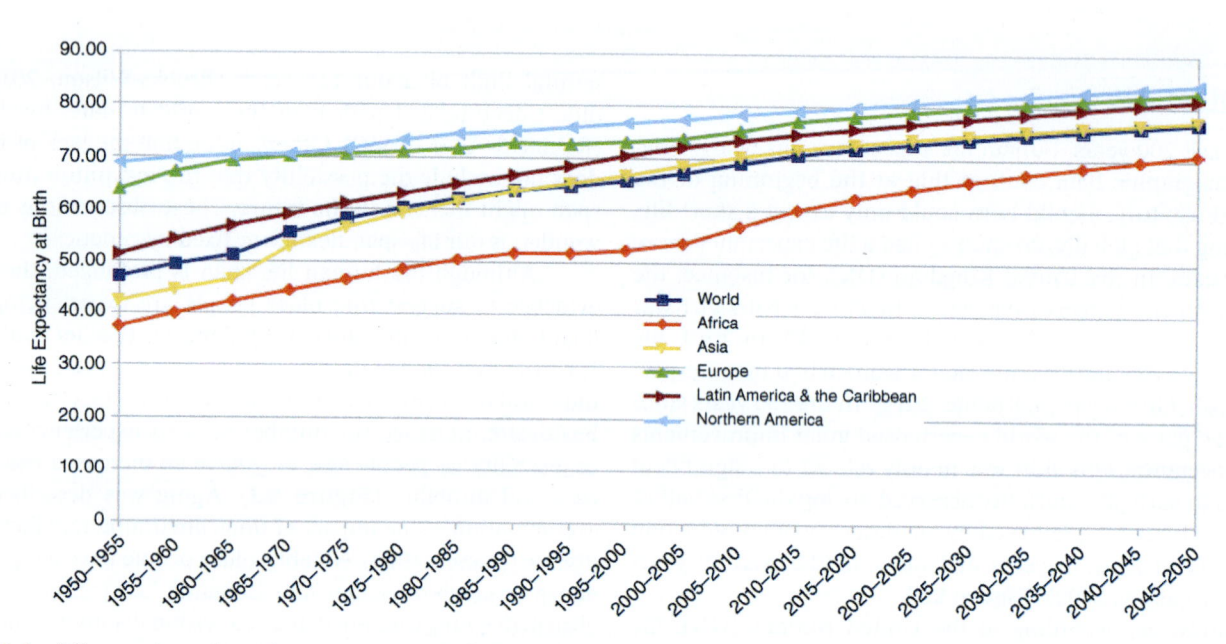

FIGURE 8.2 Life expectancy by region, 1950 to 2050. UN World Population Prospects, 2017. Source: (Adapted from Roser, 2019).

for prevention and treatment, the so-called "negative" biology, might be the wrong way to evaluate human health (Farrelly, 2012). Rather than examining what causes disease and disability, emphasizing what causes ideal health and happiness might be a priority and possibly an alternative question to answer. "Positive" biology strives to understand positive phenotypes: why some individuals live a longer and healthier life, without suffering from the diseases that most people confront much earlier in their lives. Observations of exceptional longevity (reserved for individuals aged 100 years or more, otherwise known as centenarians) might provide insights about how to obtain exemplar health and well-being; centenarians might represent an ideal healthy aging model. Undoubtedly, the basis of human longevity and healthy aging that constitute the "positive" aging and how to conquer these desirable phenotypes are a scientific milestone (Brooks-Wilson, 2013).

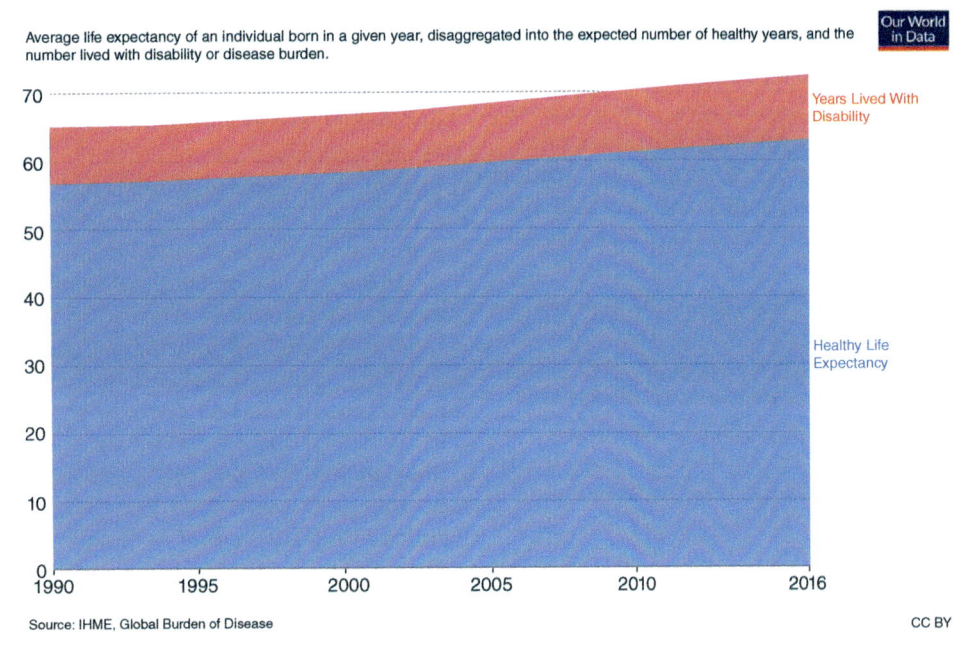

FIGURE 8.3 Worldwide healthy life expectancy and years lived with disability, 1990 to 2016. Source: (The World Bank Group, 2021).

OVERVIEW OF LONGEVITY

THE LONGEVITY BOOM

Human longevity is often defined as reaching an age of ≥85 years, but a single accepted definition does not currently exist (Murabito, Yuan, & Lunetta, 2012). Worldwide demographic data reveal that the oldest older adults, usually defined as individuals over 85-years old, are the fastest growing population group (Ritchie & Roser, 2019). As global health improves and mortality falls, people are expected to live longer than before. Consequently, the proportion of older people will substantially expand, and considering that the number of children will barely increase, for the first time in history there are more people over 60 than children under 5. The number of children under 5-years old is projected to peak and plateau for most of the twenty-first century, and as the global population of older people will continue to grow, it seems that we are moving toward an aging world.

Due to this demographic change, the UN Global Population Pyramid is undergoing a major change from the classical shape of a pyramid to a cube (Panagiotakos et al., 2011). Indeed, nonagenarians and centenarians are expanding in many countries. For instance, in Japan, the number was estimated to increase from 154 in 1963 to 36,276 in 2008 (Robine, Saito, & Jagger, 2003), a 235-fold increase in less than 50 years. The US Census bureau predicts that 834,000 centenarians will exist in the United States by the year 2050 (Velkoff, 2000). Japan, followed by Germany, Italy, Greece, Finland, and Sweden had the world's oldest populations in 2015, and by 2050, some other Asian populations, including South Korea, Hong Kong, and Taiwan are expected to experience a longevity boom (United States Census Bureau, 2015).

In 2015, Japan, Macau, Singapore, Australia, and Switzerland had the longest life expectancy at 65, with an additional 25.2 and 20 years of life for Japanese women and men, respectively. It is noticeable that among the long-lived countries, healthy life years vary between 25% and 75% of the predicted life expectancy at 65 years old, with Norway, Sweden, and Iceland having the greatest number of expected healthy years at age 65 (Sebastiani & Perls, 2012).

SEX DIFFERENCES

It is important to mention that globally, women live longer than men and account for a larger proportion of the older population, especially at exceptionally old ages. To illustrate this in the US, 1% of women born during the end of the last century lived to be 100, whereas the same percentage of men was 0.1% (Sebastiani & Perls, 2012). Furthermore, among the original 5,209 Framingham heart study participants with follow-up through 2011, there were 43 centenarian women and only 6 centenarian men. Nevertheless, men are more likely to reach extreme old age while escaping common age-related diseases, whereas women are more likely to attain 100 after surviving common morbidities (Evert, Lawler, Bogan, & Perls, 2003). Therein lies a paradox of women's survival advantage: They suffer from more illness and chronic health problems than men but die at lower rates from all the major causes of death (Austad & Bartke, 2015). The Williams evolutionary hypothesis says that the sex subjected to the greatest extrinsic hazards in the wild will evolve the more rapidly deteriorating phenotype. From this perspective, it seems that women are the superior survivors when they are old, young, and even *in utero*. Possible confounders that explain these sex discrepancies might include hormonal and immune differences as well as hemizygosity of the X-chromosome in men, among others (Brooks-Wilson, 2013).

GEOGRAPHICAL LONGEVITY CLUSTERS

There are places around the world where people live longer and probably share common behavioral and lifestyle characteristics like "family coherence, avoidance of smoking, plant-based diet, moderate and daily physical activity, social engagement, where people of all ages are socially active and integrated into the community" ("The Blue Zones", 2010). These places are defined as the "blue zones" and are a part of a large anthropologic and demographic project. More specifically, people living in Sardinia (Italy), Okinawa (Japan), Loma Linda (California), Nicoya Peninsula (Costa Rica), and Ikaria (Greece) have extremely high life expectancy, with amazing rates of people over the age of 90 compared with the average rate of high-income countries.

What makes these populations so special? Long-lived Okinawans eat a rainbow diet, based on diverse fruits and vegetables, and their daily caloric intake is substantially decreased, accounting for their low body-mass index. Additionally, Sardinian men, compared with men elsewhere, tend to live longer due to genetics as well as small, apportioned meals, handwork, and red wine. Seventh Day Adventists, a religious community residing in Loma Linda, California, are strict vegetarians, abstain from tobacco and alcohol, and exhibit significantly lower levels of stress hormones that is closely related to the weekly break from the rigors of daily life, the 24-hour Sabbath. Adventists claim this provides a time to focus on family, God and relieves their stress. The Costa Rican Nicoyan diet is based on beans and corn tortillas, people regularly perform physical jobs into old age, and have a sense of life purpose known as "plan de vida" (reason to live). Moreover, Ikarians in Greece are almost entirely free of dementia and some of the chronic diseases that affect Western communities; one in three make it to their 90s. They enjoy red wine and a relaxed pace of life that ignores clocks.

Blue Zones is a way to design the healthiest lifestyles possible for individuals and for entire communities. Over the past two decades research efforts focus on the factors associated with blue zones longevity, as well as exploring the possibility of lessons transferable to the general population (Buettner, & Skemp, 2016). Although their lifestyles differ slightly, they mostly eat a plant-based diet, exercise regularly, drink moderate amounts of alcohol, get enough sleep and have good spiritual, family and social networks. Probably, a combination of factors explains it, including geography, culture, diet, lifestyle, and a positive outlook (Pignolo, 2019; "The Blue Zones", 2010).

OVERVIEW OF THE CONCEPTS OF MORBIDITY AND MORTALITY

Along with the prolonged lifespan observed in most high-income countries, there is a growing concern about the quality of life in those living beyond 70s as well as whether the added years will be counterbalanced by increased morbidity and disability at older ages. Although amplify data indicate that lifetime medical expenses for care do not further increase at incredibly old ages, long-term care costs increase since most older adults need some form of assistance with activities of daily living (Christensen, McGue, Petersen, Jeune, & Vaupel, 2008). Consequently, questions remain whether these added years are offset by increased morbidity and disability at older ages. Therefore, it is extremely important to identify and closely examine the factors that allow long-lived individuals to be healthy and independent until the end of their lives.

There is a long debate within gerontology as to whether longer life is associated with a "compression of morbidity" or an "expansion of morbidity". According to Gruenberg (Gruenberg, 2005), the treatment of acute illnesses and the management of chronic diseases equate to living more and more frail. The theory of "failure of success" advocated that prolonging life span will prolong disease and disability. At the same theory it was argued that "the net effect of successful technical innovations used in disease control has been to raise the prevalence of certain diseases and disabilities by prolonging their average duration". Similarly, the "expansion of morbidity" advocates a pessimistic view of trading longer life with healthier years, foreseeing an increase in life expectancy through medical advances with an increase in the proportion of life spent with an underlying illness or disability (Olshansky, Rudberg, Carnes, Cassel, & Brody, 1991). People will live longer (due to reduced mortality) but with increased morbidity and duration of morbidity.

On the contrary, the "compression of morbidity" theory (Fries, 1980) states that "the burden of lifetime illness may be compressed into a shorter period before the time of death if the age of onset of the first chronic infirmity can be postponed" (**Figure 8.4**). The compression of morbidity theory was introduced as a hypothesis of healthy aging in 1980 and advocated that "the age at first appearance of symptoms of aging and chronic disease can increase more rapidly than life expectancy." In this optimistic view, changes in lifestyle can modify the risk factors for mortality and postpone the onset of morbidity. Additionally, this hypothesis strongly suggests that the net effect of primary prevention is to reduce and compress disability into a shorter period toward the end of life, decrease overall lifetime disability, and consequently, reduce the associated health care burden (Fries, Bruce, & Chakravarty, 2011).

Based on these considerations, Manton tried to bridge the gap by developing a third theory of population health change, the "dynamic equilibrium" (Manton, 1982), which is an intermediate scenario that combines the first two hypotheses: the compression and expansion hypotheses. Manton suggested an increase of life expectancy along with a constant proportion of healthy lifespan and a decrease in the severity of diseases and disabilities over time. According to this notion, the dynamic equilibrium scenario implies that "mortality reductions are at least partially, the result of reductions in the rate of chronic disease progression and is associated with a redistribution of disease and disability from more to less severe states". Regarding this possibility, the period of life span with *serious* illness or disability remains constant, whereas the time period with *moderate* disability or less severe illness increases.

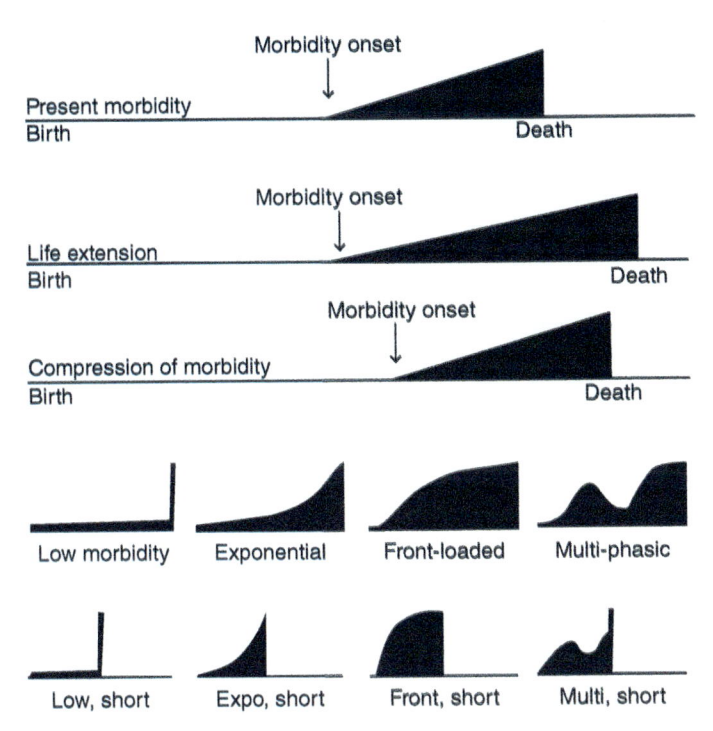

FIGURE 8.4 The compression of morbidity theory. Scenarios for future morbidity. The three major population scenarios in the upper part of the figure represent (i) depiction of a present health, (ii) a future where both life expectancy and morbidity are increased, and (iii) a future where both the time period after first morbidity and the amount of morbidity are decreased, resulting in compression of morbidity. Shaded areas under the curve represent cumulative morbidity. Source: (Fries et al., 2011 / Hindawi / CC BY-3.0).

LONGEVITY AS A HEALTHY AGING MODEL

ARE THE LONG LIVED, HEALTHY LIVED?

Over time, the likelihood of living to 100 rose from 1 in 20 million, to 1 in 50 for women in low-mortality countries, like Japan and Sweden (Pignolo, 2019). A study of centenarians (individuals aged of 100–104 years), semisupercentenarians (105–109 years), and supercentenaians (110–119 years) found that the older the age group, the greater the delay in the onset of age-related diseases (Velkoff, 2000). Lifespan and health span seem to be strongly related and individuals who live long tend to be healthier during their lives. Longevity and healthy aging are extremely complex characteristics that entail the maintenance of long-term function and disease absence or reduction (Brooks-Wilson, 2013). There lies the question. Why are some individuals long lived? What is so special about them? Observations of centenarians might give insight into why some people enjoy a long life and most of all, a life in good health.

Centenarians are generally considered a healthy aging model (Puca, Spinelli, Accardi, Villa, & Caruso, 2018). They have reduced mortality rates and are less prone to the diseases that come with aging. Some are even disease free, the so-called "escapers", while others, the "survivors" from diseases in earlier life, are frailer. Although research data indicate that 1% of Italian centenarians, for instance, are fully independent whereas 2% of the Japanese centenarians are in perfect health, defined as having no sensory problems, cognitive defects, and being independent, numerous studies suggest that centenarians were in a relatively good health 5 or 10 years previously (Robine et al., 2003). In the 1905 Danish cohort, the vast majority of those who became 100-years old in 2005, were physically independent at 92-years old, indicating only a modest decline in independent individuals' ratio between ages of 92 and 100. Additionally, individuals who survived into the highest ages had a health profile like that of individuals who were 7 or 8 years younger (Christensen et al., 2008).

Whether centenarians constitute a healthy aging prototype is an area of debate, however, living up to 100, 20 to 25 years more than the average person, is astonishing. Centenarians may represent a unique cluster for examining the genetics of the extremely long lived as well as the interaction between genes and the environment. Data from longitudinal studies reveal that centenarians were healthier than their coevals who died at younger age (Puca et al., 2018). Danish centenarians from the 1905 birth cohort study experienced fewer hospitalizations and fewer hospital days than their shorter-lived contemporaries (Engberg, Oksuzyan, Jeune, Vaupel, & Christensen, 2009). This observation might reveal two important parameters of health in the oldest older adults. First, centenarians seem to postpone critical disease into their later years of life, and second, the diseases and morbidities that centenarians suffer may be less severe or influence them to a lesser extent.

THE HERITABILITY OF LONGEVITY AND HEALTHY AGING

It is well documented that both genetics and environmental, lifestyle factors affect survival. To make it to age 100, it seems that a person must win the genetic lottery. Cumulative data indicate that to live to 100, one must inherit the right genetic variants from parents or acquire epigenetic variants through the environment (Murabito et al., 2012; Passarino, de Rango, and Montesanto, 2016). Apparently, it is strongly stated that genes affect living till old age. Longevity as well as healthy aging are highly clustered within families, but this clustering can be excluded by chance (Brooks-Wilson, 2013). Central to this notion is that the parents of centenarians were seven times more likely to have lived until 90 to 99 compared to their contemporaries, thus a centenarian's offspring show a more favorable midlife risk factor profile and a lower prevalence of age-related diseases. Notably, adults with at least one parent surviving to old age have less risk factors compared to individuals whose parents died younger; they also have clear reductions or delay in cardiovascular diseases as well as in all-cause morbidity and mortality (Brooks-Wilson, 2013).

Human longevity is, at least partially, genetically determined with an estimated heritability of 0.20 to 0.30. Additionally, the heritability of living to 100 was estimated at 0.33 and 0.48 in women and men, respectively, and increases as people age (Brooks-Wilson, 2013). The latter is consistent between several studies. For instance, the siblings of Okinawan centenarians show an increased adult survival probability that start at 55 and increases with age (Murabito et al., 2012). Long life was heritable in Icelanders aged over 70 years. Moreover, in over 20,000 Scandinavian twins, heritability of longevity was negligible from age 6 to 60 but increased with age thereafter. It is speculated that the genetic component of longevity exerts its effect for survival at much older ages, beyond the age of 90.

About 25 percent of the variation in human life span is estimated to be determined by genetics, yet candidate gene and genome-wide association studies (GWAS) have yielded few replicated longevity-gene associations to date, with the exceptions of the *ApoE* and *FOXO3A* genes (Puca et al., 2018). Specifically, there were a few shared loci in the *ApoE*, *FOXO3*, and *CETP* genes, but they are not found in all individuals with exceptional longevity (Brooks-Wilson, 2013). Interestingly, some of the gene variants that contribute to longevity are involved with cellular maintenance and function, including DNA repair, maintenance of the ends of chromosomes (regions called telomeres), and protection of cells from damage caused by unstable oxygen-containing molecules (free radicals), while some other genes are related to lipid levels and inflammation (Murabito et al., 2012). Consequently, these genetic variations, possibly inherited by long-lived parents, may predispose cells to better adapt to stress and survive an adverse environment. For instance, the longevity associated variant of BPIFB4, which is enriched in centenarians and overexpressed in healthy centenarians compared to frail ones, was reported to reduce blood pressure by activating vascular rejuvenation and promoting reparative process (Puca et al., 2018).

Moreover, it is worth mentioning that aging-related, disease-causing genes are not associated with longevity, suggesting that there are specific domains in the genome that determine longevity beyond those that determine morbidity in the population (Murabito et al., 2012). Surprisingly, centenarians do not appear to lack common complex-disease risk alleles. What is more interesting is that they have some protective genetic variants that buffer the risk alleles and allow them to remain healthy. This genetic predisposition might make individuals less prone, or more resistant, to age-related diseases as well as diseases that occur during early life (i.e., infections). For instance, in a study published in 2012 assessing the genetic variants for cancer risk along with other disease categories, Spanish centenarians, found to have lower genetic predisposition for cancer compared to matched healthy controls, possibly associated with exceptional longevity (Santos-Lozano et al., 2016).

EPIGENETIC MECHANISMS AND LONGEVITY

Human longevity is the synergistic result of random events, chance, environmental factors, and genetic predisposition. Excluding random events - events occurring without any obvious intention or cause (e.g., a war or an accident) that cannot be controlled, environmental factors are strong determinants of health and life span. Environmental factors are considered to affect probably the first seven or eight decades of life (Puca et al., 2018). After that point, genetics take control. Environmental stimuli can alter the genetic basis by promoting differential transcriptional profiles and enhancing genome stability through epigenetic mechanisms (Taormina & Mirisola, 2015).

Long life is probably inherited after the seventh or eighth decade of life, whereas during the early and midlife periods, epigenetic and environmental factors mostly affect the longevity phenotype (Taormina & Mirisola, 2015). Stochastic and non-stochastic events modulate the genetic substrate and orchestrate the establishment of a long-lived phenotype and finally lead to different outcomes (Puca et al., 2018). This observation is in accordance with the concept of developmental plasticity; the capacity to achieve lasting structural changes in response to environmental demands that are not fully met by the organism's current functional capacity. The study of epigenetic signatures of healthy aging is thought to yield insight to uncovered secrets of human longevity (Pignolo, 2019).

Changes in gene expression that occur because of molecular mechanisms that do not change the primary DNA sequence are referred to as epigenetics (see **Chapter 2**). Epigenetic mechanisms influence phenotypic expression and they are altered during development. They are also affected by the environment, diet, drugs, and aging (Taormina & Mirisola, 2015). There are many well-studied epigenetic processes, such as post-translational histone modifications, histone variants, and noncoding RNAs; however, these modifications are more of a focus in model organism research and cancer biology. One of the best studied epigenetic mechanisms called DNA methylation (DNAm), which usually results in the suppression of nearby genes, is strongly related to longevity. Epigenetic changes are cumulative with age in response to various environmental stimuli (Pignolo, 2019).

Changes in DNA methylation that occur with aging may alter normal gene expression and in turn contribute to the development of age-related diseases and functional decline (Costa, Scognamiglio, Fiorito, Benincasa, & Napoli, 2019). Methylation analysis identifies genes that are hypo- or hyper-methylated during aging (Heyn et al., 2012). After performing Whole-Genome Bisulfite Sequencing (WGBS) of newborn and centenarian genomes, Heyn et al found that DNA obtained from a 103-year-old donor was less methylated overall than DNA from the same cell type obtained from a neonate (Heyn et al., 2012). In another study, Chinese centenarians compared to middle-age controls were found to have different methylated regions that resulted in differently expressed genes correlated with age-related diseases such as type 2 diabetes, stroke, cardiovascular disease, and Alzheimer's (Xiao et al., 2015). These observations may explain why centenarians could escape from age-related diseases or their development to be delayed. Indeed, a lower level of total mean DNAm variation has been observed in Nicoyans in Costa Rica, a longevity hot spot, compared to non-Nicoyans (McEwen et al., 2017). Consequently, suppressing disease-related genes via the epigenetic modification is likely an important contributor in human longevity. However, a recent meta-analysis of 23 case control and cohort studies involving 41,607 participants, examining the interface between DNA methylation age, age-related disease, and longevity showed inconclusive outcomes and did not establish a strong association (Fransquet, Wrigglesworth, Woods, Ernst, & Ryan, 2019).

HOW TO ACHIEVE A HEALTHY AND LONG-LIFE SPAN

Numerous data indicate that dietary modification and exercise, including other healthy behaviors, such as avoiding tobacco and excessive alcohol are parameters that promote healthy aging and directly influence life span (Taormina & Mirisola, 2015). Healthy lifestyle undoubtedly influences positively both health and human longevity. This, in turn, can lead to a compression of morbidity, which has long been a goal of geriatric medicine. Conversely, poor healthy behaviors are intimately related to the increase of disease burden and along with increases in life expectancy are thought to have contributed to the rising prevalence of chronic disease and multimorbidity (Queen, Hassan, & Cao, 2020).

Dietary intervention is the most investigated nonpharmacological treatment that seems to battle against age-related diseases including obesity, atherosclerosis, diabetes, and other chronic disorders (Queen et al., 2020). A healthy diet/lifestyle along with specific dietary compounds, have found to mediate benefits on longevity and the prevention of age-related diseases (Pignolo, 2019; Queen et al., 2020). Specifically, sulforaphane - a sulfur-rich compound found in cruciferous vegetables like broccoli, bok choy, and cabbage and epigallocatechin-3-gallate—the most abundant and powerful flavonoid in green tea, act by inhibiting DNA methyltransferase and histone acetyltransferase or by modifying noncoding RNA expression and thus reducing epigenetic alterations.

Though it is not easy to examine the direct effect of a healthy lifestyle on exceptional longevity, the systematic analysis of longevity hot spots gives us insight about what it takes to be 100 ("The Blue Zones", 2010). Cumulative data support the notion that centenarians share common nutritional habits. They usually follow diets rich in fruits and vegetables, with a low glycemic load and rich antioxidant content, such as the Mediterranean diet (MD) and the Okinawan diet (Critselis & Panagiotakos, 2020; Trichopoulou & Critselis, 2004; Willcox, Scapagnini, & Willcox, 2014). These dietary patterns are associated with numerous health benefits and the prevention of several age-related disorders, such as cardiovascular disease, metabolic syndrome, and cancers as well as all-cause mortality and longevity (Critselis & Panagiotakos, 2020; Trichopoulou & Critselis, 2004). In a recent systematic review of observational studies higher adherence to the MD during midlife was associated with a 36% to 46% greater likelihood of healthy aging compared to lower adherence. Moreover, among older adults, the exclusive use of olive oil compared to no use of olive oil, was significantly associated with healthy aging and a 33% reduction in mortality risk (Critselis & Panagiotakos, 2020). Regarding the age-related outcomes, adherence to the MD seemed to protect from overall cognitive decline by 52% and reduced the risk of frailty by 68%.

Specific constituents of the MD, such as olive oil, which is rich in oleic acid and polyphenols (namely secoiridoids), impact the biological pathways implicated in the hallmarks of aging (Fernández del Río, Gutiérrez-Casado, Varela-López, & Villalba, 2016) and are associated with healthy aging (Foscolou et al., 2018). Specifically, the Mediterranean and Asian diets consist of numerous nutrients and phytochemicals which reduce inflammation and oxidative stress that consequently, may deter telomere attrition (Davinelli, Trichopoulou, Corbi, de Vivo, & Scapagnini, 2019). Likewise, the consumption of antioxidant rich diets with plentiful fruits and vegetables are associated with longer telomere length (Freitas-Simoes, Ros, & Sala-Vila, 2016) (**Table 8.1**).

Studies on Sicilian centenarians demonstrated that this population undergoes a sort of self-administered caloric restriction, with an intake of only about 1200–1300 kilocalories per day (Queen et al., 2020). Calorie restriction has a positive impact on the hallmarks of aging by improving the stress response,

Table 8.1 Epigenetic effect of some phytochemicals on aging (in different model organisms, in human beings, and in vitro).

Phytochemicals	Sources	Epigenetic targets	Findings	References
Anthocyanins	Red fruits, red onion, aubergine	NF-κB	Decrease of the plasma concentrations of several NF-κB regulated pro-inflammatory mediators.	Karlsen et al., 2007
Curcumin	Curry, turmeric	DNMT, HDAC and HAT inhibitor and miRNA modulator	Inhibition of the expression of pro-inflammatory mediators by affecting histone acetylation of transcription factors and methylation pattern of gene promoters associated with inflammatory response.	Boyanapalli and Tony Kong, 2015; Kang et al., 2006
Resveratrol	Grapes, peanuts, mulberries, cranberries, blueberries	Inhibition of HDAC inhibitor	Activation of SIRT-1 leading to deacetylation of p53, NF-κB, HSF-1, FOXO 1,3,4 and PGC-1 alpha, influencing replicative senescence, inflammation, apoptosis, metabolism and stress resistance.	Barger et al., 2008; Baur and Sinclair, 2006a, 2006b; Hubbard and Sinclair, 2014
Extra virgin olive oil	Olives	Genes involved directly or indirectly in ageing	Influence of the methylation and acetylation of genes directly or indirectly involved in ageing and metabolic diseases.	Fernández del Río et al., 2016

NF-κB: nuclear factor kappa-light-chain-enhancer of activated B cells; DNMT: DNA methyltransferase; HDAC: histone deacetylase; HAT: histone acetyltransferase; miRNA: microRNA; SIRT-1; sirtuine-1; FOXO; Forkhead box O3; HSF-1; Heat shock factor 1; PGC-1 alpha; Peroxisome proliferator-activated receptor gamma coactivator 1-alpha.
Source: (Puca et al., 2018).

DNA stability, and chromatin structure preservation, thus affecting many signaling pathways able to inhibit histone deacetylation (Pignolo, 2019; Puca et al., 2018). Nonetheless, high body-mass indices are associated with a DNA methylation profile like those of aged individuals. Similarly, an excessive calorie intake is strongly related to chronic diseases, and some argue that this change in human nutritional behavior is too recent to modulate favorably our genetics (Declerck & vanden Berghe, 2018). Moreover, the fight-or-flight response is closely related to our survival and any rapid change may promote deleterious effects in our health. The stimulation of sympathetic system that was once associated with the fight-or-flight response, nowadays has unfavorable effects on cardiovascular health (Queen et al., 2020). On the contrary, several mild stresses, such as food restriction are associated with delayed aging and promoting longevity.

Apart from following a balanced diet, blue zone centenarians are usually active. Not running a marathon but engaging in simple daily activities like gardening or walking is thought to be helpful for healthy aging ("The Blue Zones", 2010). Many Okinawans, for instance, practice martial arts, especially a dance-inspired version of tai chi. Undoubtedly, physically as well as cognitively functional centenarians certainly represent an impressive example of successful healthy aging. Moreover, physical activity positively affects the hallmarks of aging (Garatachea et al., 2015). Increased physical activity is associated with an increased life expectancy and a benefit of 4.5 years, thus combined with a normal weight, the net benefit in years added is 7.2 years (Moore et al., 2012). Physical activity, irrespective of BMI, promotes life expectancy and is a dominant factor in benefiting survival and healthy life in individuals over 74-years old (Hirsch et al., 2010). More details about the role of diet and physical activity on healthy aging will be given in **Chapters 10** and **11**.

Moreover, healthy centenarians have a strong sense of purpose. They feel needed and want to contribute to a greater good ("The Blue Zones", 2010). This strong engagement and involvement offer them a high purpose in life, which is related to better cognitive function and less disability. Conversely, a lack of social relationships is associated with a mortality risk almost equivalent to smoking (Pignolo, 2019). Long-lived, socially active individuals are more resilient to psychological stressors such as depression (Zeng & Shen, 2010). In fact, mental and emotional health are increasingly investigated in scientific studies, as they form a part of human well-being (Puca et al., 2018). An interesting analysis of the literature (Martin, MacDonald, Margrett, & Poon, n.d.) highlights three important resilience domains among centenarians: personal resilience (e.g., personality), cognitive resilience (e.g., intellectual functioning), and social and economic resilience (e.g., social support and economic resources), which suggests that a "robust" personality, cognitive reserves, and social and economic resources are resilience factors necessary for survival and optimal functioning and well-being.

Ultimately, what does it take to live "healthily" ever after? (**Table 8.2**) If we take a close look of the oldest older adults, their way of life reveals the secret of the longevity elixir. Life in small towns with little pollution, following a MD, being physically and socially active, close to family and friends, and taking a midday nap lead to happier, less stressed, healthier, and long-lived people (**Figure 8.5**) (Puca et al., 2018).

Table 8.2 Longevity factors commonly found in the blue zones.

Eating in moderation, mostly plant-based diets, with lighter meals at the end of the day
Purposeful living (hard work, work ethic, life philosophy)
Social support systems interactions with family, friends, laughter
Exercise (walking, gardening)
Nutritional Factors: goat's milk, red wine, herbal teas
Spirituality
Maintenance of a healthy body-mass index
Other possible factors: sunshine, hydration, naps

Source: (The Blue Zones, 2010).

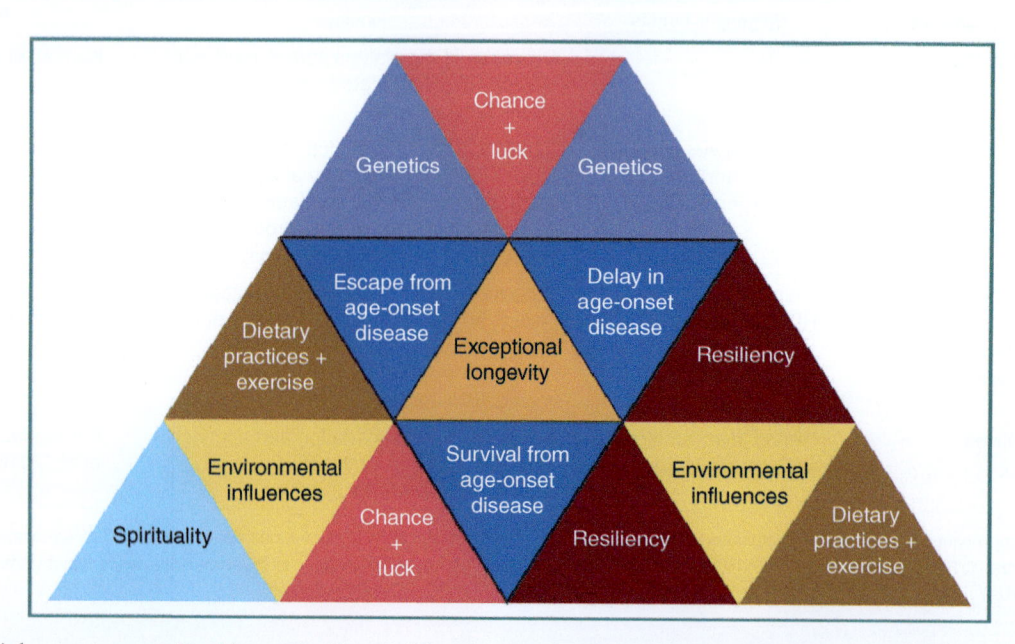

FIGURE 8.5 Multiple ways to exceptional longevity. Source: (Pignolo, 2019 / with permission of Elsevier).

KEY POINTS

- Today, we are facing a longevity revolution. An average adult can now expect to live longer than their peers in previous generations.
- Although we live longer, it does not mean that we are living healthier lives.
- Extending the lifespan through advanced medical care might prolong a life with diseases and disability. As a result, older adults may experience more disability and a poorer quality of life.
- Exceptional longevity is reserved for individuals aged 100 years or more, otherwise known as centenarians.
- Centenarians are considered, in general, a successful healthy aging model.
- Human longevity is the synergistic result of random events, chance, environmental factors, and genetic predisposition.
- Changes in DNA methylation that occur with aging may alter normal gene expression and in turn contribute to the development of age-related diseases and functional decline.
- Healthy lifestyle, including diet and physical activity impact longevity and health in old age, leading to a compression of morbidity.

SELF-ASSESSMENT QUESTIONS

1. Why are centenarians a healthy aging prototype?
2. What does it take to live to 100?
3. Longevity is inherited and expressed early in life. Is this statement accurate? Why?
4. True or False: Long-lived individuals have only favorable age-related genes.
5. Which environmental factors affect living long and healthy?
6. True or False: The secret of longevity in blue zones lies in their diet. Why?
7. Circle the correct answers. Longevity
   (a) inheritance increases with age
   (b) is epigenetically modified
   (c) is mostly genetically transmitted
   (d) all of the above
8. Complete the following statements:
   (a) Advances in medical care have prolonged human life. Nevertheless...
   (b) Positive biology studies...
   (c) The paradox of women's survival advantage is...
9. True or False: Energy restriction is associated with health improvements and increased longevity.
10. True or False: According to the compression of morbidity theory the period of life span with serious illness or disability remains constant, whereas the time period with moderate disability or less severe illness increases.

REFERENCES

Austad, S. N., & Bartke, A. (2015). Sex Differences in Longevity and in Responses to Anti-Aging Interventions: A Mini-Review. *Gerontology*, 62(1), 40–46. https://doi.org/10.1159/000381472

Buettner, D., & Skemp, S. (2016). Blue Zones: Lessons From the World's Longest Lived. *American journal of lifestyle medicine*, 10(5), 318–321. https://doi.org/10.1177/1559827616637066

Brooks-Wilson, A. R. (2013). Genetics of healthy aging and longevity. *Human Genetics*, 132(12), 1323–1338. https://doi.org/10.1007/s00439-013-1342-z

Busee, E. W. (1969). Theories of Aging. In *Behaviour and Adaptation in Later Life*. Litle Brown. Boston. MA.

Byles, J. E. (2007). Fit and Well at Eighty: Defying the Stereotypes of Age and Illness. *Annals of the New York Academy of Sciences*, 1114(1), 107–120. https://doi.org/10.1196/annals.1396.027

Calder, P. C., Carding, S. R., Christopher, G., Kuh, D., Langley-Evans, S. C., & McNulty, H. (2018). A holistic approach to healthy ageing: how can people live longer, healthier lives? *Journal of Human Nutrition and Dietetics*, 31(4), 439–450. https://doi.org/10.1111/jhn.12566

Cardona, C., & Bishai, D. (2018). The slowing pace of life expectancy gains since 1950. *BMC Public Health*, 18(1), 151. https://doi.org/10.1186/s12889-018-5058-9

Christensen, K., McGue, M., Petersen, I., Jeune, B., & Vaupel, J. W. (2008). Exceptional longevity does not result in excessive levels of disability. *Proceedings of the National Academy of Sciences*, 105(36), 13274–13279. https://doi.org/10.1073/pnas.0804931105

Costa, D., Scognamiglio, M., Fiorito, C., Benincasa, G., & Napoli, C. (2019). Genetic background, epigenetic factors and dietary interventions which influence human longevity. *Biogerontology*, 20(5), 605–626. https://doi.org/10.1007/s10522-019-09824-3

Critselis, E., & Panagiotakos, D. (2020). Adherence to the Mediterranean diet and healthy ageing: Current evidence, biological pathways, and future directions. *Critical Reviews in Food Science and Nutrition*, 60(13), 2148–2157. https://doi.org/10.1080/10408398.2019.1631752

Davinelli, S., Trichopoulou, A., Corbi, G., de Vivo, I., & Scapagnini, G. (2019). The potential nutrigeroprotective role of Mediterranean diet and its functional components on telomere length dynamics. *Ageing Research Reviews*, 49, 1–10. https://doi.org/10.1016/j.arr.2018.11.001

Declerck, K., & vanden Berghe, W. (2018). Back to the future: Epigenetic clock plasticity towards healthy aging. *Mechanisms of Ageing and Development*, 174, 18–29. https://doi.org/10.1016/j.mad.2018.01.002

Engberg, H., Oksuzyan, A., Jeune, B., Vaupel, J. W., & Christensen, K. (2009). Centenarians - a useful model for healthy aging? A 29-year follow-up of hospitalizations among 40 000 Danes born in 1905. *Aging Cell*, *8*(3), 270–276. https://doi.org/10.1111/j.1474-9726.2009.00474.x

Evert, J., Lawler, E., Bogan, H., & Perls, T. (2003). Morbidity Profiles of Centenarians: Survivors, Delayers, and Escapers. *The Journals of Gerontology Series A: Biological Sciences and Medical Sciences*, *58*(3), M232–M237. https://doi.org/10.1093/gerona/58.3.M232

Farrelly, C. (2012). 'Positive biology' as a new paradigm for the medical sciences. *EMBO Reports*, *13*(3), 186–188. https://doi.org/10.1038/embor.2011.256

Fernández del Río, L., Gutiérrez-Casado, E., Varela-López, A., & Villalba, J. (2016). Olive Oil and the Hallmarks of Aging. *Molecules*, *21*(2), 163. https://doi.org/10.3390/molecules21020163

Foscolou, A., Magriplis, E., Tyrovolas, S., Soulis, G., Bountziouka, V., Mariolis, A., . . . Panagiotakos, D. (2018). Lifestyle determinants of healthy ageing in a Mediterranean population: The multinational MEDIS study. *Experimental Gerontology*, *110*, 35–41. https://doi.org/10.1016/j.exger.2018.05.008

Fransquet, P. D., Wrigglesworth, J., Woods, R. L., Ernst, M. E., & Ryan, J. (2019). The epigenetic clock as a predictor of disease and mortality risk: a systematic review and meta-analysis. *Clinical Epigenetics*, *11*(1), 62. https://doi.org/10.1186/s13148-019-0656-7

Freitas-Simoes, T.-M., Ros, E., & Sala-Vila, A. (2016). Nutrients, foods, dietary patterns and telomere length: Update of epidemiological studies and randomized trials. *Metabolism*, *65*(4), 406–415. https://doi.org/10.1016/j.metabol.2015.11.004

Fries, J. F. (1980). Aging, Natural Death, and the Compression of Morbidity. *New England Journal of Medicine*, *303*(3), 130–135. https://doi.org/10.1056/NEJM198007173030304

Fries, J. F., Bruce, B., & Chakravarty, E. (2011). Compression of Morbidity 1980–2011: A Focused Review of Paradigms and Progress. *Journal of Aging Research*, *2011*, 1–10. https://doi.org/10.4061/2011/261702

Garatachea, N., Pareja-Galeano, H., Sanchis-Gomar, F., Santos-Lozano, A., Fiuza-Luces, C., Morán, M., . . . Lucia, A. (2015). Exercise Attenuates the Major Hallmarks of Aging. *Rejuvenation Research*, *18*(1), 57–89. https://doi.org/10.1089/rej.2014.1623

GRUENBERG, E. M. (2005). The Failures of Success. *Milbank Quarterly*, *83*(4), 779–800. https://doi.org/10.1111/j.1468-0009.2005.00400.x

Heyn, H., Li, N., Ferreira, H. J., Moran, S., Pisano, D. G., Gomez, A., . . . Esteller, M. (2012). Distinct DNA methylomes of newborns and centenarians. *Proceedings of the National Academy of Sciences*, *109*(26), 10522–10527. https://doi.org/10.1073/pnas.1120658109

Hirsch, C. H., Diehr, P., Newman, A. B., Gerrior, S. A., Pratt, C., Lebowitz, M. D., & Jackson, S. A. (2010). Physical Activity and Years of Healthy Life in Older Adults: Results From the Cardiovascular Health Study. *Journal of Aging and Physical Activity*, *18*(3), 313–334. https://doi.org/10.1123/japa.18.3.313

Manton, K. G. (1982). Changing concepts of morbidity and mortality in the elderly population. *The Milbank Memorial Fund Quarterly. Health and Society*, *60*(2), 183–244.

Martin, P., MacDonald, M., Margrett, J., & Poon, L. W. (n.d.). Resilience and longevity: In P. S. Fry & C. L. M. Keyes (Eds.), *New Frontiers in Resilient Aging* (pp. 213–238). Cambridge: Cambridge University Press. https://doi.org/10.1017/CBO9780511763151.010

McEwen, L. M., Morin, A. M., Edgar, R. D., MacIsaac, J. L., Jones, M. J., Dow, W. H., . . . Rehkopf, D. H. (2017). Differential DNA methylation and lymphocyte proportions in a Costa Rican high longevity region. *Epigenetics & Chromatin*, *10*(1), 21. https://doi.org/10.1186/s13072-017-0128-2

Moore, S. C., Patel, A. v., Matthews, C. E., Berrington de Gonzalez, A., Park, Y., Katki, H. A., . . . Lee, I.-M. (2012). Leisure Time Physical Activity of Moderate to Vigorous Intensity and Mortality: A Large Pooled Cohort Analysis. *PLoS Medicine*, *9*(11), e1001335. https://doi.org/10.1371/journal.pmed.1001335

Murabito, J. M., Yuan, R., & Lunetta, K. L. (2012). The Search for Longevity and Healthy Aging Genes: Insights From Epidemiological Studies and Samples of Long-Lived Individuals. *The Journals of Gerontology Series A: Biological Sciences and Medical Sciences*, *67A*(5), 470–479. https://doi.org/10.1093/gerona/gls089

Oeppen, J., & Vaupel, J. W. (2002). Broken Limits to Life Expectancy. *Science*, *296*(5570), 1029–1031. https://doi.org/10.1126/science.1069675

Olshansky, S. J., Rudberg, M. A., Carnes, B. A., Cassel, C. K., & Brody, J. A. (1991). Trading Off Longer Life for Worsening Health. *Journal of Aging and Health*, *3*(2), 194–216. https://doi.org/10.1177/089826439100300205

Panagiotakos, D. B., Chrysohoou, C., Siasos, G., Zisimos, K., Skoumas, J., Pitsavos, C., & Stefanadis, C. (2011). Sociodemographic and Lifestyle Statistics of Oldest Old People (>80 Years) Living in Ikaria Island: The Ikaria Study. *Cardiology Research and Practice*, *2011*, 1–7. https://doi.org/10.4061/2011/679187

Passarino, G., de Rango, F., & Montesanto, A. (2016). Human longevity: Genetics or Lifestyle? It takes two to tango. *Immunity & Ageing*, *13*(1), 12. https://doi.org/10.1186/s12979-016-0066-z

Pignolo, R. J. (2019). Exceptional Human Longevity. *Mayo Clinic Proceedings*, *94*(1), 110–124. https://doi.org/10.1016/j.mayocp.2018.10.005

Puca, A. A., Spinelli, C., Accardi, G., Villa, F., & Caruso, C. (2018). Centenarians as a model to discover genetic and epigenetic signatures of healthy ageing. *Mechanisms of Ageing and Development*, *174*, 95–102. https://doi.org/10.1016/j.mad.2017.10.004

Queen, N. J., Hassan, Q. N., & Cao, L. (2020). Improvements to Healthspan Through Environmental Enrichment and Lifestyle Interventions: Where Are We Now? *Frontiers in Neuroscience*, *14*. https://doi.org/10.3389/fnins.2020.00605

Riley, J. C. (2005). Estimates of Regional and Global Life Expectancy, 1800-2001. *Population and Development Review*, *31*(3), 537–543. https://doi.org/10.1111/j.1728-4457.2005.00083.x

Ritchie, H., & Roser, M. Age Structure. (2019). [cited 2022 October 30]. Available from https://ourworldindata.org/age-structure.

Robine, J.-M., & Allard, M. (1998). The Oldest Human. *Science*, *279*(5358), 1831–1831. https://doi.org/10.1126/science.279.5358.1831h

Robine, J.-M., Saito, Y., & Jagger, C. (2003). The emergence of extremely old people: the case of Japan. *Experimental Gerontology*, *38*(7), 735–739. https://doi.org/10.1016/S0531-5565(03)00100-1

Roser, M., Ortiz-Ospina, E., & Ritchie, H. Life expectancy. (2019). [cited 2022 October 30]. Available from https://ourworldindata.org/life-expectancy

Santos-Lozano, A., Santamarina, A., Pareja-Galeano, H., Sanchis-Gomar, F., Fiuza-Luces, C., Cristi-Montero, C., . . . Garatachea, N. (2016). The genetics of exceptional longevity: Insights from centenarians. *Maturitas*, *90*, 49–57. https://doi.org/10.1016/j.maturitas.2016.05.006

Sebastiani, P., & Perls, T. T. (2012). The Genetics of Extreme Longevity: Lessons from the New England Centenarian Study. *Frontiers in Genetics*, *3*. https://doi.org/10.3389/fgene.2012.00277

Taormina, G., & Mirisola, M. G. (2015). Longevity: epigenetic and biomolecular aspects. *Biomolecular Concepts*, *6*(2), 105–117. https://doi.org/10.1515/bmc-2014-0038

The Blue Zones. Reverse Engineering Longevity; 2008-2022. [cited 2021 March 30]. Available from: https://www.bluezones.com/2016/11/power-9/

The World Bank Group. Life expectancy at birth; 2021 review. [cited 2021 March 30]. Available from: https://data.worldbank.org/indicator/SP.DYN.LE00.IN

Trichopoulou, A., & Critselis, E. (2004). Mediterranean diet and longevity. *European Journal of Cancer Prevention*, *13*(5), 453–456. https://doi.org/10.1097/00008469-200410000-00014

United States Census Bureau. An Ageing World. 2015 [cited 2022 October 30]. https://www.census.gov/content/dam/Census/library/publications/2016/demo/p95-16-1.pdf.

Velkoff, V. (2000). Centenarians in the United States, 1990 and beyond. *Statistical Bulletin (Metropolitan Life Insurance Company: 1984)*, *81*(1), 2–9.

Willcox, D. C., Scapagnini, G., & Willcox, B. J. (2014). Healthy aging diets other than the Mediterranean: A focus on the Okinawan diet. *Mechanisms of Ageing and Development*, *136–137*, 148–162. https://doi.org/10.1016/j.mad.2014.01.002

Xiao, F.-H., He, Y.-H., Li, Q.-G., Wu, H., Luo, L.-H., & Kong, Q.-P. (2015). A Genome-Wide Scan Reveals Important Roles of DNA Methylation in Human Longevity by Regulating Age-Related Disease Genes. *PLOS ONE*, *10*(3), e0120388. https://doi.org/10.1371/journal.pone.0120388

Zeng, Y., & Shen, K. (2010). Resilience Significantly Contributes to Exceptional Longevity. *Current Gerontology and Geriatrics Research*, *2010*, 1–9. https://doi.org/10.1155/2010/525693

FURTHER READING

Bibliography

Ames B. N. (2018). Prolonging healthy aging: Longevity vitamins and proteins. *Proceedings of the National Academy of Sciences of the United States of America*, *115*(43), 10836–10844. https://doi.org/10.1073/pnas.1809045115

Acosta-Rodríguez, V. A., Rijo-Ferreira, F., Green, C. B., & Takahashi, J. S. (2021). Importance of circadian timing for aging and longevity. *Nature communications*, *12*(1), 2862. https://doi.org/10.1038/s41467-021-22922-6

Bell, C. G., Lowe, R., Adams, P. D., Baccarelli, A. A., Beck, S., Bell, J. T., Christensen, B. C., Gladyshev, V. N., Heijmans, B. T., Horvath, S., Ideker, T., Issa, J. J., Kelsey, K. T., Marioni, R. E., Reik, W., Relton, C. L., Schalkwyk, L. C., Teschendorff, A. E., Wagner, W., Zhang, K., . . . Rakyan, V. K. (2019). DNA methylation aging clocks: challenges and recommendations. *Genome biology*, *20*(1), 249. https://doi.org/10.1186/s13059-019-1824-y

Kaushik, S., Tasset, I., Arias, E., Pampliega, O., Wong, E., Martinez-Vicente, M., & Cuervo, A. M. (2021). Autophagy and the hallmarks of aging. *Ageing research reviews*, *72*, 101468. https://doi.org/10.1016/j.arr.2021.101468

Kim, S., & Jazwinski, S. M. (2018). The Gut Microbiota and Healthy Aging: A Mini-Review. *Gerontology*, *64*(6), 513–520. https://doi.org/10.1159/000490615

Links

- healthylongevitychallenge.org/
- www.bluezones.com/
- https://data.worldbank.org/indicator/SP.DYN.LE00.IN
- https://www.worldometers.info/demographics/life-expectancy/
- https://genomics.senescence.info/genes/index.html
- https://www.weforum.org/communities/gfc-on-healthy-ageing-and-longevity
- https://www.thelancet.com/journals/lanhl/home

Physiological Changes in Multiple Organ Systems Through Aging: Measuring and Monitoring Aging

CHAPTER 9

Introduction	117
Physiological Changes in Multiple Organ Systems Through Aging	119
Cardiovascular	119
Pulmonary	119
Immune System	119
Neurologic Function	120
Musculoskeletal System	120
Sarcopenia	120
Frailty	121
Measurements	122
Hand-grip Strength	122
Gait Speed	122
Balance Assessment	124
Timed Up-and-Go (TUG) Test	124
30-second Chair Stand	124
Four-stage Balance Test	124
Complex Balance Measures	124
Short Physical Performance Battery (SPPB)	124
Functionality Assessment Tools: Activities of Daily Living (ADLs) Assessment Tools	124
ADL Assessment Tool: Barthel Index	125
ADL Assessment Tool: Katz Index of Independence in Activities of Daily Living (ADL)	125
ADL Assessment Tool: Functional Independence Measure (FIM)	125
IADL Assessment Tool: ADL Profile Instrumental (IADL)	125
IADL Assessment Tool: Lawton Instrumental ADL Scale	125
IADL Assessment Tool: Performance Assessment of Self-care Skills (PASS)	125
Key Points	130
Self-assessment Questions	130
References	131
Further Reading	132
Bibliography	132
Links	132

INTRODUCTION

As mentioned in previous chapters in this unit, aging is the major risk factor for death from all age-related adult chronic diseases. By 2034, for the first time in American history, it is projected that older adults will outnumber children. A major challenge associated with advanced adult age is the relationship between significant changes in many physiologic functions, the development of several impairments, the decline in overall functional capacity, the subsequent morbidity and mortality, and the resulting loss of independence that most older adults fear more than death (Frontera, 2017).

Aging procedures in the human body are complex and yet not fully understood. At a biological level, aging is associated with the gradual accumulation of a wide variety of molecular and cellular damage. Over time, this accumulative damage increases the risk for many diseases while leading to general decline in several body functions. Ultimately, all these changes lead to death.

Prevention and Management of Cardiovascular and Metabolic Disease: Diet, Physical Activity and Healthy Aging,
First Edition. Christina N. Katsagoni, Peter Kokkinos, and Labros S. Sidossis.
© 2023 John Wiley & Sons Ltd. Published 2023 by John Wiley & Sons Ltd.

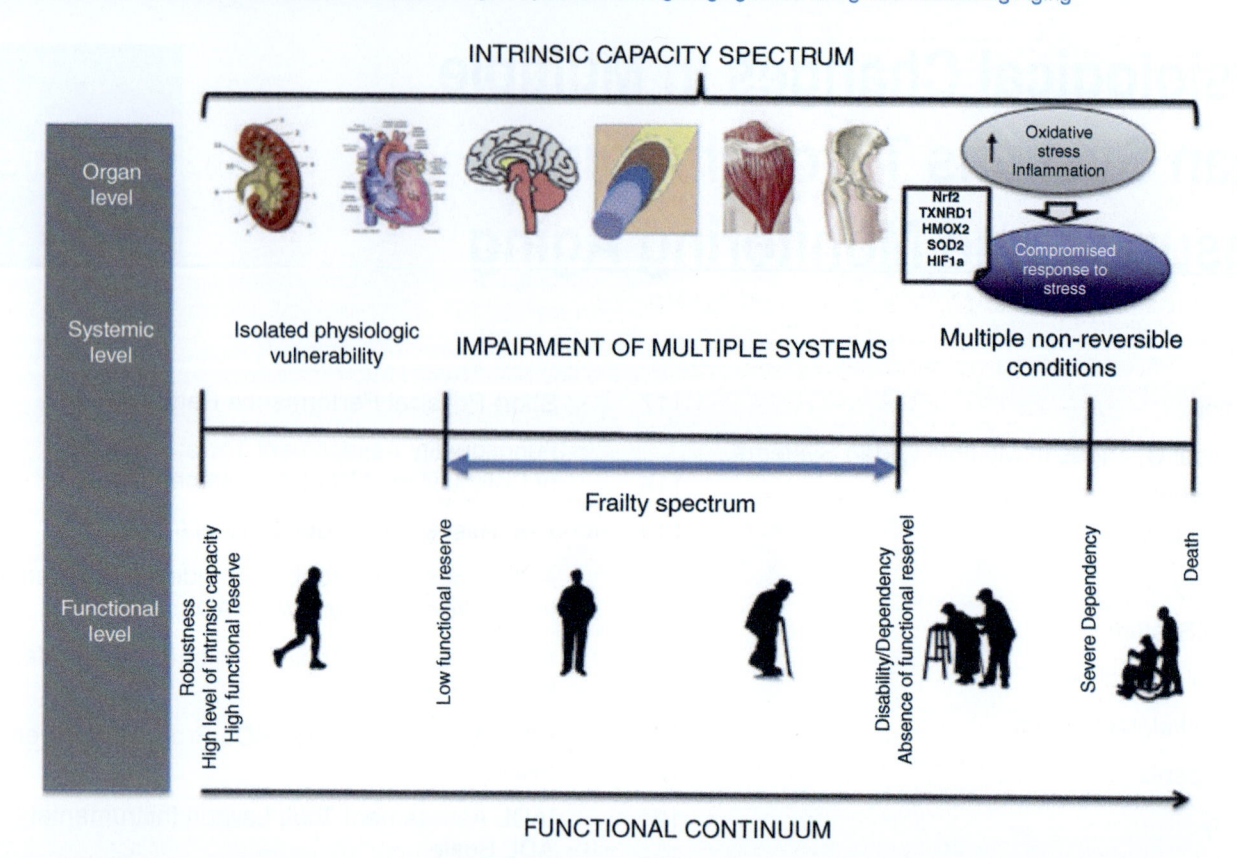

FIGURE 9.1 The spectrum of intrinsic capacity from the perspectives of organ and systemic level and their clinical manifestations. In the first stages, there are changes in isolated organs that can still be reversed and do not impact function due to a high functional reserve. As the condition progresses, other organs start to deteriorate, due to the aging processes or to accumulation of chronic diseases that share similar mechanisms of damage. At this stage, frailty status appears; there is still enough functional reserve to maintain functional autonomy, although some deterioration in performance-based tasks can be observed if carefully assessed. If the condition continues progressing, functional reserve is depleted and disability takes hold, with few chances for recovery. Source: (Angulo et al, 2020).

Progressive cellular damage is expressed as a detrimental change in maximal organ function with different trajectories across organ systems (Khan, Singer, & Vaughan, 2017). Aging affects all organs and depends on individual's genetics, developmental programming, and living or environmental conditions. All these factors combined determine the body's ability to respond to stress, hence maximal organ functionality, which explains the influence that aging has on intrinsic capacity (**Figure 9.1**) and significant differences in age-related responses between individuals (Khan et al., 2017).

As mentioned in **Chapter 7**, intrinsic capacity comprises all the mental and physical capacities that a person can draw on and includes their ability to walk, think, see, hear, and remember. For example, because maximal physiologic capacities are greatly decline with age, the ability to perform any physical task at the same absolute level of energy expenditure or muscular force becomes limited (Frontera, 2017). Aging varies from organ-to-organ and person-to-person, and it appears to be an organ-specific or organ-differential resilience and vulnerability through aging (**Figure 9.2**).

In the next paragraphs, the physiological changes observed in multiple organ systems through aging will be described.

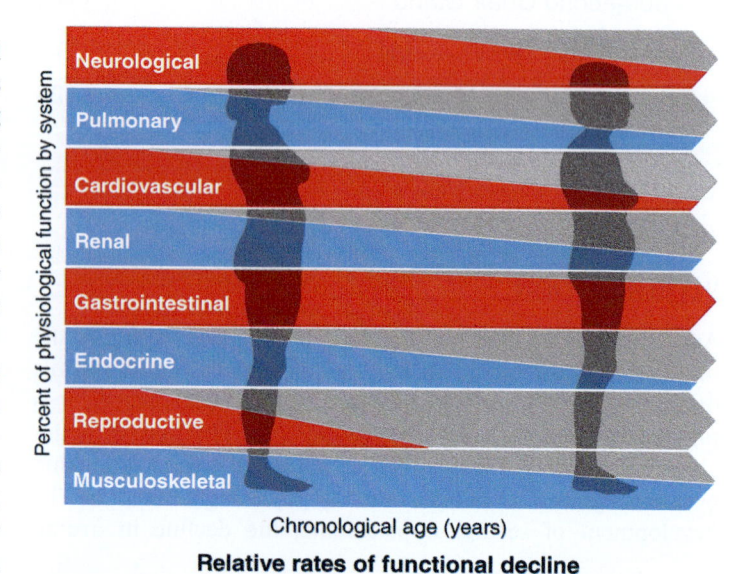

FIGURE 9.2 Relative rates of decline in maximal organ function across organ systems. Each organ system may carry a specific vulnerability to age. For example, the cardiovascular system appears to suffer biological aging more rapidly than the gastrointestinal system. Source: (Khan et al., 2017)

PHYSIOLOGICAL CHANGES IN MULTIPLE ORGAN SYSTEMS THROUGH AGING

CARDIOVASCULAR

Even though cardiovascular disease (CVD) is not necessarily related to advanced age, it is the leading cause of morbidity and mortality among older adults. The elderly are more likely to develop heart disease than younger adults due to an increased prevalence of age-associated co-morbidities such as hypertension, diabetes mellitus, and dyslipidemia. Thus, the incidence of coronary artery disease (CAD), valvular disease, rhythm disorders, and heart failure increases with age (Khan et al., 2017).

Indeed, an aging cardiovascular system has an increased level of stiffness in the aorta and large vessels in general. This results in widened pulse pressure with raised systolic blood pressure (due to an increased resistance to blood ejection from the left ventricle [LV]) and lowered diastolic pressure (due to a steep pressure drop in diastole). Consequently, changes are an increased LV afterload, mass, wall thickness, and LV end-diastolic volume. Further changes in calcium influx cause reduced LV compliance and delayed LV relaxation or decreased diastolic function as assessed by Doppler echocardiography parameters. Intrinsic heart rate also drops significantly due to both atrial pacemaker cellular loss (50% to 75% by the age of 50) and His bundle fibrosis. Fibrosis and calcification occur at the aortic valve cusp bases, annular valvular rings, and fibrous trigones. Finally, older individuals demonstrate decreased responsiveness to b-adrenergic receptor stimulation in cardiomyocytes, decreased reactivity to baroreceptor and chemoreceptor output, and increased circulating catecholamines that results in reduced exercise tolerance and decreased cardiac output.

These changes increase the heart's vulnerability to the development of age-related cardiovascular pathology such as hypertension, congestive heart failure, atrioventricular block, and aortic stenosis. Moreover, atherosclerosis is linked to premature biological aging with senescent cells identified in CAD plaques (Khan et al., 2017).

PULMONARY

Human lungs have the largest surface area in the body and represent one of the few consistently reliable physiological markers of aging. Lung cells face ongoing chemical, mechanical, biological, immunological, and xenobiotic stress over a lifetime. Aging causes progressive impairment of lung function in otherwise healthy individuals, marked by structural changes (Schneider et al., 2021).

With advancing age, peak aerobic capacity falls with a greater than 20% decline per decade after age 70. Due to loss in lung-tissue elasticity, there is a severe decrease in surface availability for gas exchange (increased anatomic dead space). Chest wall compliance decreases and dominates the increase in lung compliance, functional residual capacity decreases because of the fall in total respiratory system compliance. Forced vital capacity (FVC) declines 0.15 to 0.30 L per decade in nonsmoking men, and the forced expiratory volume in one-second (FEV1) falls 0.20–0.30 L/s per decade with a steeper decline in the seventh and eighth decades. Residual volume increases by about 10% per decade due to an increased closing volume: the lung volume at which small airways in dependent lung zones begin to collapse during exhalation. Ventilation–perfusion mismatching increases with age, as airways in the better-perfused dependent lung zones have an increased likelihood of closure during exhalation. Diffusion capacity decreases around 5% per decade, although hypoxemia does not typically develop. Further, advancing age is associated with a diminished central drive to the respiratory muscles in response to hypoxemia, hypercapnia, and mechanical load; exercise training may attenuate this hypo-responsiveness. The above changes, when combined with decreased respiratory muscle strength and reduced efficacy of mucociliary clearance, result in higher risk of pneumonia to occur (Khan et al., 2017).

IMMUNE SYSTEM

One of the most well documented consequences of aging is the decline in the immune function. The aging immune system tends to under- or malfunction over time, a condition collectively described as immunosenescence, which leads to increased vulnerability to infection, malignancy, and autoimmunity (Khan et al., 2017; Aiello et al., 2019). While elderly individuals are known to be immunodeficient, they often do not respond efficiently to novel or previously encountered antigens. For example, individuals 70 years of age and older have increased vulnerability to influenza, a situation that is exacerbated by their poor response to vaccination (Montecino-Rodriguez, Berent-Maoz, & Dorshkind, 2013).

The adaptive and innate immune systems both exhibit functional decline with aging, although innate immunity appears better preserved (Aiello et al., 2019). Regulatory T-cells lose their suppressive function and accumulate in visceral adipose tissue (Khan et al., 2017). Age-associated, chronic low-grade inflammation, "inflamm-aging", is considered a pillar of the aging process and the most common pathogenetic mechanism of age-related diseases as well as the worst prognostic factor for all causes of death (Aiello et al., 2019). Inflamm-aging is a consequence of activated inflammation-signaling networks, which are regulated by cytokines like nuclear factor κ-light-chain enhancer of activated B-cells (NF-κb) transcription factor and tumor necrosis factor (TNF)-α as well as other inflammatory stimuli such as senescent cells, obesity, circulating mitochondrial DNA, gut microbiota, and diet (Aiello et al., 2019). The aging immune system is not efficient enough to respond to chronic stimuli sufficiently, especially toward stressors that occur later in life (Aiello et al., 2019). Chronic production of pro-inflammatory cytokines is suggested to be involved in muscle atrophy that correlates with lower mobility capabilities through muscle wasting and weight loss as well as the presence of malignancies and neurodegenerative diseases in older adults (Suzuki, 2019; Aiello et al., 2019).

NEUROLOGIC FUNCTION

Cognitive decline is considered a hallmark of the aging nervous system and it is associated with increased memory loss and deteriorating mental ability, which in turn increases the risk for neurodegenerative diseases (Harman & Martín, 2020).

Cognitive decline with aging is multifactorial and related to changes in structure as well as synaptic plasticity (Khan et al., 2017). The total brain volume declines at an approximate rate of 5% per decade after the age of 40 (Panagiotou, Michel, Meijer, & Deboer, 2021). Cerebral tissue atrophy and diminished cerebral perfusion result in significant white-matter loss, but neuronal dropout varies by brain region with little or no loss in some regions (Khan et al., 2017). Notably, white-matter volume changes in aging are nonlinear with more rapid changes as age advances in humans, whereas gray matter has a smaller and more linear decrease. In addition to the prefrontal cortex, one of the most affected areas in healthy aging, the hippocampus is another greatly affected area. Advanced age is associated with widespread thinning of the cerebral cortex (Panagiotou et al., 2021). In addition, dopaminergic signaling progressively decreases via the D2 receptor. Functional MRI studies demonstrate less coordinated activation in brain regions focused on higher-order cognitive functions, which suggests a global loss of integrative function with aging. Gene expression profiling studies show that significant changes in synaptic gene expression contribute to altered higher-order integration (Khan et al., 2017; Panagiotou et al., 2021). These alterations in synaptic plasticity and loss as well as impaired neurogenesis may predispose aged individuals to neurodegenerative disorders such as Alzheimer's and Parkinson's disease (Khan et al., 2017).

MUSCULOSKELETAL SYSTEM

Alterations in structure and function of the musculoskeletal system can lead to functional loss leading to impairment and disability. If left untreated, several life-threatening complications can occur, such as falls and bone fractures associated with muscle weakness (Frontera, 2017).

The musculoskeletal system is a large group of tissues including muscles, bones, tendons, ligaments, and cartilage, which work simultaneously to ignite and maintain physical function and undergoes multiple changes with aging (Khan et al., 2017).

In older adults, type II muscle fibers or fast twitch fibers, tend to shrink in size and number. This results in lower strength and muscle tone, which lessens contractile force and therefore, limits mobility (Khan et al., 2017; Walston, 2012; Eckstrom, Neukam, Kalin, & Wright, 2020). Longitudinal studies demonstrate an up to 1.5% reduction in muscle strength per year, mainly in the lower (knee extensors and flexors), rather than the upper, limbs (Frontera, 2017). Age-related loss of muscle mass (sarcopenia) occurs involuntarily along with qualitative changes in muscle characterized by fat and connective tissue infiltration, increased levels of lipofuscin, and the accumulation of other cellular waste products (Walston, 2012; Eckstrom et al., 2020). Findings from the AGES-Reykjavik study suggest that muscle composition may be associated with mortality risk (Khan et al., 2017). Moreover, sarcopenia is also associated with acute and chronic disease states, increased insulin resistance, fatigue, and risk of falling (Eckstrom et al., 2020).

Sarcopenia

Sarcopenia (Greek "sarx" or flesh + "penia" or loss) is a highly common geriatric syndrome characterized by the involuntary loss of skeletal mass and strength that affects millions of older adults around the world (Walston, 2012). It is also considered a key component for the development of frailty in older adults (Clegg, Young, Iliffe, Rikkert, & Rockwood, 2013). In its revised definition, the European Working Group on Sarcopenia in Older People (EWGSOP2) uses low muscle strength as the primary parameter of sarcopenia; muscle strength is the most reliable measure of muscle function. Specifically, sarcopenia is probable when low muscle strength is detected. A diagnosis is confirmed by the presence of low muscle quantity or quality.

When low muscle strength, low muscle quantity/quality, and low physical performance are all detected, sarcopenia is considered severe (**Tables 9.1** and **9.2** provide the operational definition of sarcopenia and the most commonly used tools to assess the definition's criteria in clinical and research environments, respectively) (Cruz-Jentoft et al., 2019).

Untreated or underdiagnosed sarcopenia increases the risk of falls and bone fractures and impairs the ability to execute activities of daily living (ADLs). It also correlates with cardiac and respiratory disease, cognitive deterioration, ambulatory disorders, and an overall worse quality of life (Cruz-Jentoft et al., 2019). It is one of the most important causes of functional deterioration and loss of independence in older adults, since muscle mass accounts for up to 60% of body mass (Walston, 2012).

On average, 5% to 13% of older persons over 60-years old have low muscle mass, increasing up to 50% in people over the age of 80 (Morley, Anker, & von Haehling, 2014; Meier & Lee, 2020). The prevalence differs between organizations due to the lack of a universal definition (Meier & Lee, 2020). In 2016, sarcopenia was recognized as an independent condition by the ICD-10-CM Code, meaning that it is recognized as a pathological entity of its own, underlining the importance of its early diagnosis and treatment (Anker, Morley, & von Haehling, 2016). The causes of sarcopenia

Table 9.1 Concensus by the European Working Group on Sarcopenia in Older People (EWGSOP2) - 2018 operational definition of sarcopenia.

Probable sarcopenia is identified by Criterion 1.
Diagnosis is confirmed by additional documentation of Criterion 2.
If Criteria 1, 2 and 3 are all met, sarcopenia is considered severe.
(1) Low muscle strength
(2) Low muscle quantity or quality
(3) Low physical performance

Source: (Cruz-Jentoft et al., 2019).

Table 9.2 Choosing tools for sarcopenia case finding and for measurement of muscle strength, muscle mass and physical performance in clinical practice and in research.

Variable	Clinical practice	Research studies
Case finding	SARC-F questionnaire Ishii screening tool	SARC-F
Skeletal muscle strength	Grip strength Chair stand test (chair rise test)	Grip strength Chair stand test (5-times sit-to-stand)
Skeletal muscle mass or Skeletal muscle quality	Appendicular skeletal muscle mass (ASMM) by Dual-energy X-ray absorptiometry (DXA)*	ASMM by DXA
	Whole-body skeletal muscle mass (SMM) or ASMM predicted by Bioelectrical impedance analysis (BIA)[1]	Whole-body SMM or ASMM by Magnetic Resonance Imaging (MRI, total body protocol)
		Mid-thigh muscle cross-sectional area by Computed Tomography (CT) or MRI
	Lumbar muscle cross-sectional area by CT or MRI	Lumbar muscle cross-sectional area by CT or MRI
		Muscle quality by mid-thigh or total body muscle quality by muscle biopsy, CT, MRI or Magnetic resonance Spectroscopy (MRS)
Physical performance	Gait speed	Gait speed
Short physical performance battery (SPPB)	Timed-up-and-go test (TUG) 400-meter walk or long-distance corridor walk (400-m walk)	TUG 400-m walk

SARC-F = Strength, assistance with walking, rising from a chair, climbing stairs, and falls.
[1] Sometimes divided by height^2 or body-mass index (BMI) to adjust for body size.
Source: (Cruz-Jentoft et al., 2019 / with permission of Oxford University Press).

are multifactorial and include increased inflammation rates, age-related molecular changes (i.e., mitochondrial function and TGF-β pathway downregulation as well as apoptosis activation), a loss of anabolic hormones and insulin resistance, decreased size, lower total number and firing rates from motor neurons, lower activity levels, and lower energy intake (Walston, 2012).

Frailty

Frailty is a clinically recognizable condition accompanied by increased vulnerability. It is a result of the aging-related decline in maintenance and functionality across several physiological systems that define the ability to deal with everyday struggles as well as trauma or stress due to chronic disease (**Figure 9.3**) (Xue, 2011; Clegg et al., 2013). Its prevalence increases with age and reaches 9.9% in community-based older adult populations. It is estimated to be more frequent in women than in men (Sabine, 2020; Xue, 2011; Clegg et al., 2013).

Frailty often leads to reduced autonomy and independence in older adults (Nascimento et al., 2019) and increases the chances of falls, disability, and acute confusion (Clegg et al., 2013). For a diagnosis of frailty, three of five phenotypic criteria should be met: compromised energetics, low grip strength, exhaustion, slowed walking speed, low physical activity, and unintentional weight loss, which are known as the Fried phenotype score (FPS) (Xue, 2011). Detailed cutoff points for each parameter are suggested but are not the result of an overall consensus (Cederholm et al., 2017). Apart from the FPS, the frailty index is also used to screen, classify, and assess improvements made after interventions in populations that are at risk of or experience frailty (Cesari, Gambassi, Van Kan, & Vellas, 2014).

Despite their common etiologies, frailty differs from sarcopenia. The main differences lie in the loss of muscle performance, hence the amelioration of a person's functional capabilities, which is a step beyond the loss of muscle mass, strength, and

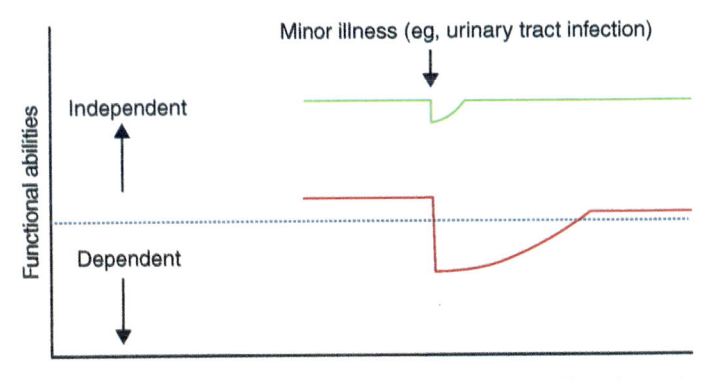

FIGURE 9.3 Vulnerability of frail elderly people to a sudden change in health status after a minor illness. Frailty is a long-established clinical expression that implies concern about an elderly person's vulnerability and outlook. The green line represents a fit elderly individual who, after a minor stressor event such as an infection, has a small deterioration in function and then returns to homeostasis. The red line represents a frail elderly individual who, after a similar stressor event, undergoes a larger deterioration, which may manifest as functional dependency and who does not return to baseline homeostasis. The horizontal dashed line represents the cutoff between dependent and independent.
Source: (Clegg et al., 2013 / with permission of Elsevier).

power alone (Nascimento et al., 2019). The presence of frailty is associated with several changes:

a. cognitive (structural, quantitative, and functional changes),
b. hormonal (decreased production and impaired signaling of growth hormone, IGF-I, sex, and sex steroid precursor hormones in parallel with a gradual rise in cortisol release), and
c. immunity downfall and dysregulation (reduced production of T lymphocytes and B cell-controlled antibody response, the phagocytic activity of neutrophils, macrophages, and natural killer cells, and the unmediated over-accumulation of inflammation markers such as interleukin 6, C reactive protein, tumor necrosis factor, and CXC chemokine ligant-10), in parallel with a loss of physiological reserve in the respiratory, cardiovascular, renal, and haemopoietic systems as a consequence of unregulated inflammation and brain-hormonal inadequacies (Clegg et al., 2013; Angulo, El Assar, Álvarez-Bustos, & Rodríguez-Mañas, 2020).

Figure 9.4 depicts in a concise manner the pathophysiology of frailty and how the interaction between age-related chronic diseases, aging process, oxidative stress, and inflammation may lead to multi-system dysfunction and frailty phenotype in older adults (Angulo et al., 2020).

MEASUREMENTS

Although aging is inevitable, the idea of healthy aging recognizes that the rate of deterioration differs amongst individuals and is modifiable through actions implemented by health policies (Green & Hillersdal, 2021). Health policy recommendations rely on scientifically approved strategies for measuring and monitoring aging (Green & Hillersdal, 2021). Physical capabilities and performance in ADLs are measured with several different assessment tools using both question- and physical performance-based tests.

In the next paragraphs, a more analytical view of the tools that directly assess the individual's physical condition will be presented. Moreover, a briefer review will include tools that assess functionality throughout everyday life activities.

HAND-GRIP STRENGTH

According to the WHO, measuring an individual's hand-grip strength is the most reliable test to assess an older person's vitality (a domain of intrinsic capacity) (**Figure 9.5**). A growing body of evidence suggests that skeletal muscle function is an important component of intrinsic capacity in older adults. The hand-grip strength procedure tests the muscular strength, or the maximum force/tension generated by one's forearm muscles. It is a simple yet powerful predictor of intrinsic capacity decline and the onset of morbidity and mortality. Multiple measurements should be taken over time to track the capacity of older people and chart trajectories. Data analysis from China, Ghana, India, Mexico, the Russian Federation, and South Africa prove a significant and consistent relationship between hand-grip strength and other parameters of intrinsic capacity across the five important domains of locomotion, psychological cognition, vitality, and sensory and underscores that this test is the most important measure of intrinsic capacity.

Major determinants of hand-grip strength are age, sex, stature, weight, nutritional status, socio-economic status, and chronic disease. To take the measurement, in a sitting position, keep your upper arm against your body and bend your elbow to 90 degrees with the palm facing in (like shaking hands), then squeeze the dynamometer as hard as possible for a few seconds (WHO, 2020). **Table 9.3** presents the cutoff values for low hand-grip strength.

GAIT SPEED

Walking is a complex ability derived from the efficient interaction of an individual's neuromuscular, cardiovascular, and cognitive systems. Walking speed correlates with independence, health status, and functional capacity and is predictive of frailty, general disability, cognitive deterioration, cardiovascular, and all-cause mortality (Forte, De Vito, & Boreham, 2021). Among the available physical performance measures, gait speed is

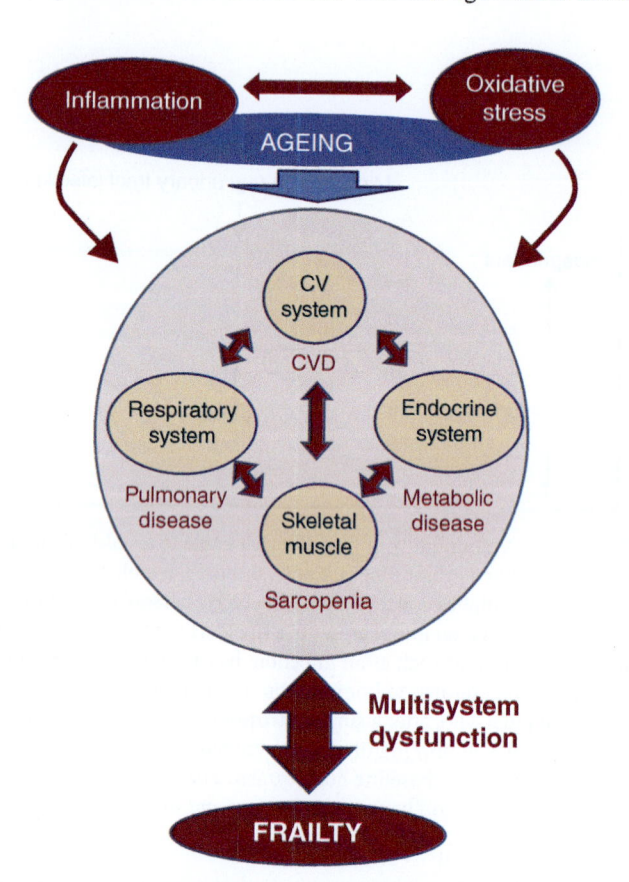

FIGURE 9.4 Pathophysiology of frailty. Aging, together with an increase in oxidative damage and chronic inflammation, is three interrelated, age-dependent processes that provide a background prone to organic systems dysfunction and age-related chronic diseases. The interaction between age-related chronic diseases, aging process, oxidative stress, and inflammation may lead to multi-system dysfunction and frailty phenotype in older adults. Source: (Angulo et al., 2020 / with permission of Elsevier).

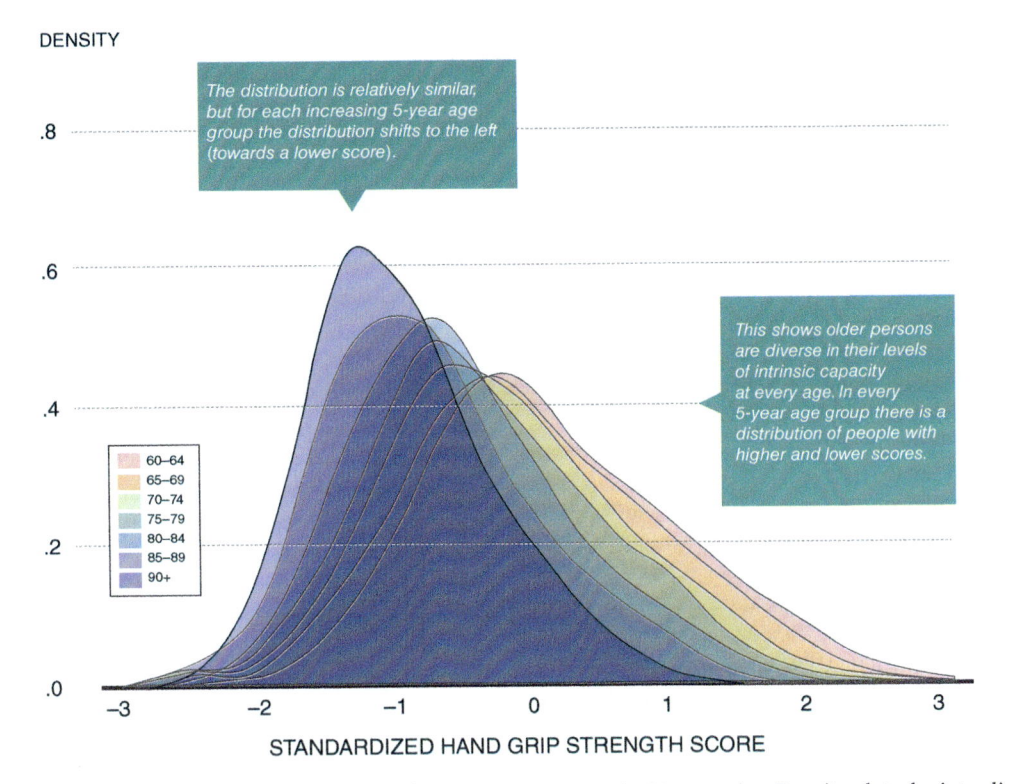

FIGURE 9.5 Vitality (hand-grip strength), score distribution by 5-year age groups, in 36 countries. Density plots depict a distribution of people and their scores. This represents more than 121,000 older persons in 36[1] countries, within seven distributions, one for each 5-year age group (60–64, 65–69, 70–74, 75–79, 80–89, 90+ years). Source: WHO, *Decade of Healthy Ageing: baseline report*. 2020.

[1]Austria, Belgium, Brazil, Bulgaria, Canada, China, Croatia, Cyprus, Czechia, Denmark, Estonia, Finland, France, Germany, Ghana, Greece, Hungary, India, Israel, Italy, Latvia, Lithuania, Luxembourg, Malaysia, Malta, Mexico, Netherlands, Poland, Portugal, Romania, Slovakia, Slovenia, South Africa, Spain, Sweden, and Switzerland.

Table 9.3 Cutoff value for low hand-grip strength. EWGSOP = the European Working Group on Sarcopenia in Older People; AWSG = the Asian Working Group for Sarcopenia; KNHANES = the Korea National Health and Nutrition Examination Survey.

	EWGSOP I	EWGSOP II	AWGS	KHANES VI
Method	-2SD	-2SD	Lower 20th percentile	Lower 25th percentile
Cutoff value (kg)				
Male	<30	<27	<26	<28
Female	<20	<16	<18	<16

Source: (S. H. Lee and H. S. Gong, 2020).

considered the most suitable for implementation in the standard clinical evaluation of older individuals, because is quick, inexpensive, highly reliable in measuring a person's functional capacity, and easy to use in clinical settings (Cesari et al., 2005).

According to a systematic review by Rydwik et al., there is a moderate association between habitual/maximum speed and performance of the ADLs. The distance the individual needs to cover to complete the trial can vary from 2 to 40 meters of flat surface, while speed is often measured as "normal"/ "self-selected"/ "habitual" and "maximum". The most used cutoff point to assess gait velocity is 1 m/s. A walking speed lower than 1 m/s indicates a high risk of health-related outcomes (persistent lower extremity limitation) in well-functioning people. Other cutoff points are also used to determine the best prognostic value. The EWGSOP2 recommends the use of a 0.8 m/s cutoff to indicate severe sarcopenia (Cruz-Jentoft et al., 2019). A cutoff point of 0.56 m/s showed a sensitivity level of 71.7% and specificity level of 74.2% for fall risk in community-dwelling frail men, while among geriatric patients in rehabilitation wards, a cutoff point of 0.15 m/s distinguished subjects requiring long-term hospital care from those who could live independently in their own home (Rydwik, Bergland, Forsén, & Frändin, 2012). Recently, tests of walking in more complex settings were proposed as a better tool to identify the ability of older subjects to adapt to everyday environmental challenges, since it is highly unlikely for older adults to walk exclusively flat paths in a mostly undisturbed manner during everyday life. These tests may better reflect functional capacity, especially in high functioning older adults. However, introducing unfamiliar actions or more than one constraint to basic walking may increase variability in performance and inconsistency among trials and reliability, especially considering the variability that already exists due to the different speeds and distances used in research and clinical settings (Forte et al., 2021).

BALANCE ASSESSMENT

Balance is the ability to keep one's body center of mass (COM) within the limits of the base of support (BOS). Balance is important for many functional activities of everyday life such as mobility and fall avoidance. Balance deterioration occurs in up to 75% of people aged 70 years and older and has a high prevalence in people with neuro-musculoskeletal disorders. Assessing balance abilities is complicated both due to their complex multifactorial nature and the wide variety of psychometrically valid, standardized tests available. Yet, the need for accurate assessment remains, since timely diagnoses of potential impairment directly affects falls risk, treatment planning, and evaluation changes over time (Sibley, Straus, Inness, Salbach, & Jaglal, 2011; Singh, Pillai, Tan, Tai, & Shahar, 2015).

There are numerous single physical performance tests implemented to screen for the risk of falls and balance impairments in older adults. Examples of these are the 30-s chair stand test, push-and-release test, single-leg stance test, and timed up-and-go (TUG) test (Singh et al., 2015; Centers for Disease Control and Prevention 2019). The CDC recommends the TUG, 30-s chair stand, or four-stage balance test as the simplest and most accurate tests to assess a patient's mobility, leg strength and endurance, and balance, respectively (Centers for Disease Control and Prevention 2019). See the Further Reading section for links to documentation about each test and relevant videos.

Timed Up-and-Go (TUG) Test

The TUG test reliably assesses the functional mobility of older adults. Participants are asked to sit on a chair (height of 46 cm and with an arm-rest height of 65 cm) placed against a wall. They are next asked to stand and walk at their normal pace until they cover a straight distance of 3 m. At the 3-m point they should turn around and walk toward the chair along the same path. The time is recorded in seconds (s) and the test ends when the participant's buttock touches the chair. The procedure is repeated three times with adequate time to rest between each session. The mean of the three times is taken as the TUG score.

30-second Chair Stand

The 30-s chair test is used to assess leg strength and endurance. Participants are requested to sit on a chair with their arms crossed over their chest, their back straight, and their feet flat on the floor. When instructed, examinees should rise to a full standing position without using their hands for help and sit back down. The procedure is repeated for 30 s and the number of full sit-ups is compared to a cutoff for fall risks based on their age (Harvard Health Letter, 2023).

Four-stage Balance Test

The four-stage balance test is used to assess static balance. The examinee is instructed in a specific sequence of progressively harder to maintain standing positions (feet side by side, one in front of the other while maintaining contact, tandem stand, and one-foot stand). The examiner stands next to the participant holding their arm until they master their balance through each position. If the individual cannot maintain their balance for 10 s without moving their feet or needing support, they are considered at a high risk for falling (Ncipc Duip, 2017).

COMPLEX BALANCE MEASURES

There are also more complex standardized balance measures that usually assess the eight components of balance (postural alignment, static and dynamic stability, reactive control, balance within functional tasks, and underlying motor, sensory, and cognitive systems/contributions). Most recognized standardized tests from the literature are the short physical performance battery (SPPB) (Bergland & Strand, 2019), balance evaluation systems test (BESTest), Berg balance scale (BBS), community balance and mobility scale (CB&M), clinical test of sensory integration in balance (CTSIB), and performance-oriented mobility assessment (POMA) (Sibley et al., 2011; Podsiadlo, D & Richardson, 1991).

Short Physical Performance Battery (SPPB)

Most frequently used is the SPPB, which is a well-established instrument to assess the overall physical performance (including balance) of community-dwelling, nursing home-dwelling, or hospitalized older individuals. The SPPB consists of a timed 4-m walk at the participant's normal pace, a timed repeated chair sit-to-stand test, and 10-s balance tests with feet side by side, semi-tandem, and full tandem. Low SPPB scores correlate with severe outcomes such as falls, mobility loss, disability, hospitalization, longer hospital stays, nursing home admissions, and death. Other data suggest that the SPPB can be used for the early detection of frailty and that a total score ≤ 9 can distinguish frail from non-frail persons (Bergland & Strand, 2019).

Both single and complex physical performance tests are more widely used in clinical settings because of their low cost, short evaluation time, and lack of obligatory equipment for most of them, compare to the gold-standard method of dynamic postural control, computerized dynamic posturography (CDP), a method requiring expensive equipment that is not widely available (Sipe, Ramey, Plisky, & Taylor, 2019).

Functionality Assessment Tools: Activities of Daily Living (ADLs) Assessment Tools

ADLs describe collectively fundamental skills that a person must acquire to be characterized as a functionally able individual. The term was first used in 1950 by Sidney Katz (Edemekong et al., 2020). ADLs are divided into two categories: basic and instrumental ADLs (IADLs). Basic or physical ADLs include skills required to deal with one's basic physical needs, including personal hygiene, grooming, dressing, toileting, transferring, or eating (Edemekong, Bomgaars, Sukumaran, & Levy, 2022). IADLs include more complex interactions between the person and the home/community that they live in. Examples include financial management, housekeeping, shopping for groceries, making telephone calls, and taking medication (Edemekong et al., 2020; Pashmdarfard & Azad, 2020). The most frequently used parameters to assess one's ability to meet their basic needs, according to the WHO, are the ability to get dressed, take medication, and manage money. The extent to which older adults can perform these activities on a day-to-day basis is strongly associated with their level of intrinsic capacity (WHO, 2020). The decline in both physical and cognitive functions that accompanies aging negatively affects the ADLs, hence affecting the person's quality of life (Edemekong et al., 2020). Performance measures can be integrated with routine clinical practice as convenient global markers for health-related risks in older adults (Studenski et al., 2003). To have a clearer view of the functional capabilities that older adults have to perform their everyday life activities and be independent, the healthcare team must have a full and accurate understanding of all types of effective ADL and IADL measures (Pashmdarfard & Azad, 2020).

The next few paragraphs will list some of the most used ADL and IADL assessment tools, a more complete listing of these tools is presented in **Table 9.4**.

ADL Assessment Tool: Barthel Index

The Barthel index (BI) was designed in 1955 and assesses 10 activities related to basic ADLs, which include: bowels, bladder, grooming, feeding, toilet use, transfer, mobility, dressing, stairs, and bathing. The estimated total score ranges between 0 (total disability and dependency) and 20 (maximum strength and independence). A total change of at least 2 points indicates a significant change in the degree of a person's (in)dependence (Pashmdarfard & Azad, 2020).

ADL Assessment Tool: Katz Index of Independence in Activities of Daily Living (ADL)

This tool was developed by Katz et al., in 1959, with the purpose of assessing the basic ADL function among older adults in the community and in all care settings. The initial version of the Katz index (KI) included eight basic ADL skills that were reduced to six including: bathing, dressing, transfer, toileting, feeding, and continence. To score this tool, if an older adult can perform an activity, they get a score of 1, and if they are unable to do so, a score of 0. The total score varies between 6 (maximum performance) and 0 (lack of performance). A score of 6 represents full function, 4 is moderate impairment, and a 2 or less indicates severe functional impairment. This tool has been translated into American English, Brazilian, and Turkish (Pashmdarfard & Azad, 2020).

ADL Assessment Tool: Functional Independence Measure (FIM)

The functional independence measure (FIM) was developed by the American Academy of Physical Medicine and Rehabilitation and the American Congress of Rehabilitation Medicine between 1984 and 1987. Keith et al., published the final product in 1987. This tool consists of 18 items that evaluate six functional areas of the individual. Thirteen of the items are Motor-FIM and five are the Cognitive-FIM. The Motor-FIM items of this tool are based on the BI. The FIM is useful for stroke patients in all age groups, but its use requires training and specialty courses under the supervision of trained professionals. This tool has been translated and validated in German, Italian, Spanish, Swedish, Finnish, Portuguese, African, Turkish, and French (Pashmdarfard & Azad, 2020).

IADL Assessment Tool: ADL Profile Instrumental (IADL)

Bottar et al., developed the IADL in 2010; it is an upgraded version of the ADL profile developed to evaluate the IADL performance of individuals with items that are closely related to the environmental performance. This tool includes 29 items in eight areas: putting on outdoor clothes, going to the grocery store, shopping for groceries, preparing a hot meal for guests, having a meal with guests, cleaning up after a meal, getting information, and making a budget. This tool is an ecological measure of an individual's autonomy in completing activities in the community and at home. The Canadian version of this tool is available and its use requires workshops held by the developer (Pashmdarfard & Azad, 2020).

IADL Assessment Tool: Lawton Instrumental ADL Scale

Lawton and Brody developed this scale in 1969 to assess the independence of older adults in IADL performance. This tool includes eight activities: the ability to use a phone, shopping, meal preparation, housekeeping, laundry, the mode of transportation, the responsibility for one's own medication, and the ability to handle finance. The scoring scale is 0 and 1, and the sum of the scores varies from 0 (low function, dependence) to 8 (high function, independence). Of the items in this tool, women should answer up to eight questions, but men may skip the three items related to meal preparation, housekeeping, and laundry. However, recent studies suggest that it is better for men to respond to these items and questions, as these three items together provide a good predictor of the independence and dependence of the older adult based on IADL performance. This scale was translated and validated in Australian English, Spanish, Malay, and Korean (Pashmdarfard & Azad, 2020).

IADL Assessment Tool: Performance Assessment of Self-care Skills (PASS)

This tool is a criterion reference, client reference, performance-based, and observational developed in 1988 by Rogers and Holm that includes 26 tasks and 163 sub-tasks. PASS assesses the IADL performance of individuals in four functional areas: functional mobility (5 items), basic ADL (3 items), ADL function with an emphasis on physical performance (4 items), and ADL function with an emphasis on cognitive function (14 items) (Pashmdarfard & Azad, 2020).

Lastly, **Table 9.5** presents a summary report on the most used measurements to assess organ-specific changes in physiological function among older adults (Khan, Singer, and Vaughan, 2017).

Table 9.4 Activities of Daily Living (ADL) and Instrumental Activities of Daily Living (IADL) assessment tools; characteristics of included measures.

PROM	Target population	Mode of administration (e.g. self-report, interview-based, parent/proxy Report etc.)	Recall period	Sub scales, Number of items	Range of scores scoring	Original language	Available translations
Barthel Index (BI) Mahoney & Bartkel (1995)	Stroke, other neuromuscular, musculoskeletal disorders, oncology patients	Self-report, direct observation.	Self-report: 2-5 minutes; direct observation: 20 minutes, also according to patient's abilities and tolerance	10 activities related to Basic ADL	0 (maximum disability and dependency) to 20 (maximum strength and independence)	English	Portuguese, British, Dutch, German, Taiwanese, Turkish, Chinese (Hong Kong), Persian.
Katz Index of Independence in Activities of Daily Living (ADL) Katz et at (1959)	Older adults in the community and all care settings	Self-report, direct observation.	Self-report: 2-5 minutes; direct observation: 20 minutes, also according to patient's abilities and tolerance	6 Basic ADL function	Total score: between 6 (maximum performance) and 0 (lack of performance). Also: score of 6 (full function), 4 (moderate impairment), and 2 or less (severe functional impairment).	American (English)	Brazilian, Turkish, Swedish, Persian
Functional Independence Measure (FIM) Instrument American Academy of Physical Medicine and Rehabilitation & American Congress of Rehabilitation Medicine Keith et al (1987)	Stroke, TBI, SCI, MS, elderly individuals undergoing inpatient rehabilitation, children as young as 7 years old	Performance based (direct observation of the evaluated function)	It take between 30-45 minutes to administer and score, with 7 minutes to gather demographic information.	18 items that evaluate 6 functional areas, The 13 items are named as Motor-FIM and its 5 items are named as Cognitive-FIM	Each item is scored on a 7-point Likert scale, and the score indicates the amount of assistance required to perform each item (1 = total assistance in all areas. 7 = total independence in all areas). A final summed score is created and ranges from 18-126 (18 represents complete dependence/total assistance, 126 represents complete independence).	English	German, Italian, Spanish, Swedish, Finnish, Portuguese, African, Turkish, French, Persian
Activities of Daily Living (ADL) Profile Dutil et al (1990)	TBI, Stroke	Performance-based evaluation (direct observation of the evaluated function), and semi-structured interviews with the person or other people (individual's caregivers)	30-60 minutes When administered in preparation for discharge from a rehabilitation hospital up to 7 hours may be required.	Assesses the ADL function of in three personal environments (with 6 items), Home (with 5 items), and the Community (with 9 items).	0 (full independency) to 3 (full dependency)	Canadian	Canadian, French

Name	Target population	Mode of administration	Recall period / time	Sub/scales, Number of items	Range of scores/scoring	Original language	Available translations
Activities of Daily Living Questionnaire (ADLQ) Johnson et al (2004)	Individual with cognitive impairment, especially Alzheimer	Informant-based	5-10 minutes	6 areas	0 (no problem) to 3 (need help for completion and long-term)	English	American, Chinese, Spanish, Brazilian, Chilean
PROM	Target population	Mode of administration (e.g. self-report, interview-based, parent/proxy Report etc.)	Recall period	Sub/scales, Number of items	Range of scores/scoring	Original language	Available translations
Australian Therapy Outcome Measures (AusTOMs) Perry et al (2004)	Client profiles and patterns of services provision across health care settings	Performance-based evaluation tool	Not mentioned	There are 6 speech pathology scales, 9 physiotherapy scales and 12 occupational therapy scales.	0 (sever impairment, complete difficulty) to 5 (no impairment, no difficulty)	Australian	English, Swedish
Melbourne Low-Vision ADL Inder (MILVAI) Haymes et al (2001)	Individuals with visual impairment	Performance-based evaluation tool (desk based clinical assessment)	Not mentioned	Consisting 18 observational items in the field of ADL functions, and 9 items for self-care activities	Scoring for each item is based on independency, speed and accuracy of performance on a five descriptive Likert scale (0-4)	English	English
Self-Assessment Parkinson's disease Disability Scale (SPDDS) Brown (1989)	Parkinson	Self-report (paper-pencil)	5 minutes	24 items that assess the ADL performance	5 (ability to do work alone and without difficulty) to 1 (unable to do activity)	English	English, Serbian
Frenchay Activities Index (FAI) Holbrook & Skilbeck (1983)	Stroke	Interview	5 minutes	15 items that cover three areas of domestic chores Work/Leisure, and Outdoor activities.	1 (lowest level of activity) to 4 (highest level of activity)	English	English, Chinese, Dutch
Activities of Daily Living (IADL) Profile Instrumental	TBI	Performance-based evaluation (direct observation of the evaluated function), and semi-structured interviews with the person or other people (individual's caregivers	30-60 minutes	29 items in 8 areas	0 (full independency) to 3 (full dependency)	English	Canadian

(Continued)

Table 9.4 (Continued)

PROM	Target population	Mode of administration (e.g. self-report, interview-based, parent/proxy Report etc.)	Recall period	Sub scales, Number of items	Range of scores scoring	Original language	Available translations
Bottar et al (2010)							
Lawton Instrumental Activities of Daily Living Scale (LLADL)	Older adults but isn't useful for institutionalized older adults	Self-report	10-15 minutes	8 activities related to IADL	Scoring scale is zero and one. Sum of the scores is varied from 0 (low function, dependence) to 8 (high function, independence)	English	Spanish, Malay, Korean, Persian
Lawton and Brody (1969)							
Performance Assessment of Self-care Skills (PASS)	Adolescence through old age	This tool is a criterion reference, client reference, performance-based and observational		26 tasks contain: 5 functional mobility (MOB), 3 (ADL), 14 IADL with a cognitive emphasis (C-IADL), 4 IADL with a physical emphasis (P-IADL).	4 point (0-3) ordinal scale.	English	English Persian
Rogers & Holm (1988)							

Source: (Pashmdarfard and Azad, 2020).

Table 9.5 Measures of organ-specific changes in physiological function.

Organ system	Measures of organ-specific function
Cardiovascular	Brachial pulse pressure
	LV mass
	Relative wall thickness
	Echocardiographic parameters (E/A, e')
	Pulse wave velocity
	Augmentation index
	Aortic valve calcification
	Heart rate variability
Respiratory	Peak aerobic capacity
	Spirometry (FEV_1, FVC, FEV_1/FVC ratio)
	Lung volumes (TLC, FRC, RV)
	DLCO
	Quantitative ventilation-perfusion scanning
Renal	Cystatin C
	Creatinine clearance
Immune	Immune risk profile (assessment of T-cell proliferation in response to mitogens, B-cell numbers, CD4:CD8 T-cell ratio, and CMV serologic status)
Bone marrow	Hemoglobin
Neurocognitive	Mini-mental status examination
	Cognitive battery
	Functional MRI
Digestive and hepatic Endocrine	Vitamin K-dependent clotting factor levels
	Thyroid biochemical tests
	Fasting glucose
	Insulin
	Circulating estrogen and testosterone levels
Musculoskeletal	Hand grip strength
	Unipedal stance test of balance
	Grooved pegboard test of fine motor coordination
	SF-36 physical functioning scale
Integumentary	Skin elasticity
	Thickness
	Wrinkle parameter
Sensory	Visual acuity
	Auditory test
	Retinal microvascular damage (arteriovenous ratio)

Source: (Khan, Singer, and Vaughan, 2017).

KEY POINTS

- Aging procedures are a wide range of accumulated molecular and cellular damage, which over time is expressed as decreased maximal organ function with different trajectories across organ systems.

- Aging can significantly influence cardiovascular functionality through mechanisms that ultimately result in the development of age-related pathological entities such as atherosclerosis, hypertension, congestive heart failure, atrioventricular block, and aortic stenosis.

- Aging elevates the risk of pneumonia as well as decreased aerobic capacity in older adults due to mechanisms that deteriorate lung-tissue elasticity and surface availability, diminish the nervous drive toward respiratory muscles in response to chemical and mechanical stimuli, and reduce muscle strength and mucociliary clearance.

- Inflamm-aging is the age-associated, chronic, low-grade inflammation that is a consequence of (hyper-)activated inflammation-signaling networks and is a risk factor for all causes of death.

- Older people experience a loss of total brain volume, decreased dopaminergic signaling, and brain plasticity, which progressively make them more susceptible to neurodegenerative diseases.

- Aging procedures affect muscle composition in a negative way, which results in an increased risk for falling, developing insulin resistance, and feeling fatigued.

- Sarcopenia and frailty are the most common and well-studied geriatric syndromes that include muscle wasting as a primary symptom, deteriorate the individual's functional and ambulatory capacity when left untreated, and threaten autonomy and quality of life.

- Sarcopenia proceeds frailty and their main difference lies in the fact that frailty also includes loss of muscle functionality as well as muscle mass and strength. Sarcopenia is characterized only by the last two.

- According to the WHO, hand-grip strength is the most reliable technique to assess vitality.

- Apart from hand-grip strength, the most used physical performance and balance tests are the gait speed, timed up-and-go, 30-s chair stand, and four-stage balance tests.

- Activities of daily living (ADLs) describe a collection of fundamental skills that a person must acquire to be characterized as a functionally able individual.

- Some of the tools used to assess levels of functionality in older people are the Barthel index, Katz index of independence in ADL, functional independence measure (FIM), ADL profile instrumental, Lawton instrumental ADL scale, and performance assessment of self-care skills (PASS).

SELF-ASSESSMENT QUESTIONS

1. Briefly describe the changes that the cardiovascular system undergoes in the context of aging.

2. Briefly describe the changes that the pulmonary system undergoes in the context of aging.

3. What is inflamm-aging and how is it correlated to the aging procedures?

4. Why is the successful management of sarcopenia and frailty of outmost importance in the context of establishing healthy aging in older populations?

5. Briefly describe the goal of the timed up-and-go test and how it is used in clinical practice.

6. Muscle mass accounts for:
   (a) Up to 40% of body mass
   (b) Up to 50% of body mass
   (c) Up to 60% of body mass

7. What is the annual reduction in muscle strength according to longitudinal studies?
   (a) 1.5%
   (b) 3%
   (c) 4.5%

8. What is the cutoff point for detecting low hand-grip strength based on EWGSOP II?
   (a) <30kg for men and <20kg for women
   (b) <27kg for men and <16kg for women
   (c) <28kg for men and <16kg for women

9. What is the gait-speed cutoff point associated with severe sarcopenia according to EWGSOP II?
   (a) 1 m/s
   (b) 0.8 m/s
   (c) 0.5 m/s

10. True or False: Aging depends on an individual's genetic predisposition and developmental programming alone.

11. True or False: Older adults show a decreased responsiveness to b-adrenergic stimuli.

12. True or False: After the age of 40, total brain volume drops at an approximate rate of 5% per decade.

13. True or False: 13% of people over the age of 80 are diagnosed with low muscle mass.

14. True or False: Hand-grip strength is the most dependable measurement for assessing muscular strength in elderly populations.

REFERENCES

Aiello, A., Farzaneh, F., Candore, G., Caruso, C., Davinelli, S., Gambino, C. M., . . . Accardi, G. (2019). Immunosenescence and its hallmarks: How to oppose aging strategically? A review of potential options for therapeutic intervention. *Frontiers in Immunology, 10*(September), 1–19. https://doi.org/10.3389/fimmu.2019.02247

Angulo, J., El Assar, M., Álvarez-Bustos, A., & Rodríguez-Mañas, L. (2020). Physical activity and exercise: Strategies to manage frailty. *Redox Biology, 35*(January), 101513. https://doi.org/10.1016/j.redox.2020.101513

Anker, S. D., Morley, J. E., & von Haehling, S. (2016). Welcome to the ICD-10 code for sarcopenia. *Journal of Cachexia, Sarcopenia and Muscle, 7*(5), 512–514. https://doi.org/10.1002/jcsm.12147

Bergland, A., & Strand, B. H. (2019). Norwegian reference values for the Short Physical Performance Battery (SPPB): The Tromsø Study. *BMC Geriatrics, 19*(1), 1–10. https://doi.org/10.1186/s12877-019-1234-8

Cederholm, T., Barazzoni, R., Austin, P., Ballmer, P., Biolo, G., Bischoff, S. C., . . . Singer, P. (2017). ESPEN guidelines on definitions and terminology of clinical nutrition. *Clinical Nutrition, 36*(1), 49–64. https://doi.org/10.1016/j.clnu.2016.09.004

Centers for Disease Control and Prevention (CDC). (2019). Algorithm for Fall Risk Screening, Assessment, and Intervention. *CDC, 2*. Retrieved from www.cdc.gov/steadi.

Cesari, M., Gambassi, G., Van Kan, G. A., & Vellas, B. (2014). The frailty phenotype and the frailty index: Different instruments for different purposes. *Age and Ageing, 43*(1), 10–12. https://doi.org/10.1093/ageing/aft160

Cesari, M., Kritchevsky, S. B., Penninx, B. W. H. J., Nicklas, B. J., Simonsick, E. M., Newman, A. B., . . . Pahor, M. (2005). Prognostic value of usual gait speed in well-functioning older people - Results from the health, aging and body composition study. *Journal of the American Geriatrics Society, 53*(10), 1675–1680. https://doi.org/10.1111/j.1532-5415.2005.53501.x

Chair Stand. *Harvard Health Letter,* (JANUARY), 1, 2023.

Clegg, A., Young, J., Iliffe, S., Rikkert, M. O., & Rockwood, K. (2013). Frailty in elderly people. *The Lancet, 381*(9868), 752–762. https://doi.org/10.1016/S0140-6736(12)62167-9

Cruz-Jentoft, A. J., Bahat, G., Bauer, J., Boirie, Y., Bruyère, O., Cederholm, T., . . . Schols, J. (2019). Sarcopenia: Revised European consensus on definition and diagnosis. *Age and Ageing, 48*(1), 16–31. https://doi.org/10.1093/ageing/afy169

Eckstrom, E., Neukam, S., Kalin, L., & Wright, J. (2020). Physical Activity and Healthy Aging. *Clinics in Geriatric Medicine, 36*(4), 671–683. https://doi.org/10.1016/j.cger.2020.06.009

Edemekong, P. F., Bomgaars, D. L., Sukumaran, S., & Levy, S. B. (2022). Activities of Daily Living. *Encyclopedia of the Neurological Sciences, 47*–48. https://doi.org/10.1016/B978-0-12-385157-4.00464-4

Edemekong, P. F., Bomgaars, D. L., Sukumaran, S., & et al. (2020). *Activities of Daily Living - StatPearls - NCBI Bookshelf.* Retrieved from https://www.ncbi.nlm.nih.gov/books/NBK470404/

Forte, R., De Vito, G., & Boreham, C. A. G. (2021). Reliability of walking speed in basic and complex conditions in healthy, older community-dwelling individuals. *Aging Clinical and Experimental Research, 33*(2), 311–317. https://doi.org/10.1007/s40520-020-01543-x

Frontera, W. R. (2017). Physiologic Changes of the Musculoskeletal System with Aging: A Brief Review. *Physical Medicine and Rehabilitation Clinics of North America, 28*(4), 705–711. https://doi.org/10.1016/j.pmr.2017.06.004

Green, S., & Hillersdal, L. (2021). Aging biomarkers and the measurement of health and risk. *History and Philosophy of the Life Sciences, 43*(1), 1–23. https://doi.org/10.1007/s40656-021-00367-w

Harman, M. F., & Martín, M. G. (2020). Epigenetic mechanisms related to cognitive decline during aging. *Journal of Neuroscience Research, 98*(2), 234–246. https://doi.org/10.1002/jnr.24436

Khan, S. S., Singer, B. D., & Vaughan, D. E. (2017). Harvard Prevention Research Center on Nutrition and Physical Activity. Molecular and physiological manifestations and measurement of aging in humans. *Aging Cell, 16*(4), 624–633. https://doi.org/10.1111/acel.12601

Meier, N. F., & Lee, D. chul. (2020). Physical activity and sarcopenia in older adults. *Aging Clinical and Experimental Research, 32*(9), 1675–1687. https://doi.org/10.1007/s40520-019-01371-8

Montecino-Rodriguez, E., Berent-Maoz, B., & Dorshkind, K. (2013). Causes, consequences, and reversal of immune system aging. *Journal of Clinical Investigation, 123*(3), 958–965. https://doi.org/10.1172/JCI64096

Morley, J. E., Anker, S. D., & von Haehling, S. (2014). Prevalence, incidence, and clinical impact of sarcopenia: facts, numbers, and epidemiology—update 2014. *Journal of Cachexia, Sarcopenia and Muscle, 5*(4), 253–259. https://doi.org/10.1007/s13539-014-0161-y

Nascimento, C. M., Ingles, M., Salvador-Pascual, A., Cominetti, M. R., Gomez-Cabrera, M. C., & Viña, J. (2019). Sarcopenia, frailty and their prevention by exercise. *Free Radical Biology and Medicine, 132*, 42–49. https://doi.org/10.1016/j.freeradbiomed.2018.08.035

Ncipc Duip, C. (2017). The 4-Stage Balance Test. *Steadi.* Retrieved from https://www.cdc.gov/steadi/pdf/4-stage_balance_test-a.pdf

Panagiotou, M., Michel, S., Meijer, J. H., & Deboer, T. (2021). The aging brain: sleep, the circadian clock and exercise. *Biochemical Pharmacology, 191*(March), 114563. https://doi.org/10.1016/j.bcp.2021.114563

Pashmdarfard, M., & Azad, A. (2020). Assessment tools to evaluate activities of daily living (ADL) and instrumental activities of daily living (IADL) in older adults: A systematic review. *Medical Journal of the Islamic Republic of Iran, 34*(1). https://doi.org/10.34171/mjiri.34.33

Podsiadlo, D & Richardson, S. (1991). The Timed Up and Go: A Test of Basic Functional Mobility for Frail Elderly Persons. *Journal of the American Geriatrics Society, 39*(2), 142–148. Retrieved from https://pubmed.ncbi.nlm.nih.gov/1991946/

Rydwik, E., Bergland, A., Forsén, L., & Frändin, K. (2012). Investigation into the reliability and validity of the measurement of elderly people's clinical walking speed: A systematic review. *Physiotherapy Theory and Practice, 28*(3), 238–256. https://doi.org/10.3109/09593985.2011.601804

Studenski, S., Perera, S., Wallace, D., Chandler, J. M., Duncan, P. W., Rooney, E., ... & Guralnik, J. M. (2003). Physical performance measures in the clinical setting. *Journal of the American Geriatrics Society, 51*(3), 314–322.

Sabine, R. (2020). Epidemiology of Frailty in Older People. *Advances in Experimental Medicine and Biology, 21*–27(1216). Retrieved from https://doi.org/10.1007/978-3-030-33330-0_3

Schneider, J. L., Rowe, J. H., Garcia-de-Alba, C., Kim, C. F., Sharpe, A. H., & Haigis, M. C. (2021). The aging lung: Physiology, disease, and immunity. *Cell, 184*(8), 1990–2019. https://doi.org/10.1016/j.cell.2021.03.005

Sibley, K. M., Straus, S. E., Inness, E. L., Salbach, N. M., & Jaglal, S. B. (2011). Balance assessment practices and use of standardized balance measures among Ontario physical therapists. *Physical Therapy*, *91*(11), 1583–1591. https://doi.org/10.2522/ptj.20110063

Singh, D. K. A., Pillai, S. G. K., Tan, S. T., Tai, C. C., & Shahar, S. (2015). Association between physiological falls risk and physical performance tests among community-dwelling older adults. *Clinical Interventions in Aging*, *10*, 1319–1326. https://doi.org/10.2147/CIA.S79398

Sipe, C. L., Ramey, K. D., Plisky, P. P., & Taylor, J. D. (2019). Y-balance test: A valid and reliable assessment in older adults. *Journal of Aging and Physical Activity*, *27*(5), 663–669. https://doi.org/10.1123/japa.2018-0330

Suzuki, K. (2019). Chronic inflammation as an immunological abnormality and effectiveness of exercise. *Biomolecules*, *9*(6), 3–7. https://doi.org/10.3390/biom9060223

Walston, J. D. (2012). Sarcopenia in older adults. *Current Opinion in Rheumatology*, *24*(6), 623–627. https://doi.org/10.1097/BOR.0b013e328358d59b

WHO. (2020). Decade of Healthy Ageing: baseline report. In *World Health Organization*.

Xue, Q. L. (2011). The Frailty Syndrome: Definition and Natural History. *Clinics in Geriatric Medicine*, *27*(1), 1–15. https://doi.org/10.1016/j.cger.2010.08.009

FURTHER READING

Bibliography

World Health Organization, *Decade of healthy ageing: Baseline report*. 2020.

World Health Organization (2020) Decade of healthy ageing: Baseline report (License: CC BY-NC-SA 3.0 IGO). Geneva: World Health Organization.

Welch, S. A., Ward, R. E., Beauchamp, M. K., et al., (2021). The Short Physical Performance Battery (SPPB): A Quick and Useful Tool for Fall Risk Stratification Among Older Primary Care Patients, *Journal of the American Medical Directors Association* 22(8): 1646–1651. doi: 10.1016/j.jamda.2020.09.038.

Links

- https://www.cdc.gov/steadi/

4-Stage Balance Test:

- https://www.cdc.gov/steadi/pdf/4-Stage_Balance_Test-print.pdf
- https://www.youtube.com/watch?v=3HvMLLIGY6c

30-Second Chair Stand:

- https://www.cdc.gov/steadi/pdf/STEADI-Assessment-30Sec-508.pdf
- https://www.youtube.com/watch?v=Ng-UOHjTejY

Katz Index of Independence in Activities of Daily Living:

- https://geriatrictoolkit.missouri.edu/funct/Katz_ADL.pdf

Lawton-Brody Instrumental Activities of Daily Living Scale (IADL):

- https://geriatrictoolkit.missouri.edu/funct/Lawton_IADL.pdf

Timed Up-and-Go Test:

- https://www.cdc.gov/steadi/pdf/TUG_test-print.pdf
- https://www.youtube.com/watch?v=BA7Y_oLElGY

The Barthel Index:

- https://www.sralab.org/sites/default/files/2017-07/barthel.pdf

The Role of Plant-based Diets on Healthy Aging

CHAPTER 10

Introduction	133
The Role of Macronutrients in Healthy Aging	134
Protein	134
Carbohydrates	137
Fat Intake	138
Plant-based Diets	142
Plant Polyphenols	143
The Mediterranean Diet	145
The Nordic Diet	148
Dietary Approaches to Stop Hypertension (DASH) Diet	149
The Okinawan Diet	150
Key Points	151
Self-assessment Questions	152
References	152
Further Reading	157
Bibliography	157
Links	157

INTRODUCTION

Human genome, the living environment, and lifestyle factors such as nutrition and physical activity are of utmost importance in determining an individual's lifespan by affecting disease risk and survival (Ekmekcioglu, 2020). Although genetic influence accounts for approximately 20% to 25% of total lifespan, the main part of healthy aging and life expectancy is determined by lifestyle and environmental factors. Improvements in several core lifestyle measures like income, nutrition, education, hygiene, medical therapy, and health care provision have made significant improvement in longevity and quality of life (QOL) (Ekmekcioglu, 2020). A large body of research indicates that nutritional and metabolic factors could also influence health span and longevity by affecting the epigenetic program (Pignatti, Adamo, Stefanelli, Flamigni, & Cetrullo, 2020). For instance, nutritional and dietary factors are postulated to affect DNA methylation by changing the availability of methyl donors and altering the activity of the DNA methyltransferase (DNMT) enzymes as described in **Chapter 2**. Folate and related B vitamins are key nutrients in 1-carbon metabolism, the main metabolic pathway that generates methyl groups for DNA methylation, are essential factors that can modify epigenetic age (Pignatti et al., 2020.).

The relationship between nutrition and healthy aging is a subject of increased interest among gerontology researchers, since dietary interventions can prevent, or at least delay, the onset of many age-related chronic conditions (Capurso, 2021). But what qualifies as a healthy diet, in terms of its macro- and micronutrients composition, that successfully extends healthy living remains an unanswered question of high priority for human nutrition research (Panagiotou, Michel, Meijer, & Deboer, 2021; Brandhorst & Longo, 2019). Defining a globally healthy diet is not a simple query, since nutritional needs vary substantially by age, sex, disease status, physical activity levels, and cultural norms (Dominguez et al., 2022). Poor nutrition has severe consequences on health that tend to accumulate over a person's lifespan and negatively influence later stages of life (Bruins, Van Dael, & Eggersdorfer, 2019; Capurso, 2021). As discussed in **Chapter 1**, according to the WHO, unhealthy diets and physical inactivity are among the main modifiable risk factors that can increase the number of non-communicable diseases (NCDs) worldwide and consequently, worsen the global burden of disease (Bruins et al., 2019). Western-like lifestyles and easy access to high-energy, low-nutrient rich foods are considered a major part of the problem. However, across countries, there is considerable variation in the consumption of nutrients and foods/food groups. For example, based on a study that compared the macro- and micronutrient intake in four European countries, as shown in **Table 10.1**, while there is a significant part of the population that consumes an excess of

---

Prevention and Management of Cardiovascular and Metabolic Disease: Diet, Physical Activity and Healthy Aging,
First Edition. Christina N. Katsagoni, Peter Kokkinos, and Labros S. Sidossis.
© 2023 John Wiley & Sons Ltd. Published 2023 by John Wiley & Sons Ltd.

Table 10.1 Percentage of adults with nutrient intakes meeting the estimated average requirement (EAR), adequate intake (AI), or exceeding the maximal reference value (MRV). E% = energy intake; MUFA = mono-unsaturated fatty acids; SFA = saturated fatty acids. The red, orange, yellow, light green, and dark green signals are ≤5%, 6–35%, 36–65%, 66–95%, and ≥96% of people meeting the EAR, respectively.

% Meeting EAR or AI	EAR or AI	Denmark n = 2025 people	Czech Republic n = 1869 people	Italy n = 2831 people	France n = 2624 people
Protein, g/d	0.66 g/kg BW	84%	88%	99%	98%
MUFA, E\%	10–20 E%	69%	92%	75%	77%
Dietary fiber, g/d	25	19%	4%	12%	9%
% exceeding MRV			MRV		
SFA, E%	<10 E%	86%	80%	62%	91%
Added sugar, E%	<10 E%	32%	21%	24%	

Sources: (Adapted from Bruins et al., 2019; Mertens et al., 2019).

energy, sugar, saturated fat, and salt, as part of the Western world, there is another significant part that fails to meet the required or adequate intake for a wide range of essential nutrients, e.g. dietary fiber (Bruins et al., 2019; Mertens et al., 2019).

This evidence aligns with data from other studies in older adults that highlight the broadly inadequate dietary patterns in terms of nutrients and food/food groups in this population compared with the current food-based recommendations. As depicted in **Figure 10.1**, most adults aged over 50-years old fall short on recommendations for the most nutritious food groups, including whole grains, seafood, vegetables, fruits, seeds, nuts, and legumes (Roberts et al., 2021).

Nevertheless, there is not an ideal dietary pattern that grants healthy aging for all individuals. However, a continuously growing body of evidence, suggests that plant-based diets are promising in decreasing all-cause mortality and furthering life expectancy, especially when compared to the effects that Western dietary patterns have on human health and aging.

THE ROLE OF MACRONUTRIENTS IN HEALTHY AGING

PROTEIN

One of the most difficult topics regarding the association between nutrition and longevity is the optimal extent/quantity of (age-dependent) human protein intake (Pignatti et al., 2020). Older adults have higher protein needs because of the anabolic resistance, a phenomenon that limits muscle maintenance and accretion. Anabolic resistance is defined as the inability of an anabolic stimulus (e.g., protein provision, hormonal stimulation, and/or muscle contraction) to stimulate muscle protein synthesis (MPS). It frequently occurs with increasing age and when someone becomes inactive or suffers a critical illness. Therefore, anabolic resistance increases protein needs to offset the elevated metabolism of inflammatory conditions such as heart failure, chronic obstructive pulmonary disease (COPD), or

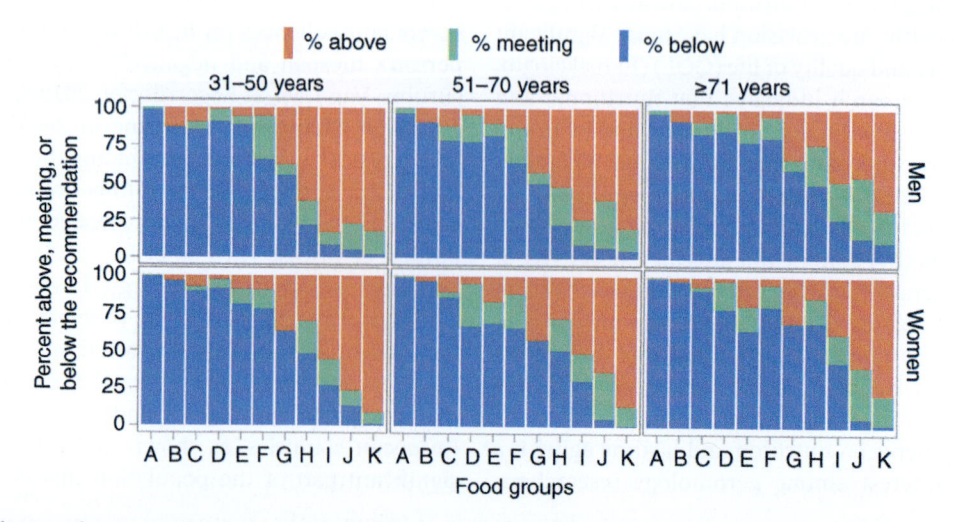

FIGURE 10.1 Dietary adequacy by age groups. Percentage of adults consuming above, below, or at the recommended intakes for food groups in the 2020–2025 Dietary Guidelines by sex and age group, based on dietary data obtained from the 2007–2010 NHANES. A = whole grains, B = dairy; C = seafood; D = vegetables; E = fruit; F = oils; G = nuts, seeds, soy; H = protein; I = meat, poultry, eggs; J = refined grains; K = SoFAS; SoFAS = solid fats and added sugars. Note: Total vegetables includes beans and peas. Protein excludes beans and peas. Source: (Roberts et al., 2021 / with permission of Oxford University Press).

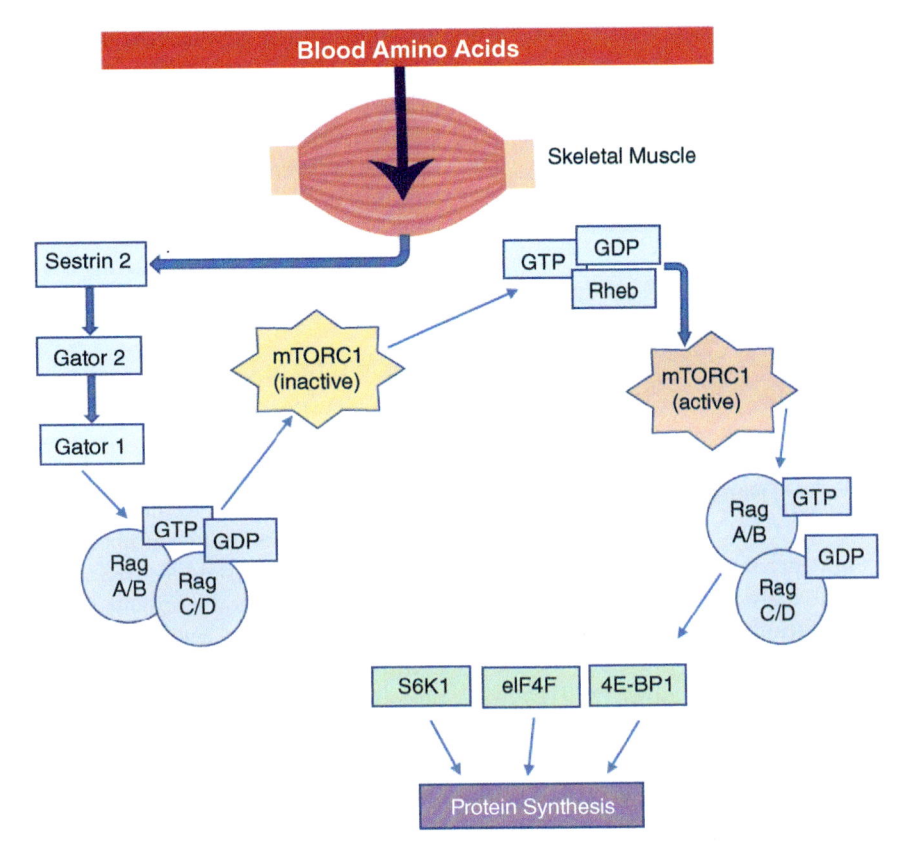

FIGURE 10.2 Overview of the mTOR signaling pathway with the basic features of mTOR involvement in regulating MPS. Amino acids (AAs) enter the muscle from the blood stream. Sestrin2 is involved in sensing and signaling the AA to the Rag GTPases. The interaction of Sestrin2 with GATOR2 inhibits mTORC1 signaling in the absence of leucine. GATOR1 is a Rag GTPase-activating protein that causes RagA/B to switch to an inactive form containing GDP, which inactivates mTORC1 in the absence of AAs. GATOR1 thus inhibits mTORC1. In the presence of AAs, GATOR2 activates RagA/B and inhibits GATOR1, which promotes activation of mTORC1. Rheb is an essential and potent kinase activator of mTORC1. Activation of mTORC1 causes phosphorylation of S6K1 and 4E-BP1, which promote protein synthesis by activating ribosomal protein S6 and causing the release of eI4F4, the translation initiation factor. Source: (Olaniyan et al., 2020 / with permission of Cambridge University Press).

chronic kidney disease (CKD) and undergoing dialysis. In healthy older adults and in a variety of diseases, protein anabolism is related to net protein intake (Deutz et al., 2014). The increased availability of amino acids (AAs), especially essential AAs through increased protein intake, stimulates MPS, by activating the mammalian target of rapamycin (mTOR) signaling pathway in muscle cells, which acts to integrate intracellular and extracellular signals that orchestrate cell growth and metabolism (**Figure 10.2**) (Olaniyan, O' Halloran, & McCarthy, 2020; Pignatti et al., 2020; Deutz et al., 2014; Olaniyan et al., 2020).

There are many reasons why older adults fail to consume enough protein. This includes a genetic predisposition to low appetite, physiological changes such as impaired sense of smell, taste, and vision, poor oral health, inadequate digestion, insulin and anabolic resistance, inflammation, decreased insulin-like growth factor IGF-I levels. Medical conditions that lead to age- and disease-associated anorexia, physical pain and mental disabilities that limit shopping and food preparation and food insecurity due to financial and social limitations are also considered possible reasons of low protein intake in older adults. (Deutz et al., 2014; Pilgrim, Robinson, Sayer, & Roberts, 2015; Olaniyan et al., 2020; Lonnie et al., 2018). Additionally, individuals with low physical activity levels have decreased rates of nitrogen retention and therefore, have increased protein requirements to maintain muscle mass tissue (Lonnie et al., 2018). Whatever the reason is, meeting protein needs on a daily basis is necessary for older individuals in order to compensate the age-related losses in skeletal muscle mass and strength as well as for maintaining physical functionality, and independence. Moreover, adequate protein is needed for preventing common clinical conditions that affect their QOL such as sarcopenia, frailty, or loss of balance (Ortolá, Struijk, García-Esquinas, Rodríguez-Artalejo, & López-García, 2020) (**Figure 10.3**).

Protein Intake: Quantity

According to the existing recommendations, protein intake in older adults should be at least 1 g per kg of body weight per day. The amount should be individually adjusted according to nutritional status, physical activity levels, disease status, and tolerance. The traditional recommendation for protein intake,

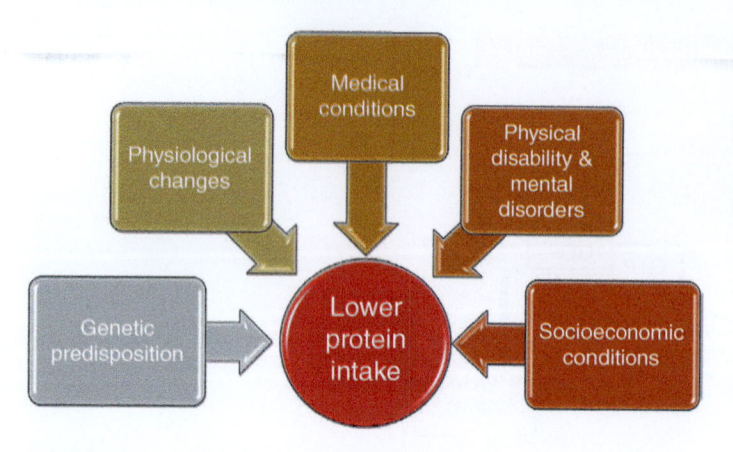

FIGURE 10.3 Protein status: factors that lead to lower protein intake in older persons. Source: (Deutz et al., 2014 / with permission of Elsevier).

that is 0.8 g/kg body of weight per day for all adults, is outdated for older persons. Instead, daily amounts of 1.0–1.2 g/kg of body weight is suggested for healthy older adults by several expert groups for its beneficial effects on muscle mass and strength, physical function, hip fracture rates, and frailty (Volkert et al., 2019; Ortolá et al., 2020). In case of illness, protein requirements may be further increased due to inflammation (including inflamm-aging), infections, and wounds, however, by how much is difficult to assess. Daily amounts of 1.2–1.5 g/kg of body weight have been also suggested for older adults with acute or chronic illness and up to 2.0 g/kg of body weight per day for severe illness, injury, or malnutrition (Volkert et al., 2019).

Although most studies agree on the elevated protein needs of older adults, there is also a non-negligible number of studies supporting a positive correlation between low-protein diets (<20% protein-derived consumed calories) and lower rates of aging-related diseases. Prospective and randomized clinical trials (RCTs) demonstrate that low-protein diets in humans enhance metabolic health, promote lean physical appearances, lower blood glucose, and decrease the risk of developing diabetes (Brandhorst & Longo, 2019). As mentioned in **Chapter 8**, observational studies conducted in so-called "blue zones" (populations with exceptional longevity rates), indicate that plant-based, low-protein dietary patterns with an emphasis on fruit, vegetable, and nut intake are preferred (Chrysohoou et al., 2016; Brandhorst & Longo, 2019; Appel, 2008). The hypothesis is that lower protein intake results in lower activity of the growth hormone (GH)/ insulin-like growth factor 1 (IGF-1) axis, which plays a protective role against the (early) onset of age-related pathologies and aging itself. Cohort studies suggest a positive correlation between high animal-based protein and fat as well as low carbohydrate consumption with higher mortality (Susan, 2007; Brandhorst & Longo, 2019). But most of these findings fail to remain statistically important when controlled for sex, age, and age group. For instance, when considering men and women more than 50-years old in the NHANES dataset, a positive correlation between protein intake and increased mortality was not supported (Levine et al., 2014; Brandhorst & Longo, 2019). In fact, individuals older than 65-years old who consumed a high-protein diet had a 28% reduction in all-cause mortality and a 60% reduction in cancer mortality compared with low-protein diets irrespectively of fat, carbohydrate intake or the protein source (Susan, 2007; Brandhorst & Longo, 2019). Overall, low-protein intake in humans may be beneficial for those 50–65-years of age but detrimental at older ages. Nonetheless, more relevant nutritional studies are necessary to have a better understanding of both the benefits and risks of different levels of protein intake during the human lifespan (Pignatti et al., 2020).

Protein Intake: Quality

Protein quality is determined by its AA composition/profile (especially leucine) and digestibility or bioavailability and has a significant impact on protein metabolism. It affects the contribution of a protein to increase the MPS following consumption. Protein digestibility and absorption kinetics are independent predictors of postprandial MPS. Protein digestibility relates to the amount of dietary protein that is effectively digested and absorbed in a form acceptable for body protein synthesis. It is influenced by protein structure, the food matrix in which a protein is contained, the presence of anti-nutritional factors (factors that can reduce the bioavailability of macro and micronutrients), and the processing method applied to a food. The digestion speed of a protein also influences postprandial protein retention and accretion. Slowly digested proteins, such as casein, are associated with slower AA absorption kinetics, which affects whole-body protein anabolism by promoting protein deposition (Olaniyan et al., 2020).

Proteins obtained after consuming animal products such as eggs, dairy, and meat, are of high nutritional value and therefore, highly digestible (>90%) (Olaniyan et al., 2020). Overall, animal-based foods are recognized as superior protein sources due to their complete AA composition (including essential AAs), which are more bioavailable and more easily digested, compared to plant-based sources (Lonnie et al., 2018). Once they become bioavailable, these AAs can help increase postprandial MPS (Olaniyan et al., 2020).

Leucine is the AA with an important role in MPS. Animal-based foods high in leucine, including chicken, lean beef, pork, and fish serve as a potent anabolic signals (Paproski, Finello, Murillo, & Mandel, 2019). Leucine is correlated to increased muscle mass, strength, and preventing age-induced muscle deterioration through activating the mTOR pathway (Paproski et al., 2019; Olaniyan et al., 2020). Consequently, leucine supplementation is used to prevent further reduction and loss of lean mass in middle-aged adults (52±1 years) during periods of bed rest. According to the recommendations of the international study group to review dietary protein needs with aging (PROT-AGE study group), 2.5–2.8 g of leucine per meal is sufficient to reach the anabolic threshold and optimize MPS (Lonnie et al., 2018).

Plant protein sources (such as oat, pea, potato) exhibit digestibility values ranging from 45% to 80% (Olaniyan et al., 2020). Studies involving plant-based proteins prove that they can instigate MPS in levels similar to dairy proteins, but only when ingested in amounts that largely exceed the RDA. This is probably because most plant-based proteins have a lower leucine content of 6% to 8%, compared to animal proteins with 8.5% to 10%, and thus, when consumed in low doses, do not increase MPS to a comparable extent. In general, plants contain a lower content of leucine (<8% of total protein) in comparison to animal-based foods (8–14%). However, some plants are still a relatively good source if consumed in larger volumes: dried seaweed (4.95 g/100 g), dry-roasted soybeans (3.22/100 g), roasted pumpkin seeds (2.39 g/100 g), dry-roasted peanuts (1.53 g/100 g), and cooked lentils (1.29 g/1 cup). Overall, when matched by leucine content or protein quantity, MPS rates do not differ between plant and animal proteins (Olaniyan et al., 2020) (Morgan et al., 2021).

While protein content and AA composition vary between plant species, in general, plant-based foods have an incomplete AA profile, which in turn obstructs the MPS process (Olaniyan et al., 2020; Morgan et al., 2021; Lonnie et al., 2018). For example protein from legumes is limited in methionine and cysteine; cereals in lysine and tryptophan; vegetables, nuts, and seeds in methionine, cysteine, lysine, threonine; and seaweed in histidine, lysine (Lonnie et al., 2018). However, plant-based food sources of protein, such as lentils, legumes, and cereals, if combined together (meaning to eat 2 or more of these incomplete proteins at the same time), they form a complementary protein—a protein that contains all the essential amino acids. Nevertheless, plant proteins, particularly soy and wheat, have a lower potential to initiate MPS because their AAs are more easily turned into urea due to essential AA insufficiency. The increased conversion of AAs to urea means that fewer plant-derived AAs become available in the systemic circulation, resulting in lower postprandial availability of AAs to stimulate MPS (Olaniyan et al., 2020). Last but not least, lower absorption rates of plant-based proteins can be attributed to dietary fiber, phytates, tannins, and saponins, which act as antinutrients by blocking protein absorption (Olaniyan et al., 2020; Morgan et al., 2021; Lonnie et al., 2018).

CARBOHYDRATES

While there is not a definite consensus on the dietary requirement for carbohydrates, the European Food Safety Authority and Nordic Nutrition Recommendations currently recommend that 45% to 60% of total energy intake should come from carbohydrates, given that total energy balance conditions are being fulfilled. Accordingly, the UK Scientific Committee on Nutrition (SACN) sets an average intake of carbohydrates that corresponds to 50% of daily energy intake. Although carbohydrates could offer a great option for older adults to increase their energy needs, when needed, both high and low in carbohydrates diets pose a threat to health. More specifically, results from the ARIC (atheroscleoris risk in communities) study that included 15,428 people and a meta-analysis that pooled ARIC data along with seven multinational prospective studies showed that both low and high carbohydrate consumption are associated with a higher all-cause mortality. However, a significant number of studies (discussed later in this chapter) indicate that the kind/quality is far more important than the quantity of carbohydrates consumed (Großkopf & Simm, 2020).

Free Sugars

Free sugars include all mono- and di-saccharides added to foods by the manufacturer, cook, or consumer plus the sugars naturally present in honey, syrups, and unsweetened fruit juices (Kehoe, Walton, & Flynn, 2019). In human cells, the presence of high glucose content negatively affects aging of endothelial progenitor cells and fibroblasts. Elevated glucose enhances various aging-related phenotypes through activation of the p38 mitogen-activated protein kinase (MAPK). For instance, the consumption of drinks high in sugar, like sugar-sweetened soda, appears to increase cell aging by 1.8 years for each 8 oz serving per day (Tucker, 2018). High glucose intakes also induce the downregulation of sirtuins, which reduces forehead box transcription factors (FOXO) activity and accelerates cellular senescence (Capurso, 2021). Lastly, conditions that cause hyperglycemia (namely insulin resistance, DM and others) exacerbate inflammation by increasing the production of reactive oxygen species (ROS) and advanced glycation end products (AGEs) leading to tissue stiffening and reduced enzyme functionality (Capurso, 2021; Großkopf & Simm, 2020). These mechanisms are thought to be at least partially responsible for many degenerative diseases, such as hypertension, diastolic heart failure, kidney dysfunction, cataract formation, dementia, and cognitive decline in general (Großkopf & Simm, 2020).

According to the WHO, free sugars intake should not exceed 10% of the total daily personal energy intake. This restriction that can reach up to 5% due to existing moderate evidence that high free sugars intake correlates with an increased risk for developing dental carries and weight management problems (Kehoe et al., 2019). The WHO guideline refers to all adult populations, underscoring the lack of data that refer specifically to older adults. Nevertheless, older individuals should make efforts to cut down on added sugars intake, since high added sugars intake is associated with increased levels of adipose tissue, development of frailty, severe pathology and relative symptoms of Alzheimer's disease and cardiovascular disease (CVD)-related mortality (Z. M. Liu, Tse, Chan, Wong, & Wong, 2018; Laclaustra et al., 2018; Valencia, Nagaraj, Osman, Rabinovitch, & Marcinek, 2021; An et al., 2018). Epidemiological evidence indicates that the mean intake of free sugars in this population ranges from 5% of the total energy intake in Spain to 11% in the UK and Netherlands, while only 31% of older people living in the Netherlands adhere to the less than 10% guideline by the WHO (Kehoe et al., 2019).

Dietary Fiber

Human health and aging procedures are significantly affected by dietary fiber intake. Data from epidemiological studies indicate that persons who consume higher amounts of fiber than their counterparts tend to live longer and healthier lives. More specifically, fiber consumption is linked to telomere length, which highly correlates with chronological age and the pathophysiology of disease and premature mortality. As age increases, telomeres become shorter by approximately 15 base pairs per year. In relevant studies, subjects who consumed bigger amounts of fiber tended to have longer telomeres. In fact, a 10 g increase in fiber per 1000 kcal equaled an extra 67 base pair telomere length, which can be translated to 4.3 fewer years of biological aging (67 extra base pairs ÷ 15.5 base pairs short per year) (Tucker, 2018). This 10 g increase in fiber intake also reduced the risk of death by 11%.

Furthermore, other diseases commonly found in older adults, like heart disease, stroke, T2D, osteoporosis, and breast cancer are also less common among those who consume higher quantities of fiber. This can be attributed to shorter telomere length and to the anti-inflammatory effect that higher fiber intake have; as fiber intake increases, inflammation and oxidative stress markers tend to decrease (Tucker, 2018). This anti-inflammatory effect is partially mediated by the improved glucose and glycemic control from significant amounts of fiber (Tucker, 2018). It can also be attributed to the fact that adequate or increased fiber intake helps preferable intestinal microbiota proliferation, which positively affects the evolution of several age-related diseases and syndromes. A poor in microbiota gut environment is linked to the early onset and progression of neurodegenerative diseases, including dementia and Parkinson's disease, via mechanisms that collectively form the so-called "gut-brain axis". More research data also suggest that the gut microbiome is involved in the complex mechanisms that lead to age-related muscle wasting and sarcopenia. The intestinal microbiota from malnourished individuals is deeply disrupted and contributes to wasting through multiple mechanisms, including anabolic resistance, malabsorption, induction of anorexia, and reduced synthesis of vitamins, as depicted in **Figure 10.4** (Strasser, Wolters, Weyh, Krüger, & Ticinesi, 2021).

Inadequate dietary fiber intake also results in impaired bowel function and constipation, commonly found conditions in older adults, that contribute to increased risk for gastrointestinal disease and adversely affect the QOL (Kehoe et al., 2019). Since dietary fiber may contribute to the normalization of bowel functions, and intake is usually low in geriatric patients, the importance of adequate dietary fiber intake is emphasized. According to the European Society for Clinical Nutrition and Metabolism (ESPEN), 25 g of fiber daily are considered adequate for normal laxation in adults and is regarded as a guiding value for older patients also (Volkert et al., 2019); the UK SACN recommends an average intake of 30 g per day. Mean intakes of dietary fiber are below the current recommendations, as seen in **Table 10.2** (Kehoe et al., 2019). Since the link between adequate fiber intake and anti-aging effects through several mechanisms is more established, attempts to promote balanced diets that focus on sources of fiber should continue to be encouraged.

FAT INTAKE

Fat, in the form of free fatty acids and triacylglycerols (triglycerides), is a macronutrient consumed by humans through their everyday diet. Fatty acids are major ingredients of triglycerides, phospholipids, and other complex lipids. Foods contain different amounts of fat and types of fatty acids, and these may be affected by processing, storage, and cooking methods (Calder, 2015). Fat plays a very important role in several bodily functions, including energy storage and release, overall metabolism regulation, lipoprotein and cell membrane formation, hormone production, and mechanical organ protection (Arnett et al., 2019). An overview of the correlation between each main category of fat lipid intake with health outcomes will be followed with a focus on older individuals.

Saturated Fat

Saturated fatty acids (SFAs) are a heterogeneous group of fatty acids that contain only carbon-to-carbon single bonds. Examples

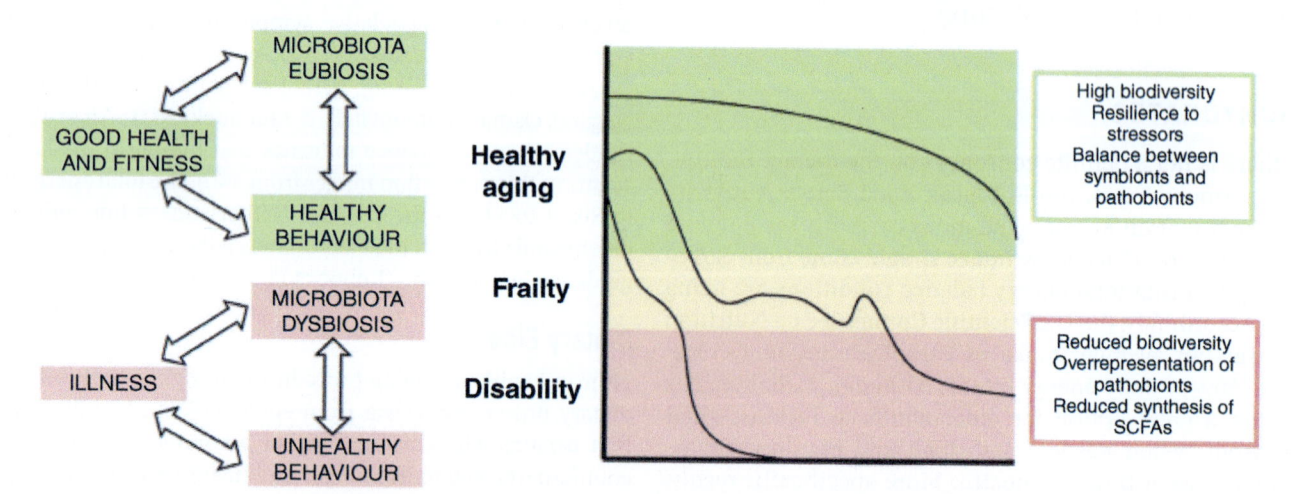

FIGURE 10.4 Hypothetical model of the possible association between microbiota and aging trajectories, based on current knowledge of the association between frailty and microbiota. Healthy aging (top curve) may be associated with the maintenance of microbiota eubiosis (i.e., balance between symbionts and pathobionts) that contributes to the overall fitness of the organism in a virtuous cycle. Aging with frailty, characterized by a general, slow decline of health status and performance following acute illness and exacerbation of chronic diseases with occasional and transitory improvements (middle curve), may be associated with a tendency toward microbiota dysbiosis (i.e., reduced species richness and increased representation of opportunistic pathogens). Disability, following an acute disruptive event or accelerated multi-morbidity (bottom curve), may be associated with severe microbiota dysbiosis, causing a vicious cycle that sustains illness and further decline of health status. Source: (Strasser et al., 2021 / MDPI / CC BY 4.0).

Table 10.2 Summary of mean intakes of macronutrients, free sugars, and dietary fiber in older European adults from National Nutrition Surveys.

Country (Reference)	Study name	Study years	Age (years)	Protein (%E)	Fat (%E)	Saturated fat (%E)	MUFA (%E)	PUFA (%E)	CHO (%E)	Free sugar (%E)	Dietary fibre (g/d)
Andorra	Evaluation of the nutritional status of Andorra population	2004–2005	65–75	18	40	13			41		17
Austria	Austrian Nutrition Report	2010–2012	65–80	15	36	16	12	7	45		20
Belgium	Belgian National Food Consumption Survey	2004	60+	17	39	17	14	7	44		
Denmark	Danish Dietary Survey	2011–2013	65–75	15	36	15	13	6	41		23
Finland	FINDIET 2012	2012	65–74	17	34	14	12	6	45		23
France	Individual and National Food Consumption Surveys	2006–2007	55–79	17	39	11	14	6	44		19
Germany	National Nutrition Survey II	2005–2007	51–80	15	36	15	12	5	47		26
Hungary	Hungarian Dietary Survey 2009	2009	60+	15	38	11			46		22
Iceland	The Diet of Icelanders 2010–2011-A national dietary survey	2010–2011	61–80	19	38	16			39		16
Ireland	National Adult Nutrition Survey	2008–2010	65+		34	14	12	6			
Italy	Italian National Food Consumption Survey	2005–2006	65+	16	34	11	17	4	46		20
Lithuania	Actual nutrition and nutrition habits of adults and elderly of Lithuania	2013–2014	65–75	15	40	12			47		15
Netherlands	Dutch National Food Consumption Survey- Older Adults	2010–2012	70+	16	34	13	11	7	43	11	21
Norway	Norkost3	2010–2011	60–70	18	35	14	12	6	42		25
Portugal	National Food and Physical Activity Survey	2015–2016	65+	20	29	10	12	5	48		20
Spain	Anthropometry, Intake and Energy Balance in Spain	2013	65+	20	29	10	12	5	48		20
Sweden	Riksmaten 2010–2011 Food and Nutrition Among Adults in Sweden	2010–2011	65–80	17	35	11	17	6	40	5	15
UK	National Diet and Nutrition Survey	2014/15–2015/16	65+	17	34	13			46	11	17

Source: (Kehoe et al., 2019).

of foods rich in SFAs are meat, especially red meat and products; butter and butter-fat; dairy foods like milk, yogurt, and cheese; animal fats such as tallow and lard; and plant oils such as cocoa butter, which is common in chocolate, coconut oil, and palm and palm kernel oils (Astrup et al., 2020). Amounts of individual SFAs vary significantly among these sources. For instance, many plant oils exhibit high concentrations of palmitic acid, as do fish and fish oils, while dairy fats are abundant in pentadecanoic acid and hexadecenoic acid. SFAs are also synthesized *de novo* in humans using either carbohydrates or AAs as substrates (Calder, 2015).

SFAs are continuously associated with a higher risk of total and cause-specific mortality (Arnett et al., 2019). Several medium and long-chain fatty acids were statistically correlated with elevated transcription factors that upregulate cholesterol, fatty acids, triglycerides, phospholipids, and lipoprotein synthesis as well as inflammation mediators (Calder, 2015; Fritsche, 2015). Additionally, even-numbered SFAs (lauric, myristic, and palmitic acids) correlate with increased levels of coagulation and insulin resistance (Calder, 2015). Given the high prevalence of CVD and mortality, the American Heart Association (AHA) proposed in its 2013 guidelines to reduce saturated fat consumption for all age groups, including older adults, to better control risk factors such as high levels of low-density lipoprotein (LDL) cholesterol. This recommendation was based upon studies indicating that when food was supplied to adults in a dietary pattern with a macronutrient composition of 5% to 6% saturated fat, 26% to 27% total fat, 15% to 18% protein, and 55% to 59% carbohydrates, LDL cholesterol was lowered by 11–13 mg/d compared with the control diet (14%–15% saturated fat, 34%–38% total fat, 13%–15% protein, and 48%–51% carbohydrate) (Eckel et al., 2014).

However, based on several other prospective studies, SFA consumption is not responsible for higher coronary heart disease (CHD) risk and mortality, since replacing them with carbohydrates did not have any relative protective action. Furthermore, several systematic reviews of cohort studies have shown no significant association between saturated fat intake and coronary artery disease or mortality, and some even suggested a lower risk of stroke with higher consumption of saturated fat (De Souza et al., 2015; Siri-Tarino, 2009; Kang, Yang, & Xiao, 2020; Zhu, Bo, & Liu, 2019).

Whereas several reports show no association between an increased intake of SFAs and risk for chronic disease, individuals with higher circulating levels of even-chain SFA (particularly palmitate) have an increased risk of developing metabolic syndrome, diabetes, CVD, heart failure, and mortality (Astrup et al., 2020). This may be due to the difference between dietary saturated fat and circulating SFAs. Moreover, there are cases in which the presence of SFAs via food consumption amplifies the association of predisposing genetic variants with increased CVD or obesity risk (Astrup et al., 2020). In these cases, the reduction of SFA consumption may be beneficial and therefore worthy of recommendation. Lastly, increased SFA intake is associated with shorter lymphocyte telomere length, which is used as an aging biomarker (Dhillon, Deo, Chua, Thomas, & Fenech, 2021).

Unsaturated Fatty Acids: Omega-3

There is a growing body of literature proving that an adequate consumption of n-3 poly-unsaturated fatty acids (PUFAs) can promote several aspects of healthy aging. More specifically, prospective cohort studies show that higher levels of long-chain, n-3 PUFAs, but not α-linolenic acid, are consistently associated with a lower likelihood of unhealthy aging. For each interquartile range, the risk of unhealthy aging was lowered by 15% (95% confidence interval, 6% to 23%) for eicosapentaenoic acid (EPA), 16% (5% to 24%) for docosapentaenoic acid (DPA) and 18% (7% to 28%) for total long-chain, n-3 PUFA (Lai et al., 2018). Apart from EPA, all other PUFAs are positively associated with telomere length (Dhillon et al., 2021). Other large prospective studies with older adults, indicate that plasma n-3 PUFA levels were associated with a 27% reduction in total mortality risk across quintiles, increasing the life expectancy of individuals in the highest quintile by about 2 years (Tessier & Chevalier, 2018). A 5-week, cross-over, placebo-controlled study proved that daily fish oil PUFA (3 g daily) was associated with significantly lower plasma triglyceride levels and systolic blood pressure (Ruxton, Derbyshire, & Toribio-Mateas, 2016). The lower triglyceride levels occurred through a combination of actions, including the diversion of hepatic fatty acids toward β-oxidation and away from triacylglycerol synthesis, inhibition of hepatic triacylglycerol synthesis, and downregulation of apolipoprotein B100 synthesis required for very low-density lipoprotein (VLDL) assembly.

EPA and docosahexaenoic acid (DHA) help increase the production of eicosanoids with vasoactive effects, the secretion of aldosterone, the generation of nitric oxide by the endothelium, vascular reactivity, and cardiac hemodynamics (Calder, 2015). Through these effects on the lipid profile, vascular function, inflammation and blood pressure, EPA and DHA reduce the likelihood of atherosclerosis and consequently, the risk of CVD in Western populations (Calder, 2015). Furthermore, adequate quantities of n-3 PUFA in the long term can significantly support muscle anabolic processes in older adults via reducing pro-inflammatory cytokines, myosteatosis, mitochondrial ROS emissions and improving insulin sensitivity (Tessier & Chevalier, 2018). Lastly, n3-PUFAs are shown to reverse age-related synaptic plasticity changes, promote neurogenesis, and maintain brain structure and functions against inflamm-aging (Cutuli, 2016).

n-3 PUFAs are essential nutrients since they cannot be synthesized *de novo* in humans. Generally, n-3 fatty acids intake falls within the acceptable macronutrient distribution range, which is 0.5% to 2% of energy intake [25]. Although fatty fish are the main and most common source of n-3 PUFAs, shellfish, seafood, seaweed, flax, soy, rapeseeds, nuts, and certain animal products (for instance, meat and eggs), can also help increase total intake (Calder, 2015). No RDA recommendations exist for n-3 PUFA; only adequate intake (AI) is established for ALA (1.6 g/day for men and 1.1 g/day for women, aged ≥14 years). However, most expert groups suggest 250–500 mg/day EPA and DHA for cardiovascular health, which translates into about 2 servings (140 g, 5 oz) of fatty fish per week.

Although older adults tend to consume more fish that are high in n-3 PUFA compared to younger adults, their intake remains suboptimal, with a mean of 0.19±0.02 oz/day (Tessier & Chevalier, 2018). This finding comes in accordance with other European surveys which report that there is a general deficit of omega-3 fatty acids in older adults, with 60.1% of people being at risk of clinical deficiency for a-linolenic acid while 46.9% risked deficiency for long-chain omega-3 PUFA (Ruxton et al., 2016).

Unsaturated Fatty Acids: Omega-6

n-6 PUFAs are most commonly found in seeds, nuts, and plant-based oils, which mainly consist of linoleic acid. Margarine-type spreads, which are also rich in n-6 PUFA, reflect the fatty acid composition of the parent vegetable oil, although some PUFAs may be lost in the hardening process. Linoleic acid also makes a significant contribution to vegetable oils that are rich in oleic acid (e.g., rapeseed, peanut, and olive oils) or palmitic acid (e.g., palm oil). Over the second half of the twentieth century, there was a move in Western countries to increase the use of vegetable oils for culinary purposes and to replace butter and other animal fats with margarine-type spreads, resulting in a marked increase in intake of linoleic acid in these populations (Calder, 2015).

Human cell membrane phospholipids, especially those found in skin ceramides, contain significant proportions of linoleic acid, which prevents skin integrity breakdown and transdermal water loss (Calder, 2015). Conversely, arachidonic acid is predominantly found in brain tissue as a structural component. In its free form, it acts as cell-signaling molecule that mediates inflammatory processes via the NF-κB pathway. Lastly, as a structural component of cell membranes, it is usually promoted as a substrate for eicosanoid synthesis (prostaglandins, thromboxanes, and leukotrienes), which regulate immune response, pain experience, bone turnover, platelet aggregation, blood clotting, smooth muscle contraction, renal function, and tumor cell proliferation.

A higher arachidonic acid content of cell membranes creates a procoagulant, pro-inflammatory, proallergic, and protumor environment equivalent to low-grade inflammation. However, overall literature findings suggest that arachidonic acid has an inverse, or even lack of association with inflammation markers like C reactive protein and TNF-α or CHD risk (Calder, 2015). In fact, in human studies, higher plasma levels of n-6 PUFAs, mainly arachidonic acid, were associated with decreased plasma levels of serum pro-inflammatory markers, particularly interleukin (IL)-6 and IL-1 receptor antagonist, and increased levels of anti-inflammatory markers, particularly transforming growth factor. When healthy volunteers were given seven times the usual intake of arachidonic acid (i.e., 1.5 g/d) in a 7-week controlled feeding study, no effects on platelet aggregation, bleeding times, the balance of vasoactive metabolites, serum lipid levels, or immune response were observed (Harris et al., 2009).

Higher plasma-PUFA levels correlate with a lower ratio of total to high-density lipoprotein (HDL) cholesterol, and epidemiologically, replacing 10% of calories from SFA with n-6 PUFA is linked to an 18-mg/dL decrease in LDL cholesterol, greater than that observed in a similar replacement with carbohydrate. These findings confirm an LDL-lowering effect of omega-6 PUFA beyond that produced by the removal of SFAs. The favorable effects of linoleic acid on cholesterol levels are well documented and predict significant reductions in CHD risk (Harris et al., 2009; Calder, 2015).

Unsaturated Fatty Acids: Trans Fatty Acids

Trans fatty acids (TFAs) may be created through metabolic processes such as microbial metabolism in the rumen, industrial procedures (for instance during biohydrogenation to harden oils into spreads), or cooking practices like using vegetable oils at high temperatures for frying. The most well-studied TFAs, in the context of human health, are elaidic acid (trans-18:1-n-9), trans vaccenic acid (trans-18:1-n-11), cis-9, trans-11 conjugated linoleic acid (CLA), and trans-10, cis-12 CLA. Ruminant milk and meat are sources of trans vaccenic acid and cis-9, trans-11 CLA, while the main sources of elaidic acid and trans-10, cis-12 CLA are industrially processed oils (Calder, 2015).

TFAs bear some resemblances to SFAs, as far as their physical properties are concerned. As a result, TFA incorporation into cell membranes makes the latter more rigid, negatively affecting membrane-protein functionality and interactivity with lipid raft formations, which lowers the quality of cell signaling. Results from a meta-analysis of RCTs show that trans-18:1 fatty acids can raise LDL cholesterol to similar levels as myristic and palmitic acid while decreasing total HDL-cholesterol levels. The latter observation is quite impressive, since no other lipid molecule has demonstrated this harmful potential (Gayet-Boyer et al., 2014). TFAs also appear to increase the levels of several inflammatory cytokines, but are not associated with elevated blood pressure or coagulation (Calder, 2015).

TFA consumption affects unfavorably the risk of developing CVD and is associated with a higher all-cause mortality (Calder, 2015; Arnett et al., 2019). Due to their negative repercussions on human health, public health providers suggest abstaining from TFA consumption. Since partially hydrogenated oils are optional food additives, their elimination has been a public health priority (Arnett et al., 2019).

Fat Intake in Older Adults

Increased fat consumption amongst older adults remains controversial. While a higher dietary fat content could be perceived as an advantage by preventing malnutrition in older adults, existing data show inconclusive results. A cohort study reported that high-energy intake from total, SFA and mono-unsaturated fatty acids (MUFA) resulted in increased risk of older adults for developing malnutrition 10 years later, especially for those with a body-mass index (BMI) less than 25 kg/m^2 at the beginning of the study (Söderström et al., 2015). In contrast, another prospective cohort study reported that higher MUFA and PUFA intake is associated with a lower risk of developing muscle weakness, while SFA consumption did not have any. Regarding PUFA intake, both n-3 and n-6 showed independent contributions to the association, probably because of their anti-inflammatory properties. n-3 fatty acids also had an inverse dose correlation with lower-extremity functional impairment (Arias-Fernández, Struijk, Rodríguez-Artalejo, López-García, & Lana, 2020). Another cross-sectional study reported that total PUFA and specific lipids such as α-linolenic acid are inversely associated with high blood pressure but positively associated with abdominal obesity in middle-aged and older adults (Julibert, Bibiloni, Mateos, Angullo, & Tur, 2019).

Furthermore, when considering the effect of different lipid intakes among middle-aged and older adults on cardiovascular risk factors and CVD incidence, results focus again on the quality of lipid consumption. An RCT compared the effects of introducing extra-virgin coconut oil (a plant-derived SFA), extra-virgin olive oil (a plant-derived MUFA), or unsalted butter (an animal-derived SFA) in participants' usual diet for 4 weeks. Butter significantly increased LDL cholesterol levels, while this did not happen with olive or coconut oil consumption. No significant changes were observed between the three intervention groups in terms of weight, BMI, central adiposity, fasting blood glucose, and blood pressure (Khaw et al., 2018). Moreover, results from a cross-sectional analysis indicated that amongst institutionalized older adults, total fat and saturated fat from meat and dairy foods were associated with higher serum

HDL-cholesterol levels. Dairy fat intake and the number of dairy servings of dairies were associated with a lower total cholesterol to HDL-cholesterol ratio (TC: HDL-cholesterol ratio). Every additional 10 g of fat and saturated fat from dairy products, and each additional serving, was associated with a lower TC:HDL-cholesterol ratio, when they remained within the recommended levels of fat consumption (Y. Liu et al., 2019).

Finally, in terms of cognitive function, a study conducted in older, community-dwelling, individuals, showed that a total increase in the quantity of fats consumed at breakfast, especially when substituting for the equivalent energy from carbohydrates, was associated with a lower rate of cognitive decline in this population. Additionally, the correlation was stronger in urban residents (Shang, Hill, Li, & He, 2021). The positive effects on cognitive decline are attributed to higher n-3 PUFA (especially α-linolenic acid), which are associated with slower deterioration rates in global cognitive function and memory. Interestingly, the intake of other fatty acids were not associated with cognitive decline according to this study, but overall, the results were drawn from a mainly middle-aged, not older, population (Nooyens, van Gelder, Bueno-de-Mesquita, van Boxtel, & Verschuren, 2018).

These findings do not alter current dietary recommendations to reduce saturated fat intake or total fat intake in general but highlight the need for further elucidation of the more nuanced relationships between different dietary fats and health.

PLANT-BASED DIETS

As research for quantifying dietary associations with health has moved from single nutrients or foods to dietary patterns, as a way to represent the totality of people's diet, plant-based diets have been shown promising results in improving all-cause mortality and furthering life expectancy.

As defined by the WHO, plant-based diets are food patterns that put emphasis on the consumption of foods that are mainly plant-derived, while lowering or even excluding the consumption of animal products (WHO/Europe, 2021). Most plant-based food patterns consist of minimally processed fruits, vegetables, whole grains, legumes, nuts, seeds, herbs, and spices (Ostfeld, 2017). Vegetarian diets are a subgroup of plant-based diets, which may exclude the consumption of some or even all forms of animal foods and products. **Table 10.3** summarizes the most common vegetarian diets. Briefly, vegan diet is the strictest form of plant-based diets, since it completely omits all animal products, including meat, dairy, fish, eggs, and (usually) honey. Daily caloric and nutrient intake is based on vegetable, fruit, nut, seed, legume, and plant-derived oil consumption. Less strict forms of vegetarian diets can include to some extent the consumption of eggs, dairy products, poultry, and fish, or a combination there of. The raw vegan diet combines veganism and raw foodism and it consists of foods that are eaten uncooked or that have not been heated above 48°C. (Dominguez et al., 2022).

Plant-based diets provide protection against premature mortality and most NCDs like cardiovascular illness or cancer. This can be explained by both the lower presence of SFAs and free sugars as well as the higher consumption of fruits and vegetables, which reaches the WHO goal for at least 400 g (5 portions) of fruits and vegetables more easily. According to the Global Burden of Disease study that evaluated the consumption of major foods and nutrients across 195 countries and assessed their impact of their suboptimal intake on NCD mortality and morbidity during 1990–2017, the leading dietary risk factors for mortality was shown to be diets low in whole grains, low in fruit, low in nuts and seeds, low in vegetables, low in n-3 fatty acids, and high in sodium and red-meat consumption (Afshin et al., 2019). Evidence suggests that vegetarian and vegan diets can significantly protect individuals from CHD as well as all forms of cancer, compared to non-vegetarians. Additionally, the Global Burden of Disease Study showed that overconsuming red or overly processed meat, with a parallel inadequate intake of fruits, vegetables, and whole grains were the main recognized global risk factors. Adopting a plant-based dietary pattern lowers the risk of obesity, T2D, and CHD. More specifically, the risk of CHD may be reduced by up to 40%, while the risk of cerebral vascular disease events by 29%. Moreover, diets rich in foods such as fruits, vegetables, legumes, grains, nuts, and seeds cut the risk of Alzheimer's disease by more than 50% (Kahleova, Levin, & Barnard, 2020). Most plant-based dietary patterns are proven to protect against common age-related diseases and conditions, such as frailty, risk of falls, sensory degradation and chronic constipation (Towery et al., 2018; Roberts et al., 2021). Finally, in terms of lengthening life expectancy, there is enough evidence to support that plant-based diets, due to their high antioxidant and anti-inflammatory effects, are positively associated with reduced attrition rates of telomeres, which is a major indicator of aging procedures (Crous-Bou, Molinuevo, & Sala-Vila, 2019).

Studies that use older adults as a target population to assess the effects of plant-based/vegetarian diets are scarce. Most of the studies that discuss this topic target older Asian individuals averaging between 50- and 60-years old. Yet, despite some contradictions, older adults can receive beneficial effects from adhering to vegetarian or plant-based dietary patterns in general. Data from the Adventist health study 2, which examined middle-aged adults, support that vegetarian diets are associated with lower all-cause mortality, with a special referencing to pescatarians, who exhibited reduced incident mortality, compared to other types

Table 10.3 Common vegetarian diets.

Common vegetarian diets

- **Vegan** diets omit all animal products, including meat, dairy, fish, eggs and (usually) honey.
- **Lacto-vegetarian** diets exclude meat, fish, poultry and eggs, but include dairy products such as milk, cheese, yoghurt and butter.
- **Lacto-ovo** vegetarian diets include eggs and dairy, but not meat or fish.
- **Ovo-vegetarian** diets exclude meat, poultry, seafood and dairy products, but allow eggs.
- **Pesco-vegetarian** (or **pescatarian**) diets include fish, dairy and eggs, but not meat.
- **Semi-vegetarian** (or **flexitarian**) diets are primarily vegetarian but include meat, dairy, eggs, poultry and fish on occasion, or in small quantities.

Source: (WHO/Europe, 2021).

that indicated no benefit (Morris et al., 2015a; Dominguez et al., 2022). Meta-analyses of prospective cohort studies indicate that the risk of CHD and stroke decrease by 4% for each additional portion of fruits and vegetables per day (Dauchet, Amouyel, Hercberg, & Dallongeville, 2006; Bazzano & Fotino, 2011). However, the same cannot be said about the risk of metabolic syndrome in older adults, since a cross-sectional study conducted in Iran, reported that plant-based diets are not significantly associated with it (Amini* et al., 2021). Furthermore, based on results from studies conducted in Seven-Day Adventist older women, adhering to a vegetarian diet was associated with improved nutrient intake and reduced blood glucose and lipid levels compared to non-vegetarian peers (Nieman et al., 1989). Greater adherence to dietary patterns consistent with vegetarianism is associated with better cognitive performance, especially in executive functioning, such as generation and processing speed, and memory capabilities (Ramey, Shields, & Yonelinas, 2022). Also, for older women, a negative association between vegetarian diets and hip-bone mineral density is observed, especially compared to omnivore individuals (Lau, Kwok, Woo, & Ho, 1998). Finally, vegetarian older adults have a 20% lower risk of developing cataracts, according to a prospective study conducted in Taiwan (Chiu, Chang, Lin, & Lin, 2021).

PLANT POLYPHENOLS

Natural biophenols are a wide group of molecules (over 8000 described so far) found only in the plant kingdom; their molecules have at least one aromatic ring, which can carry one or more hydroxyl groups. Biophenols have remarkable antioxidant power and are produced as secondary metabolites by plants for protection against bacteria, fungi, and insects. Plant polyphenols are categorized as either non–flavonoids or flavonoids; the latter are further divided into flavanols, flavanonols, flavones, anthocyanins, procyanidins, phenolic acids, stilbenes, and tannins, depending on the number of hydroxyls in the molecule as well as the nature and the position of other substituents. The main phytochemicals, phenolic compounds, and flavonoids found in fruit and vegetables are presented in **Tables 10.4, 10.5** and **10.6**, respectively (Dominguez, Di Bella, Veronese, & Barbagallo, 2021).

Plant polyphenols (and phytonutrients in general), interfere with a wide range of signaling pathways that govern protein homeostasis, DNA repair (**Figure 10.5**), metabolism adaptations, and antioxidant defenses. More specifically, polyphenols are a remarkable food ingredient for their unprecedented food antioxidant properties and their ability to reduce aggregation rates of peptides/proteins into amyloid assemblies. Both mechanisms

Table 10.4 Main phytochemicals with bioactive properties contained in fruit and vegetables.

Phytosterols	Organosulfur Compounds	Carotenoids	Alkaloids	Phenolics
• Sitosterol	• Alliin	• α-carotene	• Caffeine	• Flavonoids
• Campesterol	• γ-glutamyl-5-allyl-L-cysteine	• β-carotene	• Trigonelline	• Phenolic acids
• Stimasterol	• Glucosinolates and derivatives	• β-cryptoxant		• Lignans
• Sitostanol		• Lutein		• Stilbenes
• Campestanol		• Zeaxanthin		• Coumarins
		• Lycopene		• Tannins

Source: (Dominguez et al., 2021).

Table 10.5 Main phenolic compounds in fruit and vegetables.

Flavonols	Phenolic Acids	Lignans	Stilbenes	Tannins
• Flavonols	• Hydroxycinnamic acid derivatives	• Cinnamicacid	• Resveratrol	• Proanthocyanidins
• Flavan-3-ols	○ Caffeic acid			
• Isoflavones	○ Ferulic acid			
• Anthocyanidins	○ Curcumin			
• Flavanones				
• Flavones				

Source: (Dominguez et al., 2021).

Table 10.6 Main flavonoids in fruit and vegetables.

Flavonols	Flavan-3-ols	Isoflavones	Anthocyanidins	Flavanones	Flavones
• Quercetin	• Catechin	• Genistein	• Cyanidin	• Hesperetin	• Apigeni
• Kaempferol	• Epicatechin	• Daidzein	• Delphinidin	• Naringeni	• Luteoli
• Myricetin	• Epigallocatechin	• Biochanin A	• Malvidin	• Eriodictyol	• Baicalein
	• Epigallocatechin gallate		• Pelargonidin		
	• Epicatechin gallate				

Source: (Dominguez et al., 2021).

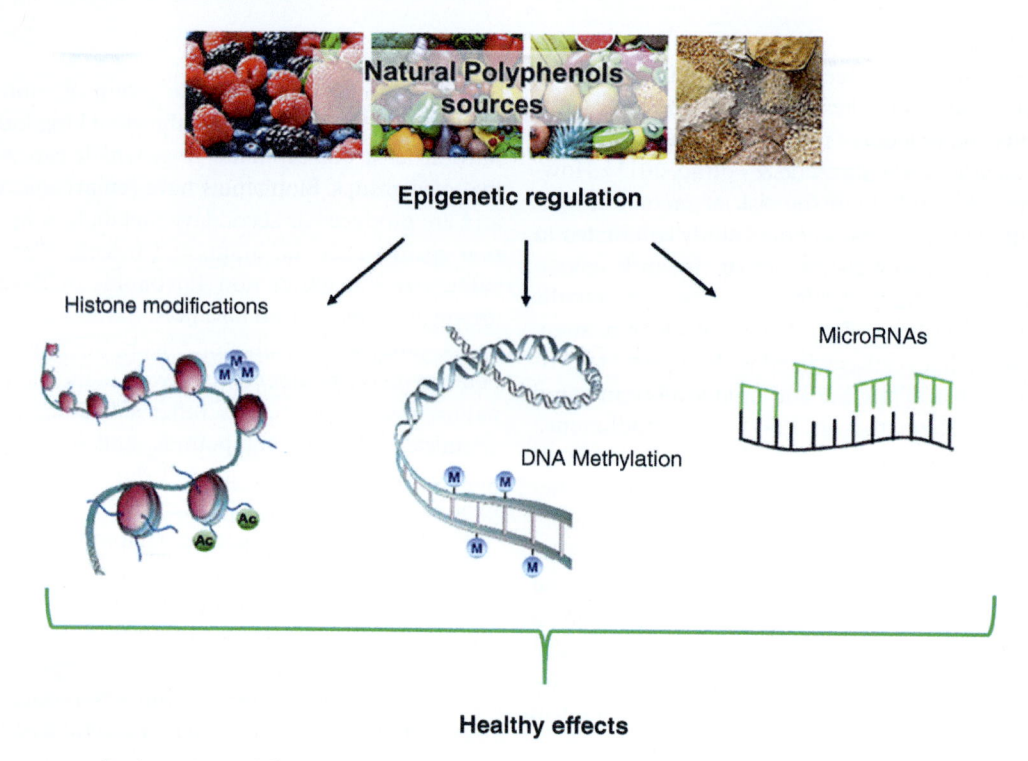

FIGURE 10.5 A summary of epigenetic modifications mediated by plant polyphenols. Source: (Leri et al., 2020 / MDPI / CC BY 4.0).

are key processes in the development of several chronic diseases, including T2D, metabolic syndrome, and Alzheimer's and Parkinson's diseases.

Plant polyphenols can also beneficially regulate glucose metabolism by lowering intestine carbohydrate digestion, glucose absorption, the stimulation of pancreatic β-cells for insulin secretion, modulation of liver glucose release, and insulin-sensitive tissue activation. These metabolic effects are mainly attributed to compounds like quercetin, myricetin, luteolin, theaflavin, and resveratrol. The protective effect most plant-based food patterns like the Mediterranean or Asian (analytically discussed later in this chapter) diets have, are mainly supported by their high phytonutrient concentrations, and therefore, their disease preventive, or even therapeutic abilities, as far as metabolic pathologies and age-related deterioration are concerned. Increasing evidence indicates that polyphenolic elements in plants such as curcumin, sulforaphane, and resveratrol act in a hermetic manner by activating adaptive stress responses.

The beneficial effects of plant derivatives, including, especially for olives (*Olea europaea-* the most extensively studied for its antioxidative properties plant), oil and leaf extracts, were known for the last couple of centuries and been scientifically investigated over several recent decades; this research has progressively led to a focus on the multitarget activity and health properties of plant polyphenols, including the anti-amyloid aggregation, antioxidant, antimicrobial, antihypertensive, hypoglycemic, and vasodilator effects. Other polyphenols found in fruits, vegetables, and red wine are associated with improved aging. Their antioxidant power modulates oxidative pathways, has direct action on enzymes, proteins, receptors, and several types of signaling paths and interferes with epigenetic modifications of chromatin (**Figures 10.6** and **10.7**) (Leri et al., 2020).

Most plant-based diets are reported to have mostly beneficial effects on the presence or effective prevention of geriatric syndromes like sarcopenia and frailty (Roberts et al., 2021). Interestingly, low meat and poultry intake does not render the daily protein intake reaching a recommended quantity completely impossible. Moreover, the rich anti-inflammatory load provided by most plant-based diets acts as a skeletal muscle preservative against inflamm-aging (Mazza et al., 2021). But, as mentioned previously, several studies do not acknowledge proteins from plant sources as equivalent to those that are animal derived.

Studies examining the specific effects of protein from different sources reported beneficial effects of higher animal protein intake on muscle mass and strength, functional performance, hip fractures (only in men), and frailty, but detrimental to catastrophic effects on T2D and cardiovascular mortality (Bradlee, Mustafa, Singer, & Moore, 2018; Fung, Meyer, Willett, & Feskanich, 2017; Sluijs et al., 2010; Song et al., 2016; McCrea, Bromley, Mcnally, O'Byrne, & Wade, 2004; McLean, Mangano, Hannan, Kiel, & Sahni, 2016; Sandoval-Insausti et al., 2016; Ortolá et al., 2020). Vegetable protein, however, is associated with a lower risk of muscle loss, frailty, hip fracture, T2D, and cardiovascular and all-cause mortality (Sluijs et al., 2010; Fung et al., 2017; Chan, Leung, & Woo, 2014; Kobayashi, Suga, & Sasaki, 2017; Lonnie et al., 2018). Replacing total animal protein, dairy protein, or meat protein with vegetable protein leads to significantly less deficit accumulation over 8.2 years (even when adjusted for fat intake changes), whereas the replacement of egg protein or fish protein did not show a statistically significant association with deficit accumulation,

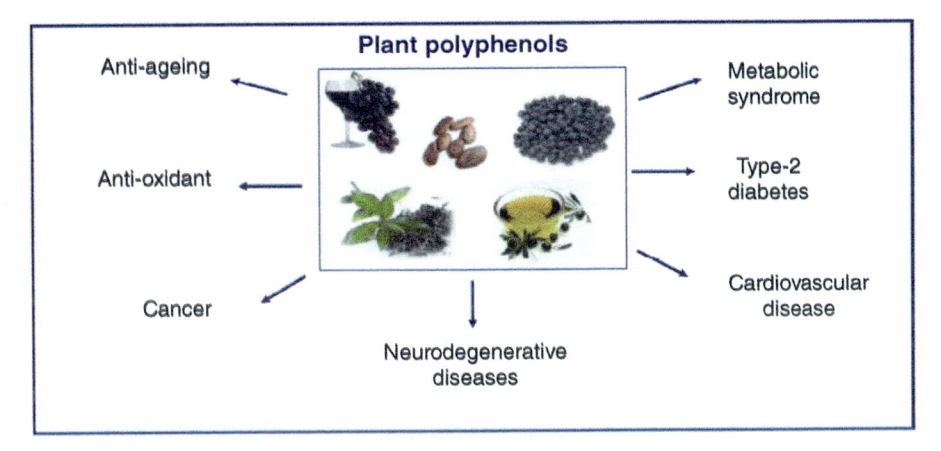

FIGURE 10.6 Plant polyphenols can help prevent/combat a number of lifestyle, metabolic, and aging associated pathologies. Source: (Leri et al., 2020 / MDPI / CC BY 4.0).

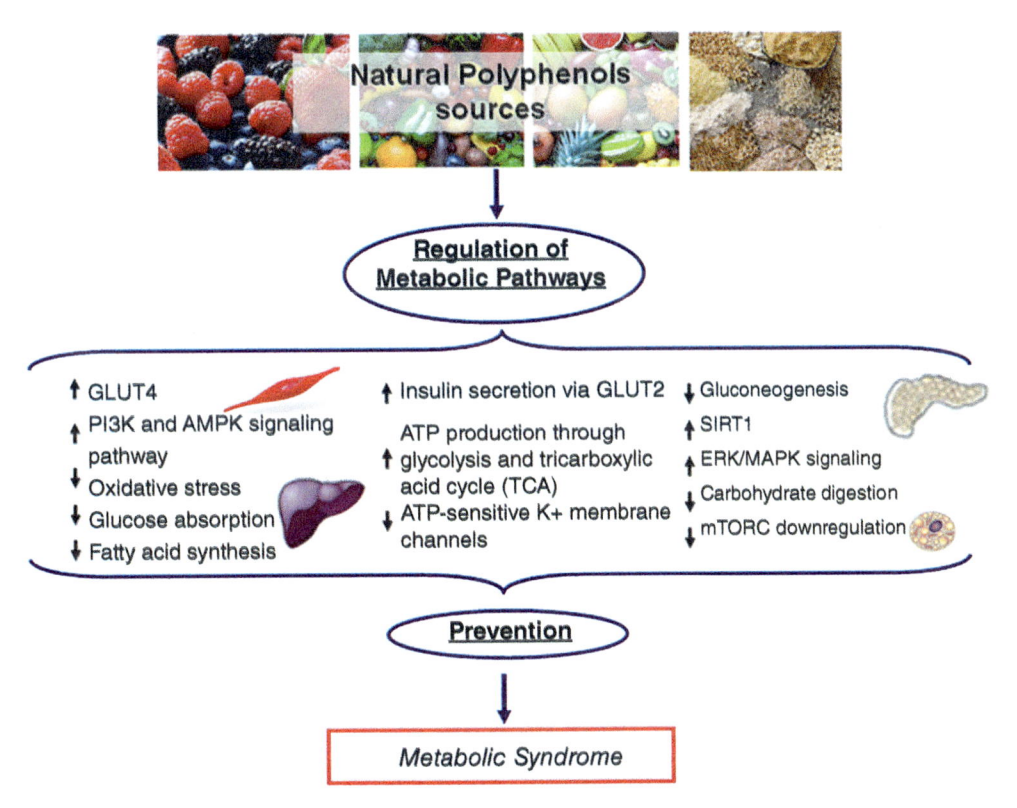

FIGURE 10.7 Schematic representation of the main metabolic pathways influenced by plant polyphenols. Activated pathways are represented with an upward arrow, while inactivated pathways with a downward one. Source: (Leri et al., 2020 / MDPI / CC BY 4.0).

according to a recent clinical research study (Ortolá et al., 2020). This evidence and the association of substituting vegetable protein for animal protein with a lower risk of mortality, underscores the importance of protein source (Ortolá et al., 2020; Morgan et al., 2021). Further investigations are needed to understand the impact and potential roles of separate nutrients/foods, animal- or plant-based, in chronic disease prevention and management by age and other lifestyle factors (Keaver et al., 2021).

THE MEDITERRANEAN DIET

The Mediterranean diet (MD) is a dietary pattern that mainly focuses on plant-derived foods that are locally and seasonally produced, while allowing the intake of animal products in small/controlled quantities (more about the MD in **Chapter 3**). An up-to-date approach of the MD is depicted in **Figure 10.8**.

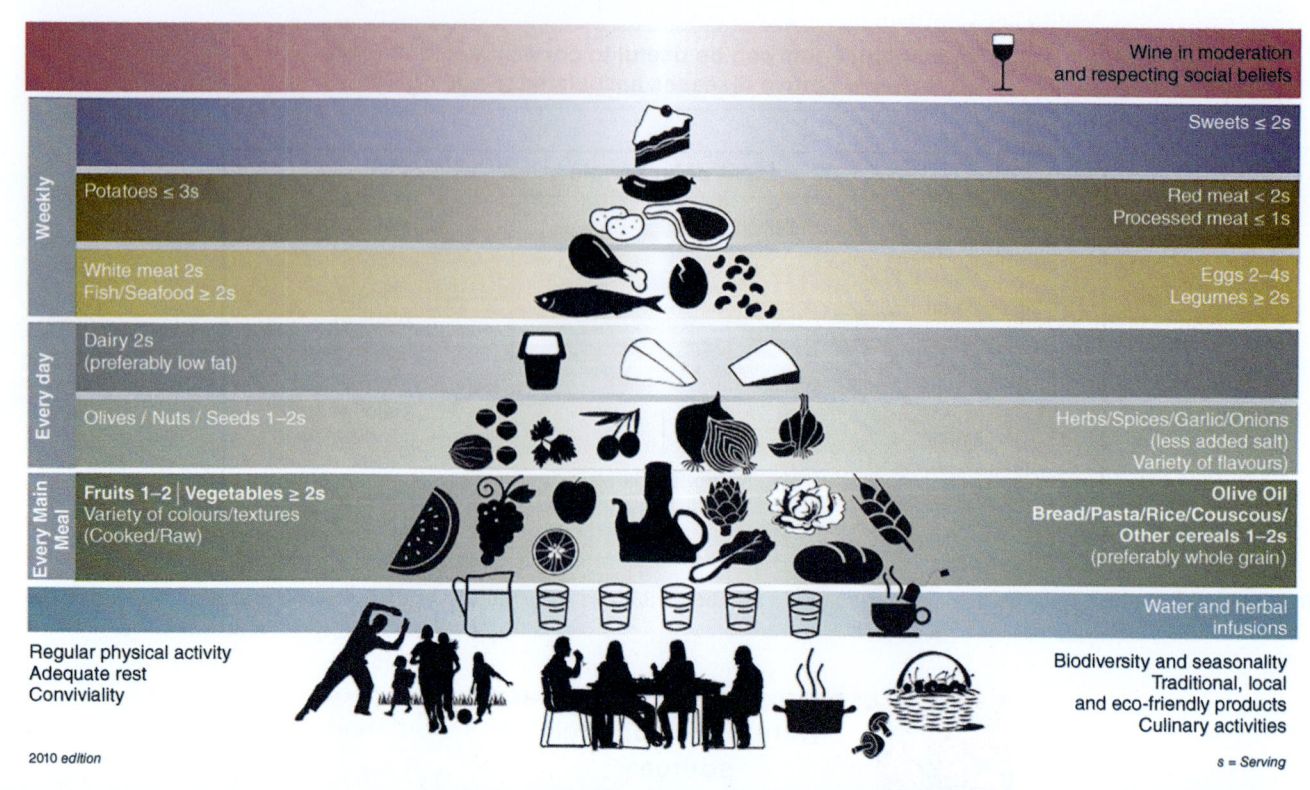

FIGURE 10.8 The Mediterranean diet pyramid: a lifestyle for today. The traditional MD pyramid has evolved to the new way of life. The new pyramid follows the previous pattern: at the base, foods that should sustain the diet, and at the upper levels, foods to be eaten in moderate amounts. Social and cultural elements characteristic of the Mediterranean way of life are also incorporated. It is not just about prioritizing some food groups over others, but also paying attention to how they are selected, cooked, and eaten. It also depicts the composition and recommended number of servings for meals. Source: (Bach-faig et al., 2011 / with permission of Cambridge University Press).

The protective properties of the MD are mainly attributed to a high intake of MUFAs and polyphenols found in olive oil and extra-virgin olive oil (EVOO), PUFAs deriving from fish, and the wide variety of antioxidants contained in fruits, legumes, vegetables, and wine (Mazza et al., 2021). Regarding olive oil consumption, analyses of Greek adults older than 50-years of age proved that exclusive olive oil intake, compared to no olive oil use, is significantly associated with healthy aging, especially among adults older than 70 years (Foscolou et al., 2019).

Throughout the scientific literature, there are several studies advocating the mechanisms and beneficial effects of adhering to the MD on health and healthy aging (**Figure 10.9**). The PREDIMED intervention proved that following an MD pattern, supplemented with EVOO or nuts, with a fairly high fat intake (35–40% of the total energy intake), decreased incidence of major CVD events by almost 30% in participants with a high CVD risk over 4.8 years of follow-up, compared to a low-fat diet, a fat intake of ≤30% of total energy intake, control. Adherence to the MD during midlife was correlated with a 36% to 46% greater likelihood of healthy aging (Critselis & Panagiotakos, 2020). This, like other MD beneficial impacts, is attributed to its proper mixture of salutary sources of fats, starches, proteins, fiber, vitamins, minerals, and countless bioactive compounds like phytosterols, terpenes, and polyphenols. The chronic consumption of these nutrients acts synergistically by biological and molecular mechanisms, to overall lessen the risk of NCDs (Dominguez et al., 2021; Keaver et al., 2021).

For older adults, there are a few studies that prove the beneficial effects of adopting the MD dietary pattern in this specific life stage. A longitudinal study conducted in a European older population found that adherence to the MD correlates with a reduced risk for all-cause mortality, while a lack of adherence leads to a population attributable risk of 60% in all-cause deaths (Knoops et al., 2004). The Uppsala longitudinal cohort study of adult men also proved that adherence to a dietary pattern similar to the MD is associated with independent aging (a mini-mental state examination score of at least 25, lack of dementia, independence in personal ADLs, no institutionalization, and ability to walk outside alone) and survival (Franzon et al., 2017). Moreover, adherence to the MD has protective effects against frailty and cognitive deterioration for older adults (Ghosh et al., 2020). Finally, a study conducted in older individuals from 26 Mediterranean islands found that adherence to the MD remains stable with increasing age (Foscolou et al., 2018).

A mechanism considered crucial for the health benefits provided by the MD is favorable modification of the gut microbiota due to high fiber consumption by those adherent to this pattern; new evidence suggests that gut microbiota composition can predispose an individual toward or away from the development of CVD, obesity, and inflammatory diseases. Regarding CVD, a high adherence to the MD was associated

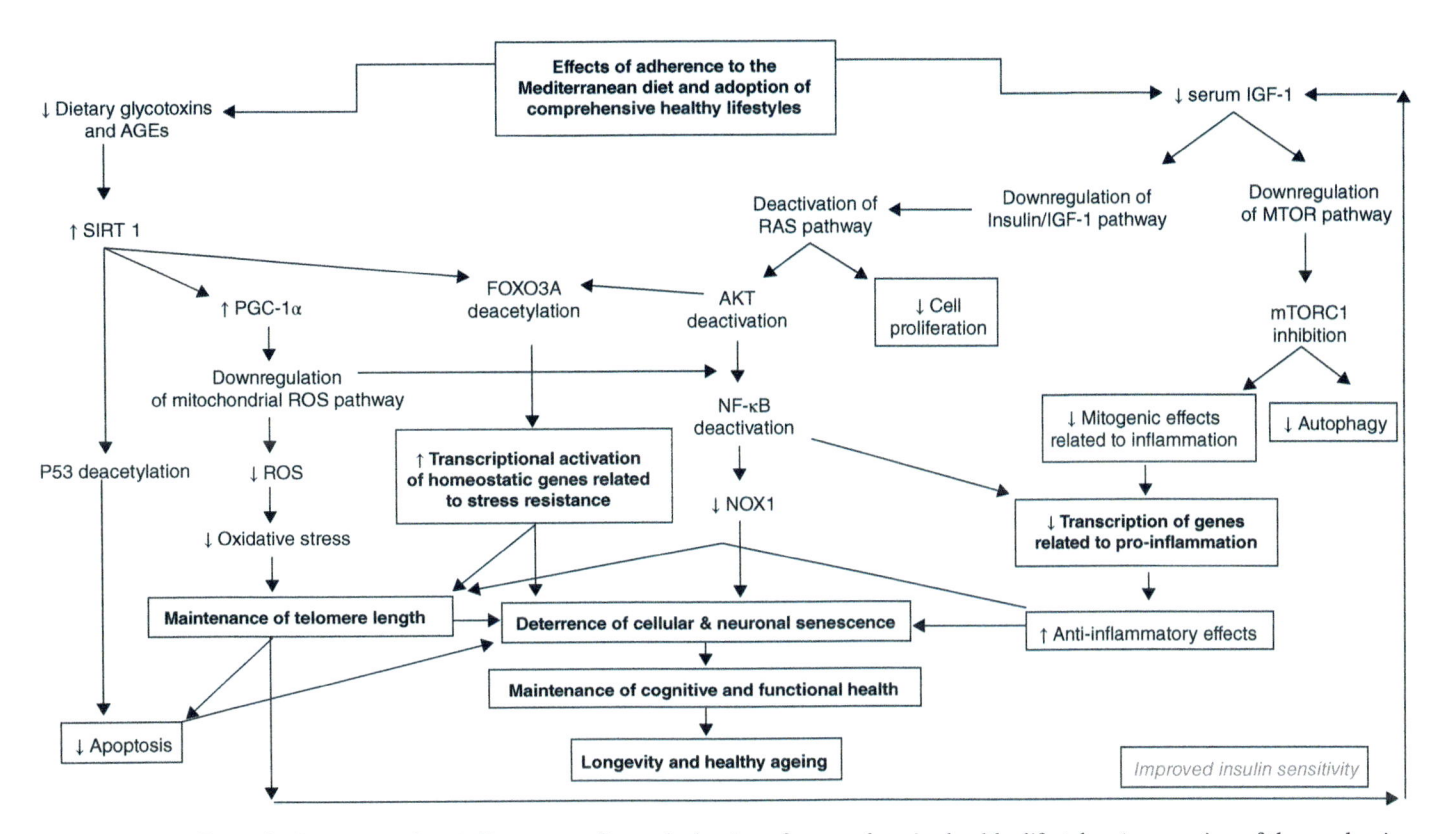

FIGURE 10.9 Effects of adherence to the Mediterranean diet and adoption of comprehensive healthy lifestyles. An overview of the mechanisms and nutrient-sensing pathways that modulate healthy aging are depicted. In brief, adherence to the MD most often entails fewer dietary glycotoxins and lower production of advanced glycation end-products (AGEs), which activate Sirtuin 1 (SIRT 1); subsequent downregulation of the mitochondrial reactive oxygen species (ROS) pathway deters telomere attrition and lowers cellular apoptosis and death. Adherence to the MD also induces lower serum IGF-1 levels, which downregulate several nutrient-sensing pathways, including the mTOR and insulin/IGF-1 pathways. In particular, mTOR pathway downregulation enhances anti-inflammatory intracellular environment and diminished cellular autophagy. Downregulating the insulin/IGF-1 pathway deactivates the AKT and NF-kB pathways, enhancing anti-inflammatory effects and deterring cellular and/or neuronal senescence. The constellation of these pathways favors the deterrence of cellular and neuronal aging, which facilitates cognitive and functional health and ultimately preserves healthy aging. Source: (Critselis & Panagiotakos, 2020 / with permission of Taylor & Francis).

with enriched Firmicutes and Bacteroidetes as well as increased fecal SCFAs. Conversely, poor adherence to the MD was associated with increased l-Ruminococcus and Streptococcus bacteria and higher urinary trimethylamine N-oxide concentrations, a marker of increased risk of CVD (De Filippis et al., 2016). Furthermore, Pisanu et al. showed that in a sample of 23 obese patients, a moderately hypocaloric MD reduced body weight, which was accompanied with an increase in several Bacteroidetes taxa and a depletion of many Firmicutes taxa after three months of intervention (Pisanu et al., 2020). Moreover, a study of 23 overweight omnivores comparing the MD with a vegetarian diet reported a significant increase in propionic-acid production, which is negatively correlated with changes to a several inflammatory cytokines in participants that followed a MD pattern (Pagliai et al., 2020). Lastly, the NU-AGE diet study, which targeted older adults from 65- to 79-years old found that adherence to the MD for 1 year can significantly reduce levels of CRP and IL-17 (Ghosh et al., 2020).

Evidence also suggests that populations strictly following the MD pattern, and therefore consuming significant amounts of polyphenols daily, show a lower all-cause mortality risk. Adherence to the MD improved endothelial function, platelet aggregation, and lipid metabolism (reducing LDL cholesterol), which provided a cardio-protective effect (Mazza et al., 2021) (Dominguez et al., 2021). Regarding cancer pathogenesis, studies have shown that women following the MD show a reduced activity of cellular mitogens like IGF-1, testosterone, and estradiol by producing more of the respective binding proteins (Dominguez et al., 2021). At a molecular level, adherence to the MD is significantly correlated with longer telomeres in many populations of different backgrounds (Crous-Bou et al., 2019; Critselis & Panagiotakos, 2020). More specifically, the polyphenolic compounds that are more than abundant in the MD actively interfere with epigenetic mechanism that govern histone methylation and acetylation as well as the rate of telomere attrition (Crous-Bou et al., 2019; Dominguez et al., 2021). For instance, polyphenols found in grapes, berries, peanuts, and EVOO correlate with the DNA methylation of genes linked to crucial tumor suppressors and promoters, while molecules like the anthocyanins found in eggplants, black grapes, and cruciferous vegetables are linked to many DNA-repair mechanisms (Dominguez et al., 2021). Moreover, antioxidant micronutrients such as vitamins C and E as well as carotenoid molecules protect the aging muscle system from chronic inflammation due to their well-known anti-inflammatory and antioxidant properties (Mazza et al., 2021; Capurso, Bellanti, Buglio, & Vendemiale, 2020). Finally, because of the reduction in vascular and cardio-metabolic risk, suppression of oxidative stress, and anti-diabetic effects, the MD is included among those dietary patterns with neuro- and cognitive protective effects (Dominguez et al., 2021; Crous-Bou et al., 2019; Chen, Maguire, Brodaty, & O'Leary, 2019).

THE NORDIC DIET

The Nordic diet (ND) (**Figure 10.10**) shares many similarities with the MD but includes foods that are traditionally used in northern European countries such as Denmark, Finland, Iceland, Norway, and Sweden (Kanerva, Kaartinen, Schwab, Lahti-Koski, & Männistö, 2014; Mithril et al., 2012).

Although the ND was developed more recently, the literature on this healthy dietary pattern has grown. In older adults, significant inverse associations exist between the ND and CVD risk factors (Galbete et al., 2018; Gunge et al., 2017; Simpson et al., 2012; Risérus, 2015), such as glucose parameters (Tertsunen, Hantunen, Tuomainen, & Virtanen, 2021), cancer risk (Kyrø et al., 2013), and mental disorders (Wu et al., 2021) (Shakersain et al., 2018) as well as all-cause mortality (Olsen et al., 2011), thus increasing overall life and health expectancies (Ratjen et al., 2017; Dominguez et al., 2022).

A cohort study showed that the lowest adherence to ND is associated with a higher risk of T2D incidence as well as higher blood glucose and insulin concentrations, after adjusting for several confounders (Tertsunen et al., 2021).The ND also has promising beneficial effects on cognitive health in older adults. According to Wu et al., participants older than 60 years who were adherent to ND had an approximate 20% higher probability to be free of dementia and disability compared to those with low ND adherence. Moreover, after adjusting for lifestyle factors and other potential confounders, those who followed a ND pattern lived an average of 1.24 years longer without the presence of dementia, compared to those with a low adherence to the ND (Wu et al., 2021). As far as disability is concerned, a longitudinal study with a 10-year follow-up showed a higher probability of mobility limitations and difficulties with self-care activities in older adults who did not follow the ND pattern, compared to those who do (Perälä et al., 2019). Another study found that a higher adherence to the ND is associated with better physical performance over a 10-year period, but only in women (Perälä et al., 2016). These improved physical performance levels reflect better aerobic

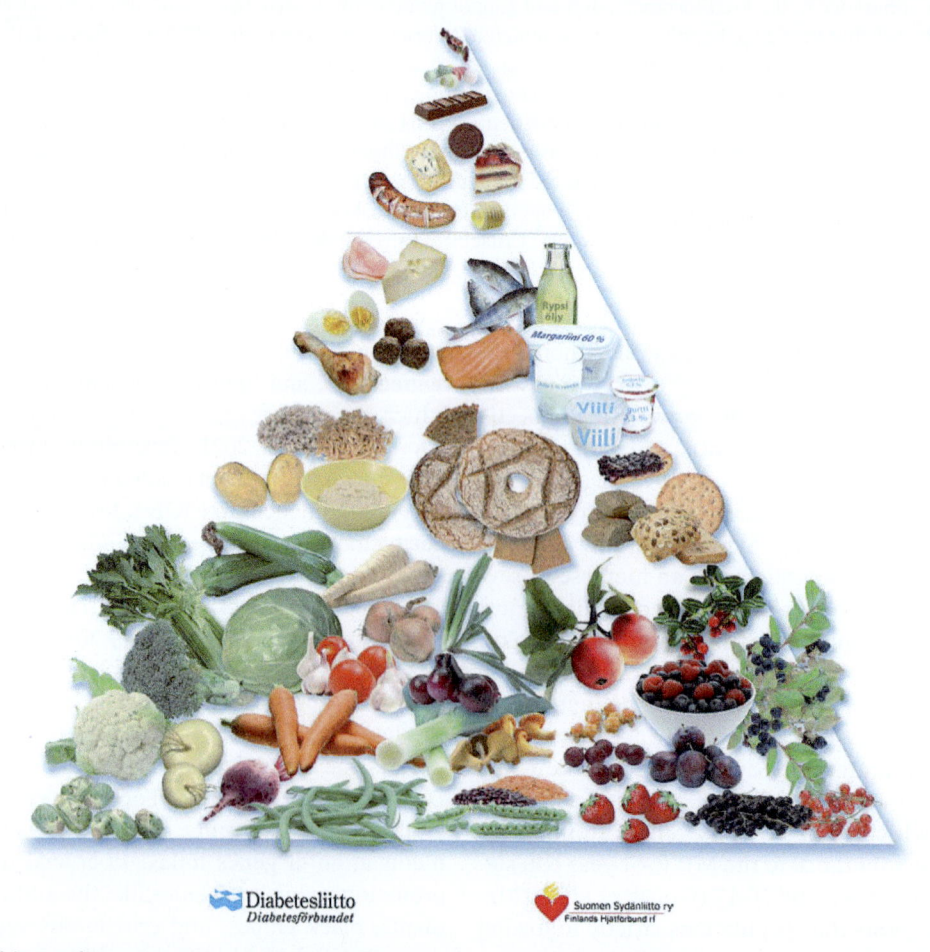

FIGURE 10.10 The Baltic Sea diet pyramid (created by the Finnish Heart Association, the Finnish Diabetes Association, and the University of Eastern Finland). Source: (Kanerva et al., 2014 / with permission of Cambridge University Press).

endurance as well as upper- and lower-body strength, as expressed through physical functionality tests such as chair-stand and 6-min walk tests (Perälä et al., 2016). Another study from the same researcher showed that adherence to the ND predicted greater hand-grip and muscle strength over a 10-year period.

Overall, the ND is suggested as a very promising dietary pattern to help decrease the burden of physical limitations among older adults. This property is mainly attributed to the anti-inflammatory effects of the ND through the frequent consumption of foods and nutrients (for instance polyphenols or carotenoids) with high antioxidant capacities that act against inflammation and inflammation-induced diseases like frailty, dementia, and CVD (Wu et al., 2021). Nevertheless, further research is needed to confirm its effects in larger, well-designed studies from other Nordic populations as well as populations of countries outside the Scandinavian nations (Renzella et al., 2018) (Dominguez et al., 2022).

DIETARY APPROACHES TO STOP HYPERTENSION (DASH) DIET

To successfully manage hypertension with methods other than drug therapy, the Dietary Approaches to Stop Hypertension (DASH) dietary pattern was proposed in 1977. As mentioned in **Chapter 3** and it will be discussed on **chapter 16**, this pattern mostly includes fruits, vegetables, low-fat dairy products, nuts, legumes, whole grains, and fish. The aforementioned food choices boost the daily consumption of fiber and micronutrients such as K, Ca, Mg, and antioxidants (**Figure 10.11**) while significantly reducing saturated fat, cholesterol, and Na consumption (Akhlaghi, 2020).

The DASH dietary pattern provides substantial health benefits in older adults on factors associated with CVD risk (Talaei, Koh, Yuan, & van Dam, 2019; Suri et al., 2019) and obesity (Suri et al., 2019), including lowering blood pressure, improving metabolic syndrome and T2D profiles (i.e., improvements in body weight, waist circumference, serum TG, VLDL-cholesterol, total- to HDL-cholesterol ratio, insulin levels, insulin resistance, insulin sensitivity index, and systolic and diastolic pressure) as well as reducing the 10-year CHD risk. Also, the DASH diet improves cognitive and functional abilities in older adults due to lowered inflammatory loads and adequate calcium intake (Chen et al., 2019; Jayanama et al., 2021; Akhlaghi, 2020; Suri et al., 2019) like frailty (Jayanama et al., 2021) and bone health (Suri et al., 2019).

Indeed, an inverse association between the DASH diet index and visceral adiposity index (a reliable estimate of visceral adiposity) was reported by Ferguson et. al., supporting the implementation of nutritional counseling for older adults regarding the DASH diet to reduce the cardio-metabolic risk of this population (Ferguson, Knol, & Ellis, 2021). Another cross-sectional study reported an inverse association between adopting the DASH dietary pattern and lower fibrinogen levels, which lowers the possibility of increased diastolic blood pressure and insulin levels (Jalilpiran, Darooghegi Mofrad, Mozaffari, Bellissimo, & Azadbakht, 2020).

The DASH dietary pattern was also inversely associated with non-alcoholic fatty liver disease in older adults living in China, especially in women and those without abdominal obesity (Xiao et al., 2020). Additionally, in older women, diet modifications toward the DASH dietary pattern favor the development of an anti-inflammatory systemic environment through elevated adiponectin levels accompanied by a favorable changes in metabolic profiles (reduced blood glucose levels and waist circumference), even with variations in abdominal obesity (Nilsson, Halvardsson, & Kadi, 2019).

Another cross-sectional study in post-menopausal Iranian women reported beneficial effects of adhering to the DASH diet on bone health, supporting that women in the highest tertile of DASH score had a lower risk of osteoporosis at the lumbar spine, but unfortunately not at the femoral neck (Shahriarpour, Nasrabadi, Shariati-Bafghi, Karamati, & Rashidkhani, 2020). Scarce evidence exists regarding the effect

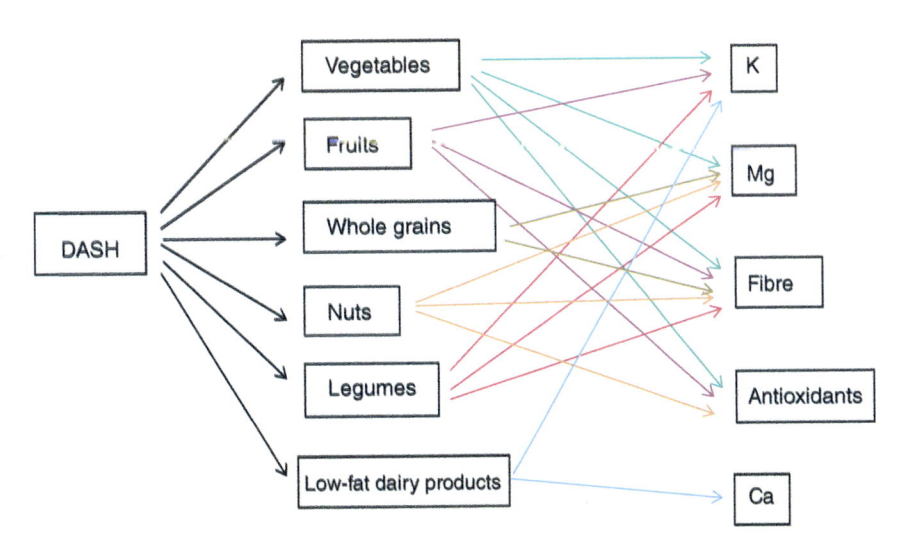

FIGURE 10.11 Major nutrients provided by components of the Dietary Approaches to Stop Hypertension (DASH) diet. Source: (Akhlaghi, 2020 / with permission of Cambridge University Press).

of the DASH dietary pattern on sarcopenia; a recent report fails to prove significant associations between adherence to the DASH diet and odds of sarcopenia in older populations after controlling for several cofounders (Soltani, Hashemi, Heshmat, Motlagh, & Esmaillzadeh, 2020), which agrees with two other relevant studies that also fail to correlate DASH-like patterns with sarcopenia (Mohseni et al., 2017; Kim, Lee, Kye, Chung, & Kim, 2015).

With regard to cognitive health, a systemic review analyzing the DASH diet among other dietary patterns such as the MD, showed that the DASH diet may help improve cognitive function outcomes, especially for those at risk of CVD (Chen et al., 2019). Longitudinal studies on middle-aged and older adults revealed that a continuously high adherence to the DASH diet is significantly associated with a lower risk of Alzheimer's disease and slower rate of decline in global cognition as well as episodic and semantic memory (Morris et al., 2015b; Tangney et al., 2014). However, there are studies with similar designs showing a partial association between adherence to the DASH diet and cognition (verbal memory over executive function/process) (Blumenthal et al., 2017) or that fail to prove any statistically important associations (Shakersain et al., 2018).

Evidence regarding kidney function, CKD, or its progression, suggests that a higher adherence to the DASH dietary pattern is associated with lower odds of CKD in older Korean adults (Lee et al., 2017). In another cohort study, participants with a higher adherence to the DASH diet had a lower risk for CKD progression (Hu et al., 2021)

THE OKINAWAN DIET

Okinawa, a Japanese prefecture also known as the Ryuku Islands, is another blue zone, due to the long life expectancy of its residents (D. Craig Willcox et al., 2009; 2014). Much of the longevity that Okinawa citizens display is related to a healthy lifestyle, which consists partly of their traditional diet that is fundamentally different from the MD pattern but is included with plant-based diets that exert beneficial effects on cardio-metabolic risk and healthy aging (D. Craig Willcox et al., 2014).

Traditional Okinawan dietary patterns are characterized by: a high consumption of vegetables and legumes (mostly soy-derived), moderate consumption of fish products, low intake of meat, dairy and meat products, and moderate alcohol consumption. Consequently, the traditional Okinawan diet includes a very low-fat intake, especially saturated fat, with a very high intake of unrefined carbohydrates through orange-yellow root vegetables, such as sweet potatoes, green leafy vegetables, and seaweeds. Spices such as bitter greens, peppers, and turmeric are preferred to salt, which along with its rich antioxidant phytonutrient content and low glycemic load, explains the significant cardio-protective effects that the Okinawan diet has (D. Craig Willcox et al., 2009).

The Okinawan pattern is low in calories yet nutritionally dense, particularly in vitamins, minerals, and phytonutrients. Additionally, the Okinawa dietary pattern differentiates itself from the traditional MD pattern by being rich in high quality carbohydrates and extra low in fat, while in the MD, carbohydrates and fats provide up to 42% and 45% of daily energy intake, respectively (D. Craig Willcox et al., 2009; 2014). The shared features, however, are more than their discrepancies and include a high intake of unrefined carbohydrates and phytonutrients, mostly from vegetables, moderate-to-high legume consumption, an emphasis on fish and/or lean meats, s healthy fat profile (increased n-3 and MUFA intake with low SFAs). The resemblances between these nutrient and food patterns are considered the key that leads to decreased rates of CVD, certain cancers, and diabetes, mainly through oxidative stress–related mechanisms (**Figure 10.12**) (D. Craig Willcox et al., 2009).

The Okinawan diet is acknowledged as an anti-inflammatory food pattern that is very likely to be related to health and longevity. Its health properties are attributed to its low caloric, yet elevated nutrient density where vitamins and phytonutrients are concerned. Vegetables, legumes, and soy-derived products, which are most abundant in the Okinawan diet, are phytonutrient dense and provide many health benefits. More specifically, they are rich in the antioxidant vitamins A, C, and E; water-soluble vitamins such as thiamine, riboflavin, and vitamin B6; anthocyanins, polyphenols, carotenoids, and flavonoids (D. Craig Willcox et al., 2009). Regarding these vitamins, Okinawans exceed their daily needs by consuming sweet potatoes as the staple accompanying carbohydrate source in everyday meals (compared to the rest of Japanese citizens who use white rice instead). Vitamin E, which is found in elevated concentrations in sweet potatoes, is a fat-soluble vitamin that possesses antioxidant properties and is truly effective at scavenging free-radical molecules that may prevent hyperphosphorylated tau protein dysfunction and Aβ protein-induced death in brain cell–derived cultures. Neuroprotective benefits via these mechanisms are being gained throughout the

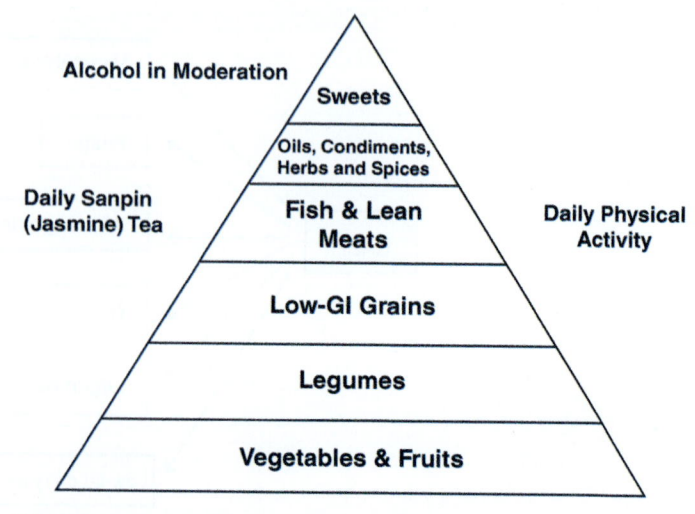

FIGURE 10.12 Traditional Okinawan diet food pyramid. Source: (Willcox, Scapagnini, and Willcox, 2014).

life course (Bruins et al., 2019). Furthermore, the vitamins mentioned provide cardio-protective actions through reducing homocysteine levels and improving endothelial function (Bruins et al., 2019).

The carotenoids that are most found in brightly colored vegetables of the Okinawan cuisine, like beta-carotene and lycopene are also high antioxidant molecules. Marine-derived carotenoids astaxanthin, fucoxanthin, and fucoidan, are found in seaweed, algae, and kelp along with lutein and zeaxanthin; these nutrients are currently discussed as core mediators of ocular function and health, since macular degeneration is a major future NCD (Bruins et al., 2019; D. Craig Willcox et al., 2009). Especially lutein and zeaxanthin, as macular pigments found in the human retina absorb high-energy, short-wavelength blue light, neutralize ROS, protecting against UV-induced peroxidation, reduce lipofuscin formation, and protect the retina from oxidative damage (Bruins et al., 2019).

These xanthophylls also influence cognitive health in older adults (Crous-Bou et al., 2019). Anthocyanins, also found in sweet potatoes, have intense anti-inflammatory properties when consumed daily (D. Craig Willcox et al., 2009). Finally, flavonoids also contribute to the management of higher inflammatory load.

Soy, which is used daily, is rich in phytochemicals such as isoflavones, saponins, and or trypsin inhibitors, which have strong anti-inflammatory effects and exhibit hermetic properties. For instance, they can activate cell-signaling pathways such as the sirtuin-FOXO pathway or act as potent activators of gene expression in FOXO3, a gene that is strongly associated with healthy aging and longevity, among other health-promoting properties. Some isoflavones are potent dual PPARa/g agonists and/or aryl hydrocarbon–receptor agonists that induce cell-cycle arrest and modulate xenobiotic metabolism (D. Craig Willcox et al., 2014).

KEY POINTS

- The main part of healthy aging and life expectancy is attributed to environmental and lifestyle factors since a genetic predisposition accounts for 20% to 25% of the total lifespan.
- Poor nutrition has severe consequences on health that tend to accumulate over a person's lifespan and influence later stages of life in a negative way.
- Although there is no ideal dietary pattern that grants healthy aging for all individuals, plant-based diets are really promising for decreasing all-cause mortality and furthering life expectancy, especially compared to the effects Western dietary patterns have on human health and aging.
- Older adults have higher protein needs because of anabolic resistance to the positive effects of dietary protein on synthesis of protein, a phenomenon that limits muscle maintenance and accretion.
- The traditional recommendation for protein intake of 0.8 g/kg of body weight per day is outdated for older adults. Daily amounts of 1.0 to 1.2 g/kg of body weight is suggested for healthy older persons, and up to 2.0 g/kg of body weight per day in cases of severe illness, injury, or malnutrition. Low protein intake in humans may be beneficial for those 50- to 65-years old but can be detrimental when at older ages.
- Studies involving plant-based proteins prove that they can instigate MPS in levels relative as to dairy proteins, but only when ingested in amounts that largely exceed the RDA.
- Plant-based foods have an incomplete AA profile, which prevent muscle synthesis from occurring.
- 45% to 60% of total energy intake should be from carbohydrates, given that total energy balance conditions are being fulfilled. Both low and high carbohydrate consumption are associated with a higher all-cause mortality.

- High glucose content enhances aging-related phenotypes and deteriorates inflammation status that can lead to the gradual progression of degenerative diseases. Consequently, free-sugar intake should not exceed 5% to 10% of the total daily personal energy intake.
- Older adults who consume bigger amounts of fiber daily have a lower risk for developing NCDs that are most common in older adults. Health organizations recommend the average consumption of 25 to 30g of fiber per day for normal laxation and anti-aging effects.
- Increased fat consumption amongst older adults remains controversial, regarding both the source/type and the quantity of fatty acids consumed, when it comes to health outcomes on older individuals. Most data on PUFA suggest their beneficial effect on health outcomes, while saturated fats remain controversial overall.
- Plant-based diets are food patterns that focus on the consumption of food that is mainly plant-derived, while lowering or even excluding the consumption of animal products.
- Older adults can enjoy beneficial effects by adhering to vegetarian or plant-based dietary patterns, although studies that address this specific population are scarce compared to those that focus on general population.
- Plant polyphenols (part of the phytonutrient group), interfere in a beneficial way with a wide range of signaling pathways that govern protein homeostasis, DNA repair, metabolism adaptations, and antioxidant defenses.
- Adherence to any plant-based dietary pattern by older individuals can grant significant benefits to the manifestation and progress of both chronic diseases and geriatric syndromes.

SELF-ASSESSMENT QUESTIONS

1. Define the plant-based diets that exist and briefly describe their main sub-groups.

2. Why do older individuals have higher protein needs?

3. Why do most health organizations recommend reducing free-sugar consumption?

4. What is the appropriate daily amount of protein for older individuals to maintain muscle mass and strength?
   (a) 0.8–1 g/kg body weight
   (b) 1.0–1.2 g/kg body weight
   (c) >2 g/kg body weight

5. Which amino acid is of most importance in terms of higher protein quality?
   (a) Leucine/
   (b) Tryptophane/
   (c) Lysine

6. Each 10 g increase in fiber per 1000 kcal equals how many extra telomere base pairs, which translates to 4.3 fewer years of biological aging?
   (a) 32 base pairs
   (b) 67 base pairs
   (c) 95 base pairs

7. What is the current recommendation regarding fiber intake in older adults?
   (a) 15–20 g/day
   (b) 20–30 g/day
   (c) >30 g/day

8. What is the average suggested daily intake of EPA and DHA for cardiovascular health?
   (a) 250–500 mg/day
   (b) 500–750 mg/day
   (c) 750–1000 mg/day

9. True or False: For healthy and disease-free aging, high-protein diets are recommended for all age groups.

10. True or False: For muscle protein synthesis to be optimized, 2.5 g to 2.8 g of leucine per meal is considered sufficient.

11. True or False: Plant-derived proteins can exert the same effect in muscle protein synthesis as animal-derived proteins under all circumstances.

12. True or False: N-3 poly-unsaturated fatty acids are classified as essential nutrients.

13. True or False: Flavanols, flavanonols, flavones, anthocyanins, procyanidins, phenolic acids, stilbenes, and tannins are the main sub-categories of non-flavonoid plant polyphenols.

14. True or False: Resveratrol is a phytonutrient that aid fat metabolism.

15. Match the food source (a–g) with the type of fat it contains (i–iv):
    (a) Palm kernel oils
    (b) Fatty fish
    (c) Red meat
    (d) Vegetable oils
    (e) Margarine-like spreads
    (f) Olive oil
    (g) Ruminant milk

    i. saturated fats
    ii. n-3 unsaturated fats
    iii. n-6 unsaturated fats
    iv. trans fats

16. Briefly describe the Mediterranean dietary (MD) pattern and the benefits it can provide to older individuals.

17. Briefly describe the Nordic dietary pattern (ND). Are there any differences between it and the MD?

18. True or False: When DASH was first launched, there was no actual limitation in salt intake.

19. True or False: One of the main three key micronutrients of the DASH dietary pattern is zinc.

20. True or False: The DASH dietary pattern has been proven to have beneficial effects on risk factors regarding CVD, diabetes, obesity, inflammation, frailty, and bone health.

21. True or False: According to the DASH diet, the daily dose of dietary potassium (K) that grants beneficial effects on human health are 4.7 g.

22. Briefly describe the Okinawan dietary pattern. How does it differentiate itself from other plant-based dietary patterns?

REFERENCES

Afshin, A., Sur, P. J., Fay, K. A., Cornaby, L., Ferrara, G., Salama, J. S., . . . Murray, C. J. L. (2019). Health effects of dietary risks in 195 countries, 1990–2017: a systematic analysis for the Global Burden of Disease Study 2017. *The Lancet, 393*(10184), 1958–1972. https://doi.org/10.1016/S0140-6736(19)30041-8

Akhlaghi, M. (2020). Dietary Approaches to Stop Hypertension (DASH): Potential mechanisms of action against risk factors of the metabolic syndrome. *Nutrition Research Reviews, 33*(1), 1–18. https://doi.org/10.1017/S0954422419000155

Amini*, M. R., Shahinfar, H., Djafari, F., Sheikhhossein, F., Naghshi, S., Djafarian, K., ... Shab-Bidar, S. (2021). The association between plant-based diet indices and metabolic syndrome in Iranian older adults. *Nutrition and Health*, 27(4), 435–444. https://doi.org/10.1177/0260106021992672

An, Y., Varma, V. R., Varma, S., Casanova, R., Dammer, E., Pletnikova, O., ... Thambisetty, M. (2018). Evidence for brain glucose dysregulation in Alzheimer's disease. *Alzheimer's and Dementia*, 14(3), 318–329. https://doi.org/10.1016/j.jalz.2017.09.011

Appel, L. J. (2008). Editorial: Dietary patterns and longevity expanding the blue zones. *Circulation*, 118(3), 214–215. https://doi.org/10.1161/CIRCULATIONAHA.108.788497

Arias-Fernández, L., Struijk, E. A., Rodríguez-Artalejo, F., López-García, E., & Lana, A. (2020). Habitual dietary fat intake and risk of muscle weakness and lower-extremity functional impairment in older adults: A prospective cohort study. *Clinical Nutrition*, 39(12), 3663–3670. https://doi.org/10.1016/j.clnu.2020.03.018

Arnett, D. K., Blumenthal, R. S., Albert, M. A., Buroker, A. B., Goldberger, Z. D., Hahn, E. J., ... Ziaeian, B. (2019). 2019 ACC/AHA Guideline on the Primary Prevention of Cardiovascular Disease: A Report of the American College of Cardiology/American Heart Association Task Force on Clinical Practice Guidelines. In *Circulation* (Vol. 140). https://doi.org/10.1161/CIR.0000000000000678

Astrup, A., Magkos, F., Bier, D. M., Brenna, J. T., de Oliveira Otto, M. C., Hill, J. O., ... Krauss, R. M. (2020). Saturated Fats and Health: A Reassessment and Proposal for Food-Based Recommendations: JACC State-of-the-Art Review. *Journal of the American College of Cardiology*, 76(7), 844–857. https://doi.org/10.1016/j.jacc.2020.05.077

Bach-faig, A., Berry, E. M., Lairon, D., Reguant, J., Trichopoulou, A., Dernini, S., ... Belahsen, R. (2011). Mediterranean diet pyramid today. Science and cultural updates. 14(1), 2274–2284. https://doi.org/10.1017/S1368980011002515

Bazzano, L. A., & Fotino, D. (2011). Fruit and Vegetable Consumption, Hypertension, and Risk of Stroke. *Nutritional and Metabolic Bases of Cardiovascular Disease*, 330–336. https://doi.org/10.1002/9781444318456.ch41

Blumenthal, J. A., Smith, P. J., Mabe, S., Hinderliter, A., Welsh-Bohmer, K., Browndyke, J. N., ... Sherwood, A. (2017). Lifestyle and Neurocognition in Older Adults with Cardiovascular Risk Factors and Cognitive Impairment. In *Psychosomatic Medicine* (Vol. 79). https://doi.org/10.1097/PSY.0000000000000474

Bradlee, M. L., Mustafa, J., Singer, M. R., & Moore, L. L. (2018). High-protein foods and physical activity protect against age-related muscle loss and functional decline. *Journals of Gerontology - Series A Biological Sciences and Medical Sciences*, 73(1), 88–94. https://doi.org/10.1093/gerona/glx070

Brandhorst, S., & Longo, V. D. (2019). Protein Quantity and Source, Fasting-Mimicking Diets, and Longevity. *Advances in Nutrition*, 10, S340–S350. https://doi.org/10.1093/advances/nmz079

Bruins, M. J., Van Dael, P., & Eggersdorfer, M. (2019). The role of nutrients in reducing the risk for noncommunicable diseases during aging. *Nutrients*, 11(1). https://doi.org/10.3390/nu11010085

Calder, P. C. (2015). Functional Roles of Fatty Acids and Their Effects on Human Health. *Journal of Parenteral and Enteral Nutrition*, 39, 18S–32S. https://doi.org/10.1177/0148607115595980

Capurso, C. (2021). Whole-grain intake in the mediterranean diet and a low protein to carbohydrates ratio can help to reduce mortality from cardiovascular disease, slow down the progression of aging, and to improve lifespan: A review. *Nutrients*, 13(8). https://doi.org/10.3390/nu13082540

Capurso, C., Bellanti, F., Buglio, A. Lo, & Vendemiale, G. (2020). The mediterranean diet slows down the progression of aging and helps to prevent the onset of frailty: A narrative review. *Nutrients*, 12(1). https://doi.org/10.3390/nu12010035

Chan, R., Leung, J., & Woo, J. (2014). *Associations of Dietary Protein Intake on Subsequent Decline*. 18(2).

Chen, X., Maguire, B., Brodaty, H., & O'Leary, F. (2019). Dietary patterns and cognitive health in older adults: A systematic review. *Journal of Alzheimer's Disease*, 67(2), 583–619. https://doi.org/10.3233/JAD-180468

Chiu, T. H. T., Chang, C. C., Lin, C. L., & Lin, M. N. (2021). A Vegetarian Diet Is Associated with a Lower Risk of Cataract, Particularly Among Individuals with Overweight: A Prospective Study. *Journal of the Academy of Nutrition and Dietetics*, 121(4), 669–677.e1. https://doi.org/10.1016/j.jand.2020.11.003

Chrysohoou, C., Pitsavos, C., Lazaros, G., Skoumas, J., Tousoulis, D., & Stefanadis, C. (2016). Determinants of All-Cause Mortality and Incidence of Cardiovascular Disease (2009 to 2013) in Older Adults. *Angiology*, 67(6), 541–548. https://doi.org/10.1177/0003319715603185

Critselis, E., & Panagiotakos, D. (2020). Adherence to the Mediterranean diet and healthy ageing: Current evidence, biological pathways, and future directions. *Critical Reviews in Food Science and Nutrition*, 60(13), 2148–2157. https://doi.org/10.1080/10408398.2019.1631752

Crous-Bou, M., Molinuevo, J. L., & Sala-Vila, A. (2019). Plant-Rich Dietary Patterns, Plant Foods and Nutrients, and Telomere Length. *Advances in Nutrition*, 10(1), S296–S303. https://doi.org/10.1093/advances/nmz026

Cutuli, D. (2016). Functional and Structural Benefits Induced by Omega-3 Polyunsaturated Fatty Acids During Aging. *Current Neuropharmacology*, 15(4), 534–542. https://doi.org/10.2174/1570159x14666160614091311

Dauchet, L., Amouyel, P., Hercberg, S., & Dallongeville, J. (2006). Fruit and vegetable consumption and risk of coronary heart disease: A meta-analysis of cohort studies. *Journal of Nutrition*, 136(10), 2588–2593. https://doi.org/10.1093/jn/136.10.2588

De Filippis, F., Pellegrini, N., Vannini, L., Jeffery, I. B., La Storia, A., Laghi, L., ... Ercolini, D. (2016). High-level adherence to a Mediterranean diet beneficially impacts the gut microbiota and associated metabolome. *Gut*, 65(11), 1–10. https://doi.org/10.1136/gutjnl-2015-309957

De Souza, R. J., Mente, A., Maroleanu, A., Cozma, A. I., Ha, V., Kishibe, T., ... Anand, S. S. (2015). Intake of saturated and trans unsaturated fatty acids and risk of all cause mortality, cardiovascular disease, and type 2 diabetes: Systematic review and meta-analysis of observational studies. *BMJ (Online)*, 351, 1–16. https://doi.org/10.1136/bmj.h3978

Deutz, N. E. P., Bauer, J. M., Barazzoni, R., Biolo, G., Boirie, Y., Bosy-Westphal, A., ... Calder, P. C. (2014). Protein intake and exercise for optimal muscle function with aging: Recommendations from the ESPEN Expert Group. *Clinical Nutrition*, 33(6), 929–936. https://doi.org/10.1016/j.clnu.2014.04.007

Dhillon, V. S., Deo, P., Chua, A., Thomas, P., & Fenech, M. (2021). Telomere length in healthy adults is positively associated with polyunsaturated fatty acids, including arachidonic acid, and negatively with saturated fatty acids. *Journals of Gerontology - Series A Biological Sciences and Medical Sciences*, 76(1), 3–6. https://doi.org/10.1093/GERONA/GLAA213

Dietary cholesterol trans fatty acids and. (1992). 1992.

Dominguez, L. J., Di Bella, G., Veronese, N., & Barbagallo, M. (2021). Impact of mediterranean diet on chronic non-communicable diseases and longevity. *Nutrients. [revista en Internet] 2021 [acceso 10 de setiembre de 2021]*; 13(6): 2028. Retrieved from https://www.ncbi.nlm.nih.gov/pmc/articles/PMC8231595/pdf/nutrients-13-02028.pdf

Dominguez, L. J., Veronese, N., Baiamonte, E., Guarrera, M., Parisi, A., Ruffolo, C., ... Barbagallo, M. (2022). Healthy Aging and Dietary Patterns. *Nutrients, 14*(4), 1–22. https://doi.org/10.3390/nu14040889

Eckel, R. H., Jakicic, J. M., Ard, J. D., De Jesus, J. M., Houston Miller, N., Hubbard, V. S., ... Yanovski, S. Z. (2014). 2013 AHA/ACC guideline on lifestyle management to reduce cardiovascular risk: A report of the American College of cardiology/American Heart Association task force on practice guidelines. *Circulation, 129*(25 SUPPL. 1), 76–99. https://doi.org/10.1161/01.cir.0000437740.48606.d1

Ekmekcioglu, C. (2020). Nutrition and longevity–From mechanisms to uncertainties. *Critical Reviews in Food Science and Nutrition, 60*(18), 3063–3082. https://doi.org/10.1080/10408398.2019.1676698

Ferguson, C. C., Knol, L. L., & Ellis, A. C. (2021). Visceral adiposity index and its association with Dietary Approaches to Stop Hypertension (DASH) diet scores among older adults: National Health and Nutrition Examination Surveys 2011–2014. *Clinical Nutrition, 40*(6), 4085–4089. https://doi.org/10.1016/j.clnu.2021.02.008

Foscolou, A., Critselis, E., Tyrovolas, S., Chrysohoou, C., Sidossis, L. S., Naumovski, N., ... Panagiotakos, D. (2019). The effect of exclusive olive oil consumption on successful aging: A combined analysis of the Attica and MEDIS epidemiological studies. *Foods, 8*(1). https://doi.org/10.3390/foods8010025

Foscolou, A., Magriplis, E., Tyrovolas, S., Soulis, G., Bountziouka, V., Mariolis, A., ... Panagiotakos, D. (2018). Lifestyle determinants of healthy ageing in a Mediterranean population: The multinational MEDIS study. *Experimental Gerontology, 110*(April), 35–41. https://doi.org/10.1016/j.exger.2018.05.008

Franzon, K., Byberg, L., Sjögren, P., Zethelius, B., Cederholm, T., & Kilander, L. (2017). Predictors of Independent Aging and Survival: A 16-Year Follow-Up Report in Octogenarian Men. *Journal of the American Geriatrics Society, 65*(9), 1953–1960. https://doi.org/10.1111/jgs.14971

Fritsche, K. L. (2015). The Science of Fatty Acids and Inflammation. *Advances in Nutrition, 6*(3), 293S–301S. https://doi.org/10.3945/an.114.006940

Fung, T. T., Meyer, H. E., Willett, W. C., & Feskanich, D. (2017). Protein intake and risk of hip fractures in postmenopausal women and men age 50 and older. *Osteoporosis International, 28*(4), 1401–1411. https://doi.org/10.1007/s00198-016-3898-7

Galbete, C., Kröger, J., Jannasch, F., Iqbal, K., Schwingshackl, L., Schwedhelm, C., ... Schulze, M. B. (2018). Nordic diet, Mediterranean diet, and the risk of chronic diseases: The EPIC-Potsdam study. *BMC Medicine, 16*(1), 1–13. https://doi.org/10.1186/s12916-018-1082-y

Gayet-Boyer, C., Tenenhaus-Aziza, F., Prunet, C., Marmonier, C., Malpuech-Brugère, C., Lamarche, B., & Chardigny, J. M. (2014). Is there a linear relationship between the dose of ruminant trans-fatty acids and cardiovascular risk markers in healthy subjects: Results from a systematic review and meta-regression of randomised clinical trials. *British Journal of Nutrition, 112*(12), 1914–1922. https://doi.org/10.1017/S0007114514002578

Ghosh, T. S., Rampelli, S., Jeffery, I. B., Santoro, A., Neto, M., Capri, M., ... O'Toole, P. W. (2020). Mediterranean diet intervention alters the gut microbiome in older people reducing frailty and improving health status: The NU-AGE 1-year dietary intervention across five European countries. *Gut, 69*(7), 1218–1228. https://doi.org/10.1136/gutjnl-2019-319654

Großkopf, A., & Simm, A. (2020). Carbohydrates in nutrition: friend or foe? *Zeitschrift Fur Gerontologie Und Geriatrie, 53*(4), 290–294. https://doi.org/10.1007/s00391-020-01726-1

Gunge, V. B., Andersen, I., Kyrø, C., Hansen, C. P., Dahm, C. C., Christensen, J., ... Olsen, A. (2017). Adherence to a healthy Nordic food index and risk of myocardial infarction in middle-aged Danes: The diet, cancer and health cohort study. *European Journal of Clinical Nutrition, 71*(5), 652–658. https://doi.org/10.1038/ejcn.2017.1

Harris, W. S., Mozaffarian, D., Rimm, E., Kris-Etherton, P., Rudel, L. L., Appel, L. J., ... Sacks, F. (2009). Omega-6 fatty acids and risk for cardiovascular disease: A science advisory from the American Heart Association nutrition subcommittee of the council on nutrition, physical activity, and metabolism; council on cardiovascular nursing; and council on epidem. *Circulation, 119*(6), 902–907. https://doi.org/10.1161/CIRCULATIONAHA.108.191627

Hu, E. A., Coresh, J., Anderson, C. A. M., Appel, L. J., Grams, M. E., Crews, D. C., ... Townsend, R. R. (2021). Adherence to Healthy Dietary Patterns and Risk of CKD Progression and All-Cause Mortality: Findings From the CRIC (Chronic Renal Insufficiency Cohort) Study. *American Journal of Kidney Diseases, 77*(2), 235–244. https://doi.org/10.1053/j.ajkd.2020.04.019

Jalilpiran, Y., Darooghegi Mofrad, M., Mozaffari, H., Bellissimo, N., & Azadbakht, L. (2020). Adherence to dietary approaches to stop hypertension (DASH) and Mediterranean dietary patterns in relation to cardiovascular risk factors in older adults. *Clinical Nutrition ESPEN, 39*, 87–95. https://doi.org/10.1016/j.clnesp.2020.07.013

Jayanama, K., Theou, O., Godin, J., Cahill, L., Shivappa, N., Hébert, J. R., ... Rockwood, K. (2021). Relationship between diet quality scores and the risk of frailty and mortality in adults across a wide age spectrum. *BMC Medicine, 19*(1), 1–13. https://doi.org/10.1186/s12916-021-01918-5

Julibert, A., Bibiloni, M. D. M., Mateos, D., Angullo, E., & Tur, J. A. (2019). Dietary fat intake and metabolic syndrome in older adults. *Nutrients, 11*(8), 1–16. https://doi.org/10.3390/nu11081901

Kahleova, H., Levin, S., & Barnard, N. D. (2020). Plant-Based Diets for Healthy Aging. *Journal of the American College of Nutrition, 0*(0), 1–2. https://doi.org/10.1080/07315724.2020.1790442

Kanerva, N., Kaartinen, N. E., Schwab, U., Lahti-Koski, M., & Männistö, S. (2014). The baltic sea diet score: A tool for assessing healthy eating in nordic countries. *Public Health Nutrition, 17*(8), 1697–1705. https://doi.org/10.1017/S1368980013002395

Kang, Z. Q., Yang, Y., & Xiao, B. (2020). Dietary saturated fat intake and risk of stroke: Systematic review and dose–response meta-analysis of prospective cohort studies. *Nutrition, Metabolism and Cardiovascular Diseases, 30*(2), 179–189. https://doi.org/10.1016/j.numecd.2019.09.028

Keaver, L., Ruan, M., Chen, F., Du, M., DIng, C., Wang, J., ... Zhang, F. F. (2021). Plant- And animal-based diet quality and mortality among US adults: A cohort study. *British Journal of Nutrition, 125*(12), 1405–1415. https://doi.org/10.1017/S0007114520003670

Kehoe, L., Walton, J., & Flynn, A. (2019). Nutritional challenges for older adults in Europe: Current status and future directions. *Proceedings of the Nutrition Society, 78*(2), 221–233. https://doi.org/10.1017/S0029665118002744

Khaw, K. T., Sharp, S. J., Finikarides, L., Afzal, I., Lentjes, M., Luben, R., & Forouhi, N. G. (2018). Randomised trial of coconut oil, olive oil or butter on blood lipids and other cardiovascular risk factors in healthy men and women. *BMJ Open, 8*(3). https://doi.org/10.1136/bmjopen-2017-020167

Kim, J., Lee, Y., Kye, S., Chung, Y. S., & Kim, K. M. (2015). Association between healthy diet and exercise and greater muscle mass in older adults. *Journal of the American Geriatrics Society, 63*(5), 886–892. https://doi.org/10.1111/jgs.13386

Knoops, K. T. B., De Groot, L. C. P. G. M., Kromhout, D., Perrin, A. E., Moreiras-Varela, O., Menotti, A., & Van Staveren, W. A. (2004). Mediterranean diet, lifestyle factors, and 10-year mortality in elderly European men and women: The HALE project. *Journal of the American Medical Association*, *292*(12), 1433–1439. https://doi.org/10.1001/jama.292.12.1433

Kobayashi, S., Suga, H., & Sasaki, S. (2017). Diet with a combination of high protein and high total antioxidant capacity is strongly associated with low prevalence of frailty among old Japanese women: A multi-center cross-sectional study. *Nutrition Journal*, *16*(1), 1–10. https://doi.org/10.1186/s12937-017-0250-9

Kyrø, C., Skeie, G., Loft, S., Overvad, K., Christensen, J., Tjønneland, A., & Olsen, A. (2013). Adherence to a healthy Nordic food index is associated with a lower incidence of colorectal cancer in women: The Diet, Cancer and Health cohort study. *British Journal of Nutrition*, *109*(5), 920–927. https://doi.org/10.1017/S0007114512002085

Laclaustra, M., Rodríguez-Artalejo, F., Guallar-Castillón, P., Banegas, J. R., Graciani, A., García-Esquinas, E., . . . López-García, E. (2018). Prospective association between added sugars and frailty in older adults. *American Journal of Clinical Nutrition*, *107*(5), 772–779. https://doi.org/10.1093/ajcn/nqy028

Lai, H. T. M., De Oliveira Otto, M. C., Lemaitre, R. N., McKnight, B., Song, X., King, I. B., . . . Mozaffarian, D. (2018). Serial circulating omega 3 polyunsaturated fatty acids and healthy ageing among older adults in the Cardiovascular Health Study: Prospective cohort study. *BMJ (Online)*, *363*, 14–23. https://doi.org/10.1136/bmj.k4067

Lau, E. M. C., Kwok, T., Woo, J., & Ho, S. C. (1998). Bone mineral density in Chinese elderly female vegetarians, vegans, lacto-vegetarians and omnivores. *European Journal of Clinical Nutrition*, *52*(1), 60–64. https://doi.org/10.1038/sj.ejcn.1600516

Lee, H. S., Lee, K. B., Hyun, Y. Y., Chang, Y., Ryu, S., & Choi, Y. (2017). DASH dietary pattern and chronic kidney disease in elderly Korean adults. *European Journal of Clinical Nutrition*, *71*(6), 755–761. https://doi.org/10.1038/ejcn.2016.240

Leri, M., Scuto, M., Ontario, M. L., Calabrese, V., Calabrese, E. J., Bucciantini, M., & Stefani, M. (2020). Healthy effects of plant polyphenols: Molecular mechanisms. In *International Journal of Molecular Sciences* (Vol. 21). https://doi.org/10.3390/ijms21041250

Levine, M. E., Suarez, J. A., Brandhorst, S., Balasubramanian, P., Cheng, C. W., Madia, F., . . . Longo, V. D. (2014). Low protein intake is associated with a major reduction in IGF-1, cancer, and overall mortality in the 65 and younger but not older population. *Cell Metabolism*, *19*(3), 407–417. https://doi.org/10.1016/j.cmet.2014.02.006

Liu, Y., Poon, S., Seeman, E., Hare, D. L., Bui, M., & Iuliano, S. (2019). Fat from dairy foods and "meat" consumed within recommended levels is associated with favourable serum cholesterol levels in institutionalised older adults. *Journal of Nutritional Science*, 1–8. https://doi.org/10.1017/jns.2019.5

Liu, Z. M., Tse, L. A., Chan, D., Wong, C., & Wong, S. Y. S. (2018). Dietary sugar intake was associated with increased body fatness but decreased cardiovascular mortality in Chinese elderly: An 11-year prospective study of Mr and Ms OS of Hong Kong. *International Journal of Obesity*, *42*(4), 808–816. https://doi.org/10.1038/ijo.2017.292

Lonnie, M., Hooker, E., Brunstrom, J. M., Corfe, B. M., Green, M. A., Watson, A. W., . . . Johnstone, A. M. (2018). Protein for life: Review of optimal protein intake, sustainable dietary sources and the effect on appetite in ageing adults. *Nutrients*, *10*(3), 1–18. https://doi.org/10.3390/nu10030360

Mazza, E., Ferro, Y., Pujia, R., Mare, R., Maurotti, S., Montalcini, T., & Pujia, A. (2021). Mediterranean Diet In Healthy Aging. *Journal of Nutrition, Health and Aging*, *25*(9), 1076–1083. https://doi.org/10.1007/s12603-021-1675-6

McCrea, L. G., Bromley, J. L., Mcnally, C. J., O'Byrne, K. K., & Wade, K. A. (2004). Houston 2001. *The Counseling Psychologist*, *32*(1), 78–88. https://doi.org/10.1177/0011000003260172

McLean, R. R., Mangano, K. M., Hannan, M. T., Kiel, D. P., & Sahni, S. (2016). Dietary Protein Intake Is Protective Against Loss of Grip Strength Among Older Adults in the Framingham Offspring Cohort. *Journals of Gerontology - Series A Biological Sciences and Medical Sciences*, *71*(3), 356–361. https://doi.org/10.1093/gerona/glv184

Mertens, E., Kuijsten, A., Dofková, M., Mistura, L., D'Addezio, L., Turrini, A., ... & Geleijnse, J. M. (2019). Geographic and socioeconomic diversity of food and nutrient intakes: a comparison of four European countries. *European journal of nutrition*, *58*, 1475–1493.

Mithril, C., Dragsted, L. O., Meyer, C., Blauert, E., Holt, M. K., & Astrup, A. (2012). Guidelines for the New Nordic Diet. *Public Health Nutrition*, *15*(10), 1941–1947. https://doi.org/10.1017/S136898001100351X

Mohseni, R., Aliakbar, S., Abdollahi, A., Yekaninejad, M. S., Maghbooli, Z., & Mirzaei, K. (2017). Relationship between major dietary patterns and sarcopenia among menopausal women. *Aging Clinical and Experimental Research*, *29*(6), 1241–1248. https://doi.org/10.1007/s40520-016-0721-4

Morgan, P. T., Harris, D. O., Marshall, R. N., Quinlan, J. I., Edwards, S. J., Allen, S. L., & Breen, L. (2021). Protein Source and Quality for Skeletal Muscle Anabolism in Young and Older Adults: A Systematic Review and Meta-Analysis. *Journal of Nutrition*, *151*(7), 1901–1920. https://doi.org/10.1093/jn/nxab055

Morris et al., 2012. (2015a). 基因的改变NIH Public Access. *Gerontology*, *61*(6), 515–525. https://doi.org/10.1001/jamainternmed.2013.6473.Vegetarian

Morris, M. C., Tangney, C. C., Wang, Y., Sacks, F. M., Bennett, D. A., & Aggarwal, N. T. (2015b). MIND diet associated with reduced incidence of Alzheimer's disease. *Alzheimer's and Dementia*, *11*(9), 1007–1014. https://doi.org/10.1016/j.jalz.2014.11.009

Nieman, D. C., Underwood, B. C., Sherman, K. M., Arabatzis, K., Barbosa, J. C., Johnson, M., & Shultz, T. D. (1989). Dietary status of Seventh-Day Adventist vegetarian and non-vegetarian elderly women. *Journal of the American Dietetic Association*, *89*(12), 1763–1769.

Nilsson, A., Halvardsson, P., & Kadi, F. (2019). Adherence to dash-style dietary pattern impacts on adiponectin and clustered metabolic risk in older women. *Nutrients*, *11*(4), 1–9. https://doi.org/10.3390/nu11040805

Nooyens, A. C. J., van Gelder, B. M., Bueno-de-Mesquita, H. B., van Boxtel, M. P. J., & Verschuren, W. M. M. (2018). Fish consumption, intake of fats and cognitive decline at middle and older age: the Doetinchem Cohort Study. *European Journal of Nutrition*, *57*(4), 1667–1675. https://doi.org/10.1007/s00394-017-1453-8

Olaniyan, E. T., O'Halloran, F., & McCarthy, A. L. (2020). Dietary Protein Considerations for Muscle Protein Synthesis and Muscle Mass Preservation in Older Adults. *Nutrition Research Reviews*. https://doi.org/10.1017/S0954422420000219

Olsen, A., Egeberg, R., Halkjær, J., Christensen, J., Overvad, K., & Tjønneland, A. (2011). Healthy aspects of the nordic diet are related to lower total mortality1,2. *Journal of Nutrition*, *141*(4), 639–644. https://doi.org/10.3945/jn.110.131375

Ortolá, R., Struijk, E. A., García-Esquinas, E., Rodríguez-Artalejo, F., & López-García, E. (2020). Changes in Dietary Intake of Animal and Vegetable Protein and Unhealthy Aging. *American Journal of Medicine*, *133*(2), 231–239.e7. https://doi.org/10.1016/j.amjmed.2019.06.051

Ostfeld, R. J. (2017). Definition of a plant-based diet and overview of this special issue. *Journal of Geriatric Cardiology*, *14*(5), 315. https://doi.org/10.11909/j.issn.1671-5411.2017.05.008

Pagliai, G., Russo, E., Niccolai, E., Dinu, M., Di Pilato, V., Magrini, A., . . . Amedei, A. (2020). Influence of a 3-month low-calorie Mediterranean diet compared to the vegetarian diet on human gut microbiota and SCFA: the CARDIVEG Study. *European Journal of Nutrition*, *59*(5), 2011–2024. https://doi.org/10.1007/s00394-019-02050-0

Panagiotou, M., Michel, S., Meijer, J. H., & Deboer, T. (2021). The aging brain: sleep, the circadian clock and exercise. *Biochemical Pharmacology*, *191*(March), 114563. https://doi.org/10.1016/j.bcp.2021.114563

Paproski, J. J., Finello, G. C., Murillo, A., & Mandel, E. (2019). The importance of protein intake and strength exercises for older adults. *Journal of the American Academy of Physician Assistants*, *32*(11), 32–36. https://doi.org/10.1097/01.JAA.0000586328.11996.c0

Perälä, M. M., von Bonsdorff, M. B., Männistö, S., Salonen, M. K., Simonen, M., Pohjolainen, P., . . . Eriksson, J. G. (2019). The Healthy Nordic Diet and Mediterranean Diet and Incidence of Disability 10 Years Later in Home-Dwelling Old Adults. *Journal of the American Medical Directors Association*, *20*(5), 511–516.e1. https://doi.org/10.1016/j.jamda.2018.09.001

Perälä, M. M., Von Bonsdorff, M., Männistö, S., Salonen, M. K., Simonen, M., Kanerva, N., . . . Eriksson, J. G. (2016). A healthy Nordic diet and physical performance in old age: Findings from the longitudinal Helsinki Birth Cohort Study. *British Journal of Nutrition*, *115*(5), 878–886. https://doi.org/10.1017/S0007114515005309

Pignatti, C., D'Adamo, S., Stefanelli, C., Flamigni, F., & Cetrullo, S. (2020). Nutrients and pathways that regulate health span and life span. *Geriatrics*, *5*(4), 95.

Pilgrim, A. L., Robinson, S. M., Sayer, A. A., & Roberts, H. C. (2015). An overview of appetite decline in older people. *Nursing Older People*, *27*(5), 29–35. https://doi.org/10.7748/NOP.27.5.29.E697

Pisanu, S., Palmas, V., Madau, V., Casula, E., Deledda, A., Cusano, R., . . . Velluzzi, F. (2020). Impact of a moderately hypocaloric mediterranean diet on the gut microbiota composition of italian obese patients. *Nutrients*, *12*(9), 1–19. https://doi.org/10.3390/nu12092707

Ramey, M. M., Shields, G. S., & Yonelinas, A. P. (2022). Markers of a plant-based diet relate to memory and executive function in older adults. *Nutritional Neuroscience*, *25*(2), 276–285. https://doi.org/10.1080/1028415X.2020.1751506

Ratjen, I., Schafmayer, C., di Giuseppe, R., Waniek, S., Plachta-Danielzik, S., Koch, M., . . . Lieb, W. (2017). Postdiagnostic mediterranean and healthy nordic dietary patterns are inversely associated with all-cause mortality in long- term colorectal cancer survivors. *Journal of Nutrition*, *147*(4), 636–644. https://doi.org/10.3945/jn.116.244129

Renzella, J., Townsend, N., Jewell, J., Roberts, N., Rayner, M., & Wickramasinghe, K. (2018). *What national and subnational interventions and policies based on*. *1*, 74. Retrieved from https://www.euro.who.int/__data/assets/pdf_file/0011/365285/hen-58-eng.pdf

Risérus, U. (2015). Healthy Nordic diet and cardiovascular disease. *Journal of Internal Medicine*, *278*(5), 542–544. https://doi.org/10.1111/joim.12408

Roberts, S. B., Silver, R. E., Das, S. K., Fielding, R. A., Gilhooly, C. H., Jacques, P. F., . . . Booth, S. (2021). Healthy Aging - Nutrition Matters: Start Early and Screen Often. *Advances in Nutrition*, *12*(4), 1438–1448. https://doi.org/10.1093/advances/nmab032

Ruxton, C. H. S., Derbyshire, E., & Toribio-Mateas, M. (2016). Role of fatty acids and micronutrients in healthy ageing: A systematic review of randomised controlled trials set in the context of European dietary surveys of older adults. *Journal of Human Nutrition and Dietetics*, *29*(3), 308–324. https://doi.org/10.1111/jhn.12335

Sandoval-Insausti, H., Pérez-Tasigchana, R. F., López-García, E., García-Esquinas, E., Rodríguez-Artalejo, F., & Guallar-Castillón, P. (2016). Macronutrients Intake and Incident Frailty in Older Adults: A Prospective Cohort Study. *Journals of Gerontology - Series A Biological Sciences and Medical Sciences*, *71*(10), 1329–1334. https://doi.org/10.1093/gerona/glw033

Shahriarpour, Z., Nasrabadi, B., Shariati-Bafghi, S. E., Karamati, M., & Rashidkhani, B. (2020). Adherence to the dietary approaches to stop hypertension (DASH) dietary pattern and osteoporosis risk in postmenopausal Iranian women. *Osteoporosis International*, *31*(11), 2179–2188. https://doi.org/10.1007/s00198-020-05450-9

Shakersain, B., Rizzuto, D., Larsson, S. C., Faxén-Irving, G., Fratiglioni, L., & Xu, W. L. (2018). The nordic prudent diet reduces risk of cognitive decline in the Swedish older adults: A population- based cohort study. *Nutrients*, *10*(2). https://doi.org/10.3390/nu10020229

Shang, X., Hill, E., Li, Y., & He, M. (2021). Energy and macronutrient intakes at breakfast and cognitive declines in community-dwelling older adults: A 9-year follow-up cohort study. *American Journal of Clinical Nutrition*, *113*(5), 1093–1103. https://doi.org/10.1093/ajcn/nqaa403

Simpson, R. J., Lowder, T. W., Spielmann, G., Bigley, A. B., LaVoy, E. C., & Kunz, H. (2012). Exercise and the aging immune system. *Ageing Research Reviews*, *11*(3), 404–420. https://doi.org/10.1016/j.arr.2012.03.003

Siri-Tarino, P. (2009). 2.7 Association of saturated fat with CVD - meta-analysis of prospective cohort studies. *The Practitioner*, *253*(1717), 5. https://doi.org/10.3945/ajcn.2009.27725.1

Sluijs, I., Beulens, J. W. J., Van Der A, D. L., Spijkerman, A. M. W., Grobbee, D. E., & Van Der Schouw, Y. T. (2010). Dietary intake of total, animal, and vegetable protein and risk of type 2 diabetes in the European Prospective Investigation into Cancer and Nutrition (EPIC)-NL study. *Diabetes Care*, *33*(1), 43–48. https://doi.org/10.2337/dc09-1321

Söderström, L., Rosenblad, A., Adolfsson, E. T., Wolk, A., Hakansson, N., & Bergkvist, L. (2015). A high energy intake from dietary fat among middle-Aged and older adults is associated with increased risk of malnutrition 10 years later. *British Journal of Nutrition*, *114*(6), 915–923. https://doi.org/10.1017/S0007114515002317

Soltani, S., Hashemi, R., Heshmat, R., Motlagh, A. D., & Esmaillzadeh, A. (2020). Association of dietary approaches to stop hypertension eating style and risk of sarcopenia. *Scientific Reports*, *10*(1), 1–9. https://doi.org/10.1038/s41598-020-76452-0

Song, M., Fung, T. T., Hu, F. B., Willett, W. C., Longo, V. D., Chan, A. T., & Giovannucci, E. L. (2016). Association of animal and plant protein intake with all-cause and cause-specific mortality. *JAMA Internal Medicine*, *176*(10), 1453–1463. https://doi.org/10.1001/jamainternmed.2016.4182

Strasser, B., Wolters, M., Weyh, C., Krüger, K., & Ticinesi, A. (2021). The effects of lifestyle and diet on gut microbiota composition, inflammation and muscle performance in our aging society. *Nutrients*, *13*(6). https://doi.org/10.3390/nu13062045

Suri, S., Kumar, V., Kumar, S., Goyal, A., Tanwar, B., Kaur, J., & Kaur, J. (2019). DASH Dietary Pattern: A Treatment for Non-communicable Diseases. *Current Hypertension Reviews*, *16*(2), 108–114. https://doi.org/10.2174/1573402115666191007144608

Susan, M. (2007). Annals of Internal Medicine Article Outcome Studies. *Annals of Internal Medicine*, (February), 941–952.

Talaei, M., Koh, W. P., Yuan, J. M., & van Dam, R. M. (2019). DASH Dietary Pattern, Mediation by Mineral Intakes, and the Risk of Coronary Artery Disease and Stroke Mortality. *Journal of the American Heart Association*, *8*(5). https://doi.org/10.1161/JAHA.118.011054

Tangney, C. C., Li, H., Wang, Y., Barnes, L., Schneider, J. A., Bennett, D. A., & Morris, M. C. (2014). Relation of DASH- and Mediterranean-like dietary patterns to cognitive decline in older persons. *Neurology*, *83*(16), 1410–1416. https://doi.org/10.1212/WNL.0000000000000884

Tertsunen, H. M., Hantunen, S., Tuomainen, T. P., & Virtanen, J. K. (2021). Adherence to a healthy Nordic diet and risk of type 2 diabetes among men: the Kuopio Ischaemic Heart Disease Risk Factor Study. *European Journal of Nutrition, 60*(7), 3927–3934. https://doi.org/10.1007/s00394-021-02569-1

Tessier, A. J., & Chevalier, S. (2018). An update on protein, leucine, omega-3 fatty acids, and vitamin d in the prevention and treatment of sarcopenia and functional decline. *Nutrients, 10*(8), 1–17. https://doi.org/10.3390/nu10081099

Towery, P., Guffey, J. S., Doerflein, C., Stroup, K., Saucedo, S., & Taylor, J. (2018). Chronic musculoskeletal pain and function improve with a plant-based diet. *Complementary Therapies in Medicine, 40*(August), 64–69. https://doi.org/10.1016/j.ctim.2018.08.001

Tucker, L. A. (2018). Dietary fiber and telomere length in 5674 US adults: An NHANES study of biological aging. *Nutrients, 10*(4), 1–16. https://doi.org/10.3390/nu10040400

Valencia, A. P., Nagaraj, N., Osman, D. H., Rabinovitch, P. S., & Marcinek, D. J. (2021). Are fat and sugar just as detrimental in old age? *GeroScience, 43*(4), 1615–1625. https://doi.org/10.1007/s11357-021-00390-6

Volkert, D., Beck, A. M., Cederholm, T., Cruz-Jentoft, A., Goisser, S., Hooper, L., . . . Bischoff, S. C. (2019). ESPEN guideline on clinical nutrition and hydration in geriatrics. *Clinical Nutrition, 38*(1), 10–47. https://doi.org/10.1016/j.clnu.2018.05.024

WHO/Europe. (2021). *Plant-based diets and their impact on health, sustainability and the environment.* 14p.

Willcox, D. Craig, Willcox, B. J., Todoriki, H., & Suzuki, M. (2009). The okinawan diet: Health implications of a low-calorie, nutrient-dense, antioxidant-rich dietary pattern low in glycemic load. *Journal of the American College of Nutrition, 28*(November 2013), 500S–516S. https://doi.org/10.1080/07315724.2009.10718117

Willcox, Donald Craig, Scapagnini, G., & Willcox, B. J. (2014). Healthy aging diets other than the Mediterranean: A focus on the Okinawan diet. *Mechanisms of Ageing and Development, 136–137*, 148–162. https://doi.org/10.1016/j.mad.2014.01.002

Wu, W., Shang, Y., Dove, A., Guo, J., Calderón-Larrañaga, A., Rizzuto, D., & Xu, W. (2021). The Nordic prudent diet prolongs survival with good mental and physical functioning among older adults: The role of healthy lifestyle. *Clinical Nutrition, 40*(8), 4838–4844. https://doi.org/10.1016/j.clnu.2021.06.027

Xiao, M. L., Lin, J. S., Li, Y. H., Liu, M., Deng, Y. Y., Wang, C. Y., & Chen, Y. M. (2020). Adherence to the Dietary Approaches to Stop Hypertension (DASH) diet is associated with lower presence of non-alcoholic fatty liver disease in middle-aged and elderly adults. *Public Health Nutrition, 23*(4), 674–682. https://doi.org/10.1017/S1368980019002568

Zhu, Y., Bo, Y., & Liu, Y. (2019). Dietary total fat, fatty acids intake, and risk of cardiovascular disease: A dose-response meta-analysis of cohort studies. *Lipids in Health and Disease, 18*(1), 1–14. https://doi.org/10.1186/s12944-019-1035-2

FURTHER READING

Bibliography

Hever, J. (2016). Plant-Based Diets: A Physician's Guide SUMMARY OF HEALTH BENEFITS. *The Permanente Journal/Perm J 2016 Summer Perm J 2016 Summer, 2020*(33), 15–82. http://dx.doi.org/10.7812/TPP/15-082

WHO. (2002). Keep fit for life: Meeting the nutritional needs of older persons. Geneva: World Health Organization, 1–83. chrome-extension://efaidnbmnnnibpcajpcglclefindmkaj/http://apps.who.int/iris/bitstream/handle/10665/42515/9241562102_annexes.pdf?sequence=2

Links

- Plant-Based Climate Summit (1st of April 2021)
- https://www.youtube.com/watch?v=dxzSfiFz3fo

Physical Activity as a Determinant of Healthy Aging

CHAPTER 11

Introduction	159	Physical Activity and Frailty	163
Physical Inactivity	159	The VIVIFRAIL Exercise Protocol	163
Physical Activity as a Determinant of Healthy Aging	161	Physical Activity Recommendations for Older Adults	164
		Key Points	165
Cardiovascular Health	161	Self-assessment Questions	166
Immune System	162	References	166
Cognitive Function	162	Further Reading	167
Musculoskeletal Health	163	Bibliography	167
Physical Activity and Sarcopenia	163		

INTRODUCTION

As described thoroughly in **Unit 2**, being physically active is of major importance for maintaining health and normal functioning (Bangsbo et al., 2019; Koehler & Drenowatz, 2019). Nowadays, there is historical recognition that physical inactivity is detrimental to health by causing significant decline in the functional capacity of most organ systems in humans, mammals, and rodents (Booth, Roberts, & Laye, 2012).

Physical inactivity is an actual cause of numerous physiological dysfunctions that cause, usually permanent, pathological changes which over time lead to overt chronic diseases, culminating as contributors to premature mortality (Booth, Roberts, Thyfault, Ruegsegger, & Toedebusch, 2017). Studies conducted in the United States indicate that older adults above 60 years of age, who live in community-based environments, spend approximately 8 to 11 hours per day being sedentary, with their most common pastimes watching television or browsing the internet (Kehler & Theou, 2019). It is important to mention, however, that physical inactivity and activity/exercise are not considered mirror images; there are different mechanisms that govern each state of body activity, and it is important to understand the difference between how inactivity causes disease and how exercise acts as a primary prevention for the same diseases (Booth et al., 2012).

PHYSICAL INACTIVITY

According to the 2020 guidelines on physical activity and sedentary behavior by the WHO, physical inactivity is defined as the incapability of an individual to follow current age-group recommendations regarding weekly levels of physical activity. This practically means 150 to 300 min of moderate-intensity or 75 to 150 min of vigorous-intensity exercise per week for people of 18 years and older (Bull et al., 2020). The Physical Activity Guidelines Advisory Committee also recognizes a strong dose-response relationship between sedentary behavior and cardiovascular disease (CVD) mortality and all-cause mortality (Chaput et al., 2020). Physical inactivity is an initiating cause of a chronic disease or condition. **Figure 11.1** presents a comprehensive view of how low physical activity correlates with all kinds of diseases.

Indeed, high levels of physical inactivity, or sedentary behavior, is linked with at least 35 chronic diseases/clinical conditions such as CVD; colon, endometrium, or lung cancer: type 2 diabetes and obesity; and increased overall mortality rates (Thyfault, Du, Kraus, Levine, & Booth, 2015; Ross et al., 2020) (**Figures 11.2** and **11.3**).

Based on the famous reduced stepping studies conducted in the 2000s, an important reduction in even the number of steps taken on daily basis by a healthy adult, could result in a 7% decrease in VO_2max, 17% decrease in peripheral insulin sensitivity,

---

Prevention and Management of Cardiovascular and Metabolic Disease: Diet, Physical Activity and Healthy Aging,
First Edition. Christina N. Katsagoni, Peter Kokkinos, and Labros S. Sidossis.
© 2023 John Wiley & Sons Ltd. Published 2023 by John Wiley & Sons Ltd.

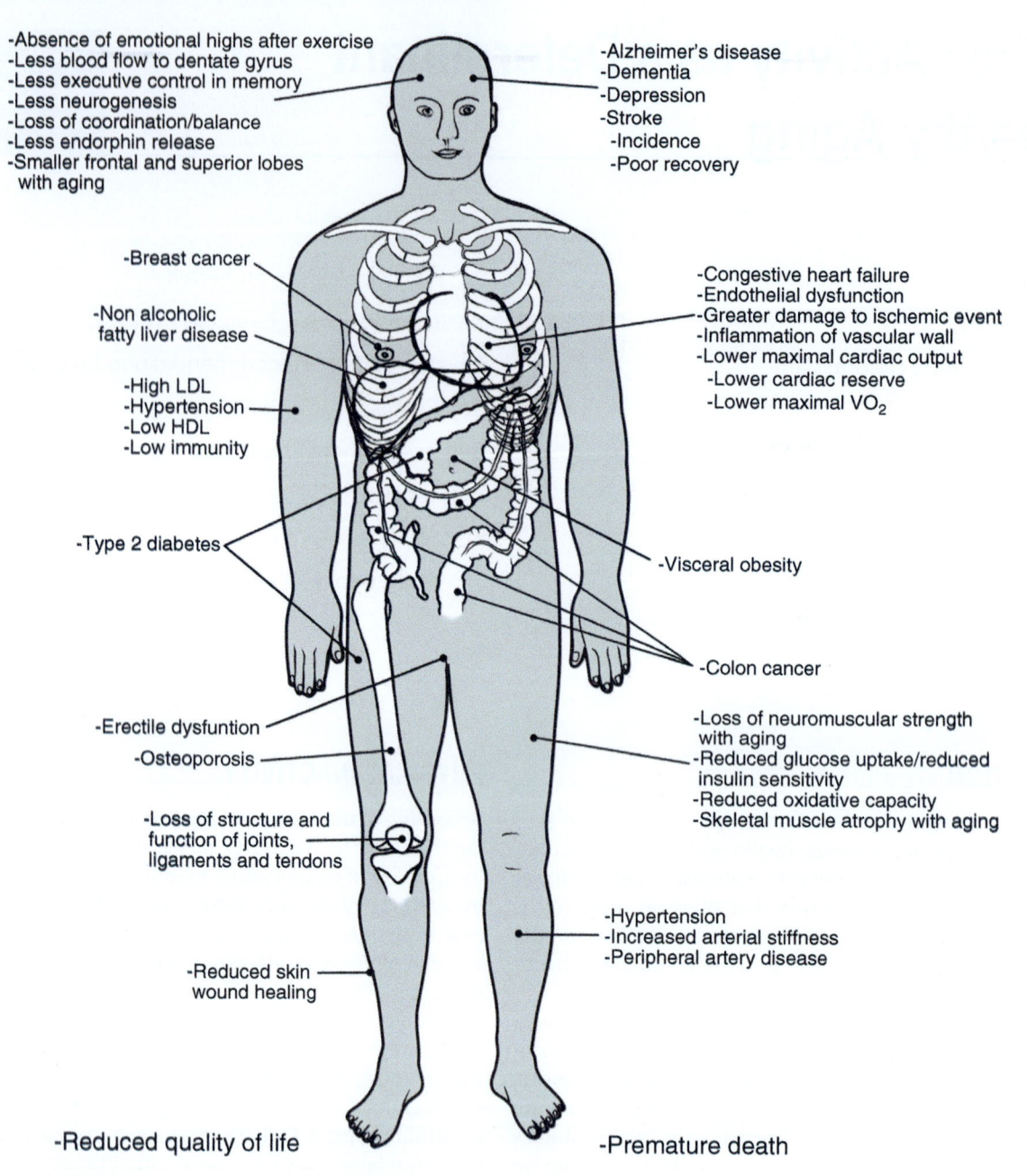

FIGURE 11.1 Health deficiencies accelerated by decreasing physical activity from higher to lower levels. Source: (Booth et al., 2012 / with permission of John Wiley & Sons).

and concurrent decreases in the insulin-stimulated ratio of pAkt-Thr/total Akt in skeletal muscle (Booth et al., 2012).

Physical inactivity uses multiple pathways to cause chronic diseases that are not necessarily similar to those through which exercise acts as a primary protector. For example, inactivity and exercise differ in the context of the time courses of structural changes in conduit arteries and change in endothelial function; inactivity leads to immediate negative remodeling of the vessel, while exercise needs up to 6 weeks to enact positive effects (Booth et al., 2012; Thijssen et al., 2010). In addition, the cardio-protective effects of exercise are due to vasodilation by the nitric oxide pathway while deconditioning activated vasoconstrictor pathways (**Figure 11.4**).

Moreover, an analysis of skeletal-muscle gene expression before bed rest, immediately after bed rest, and after 4 weeks of post-bed rest training, indicated a difference in the number of mRNAs produced. A 9-day period of bed rest altered a total of 4500 mRNAs, while a 4-week post-bed training program normalized the expression of only 80% of the original mRNA count. This finding strengthens the hypothesis that even short periods of inactivity (such as 9 days) can severely alter biological pathways relevant to an individual's health, even at the molecular level. This result agrees with the findings of Stein and Bolster, who investigated the genes that govern muscle catabolism and rebuilding. These researchers hypothesized that if physical activity were the opposite of physical inactivity, then the

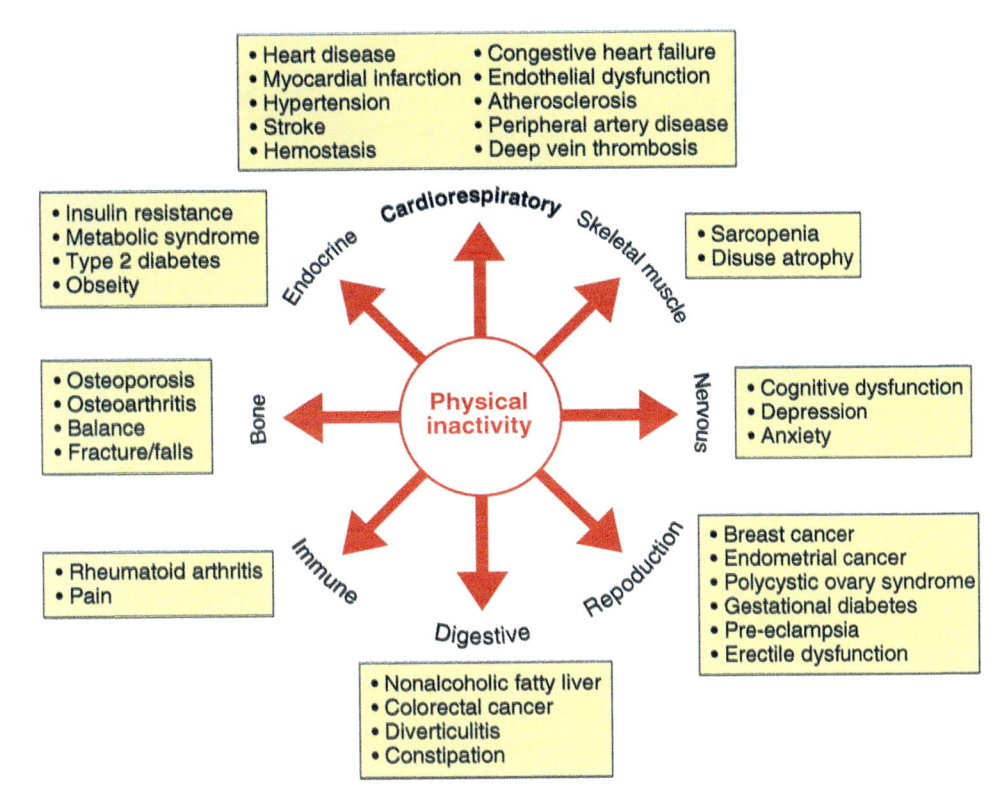

FIGURE 11.2 Physical inactivity increases 35 chronic diseases. Source: (Booth et al., 2017).

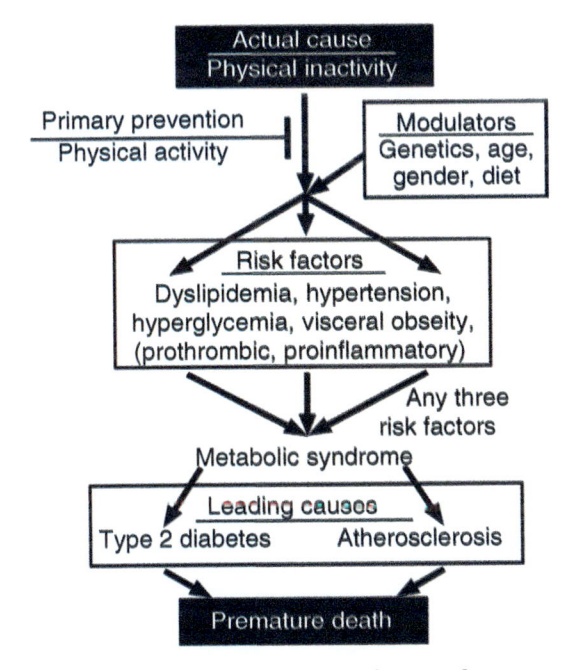

FIGURE 11.3 Physical inactivity is an actual cause of premature death by interacting with other environmental factors to increase risk factors for metabolic syndrome, which, in turn produces two "leading causes" of "premature death" (type 2 diabetes and atherosclerosis). Source: (Booth et al., 2012 / with permission of John Wiley & Sons).

expected result would be changes in many of the same genes for atrophy and regrowth. However, a comparison of these two gene lists showed virtually no genes appearing on both lists (Booth et al., 2012). Although literature suggests that the mechanisms through which exercise and inactivity impact the physiological functions are directly correlated with aging parameters, studies on the molecular neurobiology for physical inactivity are only in their infancy.

PHYSICAL ACTIVITY AS A DETERMINANT OF HEALTHY AGING

CARDIOVASCULAR HEALTH

Physical activity positively affects many physiological mechanisms related to the aging process. Evidence shows that a person's rapid/severe turn to inactivity can rapidly decrease cardio-respiratory fitness (CRF); an individual's cardiovascular (heart and blood vessels) and respiratory systems capacity to supply oxygen to the rest of the body. Higher CRF correlates with improved insulin sensitivity, lipid and lipoprotein profile, body composition, systematic inflammation, blood pressure, and autonomous nervous system functioning. Low functional capacity values for maximal aerobic capacity (VO_2max) are a risk biomarker for death as it correlates with a shorter life expectancy, independent of other risk factors. For example, the Dallas bed-rest study indicated that when healthy young men were put on a continuous 20-day bed rest, their VO_2max decreased by 27%. Regular physical activity can also, in the long term, reduce systematic inflammation, endothelial dysfunction, and common cardiovascular risks like hypertension (Booth et al., 2012; Gremeaux et al., 2012; Daskalopoulou et al., 2017). Overall,

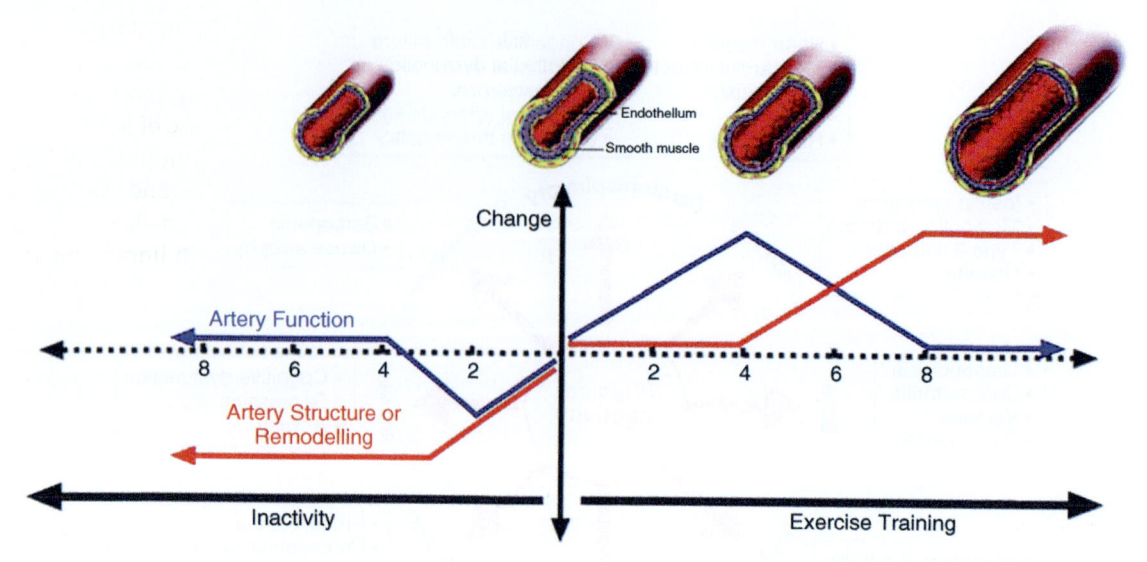

FIGURE 11.4 Hypothesized changes in artery function and structure (remodeling) in response to inactivity and exercise training in humans. Studies performed in both animals and humans suggest that rapid changes occur in artery function, including nitric oxide (NO) bioavailability, in response to exercise training and that these changes are superseded by arterial remodeling and normalization of function. Physical inactivity is associated with rapid changes in arterial diameter, with structural remodeling occurring within weeks of, for example, spinal cord injury. There is little evidence for longer term vascular dysfunction in response to inactivity. Changes in artery function and structure occur rapidly in response to activity and inactivity. Source: (Thijssen et al., 2010 / with permission of Springer Nature).

achieving and maintaining an increased CRF (and muscle strength) from young to older stages of life through regular physical exercise can delay the onset of frailty due to primary aging (Booth et al., 2012).

IMMUNE SYSTEM

Although physical activity during aging helps immune activity, most mechanisms through which exercise exerts these beneficial effects are still unknown (Simpson et al., 2012). Yet, they include multiple neuro-endocrinological factors that alter exercise-induced metabolism and metabolic factors. For instance, reductions in plasma glucose or glutamine concentrations influence lymphocyte function through alteration of stress hormone, catecholamine, growth hormone, and other cytokine levels (Pedersen & Hoffman-Goetz, 2000; Scartoni et al., 2020). Also, exercise contributes to a lower accumulation of autoreactive immune cells in a way that improves programmed cell death (Scartoni et al., 2020).

A single bout of exercise in older adults can increase natural killer (NK) cell activity and significantly decrease TNF-α, IL-6, and IL-1β levels. NK and effector-memory CD8+ T cells are mobilized into the bloodstream with acute exercise, causing a two- to threefold increase in the blood lymphocyte count. The same type of cells leave the bloodstream during the early stages of exercise recovery, although the number of cells that extravasate the blood (presumably to recirculate to the peripheral tissues), are usually bigger than the number of cells that were mobilized, which results in short-term lymphocytopenia. Given that the cell types preferentially mobilized by exercise have high effector functions (NK cells, effector-memory T cells), one possible mechanism for enhanced immunity through exercise is due to the increased trafficking of cells throughout peripheral tissues and circulation (Simpson et al., 2012). Regular moderate activity over a 2-month period also reduced the pro-inflammatory profile of older adults by decreasing TNF-α, MCP-1, and nitric oxide synthase mRNA levels in peripheral-blood mononuclear cells (PBMCs). These results were independent from a reduction in adipose tissue, suggesting that exercise has a direct anti-inflammatory effect (Simpson et al., 2012; Scartoni et al., 2020). Exercise also moderates immunosenescence and provides anti-inflammatory properties that act against inflamm-aging (Simpson et al., 2012). Age-related accumulation of late-stage differentiated T cells and/or thymic involution are key contributors to the immunosenescence process, due to induced restrictions in T cell repertoire and stress reduction (Simpson et al., 2012). Moreover, increases in the body's antioxidant capabilities with regular exercise can prevent cellular DNA and structural damage from ROS, therefore preventing the premature biological aging of specific immune cells (Pedersen & Hoffman-Goetz, 2000).

COGNITIVE FUNCTION

Physically active older adults, compared to their inactive counterparts, show benefits in terms of physical and cognitive function, depression, quality of life (QOL), and compression of disability (Bangsbo et al., 2019). Physical health (with a focus on aerobic health/fitness), is a crucial factor in improving cognition, memory, and mental health. It is also important for promoting structural and functional plasticity in the brain along the same pathways as pharmacological antidepressants (Panagiotou, Michel, Meijer, & Deboer, 2021). The neuroprotective effect of aerobic exercise was demonstrated in patients with mild cognitive impairment, dementia (Nuzum et al., 2020), and depression (Gujral, Aizenstein, Reynolds, Butters, & Erickson, 2017). Trophic factor production of brain-derived neurotrophic factor and IGF-1 is induced after exercise and, along with the increased availability of serotonin and norepinephrine as well as better HPA-axis activity, may alleviate depression through an increase in hippocampal volume.

MUSCULOSKELETAL HEALTH

Physically active older adults, compared to their inactive counterparts, show benefits in terms of physical function, intrinsic capacity, mobility, musculoskeletal pain, and risk of falls and fractures (Booth et al., 2012). A history of falls consistently correlates with the functional capacity and physical activity level of older adults, which implies that strength and balance decline affects their ability to avoid a fall after an unexpected trip or slip (Moreira, Rodacki, Pereira, & Bento, 2018). A higher prevalence of disability, premature death, and reduced QOL among the population is associated with less physical activity (Booth et al., 2012). In these terms, expert groups around the world recommend physical exercise and/or nutritional intervention to prevent and treat sarcopenia, which dramatically deteriorates an older individual's independence and QOL (as discussed below in this chapter) (Dedeyne et al., 2020).

Moreover, lifelong physically active older adults seem to have better physiological functioning of their metabolic, skeletal, cardiovascular, and immune systems than those who used to exercise irregularly or not at all. When exercise does not exceed the individual's maximal physical potential, to avoid acute inflammation caused by tissue damage, regular exercise can activate intracellular quality control systems that lead to chronic inflammation suppression (Suzuki, 2019). However, this is not discouraging for people who were not habitually physically active earlier in their lives since physical activity exerts beneficial effects even in these populations.

Physical Activity and Sarcopenia

Both prevention and treatment of sarcopenia include increased physical-activity levels (Meier Lee, 2020). A growing body of evidence suggests that resistance exercise is the first and foremost therapeutic approach to prevent and reverse sarcopenia (Morley, Anker, & von Haehling, 2014; Nascimento et al., 2019). Based on a systematic review by the International Sarcopenia Initiative (EWGSOP and IWGS) exercise interventions are in position to augment muscle strength and improve physical performance, but there are not consistent evidence about the improvement of muscle mass in sedentary, community-dwelling older individuals (Cruz-Jentoft et al., 2014). Cross-sectional studies report that older adults who remain physically active, maintain higher levels of CRF, upper and lower body strength. Moreover, avoiding sedentary time is significantly associated with reduced odds of having low muscle mass and slow gait speed and consequently, sarcopenia (Meier & Lee, 2020). Reports also state that the practice of an even 6-week- long intervention programs with focus on strength training shows increase in muscle quality and,

consequently, functional capacity, in older women, insinuating that such strategies are feasible and effective in delaying muscle quality deterioration during aging (Nascimento et al., 2019). Strength training enables the release of hypertrophic factors and hormones that increase protein synthesis. In this way, it potentially benefits both muscle mass and function (Nascimento et al., 2019). Endurance training can also provide some benefits for sarcopenic individuals, through improving maximal oxygen consumption, oxidative capacity, mitochondrial density and activity as well as insulin sensitivity (Nascimento et al., 2019; Angulo, El Assar, Álvarez-Bustos, & Rodríguez-Mañas, 2020), which translates into better functional capacity (Angulo et al., 2020).

Physical Activity and Frailty

Although frailty is more of a dynamic than a static process, a transition to a more severe frailty is more common than improvement. (Clegg, Young, Iliffe, Rikkert, & Rockwood, 2013). Thus, detecting, grading severity and managing frailty can have large benefits for individuals, their families, and the broader community.

Exercise has physiological effects on all systems affected by frailty and must be used as a treatment for this age-related condition (Angulo et al., 2020). It can significantly improve functional capacity, decrease the risk of falls, and contribute to gait ability, balance, and cardio-respiratory capacity (Nascimento et al., 2019). Recommendations on the most appropriate exercise protocol for older individuals who deal with frailty remains unclear. The most frequently proposed physical interventions target multi-component physical-activity programs that address resistance, endurance, balance, and flexibility (Dent et al., 1957; Casas-herrero et al., 2019). A gradually progressive physical-activity program beginning with flexibility and balancing training, followed by resistance and endurance training is beneficial for physical function as it can lower the prevalence of frailty by 9% when practiced for 12 months (Walston, Buta, & Xue, 2018). A schematic of how physical activity influences the development of frailty is depicted in **Figure 11.5**.

The VIVIFRAIL Exercise Protocol

The VIVIFRAIL exercise protocol offers a general guideline for designing personalized, multi-component, physical activity programs for individuals over 70-years old who are affected by frailty. The program's design depends on their functional capacity level - serious, moderate, or slight limitations as indicated by short physical performance battery (SPPB) - a walking speed test and their risk of falling. It focuses on the following components of physical fitness: arm and length strength and power, balance and coordination, flexibility, and cardiovascular endurance (Casas-herrero et al., 2019).

A clinical trial in hospitalized patients conducted by Martínez-Velilla and his colleagues included a physical exercise protocol based on VIVIFRAIL with up to two daily sessions of 20 minutes each for 5 to 7 consecutive days per week under the

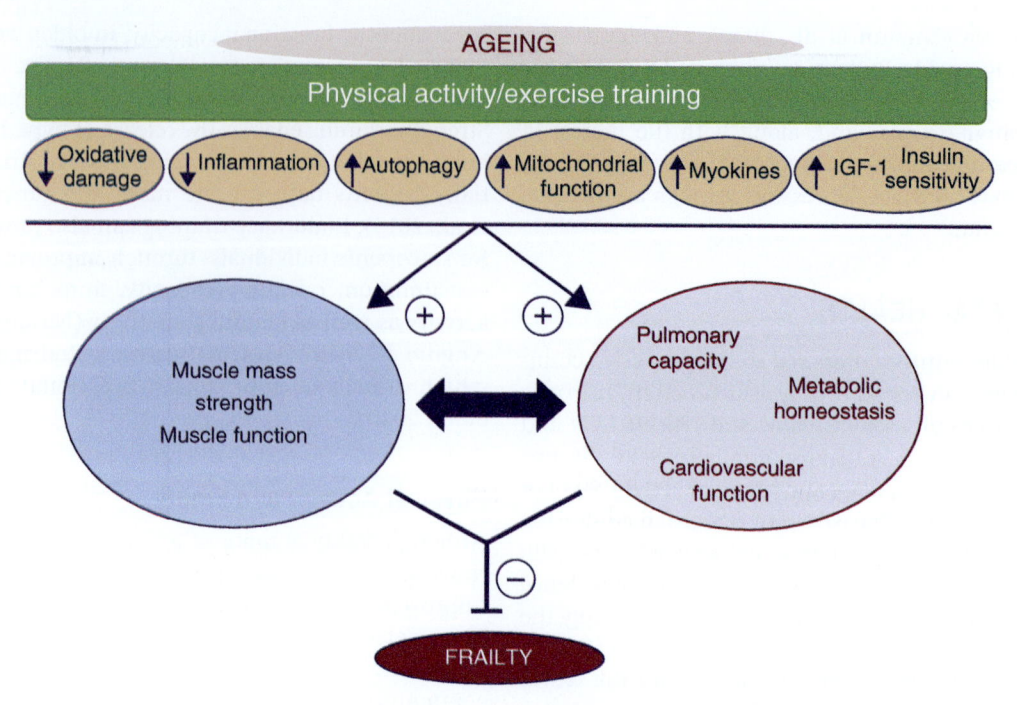

FIGURE 11.5 Physical activity/exercise training may influence the outcome of the aging process by modulating key signaling pathways. Exercising results in reduced age-related oxidative damage, reduced chronic inflammation, increased autophagy, improved mitochondrial function, improved myokine profile, augmented insulin-like growth factor-1 (IGF-1) signaling, and insulin sensitivity. These actions promote beneficial effects on skeletal muscle (muscle mass, strength, and function) but also at systemic level, inducing improvements in function of cardiovascular, respiratory, and metabolic systems. Exercise-induced improvements in muscle function as well as systemic benefits and age-related chronic diseases alleviation are all related to the improvements in physical function and frailty improvement by exercise/physical activity. Source: (Angulo et al., 2020 / with permission of Elsevier).

supervision of an experienced fitness specialist. According to the study results, the VIVIFRAIL protocol successfully prevented or minimized the risk of falling, increased normal gait speed, and improved cognitive, mood, and functional status (e.g., higher scores or performance in assessment tools like SPPB, and Barther's index) (Izquierdo et al., 2019). Interestingly, these physical exercise programs are more effective at reducing or postponing frailty when conducted in groups, highlighting an even greater positive effect of physical activity when approached as a window for social interaction (Nascimento et al., 2019).

Overall, evidence-based recommendations suggest that improvements in the physiologic and functional levels of frail populations can be reached within 8 to 48 weeks of training with a frequency of 1 to 6 sessions per week, volume of 1 to 3 sets, 6 to 15 repetitions, and an intensity of 30% to 70% maximum repetition, especially when conducted in groups (Nascimento et al., 2019).

Interventions that aim to improve the physical status of older adults, include personalized exercise programs, home modifications, or home- and community-based occupational therapy, that often include exercises to build strength, balance, coordination, flexibility, and aerobic fitness. These interventions can positively affect multiple physiological systems, functional capacity and rehabilitation in this population (Bangsbo et al., 2019). Studies show that improving individuals' performance in these domains has a high impact on reducing the number of falls and related injuries. According to the 2020 baseline report on healthy aging by the WHO, balance and functional exercises reduce the rate of falls by 24% and the number of people that experience one or more falls by 13% (WHO, 2020). These percentages are quite important, since approximately one-third of people over 65 fall annually, based on a 2020 review by Eckstrom et al. (Eckstrom, Neukam, Kalin, & Wright, 2020).

PHYSICAL ACTIVITY RECOMMENDATIONS FOR OLDER ADULTS

According to the American College of Sports Medicine (ACSM) Position Stand published in 2009, physical-activity maintenance in older adults contributes to healthier aging through better functional capabilities and better management of chronic diseases (Chodzko-Zajko et al., 2009). The guidelines for this population recommend a minimum of 150 minutes of physical activity per week to attain health benefits, since increasing the amount of physical activity through higher intensity, greater frequency, and/or longer duration confer even more benefits. The intensity and duration of physical activity should be low at the outset for older adults who are highly deconditioned, functionally limited, or have chronic conditions that affect their ability to perform physical tasks.

The progression of activities should be individual and tailored to tolerance and preference; a conservative approach may be necessary for the most deconditioned and physically limited older adults. Muscle-strengthening activities and/or balance training may need to precede aerobic training activities among very frail individuals. Older adults should exceed the recommended minimum amounts of physical activity if they desire to improve their fitness. If chronic conditions preclude activity at the recommended minimum amount, older adults should perform physical activities as tolerated so as to avoid being sedentary (Chodzko-Zajko et al., 2009).

The most current evidence from the 2020 WHO physical-activity guidelines reaffirms that all adults 18 years and older should regularly perform physical activity and that some physical activity is better than none. Recommendations regarding older adults (65 years and above) are identical to those for adults between 18 and 65 years of age as the evidence reviewed for this set of guidelines were gathered from studies without an upper age limit and therefore included adults who over the age of 65.

The adult guidelines include strong recommendations based on overall moderate-certainty evidence for weekly volumes of aerobic and muscle-strengthening physical activity. Many of the benefits of physical activity are observed within average weekly volumes of 150 to 300 min of moderate-intensity or 75 to 150 min of vigorous-intensity, or an equivalent combination of moderate-to-vigorous physical activity (MVPA). The weekly range of recommended aerobic-activity volume is a notable difference from the 2010 WHO recommendations that only specified minimum weekly thresholds. MVPA bouts of any duration now count toward these recommendations, reflecting new evidence supporting the value of total physical-activity volume, regardless of bout length. This recommendation differs from the WHO 2010 guidelines requiring bouts of at least 10 min.

In the 2020 guidelines, the WHO also stated that some physical activity is better than none. More specifically, it clarified that health benefits can be earned, even if an individual is not meeting the current recommendations (Bull et al., 2020). This agrees with the 2019 Copenhagen Consensus statement on physical activity and aging, which suggests that when it comes to physical-activity volume, benefits for older adults (i.e., better physical function and reduced premature mortality) can be reached even with lower intensity exercise than the oft-used guidelines of 150 min of moderate-to-vigorous intensity physical activity per week (Bangsbo et al., 2019). Furthermore, Canadian guidelines underscore that progression toward any of these targets will result in health benefits, even if the systematic following of these directions is expected to be challenging at times (Ross et al., 2020). Moreover, when addressing older adults in particular, the WHO suggests that they be as physically active as their current functional ability allows. It continues by emphasizing that their level of effort for physical activity should be relative to their level of fitness. As a consequence, a consult with a healthcare professional and/or a physical-activity specialist may be needed to determine the right type and amount of activity (Bull et al., 2020).

As far as older adults are concerned, the WHO declares that regular physical activity prevents falls and fall related injuries as well as declines in bone health and functional ability. This is beyond the health benefits that cover the spectrum of NCDs trajectories in older adults. For those over 65, there is a strong recommendation for weekly physical activity in the form of varied multi-component exercise programs that focus on functional balance and strength training at a moderate intensity for three or more days a week (Bull et al., 2020). This advice also aligns with direction from the Canadian 24-hour movement guidelines for adults aged 65 years or older (Ross et al., 2020). High-certainty evidence demonstrates that balance and functional exercises reduce the rate of falls and that engaging in a range of physical activities can help improve a wide range of elements of physical function. This guideline addresses all persons who are 65 years or older, which updates the 2010 guidelines that only suggested this combination of physical-activity exercises for older individuals with mobility problems (Bull et al., 2020; Chodzko-Zajko et al., 2009). For ideas on how to implement the recommended types of exercise in the everyday life of older adults, please read the Physical Activity Guidelines for Americans (see Further Reading).

KEY POINTS

- Being physically active is of major importance to maintain health and normal functions; physical inactivity causes permanent pathological changes, which leads over time to chronic diseases.
- Physical activity and inactivity are not mirror images; the first exerts its beneficial effects through different mechanisms than those used by the latter to negatively influence an individual's health outcome.
- Physical activity can significantly enhance the quality of everyday life in older adults by positively affecting cardio-respiratory fitness, immune, cognitive, and musculoskeletal function.
- To obtain health benefits in adults older than 18 years of age, public health organizations recommend that physical activity should have an average weekly volume of 150 to 300 min at a moderate intensity or 75 to 150 min at a vigorous intensity.
- For individuals older than 65, guidelines clarify that even when functional inability or other reason prevents one from meeting the recommended levels, healthy benefits can still be obtained through lower levels of physical exercise.
- For those over 65 is strongly recommended to implement at least one moderate-intensity, varied, and multi-component exercise program that focuses on functional balance, strength training, and aerobic capacity improvement on three or more days per week.
- Guidelines regarding the implementation of balance and functional training were recently updated, since these exercises were previously recommended only for older adults with mobility problems.

SELF-ASSESSMENT QUESTIONS

1. What is the current definition of physical inactivity?
2. How is the influence of physical inactivity differentiated from that of physical activity?
3. How can regular physical activity contribute to healthy aging?
4. Can physical activity be included in the therapeutic management of sarcopenia and frailty?
5. Circle the correct answer. What is the approximate percentage of people over 65 expected to experience a single fall during a one-year period?
   (a) 20%
   (b) 30%
   (c) 40%
6. Circle the correct answer. What percentage of people who experience one or more falls annually can be averted through systematic functional training?
   (a) 13%
   (b) 24%
   (c) 35%
7. Circle the correct answer. How much time is needed to gain physiologic and functional improvements through physical training in older adults?
   (a) 8–48 weeks
   (b) 4–44 weeks
   (c) 12–52 weeks
8. Circle the correct answer. What is the recommended frequency of physical-activity sessions to improve physical status in an older individual?
   (a) 1–2 days per week
   (b) 2–3 days per week
   (c) >3 days per week
9. Circle the correct answer. The VIVIFRAIL exercise protocol:
   (a) Addresses people of 70 years old and older.
   (b) Uses SPPB and hand-grip strength to assess an older person's functional ability.
   (c) Focuses on cardiovascular endurance and flexibility alone.
10. True or False: Balance and strength training is only necessary for older individuals who deal with mobility problems.
11. True or False: Aerobic training activities should precede balance or muscle-strengthening activities.
12. True or False: To gain health benefits, each physical-activity bout should last longer than 10 minutes.
13. True or False: Physical activity of any type, duration, or intensity can positively influence health and functionality.
14. True or False: The best health and functionality outcomes are acquired when the physical-activity programs are scheduled as 1:1 sessions (trainer and trainee only).

REFERENCES

Angulo, J., El Assar, M., Álvarez-Bustos, A., & Rodríguez-Mañas, L. (2020). Physical activity and exercise: Strategies to manage frailty. *Redox Biology*, *35*(January), 101513. https://doi.org/10.1016/j.redox.2020.101513

Bangsbo, J., Blackwell, J., Boraxbekk, C. J., Caserotti, P., Dela, F., Evans, A. B., . . . Viña, J. (2019). Copenhagen Consensus statement 2019: Physical activity and ageing. *British Journal of Sports Medicine*, *53*(14), 856–858. https://doi.org/10.1136/bjsports-2018-100451

Booth, F. W., Roberts, C. K., & Laye, M. J. (2012). Lack of exercise is a major cause of chronic diseases. *Comprehensive Physiology*, *2*(2), 1143–1211. https://doi.org/10.1002/cphy.c110025

Booth, F. W., Roberts, C. K., Thyfault, J. P., Ruegsegger, G. N., & Toedebusch, R. G. (2017). Role of inactivity in chronic diseases: Evolutionary insight and pathophysiological mechanisms. *Physiological Reviews*, *97*(4), 1351–1402. https://doi.org/10.1152/physrev.00019.2016

Bull, F. C., Al-Ansari, S. S., Biddle, S., Borodulin, K., Buman, M. P., Cardon, G., . . . Willumsen, J. F. (2020). World Health Organization 2020 guidelines on physical activity and sedentary behaviour. *British Journal of Sports Medicine*, *54*(24), 1451–1462. https://doi.org/10.1136/bjsports-2020-102955

Casas-herrero, A., Anton-rodrigo, I., Zambom-ferraresi, F., Asteasu, M. L. S. De, Martínez-Velilla, N., Elexpuru-estomba, J., . . . Ramon-espinoza, F. (2019). 13063_2019_Article_3426. 1–12.

Chaput, J. P., Dutil, C., Featherstone, R., Ross, R., Giangregorio, L., Saunders, T. J., . . . Carrier, J. (2020). Sleep duration and health in adults: an overview of systematic reviews. *Applied Physiology, Nutrition, and Metabolism = Physiologie Appliquee, Nutrition et Metabolisme*, *45*(10), S218–S231. https://doi.org/10.1139/apnm-2020-0034

Chodzko-Zajko, W. J., Proctor, D. N., Fiatarone Singh, M. A., Minson, C. T., Nigg, C. R., Salem, G. J., & Skinner, J. S. (2009). Exercise and physical activity for older adults. *Medicine and Science in Sports and Exercise*, *41*(7), 1510–1530. https://doi.org/10.1249/MSS.0b013e3181a0c95c

Clegg, A., Young, J., Iliffe, S., Rikkert, M. O., & Rockwood, K. (2013). Frailty in elderly people. *The Lancet*, *381*(9868), 752–762. https://doi.org/10.1016/S0140-6736(12)62167-9

Cruz-Jentoft, A. J., Landi, F., Schneider, S. M., Zúñiga, C., Arai, H., Boirie, Y., . . . Cederholm, T. (2014). Prevalence of and interventions for sarcopenia in ageing adults: A systematic review. Report of the International Sarcopenia Initiative (EWGSOP and IWGS). *Age and Ageing*, *43*(6), 48–759. https://doi.org/10.1093/ageing/afu115

Daskalopoulou, C., Stubbs, B., Kralj, C., Koukounari, A., Prince, M., & Prina, A. M. (2017). Physical activity and healthy ageing: A systematic review and meta-analysis of longitudinal cohort studies. *Ageing Research Reviews*, *38*, 6–17. https://doi.org/10.1016/j.arr.2017.06.003

Dedeyne, L., Dupont, J., Koppo, K., Verschueren, S., Tournoy, J., & Gielen, E. (2020). Exercise and Nutrition for Healthy AgeiNg (ENHANce) project – effects and mechanisms of action of combined anabolic interventions to improve physical functioning in sarcopenic older adults: study protocol of a triple blinded, randomized controlled trial. *BMC Geriatrics*, *20*(1), 1–14. https://doi.org/10.1186/s12877-020-01900-5

Dent, E., Morley, J. E., Woodhouse, L., Fried, L. P., Woo, J., Aprahamian, I., . . . Vellas, B. (1957). RAY COUNTY Memorial Hospital. *Hospital Management*, *83*(3), 44–45.

Eckstrom, E., Neukam, S., Kalin, L., & Wright, J. (2020). Physical Activity and Healthy Aging. *Clinics in Geriatric Medicine*, *36*(4), 671–683. https://doi.org/10.1016/j.cger.2020.06.009

Gremeaux, V., Gayda, M., Lepers, R., Sosner, P., Juneau, M., & Nigam, A. (2012). Exercise and longevity. *Maturitas*, *73*(4), 312–317. https://doi.org/10.1016/j.maturitas.2012.09.012

Gujral, S., Aizenstein, H., Reynolds, C. F., Butters, M. A., & Erickson, K. I. (2017). Exercise effects on depression: Possible neural mechanisms. *General Hospital Psychiatry*, *49*(April), 2–10. https://doi.org/10.1016/j.genhosppsych.2017.04.012

Izquierdo, M., Martínez-Velilla, N., Casas-Herrero, A., Zambom-Ferraresi, F., Sáez De Asteasu, M. L., Lucia, A., . . . Rodríguez-Mañas, L. (2019). Effect of Exercise Intervention on Functional Decline in Very Elderly Patients During Acute Hospitalization: A Randomized Clinical Trial. *JAMA Internal Medicine*, *179*(1), 28–36. https://doi.org/10.1001/jamainternmed.2018.4869

Kehler, D. S., & Theou, O. (2019). The impact of physical activity and sedentary behaviors on frailty levels. *Mechanisms of Ageing and Development*, *180*(November 2018), 29–41. https://doi.org/10.1016/j.mad.2019.03.004

Koehler, K., & Drenowatz, C. (2019). Integrated role of nutrition and physical activity for lifelong health. *Nutrients*, *11*(7), 10–12. https://doi.org/10.3390/nu11071437

Meier, N. F., & Lee, D. chul. (2020). Physical activity and sarcopenia in older adults. *Aging Clinical and Experimental Research*, *32*(9), 1675–1687. https://doi.org/10.1007/s40520-019-01371-8

Moreira, N. B., Rodacki, A. L. F., Pereira, G., & Bento, P. C. B. (2018). Does functional capacity, fall risk awareness and physical-activity level predict falls in older adults in different age groups? *Archives of Gerontology and Geriatrics*, *77*(March), 57–63. https://doi.org/10.1016/j.archger.2018.04.002

Morley, J. E., Anker, S. D., & von Haehling, S. (2014). Prevalence, incidence, and clinical impact of sarcopenia: facts, numbers, and epidemiology—update 2014. *Journal of Cachexia, Sarcopenia and Muscle*, *5*(4), 253–259. https://doi.org/10.1007/s13539-014-0161-y

Nascimento, C. M., Ingles, M., Salvador-Pascual, A., Cominetti, M. R., Gomez-Cabrera, M. C., & Viña, J. (2019). Sarcopenia, frailty and their prevention by exercise. *Free Radical Biology and Medicine*, *132*, 42–49. https://doi.org/10.1016/j.freeradbiomed.2018.08.035

Nuzum, H., Stickel, A., Corona, M., Zeller, M., Melrose, R. J., & Wilkins, S. S. (2020). Potential Benefits of Physical Activity in MCI and Dementia. *Behavioural Neurology*, *2020*. https://doi.org/10.1155/2020/7807856

Panagiotou, M., Michel, S., Meijer, J. H., & Deboer, T. (2021). The aging brain: sleep, the circadian clock and exercise. *Biochemical Pharmacology*, *191*(March), 114563. https://doi.org/10.1016/j.bcp.2021.114563

Pedersen, B. K., & Hoffman-Goetz, L. (2000). Exercise and the immune system: Regulation, integration, and adaptation. *Physiological Reviews*, *80*(3), 1055–1081. https://doi.org/10.1152/physrev.2000.80.3.1055

Ross, R., Chaput, J. P., Giangregorio, L. M., Janssen, I., Saunders, T. J., Kho, M. E., . . . Tremblay, M. S. (2020). Canadian 24-Hour Movement Guidelines for Adults aged 18-64 years and Adults aged 65 years or older: an integration of physical activity, sedentary behaviour, and sleep. *Applied Physiology, Nutrition, and Metabolism = Physiologie Appliquee, Nutrition et Metabolisme*, *45*(10), S57–S102. https://doi.org/10.1139/apnm-2020-0467

Scartoni, F. R., Sant'Ana, L. de O., Murillo-Rodriguez, E., Yamamoto, T., Imperatori, C., Budde, H., . . . Machado, S. (2020). Physical Exercise and Immune System in the Elderly: Implications and Importance in COVID-19 Pandemic Period. *Frontiers in Psychology*, *11*(November). https://doi.org/10.3389/fpsyg.2020.593903

Simpson, R. J., Lowder, T. W., Spielmann, G., Bigley, A. B., LaVoy, E. C., & Kunz, H. (2012). Exercise and the aging immune system. *Ageing Research Reviews*, *11*(3), 404–420. https://doi.org/10.1016/j.arr.2012.03.003

Suzuki, K. (2019). Chronic inflammation as an immunological abnormality and effectiveness of exercise. *Biomolecules*, *9*(6), 3–7. https://doi.org/10.3390/biom9060223

Thijssen, D. H. J., Maiorana, A. J., O'Driscoll, G., Cable, N. T., Hopman, M. T. E., & Green, D. J. (2010). Impact of inactivity and exercise on the vasculature in humans. *European Journal of Applied Physiology*, *108*(5), 845–875. https://doi.org/10.1007/s00421-009-1260-x

Thyfault, J. P., Du, M., Kraus, W. E., Levine, J. A., & Booth, F. W. (2015). Physiology of sedentary behavior and its relationship to health outcomes. *Medicine and Science in Sports and Exercise*, *47*(6), 1301–1305. https://doi.org/10.1249/MSS.0000000000000518

Walston, J., Buta, B., & Xue, Q. L. (2018). Frailty Screening and Interventions: Considerations for Clinical Practice. *Clinics in Geriatric Medicine*, *34*(1), 25–38. https://doi.org/10.1016/j.cger.2017.09.004

WHO. (2020). Decade of Healthy Ageing: baseline report. In *World Health Organization*.

FURTHER READING

Bibliography

B. K. Pedersen and B. Saltin, (2015). Exercise as medicine - Evidence for prescribing exercise as therapy in 26 different chronic diseases. *Scand. J. Med. Sci. Sport.*, *25*: 1–72. doi: 10.1111/sms.12581.

C. López-Otín, et al., (2013). The hallmarks of aging. *Cell 153* (6): 1194. doi: 10.1016/j.cell.2013.05.039.

US Department of Health and Human Services (2008). Physical activity guidelines for Americans, *Okla. Nurse*, *53* (4): 25. doi: 10.1249/fit.0000000000000472.

How much physical activity do older adults need? (2022, June 03). Retrieved October 25, 2022, from https://www.cdc.gov/physicalactivity/basics/older_adults/index.htm

Go4Life Exercise Videos (National Institute of Health on Aging); [Video file]. (n.d.). Retrieved October 25, 2022, from https://www.youtube.com/user/NatlInstituteOnAging

Vivifrail. (n.d.). Retrieved October 25, 2022, from https://vivifrail.com/resources/

Cardiovascular Health, Diet, and Physical Activity

UNIT 4

Heart Failure

CHAPTER 12

Introduction	171
Definition	172
Classification	172
Prevalence	173
Clinical Conditions Associated with Heart Failure	175
Obesity	175
Obesity Paradox	175
Malnutrition and Sarcopenia Heart Failure Patients	175
Diabetes and Heart Failure	176
Heart Failure in Older Adults	176
Cognitive Impairment in Patients with Heart Failure	176
Therapeutic Management of Heart Failure	176
Lifestyle Factors and Heart Failure	177
Body Weight and Caloric Restriction	177
Nutrition and Dietary Approaches	177
Sodium Restriction	177
Fluid Restriction	179
Dietary Patterns	179
DASH Diet	180
Mediterranean Diet	180
Nutritional Supplements	181
Thiamine Supplementation	181
Iron Supplementation	181
Essential Amino Acids Supplementation	181
Omega-3 Poly-unsaturated Fatty Acid Supplementation	181
Physical Activity and Exercise for Heart Failure Prevention and Therapy	182
Physical Activity and Heart Failure	182
Physical Inactivity and Heart Failure	182
Exercise Training in Heart Failure	183
Intensity of Exercise in Patients with Heart Failure	184
Type of Exercise in Patients with Heart Failure	184
Tailored Exercise Advice in Patients with Heart Failure	185
Key Points	185
Self-assessment Questions	186
Case Scenario	187
References	187
Further Reading	189
Bibliography	189
Links	189

INTRODUCTION

Heart failure (HF) is a major part of the cardiovascular disease spectrum. The American College of Cardiology/American Heart Association guidelines define HF as a "complex clinical syndrome that can result from any structural or functional cardiac disorder that impairs the ability of the ventricle to fill or eject blood." HF is a set of complex and heterogeneous conditions with underlying variability in etiology, pathophysiology, metabolic, and other individual factors that constitutes an end stage of several cardiovascular disorders, coronary heart disease (CHD) and hypertension being the most common in the Western world. The classification of HF is based on different etiologies and their associated mechanistic disturbances of

Prevention and Management of Cardiovascular and Metabolic Disease: Diet, Physical Activity and Healthy Aging,
First Edition. Christina N. Katsagoni, Peter Kokkinos, and Labros S. Sidossis.
© 2023 John Wiley & Sons Ltd. Published 2023 by John Wiley & Sons Ltd.

cardiac function. The prevalence of HF is high and is increasing over time due to an increasing older adult population and an improved survival as well as to the increase in the prevalence of relevant to HF risk factors such as obesity and diabetes. A range of interventions can help improve quality of life (QOL) as well as reduce hospital admissions and mortality in chronic heart failure (CHF), including pharmacological, medical, and lifestyle. Nutrition is a critical factor in the incidence and progression of HF. Related features to HF are obesity, sarcopenia, sarcopenia in combination with obesity or weight loss (even tissue loss of both lean and fat mass, e.g., cachexia), dietary approaches such as restricting sodium and fluids as well as dietary plans such as the Mediterranean diet (MD) and Dietary Approaches to Stop Hypertension (DASH) diet. CHF is characterized by reduced functional ability, severe exercise intolerance, reduced QOL, increased dependence to complete daily activities, and an increased risk of adverse events. Physical activity (PA), generally, has a positive effect on many CHD and HF risk factors, such as hypertension. Exercise plays an important role in the development of HF, as it seems to have a protective role by positively affecting HF in secondary prevention and influencing the prognosis of HF in the *future for HF* patients.

DEFINITION

HF is a major part of the cardiovascular disease spectrum. American College of Cardiology/American Heart Association guidelines define HF as a "complex clinical syndrome that can result from any structural or functional cardiac disorder that impairs the ability of the ventricle to fill or eject blood" (Yancy et al., 2013). HF is a set of complex and heterogeneous conditions with underlying variability in etiology, pathophysiology, metabolic, and other individual factors that constitutes an end stage of several cardiovascular disorders, CHD and hypertension being the most common in the Western world (Lindgren & Börjesson, 2021). As a clinical syndrome, the diagnosis of HF is based on three cornerstones: typical symptoms (including shortness of breath, ankle swelling, orthopnea, lower limb swelling, and chronic fatigue), signs (jugular vein stasis, pulmonary crackles, and pitting edema), and results from relevant diagnostic tests (e.g., electrocardiogram, transthoracic echocardiography, serum natriuretic peptides) that can be linked to cardiac dysfunction (Ponikowski et al., 2016), often caused by a structural and/or functional cardiac abnormality that results in reduced cardiac output and/or elevated intracardiac pressures (Ponikowski et al., 2016). It is a complicated clinical syndrome regarding the implications in terms of mortality and morbidity of patients with HF as well as the plan for medical care. Many epidemiologic studies have relied on clinical diagnostic criteria for its identification. These criteria include the Framingham, Boston, Gothenburg, and cardiovascular health study criteria, all of which have relatively similar performance characteristics for the detecting HF with a high sensitivity compared with cardiologist evaluation (Dharmarajan & Rich, 2017).

CLASSIFICATION

The classification of HF is based on different etiologies and their associated mechanistic disturbances of cardiac function. HF incidence is divided according to left ventricular ejection fraction (LVEF), an echocardiographic estimate of left ventricular systolic function. LVEF is a strong marker for underlying pathophysiology as well as a marker for sensitivity to pharmacotherapy (Lindgren & Börjesson, 2021). The classification also depends on the level of LVEF, therefore an LVEF < 40% is classified as HF-reduced ejection fraction (HFrEF), whereas an LVEF of 50% is classified as HF-preserved ejection fraction (HFpEF).

Furthermore, HF could be characterized as a chronic state or an acute state. CHF is characterized by the reduced ability of the heart to pump and/or fill with blood, which results in fatigue, dyspnea, and exercise intolerance. Patients with CHF often have reduced functional capacity and a decreased QOL; the main causes for CHF are mentioned below (**Table 12.1**) (de Gregorio, 2018).

Patients with acute heart failure (AHF) have a less well-understood presentation and management of the disease. AHF is a clinical diagnosis based on symptoms and signs of fluid overload, with or without evidence of hypoperfusion, which may be supported by radiological evidence (pulmonary congestion on chest X-ray) and biochemical markers (like B-type natriuretic peptide, BNP, or N-terminal pro-BNP). AHF is characterized by a rapid onset, with new or worsening signs and symptoms that are potentially life-threatening, and patients require immediate hospitalization. Although AHF may be the reason for hospitalization, usually a pre-existing cardiomyopathy persists that foretells a poor prognosis with a high risk of readmission and death post-discharge. For clinical and hemodynamic characteristics, older guidelines by the European Society of Cardiology classified patients with AHF into one of the below mentioned six groups (I–VI) (**Table 12.2**) (Kurmani & Squire, 2017).

Table 12.1 Main causes of chronic left heart failure.

With left ventricular ventilation
Ischemic heart disease and previous myocardial infarction
Primary or secondary dilated cardiomyopathy
Previous myocarditis
End-stage hypertensive heart disease
End-stage hypertrophic cardiomyopathy
Aortic regurgitation
Without left ventricular dilatation
Hypertensive heart disease
Ischemic heart disease
Hypertrophic cardiomyopathy
Left ventricular (pseudo)hypertrophy from storage/infiltrative/systemic disease
Restrictive cardiomyopathy

Source: (de Gregorio, 2018).

Table 12.2 Classification of patients with acute heart failure into one of six groups (I–VI), according to clinical conditions.

Category	Signs
Acute decompensated HF (ADHF) (I)	With signs and symptoms of acute heart failure (AHF), which are mild and do not complete criteria for cardiogenic shock, pulmonary oedema or hypertensive crisis.
Hypertensive AHF (II)	Of HF together with high blood pressure and relatively preserved left ventricular function with a chest radiograph compatible with acute pulmonary oedema.
AHF with pulmonary oedema (III)	Of severe respiratory distress, with crackles over the lung and orthopnoea.
Cardiogenic shock (IV)	Of reduced blood pressure (systolic BP <90 mmHg or a drop of mean arterial pressure >30 mmHg) and/or low urine output (0.5 ml/kg/h). The pulse rate is over 60 beats per minute, with or without evidence of organ congestion.
High output failure (V)	Of high cardiac output, commonly with high heart rate as a result of arrhythmias, thyrotoxicosis, anaemia, Paget's disease, iatrogenic or by other mechanisms.
Right-sided HF (VI)	Of low output syndrome with increased jugular venous pressure, liver size and hypotension.

Source: (Adapted from Kurmani & Squire, 2017).

This classification system focuses on the treatment decision of the physician to manage the underlying cause of AHF. However, AHF patients may be also classified according to their initial clinical symptoms and signs for the attending physician to identify those most at risk and direct specific interventions. A usual marker is the level of systolic blood pressure (SBP) upon admission. Less than 10% of patients present with systolic hypotension (SBP < 90 mm Hg) which carries with it a poor prognosis and thereby leads the management of these patients to higher dependency areas with more aggressive therapy. Furthermore, there are also recent guidelines from the European Society of Cardiology.

A more comprehensive method to classify patients presenting with AHF was developed by Stevenson and colleagues (Nohria et al., 2003), who used the severity of presentation rather than the underlying etiology. This method is based on the initial clinical assessment of the patient to consider signs and symptoms of congestion (orthopnea, dependent edema, elevated jugular venous pulsation) and peripheral perfusion (cold extremities, oliguria, and narrow pulse pressure). Moreover, patients are described as either 'wet' or 'dry' depending on their fluid status and either 'cold' or 'warm' depending on the assessment of their perfusion status. This combined clinical assessment identifies four groups of patients (warm and wet, warm and dry, cold and dry, and cold and wet) that not only allow for initial stratification as a guide to therapy (**Figure 12.1**) but also carries with it prognostic information. Warm and dry patients have a 6-month mortality rate of 11% compared to 40% for the cold and wet profile (Nohria et al., 2003). As a practical measure, this method of classification and risk stratification is a prudent step in AHF management. However, compared to CHF, therapy that improves long-term survival following admission with AHF, although characterized by a distinctive set of signs and symptoms, is a major challenge in classifying AHF as a single entity is that the patient population is not uniform. Most patients with AHF lie between these extremes and therefore also demonstrate a distribution of underlying pathology and precipitants, leading to the common endpoint of fluid overload.

PREVALENCE

The prevalence of HF is high and increasing over time. It was estimated that 2% to 4% of the general adult population, corresponding to more than 60 million people worldwide, have HF, and it is characterized by a low 5-year survival of 35–55% (Lindgren et al., 2017). However, there might be an underestimation of HF disease, since patients older than 65 years with asymptomatic left ventricular (LV) systolic dysfunction is 5.5% (Wickman et al., 2021). Generally, the increase in HF prevalence worldwide could be explained by an increase in older adult population and improved survival as well as an increase in the prevalence of HF-related risk factors such as increased obesity and diabetes melitus (DM) (Dharmarajan & Rich, 2017). This could also explain the increase in the prevalence of HF in younger individuals who have a high body-mass index (BMI) and characterize HF as an important component of non-communicable diseases (Groenewegen et al., 2020). According to specific age ranges from NHANES data, in men over 18 years of age and specifically between 40 and 59 years present with a proportion of HF at 1.5%, with 6.6% in ages 60 to 79 years of age, and 10.6% in people 80 years and older, whereas women in the same age ranges are 1.2%, 4.8%, and 13.5%, respectively. **Figure 12.2** shows that for women 80 years and older, HF is of higher prevalence compared to men of the same age (Dharmarajan & Rich, 2017).

Regarding the epidemiology of AHF, the data derive from large-scale registries in the USA and Europe, which demonstrate that patients are mostly men diagnosed at a mean age of more than 70 years, and thus, are related to ischemic heart disease and CHF. Additionally, 66% to 75% of these patients do not have de novo AHF, on the contrary, they already had a previous history of HF, which was identified during their hospitalization, and many also were diagnosed with a co-morbid disease such as DM (≥ 40% in some registries) and chronic obstructive pulmonary disease (COPD) (almost 20% of patients). Most of these registries show a difference in hospital mortality rate depending on the age, from 4% to 7%, which rises to 12% for

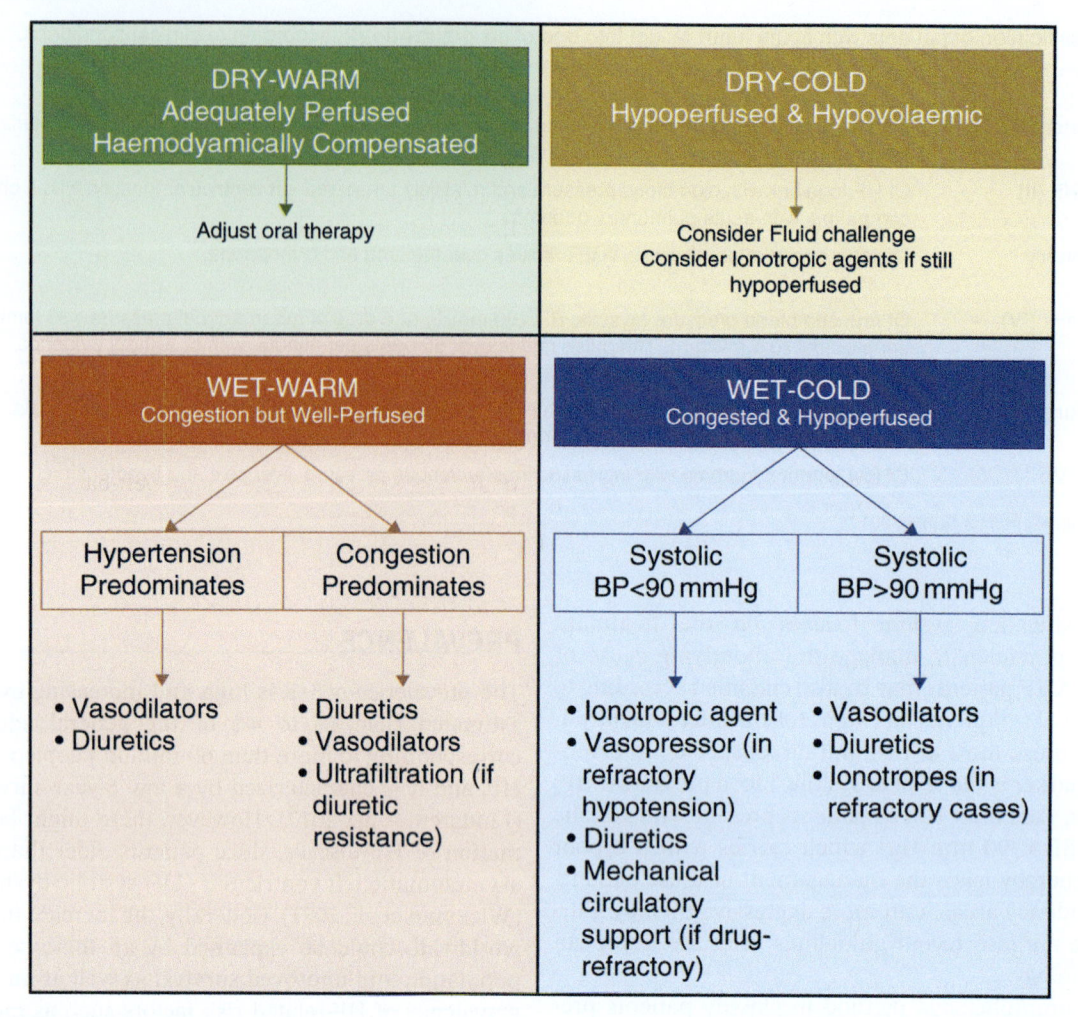

DRY-WARM Adequately Perfused Haemodyamically Compensated	DRY-COLD Hypoperfused & Hypovolaemic
↓ Adjust oral therapy	↓ Consider Fluid challenge Consider Ionotropic agents if still hypoperfused
WET-WARM Congestion but Well-Perfused	**WET-COLD** Congested & Hypoperfused
Hypertension Predominates / Congestion Predominates	Systolic BP<90 mmHg / Systolic BP>90 mmHg
• Vasodilators • Diuretics ——— • Diuretics • Vasodilators • Ultrafiltration (if diuretic resistance)	• Ionotropic agent • Vasopressor (in refractory hypotension) • Diuretics • Mechanical circulatory support (if drug-refractory) ——— • Vasodilators • Diuretics • Ionotropes (in refractory cases)

FIGURE 12.1   Layering patients with AHF according to their initial clinical presentation, and perfusion status, i.e., COLD or WARM and degree of fluid congestion (WET or DRY). Adapted from 2016 ESC guidelines.

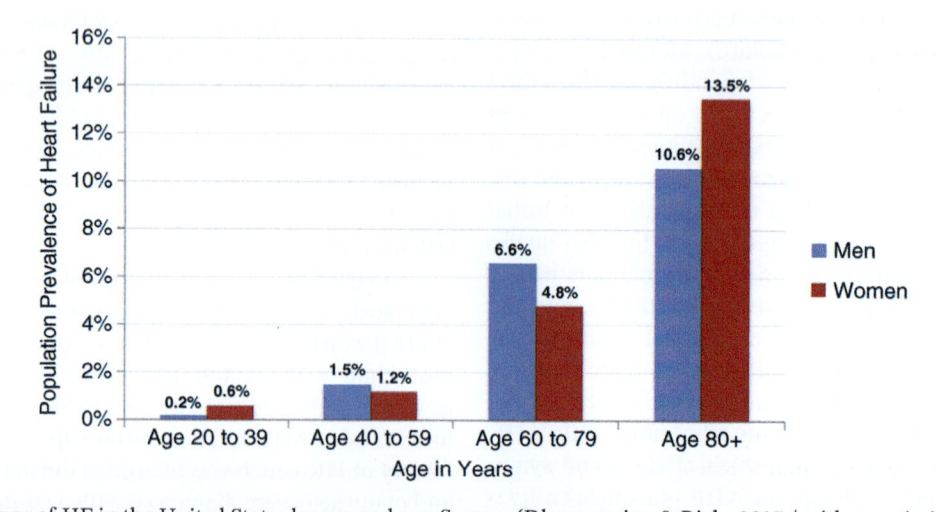

FIGURE 12.2   Prevalence of HF in the United States by age and sex. Source: (Dharmarajan & Rich, 2017 / with permission of Elsevier).

patients aged 75 years. Mortality after hospitalization was also high and appears not to have improved significantly over the past decade. Furthermore, in terms of cardiovascular death and hospitalizations, there is a difference between patients with HFpEF and HFrEF, probably due to the fact that no treatment convincingly reduces mortality or morbidity in HFpEF (Kurmani & Squire, 2017).

CLINICAL CONDITIONS ASSOCIATED WITH HEART FAILURE

Patients diagnosed with HF have a poor prognosis and are characterized by a poor nutritional status that can influence the disease's development and progression. Related features to HF are obesity, sarcopenia, sarcopenia in combination with obesity or weight loss (even tissues loss of both lean and fat mass, e.g., cachexia). Regarding the weight loss, which causes many nutritional deficiencies, it could be the result of different etiologies, including what was suggested two decades ago, that HF patients present a hypercatabolic state that results in a chronic negative energy balance and protein-calorie malnutrition (Aggarwal et al., 2018).

HFpEF is more prevalent with metabolic syndrome (MetS) and cardiac hypertrophy. Insulin resistance is involved in the development of HF and cardiac hypertrophy and is correlated with hypertension, coronary artery disease, LV hypertrophy, DM, and obesity (Aggarwal et al., 2018). HF is related to hypertension, type 2 diabetes mellitus (T2D), chronic inflammation, coronary artery disease, sarcopenia, and obesity, so it is important to study possible nutrition recommendations regarding prevention as well as HF therapy to improve clinical outcomes (Billingsley et al., 2019).

OBESITY

Overweight, obesity, and abdominal obesity, in particular, are implicated as independent risk factors for the development of cardiovascular disease, including HF. Concerning the impact of obesity on the incidence of HF, a higher BMI in midlife enhances the risk of HF in later life, and a 30% hypothetical reduction in obesity/overweight would potentially prevent 8.5% of HF events.

Moreover, the American Heart Association has recognized obesity as a qualifying risk factor for HF and released a specific scientific statement on HF prevention, thus recommending the maintenance of normal weight as one way to prevent HF.

OBESITY PARADOX

Despite the unfavorable impact that obesity has on risk factors for CHD, and other cardiovascular diseases (CVD) such as hypertension, HF and atrial fibrillation, several studies and metanalysis have demonstrated the so called "obesity paradox," which indicates that once CVD (including HF) becomes established, patients with overweight and obesity have a better prognosis than do their lean counterparts with the same CVD.

Oreopoulos et al., (Oreopoulos et al., 2008) reviewed 29,000 patients from nine major HF studies and demonstrated reductions in CVD and total mortality of 19% and 16% in those overweight, and 40% and 33% in those with obesity, compared with normal-weight patients with HF, even after adjusting for well-known risk factors. In patients with dilated cardiomyopathy at the first-onset of decompensated HF, the group with patients suffering from obesity had an improved LVEF versus patients without obesity after treatment for one year, and a multivariate regression analysis revealed that independent predictors of LVEF improvement after 12 months were nuclear diameter and absence of myofilament lysis in heart biopsies, in part from the effect of diuretics (Lavie et al., 2012).

However, even in patients with obesity, body weight could be reduced by following a well-balanced hypocaloric diet (Carbone et al., 2019).

MALNUTRITION AND SARCOPENIA HEART FAILURE PATIENTS

Normal weight is important in HF, as underweight patients or those with lean sarcopenia are associated with advanced HF and poor outcomes. These conditions may lead to a reduction of cardiac output and eventually predispose HF patients to complications, including higher rates of hospital (re)admissions and mortality. Malnutrition is a common sign in HF patients, especially in severe HF, reaching 30% to 70% of HF patients (Rahman et al., 2016). It results from a series of pathophysiological mechanisms based on an imbalance between anabolism and catabolism, neurohormonal factors, intestinal edema, sense of anorexia, and pathogenic effects of HF progression. A chronic state of malnutrition in HF patients increases the risk for developing cardiac cachexia, characterized as unintentional edema-free weight loss through loss of muscle, fat, and bone mass, which is strongly associated with decreased health-related QOL and increased mortality (Ishikawa & Sattler, 2021).

Intestinal edema-induced malabsorption and anorexia with inadequate food consumption cause a series of macronutrient and micronutrient deficiencies, e.g., in vitamins B, C, D as well as low levels of calcium, selenium, zinc, iron, and coenzyme Q10 (CoQ10) (Wickman et al., 2021). Sarcopenia that generally presents in 5% to 20% of the population greater than 60 years of age and even more (50%) in patients more than 80 years was also seen in individuals with high fat mass, a condition known as sarcopenic obesity. HF patients with sarcopenia may be in a worse situation than patients with cachexia and have a more pronounced decline in CRF and QOL. Increased protein intake, creatine, the amino acid leucine, vitamin D, and n-3 PUFA were proposed for treatment but there are still no firm recommendations (Billingsley et al., 2019). A very low BMI (< 18 kg/m^2), is linked to macro- and micronutrient deficiencies and it could be of benefit for these patients to follow a hypercaloric (35–40 kcal/kg/day), high-protein diet (1.5 g/kg body weight), with a fat content of 1.0–1.5 g/kg/body weight and a high-carbohydrate intake of almost 4–5 g/kg of body weight, in the context of a healthy diet pattern like MD or DASH diet (Bianchi, 2020).

DIABETES AND HEART FAILURE

A number of cohort studies have evaluated the associations between DM and HF, with most of them showing a positive correlation and only a few no association.

In the systematic review and meta-analysis by Aune et al., (Aune et al., 2018) conducted in 2018, 77 prospective studies (e.g., population- and patient-based studies) were included, aiming to investigate associations between diabetes and blood glucose and HF risk. According to the results, a diabetes diagnosis was associated with a twofold increase in HF risk in the general population, while in the patient-based studies, a 69% increase in the relative risk (RR) of HF. Considering the type of diabetes, T1D was associated with a 3.6-fold increase in HF risk. Moreover, the RR of HF was associated with an increase of 23% per 20mg/dl increase in blood glucose, in population-based studies. In total, a nonlinear, J-shaped association was revealed between blood glucose and HF risk. In another meta-analysis by Ohkuma et al., (Ohkuma, Komorita, Peters, & Woodward, 2019) with data from 47 cohorts including 12,142,998 individuals and 253,260 heart failure events, T2D was associated with a 9% greater HF risk in women than men (Ohkuma et al., 2019).

The mechanisms that could explain the increased risk of HF observed in patients with diabetes include risk factors that are common in diabetes and HF. In particular, diabetes increases the risk of hypertension, CHD, and atrial fibrillation, conditions that are strongly related to HF. Moreover, diabetes is linked to the development of diabetic cardiomyopathy, which is characterized by microangiopathy, myocardial fibrosis, and autonomic neuropathy and makes the heart unable function properly (Aune et al., 2018).

HEART FAILURE IN OLDER ADULTS

HF is often observed in older adults, and this seems largely related to the high prevalence of traditional cardiovascular risk factors (e.g., CHD, diabetes, obesity) in this population (Dharmarajan & Rich, 2017).

Epidemiological prospective data support an increased risk of HF in older adults that could be attributed by 13.1% to the CHD and 12.8% to the SBPs greater than 140 mm Hg found in this population. Both the atherosclerosis risk in communities study (Folsom, Yamagishi, Hozawa, & Chambless, 2009) and NHANES study (He et al., 2001) have confirmed these results, showing also that diabetes and obesity are responsible for a significant proportion of HF incidence.

The higher prevalence of HF in the elderly is also associated with age-associated changes in cardiovascular structure and function including diminishing chronotropic and inotropic responses, raising intracardiac pressures with ventricular filling, and increasing afterload. These conditions result in reducing the ability of the heart to respond to stress, whether that stress is physiologic (e.g., exercise) or pathologic (e.g., myocardial ischemia or sepsis) (Dharmarajan & Rich, 2017).

COGNITIVE IMPAIRMENT IN PATIENTS WITH HEART FAILURE

Cognitive impairment is common in HF and is approximately found in 40% of patients, in contrast to the general population where prevalence ranges from 16% to 20%.

Apart from the age-related cognitive decline that older adults are at risk of, namely Alzheimer's disease and other etiologies of dementia, they are also at risk for HF-related cognitive impairment (recently termed "cardio-cerebral syndrome"). This syndrome refers to cardiac dysfunction due to varying brain injuries, e.g., stroke. Cognitive impairment may be severe or mild severity evolving into dementia (representing a significant decline from prior level of function), and to more severe dementia (marked by significant impairment that interferes with activities of daily living) (Gorodeski et al., 2018). Cognitive impairment in patients with HF is associated with poor outcomes namely worse QOL, family member/caregiver distress, increased disability, high hospital readmission risk and mortality risk.

The mechanisms for cognitive impairment in older adults with HF are complex and involve several parameters. Some of them include reduced cardiac output; a high burden of cardiovascular risk factors; other neurohormonal, nutritional, and inflammatory mechanisms; and sleep apnea (more in **Chapter 19**) (Gorodeski et al., 2018).

Frailty (more in **Unit 3**) is extremely common in older adults with HF, and it is not related to age or functional classification. In a recent metanalysis (Denfeld et al., 2017) of 26 studies involving 6896 patients with HF, the overall estimated prevalence of frailty in HF was 44.5%, while it was not associated with age or functional class. In fact, frailty was high among studies with younger HF patients. The mechanisms through which frailty could be explained in patients with HF include interrelationships between neurohormonal dysregulation, inflammation, and skeletal muscle dysfunction, which have been noted to also parallel the pathogenesis of HF (Denfeld et al., 2017).

THERAPEUTIC MANAGEMENT OF HEART FAILURE

A range of interventions can help improve QOL, reduce hospital admissions, and mortality in CHF, such as pharmacological (e.g., angiotensin II receptor blockers, diuretics, beta-blockers, cardiac glycosides, and anticoagulants), medical (cardiac resynchronization therapy), and lifestyle (smoking cessation, dietary changes, and exercise) (Billingsley et al., 2019). According to the type, for HFrEF there is a standardized approach for treatment despite the heterogeneity of etiologies, whereas, for HFpEF there is not a specific treatment due to the difficulty in identifying phenotyping subgroups with differential responses to therapy and cohorts for personalized interventions (Wickman et al., 2021). A range of exercise frequencies, intensities, modalities, and durations are reported for the management of CHF.

Regarding AHF, to date, there is little information as to the therapy guidelines that may improve long-term outcomes since patients remain heterogeneity and present at different stages of decompensation of cardiac function. For AHF, the pharmacological treatment (loop diuretics, vasodilators, and inotropes) has remained largely unchanged since the 1970s and is predominantly aimed at correcting hemodynamic compromise and fluid overload with no standard therapy. Patients with AHF are treated according to their clinical condition and is largely based on factors such as SBP and renal function. In this case, structured exercise training is also recommended and should be an integral part of the treatment pathway (Billingsley et al., 2019).

LIFESTYLE FACTORS AND HEART FAILURE

HF patients should remain functional before and after hospitalizations and succeed at QOL. There are various factors involved to reinforce this (**Table 12.3**) (de Gregorio, 2018).

Unhealthy dietary models, body weight and consumption of low nutritional quality foods, low PA, and mental stress, may influence the rapidly changing epidemiology of HF, as shown in **Figure 12.3** (Aggarwal et al., 2018) and **Figure 12.4** (de Gregorio, 2018).

Table 12.3 Essential factors for Cardiac Rehabilitation (CR) programs.

People's need centered
Refining patient's ability and skills for daily routines
Encouraging social activities and return to work
Enabling patient's psychological course
Improving people's relationship with relatives
Responding to changes in people's needs
Taking patients part of their therapy
Helping patients to change lifestyle
Providing interdisciplinary team counseling
Reducing re-hospitalization and clinical outcomes

Source: (de Gregorio, 2018).

BODY WEIGHT AND CALORIC RESTRICTION

A high BMI results in metabolic and neurohormonal pathways that increase the risk for HF (**Figure 12.5**) (Bianchi, 2020) as well as the symptomatology, so weight loss in overweight and patients with obesity and HF may prevent further progression of the disease, improve cardiac function, improve symptoms, and decrease the possibility of hospitalization (Billingsley et al., 2019). Obesity increases specifically the risk of HFpEF, due to HF signs in the presence of a normal LVEF (Carbone et al., 2019). A review by Bianchi (Bianchi, 2020), indicates that although following a controlled diet is still inconclusive regarding heart function and clinical outcomes in patients with CHF, it is important to succeed in reducing body weight, thus insulin activity and glucose regulation on the basis of a dietary plan. Thus, HF patients with an increased BMI could attempt a reduction in body weight by an average reduction in energy intake of 20% to 30% of their usual daily caloric intake, with a macromolecule composition of 1.5 g/kg bodyweight for protein, 3–4 g/kg/body weight for carbohydrates, and 0.8–1.0 g/kg body weight for fat, because this will also improve insulin activity and glucose control. Such a diet should include lifestyle interventions and there must be great caution so as not to lose fat-free mass.

NUTRITION AND DIETARY APPROACHES

SODIUM RESTRICTION

There is strong scientific evidence from clinical trials and meta-analyses that salt restriction may prevent hypertension, stroke, and CVD, but not for the role of sodium restriction in reducing the incidence of HF. The current primary dietary approaches for HF management include sodium and fluid restriction, but individualization to patient needs is essential as multiple variables need to be considered in advanced HF. Strict

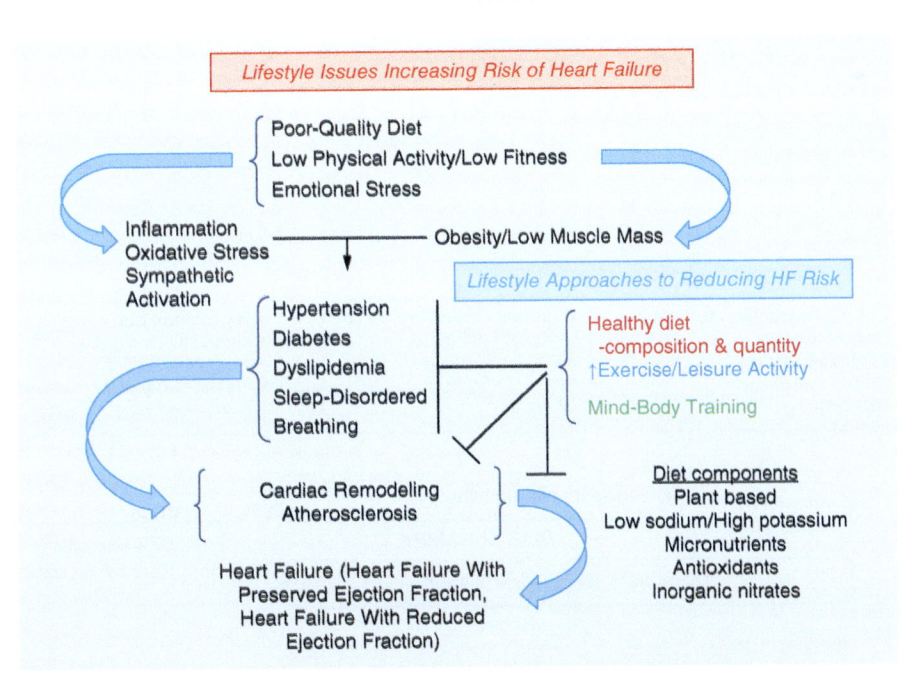

FIGURE 12.3 How lifestyle factors may influence the development of HF and possible therapeutic interventions. Source: (Aggarwal et al., 2018 / with permission of Elsevier).

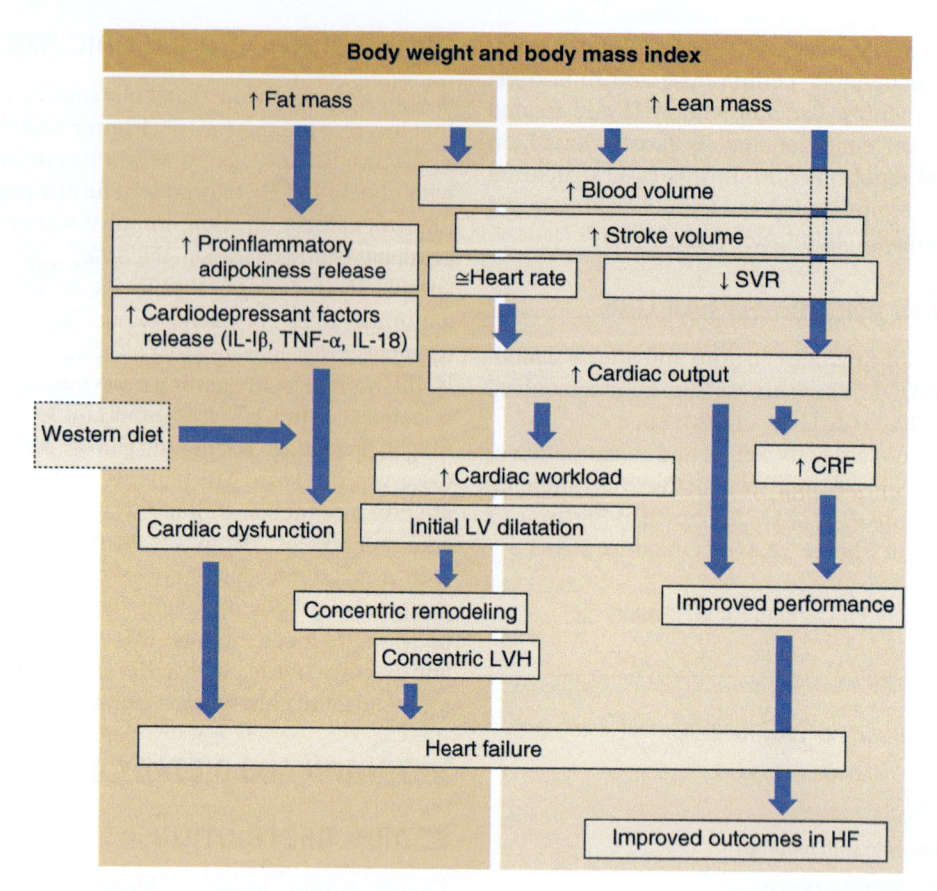

FIGURE 12.4 Proposed mechanisms for the relation between body composition and HF. Source: (Adapted from de Gregorio, 2018).

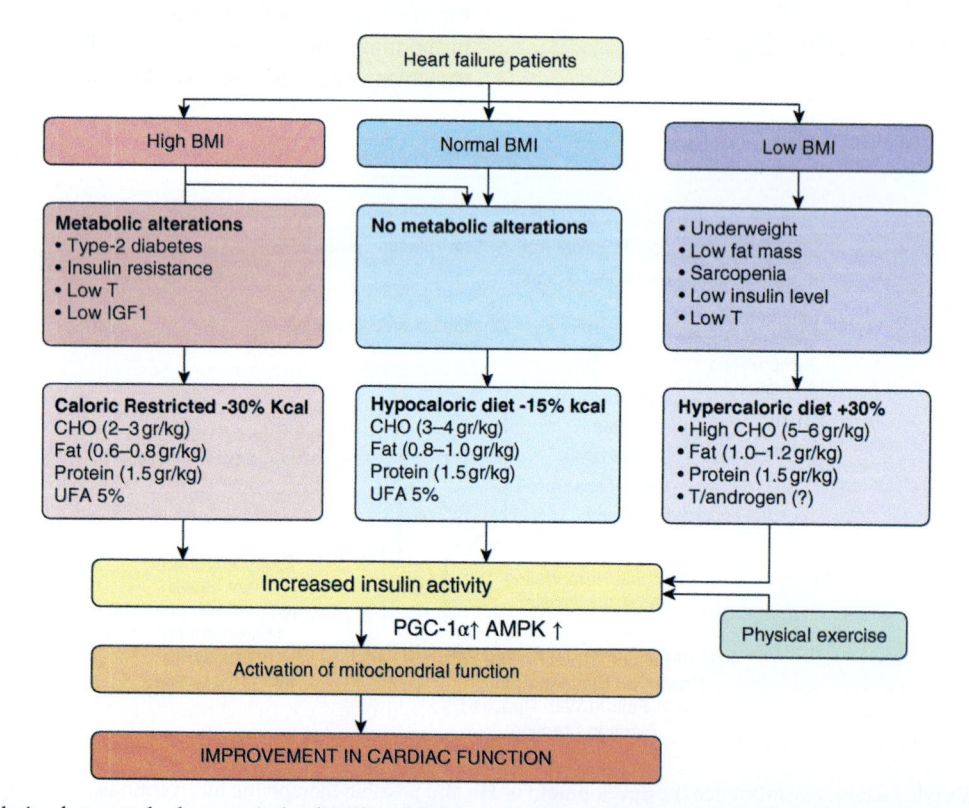

FIGURE 12.5 The relation between body-mass index (BMI) and HF. Source: (Bianchi, 2020/ with permission of Springer Nature).

low-sodium recommendations may cause adverse nutritional and physiologic situations, whereas strict to low-sodium recommendations or modest sodium intake may contribute to cardiac performance in compensated HF, and the exact level recommended should be adjusted based on the patient's clinical evaluation. On the other hand, excessive sodium and fluid intake that could reflect non-compliance may cause HF exacerbation and hospitalizations, and excessive sodium and fluid restrictions increase the perception of thirst (Wickman et al., 2021).

Various levels of sodium restriction may be recommended in clinical practice, despite a limited rationale for these levels. The level of suggested restriction in guidelines varies dramatically from <1500 mg to <3000 mg per day (Kokkinos et al., 2010). The mechanism of benefit for sodium restriction in HF could be explained by reduced fluid retention, which prevents worsening of HF signs and symptoms. However, the opposite case against sodium restriction in HF argues that a low-sodium diet may worsen HF, although the evidence is limited. Some studies show that there is a worsening in neurohormonal profile with sodium restriction in patients with HF (Aggarwal et al., 2018). Additionally, patients with HF are at an increased risk of malnutrition and sodium-restricted diets may cause a decrease in food intake, thus in macro- and micronutrients such as calcium, magnesium, zinc, iron, thiamine, vitamins D, E, and K, and folate, therefore worsening nutrition status.

Limiting sodium intake to 1.5 g/d requires consumption of reduced sodium and no salt-added versions of most foods with restricted salt use during food preparation. Additionally, potential barriers to achieving low-sodium adherence of 1.5 g/d include awareness and availability of reduced-sodium food options, familiarity with alternative flavoring options when preparing foods, and food palatability and preferences. Sodium intake of 2.3 g/d is more achievable than lower sodium levels with regular foods, avoidance of highly salted processed foods, limiting use of table salt, and modestly seasoning with salt while cooking. Even when reduced-sodium intake is achieved, however, not all individuals experience BP changes in response to sodium intake, indicating that people can be salt-sensitive or salt-resistant.

The effects of sodium restriction in patients with HF remain to be elucidated. It is very important to personalize the recommendations for sodium, according to the stage of HF and the current symptoms, whether it is HFpEF or HFrEF the LVEF, the medications affecting cardiac function and urinary output, possible co-morbidities, BMI, and current diet. In this regard, the method of patient education is important and may prevent the unintended reduction of other nutrients (Billingsley et al., 2019).

FLUID RESTRICTION

Routine fluid restriction for all patients with HF is not supported by current guidelines. The ACC/AHA HF guidelines suggest for patients with HF class D or severe hyponatremia, fluid restriction of 1.5 to 2 L/day. This is based on expert opinion since there is limited evidence on the benefits of such restriction (Billingsley et al., 2019). European Society of Cardiology (ESC) Guidelines endorse the same level of fluid restriction in severe HF to relieve symptoms and congestion; however, recommendation and level of evidence are not provided.

Hypernatremia (defined as serum sodium concentration <135 mq/L) is a metabolic abnormality in hospitalized HF patients that increases the risk of readmission and is considered a poor prognostic indicator of all-cause mortality in HF patients. Water restriction contributes in an increase in serum sodium, however, water restriction alone might be difficult to do and also is difficult to be followed after hospital discharge, due to increased thirst (Rodriguez et al., 2019). Thirst develops as a result of HF as a condition in combination with the effect of medication and anxiety contributes greatly to increased thirst in patients with heart failure and is worse in younger patients, especially in males with high symptomatology and serum urea (Waldréus et al., 2013).

There are two meta-analyses of six randomized-controlled clinical trials (RCTs) on fluid restriction in HF that found no differences in readmission or mortality rates in patients with liberal fluid intake compared to those with restricted fluid intake. One RCT included 75 adult inpatients with acute decompensated HF (ADHF), who were randomly assigned to receive a fluid restriction of less than 800 mL/day in combination with a sodium-restricted (≤800 mg/day) diet (n = 38) or a standard hospital diet (n = 37) with liberal fluid and sodium intake and followed until the seventh hospital day or discharge in patients whose length of stay was less than 7 days. Results of this study showed no between-group differences in readmission rate at 30 days.

Another RCT included hyponatremic patients with HF and randomized patients to a usual care (2000 ml/day fluid restriction, n = 26) or a 1000 mL/day fluid restriction (n = 20) intervention at discharge. Compared to patients who consumed 2000 ml of fluid per day, patients on a 1000-mL restriction showed a significant improvement in 60-day post-discharge QOL scores and a nonsignificant trend toward fewer HF emergency visits, HF rehospitalizations, and all-cause deaths at 60 days.

In the light of current evidence, it is advisable to restrict fluid intake to 2 L/day only in patients with severe HF and signs of congestion or hyponatremia. Routine strict fluid restriction in all patients with HF, regardless of type, symptoms, or severity of HF, does not appear to result in a significant benefit.

DIETARY PATTERNS

Dietary therapy for HF has been mainly focused on individual nutrients, sodium, and fluids. However, dietary patterns seem to have an important role for both preventing and treating HF.

Healthy dietary patterns, such as the DASH diet and the MD are nutrient-dense patterns that could be used for the prevention and management of HF patients. According to various studies, those patterns seem protective against the incidence of CVD and they also have been studied for the therapy of HF. Both these dietary patterns share common characteristics in terms of food groups, such as the inclusion of fruits, vegetables, whole grains, legumes, and nuts. In the below paragraphs, more information will be given for those two dietary patterns.

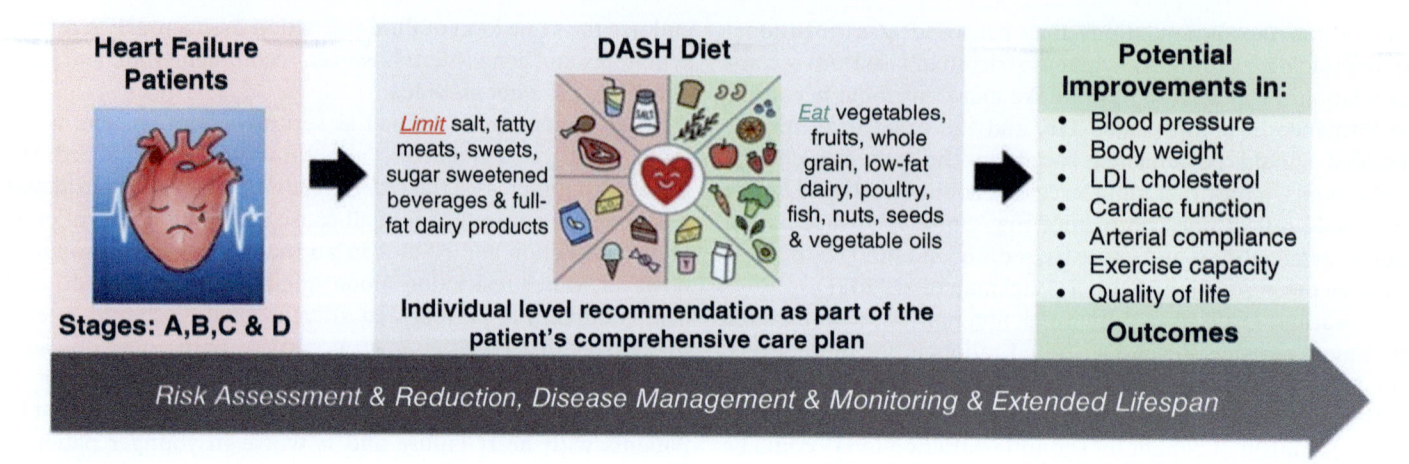

FIGURE 12.6 Using the DASH diet to manage HF. Source: (Wickman et al., 2021 / MDPI / CC BY 4.0).

DASH DIET

DASH diet has been proven to effectively reduce blood pressure and for this reason is a dietary pattern that has been investigated regarding HF. The DASH diet is characterized by increased consumption of whole grains, fruits and vegetables, low-fat dairy, lean meat, fish, poultry, nuts, seeds, and legumes, and sparse use of fats and oils (**Figure 12.6**) (Wickman et al., 2021). Such a diet is rich in antioxidants, fiber, potassium, nitrates, and low in saturated fatty acids and trans fats. These compounds can act solely or synergistically and act protectively regarding the underlying pathophysiology of HF, such as pro-inflammatory cytokines, reactive oxygen species, liver function, coagulation, endothelial function, micronutrient status, gut microbiome, and combats malnutrition (Wickman et al., 2021).

DASH diet seems to prevent the development and progression of endothelial dysfunction, which is essential for the HF development, based on epidemiological and intervention data. As DASH diet is a plant-based diet, according to a study by Lara et al. (Lara et al., 2019), such a diet is associated with a significantly lower risk of HF in a large nationally representative American cohort (hazard ratio: 0.59, 95% CI 0.41–0.86). Furthermore, Hummel et al., (Hummel et al., 2018) studied in the geriatric out-of-hospital randomized meal trial in HF (GOURMET-HF) the effect of home-delivered sodium-restricted DASH meals (DASH/SRD; 1,500 mg sodium/day) versus usual care. Patients discharged from HF hospitalization were randomized for 4 weeks to one of the two groups. According to the study results, the home-delivered DASH/SRD following HF hospitalization appeared to be safe in HF patients and affected positively their HF clinical status and 30-day re-admissions.

However, there is limited data supporting the role of this diet in slowing HF development as well as HF morbidity and mortality (Abu-Sawwa et al., 2019). More clinical trials regarding the application of DASH diet in diagnosed HF patients for HF management are needed as well as studies evaluating the effectiveness and implementation of the DASH diet for outpatient HF management.

MEDITERRANEAN DIET

The Mediterranean-type dietary patterns, namely patterns around the Mediterranean region are often characterized by a high intake of vegetables, fruits, nuts, whole grains, and extra-virgin olive oil (EVOO) with a moderate intake of fish and sometimes wine (with meals), and a low intake of dairy products, poultry, red/processed meats, and free sugars.

The Lyon diet heart study was one of the first reports that aimed to investigate the relation between the MD and HF. It was published in 1996, and it was a randomized, single-blind trial focused on the reduction in CVD complications in survivors with a first acute myocardial infarction after following the MD. This trial showed a lower number of cases developing non-fatal HF in those following a MD after 27 months versus the control group. Additionally, an extended follow up of this study showed that following a MD could significantly reduce the risk of a composite endpoint including HF by 67% (P = 0.0001) (De Lorgeril et al., 1999).

In a review by Sanches Machado d'Almeida et al., (Sanches Machado D'Almeida et al., 2018), three of the four included cohorts evaluating adherence to the MD for the primary prevention of HF, showed significant difference on the incidence of HF and/or improvements in the worsening of cardiac function parameters, for those following MD compared to those who did not adhere to MD. Of note, the same results were found for the DASH diet. Specifically, in the first cohort, 1648 post-menopausal women were included. Those who showed a high adherence to the MD, compared to the groups with lower adherence, were found to have a lower risk for developing HF (Tektonidis et al., 2015). Additionally, in a male cohort of 37,308 healthy individuals who were followed for 10.9 years, an inverse association for HF development risk was shown when there was a higher adherence to the diet, while the multivariate RR of HF mortality was 0.55 (95% CI 0.31–0.98, $p = 0.007$) and for HF incidence was 0.69 (95% CI 0.57–0.83, $p < 0.001$) (Tektonidis et al., 2016). In the third cohort, which included patients already suffering from coronary artery disease, those who developed ventricular dysfunction compared to the rest of the patients (17.8 ± 3 vs. 19.5 ± 4.7, $p < 0.001$) had a lower score on adherence to the MD (Chrysohoou et al., 2010).

In another systematic review and meta-analysis published in 2016, including 10,950 individuals, authors examined the effects of RCT-implemented Mediterranean-type interventions with control diets on vascular disease and mortality. The MD was associated with a 70% decrease in the HF incidence as well as other improvements in other vascular events (e.g., stroke and coronary events) (Liyanage et al., 2016). Additionally, considering the degree of obesity, patients of moderate BMI (i.e., 25–29.9), following a MD showed that there was a lower incidence of HF and mortality, especially when it was combined with low energy intake. In a study by Tektonidis et al. (Tektonidis et al., 2015), patients with HF who had the lowest adherence to MD had a three times greater incidence of HF and mortality compared to the highest adherence.

NUTRITIONAL SUPPLEMENTS

HF patients are also characterized by micronutrient deficiencies, which are associated with an increase in mortality in patients with HF. An example is less than 4 mmol/L potassium is significantly associated with shorter event-free survival (Abu-Sawwa et al., 2019). There are various dietary supplements that are considered useful in the treatment of HF, but more studies are needed, since none of these have been proven effective or reproducible, due to largely inconclusive results of intervention in HF patients studies examining the effect of micronutrient supplementation on HF progression, morbidity, and mortality (Abu-Sawwa et al., 2019).

THIAMINE SUPPLEMENTATION

Thiamine is a water-soluble vitamin, important for energy metabolism in the human body. Symptoms of thiamine deficiency are neurological abnormalities and congestive HF, known as dry beriberi and wet beriberi, a well characterized deficiency in patients with HF. Such a deficiency might derive from increased urinary excretion due to the use of diuretics and/or lower intake or absorption like in case of malnutrition, increased metabolic states (such as hyperthyroidism), advanced age, and frequent hospitalization (Kattoor et al., 2018). In the etiology of thiamin deficiency for HF, there is cardiac enlargement with normal rhythm, dependent edema, elevated venous pressure, peripheral neuritis or pellagra, and nonspecific electrocardiogram changes (Roman-Campos & Cruz, 2014). In such cases, it seems that there is improvement in symptoms and a reduction of heart size with vitamin supplementation. However, a small number of clinical trials have demonstrated the benefit of thiamine supplementation in improving LV systolic function in selected HF populations, particularly those receiving diuretics. Future, larger, randomized, double-blind trials will help to further elucidate the impact of thiamin on CVD events.

IRON SUPPLEMENTATION

Other HF-related micronutrient deficiencies are vitamin D, C, and E, Coenzyme Q10 (CoQ10), and iron. Currently, intravenous iron supplementation in patients with both HFrEF and iron deficiency is the only vitamin or mineral micronutrient supplementation strategy shown to definitively improve outcomes in HF, despite evidence of micronutrient deficiency being associated with poor outcomes in HF. It is possible, however, that a nutrient-dense dietary pattern providing a wealth of micronutrients along with dietary fiber, PUFA, and plant-based protein may be the supplementation strategy that most likely benefits patients with HF.

ESSENTIAL AMINO ACIDS SUPPLEMENTATION

Administration of essential amino acids (4 g/day) for 30-day also seem to improve VO_2max and exercise capacity, but there is no information provided on body weight change, caloric intake, and macronutrients due to contrasting findings from the wide differences in experimental protocols and study population. However, It is very important to decide the dietary approach based on BMI and prescribe the energy intake and macronutrient composition, although there is still a debate. (Yancy et al., 2013).

OMEGA-3 POLY-UNSATURATED FATTY ACID SUPPLEMENTATION

There is increasing interest on the effects of omega-3 poly-unsaturated fatty acids (n-3 PUFAs) in patients with HF. Results of the Gruppo Italiano per lo Studio della Sopravvivenza nell'Infarto Miocardico-HF study, the largest clinical trial assessing the effects of n-3 PUFAs in HF, suggested a modest survival advantage from dietary supplementation with 1 g/day of n-3 PUFAs [a combination of eicosapentaenoic acid (EPA)/docosahexaenoic acid (DHA)] on mortality and cardiovascular (CV) hospital admission in patients with HF. However, a recent review and a meta-analysis showed no clear benefit from n-3 PUFA supplementation on mortality or major CV events in patients at risk of or with established CV disease.

An explanation for different outcomes among RCTs is the varying doses of tested n-3 PUFAs. Indeed, even though both the ACCF/AHA (Recommendation Class IIa, Level of Evidence: B) and the ESC (Recommendation Class IIb, Level of Evidence: B) Guidelines consider n-3 PUFA supplementation an adjunctive therapy in symptomatic patients with chronic HF, no specific dose is advised, although G850 mg/day of EPA and DHA has been identified as having no effect in either HF with reduced ejection fraction or post-myocardial infarction. There is still a need to define optimal dosing and formulation of omega-3 PUFA supplements to reduce mortality and CV hospitalizations in HF.

Globally, the ESC guidelines recommend that HF patients receive education on fluids, so as to avoid excessive fluid intake and dehydration, and on a healthy diet to prevent malnutrition and maintain healthy body weight, like avoid consuming >5 g of salt daily (McDonagh et al., 2021). Dietary interventions should be studied separately for the different types of HF, namely HFrEF and HFpEF, since they differ in their risk factors and medication (Ponikowski et al., 2016). The new taxonomy of HF promotes a targeted and personalized approach to clinical care since there is a biologic interindividual variability that is still not fully understood. This variability has to do with human biologic systems and molecular pathways that present how dietary patterns, food components, social and environmental factors, genetics and host metabolic variability, gut microbiome, health, and disease status interact (Lindgren & Börjesson, 2021). It is also very important to focus on the level of adherence, for a greater effectiveness of a dietary approach. The adherence is related to factors such as taste preferences, different social and cultural norms, availability of food, social support, and self-efficacy (Lindgren & Börjesson, 2021). In order to improve efficacy and effectiveness of optimal diet patterns, the composition recommendations in HF patients should provide individualized care to improve clinical outcomes (Wickman et al., 2021). This could also be achieved by combining effective nutrition interventions with systems of care that integrate behavioral support and modification so to succeed a routine clinical care.

PA has a positive effect on many of the risk factors for CHD and HF, such as hypertension. Pandey et al. (Pandey et al., 2015), performed a large meta-analysis and showed that there is a dose-response relationship between PA and risk of HF. The consistent, linear, inverse, and dose-response association between PA and HF risk, concludes that 'more activity is better than some activity for HF prevention'. So, subjects with 500 METs-min/work of PA (the minimum guidelines recommended), had a 10% lower risk of HF compared with those with no PA, while 1000 or 2000 METs-min/work results in a 19% and 35% lower risk of HF, respectively, suggesting a re-evaluation of the actual guidelines. Furthermore, a systematic review and meta-analysis by Aune et al. (Aune et al., 2021) included 29 prospective observational studies, and there was a comparison between high versus low levels of total PA, leisure-time activity, vigorous activity, walking- and bicycling-combined occupational activity, and cardio-respiratory fitness, which showed that each was associated with a statistically significant decrease in the risk of HF.

PHYSICAL ACTIVITY AND EXERCISE FOR HEART FAILURE PREVENTION AND THERAPY

PHYSICAL ACTIVITY AND HEART FAILURE

Regular physical activity (PA) is linked to various health effects, including reduced total and cardiovascular morbidity and mortality and risk factors (**Figure 12.7**) (Lindgren et al., 2017).

PHYSICAL INACTIVITY AND HEART FAILURE

Many years of sedentary life is associated with a reduction of cardiac compliance, an adverse process that could start in middle life (Palmer et al., 2018). The mechanisms underlying the relation among HF, cardio-respiratory fitness (CRF), and physical activity/inactivity is not well defined. Low levels of CRF and inactivity correlate to obesity and MetS as well as other risk factors for CVD. Physical inactivity and low CRF are also

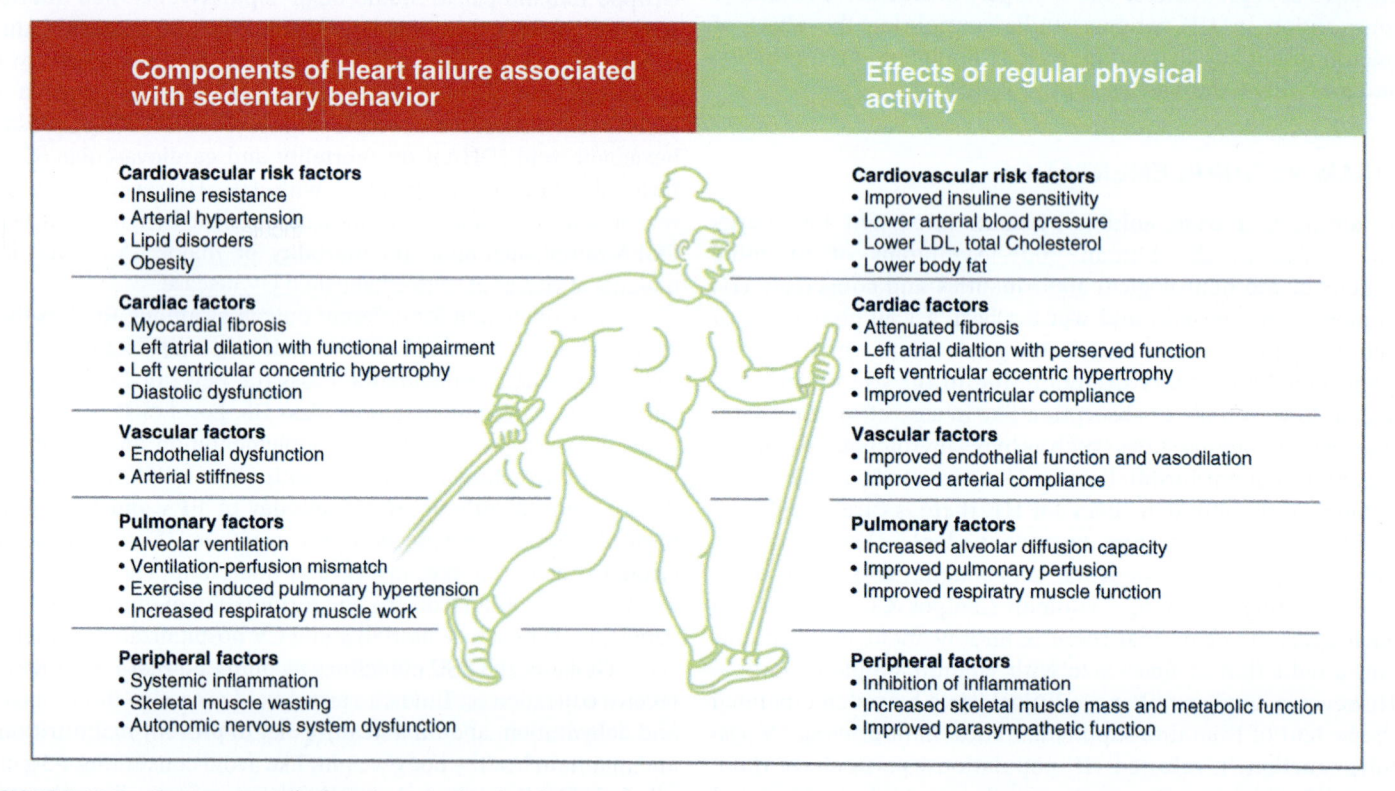

Components of Heart failure associated with sedentary behavior	Effects of regular physical activity
Cardiovascular risk factors • Insulin resistance • Arterial hypertension • Lipid disorders • Obesity	**Cardiovascular risk factors** • Improved insulin sensitivity • Lower arterial blood pressure • Lower LDL, total Cholesterol • Lower body fat
Cardiac factors • Myocardial fibrosis • Left atrial dilation with functional impairment • Left ventricular concentric hypertrophy • Diastolic dysfunction	**Cardiac factors** • Attenuated fibrosis • Left atrial dialtion with perserved function • Left ventricular eccentric hypertrophy • Improved ventricular compliance
Vascular factors • Endothelial dysfunction • Arterial stiffness	**Vascular factors** • Improved endothelial function and vasodilation • Improved arterial compliance
Pulmonary factors • Alveolar ventilation • Ventilation-perfusion mismatch • Exercise induced pulmonary hypertension • Increased respiratory muscle work	**Pulmonary factors** • Increased alveolar diffusion capacity • Improved pulmonary perfusion • Improved respiratry muscle function
Peripheral factors • Systemic inflammation • Skeletal muscle wasting • Autonomic nervous system dysfunction	**Peripheral factors** • Inhibition of inflammation • Increased skeletal muscle mass and metabolic function • Improved parasympathetic function

FIGURE 12.7 Organ system dysfunction associated with HF pathophysiology and the counteracting effects of regular PA and fitness. Source: (Adapted from Lindgren et al., 2017).

associated with obesity and increase the risk for HF in young and middle-aged populations (Lindgren et al., 2017). In such conditions, low-grade inflammation presents, thus the relevant metabolic changes cause vascular dysfunction and myocardial remodeling that may lead to HF.

CHF is characterized by reduced functional ability, severe exercise intolerance, especially for HFpEF (i.e., low peak oxygen uptake (VO_2), which limits daily activities, increased shortness of breath upon exertion, reduced QOL, increased dependence for daily activities, and increased risk of adverse events in persons living with HFrEF; EF ≤40%) (Palmer et al., 2018).

EXERCISE TRAINING IN HEART FAILURE

Exercise training is now a well-established therapy for HF patients, and in the ESC HF guideline 2016, "patients with HF are recommended to perform properly designed exercise training" (Ponikowski et al., 2016). Exercise plays an important role in three stages of HF. It affects the presentation of HF, which, it seems, has a protective role by positively affecting HF in secondary prevention and by influencing the prognosis of HF in the future for HF patients. According to different studies, exercise training can be considered as a highly effective therapy for patients with HF and shows that it can be safe, feasible, and beneficial. It increases functional capacity, resting heart rate, ventilatory efficiency, ejection fraction, and QOL and reduces the incidence of major cardiovascular events, hospitalizations, and cardiac mortality as well as the rate of new-onset atrial arrhythmias, but not ventricular arrhythmias, in patients with HF. However, as highlighted in the recent ESC guidelines on sports cardiology, exercise should be individually tailored and sporting activities may be restricted in some patients (Lindgren et al., 2017).

Exercise could be a part of cardiac rehabilitation (CR), which refers to a group of interventions needed to reassure the best physical, psychological, and social condition of HF, although accessing resources in healthcare systems are limited (de Gregorio, 2018). Generally, a CR program could be recommended early after hospital discharge, to patients after an acute CV event. CR, as a program, could be applied to a patient, according to the following data: (1) magnitude of cardiac damage and persistent ventricular dysfunction; (2) residual myocardial ischemia; (3) electrical instability; (4) clinical deterioration and co-morbidities; and (5) pulmonary function. CR could be a first-hand program for patients free of complications rather than the patients with symptoms despite intensive therapy and interventional procedures as well as when complicated by severe cardiac dysfunction, electrical instability, and/or advanced kidney disease (de Gregorio, 2018). The decision could be based on a three-level risk classification for establishing CR eligibility (**Figure 12.8**) (Billingsley et al., 2019). Stages A to D refer to the ACC HF classification reported by Hunt (2006) (de Gregorio, 2018).

LOW-RISK (all items to be satisfied):

No signs/symptoms of HF at rest (stage A or B)
No residual ischemia (resting and exercise)
Functional ability ≥6 METS
Normal HR e BP under exercise
Resting LV function ≥50% (LVEF)
No atrial fibrillation
No ventricular arrhythmias (<10 BEV/h)
No heart valve disease

INTERMEDIATE-RISK (single item):

Symptoms of HF on exertion (stage C)
Poor functional ability (4–6 METS)
Near normal HR and BP under exercise
Mid/high-exertion-induced ischemia (5–6 METS)
Mildly impaired LV function at rest (LVEF 40–45%)
Paroxysmal or permanent atrial fibrillation
Uncontrolled systolic hypertension
Mild to moderate aortic stenosis
Premature ventricular beats (> 10 BEV/h)
History of ventricular tachycardia
Adjunctive factor: advanced age

HIGH-RISK (single item):

CHF stage C or D
Resting or exertion ischemia (≤5 METS)
Low functional ability (≤ 4 METS)
Impaired LV function at rest (LVEF ≤ 35%)
History of brain ischemia
Moderate to severe aortic stenosis
Atrial fibrillation
Ventricular arrhythmias
Associated channelopathy
History of cardiac arrest or ventricular fibrillation
Adjunctive factor: advanced age

FIGURE 12.8 HF patient assessment for CR. Source: (Adapted from Billingsley et al., 2019).

The review of Palmer et al., shows that exercise training improves poor QOL and physical function in comparison to no exercise or usual care in CHF patients in the community. In order for such results to be applied further, it is of great importance to break down barriers and reinforce engagement of HF patients in exercise rather than check how it is performed (Palmer et al., 2018).

However, when a HF patient is in an unstable clinical condition, there must be great care for a CR program and high-risk patients should avoid CR until there is no instability and can then reclassify. These patients usually need to follow the entire pathway across all rehabilitation services, which includes an intensive CR program in skilled medical centers. Patients with a higher clinical risk need a safer modality of training (Palmer et al., 2018). Low-risk stable patients do not require particular attention and can be addressed to either a center-based or home-based CR. Both models have been demonstrated to ensure CV benefit and well-being.

INTENSITY OF EXERCISE IN PATIENTS WITH HEART FAILURE

The intensity of activity is classified as light-, moderate-, vigorous- or sedentary. HF patients have low rates of fulfillment of current PA guidelines, because exercising for HF patients is tough due to decreased physical health, low energy, and symptoms. Patients diagnosed with HF might present with a decline in functional capacity, even in the ability to perform daily activities.

Recommendations should include both aerobic and resistance training and include factors as seen in the **Table 12.4**, (Aggarwal et al., 2018) such as the level of intensity: the higher it is, the lower the risk of incident HF, the duration, and the frequency. Especially for the elderly and prevention of sarcopenia, strength training and, generally, muscle training should be included for improved functional capacity (Aggarwal et al., 2018).

Regarding therapy of HF, exercise is combined with CR in health care settings. CR as it was mentioned earlier, is a multifactorial model including a set of activities for managing heart disease. It provides patients generally with physical and mental activities together with social conditions, for the reduction of acute events mortality relevant to heart disease and positively influences cardiac function physical fitness and QOL in HF patients (Li et al., 2021). Until now, CR includes various exercise programs, from aerobic exercise to resistance training and peripheral muscle training. Exercise programs are also distinguished in those of continuous training (CT) and of interval training (IT) (Li et al., 2021).

Table 12.4 Exercise prescription: essential components.

Intensity	%Heart rate reserve: 70% Borg Rating of Perceived Exertion (RPE): >14 Resistance training: elastic bands, weights
Duration	30 min Shorter duration for frail Additional warm-up or cool down phase
Frequency	Daily to 5 days a week
Progression	Advance to HR/Borg RPE targets
Maintenance	Use of behavioral and nontraditional strategies

Modified with permission from L. Pinal (2010). Cardiac rehabilitation in HF: a brief review and recommendations, *Current Cardiology Reports* 12: 223–229

RPE = rate of perceived exertion; HR = heart rate
Source: (Aggarwal et al., 2018).

TYPE OF EXERCISE IN PATIENTS WITH HEART FAILURE

Aerobic exercise is recommended for patients who are in a stable condition and under optimal medical treatment (Gomes-Neto et al., 2017). Examples of such exercise are stationary bicycle, treadmill, and aerobic circuit training that can be performed for duration of 30–60 min, 3–5 times a week, for a period of 3–6 months. According to guidelines, moderate-intensity exercise (40–80% of VO_2max) is recommended initially, for stable individuals, whereas, a lower starting intensity of <40% of VO_2max is recommended for patients with more severe symptoms, which may be gradually progressed to a goal of 85% to 85% of maximum (Gomes-Neto et al., 2017).

Resistance training supplements aerobic training, and in combination increases aerobic capacity compared to aerobic exercise alone (Wickman et al., 2021). Resistance training also helps prevent sarcopenia associated with advanced HF and is recommended for 2–3 days a week in combination with aerobic training. Resistance training is also recommended in low-risk patients aiming to return to power sports, such as weightlifting.

Peripheral muscle training can be used in the initial stages of rehabilitation in patients who are characterized with muscle wasting and exercise intolerance and thus, could be recommended for HF patients with severe symptoms and reduced exercise tolerance. Such exercise includes endurance training with the use of various weights, pulleys, or resistance bands. When peripheral training increases, the patient could change to central circulatory training, including aerobic and strength training protocols (Lindgren et al., 2017). High-intensity IT typically involves short intervals of very high-intensity activity (>90% of VO_2max) alternating with recovery periods of either complete rest or low-intensity activity and can be followed by low-risk HF patients (Lindgren et al., 2017).

CT, basically known as endurance training, is characterized by a low-mid intensity, steady exercise whose duration is more than 20 min, without resting intervals, that must be completed in a considerable time (e.g., sauntering or jogging) (Li et al., 2021). It improves respiratory gas exchange, heart rate (HR) reserve, peripheral vascular resistances, and blood pressure while decreasing mortality rate. It also facilitates body weight loss but needs long-term training. Studies have shown that CT may also improve aerobic capacity, skeletal muscle function, and QOL (de Gregorio, 2018). However, CT might be difficult for a HF patient to sustain.

IT, on the contrary, is relatively high in intensity, it includes repetitions of PA but also in between there are periods of rest (Li et al., 2021). IT is increasingly used in CR for HF patients. Although it seems more risky than CT, it is as safe as low-intensity CT and is recommended by both European and American guideline committees as a safe modality of CR. Studies showed that results in cardiac improvement, even in older adult patients with stable postinfarction CHF, it is also proven and is used in individualized models of high-intensity training according to clinical condition, and it was found to improve functional capacity and atrial fibrillation recurrences in CHF patients with non-permanent atrial fibrillation following a

Table 12.5 Exercise should be individually tailored, and sporting activities may be restricted in some patients.

Mode of exercise	Intensity	Frequency	Duration (min/session)	RPE[1]
Aerobic exercise	40–80% of VO_2max[2]	3–5 days/week to daily	10–60	11–15
Peripheral muscle training	40–60% of 1RM[3]	2–3 times/week to 1 time/day	15–60	13–15
Combination of aerobic exercise and peripheral muscle training	60–80% of VO_2max, 60–80% of 1 RM	3 times/week	45–60	13–15
Hydrotherapy	40–80% of Heart rate reserve	3 times/week	45	11–15
Respiratory muscle training	30% of max. inspiratory pressure	3 times/week to daily	30–60	–
2020 ESC Guidelines on sports cardiology - Recommendations for participation in sports in heart failure		Class of recommendation	Level of evidence	
Before considering a sport activity, a preliminary optimization of HF risk factor control and therapy, including device implantation (if appropriate), is recommended.		I	C	
High-intensity power and endurance sports are not recommended in patients with HFrEF, regardless of symptoms.		III	C	

[1] RPE = Rating of perceived exertion (Borg scale 6–20)
[2] VO_2max = Maximal oxygen uptake
[3] RM = Repetition maximum. 1 RM corresponds to the maximum weight that can be lifted once through the entire exercise movement.
Sources: (Pelliccia et al., 2021; Lindgren & Börjesson, 2021).

12-month aerobic IT compared to CT (de Gregorio, 2018). In addition, IT for patients with HF appears to be more effective than CT for improving functional capacity. However, there continues to be disagreement on the effectiveness between the two exercise programs, and it cannot be distinguished which exercise program is better (Li et al., 2021).

TAILORED EXERCISE ADVICE IN PATIENTS WITH HEART FAILURE

According to ESC guidelines on sports cardiology (Pelliccia et al., 2021), exercise should be individually tailored and sporting activities may be restricted in some patients (**Table 12.5**) (Lindgren & Börjesson, 2021; Pelliccia et al., 2021). There is also a need for initial assessments and risk stratification before exercise.

Patients with HF should participate in any exercise training programs only after they have been clinically assessed including medical treatment. The initiation of exercise also delays further muscle wasting and functional decline. This assessment is achieved after clinical cardiologic evaluation for disease severity and co-morbidities must be also considered. Furthermore, a maximal exercise test is needed to assess the functional capacity of the patient. This test will show if there is for example abnormal blood pressure or arrythmias that result from exercise, and the individual will then be prescribed a specific exercise level and intensity. Especially, if a patient is considered high risk, for the exercise protocol, a close follow up is indicated at the beginning in, for example, CR programs that will continue in the future to unsupervised training sessions (Lindgren et al., 2017). However, for the influence of an exercise program, there must be also a high level of adherence. According to studies of CHF, good adherence to exercise is reinforced by strategies of behavior change (Harwood et al., 2021). Effective during the exercise periods are motivational strategies like education groups or use of standard verbal encouragement. Also, for increase in adherence, diaries and goal settings could be used to increase maintenance in exercising involved in the treatment. For sustainability of exercise, it is also helpful and easier to be prescribed, and so for the patient to get individual tailored instructions according to the suggested type of activity and intensity (Lindgren et al., 2017).

KEY POINTS

- American College of Cardiology/American Heart Association guidelines define HF as a "complex clinical syndrome that can result from any structural or functional cardiac disorder that impairs the ability of the ventricle to fill or eject blood".
- The classification of HF is based on different etiologies and associated mechanistic disturbances of cardiac function.
- HF incidence is divided according to left ventricular ejection fraction (LVEF). The classification also depends on the level of LVEF, thus for LVEF < 40%, HF is classified as HFrEF, whereas for LVEF, 50% as preserved HF (HFpEF).
- HF could characterize a chronic state or an acute state, thus chronic heart failure (CHF) or acute HF.
- The prevalence of HF is high and is increasing over time, due also to an increase in the older adult population and the prevalence of relevant to HF risk factors, e.g., obesity and DM.
- A range of interventions can help improve quality of life (QOL) and reduce hospital admissions and mortality in CHF, such as pharmacological, medical, and lifestyle.

- Unhealthy dietary models, body weight, and consumption of low nutritional quality foods, low PA, and mental stress may influence the rapidly changing epidemiology of HF.
- There is a close association between HF and body weight. A high BMI results in metabolic and neurohormonal pathways that increase the risk for HF as well as symptomatology. Underweight patients or those with lean sarcopenia are associated with advanced HF and poor outcomes.
- Malnutrition is a common sign in HF patients, especially in severe HF, reaching 30% to 70% of HF.
- The effects of sodium restriction in patients with HF remain to be elucidated. It is very important to personalize the recommendations for sodium, according to the stage of HF and the current symptoms.
- Fluid restriction is included in the management of patients with HF. In most cases, a more liberal fluid intake of 2 L per day is appropriate.
- Dietary patterns seem to have an important role in both preventing and treating HF.
- Healthy diet patterns, such as the Dietary Approaches to Stop Hypertension (DASH) diet and the Mediterranean diet (MD) provide nutrient-dense patterns and could be used for HF.
- HF patients are also characterized by micronutrient deficiencies, which have been associated with an increase in mortality in patients with HF. Although, there are various dietary supplements that have been considered useful in the treatment of HF, more studies are needed.
- To improve efficacy and effectiveness of optimal diet pattern(s), the composition recommendations for HF patients should provide individualized care to improve clinical outcomes.

- There is a dose-response relationship between PA and risk of HF.
- 'More activity is better than some activity for HF prevention'.
- Exercise plays an important role in the presentation of HF, has a protective role by positively affecting HF in secondary prevention, and influences the prognosis of HF in the *future for HF* patients.
- However, as highlighted in the recent ESC guidelines on sports cardiology, exercise should be individually tailored, and sporting activities may be restricted in some patients.
- Exercise training is a well-established therapy for HF patients, and in the European Society of Cardiology (ESC) HF guideline 2016, "patients with HF are recommended to perform properly designed exercise training" and can be part of cardiac rehabilitation (CR).
- Aerobic exercise is recommended for patients who are in a stable condition and under optimal medical treatment.
- For a HF patient in unstable clinical condition, there must be great care for CR programs, and high-risk patients should remain without CR until there is no instability and can reclassify.
- According to ESC guidelines on sports cardiology, exercise should be individually tailored, and sporting activities may be restricted in some patients. There is also the need for initial assessments and risk stratification before exercise.
- Resistance training supplements aerobic training.

SELF-ASSESSMENT QUESTIONS

1. Define HF, its characteristics, and its diagnosis.
2. How is HF categorized?
3. Why is nutrition important for patients with HF?
4. What are the major dietary factors to consider for HF. Are there specific dietary recommendations for HF patients?
5. What is the role of PA and exercise for HF. Provide an overview of the benefits of exercise in HF.
6. True or False: Patients with HF should participate in exercise training programs only after they have been clinically assessed, including medical treatment.
7. True or False: The initiation of exercise will not delay further muscle wasting and functional decline.
8. True or False: CT stands for continuous training, known as endurance training of low to moderate intensity of a steady exercise which duration is more than 20 min in continuance with no resting intervals that must be completed in a considerable time.
9. Fill in the blanks: Effective strategies for adherence are motivational strategies like _____ or use of standard verbal encouragement. Also, for increase in adherence, _____ and _____ could be used to increase maintenance in exercise involved in the treatment.
10. As a clinical syndrome, the diagnosis of HF, is based on three cornerstones:
    (a) typical symptoms, signs and results from relevant diagnostic tests that can all be linked to cardiac dysfunction, often caused by a structural and/or functional cardiac abnormality resulting in reduced cardiac output and/or elevated intracardiac pressures.
    (b) BMI, clinical symptoms and results from relevant diagnostic tests that can all be linked to cardiac dysfunction, often caused by a structural and/or functional cardiac abnormality resulting in reduced cardiac output and/or elevated intracardiac pressures.
    (c) typical symptoms, signs and spirometry that can all be linked to cardiac dysfunction, often caused by a structural and/or functional cardiac abnormality resulting in reduced cardiac output and/or elevated intracardiac pressures.
11. AHF patients may be also classified according to:
    (a) Their initial clinical symptoms and signs with systolic blood pressure (SBP) as the usual marker.
    (b) The criteria by Stevenson and colleagues who used the severity of presentation rather than the underlying etiology

and consider signs and symptoms of congestion and peripheral perfusion.
(c) a and b

12. The increase in HF prevalence worldwide could be explained by:
(a) An increase in the older adult population and an improved survival as well as an increase in the prevalence of obesity and diabetes.
(b) An increase in the older adult population, an improved survival, increase in the exercise levels above the age of 65 years of age, and an increase in heart attacks.
(c) a and b

13. For HF:
(a) PA and nutrition are important for both prevention and rehabilitation.
(b) Nutrition and body weight are important for prevention.
(c) Nutrition and normal blood pressure are important for both.

14. There is a close association between HF and body weight.
(a) A high BMI increases the risk for HF as well as the symptomatology. Weight loss in patients with overweight/obesity and HF may prevent further progression of the disease, improves cardiac function, improve symptoms, and decrease the possibility of hospitalization.
(b) "Obesity paradox" and malnutrition may also present in HF patients.
(c) a and b

15. There is a close association between HF and salt intake.
(a) Salt restriction reduces incidence of HF.
(b) A low-sodium diet may worsen HF.
(c) It is very important to personalize the recommendations for sodium, according to various factors, and patients need to be educated.

CASE SCENARIO

Ms. Griffin was diagnosed with left-sided heart failure 8 years ago, related to decades of uncontrolled hypertension. She is in skilled nursing care on oxygen by nasal cannula 24 hours a day. Ms. Griffin remains in bed or in a wheelchair because she has episodes of angina and dyspnea even at rest. Her weight has dropped from 160 pounds to 93 pounds over the past 2 years. Recently she had a PEG (percutaneous esophageal gastrostomy) feeding tube inserted.

1. Explain Ms. Griffin's classification of HF according to the New York Heart Association Functional Classification.
2. Explain how her weight loss is related to HF.
3. Explain what a sudden gain of 2 pounds may mean.
4. She manifests signs of both left-sided and right-sided HF. Explain.
5. Ms. Griffin's ejection fraction is 19%. Write a value for a normal ejection fraction and explain what an ejection fraction is.
6. Explain the types of techniques commonly used for diagnosis of HF.
7. Discuss the treatments for heart failure.

REFERENCES

Abu-Sawwa, R., Dumbar, S., Quyyumi, A., & Sattler, E. (2019). Intervención nutricional en la insuficiencia cardíaca: ¿debería recomendarse el consumo del patrón de alimentación DASH para mejorar los resultados? *Heart Fail Rev.*, 24(4), 565–573. https://doi.org/10.1007/s10741-019-09781-6.Nutrition

Aggarwal, M., Bozkurt, B., Panjrath, G., Aggarwal, B., Ostfeld, R. J., Barnard, N. D., Gaggin, H., Freeman, A. M., Allen, K., Madan, S., Massera, D., & Litwin, S. E. (2018). Lifestyle Modifications for Preventing and Treating Heart Failure. *Journal of the American College of Cardiology*, 72(19), 2391–2405. https://doi.org/10.1016/j.jacc.2018.08.2160

Aune, D., Schlesinger, S., Leitzmann, M. F., Tonstad, S., Norat, T., Riboli, E., & Vatten, L. J. (2021). Physical activity and the risk of heart failure: a systematic review and dose–response meta-analysis of prospective studies. *European Journal of Epidemiology*, 36(4), 367–381. https://doi.org/10.1007/s10654-020-00693-6

Aune, D., Schlesinger, S., Neuenschwander, M., Feng, T., Janszky, I., Norat, T., & Riboli, E. (2018). Diabetes mellitus, blood glucose and the risk of heart failure: a systematic review and meta-analysis of prospective studies. *Nutrition, Metabolism and Cardiovascular Diseases*, 28(11), 1081–1091.

Bianchi, V. E. (2020). Nutrition in chronic heart failure patients: a systematic review. *Heart Failure Reviews*, 25(6), 1017–1026. https://doi.org/10.1007/s10741-019-09891-1

Billingsley, H., Rodriguez-Miguelez, P., Del Buono, M. G., Abbate, A., Lavie, C. J., & Carbone, S. (2019). Lifestyle interventions with a focus on nutritional strategies to increase cardiorespiratory fitness in chronic obstructive pulmonary disease, heart failure, obesity, sarcopenia, and frailty. *Nutrients*, 11(12), 1–25. https://doi.org/10.3390/nu11122849

Carbone, S., Canada, J. M., Billingsley, H. E., Siddiqui, M. S., Elagizi, A., & Lavie, C. J. (2019). Obesity paradox in cardiovascular disease: Where do we stand? *Vascular Health and Risk Management*, 15, 89–100. https://doi.org/10.2147/VHRM.S168946

Chrysohoou, C., Panagiotakos, D. B., Aggelopoulos, P., Kastorini, C. M., Kehagia, I., Pitsavos, C., & Stefanadis, C. (2010). The Mediterranean diet contributes to the preservation of left ventricular systolic function and to the long-term favorable prognosis of patients who have had an acute coronary event. *American Journal of Clinical Nutrition*, 92(1), 47–54. https://doi.org/10.3945/ajcn.2009.28982

de Gregorio, C. (2018). Physical training and cardiac rehabilitation in heart failure patients. *Advances in Experimental Medicine and Biology*, 1067, 161–181. https://doi.org/10.1007/5584_2018_144

De Lorgeril, M., Salen, P., Martin, J. L., Monjaud, I., Delaye, J., & Mamelle, N. (1999). Mediterranean diet, traditional risk factors, and the rate of cardiovascular complications after myocardial infarction: Final report of the Lyon Diet Heart Study. *Circulation*, 99(6), 779–785. https://doi.org/10.1161/01.CIR.99.6.779

Denfeld, Q. E., Winters-Stone, K., Mudd, J. O., Gelow, J. M., Kurdi, S., & Lee, C. S. (2017). The prevalence of frailty in heart failure: a systematic review and meta-analysis. *International Journal of Cardiology, 236,* 283–289.

Dharmarajan, K., & Rich, M. W. (2017). Epidemiology, Pathophysiology, and Prognosis of Heart Failure in Older Adults. *Heart Failure Clinics, 13*(3), 417–426. https://doi.org/10.1016/j.hfc.2017.02.001

Folsom, A. R., Yamagishi, K., Hozawa, A., & Chambless, L. E. (2009). Absolute and attributable risks of heart failure incidence in relation to optimal risk factors. *Circulation: Heart Failure, 2*(1), 11–17.

Gomes-Neto, M., Durães, A. R., Reis, H. F. C. dos, Neves, V. R., Martinez, B. P., & Carvalho, V. O. (2017). High-intensity interval training versus moderate-intensity continuous training on exercise capacity and quality of life in patients with coronary artery disease: A systematic review and meta-analysis. *European Journal of Preventive Cardiology, 24*(16), 1696–1707. https://doi.org/10.1177/2047487317728370

Gorodeski, E. Z., Goyal, P., Hummel, S. L., Krishnaswami, A., Goodlin, S. J., Hart, L. L., . . . Alexander, K. P. (2018). Domain management approach to heart failure in the geriatric patient: present and future. *Journal of the American College of Cardiology, 71*(17), 1921–1936.

Groenewegen, A., Rutten, F. H., Mosterd, A., & Hoes, A. W. (2020). Epidemiology of heart failure. *European Journal of Heart Failure, 22*(8), 1342–1356. https://doi.org/10.1002/ejhf.1858

Harwood, A. E., Russell, S., Okwose, N. C., McGuire, S., Jakovljevic, D. G., & McGregor, G. (2021). A systematic review of rehabilitation in chronic heart failure: evaluating the reporting of exercise interventions. *ESC Heart Failure, 8*(5), 3458–3471. https://doi.org/10.1002/ehf2.13498

He, J., Ogden, L. G., Bazzano, L. A., Vupputuri, S., Loria, C., & Whelton, P. K. (2001). Risk factors for congestive heart failure in US men and women: NHANES I epidemiologic follow-up study. *Arch Intern Med, 161*(7), 996–1002.

Hummel, S. L., Karmally, W., Gillespie, B. W., Helmke, S., Teruya, S., Wells, J., Trumble, E., Jimenez, O., Marolt, C., Wessler, J. D., Cornellier, M., & Maurer, M. S. (2018). Home-delivered meals post-discharge from heart failure hospitalization: the GOURMET-HF pilot study. *Circ Heart Fail., 11*(8), 1–22. https://doi.org/10.1161/CIRCHEARTFAILURE.117.004886.Home

Ishikawa, Y., & Sattler, E. L. P. (2021). Nutrition as Treatment Modality in Heart Failure. *Current Atherosclerosis Reports, 23*(4). https://doi.org/10.1007/s11883-021-00908-5

Kattoor, A. J., Goel, A., & Mehta, J. L. (2018). Thiamine Therapy for Heart Failure: a Promise or Fiction? *Cardiovascular Drugs and Therapy, 32*(4), 313–317. https://doi.org/10.1007/s10557-018-6808-8

Kokkinos, P., Myers, J., Faselis, C., Panagiotakos, D. B., Doumas, M., Pittaras, A., Manolis, A., Kokkinos, J. P., Karasik, P., Greenberg, M., Papademetriou, V., & Fletcher, R. (2010). Exercise capacity and mortality in older men: A 20-year follow-up study. *Circulation, 122*(8), 790–797. https://doi.org/10.1161/CIRCULATIONAHA.110.938852

Kurmani, S., & Squire, I. (2017). Acute Heart Failure: Definition, Classification and Epidemiology. *Current Heart Failure Reports, 14*(5), 385–392. https://doi.org/10.1007/s11897-017-0351-y

Lara, K. M., Levitan, E. B., Gutierrez, O. M., Shikany, J. M., Safford, M. M., Judd, S. E., & Rosenson, R. S. (2019). Dietary Patterns and Incident Heart Failure in US Adults Without Known Coronary Disease. *Journal of the American College of Cardiology, 73*(16), 2036–2045. https://doi.org/10.1016/j.jacc.2019.01.067

Lavie, C., De Schutter, A., Patel, D., Church, T., Arena, R., Romero-Corra, A., . . . Milani, R. (2012). New insights into the "obesity paradox" and cardiovascular outcomes. *J Glycomics Lipidomics, 2,* e106.

Li, D., Chen, P., & Zhu, J. (2021). The effects of interval training and continuous training on cardiopulmonary fitness and exercise tolerance of patients with heart failure—a systematic review and meta-analysis. *International Journal of Environmental Research and Public Health, 18*(13). https://doi.org/10.3390/ijerph18136761

Lindgren, M., Åberg, M., Schaufelberger, M., Åberg, D., Schiöler, L., Torén, K., & Rosengren, A. (2017). Cardiorespiratory fitness and muscle strength in late adolescence and long-term risk of early heart failure in Swedish men. *European Journal of Preventive Cardiology, 24*(8), 876–884. https://doi.org/10.1177/2047487317689974

Lindgren, M., & Börjesson, M. (2021). The importance of physical activity and cardiorespiratory fitness for patients with heart failure. *Diabetes Research and Clinical Practice, 176.* https://doi.org/10.1016/j.diabres.2021.108833

Liyanage, T., Ninomiya, T., Wang, A., Neal, B., Jun, M., Wong, M. G., Jardine, M., Hillis, G. S., & Perkovic, V. (2016). Effects of the mediterranean diet on cardiovascular outcomes-a systematic review and meta-analysis. *PLoS ONE, 11*(8). https://doi.org/10.1371/journal.pone.0159252

McDonagh, T. A., Metra, M., Adamo, M., Gardner, R. S., Baumbach, A., Böhm, M., Burri, H., Butler, J., Celutkiene, J., Chioncel, O., Cleland, J. G. F., Coats, A. J. S., Crespo-Leiro, M. G., Farmakis, D., Gilard, M., & Heymans, S. (2021). 2021 ESC Guidelines for the diagnosis and treatment of acute and chronic heart failure. *European Heart Journal, 42*(36), 3599–3726. https://doi.org/10.1093/eurheartj/ehab368

Nohria, A., Tsang, S. W., Fang, J. C., Lewis, E. F., Jarcho, J. A., Mudge, G. H., & Stevenson, L. W. (2003). Clinical assessment identifies hemodynamic profiles that predict outcomes in patients admitted with heart failure. *Journal of the American College of Cardiology, 41*(10), 1797–1804. https://doi.org/10.1016/S0735-1097(03)00309-7

Ohkuma, T., Komorita, Y., Peters, S. A., & Woodward, M. (2019). Diabetes as a risk factor for heart failure in women and men: a systematic review and meta-analysis of 47 cohorts including 12 million individuals. *Diabetologia, 62*(9), 1550–1560.

Oreopoulos, A., Padwal, R., Kalantar-Zadeh, K., Fonarow, G. C., Norris, C. M., & McAlister, F. A. (2008). Body mass index and mortality in heart failure: a meta-analysis. *American heart journal, 156*(1), 13–22.

Palmer, K., Bowles, K. A., Paton, M., Jepson, M., & Lane, R. (2018). Chronic Heart Failure and Exercise Rehabilitation: A Systematic Review and Meta-Analysis. *Archives of Physical Medicine and Rehabilitation, 99*(12), 2570–2582. https://doi.org/10.1016/j.apmr.2018.03.015

Pandey, A., Garg, S., Khunger, M., Darden, D., Ayers, C., Kumbhani, D. J., Mayo, H. G., De Lemos, J. A., & Berry, J. D. (2015). Dose-Response Relationship Between Physical Activity and Risk of Heart Failure: A Meta-Analysis. *Circulation, 132*(19), 1786–1794. https://doi.org/10.1161/CIRCULATIONAHA.115.015853

Pelliccia, A., Sharma, S., Gati, S., Bäck, M., Börjesson, M., Caselli, S., Collet, J. P., Corrado, D., Drezner, J. A., Halle, M., Hansen, D., Heidbuchel, H., Myers, J., Niebauer, J., Papadakis, M., Piepoli, M. F., Prescott, E., Roos-Hesselink, J. W., Graham Stuart, A., . . . Wijns, W. (2021). 2020 ESC Guidelines on sports cardiology and exercise in patients with cardiovascular disease. *European Heart Journal, 42*(1), 17–96. https://doi.org/10.1093/eurheartj/ehaa605

Ponikowski, P., Voors, A. A., Anker, S. D., Bueno, H., Cleland, J. G. F., Coats, A. J. S., Falk, V., González-Juanatey, J. R., Harjola, V. P., Jankowska, E. A., Jessup, M., Linde, C., Nihoyannopoulos, P., Parissis, J. T., Pieske, B., Riley, J. P., Rosano, G. M. C., Ruilope, L. M., Ruschitzka, F., . . . Davies, C. (2016). 2016 ESC Guidelines for the diagnosis and treatment of acute and chronic heart failure. *European Heart Journal, 37*(27), 2129–2200m. https://doi.org/10.1093/eurheartj/ehw128

Rahman, A., Jafry, S., Jeejeebhoy, K., Nagpal, A. D., Pisani, B., & Agarwala, R. (2016). Malnutrition and Cachexia in Heart Failure.

Journal of Parenteral and Enteral Nutrition, 40(4), 475–486. https://doi.org/10.1177/0148607114566854

Rodriguez, M., Hernandez, M., Cheungpasitporn, W., Kashani, K. B., Riaz, I., Rangaswami, J., Herzog, E., Guglin, M., & Krittanawong, C. (2019). Hyponatremia in Heart Failure: Pathogenesis and Management. *Current Cardiology Reviews, 15*(4), 252–261. https://doi.org/10.2174/1573403x15666190306111812

Roman-Campos, D., & Cruz, J. S. (2014). Current aspects of thiamine deficiency on heart function. *Life Sciences, 98*(1), 1–5. https://doi.org/10.1016/j.lfs.2013.12.029

Sanches Machado D'Almeida, K., Ronchi Spillere, S., Zuchinali, P., & Corrêa Souza, G. (2018). Mediterranean diet and other dietary patterns in primary prevention of heart failure and changes in cardiac function markers: A systematic review. *Nutrients, 10*(1). https://doi.org/10.3390/nu10010058

Tektonidis, T. G., Åkesson, A., Gigante, B., Wolk, A., & Larsson, S. C. (2015). A Mediterranean diet and risk of myocardial infarction, heart failure and stroke: A population-based cohort study. *Atherosclerosis, 243*(1), 93–98. https://doi.org/10.1016/j.atherosclerosis.2015.08.039

Tektonidis, T. G., Åkesson, A., Gigante, B., Wolk, A., & Larsson, S. C. (2016). Adherence to a Mediterranean diet is associated with reduced risk of heart failure in men. *European Journal of Heart Failure, 18*(3), 253–259. https://doi.org/10.1002/ejhf.481

Waldréus, N., Hahn, R. G., & Jaarsma, T. (2013). Thirst in heart failure: A systematic literature review. *European Journal of Heart Failure, 15*(2), 141–149. https://doi.org/10.1093/eurjhf/hfs174

Wickman, B. E., Enkhmaa, B., Ridberg, R., Romero, E., Cadeiras, M., Meyers, F., & Steinberg, F. (2021). Dietary management of heart failure: Dash diet and precision nutrition perspectives. *Nutrients, 13*(12), 1–24. https://doi.org/10.3390/nu13124424

Yancy, C. W., Jessup, M., Bozkurt, B., Butler, J., Casey, D. E., Drazner, M. H., Fonarow, G. C., Geraci, S. A., Horwich, T., Januzzi, J. L., Johnson, M. R., Kasper, E. K., Levy, W. C., Masoudi, F. A., McBride, P. E., McMurray, J. J. V., Mitchell, J. E., Peterson, P. N., Riegel, B., . . . Wilkoff, B. L. (2013). 2013 ACCF/AHA guideline for the management of heart failure: A report of the american college of cardiology foundation/american heart association task force on practice guidelines. *Circulation, 128*(16), 240–327. https://doi.org/10.1161/CIR.0b013e31829e8776

FURTHER READING

Bibliography

Coats, A., Forman, D. E., Haykowsky, M., Kitzman, D. W., McNeil, A., Campbell, T. S., & Arena, R. (2017). Physical function and exercise training in older patients with heart failure. *Nature Reviews: Cardiology, 14*(9), 550–559. https://doi.org/10.1038/nrcardio.2017.70.

Felker, G. M., & Mann, D. L. (2019). Heart Failure: A Companion to Braunwald's Heart Disease E-Book. Elsevier Health Sciences.

Ferraro, K. (2015). Diet and Disease: Nutrition for Heart Disease, Diabetes, and Metabolic Stress. Momentum Press.

Gandy, J. (Ed.). (2019). Manual of dietetic practice. John Wiley & Sons.

Lehrke, M., Marx, N. (2017). Diabetes Mellitus and Heart Failure. *Am. J. Cardiol.* 120(1S):S37–S47. doi: 10.1016/j.amjcard.2017.05.014.

Slivnick, J., Lampert, B.C. (2019). Hypertension and Heart Failure. *Heart Fail Clin.* 15(4):531–541. doi: 10.1016/j.hfc.2019.06.007.

Snipelisky, D., Chaudhry, S. P., Stewart, G. C. (2019). The Many Faces of Heart Failure. *Card Electrophysiol. Clin.* 11(1):11–20. doi: 10.1016/j.ccep.2018.11.001.

Xiao, J. (Ed.). (2017). Exercise for Cardiovascular Disease Prevention and Treatment: From Molecular to Clinical, Part 2 (Vol. 1000). Springer.

Links

- https://www.cdc.gov/heartdisease/heart_failure.htm
- https://www.bsh.org.uk/
- https://ishlt.org/
- https://hfsa.org/
- https://www.escardio.org/Sub-specialty-communities/Heart-Failure-Association-of-the-ESC-(HFA)
- https://www.nicor.org.uk/category/heart-failure/
- https://www.heartlungcirc.org/article/S1443-9506(18)31777-3/fulltext
- https://www.heartfoundation.org.au/conditions/heart-failure-clinical-guidelines

Atrial/Flutter Fibrillation

CHAPTER 13

Definition	191	Physical Activity Recommendations	201
Prevalence	191	Key Points	201
Etiology	192	Self-assessment Questions	201
Complications	194	References	202
Management	195	Further Reading	204
Nutrition in Atrial Fibrillation	197	Bibliography	204
Physical Activity and Risk of Atrial Fibrillation	199	Links	204
Exercise Training and Atrial Fibrillation Management	200		

DEFINITION

Atrial fibrillation (AFib) is one of the most common types of cardiac arrhythmias, i.e., irregular heartbeats, which increases the risk of stroke, heart failure, and other cardiovascular-related complications. During AFib, the heart's two upper chambers (the atria) beat irregularly and out of coordination with the heart's two lower chambers (the ventricles). In AFib, the electrical impulses are so fast and chaotic that the atria cannot contract and squeeze blood effectively into the ventricles (Pellman & Sheikh, 2015).

Episodes of AFib may be paroxysmal/transient in which the patient's heart rhythm returns to normal automatically, or permanent, which require pharmacotherapy or other medical interventions to restore a normal heart rhythm. In some cases, AFib is caused by an underlying medical condition, such as myocardial infarction, pericarditis, pneumonia, pulmonary embolism, intravaginal thrombosis, and Wolff-Parkinson-White syndrome; however, in some patients there is no apparent reversible cause (absence of heart disease in clinical and laboratory evaluation) and AFib is considered idiopathic (Staerk, Sherer, Ko, Benjamin, & Helm, 2017). The definition and classification of AFib are presented in detail in **Table 13.1**.

PREVALENCE

The epidemiology of AFib is summarized in **Figure 13.1**. As with most heart-related diseases, the incidence and prevalence of AFib are increasing globally. According to the available epidemiological data, between 1990 and 2010, there was a modest increase in the prevalence and a major increase in the incidence of AFib. In 2010, the prevalence rates per 100,000 population were 596.2 (95% uncertainty intervals [UI]: 558.4 to 636.7) in men (5% increase since 1990) and 373.1 (95% UI: 347.9 to 402.2) in women (4% increase since 1990), while AFib incidence per 100,000 population was 77.5 (95% UI: 65.2 to 95.4) in men (28% increase from 1990) and 59.5 (95% UI: 49.9 to 74.9) in women (35% increase from 1990). The estimated number of individuals with AFib globally in 2010 was 33.5 million (20.9 million men [95% UI: 19.5–22.2 million] and 12.6 million women [95% UI: 12.0–13.7 million]). Burden associated with AFib, measured as disability-adjusted life-years, increased by 18.8% (95% UI: 15.8–19.3) in men and 18.9% (95% UI: 15.8–23.5) in women from 1990 to 2010. For both men and women, the prevalence and incidence of AFib are disproportionately higher in high-income nations compared with low-income nations (Chugh et al., 2014).

Prevention and Management of Cardiovascular and Metabolic Disease: Diet, Physical Activity and Healthy Aging,
First Edition. Christina N. Katsagoni, Peter Kokkinos, and Labros S. Sidossis.
© 2023 John Wiley & Sons Ltd. Published 2023 by John Wiley & Sons Ltd.

Table 13.1 Definition and classification of atrial fibrillation.

Term	Definition
AFib	A supraventricular tachyarrhythmia with uncoordinated atrial electrical activation and consequently ineffective atrial contraction. Electrocardiographic characteristics of AFib include: • irregular R-R intervals (when atrioventricular conduction is not impaired), • absence of distinct repeating P waves, and • irregular atrial activations.
Clinical AFib	Symptomatic or asymptomatic AFib documented by surface ECG. The minimum duration of an ECG strip required to establish the diagnosis of clinical AF is ≥30 seconds, or an entire 12-lead ECG.
AHRE, subclinical AFib	Refers to individuals without symptoms attributable to AFib, in whom clinical AFib is not previously detected (that is, there is no surface ECG tracing of AFib). **AHRE** - events fulfilling programmed or specified criteria for AHRE that are detected by CIEDs with an atrial lead allowing automated continuous monitoring of atrial rhythm and tracings storage. CIED-recorded AHRE need to be visually inspected because some AHRE may be electrical artifacts/false positives. **Subclinical AFib** includes AHRE confirmed to be AFib, AFL, or an AT, or AFib episodes detected by insertable cardiac monitor or wearable monitor and confirmed by visually reviewed intracardiac electrograms or ECG-recorded rhythm.
First diagnosed	AFib not diagnosed before, irrespective of its duration or the presence/severity of AFib-related symptoms.
Paroxysmal	AFib that terminates spontaneously or with intervention within 7 days of onset.
Persistent	AFib that is continuously sustained beyond 7 days, including episodes terminated by cardioversion (drugs or electrical cardioversion) after ≥7 days.
Long-standing persistent	Continuous AFib of >12 months' duration when decided to adopt a rhythm control strategy.
Permanent	AFib that is accepted by the patient and physician, and no further attempts to restore/maintain sinus rhythm will be undertaken. Permanent AF represents a therapeutic attitude of the patient and physician rather than an inherent pathophysiological attribute of AFib, and the term should not be used in the context of a rhythm control strategy with antiarrhythmic drug therapy or AFib ablation. Should a rhythm control strategy be adopted, the arrhythmia would be re-classified as 'long-standing persistent AFib'.

Device-programmed rate criterion for AHRE is ≥175 bpm, whereas there is no specific rate limit for subclinical AF. The criterion for AHRE duration is usually set at ≥5 min (mainly to reduce the inclusion of artifacts), whereas a wide range of subclinical AF duration cutoffs (from 10 to 20 seconds to >24 hours) is reported in studies of the association of subclinical AFib with thromboembolism. The reported duration refers to either the longest single episode or, more commonly, total duration of AHRE/subclinical AF during the specified monitoring period. Although not completely identical, the terms AHRE and subclinical AFib are often used interchangeably. Whereas a large body of high-quality evidence from RCTs informing the management of AF patients pertains exclusively to 'clinical' AF (that is, the ECG documentation of AF was a mandatory inclusion criterion in those RCTs), data on the optimal management of AHRE and subclinical AFib are lacking. For this reason, AFib is currently described as either 'clinical' or 'AHRE/subclinical', until the results of several ongoing RCTs expected to inform the management of AHRE and 'subclinical' AF are available.
AHRE = atrial high-rate episode; AFib = atrial fibrillation; ECG = electrocardiogram; AFL = atrial flutter; AT = atrial tachycardia; bpm = beats per minute; CIED = cardiac implantable electronic device; ECG = electrocardiogram; RCT = randomized controlled trial.
Source: (Adapted from Hindricks et al., 2020).

In the European Union, it is estimated that ~7.5 million people over 65 years old had AFib in 2016, and this number is expected to increase by 90%, i.e., to ~14.5 million, by 2060 (Di Carlo et al., 2019). Based on data from the Framingham heart study, the prevalence of AFib increased 3-fold over the last 50 years in the USA. The lifetime risk of AFib was estimated at about 1 in 4 in white men and women older than 40 years in 2004, while a decade later, lifetime risk estimates reached about 1 in 3 for white individuals and 1 in 5 for black individuals. In the USA, at least 3 to 6 million people have AFib, and the numbers are projected to reach 6 to 16 million by 2050 (Kornej, Borschel, Benjamin, & Schnabel, 2020). In addition, there are more than 450,000 hospitalizations with AFib as the primary diagnosis each year in the USA, which leads to approximately 158,000 deaths (Benjamin et al., 2019). Based on Centers for Disease Control and Prevention data, white people are more likely to have AFib than African Americans. With regards to gender, AFib incidence is generally lower in women than men, however, women have a higher prevalence of AFib at older ages, a fact that can be attributed to women's' higher life expectancy and a more severe disease clinical presentation and symptomatology compared to men (Mohanty, Trivedi, Gianni, & Natale, 2018). **Figure 13.2** presents important gender-specific considerations in AFib epidemiology and treatment.

ETIOLOGY

AFib is a multifactorial condition. Risk factors for AFib include increased age, hypertension, coronary artery disease, congenital heart diseases, mitral valve disease, cardiomyopathy, pericarditis, heart surgery, hyperthyroidism, obstructive sleep apnea, alcohol abuse, smoking, excessive caffeine consumption, atrial murmur, and several types of pulmonary diseases (**Table 13.2**) (Dilaveris & Kennedy, 2017; Ling, Kistler, Kalman, Schilling, & Hunter, 2016; Staerk et al., 2017).

In each patient, there may be a major mechanism that causes or maintains AFib, but often more than one mechanism coexists. In general, three mechanisms are considered predominant

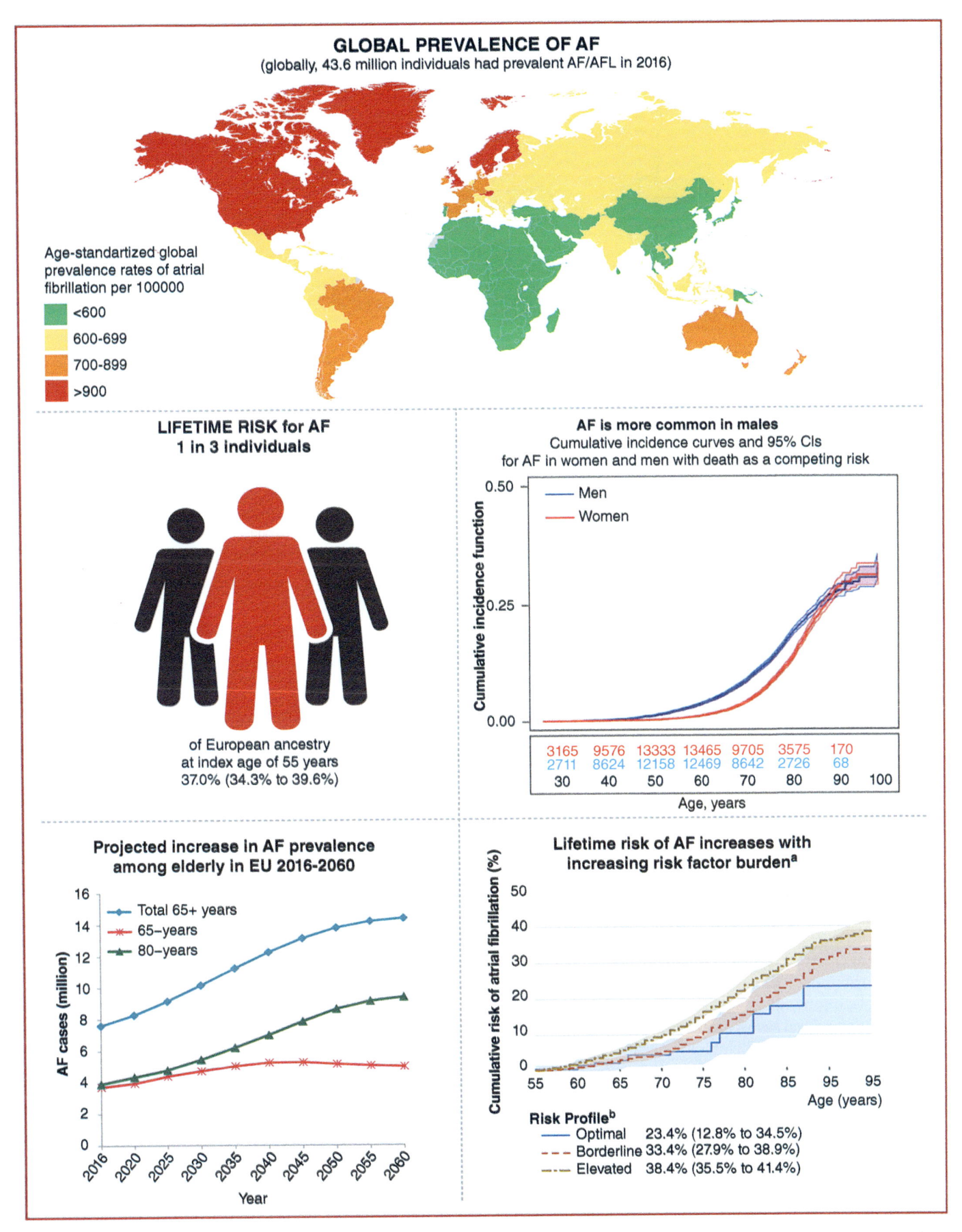

FIGURE 13.1 Epidemiology of atrial fibrillation: prevalence (upper panel); and lifetime risk and projected rise in the incidence and prevalence (lower panel). AF = atrial fibrillation; AFL = atrial flutter; BP = blood pressure; CI = confidence interval; EU = European Union. [a] Smoking, alcohol consumption, body-mass index, BP, diabetes mellitus (type 1 or 2), and history of myocardial infarction or heart failure. [b] Risk profile: optimal - all risk factors are negative or within the normal range; borderline - no elevated risk factors but >1 borderline risk factor; elevated - >1 elevated risk factor. Source: (Hindricks et al., 2020 / with permission of European Heart Journal).

Epidemiology:
Lower incidence of AF among women
After Age >75, about 60% of AF patients are females

Clinical presentation:
Women are more symptomatic than men with different symptom-profile

Long-term Outcome:
Higher prevalence of LSP AF and NPV triggers compromise the ablation success rate in women
Women with AF tend ro have poorer QOL

AF risk factors:
Older patients are more likely female
Men with first-degree relative with lone AF have higher risk of developing AF compared with women
Both high and low BMI are associated with increased AF risk in women
Low testosterone level in men and estradiol therapy in women increase the risk AF
Higher prevalence of thyroid dysfunction, hypertension and valvular heart disease in women, whereas more CAD and COPD in men
Intense physical activity lowers risk of AF in women, but is associated with higher risk in men

Gender specific Considerations In AF treatment

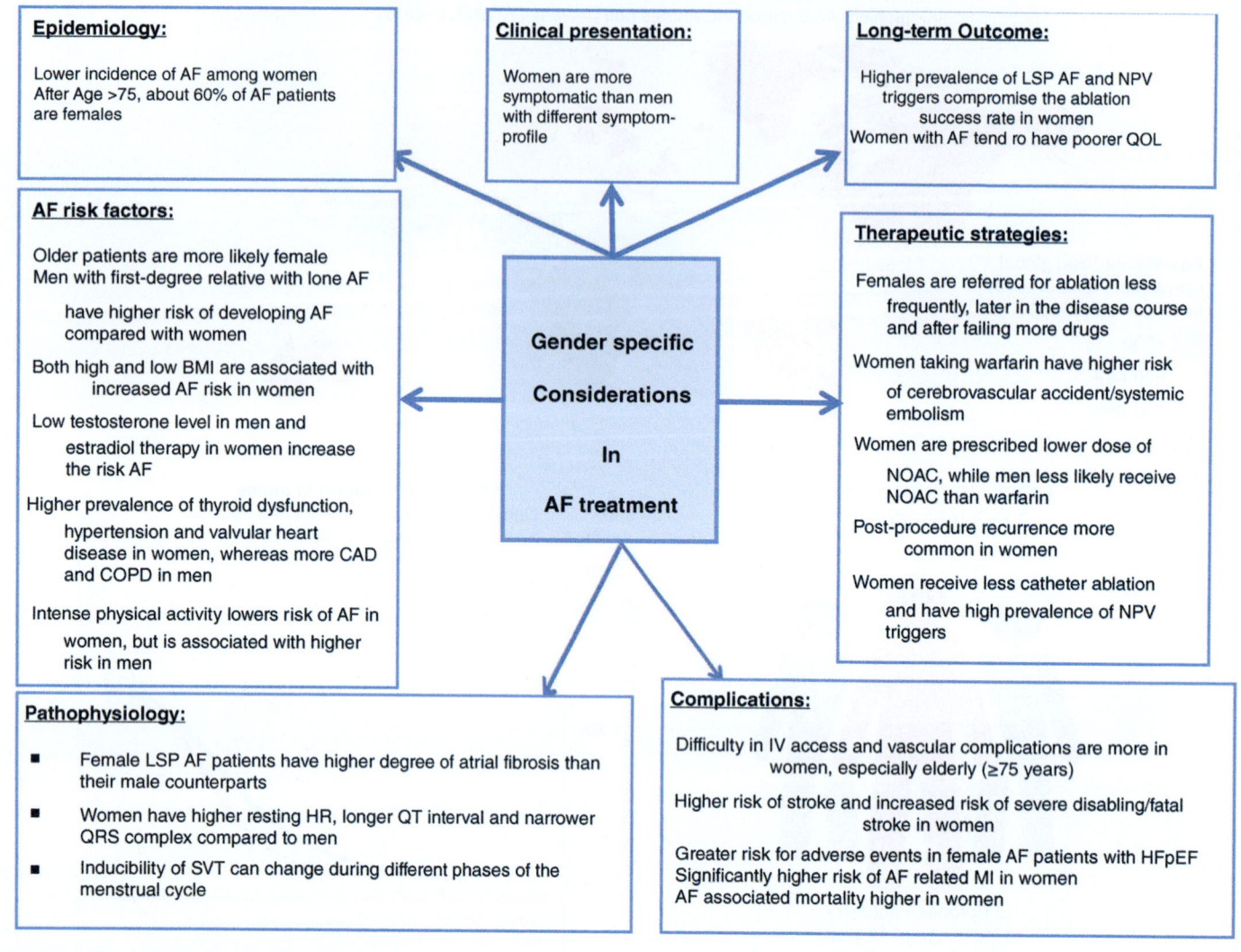

Therapeutic strategies:
Females are referred for ablation less frequently, later in the disease course and after failing more drugs
Women taking warfarin have higher risk of cerebrovascular accident/systemic embolism
Women are prescribed lower dose of NOAC, while men less likely receive NOAC than warfarin
Post-procedure recurrence more common in women
Women receive less catheter ablation and have high prevalence of NPV triggers

Pathophysiology:
- Female LSP AF patients have higher degree of atrial fibrosis than their male counterparts
- Women have higher resting HR, longer QT interval and narrower QRS complex compared to men
- Inducibility of SVT can change during different phases of the menstrual cycle

Complications:
Difficulty in IV access and vascular complications are more in women, especially elderly (≥75 years)
Higher risk of stroke and increased risk of severe disabling/fatal stroke in women
Greater risk for adverse events in female AF patients with HFpEF
Significantly higher risk of AF related MI in women
AF associated mortality higher in women

FIGURE 13.2 Gender-specific considerations in atrial fibrillation. AF = atrial fibrillation; NPV = non-PV; NOAC = novel oral anticoagulants; IV = intravenous; CAD = coronary artery disease; COPD = chronic obstructive pulmonary disease; QOL = quality of life. Source: (Mohanty et al., 2018 / with permission of Taylor & Francis).

for the initiation and progression of AFib in most patients (Al-Kaisey, Parameswaran, & Kalman, 2020; Bosch, Cimini, & Walkey, 2018; Iwasaki, Nishida, Kato, & Nattel, 2011):

- *Autonomous nervous system.* Autonomic nervous system activation can induce significant and heterogeneous changes in atrial electrophysiology and induce atrial tachyarrhythmias, including atrial tachycardia and AFib. In this context, neuromodulation may be helpful in controlling AFib. Potential therapeutic applications include ganglionated plexus ablation, renal sympathetic denervation, cervical vagal nerve stimulation, baroreflex stimulation, and cutaneous stimulation.

- *Electrophysiology of the pulmonary veins.* Rapidly spreading foci, usually located in the smooth muscle that extends into the initial part of the pulmonary veins, are responsible for AFib in a subset of patients. Ablation of these foci and electrical isolation of the pulmonary veins from the myocardium of the left atrium can effectively treat atrial fibrillation in patients whose arrhythmia is due to this mechanism. This mechanism is of high importance in young individuals without organic heart disease.

- *Substrate abnormalities, i.e., pathological changes of the atrial myocardium.* Beyond the impact of AFib itself on structural remodeling, several diseases, such as heart failure, valvular disease, hypertensive heart disease, and coronary heart disease contribute to the development of abnormal atrial substrate and create heterogeneity in the electrophysiological properties of the atrial myocardium. Promising emerging work suggests an important role for atrial substrate imaging in guiding substrate-based ablation strategies and for risk factor management in reversing atrial remodeling.

COMPLICATIONS

Patients with AFib may have various symptoms, such as palpitations, dyspnea, fatigue, chest pain, poor effort tolerance, dizziness, syncope, and disordered sleep, but ~50–90% are initially

Table 13.2 Risk factors for atrial fibrillation.

1. Increased age. AFib is closely related to age and is extremely rare in young individuals without underlying heart disease.
2. Hypertension, i.e., increased blood pressure.
3. Coronary artery disease, also known as coronary heart disease. In coronary artery disease, plaques form inside the coronary arteries, which supply the myocardium with oxygen-enriched blood.
4. Congenital heart diseases, i.e., problems with the structure of the heart that exist from birth. This includes malformations of the inner walls of the heart, valves or blood vessels that carry blood to and from the heart. Congenital abnormalities alter the normal flow of blood to the heart.
5. Mitral valve disease, i.e., abnormal blood flow from the mitral valve, from the left ventricle to the left atrium of the heart.
6. Cardiomyopathy, i.e., a serious disease in which the myocardium is inflamed or does not work as well as it should.
7. Pericarditis, i.e., inflammation of the pericardium, the protective cover that surrounds the heart.
8. Heart surgery, a significantly higher number of patients who have undergone heart surgery have AFib compared to the general population.
9. Hyperthyroidism, i.e., the disease in which the thyroid gland is overactive.
10. Obstructive sleep apnea, is a common disease in which the patient experiences breathing pauses during sleep due to obstructions of the upper airways. Obstructive sleep apnea often causes high blood pressure (hypertension), which increases the risk of cardiovascular diseases.
11. Alcohol abuse. Systematic, excessive, long-term alcohol consumption is closely associated with an increased risk of AFib. Studies have shown that the risk of atrial fibrillation is up to 45% higher in heavy drinkers compared to those who abstain from alcohol consumption.
12. Smoking. It is a well-established risk factor for AFib and other heart diseases.
13. Excessive caffeine consumption. This includes overconsumption of coffee, energy drinks, and/or soft drinks containing caffeine.
14. Atrial murmur. This is like AFib, but abnormal heart rhythms are less chaotic and better organized.
15. Chest infections and pulmonary diseases, such as pneumonia, lung cancer, emphysema, pulmonary embolism, and carbon-monoxide poisoning.

AFib = atrial fibrillation.
Sources: (Dilaveris & Kennedy, 2017; Ling et al., 2016; Staerk et al., 2017)

asymptomatic with possibly a less favorable prognosis (Hindricks et al., 2020). Although many patients with AFib can live for years without significant complications, AFib is a well-established risk factor for cardiovascular diseases, including stroke, systolic embolism, left ventricular dysfunction, and heart failure and is associated with significant declines in quality of life and functional status as well as increased risk of hospitalization, cognitive impairment/dementia, and mortality (**Figure 13.3**) (Hindricks et al., 2020).

Stroke is probably the most well-documented cardiovascular complication of AFib. In AFib, the chaotic heart rhythm may cause blood to pool in the heart's upper chambers and form clots. Once a blood clot forms, it can dislodge from the heart and travel to the brain, causing an ischemic stroke. Patients with AFib are 5 to 7 times more likely to experience a stroke compared to the general population, and AFib is estimated as the cause of 15% to 20% of total ischemic strokes (Castellano, Chinitz, Willner, & Fuster, 2014; Kamel, Okin, Elkind, & Iadecola, 2016). Cardioembolic strokes associated with AFib are usually severe, highly recurrent, and often fatal, or with permanent disability (Hindricks et al., 2020). Clots from the heart can also travel to other parts or organs of the body, such as the kidneys, the lungs, and the gastrointestinal tract and cause significant damage (Jaakkola, Kiviniemi, & Airaksinen, 2018). AFib combined with a fast heart rate for a long period of time can also lead to heart failure, a pathophysiological state in which cardiac output is insufficient to meet the needs of the body and lungs, as described in **Chapter 12** (Anter, Jessup, & Callans, 2009; Lee Park & Anter, 2013). Sharing common risk factors, AFib and heart failure often coexist, or may precipitate/exacerbate each other, which results in significantly greater mortality than either condition alone (Hindricks et al., 2020).

MANAGEMENT

The complexity of AFib requires a multifaceted, holistic, and multidisciplinary management approach, with patients and clinicians in an active partnership. Streamlining the care of patients with AFib in daily clinical practice is a challenging but essential requirement for the effective management of AFib. In recent years, substantial progress has been made in the detection of AFib and its management.

The proper management of AFib starts with an accurate diagnosis through an in-depth examination from the physician. In most patients, AFib can be easily recognized from the surface electrocardiogram with the presence of rapid, irregular fibrillatory waves, and irregular ventricular response (G. Y. Lip & Tse, 2007). After diagnosis, the atrial fibrillation better care (ABC) pathway can be used as an integrated approach for AFib management across all healthcare levels and among different specialties (G. Y. H. Lip, 2017). In the ABC pathway, A stands for "anticoagulation/avoid stroke", B for "better symptom management" and C for "comorbidity optimization". Compared with usual care, implementation of the ABC pathway has been associated with a lower risk of all-cause mortality, lower risk of a composite outcome of stroke/major bleeding/cardiovascular death and hospitalization, lower rates of cardiovascular events, and lower health-related costs (Hindricks et al., 2020).

The first step, "anticoagulation/avoid stroke", aims to identify low-risk patients who do not need antithrombotic therapy. Step 2 is to offer stroke prevention, i.e., oral anticoagulants, to those with ≥1 non-sex stroke risk factors. Step 3 is the choice of an oral anticoagulant—a non-vitamin K antagonist oral anticoagulant (given their relative effectiveness, safety, and convenience these drugs are generally the first choice as oral anticoagulant for stroke prevention in AFib) or vitamin K antagonist (Freedman, Potpara, & Lip, 2016; G. Y. Lip & Lane, 2015). The "better symptom control" step of the ABC pathway mainly focuses on heart rate control, which is an integral part of AFib

Clinical Presentation

- Asymptomatic or Silent (!)
- Symptomatic
- **Palpitations, dyspnoea, fatigue,** Chest tightness/pain, poor effort tolerance, dizziness, syncope, disorderes sleep, etc.
- **Haemodynamically unstable**
  - Syncope
  - Symptomatic hypotension
  - Acute HF, pulmonary oedema
  - Ongoing myocardial ischaemia
  - Cardiogenic shock
- Haemodynamically stable

AF-related OUTCOMES

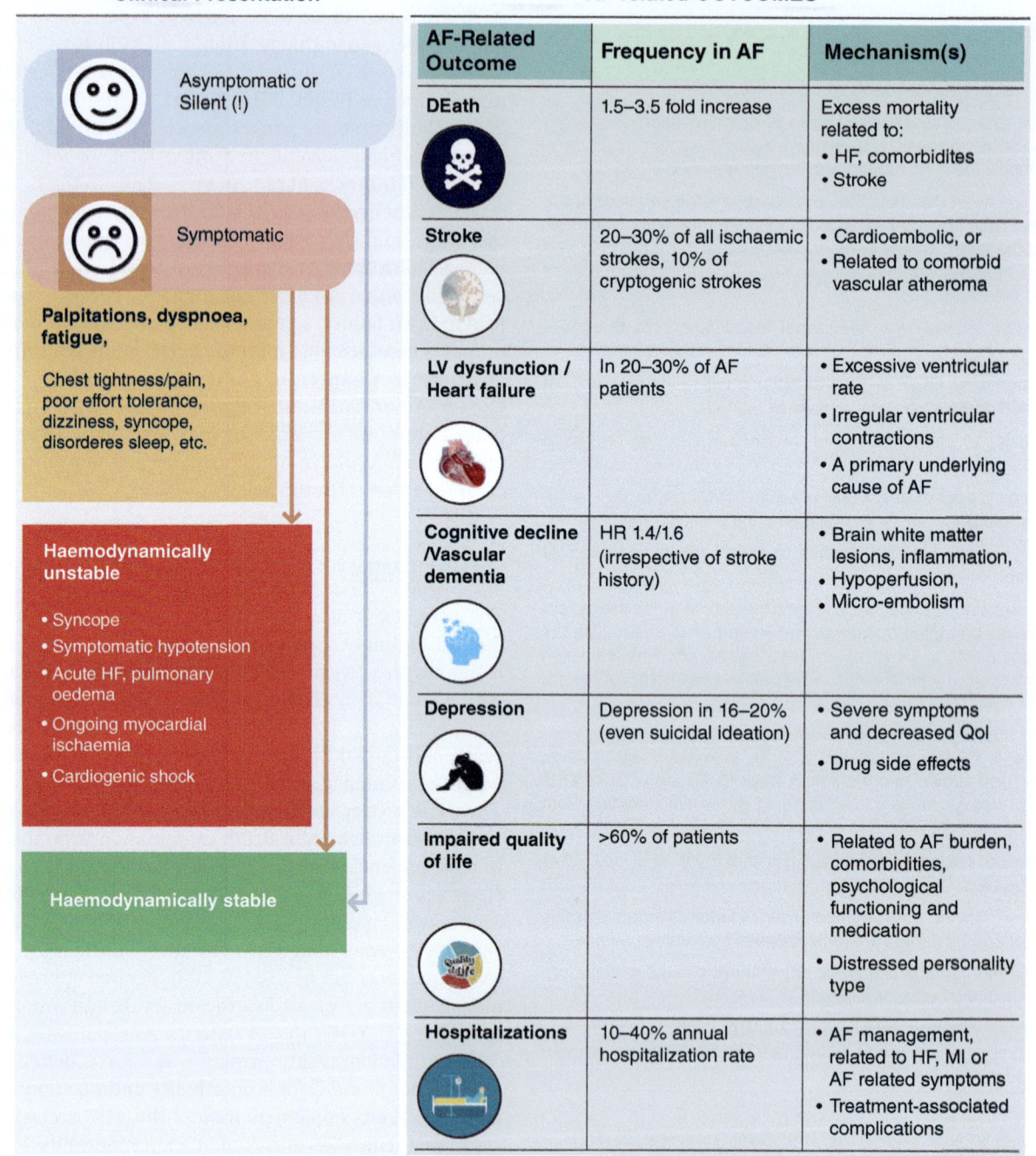

AF-Related Outcome	Frequency in AF	Mechanism(s)
DEath	1.5–3.5 fold increase	Excess mortality related to: • HF, comorbidites • Stroke
Stroke	20–30% of all ischaemic strokes, 10% of cryptogenic strokes	• Cardioembolic, or • Related to comorbid vascular atheroma
LV dysfunction / Heart failure	In 20–30% of AF patients	• Excessive ventricular rate • Irregular ventricular contractions • A primary underlying cause of AF
Cognitive decline /Vascular dementia	HR 1.4/1.6 (irrespective of stroke history)	• Brain white matter lesions, inflammation, • Hypoperfusion, • Micro-embolism
Depression	Depression in 16–20% (even suicidal ideation)	• Severe symptoms and decreased QoI • Drug side effects
Impaired quality of life	>60% of patients	• Related to AF burden, comorbidities, psychological functioning and medication • Distressed personality type
Hospitalizations	10–40% annual hospitalization rate	• AF management, related to HF, MI or AF related symptoms • Treatment-associated complications

FIGURE 13.3 Clinical presentation of atrial fibrillation and related outcomes. AF = atrial fibrillation; HF = heart failure; HR = hazard ratio; LV = left ventricle; MI = myocardial infarction; QOL = quality of life. Source: (Hindricks et al., 2020 / with permission of Elsevier).

management and is often sufficient to improve AFib-related symptoms. Drug choices for heart rate control include beta-blockers, calcium-channel blockers, and digitalis as first-line agents, with consideration of other sympatholytic in resistant cases (Hindricks et al., 2020). When pharmacotherapy is insufficient for an efficient heart rate control, other procedures can be used, most importantly cardioversion, i.e., the use of external electric shocks to restore a normal heart rhythm, and ablation (catheter or surgical), i.e., a procedure in which heart tissue responsible for abnormal electrical signals is scared or destroyed (Hindricks et al., 2020). Finally, the "comorbidity optimization" step of the ABC pathway includes the identification and management of concomitant diseases, cardio-metabolic risk factors, and unhealthy lifestyle choices. Management of risk factors and co-morbidities complements stroke prevention and reduces AFib burden and symptom severity. Interventional studies have shown that targeted therapy of underlying medical conditions significantly improves maintenance of sinus rhythm in patients with persistent AFib and heart failure (Rienstra et al., 2018).

NUTRITION IN ATRIAL FIBRILLATION

Nutrition is an important factor for the prevention and management of AFib. The available evidence shows a complex interaction between nutritional status and the risk, course, and complications of AFib (**Figure 13.4**) (Anaszewicz & Budzynski, 2017). On the one hand, overweight, obesity, and high birth mass are proposed as significant risk factors for the development of AFib, while weight loss in obese patients is linked to an improved course of AFib and reduced all-cause and cardiovascular mortality. On the other hand, a so-called obesity paradox has been observed in patients with AFib, according to which overweight patients with AFib present lower all-cause mortality compared to normal-weight and underweight patients. Overall, the relationship between nutritional status and risk of AFib and its complications is U-shaped, meaning that not only patients with obesity, but also individuals with underweight, low lean body mass, and cachexia, may have an increased risk and poor outcome of AFib.

Besides nutritional status and body habitus, data on the role of nutrition and long-term dietary habits in the prevention and management of AFib are, to date, scarce. However, it is widely accepted that the efficient management of AFib includes risk factor modification, including the treatment of underlying sleep apnea, hypertension, hyperlipidemia, and glucose intolerance (January et al., 2019), conditions tightly linked to an unhealthy lifestyle and favorably affected by the adoption of balanced dietary pattern. Therefore, besides the achievement of a healthy body weight, cardio-protective dietary modifications can be of value for patients with AFib. In this context, consistent evidence from epidemiological studies indicates that higher consumption of fruits, vegetables, nuts, legumes, fish, vegetable oils (especially olive oil), and whole grains, along with a lower/modest intake of red and processed meats, foods rich in refined carbohydrates (sugars), salt, and industrialized processed foods high in trans fatty acids, is associated with a lower incidence of cardiovascular events (**Figure 13.5**) (Mach et al., 2020). Besides individuals foods, the Prevencion con Dieta Mediterranea (PREDIMED) study, one of the few available randomized controlled clinical trials that aimed to assess the effects of diet on the primary prevention of cardiovascular disease, showed that a Mediterranean diet (emphasizing on olive oil, nuts, fresh fruits, vegetables, fish, legumes, white meat, and moderate consumption of wine with meals) supplemented with either olive oil or nuts was superior in reducing cardiovascular disease risk, compared to a low-fat diet (Estruch et al., 2006); the Mediterranean diet can therefore be recommended as a prudent dietary pattern for the prevention and management of AFib.

Patients with AFib should also consume alcohol and coffee in moderation, given their potential detrimental effects on cardiac arrythmias. Alcohol is the most common trigger of AFib reported by 35% of patients and is associated with reduced heart rate variability, sympathetic effects, and vagal stimulation (Voskoboinik et al., 2020). Binge drinking has also been associated with acute cardiac inflammation. Observational studies link regular alcohol consumption (as compared with no alcohol consumption) with dose-related increases in left atrial size, impairments in atrial mechanical and reservoir function, and adverse electrical remodeling (Voskoboinik et al., 2020). Numerous studies have also reported higher rates of recurrence of AFib after catheter ablation among regular drinkers than among non-drinkers (Voskoboinik et al., 2020). With regards to coffee, research on its relationship with arrhythmias is contradictory. Both large population studies and randomized control trials suggest that caffeine intake of up to 300 mg/day may be safe for arrhythmic patients (Voskoboinik, Kalman, & Kistler, 2018). However, there may be individual differences in susceptibility to the effects of caffeine on the factors that trigger arrhythmias in some, and up to 25% of patients report coffee as an AFib trigger (Voskoboinik et al., 2018); therefore, patients with a clear

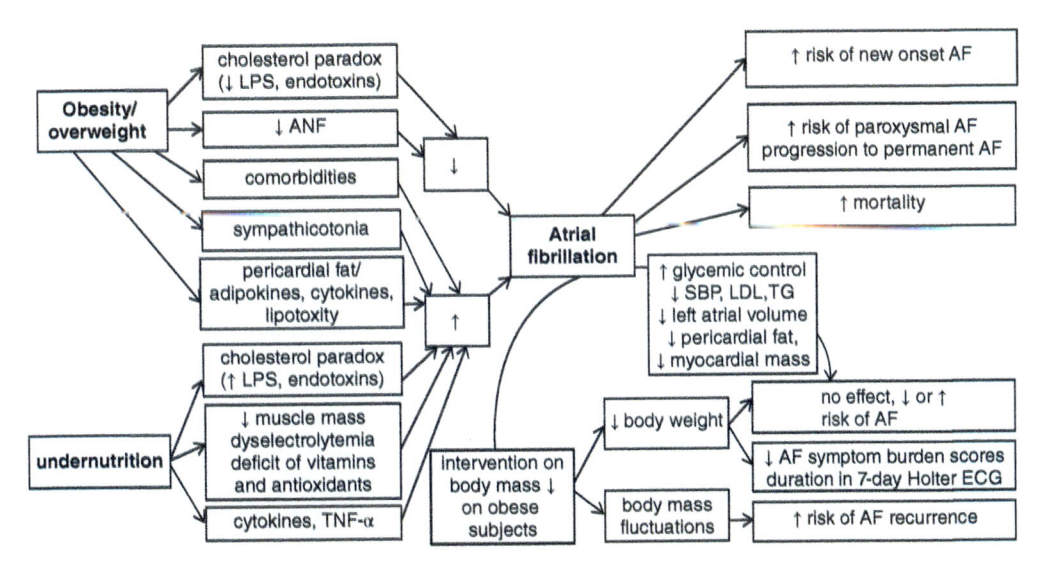

FIGURE 13.4 The role of nutritional status in the pathogenesis of atrial fibrillation. AF = atrial fibrillation; ANS = autonomic nervous system; ANF = atrial natriuretic factor; LPS = bacterial lipopolysaccharides; SBP = systolic blood pressure; LDL = low-density lipoprotein; TG = triglycerides; ↑ = unfavorable effect (increase in AF risk); ↓ = favorable effect (decrease in risk of AF and complications). Source: (Anaszewicz & Budzynski, 2017).

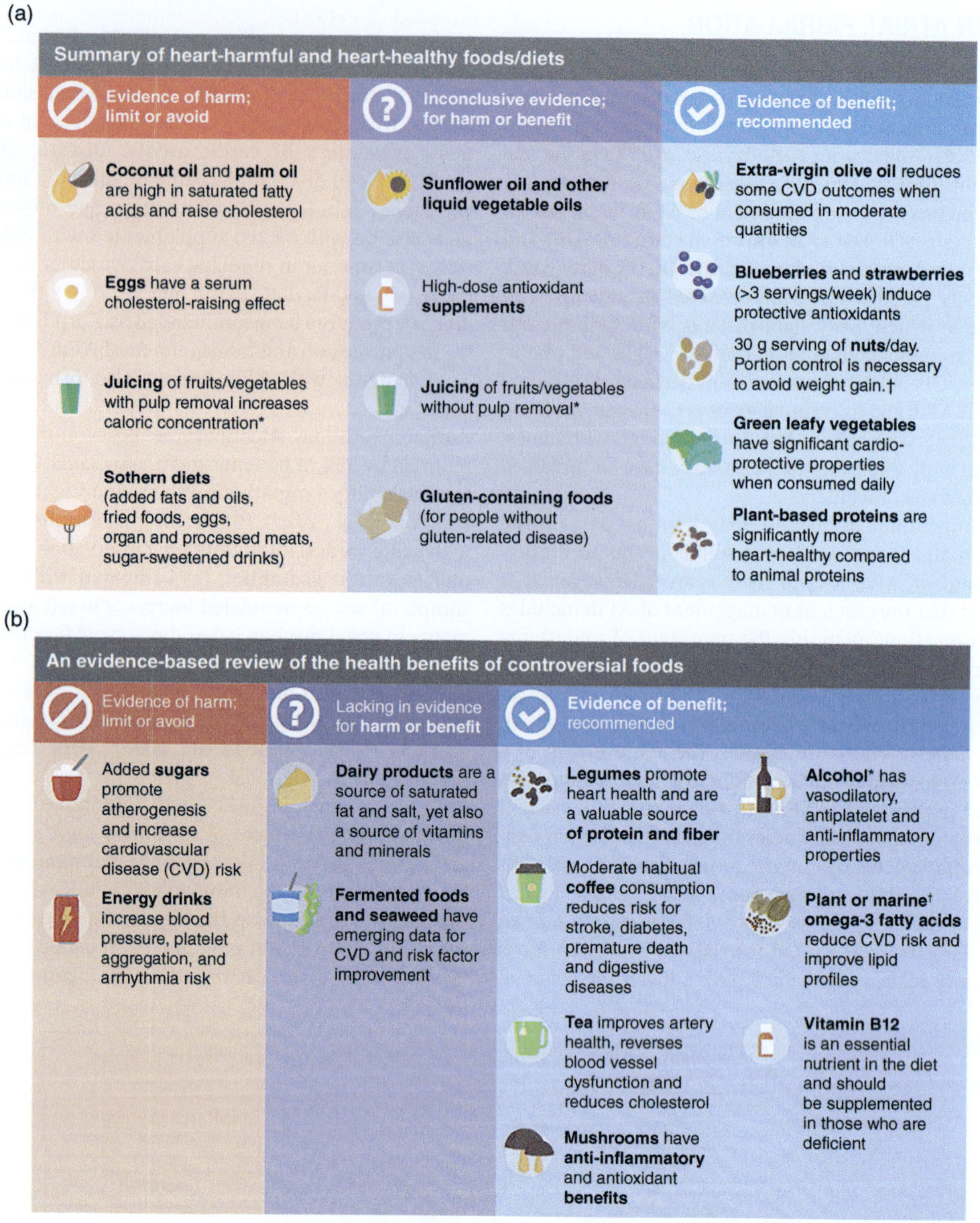

FIGURE 13.5 (a) Summary of heart-harmful and heart-healthy foods/diets. This figure summarizes the foods that should be consumed often, and others that should be avoided from a cardiovascular health perspective. *It is important to note that juicing becomes less of a benefit if calorie intake increases because of caloric concentration with pulp removal. †Moderate quantities are required to prevent caloric excess. (b) An evidence-based review of the health benefits of controversial foods. This illustration depicts the health benefits of controversial food items using the "evidence of harm," "lacking in evidence," and "evidence of benefit" designations. *It is not recommended that individuals initiate alcohol consumption for health benefit, and for those already drinking, consumption should be limited to recommended amounts and preferably consumed with meals. A patient's risk of cancers and other organ system diseases need to be weighted carefully when making recommendations. †There are some environmental and toxin (heavy metals, dioxins, polychlorinated biphenyls, and others) concerns in marine sources. Source: (Freeman et al., 2018 / with permission of Elsevier).

temporal association between coffee intake and AFib episodes should be counseled to abstain.

For patients on anticoagulation as part of their treatment, another crucial point is the dietary intake of vitamin K, as this vitamin helps blood clot and can therefore interfere with the effects of pharmacotherapy. Vitamin K is a fat-soluble vitamin that plays an important role in blood clotting, bone health, and heart health. Patients with AFib on anticoagulation medication do not need to exclude foods that contain vitamin K, but should keep the amount of these foods constant day by day (Violi, Lip, Pignatelli, & Pastori, 2016). Foods rich in vitamin K are mainly green leafy vegetables, such as cauliflower, lettuce, spinach, and cabbage, but also lentils, liver, green tea, mustard, and mayonnaise.

PHYSICAL ACTIVITY AND RISK OF ATRIAL FIBRILLATION

The relationship between physical activity and AFib is complex. On the one hand, physical activity has well-established cardioprotective properties and can help toward the prevention and/or efficient management of obesity, diabetes mellitus, hypertension, and other heart-related diseases. These beneficial effects can also offer protection against the development of AFib (Lau, Nattel, Kalman, & Sanders, 2017). On the other hand, certain modes of exercise have been positively associated with the onset of AFib and despite the health benefits of exercise, AFib is common among athletes (**Figure 13.6**) (Turagam, Flaker, Velagapudi, Vadali, & Alpert, 2015).

The benefits of exercise on cardiovascular risk are beyond doubt. At the minimum recommended physical activity level (150 min/week), the risk of mortality, coronary heart disease, and heart failure decreases significantly, while health benefits are even greater at two times the recommended level (300 min/week) (Moore et al., 2012; Sattelmair et al., 2011). Whether this protective pattern is also evident for AFib remains unclear. The study by Drca et al. (Drca, Wolk, Jensen-Urstad, & Larsson, 2014) published in 2014 examined the association between physical activity at different ages and the risk of AFib in 44,410 Swedish men aged 45 to 79 years. During a median follow up of 12 years, men who exercised >5 hours/week in their 30s had an ~20% higher relative risk for developing AFib compared to those who exercised <1 hour/week. The risk was even higher (~50%) among the men who exercised >5 hour/week at age 30 and quit exercising later in life (<1 hour/week). On the contrary, walking/bicycling for >1 hour/day at 60 years old was associated with a ~15% lower risk of AFib. Interestingly, safe levels of exercise for AFib may differ for men and women. According to an extensive meta-analysis of 22 studies, including 656,750 subjects published in 2016 (Mohanty et al., 2016), the adoption of a sedentary lifestyle was associated with a ~2.5 times higher risk of incident AFib, compared to any level of physical activity, among both men and women. In addition, women involved in moderate and intense physical activity were ~10% and ~30% less likely to develop AFib, respectively, compared to women who were physically inactive. However, in men, compared to sedentariness, only moderate-intensity physical activity was associated with a ~20% lower risk of AFib, whereas intense physical activity was associated with an ~3 times higher risk of AFib. A subsequent meta-analysis published in 2018 by Ricci et al. (Ricci et al., 2018) also revealed a complex dose-response link between physical activity and AFib risk; physical activity at volumes of 5 to 20 hours of metabolic equivalents per week was associated with a significant reduction (~10%) in AFib risk, however, no such benefit was observed for physical activity volumes exceeding 20 hours of metabolic equivalents per week.

According to available epidemiological data, avoiding sedentariness and meeting the recommended target range of physical activity is associated with the maximum benefit for AFib risk reduction in the general population. However, the dose-response relationship between physical activity and AFib risk shows a U-shaped pattern, meaning that both inactivity and a very high level of physical activity are associated with an increased risk of AFib compared to the intermediate category, i.e., a low-to-moderate physical activity level (Jin et al., 2019). Moreover, the type and intensity of physical activity may be of importance in the context of AFib risk. Although moderate-intensity aerobic exercise is beneficial, vigorous exercise and endurance athletics have not shown similar protective effects, especially in men (Mozaffarian, Furberg, Psaty, & Siscovick, 2008; Thelle et al., 2013). **Figure 13.7** provides an overview of the potential mechanisms by which exercise, especially endurance training, can lead to AFib. Although the mechanisms are not well understood, exercise-induced changes in autonomic tone alongside the development of an arrhythmogenic atrial substrate appear to contribute to AFib among athletes, despite an overall reduction in cardiovascular disease incidence (Elliott, Linz, Verdicchio, & Sanders, 2018; Mont, Elosua, & Brugada, 2009). However, in non-athletes, such mechanisms may not play a major role for the development of AFib. On the contrary, physical activity in non-athletes might reduce body weight, blood pressure, and incident diabetes mellitus, all of which are established risk factors for AFib (Ofman et al., 2013).

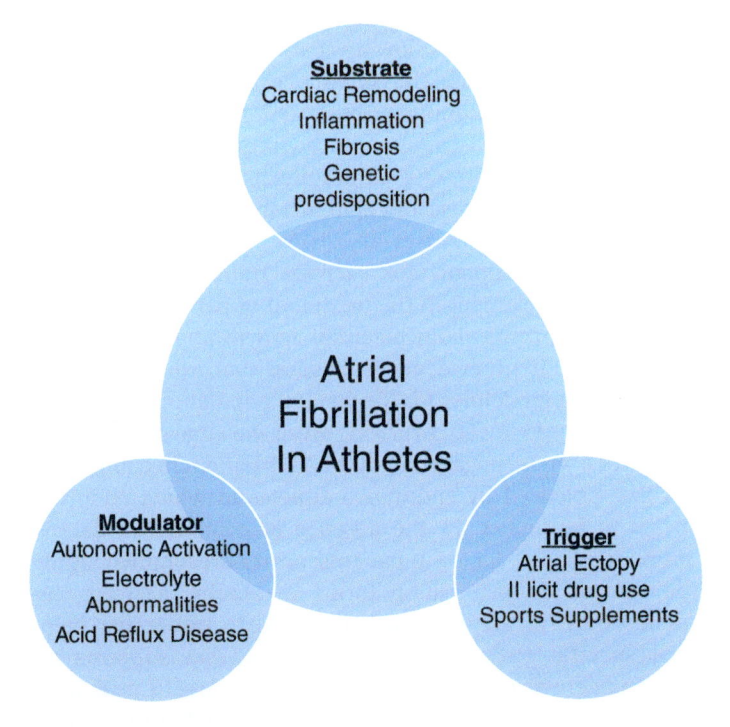

FIGURE 13.6 Schematic representation of atrial fibrillation in athletes. Source: (Adapted from Turagam et al., 2015).

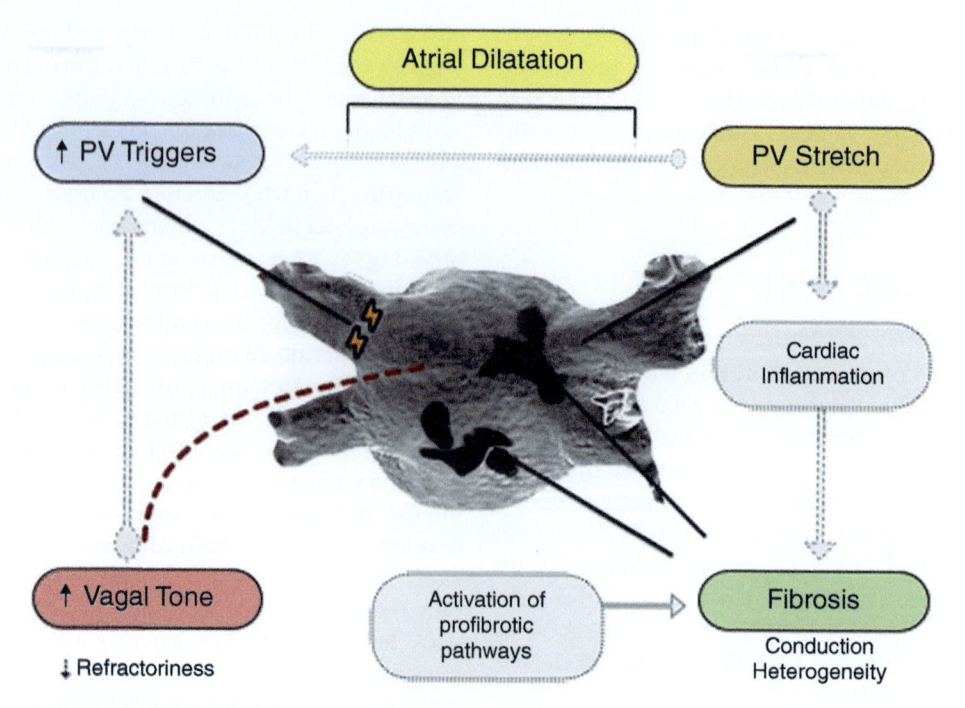

FIGURE 13.7 Summary of potential mechanisms promoting atrial arrhythmogenesis in endurance-trained athletes. PV = pulmonary vein. Source: (Elliott et al., 2018 / with permission of Elsevier).

Although the link between physical activity and AFib risk requires further investigation, cross-sectional studies have revealed that patients with AFib are characterized by low levels of physical activity, and their level of sedentariness is positively linked to the severity of AFib symptoms (Semaan et al., 2020). This observation highlights the difficulties and barriers AFib patients face when exercising, including typical AFib symptoms, such as fatigue, heart palpitations, dizziness, sweating, anxiety, and shortness of breath. These findings raise the possibility that a proportion of the poor health outcomes associated with AFib may be related to disease-associated inactivity and that the alleviation of AFib symptoms may help facilitate physical activity among those with the disease (Semaan et al., 2020).

EXERCISE TRAINING AND ATRIAL FIBRILLATION MANAGEMENT

Exercise interventions have been shown to be safe and effective for patients with a variety of metabolic and cardiovascular diseases, such as obesity, hyperlipidemia, metabolic syndrome, polycystic ovarian syndrome, type 1 and 2 diabetes mellitus, hypertension, coronary heart disease, heart failure, cerebral apoplexy, and claudication intermittent (Pedersen & Saltin, 2015). However, the effects of exercise on AFib are not so well-studied. Epidemiology supports that physically active individuals experience a modest reduction in AFib risk but doing too much exercise can considerably increase arrhythmia risk, consistent with a classic U-shaped phenomenon. Due to these findings and the fear of promoting exercise-induced cardiac arrhythmias, there is a scarcity of data regarding the effects of exercise training in patients with AFib (Elliott, Mahajan, Pathak, Lau, & Sanders, 2016).

The few available data from well-designed clinical trials support that exercise may reduce AFib burden and symptomatology, along with significant improvements in peak oxygen consumption (VO_2 peak), cardiac function, and quality of life (Malmo et al., 2016). Moreover, increases in cardio-respiratory fitness have been associated with a significant alleviation of arrhythmia burden. In specific, each 1-metabolic equivalent incremental gain in fitness has been associated with a ~10% reduction in AFib recurrence over a 4-year follow up (Pathak et al., 2015). The primary mechanisms driving the benefit of exercise on AFib include its direct effects on autonomic factors and intrinsic electrophysiological measures, and exerciseinduced improvements in cardiac structure and function, and cardio-metabolic parameters, i.e., body composition, glucose and lipid metabolism, blood pressure, and inflammation (Elliott et al., 2016). Taken together, these findings provide support for exercise training and physical activity as a key element in the treatment of patients with AFib. Despite the concerns about potential arrhythmogenic effects of exercise, there is no evidence to suggest that exercise training within current guidelines for the general population exacerbates AFib. This should not be surprising given the large differences in the dose of exercise engaged in by an AFib patient in comparison with that practiced by endurance athletes in which AFib risk appears to be higher. In the absence of comparative data of training modalities for AFib patients, current recommendations should focus on prescribing forms of aerobic exercise that patients enjoy and are most likely to adhere to, rather than being overly specific. However, the current evidence supports the efficacy of aerobic exercise activities up to, or close to, peak heart rate, if appropriate and achievable to the patient. Future research should focus on defining the optimal aerobic exercise dose for patients with AFib and establishing the role of resistance training within the exercise prescription.

PHYSICAL ACTIVITY RECOMMENDATIONS

Many studies have demonstrated the beneficial effects of moderate exercise/physical activity on cardiovascular health (Lavie, Thomas, Squires, Allison, & Milani, 2009; Menezes et al., 2015; Mont, 2010). Nevertheless, the incidence of AFib appears to be increased among elite athletes, and multiple small-scale studies have reported a relationship between AFib and vigorous physical activity, mainly related to long-term or endurance sport participation (Baldesberger et al., 2008; Karjalainen, Kujala, Kaprio, Sarna, & Viitasalo, 1998; Molina et al., 2008; Nielsen, Wachtell, & Abdulla, 2013). Based on this non-linear relationship between physical activity and AFib, the European Society of Cardiology and the European Association of Cardio-Thoracic Surgery recommend that AFib patients should be encouraged to undertake moderate-intensity exercise. They also recommend to remain physically active to prevent AFib incidence or recurrence but maybe avoid chronic excessive endurance exercise (such as marathons and long-distance triathlons, etc.), especially if aged >50 years (Hindricks et al., 2020). In this context, physical activity guidelines for the general population published by major health organizations, such as the World Health Organization (Bull et al., 2020) and the US Department of Health and Human Services (Piercy & Troiano, 2018) are suitable for the majority of AFib patients. These guidelines, as mentioned in previous chapters, recommend at least 150 minutes/week of moderate-intensity aerobic activity or 75 minutes/week of vigorous aerobic activity, or a combination of both, preferably spread throughout the week. On top of aerobic training, moderate-to-high-intensity muscle-strengthening activity on at least 2 days/week and the avoidance of sedentariness (even light-intensity activity can offset some of the risks of sedentariness) are additionally recommended for all ages.

The management of athletes with AFib is similar to general AFib management but requires a few special considerations. According to the guidelines of the European Society of Cardiology and the European Association of Cardio-Thoracic Surgery for AFib management (Kirchhof et al., 2016): (i) athletes should be counseled that long-lasting intense sports participation can promote AFib; (ii) sports with direct bodily contact or prone to trauma should be avoided in patients on oral anticoagulation; (iii) ablation should be considered to prevent recurrent AFib in athletes; (iv) the ventricular rate while exercising with AFib should be evaluated in every athlete and titrated rate control should be instituted; (v) after ingestion of pill-in-the-pocket (the patient takes a single oral dose of an antiarrhythmic drug at the time of the onset of palpitations) flecainide or propafenone (common medications prescribed to maintain sinus rhythm in patients without structural heart disease or ischemic heart disease with symptomatic recurrent atrial flutter or AFib), patients should refrain from sports as long as AFib persists and until two half-lives of the antiarrhythmic drug have elapsed.

KEY POINTS

- AFib refers to a supraventricular tachyarrhythmia with uncoordinated atrial electrical activation and consequently ineffective atrial contraction, and it is a major risk factor for cardiovascular diseases, mainly stroke and heart failure.
- Nutritional management of AFib mainly involves the adoption of a heart-healthy diet, rich in fiber-rich plant-based foods (fruits, vegetables, whole grains, and legumes), olive oil and fish, and low in salt, trans fatty acids, cholesterol, and sugars.
- Avoiding excessive amounts of alcohol and caffeine and maintaining a healthy body weight can help reduce the risk of complications associated with AFib.
- Physical activity can help prevent AFib incidence and recurrence, except for excessive endurance exercise, which may promote AFib.
- AFib is common among elite athletes. Although the mechanisms are not well understood, exercise-induced changes in autonomic tone alongside the development of an arrhythmogenic atrial substrate appear to contribute to AFib among athletes, despite an overall reduction in cardiovascular risk.
- The optimal exercise regimen for AFib patients has not yet been determined. Exercise interventions have been shown to reduce AFib burden and symptomatology, along with significant improvements in fitness and quality of life.
- AFib patients should be encouraged to undertake moderate-intensity exercise and remain physically active to prevent AFib incidence or recurrence but avoid chronic excessive endurance exercise (such as marathons and long-distance triathlons, etc.), especially if aged >50 years.

SELF-ASSESSMENT QUESTIONS

1. Define atrial fibrillation.
2. List four risk factors for atrial fibrillation.
3. What are the mechanisms of initiation and progression of atrial fibrillation in most patients?
4. What is the atrial fibrillation better care (ABC) pathway?
5. Is the Mediterranean diet recommended for the management of atrial fibrillation?
6. Explain the U-shaped relationship between physical activity and atrial fibrillation.

REFERENCES

Al-Kaisey, A. M., Parameswaran, R., & Kalman, J. M. (2020). Atrial Fibrillation Structural Substrates: Aetiology, Identification and Implications. *Arrhythm Electrophysiol Rev, 9*(3), 113–120. doi:10.15420/aer.2020.19

Anaszewicz, M., & Budzynski, J. (2017). Clinical significance of nutritional status in patients with atrial fibrillation: An overview of current evidence. *J Cardiol, 69*(5), 719–730. doi:10.1016/j.jjcc.2016.06.014

Anter, E., Jessup, M., & Callans, D. J. (2009). Atrial fibrillation and heart failure: treatment considerations for a dual epidemic. *Circulation, 119*(18), 2516–2525. doi:10.1161/CIRCULATIONAHA.108.821306

Baldesberger, S., Bauersfeld, U., Candinas, R., Seifert, B., Zuber, M., Ritter, M., . . . Attenhofer Jost, C. H. (2008). Sinus node disease and arrhythmias in the long-term follow-up of former professional cyclists. *Eur Heart J, 29*(1), 71–78. doi:10.1093/eurheartj/ehm555

Benjamin, E. J., Muntner, P., Alonso, A., Bittencourt, M. S., Callaway, C. W., Carson, A. P., . . . Stroke Statistics, S. (2019). Heart Disease and Stroke Statistics-2019 Update: A Report From the American Heart Association. *Circulation, 139*(10), e56–e528. doi:10.1161/CIR.0000000000000659

Bosch, N. A., Cimini, J., & Walkey, A. J. (2018). Atrial Fibrillation in the ICU. *Chest, 154*(6), 1424–1434. doi:10.1016/j.chest.2018.03.040

Bull, F. C., Al-Ansari, S. S., Biddle, S., Borodulin, K., Buman, M. P., Cardon, G., . . . Willumsen, J. F. (2020). World Health Organization 2020 guidelines on physical activity and sedentary behaviour. *Br J Sports Med, 54*(24), 1451–1462. doi:10.1136/bjsports-2020-102955

Castellano, J. M., Chinitz, J., Willner, J., & Fuster, V. (2014). Mechanisms of Stroke in Atrial Fibrillation. *Card Electrophysiol Clin, 6*(1), 5–15. doi:10.1016/j.ccep.2013.10.007

Chugh, S. S., Havmoeller, R., Narayanan, K., Singh, D., Rienstra, M., Benjamin, E. J., . . . Murray, C. J. (2014). Worldwide epidemiology of atrial fibrillation: a Global Burden of Disease 2010 Study. *Circulation, 129*(8), 837–847. doi:10.1161/CIRCULATIONAHA.113.005119

Di Carlo, A., Bellino, L., Consoli, D., Mori, F., Zaninelli, A., Baldereschi, M., . . . National Research Program: Progetto, F. A. I. L. F. A. i. I. (2019). Prevalence of atrial fibrillation in the Italian elderly population and projections from 2020 to 2060 for Italy and the European Union: the FAI Project. *Europace, 21*(10), 1468–1475. doi:10.1093/europace/euz141

Dilaveris, P. E., & Kennedy, H. L. (2017). Silent atrial fibrillation: epidemiology, diagnosis, and clinical impact. *Clin Cardiol, 40*(6), 413–418. doi:10.1002/clc.22667

Drca, N., Wolk, A., Jensen-Urstad, M., & Larsson, S. C. (2014). Atrial fibrillation is associated with different levels of physical activity levels at different ages in men. *Heart, 100*(13), 1037–1042. doi:10.1136/heartjnl-2013-305304

Elliott, A. D., Linz, D., Verdicchio, C. V., & Sanders, P. (2018). Exercise and Atrial Fibrillation: Prevention or Causation? *Heart Lung Circ, 27*(9), 1078–1085. doi:10.1016/j.hlc.2018.04.296

Elliott, A. D., Mahajan, R., Pathak, R. K., Lau, D. H., & Sanders, P. (2016). Exercise Training and Atrial Fibrillation: Further Evidence for the Importance of Lifestyle Change. *Circulation, 133*(5), 457–459. doi:10.1161/CIRCULATIONAHA.115.020800

Estruch, R., Martinez-Gonzalez, M. A., Corella, D., Salas-Salvado, J., Ruiz-Gutierrez, V., Covas, M.I., . . . Investigators, P. S. (2006). Effects of a Mediterranean-style diet on cardiovascular risk factors: a randomized trial. *Ann Intern Med, 145*(1), 1–11. doi:10.7326/0003-4819-145-1-200607040-00004

Freedman, B., Potpara, T. S., & Lip, G. Y. (2016). Stroke prevention in atrial fibrillation. *Lancet, 388*(10046), 806–817. doi:10.1016/S0140-6736(16)31257-0

Freeman, A. M., Morris, P. B., Aspry, K., Gordon, N. F., Barnard, N. D., Esselstyn, C. B., . . . Kris-Etherton, P. (2018). A Clinician's Guide for Trending Cardiovascular Nutrition Controversies: Part II. *J Am Coll Cardiol, 72*(5), 553–568. doi:10.1016/j.jacc.2018.05.030

Freeman, A. M., Morris, P. B., Barnard, N., Esselstyn, C. B., Ros, E., Agatston, A., . . . Kris-Etherton, P. (2017). Trending Cardiovascular Nutrition Controversies. *J Am Coll Cardiol, 69*(9), 1172–1187. doi:10.1016/j.jacc.2016.10.086

Hindricks, G., Potpara, T., Dagres, N., Arbelo, E., Bax, J. J., Blomstrom-Lundqvist, C., . . . Group, E. S. C. S. D. (2020). 2020 ESC Guidelines for the diagnosis and management of atrial fibrillation developed in collaboration with the European Association of Cardio-Thoracic Surgery (EACTS). *Eur Heart J*. doi:10.1093/eurheartj/ehaa612

Iwasaki, Y. K., Nishida, K., Kato, T., & Nattel, S. (2011). Atrial fibrillation pathophysiology: implications for management. *Circulation, 124*(20), 2264–2274. doi:10.1161/CIRCULATIONAHA.111.019893

Jaakkola, S., Kiviniemi, T. O., & Airaksinen, K. E. J. (2018). Cardioversion for atrial fibrillation - how to prevent thromboembolic complications? *Ann Med, 50*(7), 549–555. doi:10.1080/07853890.2018.1523552

January, C. T., Wann, L. S., Calkins, H., Chen, L. Y., Cigarroa, J. E., Cleveland, J. C., Jr., . . . Yancy, C. W. (2019). 2019 AHA/ACC/HRS Focused Update of the 2014 AHA/ACC/HRS Guideline for the Management of Patients With Atrial Fibrillation: A Report of the American College of Cardiology/American Heart Association Task Force on Clinical Practice Guidelines and the Heart Rhythm Society in Collaboration With the Society of Thoracic Surgeons. *Circulation, 140*(2), e125–e151. doi:10.1161/CIR.0000000000000665

Jin, M. N., Yang, P. S., Song, C., Yu, H. T., Kim, T. H., Uhm, J. S., . . . Joung, B. (2019). Physical Activity and Risk of Atrial Fibrillation: A Nationwide Cohort Study in General Population. *Sci Rep, 9*(1), 13270. doi:10.1038/s41598-019-49686-w

Kamel, H., Okin, P. M., Elkind, M. S., & Iadecola, C. (2016). Atrial Fibrillation and Mechanisms of Stroke: Time for a New Model. *Stroke, 47*(3), 895–900. doi:10.1161/STROKEAHA.115.012004

Karjalainen, J., Kujala, U. M., Kaprio, J., Sarna, S., & Viitasalo, M. (1998). Lone atrial fibrillation in vigorously exercising middle aged men: case-control study. *BMJ, 316*(7147), 1784–1785. doi:10.1136/bmj.316.7147.1784

Kirchhof, P., Benussi, S., Kotecha, D., Ahlsson, A., Atar, D., Casadei, B., . . . Group, E. S. C. S. D. (2016). 2016 ESC Guidelines for the management of atrial fibrillation developed in collaboration with EACTS. *Eur Heart J, 37*(38), 2893–2962. doi:10.1093/eurheartj/ehw210

Kornej, J., Borschel, C. S., Benjamin, E. J., & Schnabel, R. B. (2020). Epidemiology of Atrial Fibrillation in the 21st Century: Novel Methods and New Insights. *Circ Res, 127*(1), 4–20. doi:10.1161/CIRCRESAHA.120.316340

Lau, D. H., Nattel, S., Kalman, J. M., & Sanders, P. (2017). Modifiable Risk Factors and Atrial Fibrillation. *Circulation, 136*(6), 583–596. doi:10.1161/CIRCULATIONAHA.116.023163

Lavie, C. J., Thomas, R. J., Squires, R. W., Allison, T. G., & Milani, R. V. (2009). Exercise training and cardiac rehabilitation in primary and secondary prevention of coronary heart disease. *Mayo Clin Proc, 84*(4), 373–383. doi:10.1016/S0025-6196(11)60548-X

Lee Park, K., & Anter, E. (2013). Atrial Fibrillation and Heart Failure: A Review of the Intersection of Two Cardiac Epidemics. *J Atr Fibrillation*, *6*(1), 751. doi:10.4022/jafib.751

Ling, L. H., Kistler, P. M., Kalman, J. M., Schilling, R. J., & Hunter, R. J. (2016). Comorbidity of atrial fibrillation and heart failure. *Nat Rev Cardiol*, *13*(3), 131–147. doi:10.1038/nrcardio.2015.191

Lip, G. Y., & Lane, D. A. (2015). Stroke prevention in atrial fibrillation: a systematic review. *JAMA*, *313*(19), 1950–1962. doi:10.1001/jama.2015.4369

Lip, G. Y., & Tse, H. F. (2007). Management of atrial fibrillation. *Lancet*, *370*(9587), 604–618. doi:10.1016/S0140-6736(07)61300-2

Lip, G. Y. H. (2017). The ABC pathway: an integrated approach to improve AF management. *Nat Rev Cardiol*, *14*(11), 627–628. doi:10.1038/nrcardio.2017.153

Mach, F., Baigent, C., Catapano, A. L., Koskinas, K. C., Casula, M., Badimon, L., . . . Group, E. S. C. S. D. (2020). 2019 ESC/EAS Guidelines for the management of dyslipidaemias: lipid modification to reduce cardiovascular risk. *Eur Heart J*, *41*(1), 111–188. doi:10.1093/eurheartj/ehz455

Malmo, V., Nes, B. M., Amundsen, B. H., Tjonna, A. E., Stoylen, A., Rossvoll, O., . . . Loennechen, J. P. (2016). Aerobic Interval Training Reduces the Burden of Atrial Fibrillation in the Short Term: A Randomized Trial. *Circulation*, *133*(5), 466–473. doi:10.1161/CIRCULATIONAHA.115.018220

Menezes, A. R., Lavie, C. J., De Schutter, A., Milani, R. V., O'Keefe, J., DiNicolantonio, J. J., . . . Abi-Samra, F. M. (2015). Lifestyle modification in the prevention and treatment of atrial fibrillation. *Prog Cardiovasc Dis*, *58*(2), 117–125. doi:10.1016/j.pcad.2015.07.001

Mohanty, S., Mohanty, P., Tamaki, M., Natale, V., Gianni, C., Trivedi, C., . . . Natale, A. (2016). Differential Association of Exercise Intensity With Risk of Atrial Fibrillation in Men and Women: Evidence from a Meta-Analysis. *J Cardiovasc Electrophysiol*, *27*(9), 1021–1029. doi:10.1111/jce.13023

Mohanty, S., Trivedi, C., Gianni, C., & Natale, A. (2018). Gender specific considerations in atrial fibrillation treatment: a review. *Expert Opin Pharmacother*, *19*(4), 365–374. doi:10.1080/14656566.2018.1434144

Molina, L., Mont, L., Marrugat, J., Berruezo, A., Brugada, J., Bruguera, J., . . . Elosua, R. (2008). Long-term endurance sport practice increases the incidence of lone atrial fibrillation in men: a follow-up study. *Europace*, *10*(5), 618–623. doi:10.1093/europace/eun071

Mont, L. (2010). Arrhythmias and sport practice. *Heart*, *96*(5), 398–405. doi:10.1136/hrt.2008.160903

Mont, L., Elosua, R., & Brugada, J. (2009). Endurance sport practice as a risk factor for atrial fibrillation and atrial flutter. *Europace*, *11*(1), 11–17. doi:10.1093/europace/eun289

Moore, S. C., Patel, A. V., Matthews, C. E., Berrington de Gonzalez, A., Park, Y., Katki, H. A., . . . Lee, I. M. (2012). Leisure time physical activity of moderate to vigorous intensity and mortality: a large pooled cohort analysis. *PLoS Med*, *9*(11), e1001335. doi:10.1371/journal.pmed.1001335

Mozaffarian, D., Furberg, C. D., Psaty, B. M., & Siscovick, D. (2008). Physical activity and incidence of atrial fibrillation in older adults: the cardiovascular health study. *Circulation*, *118*(8), 800–807. doi:10.1161/CIRCULATIONAHA.108.785626

Nielsen, J. R., Wachtell, K., & Abdulla, J. (2013). The Relationship Between Physical Activity and Risk of Atrial Fibrillation-A Systematic Review and Meta-Analysis. *J Atr Fibrillation*, *5*(5), 789. doi:10.4022/jafib.789

Ofman, P., Khawaja, O., Rahilly-Tierney, C. R., Peralta, A., Hoffmeister, P., Reynolds, M. R., . . . Djousse, L. (2013). Regular physical activity and risk of atrial fibrillation: a systematic review and meta-analysis. *Circ Arrhythm Electrophysiol*, *6*(2), 252–256. doi:10.1161/CIRCEP.113.000147

Pathak, R. K., Elliott, A., Middeldorp, M. E., Meredith, M., Mehta, A. B., Mahajan, R., . . . Sanders, P. (2015). Impact of CARDIOrespiratory FITness on Arrhythmia Recurrence in Obese Individuals With Atrial Fibrillation: The CARDIO-FIT Study. *J Am Coll Cardiol*, *66*(9), 985–996. doi:10.1016/j.jacc.2015.06.488

Pedersen, B. K., & Saltin, B. (2015). Exercise as medicine - evidence for prescribing exercise as therapy in 26 different chronic diseases. *Scand J Med Sci Sports*, 25 Suppl 3, 1–72. doi:10.1111/sms.12581

Pellman, J., & Sheikh, F. (2015). Atrial fibrillation: mechanisms, therapeutics, and future directions. *Compr Physiol*, *5*(2), 649–665. doi:10.1002/cphy.c140047

Piercy, K. L., & Troiano, R. P. (2018). Physical Activity Guidelines for Americans From the US Department of Health and Human Services. *Circ Cardiovasc Qual Outcomes*, *11*(11), e005263. doi:10.1161/CIRCOUTCOMES.118.005263

Ricci, C., Gervasi, F., Gaeta, M., Smuts, C. M., Schutte, A. E., & Leitzmann, M. F. (2018). Physical activity volume in relation to risk of atrial fibrillation. A non-linear meta-regression analysis. *Eur J Prev Cardiol*, *25*(8), 857–866. doi:10.1177/2047487318768026

Rienstra, M., Hobbelt, A. H., Alings, M., Tijssen, J. G. P., Smit, M. D., Brugemann, J., . . . Investigators, R. (2018). Targeted therapy of underlying conditions improves sinus rhythm maintenance in patients with persistent atrial fibrillation: results of the RACE 3 trial. *Eur Heart J*, *39*(32), 2987–2996. doi:10.1093/eurheartj/ehx739

Sattelmair, J., Pertman, J., Ding, E. L., Kohl, H. W., 3rd, Haskell, W., & Lee, I. M. (2011). Dose response between physical activity and risk of coronary heart disease: a meta-analysis. *Circulation*, *124*(7), 789–795. doi:10.1161/CIRCULATIONAHA.110.010710

Semaan, S., Dewland, T. A., Tison, G. H., Nah, G., Vittinghoff, E., Pletcher, M. J., . . . Marcus, G. M. (2020). Physical activity and atrial fibrillation: Data from wearable fitness trackers. *Heart Rhythm*, *17*(5 Pt B), 842–846. doi:10.1016/j.hrthm.2020.02.013

Staerk, L., Sherer, J. A., Ko, D., Benjamin, E. J., & Helm, R. H. (2017). Atrial Fibrillation: Epidemiology, Pathophysiology, and Clinical Outcomes. *Circ Res*, *120*(9), 1501–1517. doi:10.1161/CIRCRESAHA.117.309732

Thelle, D. S., Selmer, R., Gjesdal, K., Sakshaug, S., Jugessur, A., Graff-Iversen, S., . . . Nystad, W. (2013). Resting heart rate and physical activity as risk factors for lone atrial fibrillation: a prospective study of 309,540 men and women. *Heart*, *99*(23), 1755–1760. doi:10.1136/heartjnl-2013-303825

Turagam, M. K., Flaker, G. C., Velagapudi, P., Vadali, S., & Alpert, M. A. (2015). Atrial Fibrillation In Athletes: Pathophysiology, Clinical Presentation, Evaluation and Management. *J Atr Fibrillation*, *8*(4), 1309. doi:10.4022/jafib.1309

Violi, F., Lip, G. Y., Pignatelli, P., & Pastori, D. (2016). Interaction Between Dietary Vitamin K Intake and Anticoagulation by Vitamin K Antagonists: Is It Really True?: A Systematic Review. *Medicine (Baltimore)*, *95*(10), e2895. doi:10.1097/MD.0000000000002895

Voskoboinik, A., Kalman, J. M., De Silva, A., Nicholls, T., Costello, B., Nanayakkara, S., . . . Kistler, P. M. (2020). Alcohol Abstinence in Drinkers with Atrial Fibrillation. *N Engl J Med*, *382*(1), 20–28. doi:10.1056/NEJMoa1817591

Voskoboinik, A., Kalman, J. M., & Kistler, P. M. (2018). Caffeine and Arrhythmias: Time to Grind the Data. *JACC Clin Electrophysiol*, *4*(4), 425–432. doi:10.1016/j.jacep.2018.01.012

FURTHER READING

Bibliography

Anaszewicz, M., and Budzynski, J. (2017). Clinical significance of nutritional status in patients with atrial fibrillation: An overview of current evidence. *Journal of Cardiology 69*(5): 719–730. doi: 10.1016/j.jjcc.2016.06.014.

Freeman, A.M., Morris, P.B., Aspry, K., et al. (2018). A clinician's guide for trending cardiovascular nutrition controversies: Part II. *Journal of the American College of Cardiology. 72*(5): 553–68. doi: 10.1016/j.jacc.2018.05.030.

Garnvik LE, Malmo V, Janszky I, et al. (2020). Physical activity, cardiorespiratory fitness, and cardiovascular outcomes in individuals with atrial fibrillation: the HUNT study. *European Heart Journal 41*: 1467.

Papanastasiou CA, Theochari CA, Zareifopoulos N, et al. (2021). Atrial fibrillation Is associated with cognitive impairment, all-cause dementia, vascular dementia, and Alzheimer's disease: A systematic review and meta-analysis. *Journal of General Internal Medicine 36*: 3122.

Perez, M.V., Mahaffey, K.W., Hedlin, H., et al. (2019). Large-scale assessment of a smartwatch to identify atrial fibrillation. *New England Journal of Medicine 381*: 1909.

Links

- https://www.cdc.gov/heartdisease/atrial_fibrillation.htm
- https://www.bhf.org.uk/informationsupport/conditions/atrial-fibrillation
- https://www.heart.org/en/health-topics/atrial-fibrillation
- https://www.stopafib.org/

Endothelial Function

CHAPTER 14

Introduction	205	Vasodilation	211
Endothelial Dysfunction	206	Oxidative Stress	212
Description	207	Fibrinolysis	213
Assessment	207	Angiogenesis	214
Management	208	Inflammation	214
Nutrition and Endothelial Function	208	Key Points	215
Obesity and Weight Loss	208	Self-assessment Questions	216
Nutrients and Foods	209	References	216
Dietary Patterns	209	Further Reading	220
Physical Activity and Endothelial Function	210	Bibliography	220
Exercise Training and Endothelial Function	211	Link	220

INTRODUCTION

The epithelium is a type of tissue made up of densely packed cells that rest on a basement membrane (Kurn & Daly, 2020). It is one of the five main types of animal tissues—the other four are nerve tissue, connective tissue, muscle tissue, and vascular tissue—and it serves as a covering or lining of various bodily surfaces and cavities. The epithelium may be classified according to the number of its layers as simple, stratified, or pseudostratified (Kurn & Daly, 2020).

The endothelium is a special type of epithelium that lines the blood and lymphatic vessels (Aird, 2013). It consists of a single layer of smooth thin cells that form an interface between circulating blood or lymph in the lumen and the rest of the vessel wall (Aird, 2013) (**Figure 14.1**).

The endothelium is characterized as a spatially distributed organ, with a weight of ~1 kg in the average individual that covers a total surface area of 4000 to 7000 m^2 (Aird, 2013). Endothelial cells in contact with blood are called vascular endothelial cells, whereas those in contact with lymph are known as lymphatic endothelial cells. Vascular endothelial cells line the entire circulatory system, from the heart to the smallest capillaries, where they perform several fundamental functions (Aird, 2013).

Although traditionally considered an inert, static layer in the circulatory system, the vascular endothelium is now acknowledged as a complex organ with important autocrine and paracrine functions, producing a large number of substances that regulate vasodilation, cell proliferation, angiogenesis, and hemostasis (**Table 14.1**).

First of all, endothelial cells form a semipermeable membrane that mediates transfer of ions, solutes, and fluids between the blood and interstitial compartments (Rosenberg & Aird, 1999). As a general rule, gases pass through the endothelium via simple diffusion, whereas ions, solutes, and fluids require convective flow between endothelial cells (paracellular route) or through the endothelial cell (transcellular route) (Rosenberg & Aird, 1999). However, barrier properties differ significantly between different vascular endothelia. For example, the blood-brain barrier forms a highly efficient barrier due to its tight junctional complexes and paucity of caveolae, which limits both paracellular and transcellular transport, while the liver sinusoidal endothelium possesses a discontinuous basement membrane that is highly permeable (Rosenberg & Aird, 1999).

The endothelium also regulates the traffic of leukocytes between blood and underlying tissue. Under normal conditions, constitutive trafficking of lymphocytes from blood to lymph

Prevention and Management of Cardiovascular and Metabolic Disease: Diet, Physical Activity and Healthy Aging,
First Edition. Christina N. Katsagoni, Peter Kokkinos, and Labros S. Sidossis.
© 2023 John Wiley & Sons Ltd. Published 2023 by John Wiley & Sons Ltd.

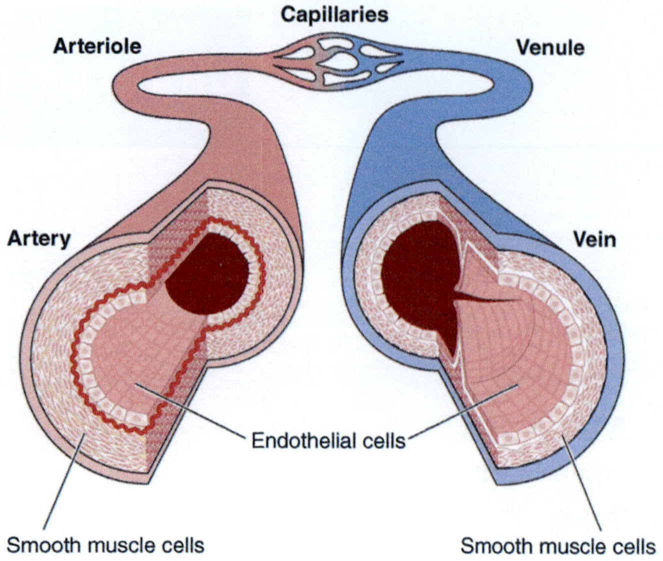

FIGURE 14.1 The endothelium. The endothelial cells form a one-cell, thick-walled layer that lines all blood vessels—including arteries, arterioles, venules, veins, and capillaries. Smooth muscle cells layer beneath endothelial cells to form the blood vessel.

Table 14.1 Autocrine and paracrine substances released from the endothelium.

Vasodilators	Vasoconstrictors
Nitric oxide, prostacyclin, endothelium-derived hyperpolarizing factor, bradykinin, adrenomedullin, C-natriuretic peptide	Endothelin-1, angiotensin-II, thromboxane A2, oxidant radicals, prostaglandin H2
Antiproliferative	**Pro-proliferative**
Nitric oxide, prostacyclin, transforming growth factor-b, heparan sulfate	Endothelin-1, angiotensin-II, oxidant radicals, platelet-derived growth factor, basic fibroblast growth factor, insulin-like growth factor, interleukins
Antithrombotic	**Prothrombotic**
Nitric oxide, prostacyclin, plasminogen-activator, protein C, tissue factor inhibitor, von Willebrand factor	Endothelin-1, oxidant radicals, plasminogen-activator inhibitor-1, thromboxane A2, fibrinogen, tissue factor
Angiogenesis	**Inflammatory markers**
Vascular endothelial growth factor	Cell adhesion molecules (P- and E-selectin, intercellular adhesion molecule, vascular cell adhesion molecule), chemokines, nuclear factor-kB

Source: (Di Francescomarino et al., 2009).

nodes occurs via specialized blood vessels, called high endothelial venules (Chi et al., 2003). In states of inflammation, endothelial cells in postcapillary venules (in nonlymphoid tissue) mediate the adhesion and trans endothelial migration of leukocytes to the extravascular space (Lacorre et al., 2004). This process involves a highly orchestrated multistep adhesion cascade that begins with initial attachment, rolling, arrest, and ends with diapedesis through the endothelium and migration through tissues (Lacorre et al., 2004). This cascade is mediated by specific molecules, such as E-selectin, P-selectin, L-selectin, and endothelial intercellular adhesion molecule-1 (ICAM-1). In addition to regulating leukocyte transfer, the endothelium plays other roles in the innate immune response. For example, activated endothelial cells may express and/or release a multitude of inflammatory mediators, such as tumor necrosis factor alpha (TNF-α), interleukin 1 (IL-1), and interferon gamma (IFN-γ).

The endothelium plays a key role in mediating vasomotor tone. Endothelial cells express several molecules that influence blood vessel diameter and flow dynamics, most notably nitric oxide (NO). The enzyme responsible for endothelial production of NO is endothelial nitric oxide synthase (eNOS), which is modulated by many extracellular signals, including (but not limited to) shear stress and growth factors (Regan & Aird, 2012). Other vasomotor molecules released by the endothelium include carbon monoxide, endothelin 1, epoxyeicosatrienoic acids, and prostaglandins. These molecules regulate the narrowing and enlargement of the blood vessels, usually referred to as vasoconstriction and vasodilation, respectively, and hence the control of blood pressure.

Finally, the vascular endothelium has a fundamental role in hemostasis. The endothelium can produce a wide variety of procoagulant and anticoagulant molecules. On the procoagulant side, endothelial cells synthesize plasminogen-activator inhibitor-1 (PAI-1), von Willebrand factor, protease activated receptors, and rarely tissue factor (TF). On the anticoagulant side, endothelial cells express, synthesize, and/or release tissue factor pathway inhibitor (TFPI), thrombomodulin (TM), endothelial protein C receptor (EPCR), tissue-type plasminogen activator (tPA), and heparan (Aird, 2013). The endothelium normally provides a surface on which blood does not clot due to the enhanced expression of anticoagulant substances; however, in pathological conditions, a shift in the hemostatic balance to one or the other side may result in increased risk of bleeding or thrombosis.

ENDOTHELIAL DYSFUNCTION

Endothelial dysfunction, i.e., the loss of normal endothelial function, is a hallmark of vascular diseases and is recognized as a key early event in the development of atherosclerosis (Hadi, Carr, & Al Suwaidi, 2005; Versari, Daghini, Virdis, Ghiadoni, & Taddei, 2009). Impaired endothelial function is often present in patients with cardio-metabolic diseases, such as coronary artery disease, diabetes mellitus, chronic kidney disease, and inflammatory diseases (e.g., rheumatoid arthritis and systemic lupus erythematosus) and is predictive of target organ damage, adverse atherosclerotic and thromboembolic cardiovascular events, including myocardial infarction, and cardiovascular mortality (Hadi et al., 2005; Versari et al., 2009). Deleterious alterations of endothelial physiology represent a key step in atherogenesis, and the endothelium is increasingly becoming a surrogate end point of therapeutic approaches to lower cardiovascular risk (Hadi et al., 2005; Versari et al., 2009).

DESCRIPTION

Endothelial dysfunction is characterized by reduction of the bioavailability of vasodilators, particularly NO, and/or an increase in endothelium-derived contracting factors (Lerman & Burnett, 1992). The resulting imbalance leads to an impairment of endothelium-dependent vasodilation, which is the functional characteristic of endothelial dysfunction. In addition to impaired endothelium-dependent vasodilation, endothelial dysfunction also comprises a specific state of endothelial activation, which is characterized by a proinflammatory, proliferative, oxidative, and procoagulatory state that favors all stages of atherogenesis (Anderson, 1999). Under normal conditions, the vascular endothelium maintains vascular tone and blood fluidity with no or little expression of proinflammatory factors. However, various traditional and novel cardiovascular risk factors, including smoking, aging, obesity, dyslipidemia, hypertension, hyperglycemia, systemic inflammation, oxidative stress, and genetic predisposition to premature atherosclerotic disease, are all associated with unfavorable alterations in endothelial function. This includes a state of chronic inflammation accompanied by a loss of antithrombotic factors and an increase in vasoconstrictor and prothrombotic products, in addition to abnormal vasoreactivity, therefore elevating the risk of cardiovascular events (Bonetti, Lerman, & Lerman, 2003). Reactive oxygen species (ROS) are generated at sites of inflammation and injury and at low concentrations can function as signaling molecules participating in the regulation of fundamental cell activities, such as cell growth and cell adaptation responses, whereas at higher concentrations, ROS can cause cellular injury and death. The vascular endothelium, which regulates the passage of macromolecules and circulating cells from blood to tissues, is a major target of oxidative stress, playing a critical role in the pathophysiology of several vascular diseases and disorders. Specifically, oxidative stress increases vascular endothelial permeability and promotes leukocyte adhesion, which is coupled with alterations in endothelial signal transduction and redox-regulated transcription factors, such as activator protein-1 (AP-1) and nuclear factor-kappa B (NF-κB) (Lum & Roebuck, 2001).

ASSESSMENT

Despite its prominent role in cardiovascular health, endothelial function is not easy to assess. This is because (i) few symptoms are directly referable or specific to the endothelium; (ii) the endothelium is hidden from view and not amenable to traditional physical diagnostic procedures; and (iii) the endothelium is not spatially confined and is therefore difficult to image using anatomic imaging methodologies. **Table 14.2** presents an overview of available diagnostic markers/procedures for the endothelium (Aird, 2013).

To date, the gold standard for diagnosing endothelial dysfunction is the physiologic assessment of vasomotor tone. This can be carried out invasively (e.g., using angiography) or noninvasively (e.g., using imaging or flow studies). The most commonly used diagnostic assay for endothelial function in clinical practice is the noninvasive flow-mediated vasodilation

Table 14.2 Diagnostic procedures and markers for endothelium.

Procedure/marker	Comments
Pathology	Not readily available except for skin biopsies; results from skin biopsies may not extrapolate to other vascular beds
Soluble mediators	
Intercellular adhesion molecule 1	Not specific to endothelial cells
Vascular cell adhesion molecule 1	Not specific to endothelial cells
P-selectin	Not specific to endothelial cells
E-selectin	Specific to endothelial cells
Thrombomodulin	Specific to endothelial cells
Tissue plasminogen activator	Not specific to endothelial cells
Plasminogen-activator inhibitor 1	Not specific to endothelial cells
von Willebrand factor	Not specific to endothelial cells
Endothelial protein C receptor	Specific to endothelial cells
Cell-based mediators	
Circulating endothelial cells	May be quantified and phenotyped; limited by small numbers in blood
Microparticles	May be quantified and phenotyped
Endothelial progenitor cells	May be quantified and phenotyped; hematopoietic in origin
Molecular imaging	Holds promise for vascular bed-specific diagnosis
Flow studies	Gold standard method in clinical mainstream

Source: (Aird, 2013).

(FMD), which measures endothelial-mediated vasorelaxation of the brachial artery in response to the release of external compression (Al-Qaisi, Kharbanda, Mittal, & Donald, 2008; Corretti et al., 2002; Edmundowicz, 2002). An increase in flow in the brachial artery is achieved by inflation of a pneumatic cuff (placed on the forearm, distal to the ultrasound imaging site) to suprasystolic pressure for 5 min. Upon deflation of the cuff, the increased flow results in shear stress, which activates eNOS to release NO via the L-arginine pathway. The NO diffuses to the smooth muscle cells causing them to relax, resulting in vasodilatation, and FMD is measured as the percentage change in brachial artery diameter from baseline in response to the increased flow. Noninvasive ultrasound FMD of the brachial artery is an alternate technique also widely used in the literature. Studies have demonstrated that abnormal FMD correlates with coronary artery disease and predicts future disease progression, including acute vascular events (Patel et al., 2004). Therefore, FMD represents a noninvasive measure of pre-clinical cardiovascular risk in populations with and without obvious risk factors.

Circulating biomarkers for the endothelium include soluble and cell-based assays. Soluble mediators consist of endothelial-derived factors involved in hemostasis, cell adhesion, vasomotor and permeability/angiogenesis. Biomarkers for endothelial dysfunction that are released by other cell types include asymmetric dimethylarginine (ADMA), lipoprotein-associated phospholipase A2, and C-reactive protein (CRP). Although there are many studies reporting the association of one or another of these mediators in different patient populations, few if any of these markers can consistently and reliably predict the presence/stage of disease, prognosis, or response to therapy in individual patients (Aird, 2013). With regard to cell-based assays, several types of cells, including circulating mature endothelial cells (CEC), endothelial microparticles (EMPs) and endothelial progenitor cells (EPCs) have been linked to endothelial function; although these cells hold promising value in detecting endothelial damage and predicting its adverse health effects, there is a need for standardization of their quantification and phenotyping methodology and a better understanding of their correlation with underlying disease state (Goon, Boos, & Lip, 2005; Horstman, Jy, Jimenez, & Ahn, 2004; Werner & Nickenig, 2007). The use of noninvasive molecular imaging to visualize biological processes at the molecular and cellular levels within the intact endothelium is another promising diagnostic procedure that remains at an investigational stage (Kaufmann et al., 2007; Kelly et al., 2005).

MANAGEMENT

Management of endothelial dysfunction mainly aims at ameliorating endothelial function, through targeting cellular output (i.e., phenotype) and/or intracellular coupling mechanisms (Aird, 2013). Examples of targeting the output include the use of neutralizing antibodies against adhesion molecules, such as ICAM-1 or VCAM-1; inducing the expression/synthesis of anticoagulants, such as TM, EPCR, TFPI, and orheparan sulfate; or increasing barrier function (Aird, 2013). Examples of modulating intracellular coupling mechanisms include neutralizing cell surface receptors (e.g., antibodies against the vascular endothelial growth factor [VEGF] receptor) and administration of antioxidants or inhibitors of NFκB signaling (Aird, 2013).

There is increasing evidence that certain approved drugs exert their beneficial effect—at least in part—by attenuating endothelial dysfunction. Experimental and clinical studies have demonstrated that a variety of currently used or investigational drugs, such as angiotensin-converting enzyme inhibitors, angiotensin AT1 receptors blockers, angiotensin-(1-7), antioxidants, beta-blockers, calcium-channel blockers, endothelial NO synthase enhancers, phosphodiesterase-5 inhibitors, sphingosine-1-phosphate, and statins exert endothelial protective effects (Su, 2015). Given the remarkable capacity of the endothelium to sense and respond to its extracellular environment, it is likely that most if not all systemically administered drugs will alter endothelial phenotype. Due to the difference in mechanisms of action, these drugs need to be used according to specific mechanisms underlying disease-specific endothelial dysfunction.

NUTRITION AND ENDOTHELIAL FUNCTION

Nutrition is widely recognized as a strong determinant of cardiovascular health (Chareonrungrueangchai, Wongkawinwoot, Anothaisintawee, & Reutrakul, 2020; Liyanage et al., 2016; Onvani, Haghighatdoost, Surkan, Larijani, & Azadbakht, 2017; Schwingshackl & Hoffmann, 2015; Studer, Briel, Leimenstoll, Glass, & Bucher, 2005). Although data on the relationship between diet and the endothelium are limited, growing evidence suggests that dietary factors play a role in modulating endothelial function.

OBESITY AND WEIGHT LOSS

Obesity is considered an important and modifiable risk factor for endothelial dysfunction. A chronic inflammatory state in obesity causes dysregulation of the endocrine and paracrine actions of adipocyte-derived factors, which disrupt vascular homeostasis and contribute to endothelial vasodilator dysfunction and subsequent hypertension (Engin, 2017; Schinzari, Tesauro, & Cardillo, 2017). While normal healthy perivascular adipose tissue ensures the dilation of blood vessels, obesity-associated perivascular adipose tissue leads to a change in profile of the released adipo-cytokines, resulting in a decreased vaso-relaxing effect (Engin, 2017; Schinzari et al., 2017). Adipose tissue inflammation, NO bioavailability, insulin resistance, and oxidized low-density lipoproteins are the main participating factors in endothelial dysfunction of obesity (Engin, 2017; Schinzari et al., 2017). Given the close relationship between obesity and endothelial dysfunction, weight loss, achieved through either diet alone or its combination with aerobic exercise, is linked with improved endothelial function as assessed by FMD in overweight and obese individuals (Ades et al., 2011; Bigornia et al., 2010; Brook et al., 2004; Mavri et al., 2011; Pierce et al., 2008; Skilton et al., 2008). This beneficial effect has been attributed to both the favorable metabolic changes associated with weight loss, including improvements in lipidemic profile indices, glucose metabolism, inhibition of thrombosis, amelioration of inflammation, and the degree of weight reduction (**Figure 14.2**) (Shankar & Steinberg, 2008). The results of available clinical trials are highly encouraging and indicate that endothelial dysfunction is at least partially reversible by weight loss. Thus, it makes sense that all obese individuals with endothelial dysfunction should be encouraged to lose weight, preferably through lifestyle modification, to improve endothelial function and cardio-metabolic health in general. However, many questions in this topic remain unanswered.

First, the optimal degree of weight loss needed for a clinically meaningful improvement in endothelial function has not been determined. Most, clinical trials of improvement in endothelial function associated with weight reduction suggest that a weight loss of ≥10% may be required before an improvement in endothelial function can be detected (Shankar & Steinberg, 2008); nevertheless, even a smaller degree of weight loss, i.e., <5%, has been shown to result in improvements in cardio-metabolic risk and can be a more suitable, realistic, and sustainable goal for most obese patients in clinical practice,

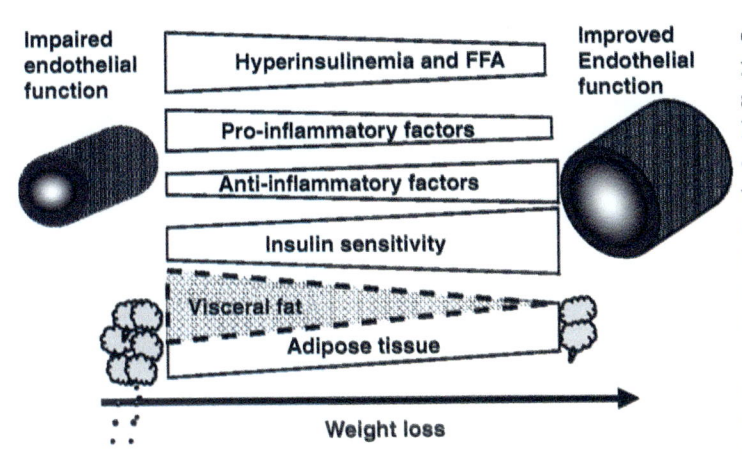

FIGURE 14.2 Simplified scheme of processes during weight loss that lead to improved vascular function. It is unknown at what degree of weight loss these processes occur and whether they are independent. FFA = free fatty acids. Source: (Shankar & Steinberg, 2008).

especially for obese patients with high cardiovascular risk or established obesity-related disorders (Jensen et al., 2014; Yumuk et al., 2015). Moreover, the optimal rate of weight loss for the endothelium remains unknown. If caloric restriction alone was sufficient to improve endothelial function, one should be able to see an early effect in patients undergoing bariatric surgery. If, however, there is persistence in the generation of various mediators responsible for the endothelial dysfunction, these factors may make it difficult to detect any significant improvements in endothelial function for long periods. This is consistent with persistent elevations in the levels of markers of endothelial activation and inflammation for several months after bariatric surgery (Vazquez et al., 2005). Therefore, it is reasonable to postulate that patients with lesser degrees of overweight/obesity, without other co-morbidities, will experience a significant improvement in endothelial function over time if they achieve significant weight loss, even if the rate of weight loss is not exceptionally rapid. Finally, the macronutrient composition of a diet may affect endothelial function independent of the effect of the weight loss itself. A clinical trial comparing the effects of a low-carbohydrate versus a low-fat diet showed that despite similar degrees of weight loss, the low-fat diet group exhibited a significant improvement in endothelial function, whereas the low-carbohydrate diet group showed no change in endothelial dysfunction (Phillips et al., 2008). Furthermore, it is highly likely that sodium intake is also reduced in proportion with the caloric restriction. From a vascular function perspective, a reduction in sodium intake is likely to affect endothelial function, either directly or indirectly, and this factor should be considered when evaluating the effects of dietary interventions on vascular function.

NUTRIENTS AND FOODS

Data on the effect of dietary components on the vascular endothelium remain scarce and conflicting. Among the various dietary components, dietary fat appears to affect endothelial function in a complex way. With regard to fat quantity, several short-term feeding trials have shown a detrimental effect of a high-fat meal on postprandial endothelial function, but this observation has not been confirmed in all available studies (Cuevas & Germain, 2004; Davis, Katz, & Wylie-Rosett, 2007). Fat quality might also be important for endothelial function; both *in vitro* and *in vivo* studies suggest that trans and saturated fatty acids result in impairments in endothelial function, whereas mono-unsaturated and omega-3 poly-unsaturated fatty acids can contrariwise improve endothelial function (Cuevas & Germain, 2004; Davis et al., 2007). Although more research is needed, this observation might suggest that a diet rich in foods with unsaturated fat, such as vegetable oils, nuts, and fish, can be beneficial for the endothelium when compared to foods rich in saturated and trans fat, such as red and processed meat, butter, stick margarine, and high-processed foods.

Besides dietary fat, polyphenols, especially flavonoids, have recently emerged as important non-nutritive substances for the cardiovascular system. Several clinical trials have demonstrated a significant increase in FMD after the consumption of foods rich in polyphenols, such as tea, grape juice, and red wine (Cuevas & Germain, 2004; Davis et al., 2007); however, it is still unclear whether it is through the effect on endothelial function, their antioxidant properties, or potential anti-inflammatory properties that polyphenols improve cardiovascular risk.

Folic acid has also been attributed with beneficial properties for endothelium; some clinical trials using folic acid supplements have shown improvements in endothelium-dependent vasodilation, whereas others have not, and this discrepancy may be attributed to the dosage and duration of supplementation (Cuevas & Germain, 2004; Davis et al., 2007). Finally, antioxidants, such as vitamins C and E have also been shown to improve endothelial function in some trials, however, data so far are controversial and inadequate to support antioxidant supplementation as a strategy to manage endothelial dysfunction in clinical practice (Cuevas & Germain, 2004; Davis et al., 2007).

DIETARY PATTERNS

As indicated in previous chapters, evaluating the impact of a single dietary factor independently of any other changes in the diet is problematic. In fact, as foods are mixtures of different nutrients and other components that show strong synergistic or antagonistic effects, it is not appropriate to attribute the health effects of a food to only one of its components. Moreover, if total energy intake is kept constant, eating less of one macronutrient implies necessarily eating more of others, and the quality of the replacement can also influence the effect observed. All these limitations require caution in interpreting the results of studies in relation to the effect of a single dietary change on cardiovascular risk. In recent years, nutrition research and epidemiology have focused on the relationship between health/disease on the one hand, and foods and dietary patterns—rather than single nutrients—on the other (Hodge & Bassett, 2016; Hu, 2002; Ocke, 2013; Willett & McCullough, 2008).

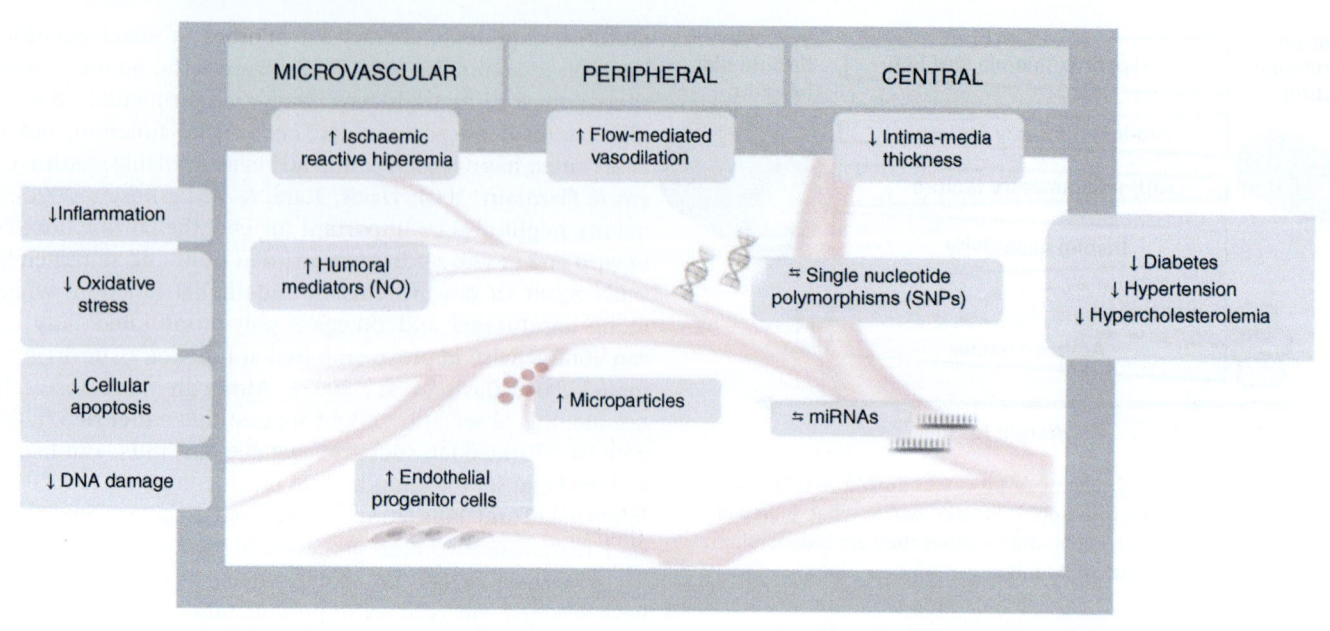

FIGURE 14.3 Effects of the Mediterranean diet on endothelial dysfunction. ↓ = decrease; ↑ = increase; ⇆ = interacts. Source: (Torres-Pena et al., 2020 / MDPI / CC BY 4.0).

Consistent evidence from epidemiological studies indicates that the adoption of "prudent" or "healthy" dietary patterns, characterized by a higher consumption of fruits, vegetables, nuts, legumes, fish, vegetable oils (especially olive oil), and whole grains, along with a lower/modest intake of red and processed meats, foods rich in refined carbohydrates (sugars), salt, and industrialized processed foods high in trans fatty acids, is associated with a lower incidence of cardiovascular disease and morality (Freeman et al., 2018; Freeman et al., 2017; Mach et al., 2020). With regard to the endothelium, there is also some epidemiological evidence that, regardless of traditional risk factors such as age, smoking, and body weight, individuals who consume a prudent diet exhibit lower levels of soluble E-selectin, a serum marker for endothelial dysfunction; conversely, adoption of a Western diet, rich in red meat, processed meat, refined grains, and French fries correlate positively with E-selectin, sI-CAM-1, and sVCAM-1, which are indicative of endothelial dysfunction and a significant role in the pathogenesis of cardiovascular disease (Lopez-Garcia et al., 2004).

Among the various healthy dietary patterns, the Mediterranean diet (MD) is well-known for its various health benefits, mainly in relation to reducing the risk of all-cause mortality, cardiovascular disease, cancer, neurodegenerative diseases, diabetes mellitus, and hypertension (Kastorini et al., 2011; Sofi, Macchi, Abbate, Gensini, & Casini, 2014). The MD can be described as a dietary pattern characterized by high consumption of olive oil (as the main edible fat), vegetables, legumes, whole grains, fruits, and nuts, a moderate consumption of poultry and fish, a low consumption of full fat dairy products and red meat, and a low-to-moderate consumption of wine as the main source of alcohol accompanying meals (Sofi, 2009). The remarkable health benefits of the MD have been attributed to its strong anti-inflammatory and antioxidant properties, deriving from the complex synergistic effects of the combination of its individual foods and their nutrients (Bullo, Lamuela-Raventos, & Salas-Salvado, 2011; Kontogianni, Zampelas, & Tsigos, 2006). Moreover, a long-term adherence to the MD is associated with a reduced risk of obesity and better weight control, compared to other dietary patterns (such as a low-fat diet), when combined with energy restriction (more in **Unit 5**) (Buckland, Bach, & Serra-Majem, 2008; Esposito, Kastorini, Panagiotakos, & Giugliano, 2011). Given that obesity, inflammation, and oxidative stress are implicated in the pathogenesis of endothelial dysfunction, the MD could constitute the first-line dietary pattern for enhancing endothelial function (**Figure 14.3**) (Torres-Pena, Rangel-Zuniga, Alcala-Diaz, Lopez-Miranda, & Delgado-Lista, 2020). This is supported by clinical trials showing significant improvements in FMD by approximately 2% after a dietary intervention based on the MD both in healthy individuals and patients with high cardiovascular risk (e.g., those with dyslipidemia, metabolic syndrome, and diabetes) (Esposito et al., 2004; Fuentes et al., 2001; Shannon et al., 2020).

PHYSICAL ACTIVITY AND ENDOTHELIAL FUNCTION

Several cross-sectional epidemiological studies have highlighted the beneficial role of physical activity in the endothelium. Although this methodological study design cannot explore etiological associations, epidemiological observations serve as the first evidence of a favorable association between physical activity and endothelial function. Habitual physical activity has been shown to positively correlate with FMD in children aged 5 to 10 years old and be a stronger predictor of vascular dilation compared to age, gender, percentage body fat, baseline arterial diameter, and ponderal index (Abbott, Harkness, & Davies, 2002). A similar positive association between leisure-time physical activity and FMD has also been observed in adolescents, even after adjustment for body habits, lipidemic profile indices, blood pressure, and inflammatory markers. Indeed, a difference of about 50 MET h/week corresponding to ~10 hours of moderate-intensity activity weekly has been associated an ~1% unit difference in maximum FMD (Pahkala et al., 2008). In young adults (aged 20–30 years old), the available evidence is conflicting, since some studies have revealed a positive correlation between physical activity level and FMD (Kingwell, Tran, Cameron, Jennings, & Dart, 1996), while other studies have shown similar FMD values between sedentary and physically active young adults, including athletes (DeSouza et al., 2000; Moe, Hoven, Hetland, Rognmo, & Slordahl, 2005; Taddei et al., 2000). This observation might suggest that endothelial function is well preserved in young healthy adults and is unlikely to be significantly affected by potentially beneficial interventions, such as aerobic exercise.

The protective role of physical activity in endothelial function is more evident in higher age groups, in which age-related endothelial dysfunction is common (Celermajer et al., 1994; Eskurza, Monahan, Robinson, & Seals, 2004). Indeed, several cross-sectional studies have shown that both middle-aged and older adults regularly participating in exercise of various types exhibit higher FMD values compared to sedentary ones, regardless of sex, body habitus, and the presence of co-morbidities (Franzoni et al., 2005; Klonizakis, Hunt, & Woodward, 2020; Payvandi et al., 2009; Siasos et al., 2013); these data suggest that exercise can be of value for older adults in whom the impairment of endothelium-dependent vasodilation is caused by a decreased production of NO or an increased degradation of NO due to the presence of age-related oxidative stress (Cernadas et al., 1998; Chou, Yen, Li, & Ding, 1998; Mutlu-Turkoglu et al., 2003; Stadtman, 1992).

EXERCISE TRAINING AND ENDOTHELIAL FUNCTION

Exercise has been advocated for the promotion of health and the non-pharmacological treatment of cardiovascular diseases. Regular practice of exercise results in numerous cardio metabolic health benefits, including improvements in body composition, lipoprotein profile, carbohydrate metabolism, insulin sensitivity, blood pressure, inflammation, and antioxidant status as well as improvements in physical fitness, quality of life, and wellness (Vina, Sanchis-Gomar, Martinez-Bello, & Gomez-Cabrera, 2012; D. E. Warburton, Nicol, & Bredin, 2006; D. E. R. Warburton & Bredin, 2017). All of the above-mentioned effects can favorably affect cardiovascular risk, and adequate physical activity has been consistently associated with significant reductions in cardio-metabolic morbidity and mortality (Jeong et al., 2019; Lear et al., 2017; Zhang, Cash, Bower, Focht, & Paskett, 2020). As a result, the adoption of a physically active way of living is universally recommended as a strategy to reduce cardio-metabolic risk and prevent cardiovascular diseases, along with other healthy lifestyle practices (Bull et al., 2020; Piercy & Troiano, 2018). Although the effect of exercise on the endothelium is less well-studied, the available evidence suggests that exercise can improve endothelial function and result in a favorable vascular remodeling through a variety of mechanisms, including vasodilation, a favorable effect on the oxidative balance of the endothelium, the promotion of fibrinolysis and angiogenesis, and a chronic anti-inflammatory effect.

VASODILATION

NO is the main vasodilator substance released by the endothelium. It is a labile, lipid-soluble gas synthesized from L-arginine through the action of eNOS following stimulation by either shear stress/increased flow through the vessel lumen or endothelial agonists. The endothelium is constantly exposed to hemodynamic forces varying in magnitude and direction, depending on the anatomy of the blood vessel and the viscous drag from the blood flow. The blood flow-linked forces that act on the arterial wall can be divided into two principal vectors: one perpendicular to the wall and the other parallel to it. Together, they create a frictional force that exerts shear stress on the surface of the endothelium. This shear stress is an important stimulus to the endothelium to produce NO, vascular remodeling, and blood vessel formation (Resnick et al., 2003).

It is well established that exercise has a strong vasodilating effect. Both animal and human studies have shown that exercise augments blood flow and shear stress in the endothelium (Di Francescomarino, Sciartilli, Di Valerio, Di Baldassarre, & Gallina, 2009; Green, Maiorana, O'Driscoll, & Taylor, 2004; McAllister & Laughlin, 2006). Exercise-induced shear stress results in upregulation of eNOS (increases in eNOS gene transcription, mRNA stability, and protein translation) and consequently increased NO production (Di Francescomarino et al., 2009; Green et al., 2004; McAllister & Laughlin, 2006). Increased NO bioactivity with exercise training has been readily and consistently demonstrated in subjects with cardiovascular disease and risk factors, in whom endothelial dysfunction exists (Di Francescomarino et al., 2009; Green et al., 2004; McAllister & Laughlin, 2006). These conditions are characterized by increased levels of oxidative stress indices, which impact NO synthase activity, and with which NO reacts; repeated exercise redresses this radical imbalance, hence leading to a greater potential for NO bioavailability. Similar exercise-induced improvements in NO vasodilator function have been less frequently found in healthy subjects, in whom a higher level of training may be needed (Di Francescomarino et al., 2009; Green et al., 2004; McAllister & Laughlin, 2006).

It must be noted that the type and duration of exercise affect the impact on NO-dependent vasodilation. For example, the ability of exercise to augment vasodilatation seems to depend upon the muscle mass subjected to training; with forearm exercise, changes are restricted to the forearm vessels, while lower body training (e.g., running and cycling) can induce a generalized whole-body benefit, even in the untrained upper limbs (Di Francescomarino et al., 2009; Green et al., 2004; McAllister

& Laughlin, 2006). Moreover, the shear stress-mediated effects of exercise on the production and bioactivity of NO differ according to exercise duration. In the untrained vessel, baseline release of NO causes subjacent smooth muscle cell vasodilation, which acts to homeostatically regulate wall shear. In response to short- and medium-term exercise training, acute increase in shear stress, associated with repetitive exposure to increased flow during exercise, stimulates increased endothelial NO production, which acts to homeostatically regulate the shear stress associated with exercise, and leads to vasodilation (Di Francescomarino et al., 2009; Green et al., 2004; McAllister & Laughlin, 2006). However, following long-term exercise training, the short-term functional adaptation is succeeded by NO-dependent structural changes, leading to arterial remodeling (increase in vessel caliber) and structural normalization of shear, while NO function gradually decreases (**Figure 14.4**) (Di Francescomarino et al., 2009; Green et al., 2004; McAllister & Laughlin, 2006). This process constitutes a longer-term mechanism for reducing shear stress, allowing NO bioactivity to return toward pre-training levels.

OXIDATIVE STRESS

Oxidative stress has emerged as a fundamental factor in the pathogenesis of endothelial dysfunction. The susceptibility of vascular cells to oxidative stress depends on the overall balance between the degree of oxidative stress and the antioxidant defense capability. Generation of ROS is a normal process in the life of aerobic organisms. Under physiological conditions, these deleterious species are mostly removed by cellular antioxidant systems, which include antioxidant vitamins, protein and non-protein thiols, and antioxidant enzymes. However, under certain conditions, such as obesity, dyslipidemia, hypertension, and insulin resistance, an imbalance between free radicals and antioxidants in favor of the former leads to a state of increased oxidative stress, which if maintained in the long term, can lead to significant damage, including lipid peroxidation and oxidative modifications of proteins and nucleic acids (Forstermann, Xia, & Li, 2017; Li, Horke, & Forstermann, 2014). Oxidative stress and the associated oxidative damage are mediators of inflammation, vascular injury, and atherosclerosis and have emerged as important factors in the pathogenesis of most cardio-metabolic diseases (Forstermann et al., 2017; Li et al., 2014).

In the vascular wall, ROS are produced by several enzyme systems including nicotinamide adenine dinucleotide phosphate (NADPH) oxidase, xanthine oxidase, uncoupled eNOS, and the mitochondrial electron transport chain. On the other hand, the vasculature is protected by antioxidant enzyme systems, including superoxide dismutases, catalase,

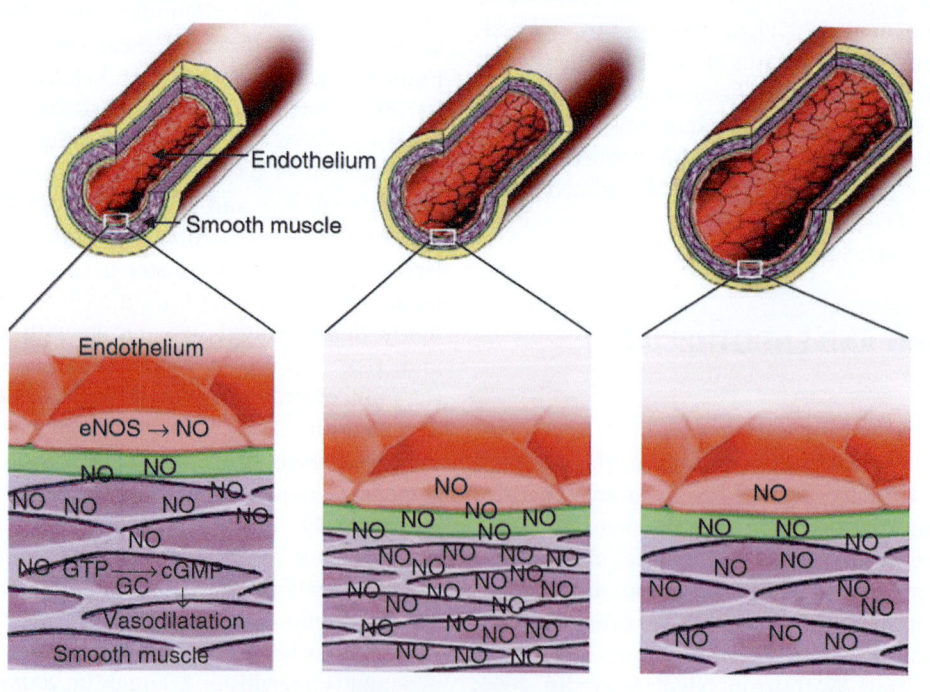

FIGURE 14.4 Hypothesized response of arteries to increased flow and shear stress following varying durations of exercise training. In the untrained vessel (left), basal release of NO causes smooth muscle cell vasodilatation which acts to homeostatically regulate wall shear. In response to medium-term exercise training (middle), an acute increase in shear stress, associated with repetitive exposure to increased flow during bouts of exercise, stimulates increased endothelial NO production and consequent vasodilatation. Upregulation of the NO-dilator system, including eNOS expression, occurs to buffer increased shear stress. Following long-term exercise training (right), structural adaptation occurs, possibly in part due to NO-mediated remodeling, resulting in a chronic increase in vessel caliber, which structurally normalizes shear stress. NO function returns to baseline levels. CGMP = cyclic guanosine monophosphate; eNOS = endothelial nitric oxide synthase; GC = guanylate cyclase; GTP = guanosine triphosphate; NO = nitric oxide. Sources: (Di Francescomarino et al., 2009; Green et al., 2004).

glutathione peroxidases, and paraoxonases, which detoxify ROS (Li et al., 2014; Soccio, Toniato, Evangelista, Carluccio, & De Caterina, 2005).

Exercise has been shown to affect the redox balance of the endothelium in a complex way. Although exercise, especially that of high intensity, is known to induce an initial period of increased oxidative stress, it also enhances the antioxidant capacity; this can be considered a cellular defensive mechanism under oxidative stress. Research has shown that an acute bout of exercise can stimulate the activity of antioxidant enzymes (Franke, Stephens, & Schmid, 1998), while chronic exercise training can promote antioxidant capacity (Chakraphan et al., 2005; Hollander et al., 2001) and inhibit the age-related decline in antioxidant defenses (Golden, Hinerfeld, & Melov, 2002; Ji et al., 1998). Specifically, exercise training has been found to augment the activity of superoxide dismutases and glutathione peroxidases as well as attenuate the activity of NADPH oxidase. These effects contribute to ROS detoxification, ultimately reducing the degradation of NO, a fact that can partially explain the vasodilating effects of exercise (**Figure 14.5**) (Fukai et al., 2000; Walther, Gielen, & Hambrecht, 2004). Presumably, these adaptations result from cumulative effects of repeated exercise bouts on the gene expression of antioxidant enzymes (Allen & Tresini, 2000). Thus, exercise-induced oxidative stress serves as an important signal to stimulate adaptation of antioxidant systems via activation of the redox-sensitive signaling pathways (Franzoni et al., 2004).

FIBRINOLYSIS

The relationship between exercise and the coagulation system is complex. On the one hand, acute exercise may lead to a prothrombotic state as indicated by an increase in fibrinogen, generation of thrombin, activation of platelets, and hemoconcentration (Koenig & Ernst, 2000). In healthy subjects, this is counteracted by a rapid increase in fibrinolytic activity. However, certain subgroups, such as patients with coronary heart disease, and especially those with exercise-induced ischemia, may be at an increased risk for an acute coronary event if exposed to unaccustomed physical exertion (Willich et al., 1993); in these patients exercise prescription should focus on light-to-moderate intensity physical activity under the supervision of specialized health professionals. On the other hand, several interventional studies have consistently found an inverse relationship between various measures of regular sport or recreational physical activity and plasma levels of fibrinogen, one of the most important clotting factors that has been convincingly shown to be an independent cardiovascular risk factor (Koenig & Ernst, 2000). The magnitude of this exercise-induced fibrinogen-lowering effect might be associated with a sizable reduction in major coronary events.

Endothelial cells are the primary site of synthesis and release of t-PA, the main thrombolytic agent that is involved in the breakdown of blood clots (Lijnen & Collen, 1997). The ability of the endothelium to locally release t-PA is critical to the fibrinolytic process. Research has shown that the capacity of the endothelium to release t-PA antigen declines significantly with age; however endothelial t-PA antigen release is well preserved in individuals who perform regular endurance exercise, and that even a brief period of aerobic exercise training can reverse the age-associated loss in the capacity of the endothelium to release t-PA in previously sedentary individuals (Shatos, Doherty, Stump, Thompson, & Collen, 1990).

Although the underlying mechanisms for this exercise-induced increase in t-PA release remain party elucidated, it is possible that mechanical alteration/deformation of the endothelium during exercise because of increased arterial pressure and pulsatile flow may upregulate t-PA mRNA expression and secretion. Mechanical shear stress was shown to be a potent stimulator of t-PA transcription and protein production (Diamond, Eskin, & McIntire, 1989; Diamond et al., 1990). Moreover, physical exercise improves endothelial intracellular calcium concentrations. Since an increase in cytoplasmic calcium can induce acute t-PA release (Kooistra, Schrauwen, Arts, & Emeis, 1994), regular exercise may also contribute to a greater capacity to release t-PA (Laughlin, Oltman, & Bowles, 1998). Reduced oxidative stress with exercise is also an attractive hypothesis, given that *in vitro* studies have shown that oxidative stress significantly inhibits t-PA release from cultured endothelial cells (Shatos et al., 1990). Although further research is needed, the available data suggest that exercise has a favorable

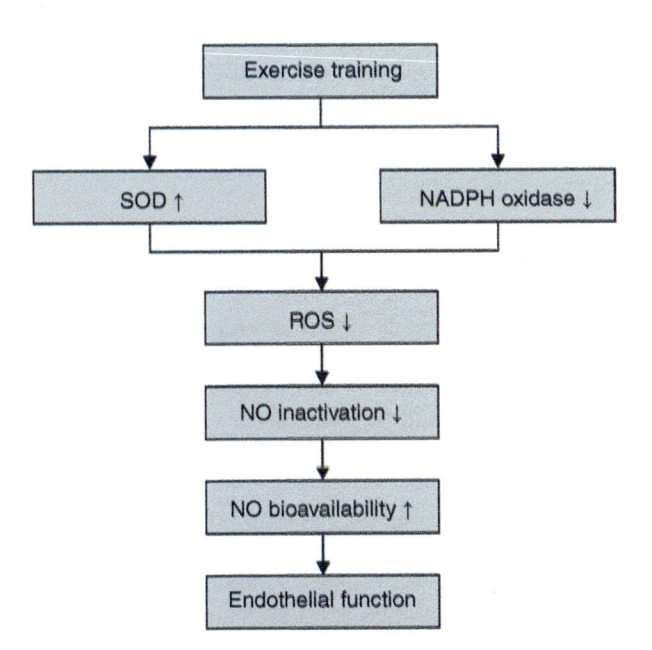

FIGURE 14.5 Nitric oxide bioavailability and exercise training. Putative mechanism by which exercise training improves endothelial function through an increase in NO bioavailability; a decrease in NO inactivation, an increase in SOD, and a decrease in NADH/NADPH oxidase activity are involved in the reduction of ROS, which leads to a decrease in NO inactivation. A decrease in NO inactivation leads to an increase in NO bioavailability. NADH/NADPH = nicotinamide adenine dinucleotide/nicotinamide adenine dinucleotide phosphate; NO = nitric oxide; ROS = reactive oxygen species; SOD = superoxide dismutase. Source: (Di Francescomarino et al., 2009).

effect on the anticoagulant capacity of the endothelium, which can explain part of its cardiovascular benefits.

ANGIOGENESIS

Angiogenesis is the physiological process through which new blood vessels are created from pre-existing vessels, formed in the earlier stage of vasculo-genesis, i.e., the process of blood vessel formation in the embryo through the de novo production of endothelial cells (Adair & Montani, 2010). Angiogenesis continues the growth of the vasculature by processes of sprouting and splitting. It is also vital for the growth and development as well as for wound healing and the formation of granulation tissue (the new connective tissue and microscopic blood vessels that form on the surface of a wound) (Adair & Montani, 2010). All tissues of the body require a continuous supply of oxygen to use metabolic substrates and produce energy. Oxygen is transferred to these tissues by blood capillaries. More capillaries can improve tissue oxygenation and thus enhance energy production, while fewer capillaries can lead to hypoxia or even anoxia. Therefore, the control of angiogenesis is important to improve the survival of poorly perfused tissues that are essential to the body (e.g., the heart, the brain, and skeletal muscles) and to rid the body of unwanted tissues (e.g., tumors) (Adair & Montani, 2010).

Angiogenesis, a component of the multifactorial adaptation to exercise training, is largely mediated by VEGF. A significant increase in VEGF mRNA abundance in human skeletal muscle in response to an acute exercise stimulus has been demonstrated (Gustafsson, Puntschart, Kaijser, Jansson, & Sundberg, 1999; Richardson et al., 1999). VEGF functions as a direct angiogenic factor with a high specificity for vascular endothelial cells, and it is involved in the formation of new blood vessels within human skeletal muscles in response to exercise (Brodal, Ingjer, & Hermansen, 1977; Hang, Kong, Gu, & Adair, 1995; Ingjer & Brodal, 1978). This represents an adaptive response in skeletal muscle to repeated exercise (i.e., training) that results in an increase in the number of capillaries per muscle fiber, which enhances oxygen transport conductance between microcirculation and mitochondria to support the enhanced oxygen needs and energy metabolism during exercise. However, after significant adaptations to exercise training, including angiogenesis, the previously large VEGF mRNA response to acute exercise is significantly attenuated; this represents a typical example of a negative feedback mechanism to reduce the level of VEGF gene expression as exercise adaptation occurs and there is no further significant need for angiogenesis (Richardson et al., 2000). Besides VEGF, bone marrow–derived EPCs have also been shown to enhance angiogenesis, promote vascular repair, and improve endothelial function (Dimmeler et al., 2001; Strehlow et al., 2003). The increased NO production during exercise is proposed to be the main stimulator for the release of EPCs (Haram, Kemi, & Wisloff, 2008).

INFLAMMATION

Inflammation has emerged as a significant determinant of endothelial dysfunction. Cell adhesion molecules (CAMs) are expressed on the surface of endothelial cells and leukocytes in response to endothelial dysfunction (Verma & Anderson, 2002). Some of these molecules are released into the plasma as soluble forms, the presence of which indicates the degree of vascular endothelial activation or dysfunction. Increased concentrations of soluble adhesion molecules are thought to hamper the immune response and mediate the atherosclerotic inflammatory process. The three major classes of CAMs include the selectins (P-selectin, L-selectin, E-selectin), the b2 integrins (CD11/CD18), and immunoglobins (intercellular adhesion molecule-1 [ICAM-1], vascular CAM-1 [VCAM-1] and platelet endothelial CAM-1 [PECAM-1]).

A growing amount of literature supports that engaging in exercise induces an anti-inflammatory phenotype in the general population, both acutely and in the long term (**Figure 14.6**), even though this may be preceded by an acute inflammatory load. The effects of acute exercise on inflammation have been mainly investigated in the muscle by assessing muscle-derived cytokines termed 'myokines', while the long-term effects of exercise on inflammation are mainly observed in adipose tissue with adipose tissue-derived cytokines termed 'adipokines'. During acute exercise, muscle contraction is thought to be the main trigger for overexpression of some inflammatory molecules, mainly IL-6; exercise-induced IL-6 mRNA within the muscle increases IL-6 in the circulation, which then acts as a trigger to activate hepatic glycogenolysis and lipolysis; this occurs because energy within the muscle is quickly depleted with exercise, so this mechanism triggers pathways to provide additional energy to the exercising muscles (Metsios, Moe, & Kitas, 2020). However, this overproduction of IL-6 occurs without the presence of TNF-a or NF-kB activation and is not thought to induce systemic inflammation (Metsios et al., 2020). In the long term, regular exercise has been consistently found to reduce several inflammatory markers, with most data referring to CRP levels both in healthy individuals and patients with chronic diseases, including heart disease and type 2 diabetes mellitus, even in the absence of weight loss (Fedewa, Hathaway, & Ward-Ritacco, 2017; Hammonds, Gathright, Goldstein, Penn, & Hughes, 2016; Hayashino et al., 2014). Although the mechanisms linking exercise to anti-inflammation remain partly elucidated, exercise can attenuate the age-associated increase in oxidative stress and NF-kB activation to reduce toll-like receptor (TRL) 4 signaling and to enhance the expression of peroxisome proliferator-activated receptor gamma co-activator (PGC)-1, which may explain its chronic anti-inflammatory effects (Di Francescomarino et al., 2009; Febbraio, 2007).

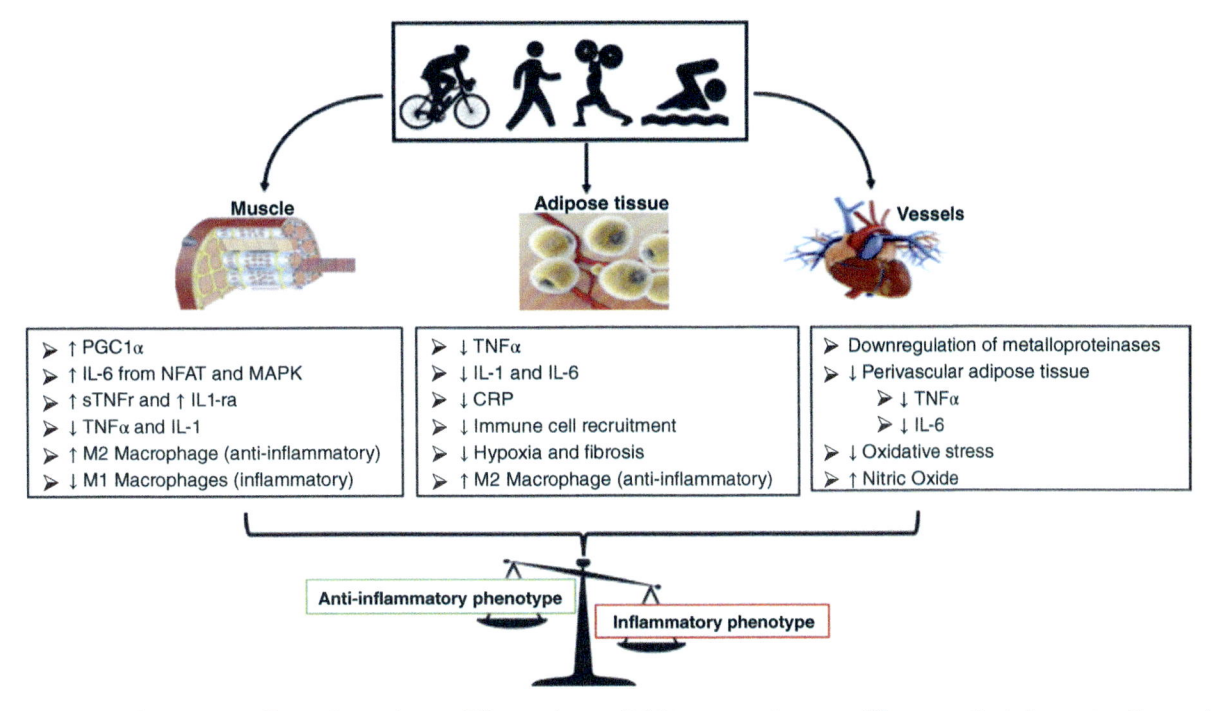

FIGURE 14.6 Anti-inflammatory effects of exercise on different tissues. PGC1a = peroxisome proliferator-activated receptor G co-activator 1a; IL-6 = interleukin 6; NFAT = nuclear factor of activated T-cells; MAPK = mitogen-activated protein kinase; sTNFr = soluble tumor necrosis factor receptors; IL-1ra = interleukin-1 receptor antagonist; TNFa = tumor necrosis factor alpha; IL-1 = interleukin 1; CRP = C-reactive protein. Source: (Metsios et al., 2020).

KEY POINTS

- The endothelium is a special type of epithelium that lines the blood and lymphatic vessels. It consists of a single layer of smooth thin cells that form an interface between circulating blood or lymph in the lumen and the rest of the vessel wall.

- Although traditionally considered a mere selectively permeable barrier between the blood stream and the outer vascular wall, the endothelium is now recognized as a crucial homeostatic organ, fundamental for the regulation of the vascular tone and structure. Improvement of endothelial function is increasingly recognized as a strategy for the prevention of cardiovascular morbidity and mortality.

- Deleterious alterations of endothelial physiology represent a key early step in the development of atherosclerosis and are involved in plaque progression and the occurrence of atherosclerotic complications and cardiovascular events.

- Obesity is considered an important and modifiable risk factor for endothelial dysfunction. Weight loss, achieved through either diet alone or its combination with aerobic exercise, has been linked with improved endothelial function and should be recommended to all obese patients with endothelial dysfunction.

- Data on the effect of dietary components on the vascular endothelium are limited. Several nutrients, such as unsaturated fats, polyphenols, and antioxidants have been correlated to improved endothelial function; however, the evidence is inconclusive and specific dietary recommendations for improving endothelial function are not available.

- Patients with endothelial dysfunction are expected to benefit from the adoption of a cardio-protective dietary pattern, characterized by a higher consumption of fruits, vegetables, nuts, legumes, fish, vegetable oils (especially olive oil), and whole grains, along with a lower/modest intake of red and processed meats, foods rich in refined carbohydrates, salt, and industrialized processed foods high in trans fatty acids.

- Given that obesity, inflammation, and oxidative stress are implicated in the pathogenesis of endothelial dysfunction, the Mediterranean diet could constitute the first-line dietary pattern for enhancing endothelial function, given its strong anti-inflammatory, antioxidant, and cardio-protective properties.

- While exercise acutely induces a pro-oxidant and inflammatory environment, regular exercise can improve endothelial function via several mechanisms; it augments blood flow and laminar shear stress, which result in increased NO production and bioavailability, thereby enhancing vasodilation; it favorably affects the endothelium through the synthesis of molecular mediators, changes in neurohormonal release and improvements in antioxidant capacity, and it elicits systemic molecular pathways connected with angiogenesis as well as a chronic anti-inflammatory effect.

- Exercise can be of special value for older adults in whom endothelial dysfunction is common due to age-related impairments in vasodilation and a state of increased oxidative stress.

SELF-ASSESSMENT QUESTIONS

1. What are the five main types of animal tissue?
2. What is endothelium and what does it consist of?
3. Define endothelial dysfunction.
4. Is it easy to assess endothelial dysfunction? Why or why not?
5. Fill in the blank: Epidemiological observations suggest a(n) _____ association between physical activity and endothelial function.
6. What are the main nutritional strategies that someone could follow to improve endothelial function?
7. What are the mechanisms by which exercise affects endothelial function?

REFERENCES

Abbott, R. A., Harkness, M. A., & Davies, P. S. (2002). Correlation of habitual physical activity levels with flow-mediated dilation of the brachial artery in 5-10 year old children. *Atherosclerosis*, *160*(1), 233–239. doi:10.1016/s0021-9150(01)00566-4

Adair, T. H., & Montani, J. P. (2010). In *Angiogenesis*. San Rafael (CA).

Ades, P. A., Savage, P. D., Lischke, S., Toth, M. J., Harvey-Berino, J., Bunn, J. Y., . . . Schneider, D. J. (2011). The effect of weight loss and exercise training on flow-mediated dilatation in coronary heart disease: a randomized trial. *Chest*, *140*(6), 1420–1427. doi:10.1378/chest.10-3289

Aird, W. C. (2013). 3 - Endothelium. In C. S. Kitchens, C. M. Kessler, & B. A. Konkle (Eds.), *Consultative Hemostasis and Thrombosis (Third Edition)* (pp. 33–41). Philadelphia: W.B. Saunders.

Al-Qaisi, M., Kharbanda, R. K., Mittal, T. K., & Donald, A. E. (2008). Measurement of endothelial function and its clinical utility for cardiovascular risk. *Vasc Health Risk Manag*, *4*(3), 647–652. doi:10.2147/vhrm.s2769

Allen, R. G., & Tresini, M. (2000). Oxidative stress and gene regulation. *Free Radic Biol Med*, *28*(3), 463–499. doi:10.1016/s0891-5849(99)00242-7

Anderson, T. J. (1999). Assessment and treatment of endothelial dysfunction in humans. *J Am Coll Cardiol*, *34*(3), 631–638. doi:10.1016/s0735-1097(99)00259-4

Bigornia, S. J., Mott, M. M., Hess, D. T., Apovian, C. M., McDonnell, M. E., Duess, M. A., . . . Gokce, N. (2010). Long-term successful weight loss improves vascular endothelial function in severely obese individuals. *Obesity (Silver Spring)*, *18*(4), 754–759. doi:10.1038/oby.2009.482

Bonetti, P. O., Lerman, L. O., & Lerman, A. (2003). Endothelial dysfunction: a marker of atherosclerotic risk. *Arterioscler Thromb Vasc Biol*, *23*(2), 168–175. doi:10.1161/01.atv.0000051384.43104.fc

Brodal, P., Ingjer, F., & Hermansen, L. (1977). Capillary supply of skeletal muscle fibers in untrained and endurance-trained men. *Am J Physiol*, *232*(6), H705–712. doi:10.1152/ajpheart.1977.232.6.H705

Brook, R. D., Bard, R. L., Glazewski, L., Kehrer, C., Bodary, P. F., Eitzman, D. L., & Rajagopalan, S. (2004). Effect of short-term weight loss on the metabolic syndrome and conduit vascular endothelial function in overweight adults. *Am J Cardiol*, *93*(8), 1012–1016. doi:10.1016/j.amjcard.2004.01.009

Buckland, G., Bach, A., & Serra-Majem, L. (2008). Obesity and the Mediterranean diet: a systematic review of observational and intervention studies. *Obes Rev*, *9*(6), 582–593. doi:10.1111/j.1467-789X.2008.00503.x

Bull, F. C., Al-Ansari, S. S., Biddle, S., Borodulin, K., Buman, M. P., Cardon, G., . . . Willumsen, J. F. (2020). World Health Organization 2020 guidelines on physical activity and sedentary behaviour. *Br J Sports Med*, *54*(24), 1451–1462. doi:10.1136/bjsports-2020-102955

Bullo, M., Lamuela-Raventos, R., & Salas-Salvado, J. (2011). Mediterranean diet and oxidation: nuts and olive oil as important sources of fat and antioxidants. *Curr Top Med Chem*, *11*(14), 1797–1810. Retrieved from http://www.ncbi.nlm.nih.gov/pubmed/21506929

Celermajer, D. S., Sorensen, K. E., Spiegelhalter, D. J., Georgakopoulos, D., Robinson, J., & Deanfield, J. E. (1994). Aging is associated with endothelial dysfunction in healthy men years before the age-related decline in women. *J Am Coll Cardiol*, *24*(2), 471–476. doi:10.1016/0735-1097(94)90305-0

Cernadas, M. R., Sanchez de Miguel, L., Garcia-Duran, M., Gonzalez-Fernandez, F., Millas, I., Monton, M., . . . Lopez, F. (1998). Expression of constitutive and inducible nitric oxide synthases in the vascular wall of young and aging rats. *Circ Res*, *83*(3), 279–286. doi:10.1161/01.res.83.3.279

Chakraphan, D., Sridulyakul, P., Thipakorn, B., Bunnag, S., Huxley, V. H., & Patumraj, S. (2005). Attenuation of endothelial dysfunction by exercise training in STZ-induced diabetic rats. *Clin Hemorheol Microcirc*, *32*(3), 217–226. Retrieved from http://www.ncbi.nlm.nih.gov/pubmed/15851841

Chareonrungrueangchai, K., Wongkawinwoot, K., Anothaisintawee, T., & Reutrakul, S. (2020). Dietary Factors and Risks of Cardiovascular Diseases: An Umbrella Review. *Nutrients*, *12*(4). doi:10.3390/nu12041088

Chi, J. T., Chang, H. Y., Haraldsen, G., Jahnsen, F. L., Troyanskaya, O. G., Chang, D. S., . . . Brown, P. O. (2003). Endothelial cell diversity revealed by global expression profiling. *Proc Natl Acad Sci U S A*, *100*(19), 10623–10628. doi:10.1073/pnas.1434429100

Chou, T. C., Yen, M. H., Li, C. Y., & Ding, Y. A. (1998). Alterations of nitric oxide synthase expression with aging and hypertension in rats. *Hypertension*, *31*(2), 643–648. doi:10.1161/01.hyp.31.2.643

Corretti, M. C., Anderson, T. J., Benjamin, E. J., Celermajer, D., Charbonneau, F., Creager, M. A., . . . International Brachial Artery Reactivity Task, F. (2002). Guidelines for the ultrasound assessment of endothelial-dependent flow-mediated vasodilation of the brachial artery: a report of the International Brachial Artery Reactivity Task Force. *J Am Coll Cardiol*, *39*(2), 257–265. doi:10.1016/s0735-1097(01)01746-6

Cuevas, A. M., & Germain, A. M. (2004). Diet and endothelial function. *Biol Res*, *37*(2), 225–230. doi:10.4067/s0716-97602004000200008

Davis, N., Katz, S., & Wylie-Rosett, J. (2007). The effect of diet on endothelial function. *Cardiol Rev, 15*(2), 62-66. doi:10.1097/01.crd.0000218824.79018.cd

DeSouza, C. A., Shapiro, L. F., Clevenger, C. M., Dinenno, F. A., Monahan, K. D., Tanaka, H., & Seals, D. R. (2000). Regular aerobic exercise prevents and restores age-related declines in endothelium-dependent vasodilation in healthy men. *Circulation, 102*(12), 1351-1357. doi:10.1161/01.cir.102.12.1351

Di Francescomarino, S., Sciartilli, A., Di Valerio, V., Di Baldassarre, A., & Gallina, S. (2009). The effect of physical exercise on endothelial function. *Sports Med, 39*(10), 797-812. doi:10.2165/11317750-000000000-00000

Diamond, S. L., Eskin, S. G., & McIntire, L. V. (1989). Fluid flow stimulates tissue plasminogen activator secretion by cultured human endothelial cells. *Science, 243*(4897), 1483-1485. doi:10.1126/science.2467379

Diamond, S. L., Sharefkin, J. B., Dieffenbach, C., Frasier-Scott, K., McIntire, L. V., & Eskin, S. G. (1990). Tissue plasminogen activator messenger RNA levels increase in cultured human endothelial cells exposed to laminar shear stress. *J Cell Physiol, 143*(2), 364-371. doi:10.1002/jcp.1041430222

Dimmeler, S., Aicher, A., Vasa, M., Mildner-Rihm, C., Adler, K., Tiemann, M., . . . Zeiher, A. M. (2001). HMG-CoA reductase inhibitors (statins) increase endothelial progenitor cells via the PI 3-kinase/Akt pathway. *J Clin Invest, 108*(3), 391-397. doi:10.1172/JCI13152

Edmundowicz, D. (2002). Noninvasive Studies of Coronary and Peripheral Arterial Blood-flow. *Curr Atheroscler Rep, 4*(5), 381-385. doi:10.1007/s11883-002-0076-5

Engin, A. (2017). Endothelial Dysfunction in Obesity. *Adv Exp Med Biol, 960*, 345-379. doi:10.1007/978-3-319-48382-5_15

Eskurza, I., Monahan, K. D., Robinson, J. A., & Seals, D. R. (2004). Effect of acute and chronic ascorbic acid on flow-mediated dilatation with sedentary and physically active human ageing. *J Physiol, 556*(Pt 1), 315-324. doi:10.1113/jphysiol.2003.057042

Esposito, K., Kastorini, C. M., Panagiotakos, D. B., & Giugliano, D. (2011). Mediterranean diet and weight loss: meta-analysis of randomized controlled trials. *Metab Syndr Relat Disord, 9*(1), 1-12. doi:10.1089/met.2010.0031

Esposito, K., Marfella, R., Ciotola, M., Di Palo, C., Giugliano, F., Giugliano, G., . . . Giugliano, D. (2004). Effect of a mediterranean-style diet on endothelial dysfunction and markers of vascular inflammation in the metabolic syndrome: a randomized trial. *JAMA, 292*(12), 1440-1446. doi:10.1001/jama.292.12.1440

Febbraio, M. A. (2007). Exercise and inflammation. *J Appl Physiol (1985), 103*(1), 376-377. doi:10.1152/japplphysiol.00414.2007

Fedewa, M. V., Hathaway, E. D., & Ward-Ritacco, C. L. (2017). Effect of exercise training on C reactive protein: a systematic review and meta-analysis of randomised and non-randomised controlled trials. *Br J Sports Med, 51*(8), 670-676. doi:10.1136/bjsports-2016-095999

Forstermann, U., Xia, N., & Li, H. (2017). Roles of Vascular Oxidative Stress and Nitric Oxide in the Pathogenesis of Atherosclerosis. *Circ Res, 120*(4), 713-735. doi:10.1161/CIRCRESAHA.116.309326

Franke, W. D., Stephens, G. M., & Schmid, P. G., 3rd. (1998). Effects of intense exercise training on endothelium-dependent exercise-induced vasodilatation. *Clin Physiol, 18*(6), 521-528. doi:10.1046/j.1365-2281.1998.00122.x

Franzoni, F., Ghiadoni, L., Galetta, F., Plantinga, Y., Lubrano, V., Huang, Y., . . . Salvetti, A. (2005). Physical activity, plasma antioxidant capacity, and endothelium-dependent vasodilation in young and older men. *Am J Hypertens, 18*(4 Pt 1), 510-516. doi:10.1016/j.amjhyper.2004.11.006

Franzoni, F., Plantinga, Y., Femia, F. R., Bartolomucci, F., Gaudio, C., Regoli, F., . . . Galetta, F. (2004). Plasma antioxidant activity and cutaneous microvascular endothelial function in athletes and sedentary controls. *Biomed Pharmacother, 58*(8), 432-436. doi:10.1016/j.biopha.2004.08.009

Freeman, A. M., Morris, P. B., Aspry, K., Gordon, N. F., Barnard, N. D., Esselstyn, C. B., . . . Kris-Etherton, P. (2018). A Clinician's Guide for Trending Cardiovascular Nutrition Controversies: Part II. *J Am Coll Cardiol, 72*(5), 553-568. doi:10.1016/j.jacc.2018.05.030

Freeman, A. M., Morris, P. B., Barnard, N., Esselstyn, C. B., Ros, E., Agatston, A., . . . Kris-Etherton, P. (2017). Trending Cardiovascular Nutrition Controversies. *J Am Coll Cardiol, 69*(9), 1172-1187. doi:10.1016/j.jacc.2016.10.086

Fuentes, F., Lopez-Miranda, J., Sanchez, E., Sanchez, F., Paez, J., Paz-Rojas, E., . . . Perez-Jimenez, F. (2001). Mediterranean and low-fat diets improve endothelial function in hypercholesterolemic men. *Ann Intern Med, 134*(12), 1115-1119. doi:10.7326/0003-4819-134-12-200106190-00011

Fukai, T., Siegfried, M. R., Ushio-Fukai, M., Cheng, Y., Kojda, G., & Harrison, D. G. (2000). Regulation of the vascular extracellular superoxide dismutase by nitric oxide and exercise training. *J Clin Invest, 105*(11), 1631-1639. doi:10.1172/JCI9551

Golden, T. R., Hinerfeld, D. A., & Melov, S. (2002). Oxidative stress and aging: beyond correlation. *Aging Cell, 1*(2), 117-123. doi:10.1046/j.1474-9728.2002.00015.x

Goon, P. K., Boos, C. J., & Lip, G. Y. (2005). Circulating endothelial cells: markers of vascular dysfunction. *Clin Lab, 51*(9-10), 531-538. Retrieved from http://www.ncbi.nlm.nih.gov/pubmed/16285476

Green, D. J., Maiorana, A., O'Driscoll, G., & Taylor, R. (2004). Effect of exercise training on endothelium-derived nitric oxide function in humans. *J Physiol, 561*(Pt 1), 1-25. doi:10.1113/jphysiol.2004.068197

Gustafsson, T., Puntschart, A., Kaijser, L., Jansson, E., & Sundberg, C. J. (1999). Exercise-induced expression of angiogenesis-related transcription and growth factors in human skeletal muscle. *Am J Physiol, 276*(2), H679-685. doi:10.1152/ajpheart.1999.276.2.H679

Hadi, H. A., Carr, C. S., & Al Suwaidi, J. (2005). Endothelial dysfunction: cardiovascular risk factors, therapy, and outcome. *Vasc Health Risk Manag, 1*(3), 183-198. Retrieved from http://www.ncbi.nlm.nih.gov/pubmed/17319104

Hammonds, T. L., Gathright, E. C., Goldstein, C. M., Penn, M. S., & Hughes, J. W. (2016). Effects of exercise on c-reactive protein in healthy patients and in patients with heart disease: A meta-analysis. *Heart Lung, 45*(3), 273-282. doi:10.1016/j.hrtlng.2016.01.009

Hang, J., Kong, L., Gu, J. W., & Adair, T. H. (1995). VEGF gene expression is upregulated in electrically stimulated rat skeletal muscle. *Am J Physiol, 269*(5 Pt 2), H1827-1831. doi:10.1152/ajpheart.1995.269.5.H1827

Haram, P. M., Kemi, O. J., & Wisloff, U. (2008). Adaptation of endothelium to exercise training: insights from experimental studies. *Front Biosci, 13*, 336-346. doi:10.2741/2683

Hayashino, Y., Jackson, J. L., Hirata, T., Fukumori, N., Nakamura, F., Fukuhara, S., . . . Ishii, H. (2014). Effects of exercise on C-reactive protein, inflammatory cytokine and adipokine in patients with type 2 diabetes: a meta-analysis of randomized controlled trials. *Metabolism, 63*(3), 431-440. doi:10.1016/j.metabol.2013.08.018

Hodge, A., & Bassett, J. (2016). What can we learn from dietary pattern analysis? *Public Health Nutr, 19*(2), 191-194. doi:10.1017/S1368980015003730

Hollander, J., Fiebig, R., Gore, M., Ookawara, T., Ohno, H., & Ji, L. L. (2001). Superoxide dismutase gene expression is activated by a single bout of exercise in rat skeletal muscle. *Pflugers Arch, 442*(3), 426-434. doi:10.1007/s004240100539

Horstman, L. L., Jy, W., Jimenez, J. J., & Ahn, Y. S. (2004). Endothelial microparticles as markers of endothelial dysfunction. *Front Biosci, 9,* 1118–1135. doi:10.2741/1270

Hu, F. B. (2002). Dietary pattern analysis: a new direction in nutritional epidemiology. *Curr Opin Lipidol, 13*(1), 3–9. Retrieved from http://www.ncbi.nlm.nih.gov/pubmed/11790957

Ingjer, F., & Brodal, P. (1978). Capillary supply of skeletal muscle fibers in untrained and endurance-trained women. *Eur J Appl Physiol Occup Physiol, 38*(4), 291–299. doi:10.1007/BF00423112

Jensen, M. D., Ryan, D. H., Apovian, C. M., Ard, J. D., Comuzzie, A. G., Donato, K. A., . . . Obesity, S. (2014). 2013 AHA/ACC/TOS guideline for the management of overweight and obesity in adults: a report of the American College of Cardiology/American Heart Association Task Force on Practice Guidelines and The Obesity Society. *Circulation, 129*(25 Suppl 2), S102–138. doi:10.1161/01.cir.0000437739.71477.ee

Jeong, S. W., Kim, S. H., Kang, S. H., Kim, H. J., Yoon, C. H., Youn, T. J., & Chae, I. H. (2019). Mortality reduction with physical activity in patients with and without cardiovascular disease. *Eur Heart J, 40*(43), 3547–3555. doi:10.1093/eurheartj/ehz564

Ji, L. L., Leeuwenburgh, C., Leichtweis, S., Gore, M., Fiebig, R., Hollander, J., & Bejma, J. (1998). Oxidative stress and aging. Role of exercise and its influences on antioxidant systems. *Ann N Y Acad Sci, 854,* 102–117. doi:10.1111/j.1749-6632.1998.tb09896.x

Kastorini, C. M., Milionis, H. J., Esposito, K., Giugliano, D., Goudevenos, J. A., & Panagiotakos, D. B. (2011). The effect of Mediterranean diet on metabolic syndrome and its components: a meta-analysis of 50 studies and 534,906 individuals. *J Am Coll Cardiol, 57*(11), 1299–1313. doi:10.1016/j.jacc.2010.09.073

Kaufmann, B. A., Sanders, J. M., Davis, C., Xie, A., Aldred, P., Sarembock, I. J., & Lindner, J. R. (2007). Molecular imaging of inflammation in atherosclerosis with targeted ultrasound detection of vascular cell adhesion molecule-1. *Circulation, 116*(3), 276–284. doi:10.1161/CIRCULATIONAHA.106.684738

Kelly, K. A., Allport, J. R., Tsourkas, A., Shinde-Patil, V. R., Josephson, L., & Weissleder, R. (2005). Detection of vascular adhesion molecule-1 expression using a novel multimodal nanoparticle. *Circ Res, 96*(3), 327–336. doi:10.1161/01.RES.0000155722.17881.dd

Kingwell, B. A., Tran, B., Cameron, J. D., Jennings, G. L., & Dart, A. M. (1996). Enhanced vasodilation to acetylcholine in athletes is associated with lower plasma cholesterol. *Am J Physiol, 270*(6 Pt 2), H2008–2013. doi:10.1152/ajpheart.1996.270.6.H2008

Klonizakis, M., Hunt, B. E., & Woodward, A. (2020). The Association Between Cardiovascular Function, Measured as FMD and CVC, and Long-Term Aquatic Exercise in Older Adults (ACELA Study): A Cross-Sectional Study. *Front Physiol, 11,* 603435. doi:10.3389/fphys.2020.603435

Koenig, W., & Ernst, E. (2000). Exercise and thrombosis. *Coron Artery Dis, 11*(2), 123–127. doi:10.1097/00019501-200003000-00006

Kontogianni, M. D., Zampelas, A., & Tsigos, C. (2006). Nutrition and inflammatory load. *Ann N Y Acad Sci, 1083,* 214–238. doi:10.1196/annals.1367.015

Kooistra, T., Schrauwen, Y., Arts, J., & Emeis, J. J. (1994). Regulation of endothelial cell t-PA synthesis and release. *Int J Hematol, 59*(4), 233–255. Retrieved from http://www.ncbi.nlm.nih.gov/pubmed/8086618

Kurn, H., & Daly, D. T. (2020). Histology, Epithelial Cell. In *StatPearls*. Treasure Island (FL).

Lacorre, D. A., Baekkevold, E. S., Garrido, I., Brandtzaeg, P., Haraldsen, G., Amalric, F., & Girard, J. P. (2004). Plasticity of endothelial cells: rapid dedifferentiation of freshly isolated high endothelial venule endothelial cells outside the lymphoid tissue microenvironment. *Blood, 103*(11), 4164–4172. doi:10.1182/blood-2003-10-3537

Laughlin, M. H., Oltman, C. L., & Bowles, D. K. (1998). Exercise training-induced adaptations in the coronary circulation. *Med Sci Sports Exerc, 30*(3), 352–360. doi:10.1097/00005768-199803000-00004

Lear, S. A., Hu, W., Rangarajan, S., Gasevic, D., Leong, D., Iqbal, R., . . . Yusuf, S. (2017). The effect of physical activity on mortality and cardiovascular disease in 130 000 people from 17 high-income, middle-income, and low-income countries: the PURE study. *Lancet, 390*(10113), 2643–2654. doi:10.1016/S0140-6736(17)31634-3

Lerman, A., & Burnett, J. C., Jr. (1992). Intact and altered endothelium in regulation of vasomotion. *Circulation, 86*(6 Suppl), III12-19. Retrieved from http://www.ncbi.nlm.nih.gov/pubmed/1424046

Li, H., Horke, S., & Forstermann, U. (2014). Vascular oxidative stress, nitric oxide and atherosclerosis. *Atherosclerosis, 237*(1), 208–219. doi:10.1016/j.atherosclerosis.2014.09.001

Lijnen, H. R., & Collen, D. (1997). Endothelium in hemostasis and thrombosis. *Prog Cardiovasc Dis, 39*(4), 343–350. doi:10.1016/s0033-0620(97)80032-1

Liyanage, T., Ninomiya, T., Wang, A., Neal, B., Jun, M., Wong, M. G., . . . Perkovic, V. (2016). Effects of the Mediterranean Diet on Cardiovascular Outcomes-A Systematic Review and Meta-Analysis. *PLoS One, 11*(8), e0159252. doi:10.1371/journal.pone.0159252

Lopez-Garcia, E., Schulze, M. B., Fung, T. T., Meigs, J. B., Rifai, N., Manson, J. E., & Hu, F. B. (2004). Major dietary patterns are related to plasma concentrations of markers of inflammation and endothelial dysfunction. *Am J Clin Nutr, 80*(4), 1029–1035. doi:10.1093/ajcn/80.4.1029

Lum, H., & Roebuck, K. A. (2001). Oxidant stress and endothelial cell dysfunction. *Am J Physiol Cell Physiol, 280*(4), C719–741. doi:10.1152/ajpcell.2001.280.4.C719

Mach, F., Baigent, C., Catapano, A. L., Koskinas, K. C., Casula, M., Badimon, L., . . . Group, E. S. C. S. D. (2020). 2019 ESC/EAS Guidelines for the management of dyslipidaemias: lipid modification to reduce cardiovascular risk. *Eur Heart J, 41*(1), 111–188. doi:10.1093/eurheartj/ehz455

Mavri, A., Poredos, P., Suran, D., Gaborit, B., Juhan-Vague, I., & Poredos, P. (2011). Effect of diet-induced weight loss on endothelial dysfunction: early improvement after the first week of dieting. *Heart Vessels, 26*(1), 31–38. doi:10.1007/s00380-010-0016-1

McAllister, R. M., & Laughlin, M. H. (2006). Vascular nitric oxide: effects of physical activity, importance for health. *Essays Biochem, 42,* 119–131. doi:10.1042/bse0420119

Metsios, G. S., Moe, R. H., & Kitas, G. D. (2020). Exercise and inflammation. *Best Pract Res Clin Rheumatol, 34*(2), 101504. doi:10.1016/j.berh.2020.101504

Moe, I. T., Hoven, H., Hetland, E. V., Rognmo, O., & Slordahl, S. A. (2005). Endothelial function in highly endurance-trained and sedentary, healthy young women. *Vasc Med, 10*(2), 97–102. doi:10.1191/1358863x05vm592oa

Mutlu-Turkoglu, U., Ilhan, E., Oztezcan, S., Kuru, A., Aykac-Toker, G., & Uysal, M. (2003). Age-related increases in plasma malondialdehyde and protein carbonyl levels and lymphocyte DNA damage in elderly subjects. *Clin Biochem, 36*(5), 397–400. doi:10.1016/s0009-9120(03)00035-3

Ocke, M. C. (2013). Evaluation of methodologies for assessing the overall diet: dietary quality scores and dietary pattern analysis. *Proc Nutr Soc, 72*(2), 191–199. doi:10.1017/S0029665113000013

Onvani, S., Haghighatdoost, F., Surkan, P. J., Larijani, B., & Azadbakht, L. (2017). Adherence to the Healthy Eating Index and Alternative Healthy

Eating Index dietary patterns and mortality from all causes, cardiovascular disease and cancer: a meta-analysis of observational studies. *J Hum Nutr Diet, 30*(2), 216–226. doi:10.1111/jhn.12415

Pahkala, K., Heinonen, O. J., Lagstrom, H., Hakala, P., Simell, O., Viikari, J. S., . . . Raitakari, O. T. (2008). Vascular endothelial function and leisure-time physical activity in adolescents. *Circulation, 118*(23), 2353–2359. doi:10.1161/CIRCULATIONAHA.108.791988

Patel, S. N., Rajaram, V., Pandya, S., Fiedler, B. M., Bai, C. J., Neems, R., . . . Feinstein, S. B. (2004). Emerging, noninvasive surrogate markers of atherosclerosis. *Curr Atheroscler Rep, 6*(1), 60–68. doi:10.1007/s11883-004-0117-3

Payvandi, L., Dyer, A., McPherson, D., Ades, P., Stein, J., Liu, K., . . . McDermott, M. M. (2009). Physical activity during daily life and brachial artery flow-mediated dilation in peripheral arterial disease. *Vasc Med, 14*(3), 193–201. doi:10.1177/1358863X08101018

Phillips, S. A., Jurva, J. W., Syed, A. Q., Syed, A. Q., Kulinski, J. P., Pleuss, J., . . . Gutterman, D. D. (2008). Benefit of low-fat over low-carbohydrate diet on endothelial health in obesity. *Hypertension, 51*(2), 376–382. doi:10.1161/HYPERTENSIONAHA.107.101824

Pierce, G. L., Beske, S. D., Lawson, B. R., Southall, K. L., Benay, F. J., Donato, A. J., & Seals, D. R. (2008). Weight loss alone improves conduit and resistance artery endothelial function in young and older overweight/obese adults. *Hypertension, 52*(1), 72–79. doi:10.1161/HYPERTENSIONAHA.108.111427

Piercy, K. L., & Troiano, R. P. (2018). Physical Activity Guidelines for Americans From the US Department of Health and Human Services. *Circ Cardiovasc Qual Outcomes, 11*(11), e005263. doi:10.1161/CIRCOUTCOMES.118.005263

Regan, E. R., & Aird, W. C. (2012). Dynamical systems approach to endothelial heterogeneity. *Circ Res, 111*(1), 110–130. doi:10.1161/CIRCRESAHA.111.261701

Resnick, N., Yahav, H., Shay-Salit, A., Shushy, M., Schubert, S., Zilberman, L. C., & Wofovitz, E. (2003). Fluid shear stress and the vascular endothelium: for better and for worse. *Prog Biophys Mol Biol, 81*(3), 177–199. doi:10.1016/s0079-6107(02)00052-4

Richardson, R. S., Wagner, H., Mudaliar, S. R., Henry, R., Noyszewski, E. A., & Wagner, P. D. (1999). Human VEGF gene expression in skeletal muscle: effect of acute normoxic and hypoxic exercise. *Am J Physiol, 277*(6), H2247–2252. doi:10.1152/ajpheart.1999.277.6.H2247

Richardson, R. S., Wagner, H., Mudaliar, S. R., Saucedo, E., Henry, R., & Wagner, P. D. (2000). Exercise adaptation attenuates VEGF gene expression in human skeletal muscle. *Am J Physiol Heart Circ Physiol, 279*(2), H772–778. doi:10.1152/ajpheart.2000.279.2.H772

Rosenberg, R. D., & Aird, W. C. (1999). Vascular-bed-specific hemostasis and hypercoagulable states. *N Engl J Med, 340*(20), 1555–1564. doi:10.1056/NEJM199905203402007

Schinzari, F., Tesauro, M., & Cardillo, C. (2017). Endothelial and Perivascular Adipose Tissue Abnormalities in Obesity-Related Vascular Dysfunction: Novel Targets for Treatment. *J Cardiovasc Pharmacol, 69*(6), 360–368. doi:10.1097/FJC.0000000000000469

Schwingshackl, L., & Hoffmann, G. (2015). Diet quality as assessed by the Healthy Eating Index, the Alternate Healthy Eating Index, the Dietary Approaches to Stop Hypertension score, and health outcomes: a systematic review and meta-analysis of cohort studies. *J Acad Nutr Diet, 115*(5), 780–800 e785. doi:10.1016/j.jand.2014.12.009

Shankar, S. S., & Steinberg, H. O. (2008). Weight loss and vascular function: the good and the unknown. *Hypertension, 52*(1), 57–58. doi:10.1161/HYPERTENSIONAHA.108.112441

Shannon, O. M., Mendes, I., Kochl, C., Mazidi, M., Ashor, A. W., Rubele, S., . . . Siervo, M. (2020). Mediterranean Diet Increases Endothelial Function in Adults: A Systematic Review and Meta-Analysis of Randomized Controlled Trials. *J Nutr, 150*(5), 1151–1159. doi:10.1093/jn/nxaa002

Shatos, M. A., Doherty, J. M., Stump, D. C., Thompson, E. A., & Collen, D. (1990). Oxygen radicals generated during anoxia followed by reoxygenation reduce the synthesis of tissue-type plasminogen activator and plasminogen activator inhibitor-1 in human endothelial cell culture. *J Biol Chem, 265*(33), 20443–20448. Retrieved from http://www.ncbi.nlm.nih.gov/pubmed/2122975

Siasos, G., Chrysohoou, C., Tousoulis, D., Oikonomou, E., Panagiotakos, D., Zaromitidou, M., . . . Stefanadis, C. (2013). The impact of physical activity on endothelial function in middle-aged and elderly subjects: the Ikaria study. *Hellenic J Cardiol, 54*(2), 94–101. Retrieved from http://www.ncbi.nlm.nih.gov/pubmed/23557608

Skilton, M. R., Sieveking, D. P., Harmer, J. A., Franklin, J., Loughnan, G., Nakhla, S., . . . Celermajer, D. S. (2008). The effects of obesity and non-pharmacological weight loss on vascular and ventricular function and structure. *Diabetes Obes Metab, 10*(10), 874–884. doi:10.1111/j.1463-1326.2007.00817.x

Soccio, M., Toniato, E., Evangelista, V., Carluccio, M., & De Caterina, R. (2005). Oxidative stress and cardiovascular risk: the role of vascular NAD(P)H oxidase and its genetic variants. *Eur J Clin Invest, 35*(5), 305–314. doi:10.1111/j.1365-2362.2005.01500.x

Sofi, F. (2009). The Mediterranean diet revisited: evidence of its effectiveness grows. *Curr Opin Cardiol, 24*(5), 442–446. doi:10.1097/HCO.0b013e32832f056e

Sofi, F., Macchi, C., Abbate, R., Gensini, G. F., & Casini, A. (2014). Mediterranean diet and health status: an updated meta-analysis and a proposal for a literature-based adherence score. *Public Health Nutr, 17*(12), 2769–2782. doi:10.1017/S1368980013003169

Stadtman, E. R. (1992). Protein oxidation and aging. *Science, 257*(5074), 1220–1224. doi:10.1126/science.1355616

Strehlow, K., Werner, N., Berweiler, J., Link, A., Dirnagl, U., Priller, J., . . . Nickenig, G. (2003). Estrogen increases bone marrow-derived endothelial progenitor cell production and diminishes neointima formation. *Circulation, 107*(24), 3059–3065. doi:10.1161/01.CIR.0000077911.81151.30

Studer, M., Briel, M., Leimenstoll, B., Glass, T. R., & Bucher, H. C. (2005). Effect of different antilipidemic agents and diets on mortality: a systematic review. *Arch Intern Med, 165*(7), 725–730. doi:10.1001/archinte.165.7.725

Su, J. B. (2015). Vascular endothelial dysfunction and pharmacological treatment. *World J Cardiol, 7*(11), 719–741. doi:10.4330/wjc.v7.i11.719

Taddei, S., Galetta, F., Virdis, A., Ghiadoni, L., Salvetti, G., Franzoni, F., . . . Salvetti, A. (2000). Physical activity prevents age-related impairment in nitric oxide availability in elderly athletes. *Circulation, 101*(25), 2896–2901. doi:10.1161/01.cir.101.25.2896

Torres-Pena, J. D., Rangel-Zuniga, O. A., Alcala-Diaz, J. F., Lopez-Miranda, J., & Delgado-Lista, J. (2020). Mediterranean Diet and Endothelial Function: A Review of its Effects at Different Vascular Bed Levels. *Nutrients, 12*(8). doi:10.3390/nu12082212

Vazquez, L. A., Pazos, F., Berrazueta, J. R., Fernandez-Escalante, C., Garcia-Unzueta, M. T., Freijanes, J., & Amado, J. A. (2005). Effects of changes in body weight and insulin resistance on inflammation and endothelial function in morbid obesity after bariatric surgery. *J Clin Endocrinol Metab, 90*(1), 316–322. doi:10.1210/jc.2003-032059

Verma, S., & Anderson, T. J. (2002). Fundamentals of endothelial function for the clinical cardiologist. *Circulation, 105*(5), 546–549. doi:10.1161/hc0502.104540

Versari, D., Daghini, E., Virdis, A., Ghiadoni, L., & Taddei, S. (2009). Endothelial dysfunction as a target for prevention of cardiovascular disease. *Diabetes Care, 32* Suppl 2, S314–321. doi:10.2337/dc09-S330

Vina, J., Sanchis-Gomar, F., Martinez-Bello, V., & Gomez-Cabrera, M. C. (2012). Exercise acts as a drug; the pharmacological benefits of exercise. *Br J Pharmacol, 167*(1), 1–12. doi:10.1111/j.1476-5381.2012.01970.x

Walther, C., Gielen, S., & Hambrecht, R. (2004). The effect of exercise training on endothelial function in cardiovascular disease in humans. *Exerc Sport Sci Rev, 32*(4), 129–134. doi:10.1097/00003677-200410000-00002

Warburton, D. E., Nicol, C. W., & Bredin, S. S. (2006). Health benefits of physical activity: the evidence. *CMAJ, 174*(6), 801–809. doi:10.1503/cmaj.051351

Warburton, D. E. R., & Bredin, S. S. D. (2017). Health benefits of physical activity: a systematic review of current systematic reviews. *Curr Opin Cardiol, 32*(5), 541–556. doi:10.1097/HCO.0000000000000437

Werner, N., & Nickenig, G. (2007). Endothelial progenitor cells in health and atherosclerotic disease. *Ann Med, 39*(2), 82–90. doi:10.1080/07853890601073429

Willett, W. C., & McCullough, M. L. (2008). Dietary pattern analysis for the evaluation of dietary guidelines. *Asia Pac J Clin Nutr, 17* Suppl 1, 75–78. Retrieved from http://www.ncbi.nlm.nih.gov/pubmed/18296306

Willich, S. N., Lewis, M., Lowel, H., Arntz, H. R., Schubert, F., & Schroder, R. (1993). Physical exertion as a trigger of acute myocardial infarction. Triggers and Mechanisms of Myocardial Infarction Study Group. *N Engl J Med, 329*(23), 1684–1690. doi:10.1056/NEJM199312023292302

Yumuk, V., Tsigos, C., Fried, M., Schindler, K., Busetto, L., Micic, D., . . . Obesity Management Task Force of the European Association for the Study of, O. (2015). European Guidelines for Obesity Management in Adults. *Obes Facts, 8*(6), 402–424. doi:10.1159/000442721

Zhang, X., Cash, R. E., Bower, J. K., Focht, B. C., & Paskett, E. D. (2020). Physical activity and risk of cardiovascular disease by weight status among U.S adults. *PLoS One, 15*(5), e0232893. doi:10.1371/journal.pone.0232893

FURTHER READING

Bibliography

Amarasekera, A.T., Chang, D., Schwarz, P., and Tan, T.C. (2021). Does vascular endothelial dysfunction play a role in physical frailty and sarcopenia? A systematic review. *Age and ageing 50*(3): 725–732.

Chrysohoou, C., Kollia, N., and Tousoulis, D. (2018). The link between depression and atherosclerosis through the pathways of inflammation and endothelium dysfunction. *Maturitas 109*: 1–5.

Lee, J.H., Lee, R., Hwang, M.H., et al. (2018). The effects of exercise on vascular endothelial function in type 2 diabetes: a systematic review and meta-analysis. *Diabetology & Metabolic Syndrome 10*: 15. doi: 10.1186/s13098-018-0316-7.

Rezazadeh, L., Gargari, B.P., Jafarabadi, M.A., and Alipour, B. (2019). Effects of probiotic yogurt on glycemic indexes and endothelial dysfunction markers in patients with metabolic syndrome. *Nutrition 62*: 162–168.

Link

- https://www.ncbi.nlm.nih.gov/books/NBK57149/

Cardio-metabolic Health, Diet, and Physical Activity

UNIT 5

Diabetes Mellitus

CHAPTER 15

Definition	223
Epidemiology	223
Types of Diabetes	225
Diagnosis of Diabetes Mellitus	226
Prediabetes	226
Complications	228
Heart Disease and Stroke	228
High Blood Pressure	228
Diabetic Retinopathy	228
Diabetic Kidney Disease	228
Diabetic Neuropathy	229
Amputations	229
Dental Disease	229
Complications of Pregnancy	230
Other Complications	230
Physiology and Pathophysiology	230
Physical Inactivity/Sedentary Behavior and Diabetes Mellitus	230
Obesity, Diabetes Mellitus and Mortality	232
Prevention or Delay of Diabetes Mellitus	232
Non-pharmacological Management of Diabetes Mellitus	232
Nutrition-based Interventions	232
Nutrition Interventions for Older Adults with Diabetes	233
Physiology of Exercise in Type 1 Diabetes	234
Physiology of Exercise in Type 2 Diabetes	234
Benefits of Physical Activity	234
Benefits of Reducing Sedentary Time	235
Exercise-based Interventions	235
Nutrition and Exercise: Combined Interventions	236
Exercise Guidelines for Diabetes Mellitus Patients	236
Key Points	237
Self-assessment Questions	237
References	238
Further Reading	240
Bibliography	240
Links	240

DEFINITION

According to the WHO 2019 updated and published guidance on how to classify diabetes mellitus (DM) (World Health Organization, 2019) and the Expert Committee on the Diagnosis and Classification of Diabetes Mellitus ("Diagnosis and Classification of Diabetes Mellitus," 2014; "Report of the Expert Committee on the Diagnosis and Classification of Diabetes Mellitus," 1998), DM can be defined as a group of metabolic disorders characterized by chronic hyperglycemia (i.e., high concentrations of blood glucose) resulting from defects in insulin production, insulin action, or both and associated with disturbances in glucose, lipid, and protein metabolism. As it will be discussed below in this chapter, long-term effects of the chronic hyperglycemia on health include damage, dysfunction, and failure of organs like the eyes, kidneys, nerves, heart, and blood vessels.

EPIDEMIOLOGY

According to the 2017 Atlas of the International Federation of Diabetes, almost 50% of the adults 20 to 79 years old living with diabetes are undiagnosed. This translates to 212.4 million people who are uninformed about their disease. Approximately 27.7 million Americans have diabetes are unaware of the diagnosis. In the last few decades, the prevalence of type 2 diabetes

Prevention and Management of Cardiovascular and Metabolic Disease: Diet, Physical Activity and Healthy Aging,
First Edition. Christina N. Katsagoni, Peter Kokkinos, and Labros S. Sidossis.
© 2023 John Wiley & Sons Ltd. Published 2023 by John Wiley & Sons Ltd.

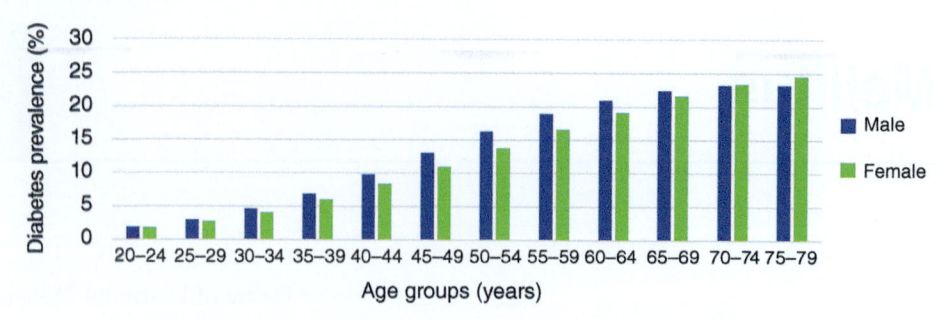

FIGURE 15.1 The prevalence of diabetes by age and gender in 2021. Source: (Sun et al., 2022 / with permission of Elsevier).

(T2D) has alarmingly grown in children and adolescents. Physical inactivity, adherence to bad dietary habits, and obesity are the culprits for this increase (*IDF Diabetes Atlas - 8th Edition*, 2017).

In 2019, the prevalence of diabetes for adults aged 20 to 79 years old worldwide was estimated to be 9.3% and is projected to be 10.2% in 2030 and 10.9% in 2045 (Saeedi et al., 2019). The prevalence of diabetes by age and gender in 2021 is shown in **Figure 15.1** (Sun et al. 2022).

The total number of patients worldwide with diabetes over the next two to three decades is projected to rise from 463 million in 2019 to 700 million in 2045 (**Table 15.1**) (Saeedi et al., 2019).

The number of patients aged 20 to 79 years with diabetes, according to region, in 2019 and the projection in 2045, is presented in **Figure 15.2** (International Diabetes Federation, 2021).

Table 15.1 Estimated prevalence of diabetes of any type for adults 20 to 79 years.

Year	Estimate number of cases worldwide
2019	463 million
2030	578 million
2045	700 million
Annual deaths due to diabetes	4 million (in 2017)

Source: (Adapted from Saeedi et al., 2019).

In 2019, diabetes was the ninth leading cause of death with an estimated of 1.5 million deaths directly attributed to diabetes (WHO, 2018). Overall, the risk for death among people with diabetes is about twice that of people without diabetes of similar age.

Number of adults (20–79 years) with diabetes worldwide

North America & Caribbean
- 2045: 63 million
- 2030: 56 million
- 2019: 48 million
- 33% increase
- 1 in 6 adults in this Region is at risk of type 2 diabetes
- 43% of global diabetes-related health expenditure occurs in this Region

South & Central America
- 2045: 49 million
- 2030: 40 million
- 2019: 32 million
- 55% increase
- 2 in 5 people with diabetes were undiagnosed
- Only 9% of global diabetes-related health expenditure for diabetes is spent in this Region

Africa
- 2045: 47 million
- 2030: 29 million
- 2019: 32 million
- 143% increase
- 3 in 5 people with diabetes were undiagnosed
- 3 in 4 deaths due to diabetes were in people under the age of 60

Middle East & North Africa
- 2045: 108 million
- 2030: 76 million
- 2019: 55 million
- 96% increase
- 1 in 8 people have diabetes
- 1 in 2 deaths due to diabetes were in people under the age of 60

South-East Asia
- 2045: 153 million
- 2030: 115 million
- 2019: 88 million
- 74% increase
- 1 in 5 adults with diabetes lives in this Region
- 1 in 4 live births are affected by hyperglycaemia in pregnancy

WORLD
- 2045: 700 million
- 2030: 578 million
- 2019: 463 million
- 51% increase

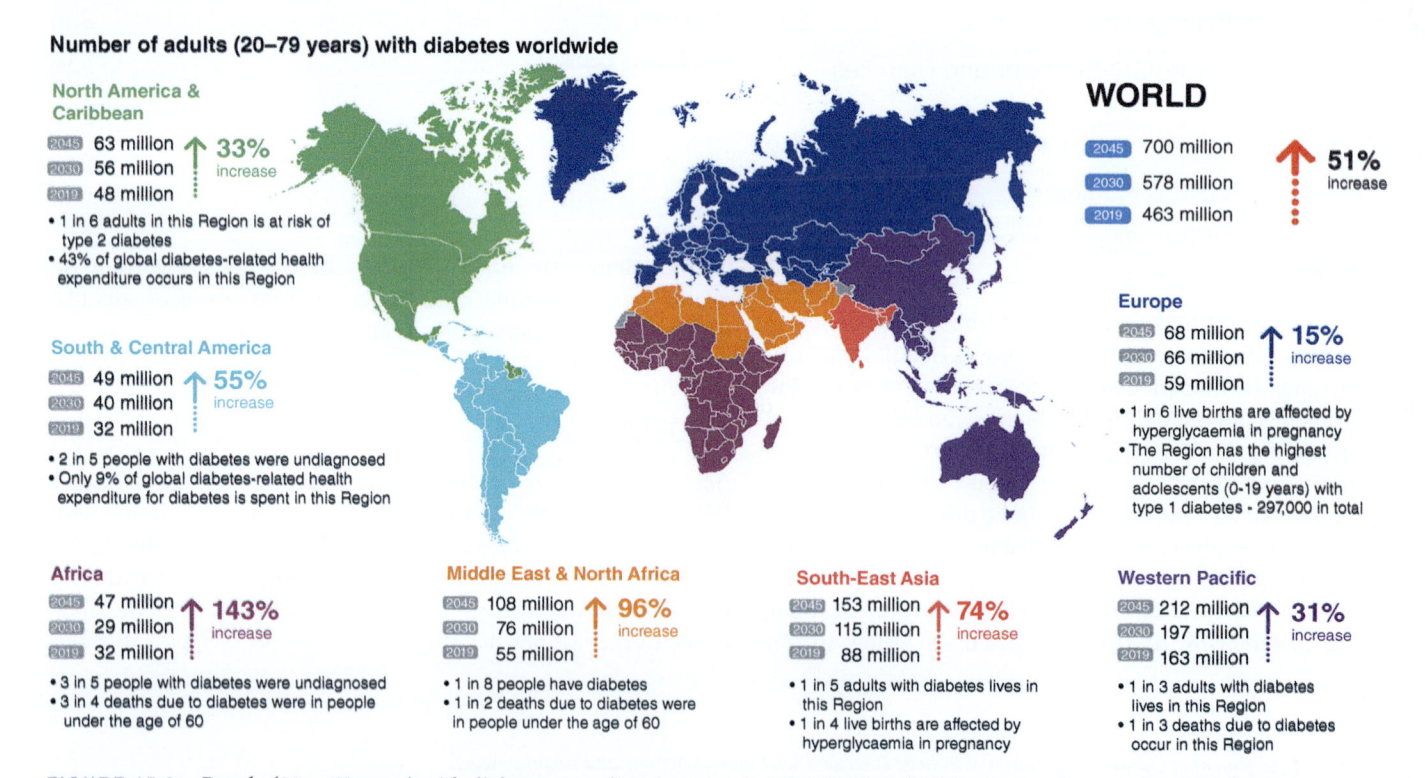

Europe
- 2045: 68 million
- 2030: 66 million
- 2019: 59 million
- 15% increase
- 1 in 6 live births are affected by hyperglycaemia in pregnancy
- The Region has the highest number of children and adolescents (0-19 years) with type 1 diabetes - 297,000 in total

Western Pacific
- 2045: 212 million
- 2030: 197 million
- 2019: 163 million
- 31% increase
- 1 in 3 adults with diabetes lives in this Region
- 1 in 3 deaths due to diabetes occur in this Region

FIGURE 15.2 People (20 to 79 years) with diabetes according to region in 2019, 2030, and 2045. Source: (International Diabetes Federation, 2021).

In 2017, the IDF estimates that the total medical cost attributable to diabetes was USD $850 billion, for patients older than 18 years, of which USD $727 billion were spent for patients aged 20 to 79 years old. Specifically in the US, healthcare expenditure for diabetes was $348 billion dollars (*IDF Diabetes Atlas - 8th Edition*, 2017). In 2045, global healthcare expenditure on diabetes is expected to reach USD $958 billion for adult patients (*IDF Diabetes Atlas - 8th Edition*, 2017).

TYPES OF DIABETES

According to published clinical practice guidelines from several organizations [e.g., American Diabetes Association (ADA), WHO, Canadian Diabetes Association], most cases can be classified into two categories, type 1 and type 2 DM, although gestational DM (i.e., diabetes with onset or first recognition during pregnancy in the second or third trimester), and other uncommon types also exist ("2. Classification and Diagnosis of Diabetes: Standards of Medical Care in Diabetes-2019," 2019; Adler et al., 2021; American Diabetes Association, 2020; World Health Organization, 2019):

1. Type 1 diabetes mellitus (T1D)
2. Type 2 diabetes mellitus (T2D)
3. Gestational diabetes mellitus (GDM)
4. Specific types of diabetes due to other causes

More specifically, T1D, formerly referred to as insulin-dependent diabetes mellitus (IDDM), accounts for 5% to 10% of all diagnosed cases of diabetes. It typically occurs in children and adolescents. However, new onset T1D can occur in all age groups with a global prevalence of 5.9 per 10,000 (Holt et al., 2021). It is an autoimmune disease and most often the result of irreparable damage to the insulin-producing cells (β-cells) of the pancreas from antibody attacks (Atkinson & Maclaren, 1994). It is characterized by an absolute deficiency of insulin, the hormone that regulates blood glucose. The rate of the pancreatic β-cell destruction varies between individuals; it occurs rapidly, mainly in infants and children, or slower, mainly in adult patients ("2. Classification and Diagnosis of Diabetes: Standards of Medical Care in Diabetes-2019," 2019). The symptoms of T1D usually include abnormal thirst and dry mouth, frequent urination, constant hunger, lack of energy and fatigue, sudden weight loss, and blurred vision (*IDF Diabetes Atlas - 8th Edition*, 2017). The clinical features distinguishing T1D, T2D, and monogenic diabetes are shown in **Table 15.2**.

T2D, formerly referred to as non-insulin-dependent diabetes mellitus (NIDDM), accounts for about 90% to 95% of diagnosed diabetes cases, usually after the age of 40 and in families. In prediabetes, characterized by insulin resistance, the insulin signaling leading to efficient transport glucose across the cell membrane is diminished. Consequently, the amount of insulin required to transport a certain amount of glucose into the cells is higher and insulin levels in these individuals are elevated (**Figure 15.3**) (Bar-Tana, 2020). As the degree of resistance increases, the need for insulin also rises. Gradually, the pancreas loses its ability to produce it. By the time T2D has appeared, insulin secretion has become defective and is not adequate to compensate for the insulin resistance (Polonsky, Sturis, & Bell, 1996). Most of the individuals with T2D are suffering from obesity, which, at least in part, is responsible for some degree of insulin resistance (Bogardus, Lillioja, Mott, Hollenbeck, & Reaven, 1985; Kolterman et al., 1981). The symptoms of T2D may be excessive thirst and dry mouth, frequent and abundant urination, lack of energy and extreme tiredness, tingling or

Table 15.2 Clinical features distinguishing type 1 diabetes, type 2 diabetes, and monogenic diabetes.

Clinical features	Type 1 diabetes	Type 2 diabetes	Monogenic diabetes
Age of onset (years)	Most <25 but can occur at any age (but not before the age of 6 months)	Usually >25 but incidence increasing in adolescents, paralleling increasing rate of obesity in children and adolescents	Usually <25; neonatal diabetes <6 months*
Weight	Usually thin, but, with obesity epidemic, can have overweight or obesity	>90% at least overweight	Similar to the general population
Islet autoantibodies	Usually present	Absent	Absent
C-peptide	Undetectable/low	Normal/high	Normal
Insulin production	Absent	Present	Usually present
First-line treatment	Insulin	Noninsulin antihyperglycemic agents, gradual dependence on insulin may occur	Depends on subtype
Family history of diabetes	Infrequent (5–10%)	Frequent (75–90%)	Multigenerational, autosomal pattern of inheritance
DKA	Common	Rare	Rare (except for neonatal diabetes[1])

[1] Neonatal diabetes is a form of diabetes with onset at <6 months of age, requires genetic testing, and may be amenable to therapy with oral sulfonylurea in place of insulin therapy. DKA = diabetic ketoacidosis
Source: (Punthakee, Goldenberg, & Katz, 2018).

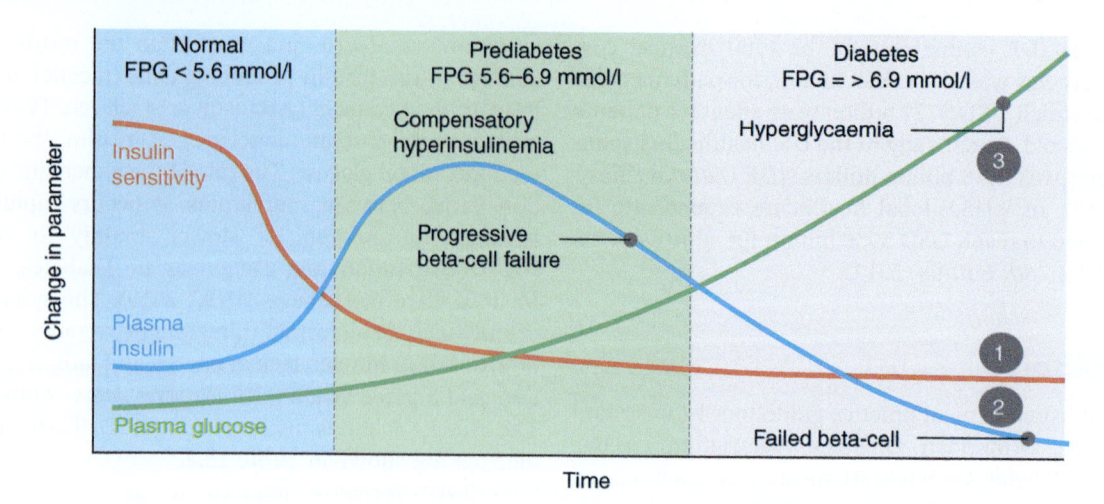

FIGURE 15.3 Insulin requirements for normal, prediabetes, and diabetes. FPG = fasting plasma glucose. Source: (Bar-Tana, 2020 / with permission of Springer Nature).

numbness in hands and feet, frequent fungal skin infections, slow healing wounds, and blurred vision (*IDF Diabetes Atlas - 8th Edition*, 2017).

GDM is a type of diabetes first diagnosed in the second or third semester of pregnancy without any prior diagnosis of T1D or T2D. Pregnant women who have not had diabetes before pregnancy should be tested for GDM at 24 to 28 weeks of pregnancy. Those diagnosed with GDM should be screened for diabetes or prediabetes at least every 3 years during their lifetime ("2. Classification and Diagnosis of Diabetes: Standards of Medical Care in Diabetes-2019," 2019).

Diabetes may be related to other causes, such as specific diseases or health conditions. Disease of the exocrine pancreas, such as pancreatitis and cystic fibrosis are examples of such diseases ("2. Classification and Diagnosis of Diabetes: Standards of Medical Care in Diabetes-2019," 2019). Cystic fibrosis-related diabetes is very common in patients with the disease, especially in adults (Moran et al., 2018), and it is mainly linked to loss of pancreatic cells resulting in both insulin and glucagon deficiency ("2. Classification and Diagnosis of Diabetes: Standards of Medical Care in Diabetes-2019," 2019). Diabetes following an organ transplant is another cause of the disease. The use of glucocorticoids after a transplant, for example, or for the treatment of HIV/AIDS may contribute to drug- or chemical-induced diabetes. Finally, monogenic diabetes syndromes, such as neonatal diabetes and maturity-onset diabetes of the young (MODY) count for a small percentage of the diabetes cases.

As many people do not fit into one category, the 2019 WHO guidance for diabetes suggested a classification system aiming in clinical care and in helping health professionals to choose appropriate treatments (**Figure 15.4**).

DIAGNOSIS OF DIABETES MELLITUS

Diagnosis of diabetes is based on blood-glucose levels. Fasting plasma glucose (FPG) or plasma glucose (PG) after a 2-hour, 75-g oral glucose tolerance test (OGTT) or HbA1c, criteria are used for setting the diagnosis with equal effectiveness, at least for T2D ("2. Classification and Diagnosis of Diabetes: Standards of Medical Care in Diabetes, 2019).

To assess FPG, there should be at least an 8-hour fast. Measurements of FPG ≥126 mg/dL (7.0 mmol/L) can set the diagnosis of diabetes. OGTT should be performed in accordance with the instruction for OGTT by the WHO. Glucose should be 75 g of anhydrous glucose and dissolved in water. If 2-h PG is ≥ 200 mg/dL (11.1 mmol/L) during OGTT, the individual is diagnosed with diabetes. When measuring HbA1c, an National Glycohemoglobin Standardization Program (NGSP)-certified and standardized, or traceable to the diabetes control and complications trial (DCCT) assay is needed to avoid variations between different laboratories. An HbA1c ≥ 6.5% (48 mmol/mol) is the cutoff point for diabetes. Finally, when the patients has symptoms of classic hyperglycemia or a hyperglycemic crisis, the diagnosis may be set when a random PG measurement is ≥ 200 mg/dL (11.1 mmol/L) (**Table 15.3**) ("2. Classification and Diagnosis of Diabetes: Standards of Medical Care in Diabetes, 2019).

PREDIABETES

Prediabetes is a condition characterized by blood-glucose levels that are higher than normal, but not high enough to be classified as diabetes. Individuals with prediabetes have impaired fasting glucose (IFG) and/or impaired glucose tolerance (IGT) and/or an HbA1c of 5.7% to 6.4% (39–47 mmol/mol). This condition may lead to T2D and may contribute to an increased risk of cardiovascular disease ("2. Classification and Diagnosis of Diabetes: Standards of Medical Care in Diabetes, 2019).

IFG is a condition in which the fasting blood-glucose level is 100 to 125 milligrams per deciliter (mg/dL), after an overnight fast ("Diagnosis and Classification of Diabetes Mellitus," 2014; "Follow-up Report on the Diagnosis of Diabetes Mellitus," 2003). The level is higher than the normal blood-glucose levels of 70 to 99 mg/dL, but not high enough to be classified as diabetes.

IGT is a condition in which the blood-glucose level is 140 to 199 mg/dL (7.8 to 11.0 mmol/L) after a 2-hour OGTT.

Type of diabetes	Brief description	Change from previous classification
Type 1 diabetes	β-cell destruction (mostly immune-mediated) and absolute insulin deficiency; onset most common in childhood and early adulthood	Type 1 sub-classes removed
Type 2 diabetes	Most common type, various degrees of β-cell dysfunction and insulin resistance; commonly associate with overweight and obesity	Type 2 sub-classes removed
Hybrid forms of diabetes		New type of diabetes
Slowly evolving, immune-mediated diabetes of adults	Similar to slowly evolving type 1 in adults but more often has features of the metabolic syndrome, a single GAD autoantibody and retains greater β-cell function	Nomenclature changed–previously referred to as latent autoimmune diabetes of adults (LADA)
Ketosis-prone type 2 diabetes	Presents with ketosis and insulin deficiency but later does not require insulin; common episodes of ketosis, not immune-mediated	No change
Other specific types		
Monogenic diabetes - Monogenic defects of β-cell function	Caused by specific gene mutations, has several clinical manifestations requiring different treatment, some occurring in the neonatal period, others by early adulthood	Updated nomenclature for specific genetic defects
- Monogenic defects in insulin action	Caused by specific gene mutations; has features of severe insulin resistance without obesity; diabetes develops when β-cells do not compensate for insulin resistance	
Diseases of the exocrine pancreas	Various conditions that affect the pancreas can result in hyperglycaemia (trauma, tumor, inflammation, etc.)	No change
Endocrine disorders	Occurs in diseases with excess secretion of hormones that are insulin antagonists	No change
Drug- or chemical-induced	Some medicines and chemicals impair insulin secretion or action, some can destroy β-cells	No change
Infection-related diabetes	Some viruses have been associated with direct β-cell destruction	No change
Uncommon specific forms of immune-mediated diabetes	Associated with rare immune-mediated diseases	No change
Other genetic syndromes sometimes associated with diabetes	Many genetic disorders and chromosomal abnormalities increase the risk of diabetes	No change
Unclassified diabetes	Used to describe diabetes that does not clearly fit into other categories. This category should be used temporarily when there is not a clear diagnostic category especially close to the time of diagnosis	New types of diabetes
Hyperglycaemia first detected during pregnancy		
Diabetes mellitus in pregnancy	Type 1 or type 2 diabetes first diagnosed during pregnancy	No change
Gestational diabetes mellitus	Hyperglycaemia below diagnostic thresholds for diabetes in pregnancy	Defined by 2013 diagnostic criteria
Diagnostic criteria for diabetes: fasting plasma glucose ≥ 7.0 mmol/L or 2-hour post-load plasma glucose > 11.1 mmol/L or Hba1 c ≥ 48 mmol/mol		
Diagnostic criteria for gestational diabetes: fasting plasma glucose 5.1–6.9 mmol/L or 1-hour post-load plasma glucose ≥ 10.0 mmol/L or 2-hour post-load plasma glucose 8.5–11.0 mmol/L		

FIGURE 15.4 Types of diabetes according to the 2019 WHO report on the classification of diabetes mellitus. Source: (World Health Organization, 2019).

Table 15.3 Diabetes and prediabetes diagnostic criteria.

Biochemical marker	Normal levels	Prediabetes		Diabetes mellitus
Hemoglobin A1C [HbA1c (%)]	<5.7% (39 mmol/mol)	5.7–6.4% (39–47 mmol/mol)		≥6.5% (48 mmol/mol)
		Impaired fasting glucose (IFG)	Impaired glucose tolerance (IGT)	
Fasting plasma glucose (FPG)	<100 mg/dL (5.6 mmol/L)	100 to 125 mg/dL (5.6–6.9 mmol/L)		≥126 mg/dL (7.0 mmol/L)
Oral glucose tolerance test (OGTT)	<140 mg/dL (7.8 mmol/L)		140 to 199 mg/dL (7.8-11.0 mmol/L) after a glucose load of 75 g anhydrous glucose dissolved in water	≥200 mg/dL (11.1 mmol/L)
Random plasma glucose				≥200 mg/dL (11.1 mmol/L)

Source: (American Diabetes Association, 2020).

This level is higher than normal but not high enough to be classified as diabetes ("Report of the Expert Committee on the Diagnosis and Classification of Diabetes Mellitus," 1997). The risk for progression to diabetes among those with prediabetes is high, but not inevitable.

Diabetes and prediabetes diagnostic criteria are summarized in **Table 15.3** (American Diabetes Association, 2020).

COMPLICATIONS

The National Institute of Diabetes and Digestive and Kidney Diseases, the International Diabetes Federation, and the ADA list several co-morbidities attributed to diabetes that include, but are not limited to, heart disease and stroke, high blood pressure, diabetic retinopathy, kidney disease, nervous system disease, amputations, dental disease, and complications of pregnancy. These complications can be categorized as chronic macrovascular complications, such as cardiovascular disease and diabetic foot, or chronic microvascular complications, such as kidney disease, neuropathy, and retinopathy (International Diabetes Federation, 2021; *IDF Diabetes Atlas - 8th Edition*, 2017) (**Figure 15.5**).

HEART DISEASE AND STROKE

- According to the National Institute of Diabetes and Digestive and Kidney Diseases, people with diabetes tend to develop heart disease at a younger age compared to people without diabetes (Barrett-Connor, Wingard, Wong, & Goldberg, 2018), while they have twice the risk of heart disease or stroke as adults without diabetes.

- Based on statistics published by the WHO, adults with diabetes have heart disease and stroke death rates about 2 to 3 times higher than adults without diabetes (WHO, 2018).

- In patients with diabetes, cardiovascular disease is a major cause of death and disability (*IDF Diabetes Atlas - 8th Edition*, 2017).

HIGH BLOOD PRESSURE

- Hypertension is a major risk factor for atherosclerotic cardiovascular disease and microvascular complications (American Diabetes Association, 2020).

- In patients with diabetes, sex (male), family history, age, and body-mass index (BMI) continue to be independent risk factors. The duration of diabetes increases the risk, whereas good renal function is protective (Tsimihodimos, González-Villalpando, Meigs, & Ferrannini, 2018).

- About two-thirds of adults with diabetes have a blood pressure greater than 130/80 mm Hg or use prescription medications for hypertension.

DIABETIC RETINOPATHY

- Diabetes is the main cause of new cases of blindness among adults aged 20 to 74 years (Centers for Disease Control and Prevention, 2011).

- The incidence of diabetic retinopathy ranges from 2.2% to 12.7% among patients with diabetes, while the annual progression estimates a range from 3.4% to 12.3% with the highest ranges found in US after 2000 (Sabanayagam et al., 2019).

- Optimization of glycemic control, blood pressure, and lipid profile may help reduce the risk or slow the progress of the diabetic retinopathy (American Diabetes Association, 2020).

DIABETIC KIDNEY DISEASE

- According to the National Kidney Foundation, 30% of patients with T1D and 10% to 40% of those with T2D will suffer from kidney failure.

- In high-income countries, 50% of cases of end-stage kidney disease are attributed to diabetic kidney disease (Tuttle et al., 2014).

CHRONIC COMPLICATIONS OF DIABETES

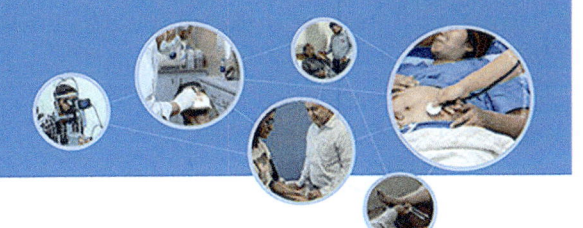

Diabetic eye disease
In most countries, *diabetic retinopathy* continues to be the leading cause of blindness in the working age population.

Diabetes and oral health
Diabetes and poor oral health negatively affect each other in a two-way relationship.

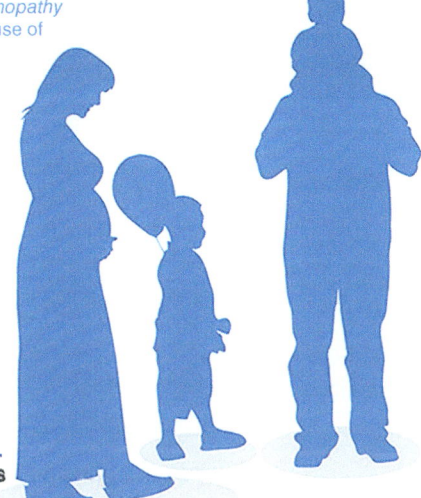

Diabetes-related complications of pregnancy
An estimated 15.8% (20.4 million) of live births were affected by *hyperglycaemia* in pregnancy in 2019.

Diabetes and cardiovascular diseases
Cardiovascular diseases account for, from one-third, to half of all, diabetes-related deaths.

Diabetic kidney disease
Diabetes, *hypertension* (high blood pressure), or a combination of both, cause 80% of *end-stage kidney disease* globally.

Nerve and/or vascular damage and diabetic foot complications
Diabetic foot and lower limb complications affect between 40 and 60 million people with diabetes globally.

FIGURE 15.5 Chronic complications of diabetes. Source: (International Diabetes Federation, 2019).

- The prevalence of end-stage kidney disease is 10 times higher in individuals with diabetes (*IDF Diabetes Atlas - 8th Edition*, 2017).
- According to a meta-analysis of cohort studies (8 cohorts of general population [1,285,045 participants] and five cohorts of chronic kidney disease [CKD; 79,519 participants] with a mean follow up of 4 years), patients with diabetes were at a higher risk of developing acute kidney injury compared to individuals without diabetes (James et al., 2015).

DIABETIC NEUROPATHY

- About 60% to 70% of people with diabetes in the US have mild to severe forms of nervous system damage. The results include damage to sensory, motor, and autonomic nerves causing symptoms such as numb, tingling, or burning feet, one-sided sharp pain (National Institute of Neurological Disorders and Stroke, 2022) as well as other problems such as depression, anxiety, and memory impairments. Gut microbiota seems to influence the release of some of the major brain neurotransmitters that act in the gut-brain axis (Thakur, Tyagi, & Shekhar, 2019).
- Gastrointestinal neuropathies include esophageal dysmotility, gastroparesis, constipation, diarrhea, and fecal incontinence (American Diabetes Association, 2020).

- Severe forms of diabetic nerve disease lead to the development of ulcers (*IDF Diabetes Atlas - 8th Edition*, 2017) and therefore, are a major contributing cause of lower-extremity amputations.

AMPUTATIONS

- The global prevalence of the diabetic foot is 6.4%, and it is higher for men. In high-income countries, the annual incidence of the disease is 2% (*IDF Diabetes Atlas - 8th Edition*, 2017).
- Among patients with diabetes, after a 43% decline between 2000 and 2009, amputation (both major and minor) rates increased by 50% from 2009 to 2015 (Creager et al., 2021).

DENTAL DISEASE

- Periodontal (gum) disease is more common in people with diabetes. Among young adults, those with diabetes compared to those without diabetes have about twice the risk (Centers for Disease Control and Prevention, 2011).
- Almost one-third of people with diabetes have severe periodontal diseases with loss of attachment of the gums to the teeth measuring 5 mm or more (Centers for Disease Control and Prevention, 2011).

- Periodontal disease is a major cause of tooth loss and is associated with an increased risk of cardiovascular disease (*IDF Diabetes Atlas - 8th Edition*, 2017).

COMPLICATIONS OF PREGNANCY

- High blood glucose during pregnancy may have consequences for both the mother and the offspring. It is possible to increase the risk for fetal loss, congenital malformations, stillbirth, perinatal death, preeclampsia, eclampsia, obstetric complications, and maternal morbidity and pregnancy related mortality. Concerning the baby, high blood glucose can cause macrosomia, or low birth weight, and shoulder dystocia during delivery (*IDF Diabetes Atlas - 8th Edition*, 2017).

- Poorly controlled diabetes before conception and during the first trimester of pregnancy can cause major birth defects in 5% to 10% of pregnancies and spontaneous abortions in 15% to 20% of pregnancies (Centers for Disease Control and Prevention, 2011).

- Poorly controlled diabetes during the second and third trimesters of pregnancy can result in excessively large babies, posing a risk to both mother and child (Centers for Disease Control and Prevention, 2011).

- Children of women with diabetes during pregnancy are at high risk of suffering from transgenerational effects such obesity, diabetes, hypertension, and kidney disease (*IDF Diabetes Atlas - 8th Edition*, 2017).

OTHER COMPLICATIONS

- Biochemical imbalances caused by uncontrolled diabetes can lead to acute life-threatening events, such as diabetic ketoacidosis and coma (Centers for Disease Control and Prevention, 2011).

- People with diabetes are more vulnerable to many other illnesses and often with worse prognoses. For example, they are more likely to die with pneumonia or influenza than people who do not have diabetes (Centers for Disease Control and Prevention, 2011).

- Diabetes is associated with an increased risk of cancer, cognitive impairment, dementia, and autoimmune diseases (for T1D only), such as autoimmune thyroid disease and celiac disease (American Diabetes Association, 2020).

- People with diabetes aged 60 years or older are 2–3 times more likely to report an inability to walk one-quarter of a mile, climb stairs, or do housework compared with people without diabetes in the same age group.

PHYSIOLOGY AND PATHOPHYSIOLOGY

The last century has been characterized by remarkable advances in our understanding of the mechanisms that lead to hyperglycemia in DM. A pathophysiological view that overcomes the historical and simplistic 'glucocentric' view could result in a better patient phenotyping and therapeutic approach (Zaccardi, Webb, Yates, & Davies, 2016).

In T2D, a combination of genetic, metabolic, and environmental factors that interact with one another including non-modifiable (ethnicity and family history/genetic predisposition) and modifiable risk factors (obesity, low physical activity, and an unhealthy diet) result in a complex network of pathological changes leading to insulin dysfunction (**Figure 15.6**).

Moreover, in T1D, several factors could trigger islet autoimmunity, while others might be protective. Islet autoimmunity is defined by the persistent presence of autoantibodies to pancreatic islet antigens. Prenatal factors such as infections, cesarean section, etc. and postnatal factors, namely dietary factors, gut dysbiosis, etc. could lead to the development of two or more islet autoantibodies, while promoters of progression from autoimmunity to overt T1D include overweight and obesity, high consumption of foods with high glycemic load and fructose content (**Figure 15.7**). These factors seem to have their effect mainly in genetically predisposed individuals (Rewers & Ludvigsson, 2016).

PHYSICAL INACTIVITY/SEDENTARY BEHAVIOR AND DIABETES MELLITUS

Numerous epidemiological studies and meta-analyses (Patterson et al., 2018; Wilmot et al., 2012) (Sgrò, Emerenziani, Antinozzi, Sacchetti, & Di Luigi, 2021) have documented strong and consistent associations between sedentary behavior (defined as waking behavior of ≤1.5 metabolic equivalent of task [MET]) as well as physical inactivity (i.e., not meeting specified physical-activity guidelines) with an increased risk of T2D onset and other chronic diseases (González, Fuentes, & Márquez, 2017). Indeed, in individuals with or at risk for developing T2D, high sedentary time is linked to poorer glycemic control and clustered metabolic risk.

In a meta-analysis (Grøntved & Hu, 2011) of prospective cohort studies to determine the association between TV viewing and risk of T2D among other chronic diseases, it was found that every 2 hours per day watching television was related to 176 cases of T2D per 100,000 individuals per year. Likewise, in another meta-analysis of 10 studies (6 prospective / 4 cross-sectional) including 505,045 participants (Wilmot et al., 2012), researchers showed that there was a 112% greater pooled relative risk of diabetes associated with higher versus lower amounts of TV time. Notably, both meta-analyses showed that the relationships between TV viewing time and T2D were independent of total physical-activity time, suggesting that the deleterious effects of higher levels of sedentary behavior are unrelated and are not mediated through the time people engage in moderate-to-vigorous physical-activity. Physical inactivity has been also related to higher risk of developing T2D, regardless of age, gender, ethnicity, or BMI (Admiraal et al., 2011).

Excess body fat may explain in part why TV time or other sedentary behaviors and physical inactivity are associated with increased diabetes risk (González et al., 2017; Sgrò et al., 2021). Other studies highlight that sitting time across the lifespan appears to be associated with diabetes independent of BMI (Hamilton, Hamilton, & Zderic, 2014), and therefore, other

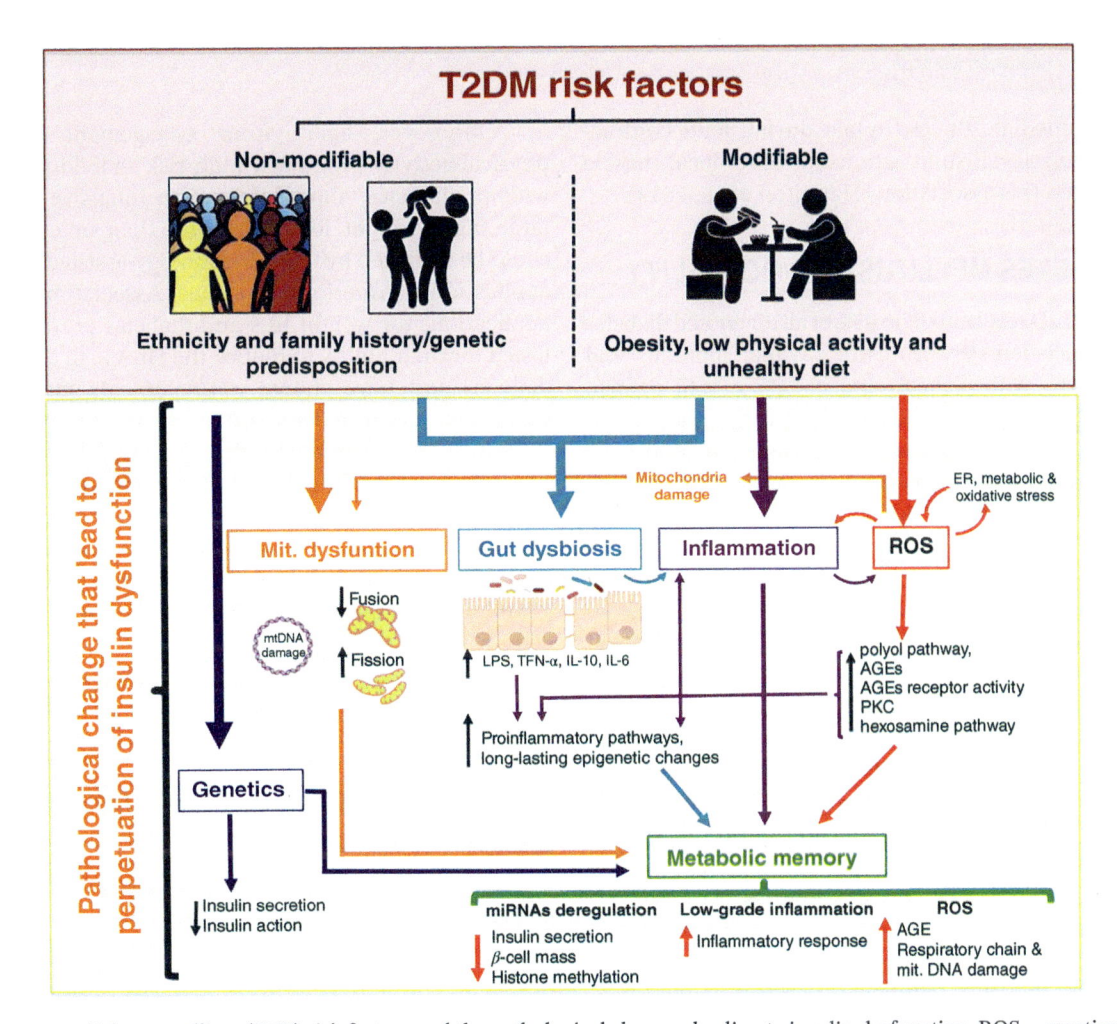

FIGURE 15.6 Type 2 diabetes mellitus (T2D) risk factors and the pathological changes leading to insulin dysfunction. ROS = reactive oxygen species; ER = endoplasmic reticulum; AGEs = advanced glycation end products; PKC = protein kinase C; LPS = lipopolysaccharide; miRNA = microRNA. Source: (Galicia-Garcia et al., 2020 / MDPI / CC BY 4.0).

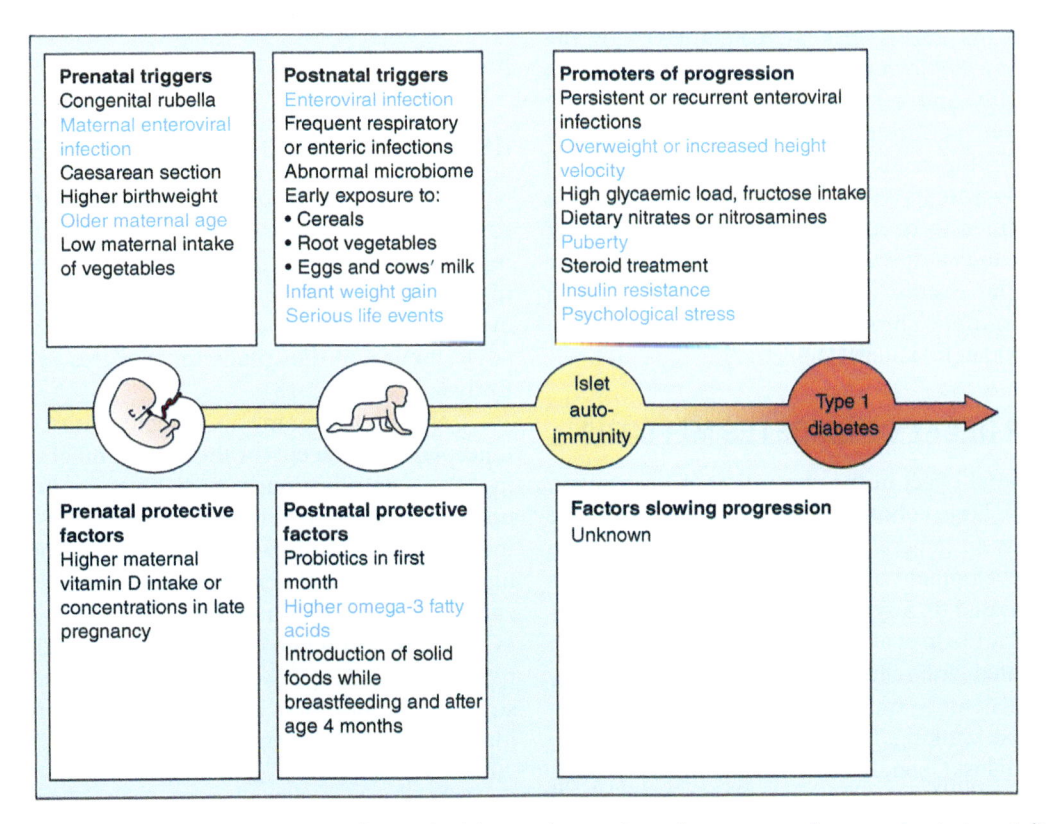

FIGURE 15.7 Environmental triggers and protective factors for islet autoimmunity and promoters of progression to type 1 diabetes. Source: (Rewers & Ludvigsson, 2016 / with permission of Elsevier).

reasons such as immediate glucose uptake during acute contractions of skeletal muscles, insulin actions, or other local muscle factors could explain this association (Hamilton et al., 2014).

OBESITY, DIABETES MELLITUS AND MORTALITY

Obesity-associated T2D reaches 90% to 95% of all diagnosed diabetes in adults. The association between cardiovascular mortality and morbidity in patients with diabetes and obesity is well defined (Scherer & Hill, 2016), as insulin resistance and diabetes are important predictors of death for cardiovascular diseases. The underline pathophysiology is very complex. Briefly, obesity and diabetes increase systemic inflammation leading to constant metabolic stress on the heart vessels and progressively to atherosclerotic disease. Therefore, early therapeutic interventions including diet and exercise are required to prevent or delay those conditions.

Physical activity is a well-known therapeutic approach that improves metabolic profile in obesity and diabetes. Several epidemiological and intervention data have consistently shown improvements in glycemic control, lipid profile, cardiovascular fitness, antioxidant status, quality of life and reduced inflammatory markers, adiposity and atherogenic progression, establishing physical activity as an evidence-based treatment modality to combat diabesity. Aerobic activity is associated with lower cardiovascular and all-cause mortality risks in both T1D and T2D. A prospective cohort study including 5859 women and men with diabetes (no information was available to distinguish T1D and T2D) from the EPIC (European Prospective Investigation Into Cancer and Nutrition) study concluded that patients who engaged in physical activity, compared to inactive patients, had a lower risk of total and CVD mortality. Leisure time activity contributed to a lower risk of all-cause mortality, while walking was associated with lower CVD risk. A meta-analysis by the same authors showed a 40% lower risk of all-cause mortality and 39% of CVD mortality and a similar decrease when leisure activity or walking were performed (Sluik et al., 2012).

Moreover, according to a recent prospective observational study, including 2,639 patients with T1D, with or without kidney disease, exercise seemed to be associated with a lower risk of premature all-cause and cardiovascular mortality, in an 11-year follow-up period. The results were showed benefit in both patients with T1D without chronic kidney disease and those with the disease (Tikkanen-Dolenc et al., 2017).

PREVENTION OR DELAY OF DIABETES MELLITUS

Exercise has a profound effect in the prevention of the disease. Strong evidence from large cohort studies support that exercise (and physical activity in general), is a highly effective way to delay or avert the development of diabetes (American Diabetes Association, 2015). Based on a systematic review of 10 prospective cohort studies from Jeon et al., physical activity of moderate intensity was associated with reduced risk of developing T2D by 31%, compared to sedentary individuals. A similar reduction was observed for brisk walking. Importantly, these changes are not affected by weight loss (Jeon, Lokken, Hu, & van Dam, 2007).

Moreover, apart from engagement with scheduled physical-activity programs, high-risk individuals, e.g., subjects with prediabetes, should follow an intensive dietary program targeting a weight loss of greater than or equal to 5%. This could be achieved by using technology-assisted tools and mobile applications (American Diabetes Association, 2015). Mobile applications for weight loss and diabetes prevention have been tested for their ability to reduce the HbA1c in the context of prediabetes and have shown improvements maintained even 2 years after the initial reductions in weight and HbA1c levels (Sepah, Jiang, & Peters, 2015).

In the USA and worldwide, successful T2D prevention strategies are being implemented through the National Diabetes Prevention Program (DPP). The goals of the US DPP trial's lifestyle change program are: i) a weight loss after 12 months of a minimum 5% of initial body weight, ii) physical activity of ≥150 min per week, and iii) attendance throughout the 12-month program with an emphasis on self-efficacy (Gruss et al., 2019).

NON-PHARMACOLOGICAL MANAGEMENT OF DIABETES MELLITUS

The non-pharmacological management of DM is mainly focused on lifestyle modifications including physical activity and diet alterations. The beneficial effects of lifestyle changes in those patients include improvements in anthropometric parameters such as body weight, BMI, and waist circumference as well as parameters associated with fat and glucose metabolism. Moreover, regular physical activity reduces the needs and dose of antidiabetic drugs and insulin dosage (Cannata et al., 2020).

In the following paragraphs, we will discuss the benefits of lifestyle modifications, namely diet and physical activity, on DM.

NUTRITION-BASED INTERVENTIONS

Nutrition is a highly important aspect of the medical care of patients with diabetes. Changes in patient's lifestyle, including nutrition, can promote better outcomes and quality of life. Patients should have access to a skilled registered dietitian-nutritionist who can provide them individualized advisement and diet plans for diabetes management (Briggs Early & Stanley, 2018)

Nutrition therapy in diabetes aims to help patients in multiple ways. Except for the major aim of delaying or preventing the complications of diabetes, nutrition therapy can improve overall health, help the patient to achieve and/or maintain a healthy weight, improve glucose management, blood pressure, and control blood lipids by promoting healthy eating patterns with a variety of nutrient-dense foods. Moreover, it focuses on behavioral aspects of eating, in order for the patient to avoid feeling guilty about food choices or focusing on single foods and their macro- or micronutrients. ("5. Lifestyle Management: Standards of Medical Care in Diabetes-2019," 2019).

According to the latest report of the ADA, an ideal percentage of calories from carbohydrates, protein, and lipids does not exist for every patient with diabetes. On the contrary, it is important to individualize the energy distribution based on each patient's habits and culture ("5. Lifestyle Management: Standards of Medical Care in Diabetes-2019," 2019).

Recommendations about carbohydrate intake do not differ substantially from those for the general population. In fact, people with diabetes are advised to consume mostly nutrient-dense carbohydrate sources that are high in fiber, including vegetables, fruits, legumes, whole grains, and dairy products. Consumption of sugar-sweetened beverages and fruit juices is discouraged. What is important when managing diabetes patients undergoing insulin replacement, (all T1D and some T2D patients), is to train them on the carbohydrate counting technique, when they have flexible insulin program or keep a similar daily carbohydrate consumption when the patient's insulin dose is fixed, to achieve better glycemic control ("5. Lifestyle Management: Standards of Medical Care in Diabetes, 2019).

Protein intake should be adjusted based on the individual's needs, and there is no need to reduce its consumption when diabetic kidney disease is not present. In that case, a patients' goal should be to maintain protein intake at the recommended daily allowance of 0.8 g/kg body weight/day ("5. Lifestyle Management: Standards of Medical Care in Diabetes, 2019).

The ideal amount of fat that patients with diabetes should consume is not set yet. What is known, is that the type of dietary fat plays an important role in diabetes management. A diet low in saturated and high in mono-unsaturated and poly-unsaturated fat, resembling the Mediterranean diet, instead of a diet low in total fat and high in carbohydrates, is recommended by the ADA for improving glucose metabolism and lowering cardiovascular disease risk. Similar to the general population, patients with diabetes are advised to avoid trans fatty acids ("5. Lifestyle Management: Standards of Medical Care in Diabetes, 2019).

There are several dietary patterns that individuals with diabetes could follow. As reported previously, the ADA promotes a dietary pattern that resembles the Mediterranean diet ("5. Lifestyle Management: Standards of Medical Care in Diabetes, 2019). According to a systematic review and meta-analysis by Ajala et al. that compared low-carbohydrate, vegetarian, vegan, low-glycemic index, high fiber, Mediterranean, and high-protein diets with control diets, it was shown that the low-carbohydrate, low-glycemic index, Mediterranean, and high-protein diets were more effective at improving glycemic control and increasing HDL-cholesterol, except for the high-protein diet, which did not increased HDL compared to the control diets. The Mediterranean diet had the most favorable outcomes, including weight loss (Ajala, English, & Pinkney, 2013). A more recent meta-analysis published in 2019, comparing different dietary interventions in patients with T2D showed interesting results. Reviewers examined 10 randomized controlled trials (RCTs) comparing the effects of the Mediterranean diet, low-fat diet (<30% of daily energy from fat and less than 10% from saturated fat), low-carbohydrate diet (<130 g carbohydrates/day), high-carbohydrate diet (55% of daily energy derived from carbohydrates), and a regular diet on glycemic control, cardiovascular risk, and weight loss. The Mediterranean diet showed a more beneficial effect on glycemic control, weight loss, and cardiovascular risk compared to the low-fat diet, and a significant reduction in HbA1c, compared to the regular diet, but no difference when compared to the low-carbohydrate diet (Pan et al., 2019).

GDM is a special type of diabetes, and proper lifestyle management is believed to be the most effective mean of treating it. The registered dietitian who manages women with GDM should focus on providing individualized nutrition plans, which must be sufficient in calories to provide enough energy for the mother and the fetus, improve glycemic control, and help the mother gain the appropriate gestational weight. According to the dietary reference intakes (DRIs) for all pregnant women, their diet should contain a minimum of 175 g of carbohydrates, a minimum of 71 g of protein, and 28 g of fiber. Moreover, their energy needs do not seem to differ from those of pregnant women without GDM. What is different because of the diabetes and is possible to change in the nutrition plan is the type of carbohydrate consumed, since they can impact glucose levels ("14. Management of Diabetes in Pregnancy: Standards of Medical Care in Diabetes, 2019).

NUTRITION INTERVENTIONS FOR OLDER ADULTS WITH DIABETES

The increase in diabetes prevalence in the elderly has contributed to a better understanding of geriatric diabetes care and the fundamentals of management. According to the clinical practice guidelines published in 2019 from the endocrine society, lifestyle modification is considered as the first-line treatment of hyperglycemia for patients aged 65 years and older with diabetes who are ambulatory (LeRoith, D., Biessels, G. J., Braithwaite et al., 2019). Indeed, a balanced diet and regular exercise are essential to patients' health. However, diabetes in older adults has been linked with increased rates of several nutrition related conditions, such as malnutrition and frailty.

The prevalence or risk of malnutrition in elderly patients with diabetes has been found to be greater than 50%. This has been associated with decreases in basic activities of daily life (ADL), grip strength, physical performance of the lower limbs (stand-up test from the chair), and quality of life (QOL), longer hospitalization, and increased rates of institution and mortality (Tamura, Y., Omura, T., Toyoshima, K., & Araki, A, 2020). Therefore, assessing nutritional status of older-adult patients is a hallmark for detecting and managing malnutrition. The assessment can be made using validated tools such as the Mini Nutritional Assessment and Short Nutritional Assessment Questionnaire (LeRoith, D., Biessels, G. J., Braithwaite et al., 2019). Diets rich in protein and energy to prevent malnutrition and weight loss are suggested for treating frailty and malnutrition in older adults with diabetes. Patients should also avoid the use of restrictive diets and instead limit the consumption of simple sugars (LeRoith, D., Biessels, G. J., Braithwaite et al, 2019).

PHYSIOLOGY OF EXERCISE IN TYPE 1 DIABETES

Exercise is well known to promote glucose uptake by the working cells. Patients with T1D require relatively less insulin to transport the same amount of glucose from the blood into the cells. Therefore, regular exercise is likely to reduce the insulin requirements of patients with T1D.

In addition to the reduction in insulin requirements, regular exercise also leads to improved physical fitness in individuals with T1D. Consequently, the patient's sense of well-being and ability to cope with physical and psychological stresses associated with the disease can be enhanced.

Due to the strong interaction between exercise, diet, and insulin it is important to keep a balance among these three factors. Each patient is different and might have a different diet, thus exercise should be tailored specifically for each patient. Furthermore, in certain conditions, exercise can be harmful and therefore, should not be recommended (**Figure 15.8**).

Because of the personalized exercise program required for such patients, only general guidelines for exercise can be addressed here. Such programs must take into consideration the following:

1. The amount of insulin the individual is using.
2. The individual's diet before and after exercise.
3. Their musculoskeletal and body weight limitations.
4. The time of day the individual exercises.
5. The type, intensity, and duration of exercise.
6. The weather conditions during exercise.
7. Their access to exercise facilities.
8. Their co-morbidities.

PHYSIOLOGY OF EXERCISE IN TYPE 2 DIABETES

Exercise recommendations for the patient with T2D are like those presented for patients with T1D, apart from the concerns of hypoglycemia in those who are taking insulin.

The effects of exercise on glucose metabolism diminish after 24 to 48 hours. Therefore, patients should perform some form of physical activity almost every day. However, sedentary individuals should not begin exercising 5 to 6 days a week, initially. Instead, the duration, frequency, and intensity of the program should progress slowly and carefully until the individual can be physically active on most days of the week.

BENEFITS OF PHYSICAL ACTIVITY

Among several benefits, aerobic training improves insulin sensitivity and insulin resistance while moderate- to high-intensity training are associated with lower overall mortality risks in both T1D and T2D.

Resistance training has many benefits in adults; e.g. improvements in muscle mass, body composition, strength, physical function, insulin sensitivity, blood pressure, lipid profile, and cardiovascular health (Colberg et al., 2016). In patients with T2D, resistance exercise improves glycemic control, insulin resistance, fat mass, blood pressure, strength, and lean body mass. Consequently, both aerobic and resistance exercise training are very useful, in terms of glucose management, cardiovascular risk factors, and safety; therefore, doing any type of exercise is better than doing no exercise for patients with T2D (Yang, Scott, Mao, Tang, & Farmer, 2014).

Regarding T1D, it is not known whether resistance exercise has an effect on glycemic control, although it seems that it can limit the risk of exercise-induced hypoglycemia (**Table 15.4**) (Cannata et al., 2020). Indeed, resistance training lessens the decrease in blood glucose during training and smaller changes

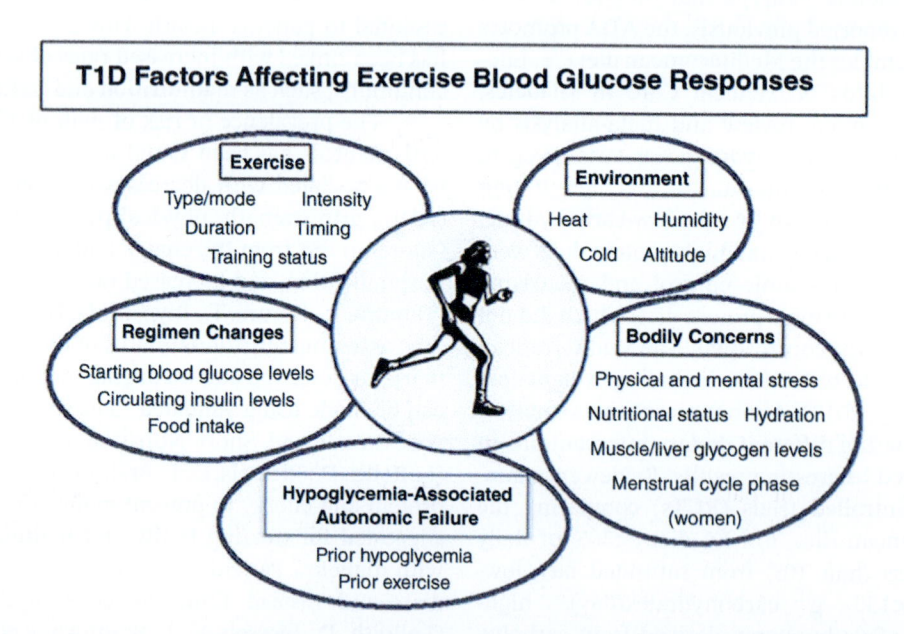

FIGURE 15.8 Type 1 diabetes factors affecting exercise blood-glucose responses. Source: (Colberg, Laan, Dassau, & Kerr, 2015).

Table 15.4 Differences in physical-activity types and their recommendation in type-1 and type-2 diabetes patients.

Patients	Aerobic	Resistance	High-intensity interval training (HIIT)
Type 1 diabetes		↑ muscular strength	
	↑ lipid metabolism		↑ cardio-protective
		↑ lipid profile	
	↓ insulin resistance		↑ metabolic benefits
		↑ better control of blood-glucose levels	
		↓ dose of insulin	
Recommendations	150 min/week at moderate-to-vigorous intensity	Engaging in 2–3 non-consecutive days/week	In younger when vigorously performed for 75 min/week
	↓ blood pressure	↑ blood pressure	↑ insulin sensitivity
	↓ triglycerides	↑ muscle mass and strength	↑ metabolic control
	↓ insulin resistance	↑ insulin responsiveness	
	↓ A1C	↑ metabolic control	
		↑ lipid profile	
		↑ cardiovascular disease	
Recommendations	150 min/week at moderate-to-vigorous intensity	Perform both flexibility and balance activities for 2 or more sessions/week.	In physically fit patients when vigorously performed for 75 min/week.

Legends ↑ increase–↓ reduction.

Source: (Cannata et al., 2020).

after the training session. This may diminish patients' fear of hypoglycemia during or after exercise in patients with T1D (Yardley et al., 2013).

For older adults, flexibility and balance exercises seem to improve motion around joints without affecting glycemic control. Balance exercises can reduce fall risk, even in patients with peripheral neuropathy. Other types of exercise, such as yoga or tai chi, are thought to improve glycemic control, although more high quality studies are needed (Colberg et al., 2016).

BENEFITS OF REDUCING SEDENTARY TIME

In sedentary individuals with overweight/obesity, glycemic control can be improved by interrupting prolonged sitting by short (≤5 min) bouts of standing or light-intensity exercises every 20 to 30 mins. Adults with T2D should interrupt prolonged sitting every 30 mins with 15 min post-meal walking and with 3 min of light walking and resistance activities (Colberg et al., 2016).

EXERCISE-BASED INTERVENTIONS

Exercise training is an important part of the treatment of diabetes, especially T2D. Aerobic exercise is the most suggested type of exercise for T2D patients, but resistance exercise has also proved to be beneficial (Buresh & Berg, 2018; Thent, Das, & Henry, 2013). An RCT with 43 T2D patients evaluated a combination of aerobic and resistance training program (3 weekly sessions, 60 minutes each), compared to a non-exercising control group, for a 12-week period. Intervention resulted in improved muscle strength and lowered fatigue, a decrease of 18% in HbA1c, and an improved overall health-related QOL (Tomas-Carus et al., 2016).

What is novel in exercise and diabetes treatment for people with T2D is that, in recent studies, interval exercise seems to be effective in promoting glycemic control, improving body composition, insulin sensitivity, aerobic capacity, and reducing oxidative stress more effectively than continuous exercise. This type of exercising should be suggested with caution, at least until more studies are available on its safety, especially for high-risk individuals such as older adults with diabetes or patients with cardiovascular disease (Buresh & Berg, 2018; Hamasaki, 2018).

Exercise is of great importance in T1D too. A recent systematic review and meta-analysis of studies that examined the effect of exercise on adults with diabetes and children with T1D showed beneficial effects on several outcomes. In adults, exercise training improved BMI, peak VO_2, and LDL-cholesterol. In children, engaging in exercise reduced insulin dose, waist circumference, LDL-cholesterol, and triglycerides. In both age groups, exercise resulted in no difference in the HbA1c%, fasting blood glucose, resting heart rate, resting systolic blood pressure, or HDL-cholesterol (Ostman, Jewiss, King, & Smart, 2018).

Physical activity was also studied in women with GDM. A meta-analysis including eight RCTs compared usual prenatal care with interventions of usual prenatal care plus weekly supervised exercise or physical-activity counseling in women with GDM.

The overall effect of exercise and physical activity on fasting blood glucose levels was not significant compared to usual prenatal care. Interestingly, when researchers compared the two types of interventions with usual prenatal care separately, physical-activity counseling showed a significant decrease of 3.88 mg/dL in fasting blood-glucose concentrations. This could be because physical-activity counseling interventions lasted longer than the weekly supervised exercise. Another explanation could be the starting point of each intervention; physical-activity counseling started early in the pregnancy while weekly supervised exercise started after the diagnosis for GDM was made, and thus, some metabolic problems may have already been present at the beginning of the intervention (Bgeginski, Ribeiro, Mottola, & Ramos, 2017).

While exercise is proved to be effective for diabetes, patients are not always engaged in sufficient exercise. One possible reason is that medical and nutritional therapy are usually a priority over exercise, when it comes to diabetes (O'Hagan, De Vito, & Boreham, 2013). Other explanations could be the fear of doing any harm during training or a lack of time (Buresh & Berg, 2018). Physicians and health practitioners need to promote healthy lifestyles that include exercise training based on the individual needs of each patient with diabetes.

NUTRITION AND EXERCISE: COMBINED INTERVENTIONS

Lifestyle interventions including diet and physical activity are commonly used for the prevention or treatment of diabetes and its complications, mostly T2D.

Johansen et al. (Johansen et al., 2017) conducted an RCT to assess the effectiveness of an intensive lifestyle intervention on glycemic control, compared to standard care, in patients with T2D. Standard care included medical counseling, education in T2D, and lifestyle advice by the study nurse at baseline and every 3 months for 12 months. The target for HbA1c level was set at 6.5%, and medication was adjusted accordingly. In addition to all these, participants in the lifestyle intervention group were assigned to perform 5 to 6 weekly aerobic sessions (duration 30–60 minutes), of which 2 to 3 sessions were combined with resistance training. They were also offered dietary counseling by clinical dietitians and given an individual dietary plan with a macronutrient distribution of 45% to 60% carbohydrate, 15% to 20% protein, and 20% to 35% fat, with less than 7% saturated fat. Furthermore, participants were encouraged to be physically active in their leisure time, which translated into more than 10,000 steps per day. Participants were followed for 12 months. The primary outcome was a change in HbA1c levels from baseline to the 12-month follow up, and the secondary outcome was a reduction in glucose-lowering medication in the same time period. Exploratory outcomes included changes in total cholesterol, LDL-cholesterol, HDL-cholesterol, TGs, blood pressure, fasting insulin, fasting glucose, 2-hour glucose concentration following an OGTT, $\dot{V}O_2$max, weight, BMI, fat mass (total and abdominal), lean body mass, and a possible reduction in blood pressure and lipid-lowering medication (Johansen et al., 2017).

The study failed to indicate that the lifestyle intervention was equivalent to the standard care, since the difference in change for HbA1c level at 12 months was not within the predefined equivalence margin. However, the analysis of the secondary outcome demonstrated that 73% of the participants who reduced the use of glucose-lowering medication belonged to the lifestyle intervention group. According to the authors, these results suggest that even if lifestyle intervention failed to be equal with standard care, it led to improved glycemic control (Johansen et al., 2017).

Lifestyle intervention for patients with T2D may also have beneficial effects on cardiovascular disease risk factors. The Look AHEAD trial was a study of 5145 overweight/obese T2D participants, aged 45 to 76 years who were randomly assigned to either an intensive lifestyle intervention group (diet and physical activity) aiming for weight loss or a control group, including standard diabetes support and education. Participants in the lifestyle intervention who lost more than 10% of their initial weight during the intervention had a 21% lower risk for a major cardiovascular event. This suggests that, in patients with T2D, the extent of weight loss is associated with the risk of cardiovascular disease (Zhang et al., 2016). Moreover, a meta-analysis evaluated 16 RCTs on patients with diabetes that compared a lifestyle intervention group with a standard care group (control group). Lifestyle interventions included increased physical activity, reduce caloric intake, dietary education and counseling, and education regarding treatment adherence or disease monitoring. Results showed a reduction in cardiovascular risk factors, such as BMI, HbA1c, and both systolic and diastolic blood pressure in intervention groups compared to control groups, but no difference in HDL-cholesterol or LDL-cholesterol (Chen et al., 2015).

EXERCISE GUIDELINES FOR DIABETES MELLITUS PATIENTS

According to the latest guidelines of the ADA adults with T1D, T2D, or prediabetes should perform aerobic exercise for 150 minutes or more on a weekly basis, at a moderate-to-vigorous intensity, for at least 3 times a week and once in 2 days. For the younger and more physically active individuals, 75 minutes per week of vigorous exercise or interval training might be enough. Adult patients should also engage in resistance training 2 to 3 times per week, but not for consecutive days.

For all adults, and especially those who have T2D, it is suggested they decrease their sedentary activities. Concerning children and adolescents with any type of diabetes or prediabetes, they should exercise at a moderate- or vigorous-intensity for at least 60 minutes per day and perform vigorous muscle-strengthening and bone-strengthening activities for at least 3 days per week ("5. Lifestyle Management: Standards of Medical Care in Diabetes, 2019).

Exercise in patients with diabetes must be carefully monitored. Exercise, diet, and insulin must interact precisely to bring the desired outcome. Because exercise has an insulin-like effect, hypoglycemia during and after exercise is the most common problem in patients who engage in physical activity. This problem is more common in patients with T1D who take insulin and less common in patients with T2D on oral hypoglycemic agents. Excessive insulin or the accelerated absorption of insulin from the ejection site may both cause hypoglycemia. It is also important to realize that hypoglycemia can occur during exercise and the 4 to 6 hours following exercise.

KEY POINTS

- DM can be defined as a group of metabolic disorders characterized by chronic hyperglycemia (i.e., high concentrations of blood glucose) resulting from defects in insulin production, insulin action, or both that is associated with disturbances in glucose, lipid, and protein metabolism.

- According to published clinical practice guidelines from several organizations (e.g., ADA WHO, Canadian Diabetes Association), most cases can be classified into two categories, type-1 and type-2 DM, although GDM (i.e., diabetes with onset or first recognition during pregnancy in the second or third trimester), and other uncommon types also exist.

- T1D, accounts for 5% to 10% of all diagnosed cases of diabetes. It typically occurs in children and adolescents. However, new onset T1D can occur in all age groups.

- Prediabetes is characterized by insulin resistance. As the degree of resistance increases, the need for insulin also rises. Gradually, the pancreas loses its ability to produce it.

- By the time T2D has appeared, insulin secretion has become defective and is not adequate to compensate for the insulin resistance.

- GDM is a type of diabetes first diagnosed in the second or third semester of pregnancy, without any prior diagnosis of T1D or T2D.

- The diagnosis of diabetes is based on blood-glucose levels. FPG or PG after a 2-hour, 75-g OGTT or HbA1c criteria are used to make the diagnosis with equal effectiveness, at least for T2D.

- Numerous co-morbidities attributed to diabetes include heart disease and stroke, high blood pressure, diabetic retinopathy, kidney disease, nervous system disease, amputations, dental disease, and pregnancy complications.

- Sedentary behavior (defined as waking behavior of ≤1.5 Metabolic Equivalent of Task [MET]) as well as physical inactivity (i.e., not meeting specified physical-activity guidelines) increases the risk for T2DM onset and other chronic diseases.

- The association between cardiovascular mortality and morbidity in patients with diabetes and obesity is well defined, as insulin resistance and diabetes are important predictors of death from cardiovascular diseases.

- Strong evidence from large cohort studies supports exercise and physical activity in general, providing a highly effective way to delay or avert the development of diabetes.

- The non-pharmacological therapy of DM is mainly focused on lifestyle modifications including physical activity and diet alterations.

- Aerobic training improves insulin sensitivity and insulin resistance, while moderate to high intensity has been associated with lower overall mortality risks in both T1D and T2D.

- In patients with T2D, resistance exercise improves glycemic control, insulin resistance, fat mass, blood pressure, strength, and lean body mass.

- In T1D, it is not known whether resistance exercise influences glycemic control, although it seems that it can limit the risk of exercise-induced hypoglycemia.

- Nutrition therapy can improve overall health, help the patient to achieve and/or maintain a healthy weight, improve glucose management, blood pressure, and blood lipid control by promoting healthy eating patterns with variety of nutrient-dense foods.

- Nutrition in diabetes should be individualized for each patient, and it should be aimed at preventing diabetes complications. The Mediterranean diet seems to have benefits according to many studies in the current literature.

- Adults with T1D, T2D or prediabetes should perform aerobic exercise for 150 minutes or more on a weekly basis, at a moderate-to-vigorous intensity, for at least 3 times a week and once in 2 days. For the younger and more physically active individuals, 75 minutes per week of vigorous exercise or interval training might be enough.

SELF-ASSESSMENT QUESTIONS

1. Define DM.
2. What are the two main types of DM?
3. What are the main procedures to diagnose DM?
4. List four co-morbidities associated with DM:
5. How do physical inactivity and sedentary behavior affect the onset of DM?
6. How does resistance exercise affect patients with T1D?
7. Is there an ideal percentage of calories that should be acquired from macronutrients for patients with diabetes?
8. According to the ADA, what are the recommendations for adults with diabetes?

REFERENCES

Classification and Diagnosis of Diabetes: Standards of Medical Care in Diabetes-2019. (2019). *Diabetes Care, 42*(Suppl 1), S13–S28. doi:10.2337/dc19-S002

American Diabetes Association. (2020). 4. Comprehensive medical evaluation and assessment of comorbidities: Standards of Medical Care in Diabetes—2020. *Diabetes care, 43*(Supplement_1), S37–S47.

Lifestyle Management: Standards of Medical Care in Diabetes-2019. (2019). *Diabetes Care, 42*(Suppl 1), S46–S60. doi: 10.2337/dc19-S005

American Diabetes Association. (2020). 10. Cardiovascular disease and risk management: Standards of Medical Care in Diabetes—2020. *Diabetes care, 43*(Supplement_1), S111–S134.

American Diabetes Association. (2020). 11. Microvascular complications and foot care: standards of medical care in diabetes– 2020. *Diabetes care, 43*(Supplement_1), S135–S151.

Management of Diabetes in Pregnancy: Standards of Medical Care in Diabetes-2019. (2019). *Diabetes Care, 42*(Suppl 1), S165–S172. doi:10.2337/dc19-S014

Adler, A., Bennett, P., Colagiuri Chair, S., Gregg, E., Venkat Narayan, K. M., Inês Schmidt, M., . . . Hocking, S. (2021). REPRINT OF: CLASSIFICATION OF DIABETES MELLITUS. *Diabetes Research and Clinical Practice, 108972*. doi: 10.1016/j.diabres.2021.108972

Admiraal, W. M., van Valkengoed, I. G., JS, L. d. M., Stronks, K., Hoekstra, J. B., & Holleman, F. (2011). The association of physical inactivity with Type 2 diabetes among different ethnic groups. *Diabet Med, 28*(6), 668–672. doi:10.1111/j.1464-5491.2011.03248.x

Ajala, O., English, P., & Pinkney, J. (2013). Systematic review and meta-analysis of different dietary approaches to the management of type 2 diabetes. *Am J Clin Nutr, 97*(3), 505–516. doi:10.3945/ajcn.112.042457

American Diabetes Association, (2015). 4. Prevention or Delay of Type 2 Diabetes. *Diabetes Care, 39*(Supplement_1), S36–S38. doi: 10.2337/dc16-S007

American Diabetes Association, (2020). 2. Classification and Diagnosis of Diabetes: Standards of Medical Care in Diabetes—2021. *Diabetes Care, 44*(Supplement_1), S15–S33. doi:10.2337/dc21-S002

Atkinson, M. A., & Maclaren, N. K. (1994). The pathogenesis of insulin-dependent diabetes mellitus. *N Engl J Med, 331*(21), 1428–1436. doi:10.1056/nejm199411243312107

Bar-Tana, J. (2020). Type 2 diabetes – unmet need, unresolved pathogenesis, mTORC1-centric paradigm. *Reviews in Endocrine and Metabolic Disorders, 21*(4), 613–629. doi:10.1007/s11154-020-09545-w

Barrett-Connor, E., Wingard, D., Wong, N., & Goldberg, R. (2018). Chapter 18: Heart disease and diabetes. *Diabetes in America,* 18–11.

Bgeginski, R., Ribeiro, P. A. B., Mottola, M. F., & Ramos, J. G. L. (2017). Effects of weekly supervised exercise or physical activity counseling on fasting blood glucose in women diagnosed with gestational diabetes mellitus: A systematic review and meta-analysis of randomized trials. *J Diabetes, 9*(11), 1023–1032. doi:10.1111/1753-0407.12519

Bogardus, C., Lillioja, S., Mott, D. M., Hollenbeck, C., & Reaven, G. (1985). Relationship between degree of obesity and in vivo insulin action in man. *Am J Physiol, 248*(3 Pt 1), E286–291. doi:10.1152/ajpendo.1985.248.3.E286

Briggs Early, K., & Stanley, K. (2018). Position of the Academy of Nutrition and Dietetics: The Role of Medical Nutrition Therapy and Registered Dietitian Nutritionists in the Prevention and Treatment of Prediabetes and Type 2 Diabetes. *J Acad Nutr Diet, 118*(2), 343–353. doi: 10.1016/j.jand.2017.11.021

Buresh, R., & Berg, K. (2018). Exercise for the management of type 2 diabetes mellitus: factors to consider with current guidelines. *J Sports Med Phys Fitness, 58*(4), 510–524. doi:10.23736/s0022-4707.17.06969-9

Cannata, F., Vadalà, G., Russo, F., Papalia, R., Napoli, N., & Pozzilli, P. (2020). Beneficial Effects of Physical Activity in Diabetic Patients. *Journal of functional morphology and kinesiology, 5*(3), 70. doi:10.3390/jfmk5030070

Chen, L., Pei, J. H., Kuang, J., Chen, H. M., Chen, Z., Li, Z. W., & Yang, H. Z. (2015). Effect of lifestyle intervention in patients with type 2 diabetes: a meta-analysis. *Metabolism, 64*(2), 338–347. doi: 10.1016/j.metabol.2014.10.018

Centers for Disease Control and Prevention. (2011). National diabetes fact sheet: national estimates and general information on diabetes and prediabetes in the United States, 2011. *Atlanta, GA: US department of health and human services, centers for disease control and prevention, 201*(1), 2568–2569.

Colberg, S. R., Laan, R., Dassau, E., & Kerr, D. (2015). Physical activity and type 1 diabetes: time for a rewire? *Journal of diabetes science and technology, 9*(3), 609–618. doi:10.1177/1932296814566231

Colberg, S. R., Sigal, R. J., Yardley, J. E., Riddell, M. C., Dunstan, D. W., Dempsey, P. C., . . . Tate, D. F. (2016). Physical Activity/Exercise and Diabetes: A Position Statement of the American Diabetes Association. *Diabetes Care, 39*(11), 2065–2079. doi:10.2337/dc16-1728

Creager, M. A., Matsushita, K., Arya, S., Beckman, J. A., Duval, S., Goodney, P. P., . . . Pollak, A. W. (2021). Reducing nontraumatic lower-extremity amputations by 20% by 2030: time to get to our feet: a policy statement from the American Heart Association. *Circulation, 143*(17), e875–e891.

Diagnosis and Classification of Diabetes Mellitus. (2014). *Diabetes Care, 37*(Supplement 1), S81–S90. doi:10.2337/dc14-S081

National Institute of Neurological Disorders and Stroke. (2022). Peripheral Neuropathy Fact Sheet. Retrieved from https://www.ninds.nih.gov/Disorders/Patient-Caregiver-Education/Fact-Sheets/Peripheral-Neuropathy-Fact-Sheet

International Diabetes Federation, (2020, 22/05/2020). Diabetes complications. Retrieved from https://www.idf.org/aboutdiabetes/complications.html

International Diabetes Federation, (2021). IDF Diabetes Atlas. Retrieved from Belgium: https://www.diabetesatlas.org

Follow-up Report on the Diagnosis of Diabetes Mellitus. (2003). *Diabetes Care, 26*(11), 3160–3167. doi:10.2337/diacare.26.11.3160

Galicia-Garcia, U., Benito-Vicente, A., Jebari, S., Larrea-Sebal, A., Siddiqi, H., Uribe, K. B., . . . Martín, C. (2020). Pathophysiology of Type 2 Diabetes Mellitus. *International Journal of Molecular Sciences, 21*(17), 6275. Retrieved from https://www.mdpi.com/1422-0067/21/17/6275

González, K., Fuentes, J., & Márquez, J. L. (2017). Physical Inactivity, Sedentary Behavior and Chronic Diseases. *Korean J Fam Med, 38*(3), 111–115. doi:10.4082/kjfm.2017.38.3.111

Grøntved, A., & Hu, F. B. (2011). Television viewing and risk of type 2 diabetes, cardiovascular disease, and all-cause mortality: a meta-analysis. *JAMA, 305*(23), 2448–2455. doi:10.1001/jama.2011.812

Gruss, S. M., Nhim, K., Gregg, E., Bell, M., Luman, E., & Albright, A. (2019). Public Health Approaches to Type 2 Diabetes Prevention: the US National Diabetes Prevention Program and Beyond. *Current Diabetes Reports, 19*(9), 78. doi:10.1007/s11892-019-1200-z

Hamasaki, H. (2018). Interval Exercise Therapy for Type 2 Diabetes. *Curr Diabetes Rev, 14*(2), 129–137. doi:10.2174/1573399812666161101103655

Hamilton, M. T., Hamilton, D. G., & Zderic, T. W. (2014). Sedentary behavior as a mediator of type 2 diabetes. *Medicine and sport science, 60*, 11–26. doi:10.1159/000357332

Holt, R. I. G., DeVries, J. H., Hess-Fischl, A., Hirsch, I. B., Kirkman, M. S., Klupa, T., . . . Peters, A. L. (2021). The management of type 1 diabetes in adults. A consensus report by the American Diabetes Association (ADA) and the European Association for the Study of Diabetes (EASD). *Diabetologia, 64*(12), 2609–2652. doi:10.1007/s00125-021-05568-3

IDF Diabetes Atlas - 8th Edition. (2017). Retrieved from

James, M. T., Grams, M. E., Woodward, M., Elley, C. R., Green, J. A., Wheeler, D. C., . . . Sarnak, M. J. (2015). A Meta-analysis of the Association of Estimated GFR, Albuminuria, Diabetes Mellitus, and Hypertension With Acute Kidney Injury. *Am J Kidney Dis, 66*(4), 602–612. doi: 10.1053/j.ajkd.2015.02.338

Jeon, C. Y., Lokken, R. P., Hu, F. B., & van Dam, R. M. (2007). Physical Activity of Moderate Intensity and Risk of Type 2 Diabetes. *A systematic review, 30*(3), 744–752. doi:10.2337/dc06-1842

Johansen, M. Y., MacDonald, C. S., Hansen, K. B., Karstoft, K., Christensen, R., Pedersen, M., . . . Ried-Larsen, M. (2017). Effect of an Intensive Lifestyle Intervention on Glycemic Control in Patients With Type 2 Diabetes: A Randomized Clinical Trial. *JAMA, 318*(7), 637–646. doi:10.1001/jama.2017.10169

Kolterman, O. G., Gray, R. S., Griffin, J., Burstein, P., Insel, J., Scarlett, J. A., & Olefsky, J. M. (1981). Receptor and postreceptor defects contribute to the insulin resistance in noninsulin-dependent diabetes mellitus. *J Clin Invest, 68*(4), 957–969. doi:10.1172/jci110350

LeRoith, D., Biessels, G. J., Braithwaite, S. S., Casanueva, F. F., Draznin, B., Halter, J. B., . . . & Sinclair, A. J. (2019). Treatment of diabetes in older adults: an Endocrine Society clinical practice guideline. *The Journal of Clinical Endocrinology & Metabolism, 104*(5), 1520–1574.

Moran, A., Pillay, K., Becker, D., Granados, A., Hameed, S., & Acerini, C. L. (2018). ISPAD Clinical Practice Consensus Guidelines 2018: Management of cystic fibrosis-related diabetes in children and adolescents. *Pediatric Diabetes, 19*(S27), 64–74. doi:10.1111/pedi.12732

O'Hagan, C., De Vito, G., & Boreham, C. A. (2013). Exercise prescription in the treatment of type 2 diabetes mellitus: current practices, existing guidelines and future directions. *Sports Med, 43*(1), 39–49. doi:10.1007/s40279-012-0004-y

World Health Organization, (2019). Classification of diabetes mellitus.

Ostman, C., Jewiss, D., King, N., & Smart, N. A. (2018). Clinical outcomes to exercise training in type 1 diabetes: A systematic review and meta-analysis. *Diabetes Res Clin Pract, 139*, 380–391. doi: 10.1016/j.diabres.2017.11.036

Pan, B., Wu, Y., Yang, Q., Ge, L., Gao, C., Xun, Y., . . . Ding, G. (2019). The impact of major dietary patterns on glycemic control, cardiovascular risk factors, and weight loss in patients with type 2 diabetes: A network meta-analysis. *Journal of Evidence-Based Medicine, 12*(1), 29–39. doi:10.1111/jebm.12312

Patterson, R., McNamara, E., Tainio, M., de Sá, T. H., Smith, A. D., Sharp, S. J., . . . Wijndaele, K. (2018). Sedentary behaviour and risk of all-cause, cardiovascular and cancer mortality, and incident type 2 diabetes: a systematic review and dose response meta-analysis. *European Journal of Epidemiology, 33*(9), 811–829. doi:10.1007/s10654-018-0380-1

Polonsky, K. S., Sturis, J., & Bell, G. I. (1996). Seminars in Medicine of the Beth Israel Hospital, Boston. Non-insulin-dependent diabetes mellitus - a genetically programmed failure of the beta cell to compensate for insulin resistance. *N Engl J Med, 334*(12), 777–783. doi:10.1056/nejm199603213341207

Punthakee, Z., Goldenberg, R., & Katz, P. (2018). Definition, classification and diagnosis of diabetes, prediabetes and metabolic syndrome. *Canadian journal of diabetes, 42*, S10–S15.

Report of the Expert Committee on the Diagnosis and Classification of Diabetes Mellitus. (1997). *Diabetes Care, 20*(7), 1183–1197. doi:10.2337/diacare.20.7.1183

Report of the Expert Committee on the Diagnosis and Classification of Diabetes Mellitus. (1998). *Diabetes Care, 21*(Supplement 1), S5–S19. doi:10.2337/diacare.21.1.S5

Rewers, M., & Ludvigsson, J. (2016). Environmental risk factors for type 1 diabetes. *Lancet (London, England), 387*(10035), 2340–2348. doi:10.1016/S0140-6736(16)30507-4

Sabanayagam, C., Banu, R., Chee, M. L., Lee, R., Wang, Y. X., Tan, G., . . . Wong, T. Y. (2019). Incidence and progression of diabetic retinopathy: a systematic review. *The Lancet Diabetes & Endocrinology, 7*(2), 140–149. doi:10.1016/S2213-8587(18)30128-1

Saeedi, P., Petersohn, I., Salpea, P., Malanda, B., Karuranga, S., Unwin, N., . . . Ogurtsova, K. (2019). Global and regional diabetes prevalence estimates for 2019 and projections for 2030 and 2045: Results from the International Diabetes Federation Diabetes Atlas. *Diabetes Research and Clinical Practice, 157*, 107843.

Scherer, P. E., & Hill, J. A. (2016). Obesity, Diabetes, and Cardiovascular Diseases: A Compendium. *Circulation research, 118*(11), 1703–1705. doi:10.1161/CIRCRESAHA.116.308999

Sepah, S. C., Jiang, L., & Peters, A. L. (2015). Long-Term Outcomes of a Web-Based Diabetes Prevention Program: 2-Year Results of a Single-Arm Longitudinal Study. *J Med Internet Res, 17*(4), e92. doi:10.2196/jmir.4052

Sgrò, P., Emerenziani, G. P., Antinozzi, C., Sacchetti, M., & Di Luigi, L. (2021). Exercise as a drug for glucose management and prevention in type 2 diabetes mellitus. *Current Opinion in Pharmacology, 59*, 95–102. doi: 10.1016/j.coph.2021.05.006

Sluik, D., Buijsse, B., Muckelbauer, R., Kaaks, R., Teucher, B., Johnsen, N. F., . . . Nothlings, U. (2012). Physical Activity and Mortality in Individuals With Diabetes Mellitus: A Prospective Study and Meta-analysis. *Arch Intern Med, 172*(17), 1285–1295. doi:10.1001/archinternmed.2012.3130

Sun, H., Saeedi, P., Karuranga, S., Pinkepank, M., Ogurtsova, K., Duncan, B. B., . . . Mbanya, J. C. (2022). IDF Diabetes Atlas: Global, regional and country-level diabetes prevalence estimates for 2021 and projections for 2045. *Diabetes Research and Clinical Practice, 183*, 109119.

Tamura, Y., Omura, T., Toyoshima, K., & Araki, A. (2020). Nutrition management in older adults with diabetes: a review on the importance of shifting prevention strategies from metabolic syndrome to frailty. *Nutrients, 12*(11), 3367.

Thakur, A. K., Tyagi, S., & Shekhar, N. (2019). Comorbid brain disorders associated with diabetes: therapeutic potentials of prebiotics, probiotics and herbal drugs. *Translational Medicine Communications, 4*(1), 12. doi:10.1186/s41231-019-0043-6

Thent, Z. C., Das, S., & Henry, L. J. (2013). Role of exercise in the management of diabetes mellitus: the global scenario. *PLoS One, 8*(11), e80436. doi: 10.1371/journal.pone.0080436

Tikkanen-Dolenc, H., Wadén, J., Forsblom, C., Harjutsalo, V., Thorn, L. M., Saraheimo, M., . . . Groop, P.-H. (2017). Physical Activity Reduces Risk of Premature Mortality in Patients With Type 1 Diabetes With and Without Kidney Disease. *Diabetes Care, 40*(12), 1727–1732. doi:10.2337/dc17-0615

Tomas-Carus, P., Ortega-Alonso, A., Pietilainen, K. H., Santos, V., Goncalves, H., Ramos, J., & Raimundo, A. (2016). A randomized controlled trial on the effects of combined aerobic-resistance exercise on muscle strength and fatigue, glycemic control and health-related quality of life of type 2 diabetes patients. *J Sports Med Phys Fitness, 56*(5), 572–578.

Tsimihodimos, V., González-Villalpando, C., Meigs, J. B., & Ferrannini, E. (2018). Hypertension and diabetes mellitus: coprediction and time trajectories. *Hypertension, 71*(3), 422–428.

Tuttle, K. R., Bakris, G. L., Bilous, R. W., Chiang, J. L., de Boer, I. H., Goldstein-Fuchs, J., . . . Molitch, M. E. (2014). Diabetic Kidney Disease: A Report From an ADA Consensus Conference. *Diabetes Care, 37*(10), 2864–2883. doi:10.2337/dc14-1296

WHO. (2018). Global Health Estimates 2016: Deaths by Cause, Age, Sex, by Country and by Region, 2000-2016. Retrieved from Geneva:

Wilmot, E. G., Edwardson, C. L., Achana, F. A., Davies, M. J., Gorely, T., Gray, L. J., . . . Biddle, S. J. H. (2012). Sedentary time in adults and the association with diabetes, cardiovascular disease and death: systematic review and meta-analysis. *Diabetologia, 55*(11), 2895–2905. doi:10.1007/s00125-012-2677-z

Yang, Z., Scott, C. A., Mao, C., Tang, J., & Farmer, A. J. (2014). Resistance exercise versus aerobic exercise for type 2 diabetes: a systematic review and meta-analysis. *Sports Med, 44*(4), 487–499. doi:10.1007/s40279-013-0128-8

Yardley, J. E., Kenny, G. P., Perkins, B. A., Riddell, M. C., Balaa, N., Malcolm, J., . . . Sigal, R. J. (2013). Resistance Versus Aerobic Exercise. *Acute effects on glycemia in type 1 diabetes, 36*(3), 537–542. doi:10.2337/dc12-0963

Zaccardi, F., Webb, D. R., Yates, T., & Davies, M. J. (2016). Pathophysiology of type 1 and type 2 diabetes mellitus: a 90-year perspective. *Postgraduate medical journal, 92*(1084), 63–69.

Zhang, P., Hire, D., Espeland, M. A., Knowler, W. C., Thomas, S., Tsai, A. G., . . . Look, A. R. G. (2016). Impact of intensive lifestyle intervention on preference-based quality of life in type 2 diabetes: Results from the Look AHEAD trial. *Obesity (Silver Spring, Md.), 24*(4), 856–864. doi: 10.1002/oby.21445

FURTHER READING

Bibliography

American Diabetes Association. (2022). *Standards of Medical Care in Diabetes—2022 Abridged for Primary Care Providers. Clinical Diabetes 40*(1): 10–38. doi: 10.2337/cd22-as01.

Holt, R.I.G., DeVries, J.H., Hess-Fischl, A., et al. (2021). The management of type 1 diabetes in adults. A consensus report by the American Diabetes Association (ADA) and the European Association for the Study of Diabetes (EASD). *Diabetologia. 64*(12): 2609–2652. doi: 10.1007/s00125-021-05568-3.

Scherer, P.E., and Hill, J.A. (2016). Obesity, diabetes, and cardiovascular diseases: A compendium. *Circulation Research, 118*(11): 1703–1705. doi: 10.1161/CIRCRESAHA.116.308999

Sgrò, P., Emerenziani, G.P., Antinozzi, C., et al. (2021). Exercise as a drug for glucose management and prevention in type 2 diabetes mellitus. *Current Opinion in Pharmacology. 59*: 95–102. doi: 10.1016/j.coph.2021.05.006.

Sigal, R.J., Armstrong, M.J., Bacon, S.L., et al. (2018). Physical Activity and Diabetes. Diabetes Canada Clinical Practice Guidelines Expert Committee. *Canadian Journal of Diabetes. 42*(Suppl 1): S54–S63. doi: 10.1016/j.jcjd.2017.10.008.

World Health Organization. (2019). Classification of diabetes mellitus.

Links

- https://www.diabetes.org/
- https://www.easd.org/
- https://idf.org/
- https://diabetesjournals.org/care
- https://diabetesjournals.org/clinical
- https://www.diabetes.ca/
- https://www.joslin.org/
- http://diabetesatwork.org/

Hypertension

CHAPTER 16

Introduction	241
Definition	242
Prevalence	242
Risk Factors	242
Unhealthy/Poor Diets	243
Sodium Intake	243
Alcohol Intake	243
Physical Inactivity	244
Body-Mass Index/Obesity	244
Co-morbidities and Complications	244
Lifestyle Modifications for the Prevention and Management of Hypertension	244
Treatment Goals for Patients with Hypertension	244
Dietary Strategies to Prevent and Manage Hypertension	244
Weight Loss	244
Sodium Restriction	245
Potassium Intake	246
Magnesium Intake	246
Calcium Intake	246
Omega-3 Fatty Acids	246
Caffeine	247
Alcohol	247
Dietary Patterns	247
DASH Diet	247
Mediterranean Diet	248
Vegetarian Diets	249
Nordic Diet	249
Physical Activity, Fitness, and Hypertension	250
Physical Activity Guidelines for Hypertension	250
Nutrition and Exercise: Combined Interventions	251
Other strategies	252
Key Points	252
Self-assessment Questions	252
Case Scenario	253
References	253
Further Reading	258
Bibliography	258
Links	258

INTRODUCTION

Hypertension was not recognized as a menace of health until the latter part of the twentieth century. In fact, even up until the 1960s, some experts in the field believed that arterial disease was the cause of hypertension and not the result (Freis ED, 1995). The use of drugs to lower blood pressure (BP) was scoffed at as "treatment of the manometer rather than of the patient". The prevailing belief among physicians was that the rise in BP was an essential compensatory mechanism (and, thus, essential blood pressure) to maintain adequate perfusion as the individuals were advanced in age. Attempts to lower BP were therefore discouraged (Freis ED, 1995).

Pioneering research by Dr. Edward Freis from the 1940s to the 1970s, however, challenged the prevailing opinion among the medical community that reduction in elevated BP per se was not beneficial. Freis and the Veterans Administration study group in the mid-1960s to early 1970s proved conclusively that treatment of hypertension reduces strokes and cardiovascular complications (Freis, 1958, 1959, 1969, 1974; Poblete et al., 1973). Since then, several large-scale trials have

Prevention and Management of Cardiovascular and Metabolic Disease: Diet, Physical Activity and Healthy Aging,
First Edition. Christina N. Katsagoni, Peter Kokkinos, and Labros S. Sidossis.
© 2023 John Wiley & Sons Ltd. Published 2023 by John Wiley & Sons Ltd.

been implemented that have significantly enhanced our knowledge of the diagnosis and treatment of hypertension.

Chronic hypertension is now recognized as a major and the most common risk factor for developing cardiovascular disease (Chobanian, A.V., 2003; MacMahon, S., 1990; Stamler, J., R. Stamler, 1993; "The sixth report of the Joint National Committee on prevention, detection, evaluation, and treatment of high blood pressure.," 1997). This relationship is direct, strong, continuous, graded, consistent, predictive, and independent (Roccella, 1993). The risk of cardiovascular morbidity and mortality increases progressively and linearly as BP rises with no evidence of a plateau (Collins, R., 1990; MacMahon, S., 1990; "The sixth report of the Joint National Committee on prevention, detection, evaluation, and treatment of high blood pressure.," 1997). The mortality risk doubles for every 20 mm Hg increase in systolic blood pressure (SBP) above the threshold of 115 mm Hg and for every 10 mm Hg increase in diastolic blood pressure (DBP) above the threshold of 75 mm Hg (Vasan, R.S., 2001).

DEFINITION

The maximum pressure generated in the aorta by the left ventricle when the heart contracts (approximately 120 mm Hg) is known as the SBP. The minimum pressure that the blood exerts in the aorta during diastole of heart (the relaxing phase of the heart) is known as the DBP (approximately 80 mm Hg) (Travis D. Homan, Stephen Bordes, 2021).

Hypertension is characterized by persistent elevated BP in system arteries (Oparil et al., 2018). According to the 2018 European Society of Cardiology and the European Society of Hypertension (ESC/ESH) guidelines, hypertension is defined as office SBP values equal to or greater than 140 mm Hg and/or DBP equal to or greater than 90 mm Hg following repeated examination. **Table 16.1** provides a classification of BP based on office BP measurement. The same classification is used in all adults (>18 years) (Unger et al., 2020; Williams et al., 2018). Conversely, the 2017 American College of Cardiology and American Heart Association (ACC/AHA) Guidelines for the prevention and management of hypertension revised the definition of hypertension as SBP >130 mm Hg or DBP >80 mm Hg (Whelton et al., 2018).

PREVALENCE

Hypertension is a worldwide public-health issue. The global prevalence of hypertension was estimated at 1.13 billion in 2015, with a global age-standardized prevalence of 24.1% and 20.1% in men and women, respectively (Zhou et al., 2017), and irrespective of income status, i.e., in lower-, middle-, and higher-income countries (Chow et al., 2013). This has changed according to the new definition criteria of hypertension. Indeed, the prevalence of hypertension increased from 18.9% with >140/90 mm Hg to 43.5% with >130/80 mm Hg (Al Ghorani, Kulenthiran, Lauder, Böhm, & Mahfoud, 2021).

Hypertension progressively increases with age, with a prevalence of >60% among people over 60 years of age (Chow et al., 2013), while about 65% of men and 75% of women develop elevated BP by the age of 70 years old (Franklin et al., 2001). Moreover, several lifestyle risk factors such as an unhealthy diet, high dietary sodium intake, low dietary potassium intake, and a lack of physical activity have been linked with increased prevalence of hypertension (Mills, Stefanescu, & He, 2020). It is estimated that the adult population with hypertension will increase to 29% by 2025 (Kearney et al., 2005; Oliveros et al., 2020).

RISK FACTORS

Primary hypertension (i.e., not resulting from a medical condition) can be identified in 90% to 95% of patients (Oparil et al., 2018). The remaining 5% to 10% of cases are secondary hypertension due to a specific cause, usually endocrine. Most people suffering from secondary hypertension have primary renal parenchyma, aldosteronism, or renal vascular disease, whereas the others have unusual endocrine disorders or drug- or alcohol-induced hypertension (Carey, Muntner, Bosworth, & Whelton, 2018).

The major pathophysiological determinants of BP in primary hypertension are shown in **Figure 16.1**. The cause of primary hypertension remains unknown and involves a combination of genetic and environmental factors, including the aging process on renal function and peripheral resistance, vascular inflammation, gene expression, and environmental influences, such as obesity and poor diet, physical inactivity,

Table 16.1 Classification of office blood pressure and definitions of hypertension grade

SBP (mm Hg)		DBP (mm Hg)	ISH, 2020 (Unger et al., 2020)	ESH/ESC, 2018 (Williams et al., 2018)	AHA/ACC, 2017 (Whelton et al., 2018)
<120	and	<80	Normal	Optimal	Normal
120–129	and/or	80–84		Normal	Elevated
130–139	and/or	85–89	High normal	High normal	Grade 1 hypertension
140–159	and/or	90–99	Grade 1 hypertension	Grade 1 hypertension	Grade 2 hypertension
160–179	and/or	100–109	Grade 2 hypertension	Grade 2 hypertension	
≥180	and/or	≥110		Grade 3 hypertension	
≥140	and	<90		Isolated systolic hypertension	

Sources: (AHA/ACC, 2017; ESH/ESC, 2018; and ISH, 2020).

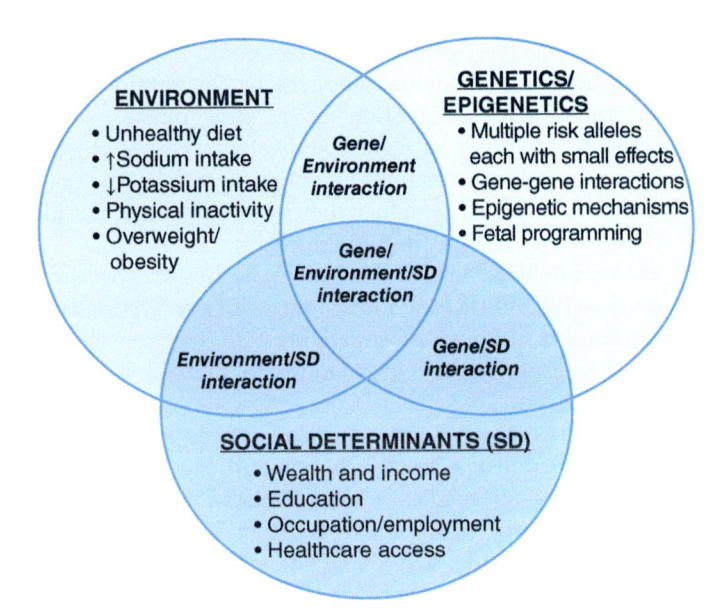

FIGURE 16.1 The major determinants of BP in primary hypertension and their interaction in adults. ↑ = increased, ↓ = decreased, BP = blood pressure, SD = social determinants. Source: (Carey et al., 2018 / with permission of Elsevier).

smoking and stress (J. E. Hall et al., 2012). Unhealthy diet and insufficient physical activity appear to be the main reversible environmental causes. The heritability of hypertension is 30% to 50% (Carey et al., 2018).

UNHEALTHY/POOR DIETS

There is accumulating evidence that links the high red meat consumption with a higher risk of poorly controlled BP and hypertension (Allen, Bhatia, Wood, Momin, & Allison, 2022). A systematic review and meta-analysis of 28 prospective studies indicated a positive association between red meat, processed meat consumption as well as sugar-sweetened beverages with the risk of hypertension. Indeed, an intake of 170 g/d of red meat, 35 g/d of processed meat, and 500 mL/d of sugar-sweetened beverages was associated with a 78% increased risk of hypertension, compared to non-consumption (Schwingshackl et al., 2017). Nevertheless, research on this subject was criticized for important methodological limitations (i.e., reverse causality, residual confounding, recall and reporting biases) (Allen et al., 2022).

The Western diet characterized by a high intake of saturated fats, refined carbohydrates, and sodium and a low intake of potassium is likely to lead to the development of hypertension through different mechanisms (Canale et al., 2021; Jama, Beale, Shihata, & Marques, 2019). The mechanisms that have been proposed include the vasoconstriction, impaired vasodilation, extracellular volume expansion, inflammation, increased sympathetic nervous system activity as well as gut dysbiosis. However, in a meta-analysis of 27 studies (16 cohort studies and 11 cross-sectional studies), the Western-style pattern (high intake of red and/or processed meat, refined grains, sweets, high-fat dairy products, butter, potatoes, and high-fat gravy, and low intake of fruits and vegetables) was not associated with an increased risk of hypertension (Wang, Shen, & Liu, 2016). Researchers showed that body-mass index (BMI) mediated the association between Western-style pattern and the risk of hypertension, while supporting that other unknown or unmeasured potential confounders, which were not considered in their analyses could also affect this association (Wang et al., 2016).

SODIUM INTAKE

Globally, sodium intake ranges between 3.5 and 5.5 g/d (9–12 g/d of salt), with marked differences among countries (Grillo, Salvi, Coruzzi, Salvi, & Parati, 2019). About 11% of sodium intake results from salt added during cooking or at the table, while more than 75% is derived from salt added during the processing of foods (i.e., bread, salted meats, cereals, canned goods) and food preparation (i.e., fast-food and restaurants) (Carey et al., 2018; Samadian, Dalili, & Jamalian, 2016). Although sodium is an essential nutrient for all humans, excessive sodium intake is an important determinant of hypertension (M. O'Donnell, Mente, & Yusuf, 2015; Whelton et al., 2012). Specifically, available evidence suggests a causal relationship between sodium intake and BP. Excessive sodium intake (>5 g/d sodium, i.e., 1 teaspoon/d of salt) is associated with an increased prevalence of hypertension and its cardiovascular complications (Grillo et al., 2019).

Excess sodium intake affects molecular pathways, thus leading to an increase in BP. Evidence shows that the BP response is based on the sensitivity in salt intake of individuals in the general population. This phenomenon is defined as salt-sensitivity, and it is based on an increase or neutral effect in BP with a high salt diet. Research has shown that approximately 50% of patients with hypertension and 25% of people with normotension are salt-sensitive. Many factors determine whether an individual is salt-sensitive or salt-resistant, such as co-morbidities like kidney dysfunction and diabetes mellitus as well as older age, genetics, quality of diet, ethnicity, or body mass. Evidence supports that salt-sensitivity is associated with an increased cardiovascular risk in both normotensive and hypertensive individuals (Bouchard et al., 2022; Grillo et al., 2019).

ALCOHOL INTAKE

There is a well-documented positive linear association between alcohol abuse, BP, the prevalence of hypertension, and cardiovascular disease (Roerecke et al., 2017). Excess alcohol intake (>3 drinks/d for men and >2 drinks/d for women) is responsible for 5% to 30% of hypertension. Alcohol consumption is directly correlated with elevated BP (Mahmood et al., 2019). It seems that there are sex-specific associations between alcohol consumption and the risk of hypertension. Indeed, several studies have documented that any alcohol consumption is associated with an increase hypertension risk in men, whereas 1-2 drinks/day in women may not be that harmful, as there is an increased risk for higher consumption levels (Briasoulis, Agarwal, & Messerli, 2012; Fernández-Solà, 2015; Roerecke et al., 2018).

PHYSICAL INACTIVITY

Physical inactivity is reportedly responsible for 5% to 13% of hypertension (Samadian et al., 2016). The absence of leisure and occupational moderate-to-vigorous physical activity has been associated with a higher risk of hypertension (Medina et al., 2018). Self-reported time spent in sedentary behavior is also associated with BP (P. H. Lee & Wong, 2015). A meta-analysis of 24 (1 cohort and 13 cross-sectional) studies demonstrated a linear association between total sedentary behavior and hypertension. The risk increased by 4% for hypertension for each hour per day that total sedentary behavior increased (Guo et al., 2020). This is because excess sedentary behavior leads to reduced energy expenditure, which is inversely associated with BP (Guo et al., 2020).

BODY-MASS INDEX/OBESITY

Epidemiological data support a linear association of BMI with BP (J. E. Hall, 2003). Increasing anthropometric measurements (waist circumference, waist-to-hip ratio, and waist-to-height ratio) in parallel with BMI leads to an increase in the risk of hypertension (A. Jayedi, Rashidy-Pour, Khorshidi, & Shab-Bidar, 2018). The prevalence of hypertension is highest among people with obesity (~36%) (Egan, Li, Hutchison, & Ferdinand, 2014; Saydah et al., 2014). Obesity is a major cause of hypertension through several mechanisms, including insulin and leptin resistance, oxidative stress, neurohormonal activation, inflammation, and kidney dysfunction (DeMarco, Aroor, & Sowers, 2014; J. E. Hall, Do Carmo, Da Silva, Wang, & Hall, 2015). In addition, people with obesity require more antihypertensive medication and are more commonly resistant to treatment than individuals with normal weight (Jordan, Kurschat, & Reuter, 2018).

CO-MORBIDITIES AND COMPLICATIONS

Hypertension is a major risk factor for stroke, heart failure, and chronic obstructive pulmonary disease (COPD) and is the most frequent comorbidity in people with COPD (M. J. O'Donnell et al., 2010; Unger et al., 2020). The increased risk of cardiovascular diseases is associated with both SBP and DBP. Moreover, hypertension is associated with the development and progression of albuminuria and any form of chronic kidney disease (CKD) (more on **Chapter 20**) (Drawz et al., 2016). Inflammatory rheumatic diseases are associated with an increased prevalence of underdiagnosed and poorly controlled hypertension (Agca et al., 2016; Ikdahl et al., 2019). In this regard, hypertension is considered one of the most important causes of premature morbidity and mortality worldwide (NICE guideline, 2019).

LIFESTYLE MODIFICATIONS FOR THE PREVENTION AND MANAGEMENT OF HYPERTENSION

Strong evidence supports the benefits of lifestyle modification for the prevention and management of hypertension. As shown in the next paragraphs, according to 2020 International Society of Hypertension (ISH) guidelines (Unger et al., 2020), adopting a healthy lifestyle (i.e., salt restriction, high consumption of vegetables and fruits, moderation of alcohol intake, weight reduction, maintaining an ideal body weight, regular physical activity, and smoking cessation) can prevent or delay the onset of hypertension as well as reduce the risk of cardiovascular disease (Oparil et al., 2018; Perumareddi, 2019).

Moreover, lifestyle modification is a well-established strategy to lower BP and treating individuals with pre-hypertension or hypertension, although most patients with hypertension will also require drug therapy in addition to lifestyle treatment (**Figure 16.2**).

As far as older adults are concerned, strategies for managing hypertension in this population may include the degree of frailty, the medical co-morbidities and psychosocial factors of the elderlies, and thus each patient should be individualized (Oliveros et al., 2020). The challenge in management and holistic care is making decisions based not only on age, but also on the overall medical, physical, social, and mental characteristics of older people. Management should begin with lifestyle modification initially, taking into consideration issues such as cognitive impairment, other medical health problems, polypharmacy, falls, gait speed, incontinence, fatigue, visual and auditory limitations, social support, caretaker availability, and frailty (Abdelhafiz, Marshall, Kavanagh, & El-Nahas, 2018; Oliveros et al., 2020).

TREATMENT GOALS FOR PATIENTS WITH HYPERTENSION

According to the 2018 ESC/ESH, optimal goals for BP treatment are <140/90 mm Hg for most patients. If the treatment is well tolerated, BP values should be targeted at ≤130/80 mm Hg. For older patients (≥65 years) receiving BP-lowering drugs, a BP range of 130/70 to 139/79 mm Hg is recommended (Williams et al., 2018). Based on 2017 ACC/AHA guidelines, the BP goal is <130/80 mm Hg for both most patients and older people (Whelton et al., 2018). Moreover, for patients at high risk, BP should be targeted at <130/80 mm Hg but >120/70 mm Hg, because over-aggressive BP reduction (<120/70 mm Hg) causes more side effects without a further reduction of cardiovascular events (Jordan et al., 2018; Williams et al., 2018).

DIETARY STRATEGIES TO PREVENT AND MANAGE HYPERTENSION

WEIGHT LOSS

Weight loss either by adhering to a healthy diet, increasing physical activity, or reducing sedentariness, is considered a vital strategy for preventing or managing hypertension in adults with overweight and obesity and hypertension. Weight loss can attenuate the risks of hypertension and related co-morbidities in this population, but further evidence is needed on the long-term efficacy of this strategy (Valenzuela et al., 2021).

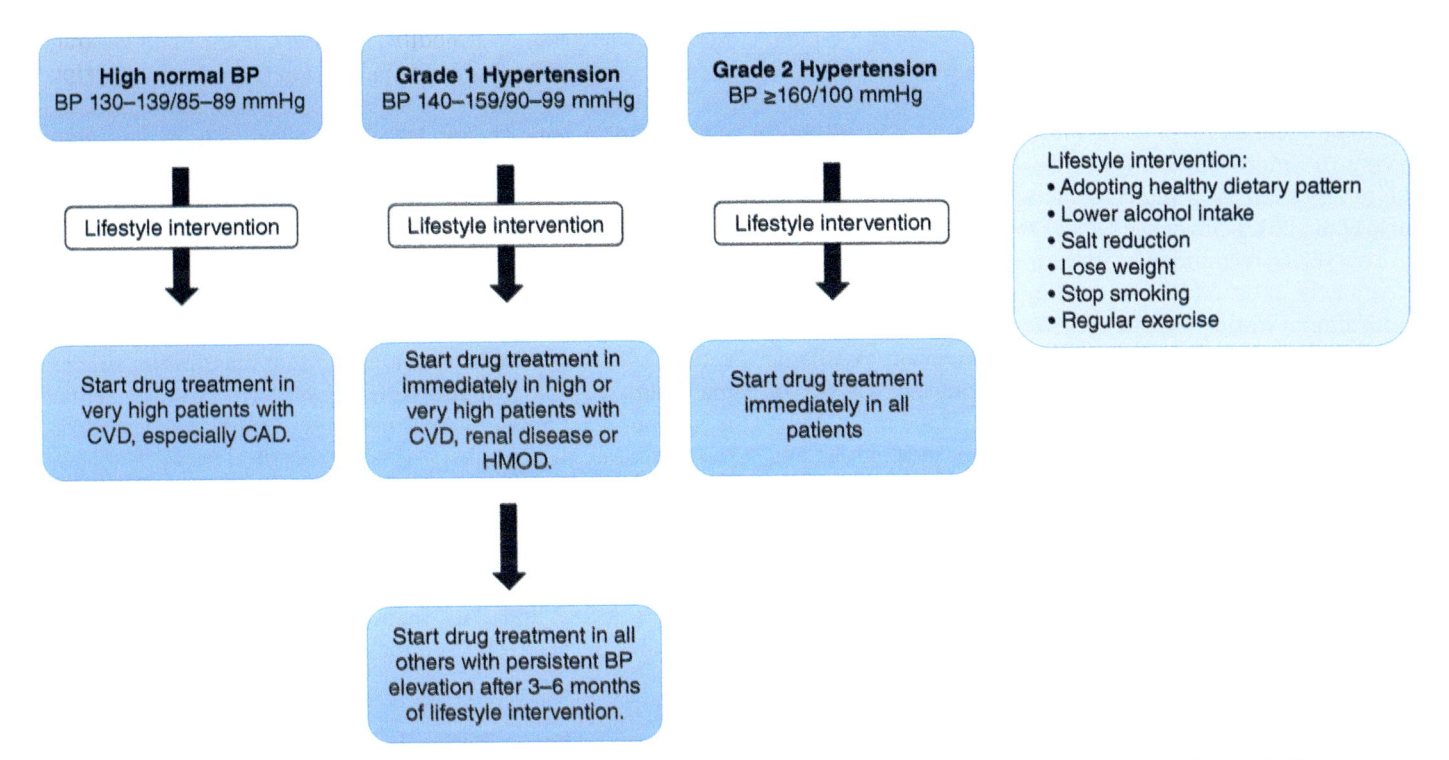

FIGURE 16.2 Initiation of blood pressure-lowering treatment (lifestyle treatment and medication) at different initial levels of office BP. BP = blood pressure; CAD = coronary artery disease; CVD = cardiovascular disease; HMOD = hypertension-mediated organ damage. Sources: (Unger et al., 2020; Williams et al., 2018).

A 2% to 3% weight loss may lead to improvements in cardiovascular disease risk factors (M. E. Hall et al., 2021). Achieving 5% to 10% of weight loss can lead to >5 and 4 mm Hg reduction in SBP and DBP, respectively (M. E. Hall et al., 2021; Unger et al., 2020). In a meta-analysis of 25 RCTs including 4874 participants, a weight reduction of 5.1 kg reduced SBP by 4.4 mm Hg and DBP by 3.6 mm Hg (Neter, Stam, Kok, Grobbee, & Geleijnse, 2003). The expected reduction in SBP is 1 mm Hg for every kilogram of body weight lost (Neter et al., 2003).

The aim is to reduce body weight so as to achieve a normal BMI (approximately 20–25 kg/m² in individuals <60 years of age; higher in older patients) or an ideal body weight but even reduction of 1 Kg might be beneficial for lowering BP or managing hypertension for adults with overweight or obesity (Whelton et al., 2018; Perumareddi, 2019; Williams et al., 2018). Indeed, every 1 kg of weight loss may lead to 1 mm Hg reduction in BP (Stevens et al., 2001). Although the optimal BMI is unclear, maintenance of healthy body weight (BMI of approximately 20–25 kg/m² in individuals <60 years of age; higher in older patients) and waist circumference (<94 cm for men and <80 cm for women) is recommended for the treatment of hypertension. Weight loss can also improve the efficacy of medications for hypertension (Piepoli et al., 2016).

However, the evidence on the actual long-term sustainability of lifestyle interventions aimed at reducing body weight is unclear, although combining energy-restrictive diets and exercise interventions seems to maximize the likelihood of maintaining body-weight reduction (Valenzuela et al., 2021).

SODIUM RESTRICTION

Sodium restriction not only decreases BP and hypertension incidence but is also associated with a reduction in cardiovascular morbidity and mortality (Whelton & He, 2014). Sodium reduction is highly recommended for preventing and managing hypertension. A meta-analysis of 34 RCTs including 3230 participants showed that a mean reduction of 1.75 g/d sodium (4.4 g/d salt) caused a mean reduction of 4.2/2.1 mm Hg in SBP/DBP, with a more pronounced effect (−5.4/−2.8 mm Hg) in individuals with hypertension (F. J. He, Li, & MacGregor, 2013). Even lower amounts of sodium intake have been tried in otherwise healthy individuals for assessing the role of sodium restriction on BP. In a systematic review and meta-analysis of 37 RCTs, reducing sodium intake (<2 g/day) led to a reduction of SBP and DBP by 3.5 and 1.8 mm Hg, respectively, with no significant adverse effect on blood lipids, catecholamines or renal function (Aburto et al., 2013). Moreover, in a meta-analysis of 133 RCTs including 12,197 participants, each 50 mmol reduction in 24 hour sodium excretion was associated with a 1.10 mm Hg reduction in SBP and a 0.33 mm Hg reduction in DBP. Researchers showed a dose-response relationship between the sodium restriction and the fall in BP, but this association was more pronounced in older people, those with higher initial BP, and non-white populations (Huang et al., 2020).

In older adults with overweight or obesity, reduction in sodium intake (~1000 mg/d) combined with weight loss can also improve BP (Whelton et al., 1998). However, weight loss in the elderlies as mentioned in **Chapter 10**, should be made with caution as it may lead to loss of lean body mass and subsequent functional decline. Nevertheless, nonpharmacologic interventions in the elderly (TONE) including weight loss are not associated with an increase in all-cause mortality and can be used for achieving BP improvements (Shea et al., 2011). Lowering salt intake to less than 1200 mg/d seems to be safe and beneficial (Aburto et al., 2013; Oliveros et al., 2020).

The WHO recommends sodium intake to be limited to approximately 2.0 g/d (5.0 g/d salt) in the general population (Organization World Health & World Health Organization, 2012), as well as to those with hypertension (Williams et al., 2018). According to the 2017 guidelines of the ACC/AHA, the optimal goal sodium intake is defined as <1500 mg/d, but a reduction of at least 1000 mg/d is desirable for most adults and especially for those with hypertension (Whelton et al., 2018).

Effective sodium reduction is not easy, and it is often difficult to determine which foods contain high salt levels. Patients with hypertension should be guided to reduce salt added when preparing foods and at the table and avoid consumption of salty foods (i.e., fast foods, soy sauce, canned foods, cheeses, bread, nuts, chips, and tomato sauces and many processed foods) (Perumareddi, 2019; Bouchard et al., 2022; Williams et al., 2018).

POTASSIUM INTAKE

Potassium excretion, as a marker of dietary intake, is inversely associated with BP. Increasing potassium intake either from diet or through a supplement can reduce BP in people with hypertension, without adverse effects (Burnier, 2019; Samadian et al., 2016).

Adults with hypertension should consume adequate amounts of dietary potassium to meet the dietary reference intake (DRI). Indeed, the 2017 ACC/AHA guidelines propose an increase in potassium intake, ideally through dietary modification (i.e., preference for foods high in potassium such as the consumption of meat, milk, fruits, and vegetables (Oparil et al., 2018; Samadian et al., 2016) and not from supplements (Whelton et al., 2018)). The suggested intake is 3500 to 5000 mg/d (Whelton et al., 2018).

However, if patients with hypertension are unable to meet the DRI for potassium through diet alone and there are no other co-morbidities, potassium supplementation of up to 3700 mg/d may be recommended to reduce elevated BP (Lennon et al., 2017). Indeed, potassium supplementation up to approximately 3700 mg/d can reduce SBP and DBP by 3 to 13 and 0 to 8 mm Hg, respectively, in individuals with hypertension (Lennon et al., 2017). A meta-analysis of 33 RCTs including 2609 participants demonstrated that potassium supplementation (≥60 mmol/d) reduced SBP and DBP by 4.4 mm Hg and 2.5 mm Hg, respectively, in individuals with hypertension (Whelton et al., 1998).

MAGNESIUM INTAKE

A meta-analysis of nine prospective cohort studies including 180,566 participants supported an inverse dose-response relationship between dietary magnesium intake and the risk of hypertension (Han et al., 2017). Similarly, inadequate levels of potassium may contribute to hypertension (Perumareddi, 2019).

Adequate amounts of dietary potassium are considered 3.5 to 5 g/d. In order to meet DRI and to control BP, patients with hypertension are recommended to consume foods high in potassium such as whole grains, green leafy vegetables, and nuts. However, the evidence assessing the relationship between magnesium intake either from food sources or via supplementation and BP in individuals with hypertension is weak. Based on an umbrella review of 16 meta-analysis (36 RCTs and 19 observational studies), clinical data showed that magnesium supplementation was able to reduce SBP and DBP by ~2 mm Hg, which is probably of limited clinical meaning. Results from observational studies showed also a weak association between dietary intake of magnesium and incidence of hypertension. (Veronese et al., 2020). Nevertheless, magnesium supplementation of 240 to 1000 mg/d may be considered for patients who are unable to meet the DRI with food sources alone (Lennon et al., 2017), achieving a SBP and DBP reduction by 1.0 to 5.6 and 1.0 to 2.8 mm Hg, respectively (Lennon et al., 2017).

CALCIUM INTAKE

Several reviews have shown an inverse association between the intake of calcium and BP or hypertension (Cormick, Ciapponi, Cafferata, Cormick, & Belizán, 2022). An adequate intake of calcium should be encouraged to prevent hypertension (van Mierlo et al., 2006).

A meta-analysis of eight prospective cohort studies including 248,398 participants with a follow-up duration ranging from 2 to 10 years showed that higher dietary calcium intake is associated slightly with a lower risk of developing hypertension (Ahmad Jayedi & Zargar, 2019). A dietary calcium intake of ≥800 mg/d may lead to a reduction of SBP >4 mm Hg and DBP >2 mm Hg in individuals with hypertension, whereas calcium supplementation of 1000 to 1500 mg/d reduces SBP/DBP >3.0/2.5 mm Hg in individuals with hypertension.

Patients with hypertension should consume adequate amounts of dietary calcium, such as milk, yogurt, cheese, and almonds, to meet the DRI in order to control BP. Calcium supplementation of 1000 to 1500 mg/d may be considered for patients unable to meet the DRI with diet alone (Lennon et al., 2017).

OMEGA-3 FATTY ACIDS

Many cohort studies and RCTs have shown associations between increased consumption of omega-3 fatty acids and lowered BP in individuals with hypertension (Bercea, Cottrell, Tamagnini, & McNeish, 2021; Colussi, Catena, Novello, Bertin, & Sechi, 2017). A meta-analysis of 70 RCTs examined the long-chain omega-3 fatty acids eicosapentaenoic acid (EPA; 20:5 n-3) and docosahexaenoic acid (DHA; 22:6 n-3) in relation to BP. Provision of ≥2 g/d EPA+DHA may lead to a reduction in SBP and DBP, with the strongest benefits observed among individuals with hypertension who are not on antihypertensive medication (Miller, Van Elswyk, & Alexander, 2014).

CAFFEINE

According to the European Food Safety Authority (EFSA) (Panel & Nda, 2015), single doses of caffeine consumption ranging from 80 to 300 mg induce a mean increase in SBP and DBP of about 3 to 8 mm Hg and 4 to 6 mm Hg, respectively, with high interindividual variability. Moreover, the available data suggest that BP generally increases 30 min after the intake of caffeine, reaches a peak after 60 to 90 min, and returns to baseline after about 2 to 4 h (Panel & Nda, 2015). The role of caffeine in regulating BP levels is controversial, and there is a debate about the possible association between the habitual consumption of coffee and the risk of hypertension (De Giuseppe, Di Napoli, Granata, Mottolese, & Cena, 2019). However, a dose-response meta-analysis of four prospective studies showed that habitual moderate coffee intake (1 or 2 cups/d) was not associated with a higher risk of hypertension in the general population and that regular coffee intake (3–7 cups/d) was associated with apparent protection against the development of hypertension, compared with no coffee consumption, through a non-linear relationship (D'Elia, La Fata, Galletti, Scalfi, & Strazzullo, 2019). According to the 2018 ESC/ESH guidelines for the management of hypertension, there is no specific recommendation for coffee consumption due to the insufficient quality of most studies (Williams et al., 2018). Apart from coffee, other sources of caffeine are tea, caffeinated soft drinks, and chocolate (De Giuseppe et al., 2019).

As far as tea consumption is concerned, its use, including black and green tea, is a widely prevalent habit worldwide and is usually the major source of flavonoid intake. The caffeine content is greater in black tea compared to green tea, whereas the latter compared to black tea, has the greatest total phenolic and flavonoid content, which are known to have antioxidant capacities (G. Liu et al., 2014; Mahdavi-Roshan, Salari, Ghorbani, & Ashouri, 2020). A meta-analysis of 5 RCTs including 408 participants showed that the regular intake of tea resulted in SBP and DBP reductions by about 4.81 and 1.98 mm Hg, respectively, in individuals with elevated BP or hypertension (Mahdavi-Roshan et al., 2020). A meta-analysis of 13 RCTs including 1115 participants suggested that black tea supplementation reduced SBP and DBP by 1.04 mm Hg and 0.59 mm Hg, respectively (Ma, Zheng, Yang, & Bu, 2021), while a meta-analysis of 24 RCTs including 1697 individuals showed that green tea lowered the SBP and DBP by 1.17 mm Hg and 1.24 mm Hg, respectively (Xu, Yang, Ding, & Chen, 2020).

With regard to cocoa consumption, cocoa flavonoids exhibit antioxidative and cardio-protective properties (Haber & Gallus, 2012). Dark chocolate may modestly reduce BP in individuals with hypertension (Haber & Gallus, 2012). A recent meta-analysis of 13 RCTs with 758 participants demonstrated a significant reduction in SBP and DBP by 2.8 mm Hg and 1.5 mm Hg, respectively, after cocoa consumption in middle-aged and older individuals (Jafarnejad, Salek, & Clark, 2020).

ALCOHOL

Strong evidence supports the detrimental effects of excessive alcohol intake on BP, the prevalence of hypertension, and cardiovascular risk. (Puddey, Mori, Barden, & Beilin, 2019; Valenzuela et al., 2021).

A meta-analysis of nine prospective cohort studies including 394,840 participants showed that low-to-moderate (0–26 g/d) alcohol consumption was inversely associated with the risk of cardiovascular disease and all-cause mortality in people with hypertension (He, 2014). Especially, <20 g/d (about 2 drinks/day) alcohol intake was associated with a 19% to 28% reduction in the overall risk of cardiovascular disease. Researchers observed a J-shaped relationship between alcohol consumption and all-cause mortality, suggesting that alcohol intake of no more than 26 g/d (2–3 drinks/d) will benefit patients with hypertension and alcohol consumption of 8 to 10 g/d will have the greatest benefit (He, 2014).

According to the 2017 ACC/AHA (Whelton et al., 2018) and the 2018 ESC/ESH guidelines (Williams et al., 2018), alcohol consumption should be limited to 1 drink per day for women and 2 drinks per day for men, whereas the 2020 ISH (Unger et al., 2020) recommended 1.5 standards drinks for women and two for men (10 g alcohol/ standard drink). Moreover, binge drinking (episodic drinking of large amounts of alcohol, often manifested by events such as drunkenness, hangovers, difficulties with work) should be avoided by patients with hypertension (Britton & McKee, 2000; Unger et al., 2020; Whelton et al., 2018; Williams et al., 2018).

DIETARY PATTERNS

Adopting a healthy/prudent diet reduces the possibility as well as the risk of hypertension. Specifically, a meta-analysis of 27 studies (16 cohort studies and 11 cross-sectional studies) demonstrated that the healthy/prudent dietary pattern (high consumption of vegetables, fruits, whole grains, olive oil, fish, soy, poultry, and low-fat dairy) was associated with reduced odds of having hypertension (Wang et al., 2016). Many dietary approaches, such as the Dietary Approach to Stop Hypertension (DASH diet), Mediterranean diet (MD), Vegetarian diets, and Nordic Diet (ND) have been used for the control of elevated BP or the management of hypertension. However, their effectiveness in reducing BP differs.

DASH Diet

As mentioned in previous chapters, the DASH dietary pattern is the most effective and well-known dietary strategy, while safe and broadly acceptable to both prevent and treat hypertension (Appel, 2017; Perumareddi, 2019). People with a high adherence to the DASH diet have reported a 44% decrease in the risk of hypertension incidence (Lelong et al., 2017). The DASH diet is rich in fruits, vegetables, whole grains, nuts, legumes, lean protein, and low-fat dairy products (**Table 16.2**) (Appel et al., 1997). Moreover, it provides approximately 4.7 g/d of potassium and it is rich in magnesium, calcium, and fiber but lower in sugar, total fat, saturated fat, and cholesterol (Appel, 2017).

In a meta-analysis of 67 RCTs that included 17,230 participants, researchers examined the effects of different dietary

Table 16.2 Characteristics of the DASH (dietary approaches to stop hypertension) dietary plan.

Food group	Servings[1]	Examples of serving
Whole grains	6–8/d	1 slice of whole-grain bread
Vegetables	4–5/d	1 cup of raw leafy vegetables
Fruits	4–5/d	1 medium fruit
Dairy products (low-fat or fat-free)	2–3/d	1 cup of milk or yogurt
Lean meat, poultry, and fish	2–3/d	2 ounces of cooked meats, chicken, or fish
Nuts, seeds, and legumes	4–5 per week	• 1/3 cup of nuts or • 2 tablespoons of peanut butter or • 2 tablespoons of seeds or • 1/2 cup of cooked peas or beans
Candy and added sugars	≤5 per week	• 1 tablespoon of sugar, jelly, or jam or • 1 cup of lemonade

[1] Recommended daily and weekly servings for a 2000-calorie/day diet.
Source: (Oparil et al., 2018).

Table 16.3 Dietary approaches included in the Schwingshackl et al. meta-analysis. DASH = Dietary Approach to Stop Hypertension.

Name	Description
DASH diet	• High intake of fruits & vegetables, low-fat dairy products, and whole grains • Low in sodium
Mediterranean dietary pattern	• High consumption of fruit, vegetables, olive oil, legumes, cereals, fish • Moderate intake of red wine during meals
Low-carbohydrate diet	• <25% carbohydrates of total energy intake • High intake of animal and/or plant protein • Often high intake of fat
Paleolithic diet	• Included: Lean meat, fish, fruit, leafy and cruciferous vegetables, root vegetables, eggs, and nuts • Excluded: Dairy products, cereal grains, beans, refined fats, sugar, candy, soft drinks, beer, and extra addition of salt
Moderate-carbohydrate diet	• 25–45% carbohydrates of total energy intake • 10–20% protein intake
High-protein diet	• >20% protein intake of total energy intake • High intake of animal and/or plant protein • <35% fat
Nordic diet	• Whole-grain products, abundant use of berries, fruit and vegetables, rapeseed oil, three fish meals per week, low-fat dairy products, and avoidance of sugar-sweetened products
Tibetan diet	• High-protein and vitamin-rich food, preferably cooked and warm food
Low-fat diet	• <30% fat of total energy intake • High intake of cereals & grains • 10–15% protein intake
Low glycemic index/load (LGI/LGL) diet	• Low glycemic index/load food selection
Vegetarian/Vegan diet	• No meat and fish (vegetarian) • no animal products (vegan)
Low-sodium diet	-
Control diet	• A usual diet

Source: (Schwingshackl et al., 2019).

approaches in SBP and DBP, as shown in **Table 16.3**. The most effective diet for reducing BP was proven to be the DASH diet. Compared to the control diet (usual diet), the DASH, MD, low-carbohydrate, Paleolithic, high-protein, low glycemic index, low-sodium, and low-fat diets were all able to significantly reduce SBP (reduction range of 8.73–2.32 mm Hg) and DBP (reduction range of 4.85–1.27 mm Hg) (Schwingshackl et al., 2019).

Evidence from RCTs seems to agree that the DASH dietary approach is the most effective dietary pattern for reducing elevated BP (Fu et al., 2020). The extent to which the DASH improves BP may be influenced by various factors. Based on a meta-analysis of 17 RCTs, DASH diet significantly reduced SBP by a mean value of 6.74 mm Hg and DBP by 3.54 mm Hg. Yet, the most prominent decrease in both SBP and DBP were observed in individuals following DASH diet with an energy restriction or individuals who were already diagnosed with hypertension (baseline BP influenced the result in RCTs) (Saneei, Salehi-Abargouei, Esmaillzadeh, & Azadbakht, 2014). Moreover, the combination of the DASH diet and low-sodium intake lead to a greater reduction in BP than the DASH diet or the low-sodium diet alone (Juraschek, Miller, Weaver, & Appel, 2017; Sacks et al., 2001).

Mediterranean Diet

The MD is characterized by the low consumption of red and processed meat, moderate consumption of dairy products, and high consumption of olive oil, fruits, vegetables, cereals (mainly unrefined), nuts, and legumes (**Figure 16.3**) (Bach-Faig et al., 2011).

The MD has been proven an effective dietary pattern to reduce BP as well as hypertension and cardiovascular risk (Cowell et al., 2021; De Pergola & D'alessandro, 2018). A 2019 Cochrane review of 30 RCTs with 12,461 participants showed that the MD had a significant beneficial effect on SBP and DBP (reduction of 3.0 mm Hg and 2.0 mm Hg, respectively) (Rees et al., 2019). In a systematic review and meta-analysis of 35 RCTs, including 13,943 participants, the MD led to a small but significant BP reduction among individuals with hypertension, while their initially elevated SBP levels (≥130 mm Hg) and the longer duration of intervention (≥16 weeks) were factors that associated with a greater reduction of BP compared to lower levels of SBP and lower duration of intervention (Filippou et al., 2021).

In addition, evidence (from observational and clinical studies) demonstrates that foods typical of the MD, such as extra virgin olive oil, fruits, vegetables, nuts, and whole grain, have a favorable effect on the risk of hypertension (De Pergola & D'alessandro, 2018). Olive oil, due to polyphenols, has a protective effect on BP by increasing the endothelial synthesis of

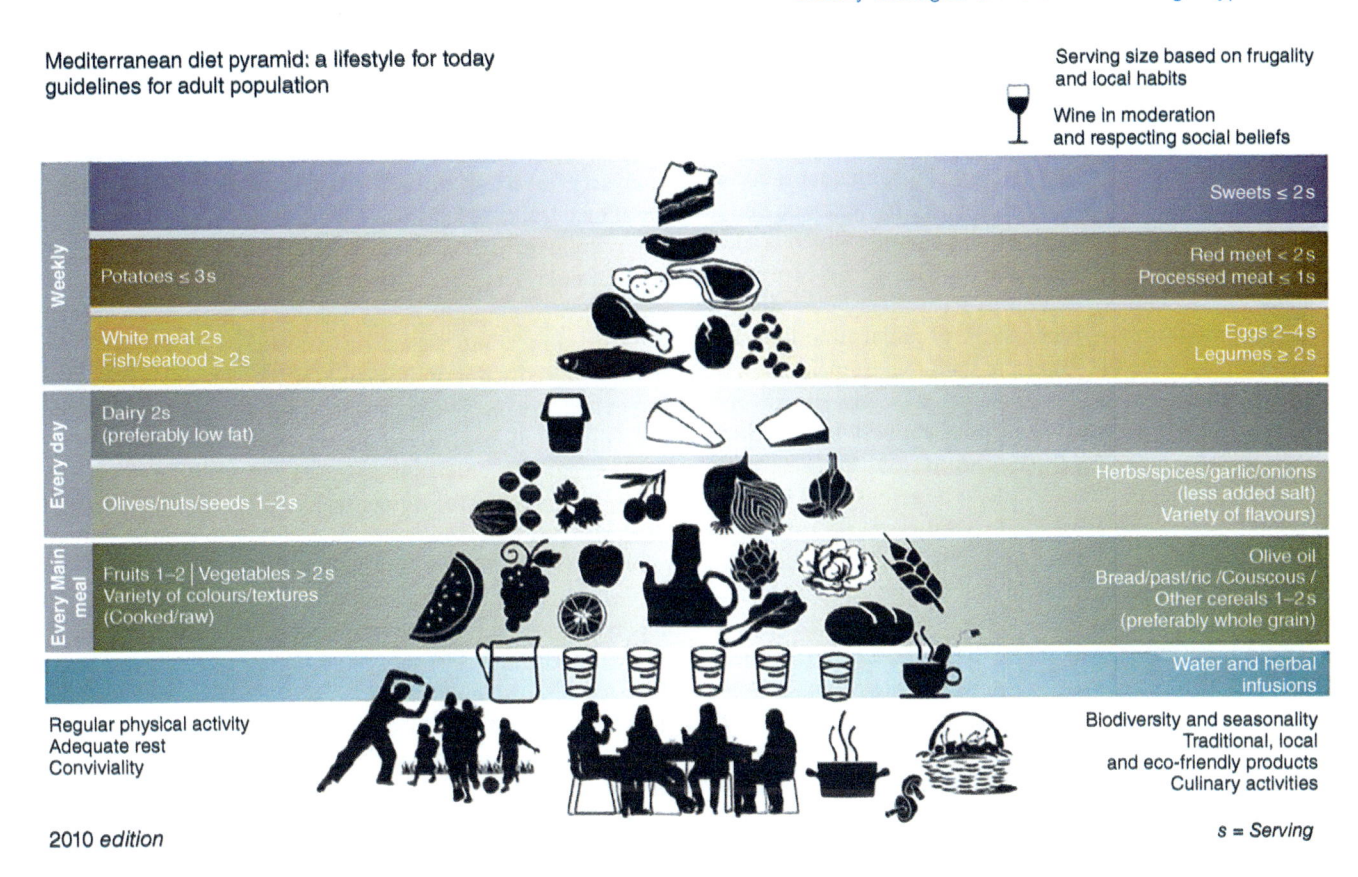

FIGURE 16.3 Mediterranean diet pyramid: a lifestyle for today. Source: (Bach-Faig et al., 2011 / with permission of Cambridge University Press).

nitric oxide and the response mediated by the endothelium-derived hyperpolarization factor. Moreover, dietary fibers increase insulin sensitivity and improve endothelial function. The content of nuts in magnesium and poly-unsaturated fatty acid may explain their protective effect on BP (Lelong et al., 2017).

Vegetarian Diets

Vegetarian diets are shown to lessen BP. People who adopt a vegetarian diet tend to have a lower BP than nonvegetarians. Several aspects of a vegetarian lifestyle may contribute to lower BP, such as low sodium along with high potassium intake, weight management, alcohol, high fiber intake, and the absence of meat and physical activity (Appel, 2017). The lowering effect of vegetarian diets on BP may be explained by several mechanisms. The emphasis on consuming vegetables, fruits, legumes, nuts, and whole grains leads to a higher intake of dietary fiber which exhibits a lower energy density and has a positive effect on satiety, so this may lead to a decrease in daily calorie intake. Moreover, fruits and vegetables are rich in antioxidants that may eliminate excess superoxide to promote the action of nitric oxide, thus lowering BP (Niu, Cao, Zhou, Cao, & Wang, 2022). In a meta-analysis of seven control trials and 32 cohort studies, vegetarian diets were associated with lower SBP (-6.9 mm Hg) and DBP (-4.7 mm Hg), compared to omnivorous diets (Yokoyama et al., 2014). Similarly, a meta-analysis of 15 RCTs published in 2020 that included 856 participants demonstrated that vegetarian diets lowered SBP and DBP by 2.7 mm Hg and 1.7 mm Hg, respectively, compared to omnivorous diets (K. W. Lee, Loh, Ching, Devaraj, & Hoo, 2020).

Nordic Diet

The ND was adopted by people who lived in Nordic countries and is based on whole grains, rapeseed oil, berries, fruits, vegetables, fish, eggs, nuts, and vegetable fat with low intake of meat products, dairy products, sweets, desserts, and alcoholic beverages. Current data from clinical studies support that ND can reduce SBP and DBP levels.

A meta-analysis of 17 RCTs, including 5014 participants, showed that ND significantly reduce SBP and DBP by 5.20 mm Hg and 3.9 mm Hg, respectively (Ndanuko, Tapsell, Charlton, Neale, & Batterham, 2016). The pooled effect of three subsequent RCTs showed that the ND is associated with a mean reduction in SBP of 4.47 mm Hg and 2.32 mm Hg in DBP, which is a relatively moderate effect compared with the consumption of comparator diets (Gibbs, Gaskin, Ji, Miller, & Cappuccio, 2021). The findings from clinical studies regarding the effect of ND on BP are of great significance as they show that complete eradication of animal products from one's diet is not necessary to produce significant improvements in BP.

Berries, which are one of the characteristics of the ND, are rich in polyphenols, especially flavonoids and may contribute to BP improvements (Basu et al., 2010; Ndanuko et al., 2016). However, further research is warranted on the effect of the ND on elevated BP (Basu et al., 2010).

PHYSICAL ACTIVITY, FITNESS, AND HYPERTENSION

The benefits of regular physical activity and exercise for the prevention and management of hypertension are well documented. Based on the 2016 WHO report, physical activity was reported to beneficially effect incident hypertension in adults, which is a key risk factor for cardiovascular disease (WHO, 2016). Moreover, physical activity is known to improve cardiovascular disease mortality, progression of hypertension, physical function, and health-related quality of life in people with hypertension.

Indeed, there is strong evidence showing an inverse dose-response relationship between physical activity and incident hypertension amongst people with normal BP (Pescatello et al., 2019), while higher levels of physical activity and improving fitness, especially cardio-respiratory fitness (CRF), decrease BP levels and the risk of hypertension (Bakker, Sui, Brellenthin, & Lee, 2018). Regular physical activity leading to an increase in CRF reduces the progressive increase in BP and prevents hypertension (Kokkinos, 2014). A meta-analysis of 22 cohort studies, including 330,222 participants, demonstrated an inverse dose-response relation between physical activity and incident hypertension (X. Liu et al., 2017). Specifically, the risk of hypertension was reduced by 6% with each 10 metabolic equivalent of task (MET) h/week increment of leisure-time physical activity. Moreover, the risk of hypertension was reduced by 6% in people who met the recommended minimum physical activity levels of 150 min/week, compared to inactive people (X. Liu et al., 2017).

Moreover, habitual physical activity (peak MET level 6.1–8.0) has therapeutic benefits for individuals with hypertension (Pescatello et al., 2019) and reduces BP levels (Oparil et al., 2018) and the risk of all-cause and CVD mortality, independently of other risk factors (Kokkinos, 2014). Both aerobic and resistance exercises are beneficial in preventing and treating hypertension ("Physical activity guidelines for Americans.," 2008) (Whelton et al., 2018).

A meta-analysis of 27 RCTs including 1480 participants showed that regular medium-to-high-intensity aerobic activity reduced SBP and DBP by a mean of 11 mm Hg and 5 mm Hg, respectively, in individuals with hypertension (Borjesson, Onerup, Lundqvist, & Dahlof, 2016). In a recent systematic review, meta-analysis and meta-regression of 24 clinical trials including 1207 participants, aerobic training with and without progression, led to a reduction in SBP and DBP by 11 mm Hg and 5.5 mm Hg, respectively, in individuals with hypertension (de Barcelos et al., 2022). Moreover, aerobic exercises decreased all ambulatory BP measures (24-h, daytime, and nighttime) yet with no significant effects for resistance exercise or combined (i.e., aerobic and resistance) exercise for any ambulatory BP measure in individuals with hypertension. Vigorous aerobic exercise also tended to have the most significant impact (Saco-Ledo et al., 2021).

As far as resistance exercise is concerned, based on a meta-analysis of 93 RCTs including 55,223 participants, endurance training as well as dynamic resistance exercise and isometric resistance training were able to lower both SBP and DBP to different extents, while combined endurance and resistance training was only able to lower DBP (Cornelissen & Smart, 2013). A meta-analysis of 30 RCTs including 646 participants demonstrated that a single bout of resistance exercise induced small-to-moderate reductions in BP that lasted for up to 24 hr (Casonatto, Goessler, Cornelissen, Cardoso, & Polito, 2016). Also, this reduction was greater in patients with hypertension and in those who used larger muscle groups (Casonatto et al., 2016). Moreover, a meta-analysis of 64 RCTs with 2344 participants showed that dynamic resistance training led to a reduction in BP that was comparable to or greater than what was achieved with aerobic training (MacDonald et al., 2016). Regarding isometric resistance training, a meta-analysis of 24 RCTs with 1143 participants demonstrated that isometric resistance training induced a significant reduction in SBP and DBP by 7 mm Hg and 5 mm Hg, respectively, especially among older people (aged ≥65 years) (Hansford et al., 2021).

Regarding older adults (aged ≥65 years), exercise is a key strategy for successful BP control. A meta-analysis of 69 clinical trials showed that exercise (any bodily activity that enhances or maintains physical fitness and overall health and wellness) led to a significant reduction of both SBP and DBP in older adults with hypertension. With regard to the type of exercise, subgroup analysis showed that resistance exercises reduced SBP and DBP by 0.69 ± 0.1 mm Hg and 0.73 ± 0.16 mm Hg, respectively, more than aerobic exercise (Kazeminia et al., 2020). Aerobic exercise in combination with resistance training seems to improve the extensive health needs of older adults with hypertension that go beyond BP reduction. Specifically, the benefits conferred by combined exercise are extensive and encompass CRF, muscular fitness, and blood lipid profile improvements (Sardeli, Griffth, dos Santos, Ito, & Chacon-Mikahil, 2021). In a meta-analysis of 53 RCTs, aerobic exercise training, dynamic resistance exercise training, and both performed together regularly for at least 3 months, led to a reduction in SBP and DBP of approximately 5 to 6 mm Hg and 2 to 3.5 mm Hg, respectively, in older individuals (Herrod et al., 2018). Similarly, a meta-analysis of 22 RCTs showed that both aerobic training and resistance training reduced SBP and DBP in older individuals, whereas the effects of combined training on BP remained unclear (Sardeli et al., 2020). A meta-analysis of 10 RCTs with 266 participants published in 2022 demonstrated that high-intensity interval training reduced SBP and DBP by 7.4 mm Hg and 5.5 mm Hg, respectively, in older adults (Carpes, Costa, Schaarschmidt, Reichert, & Ferrari, 2022).

PHYSICAL ACTIVITY GUIDELINES FOR HYPERTENSION

According to a 2020 WHO report, adults (aged 18 to 64 years) should complete at least 150 to 300 min of moderate-intensity aerobic physical activity (walking, jogging, cycling, yoga, or swimming), at least 75 to 150 min of vigorous-intensity aerobic physical activity, or an equivalent combination throughout the week. In addition, muscle-strengthening activities at a moderate or greater intensity that involve all major muscle groups on at least 2 d/week offer additional health benefits for adults (WHO, 2020).

Older people should also do varied multi-component physical activity that emphasizes functional balance and strength training (i.e., circuit training) at moderate or greater intensity, at least 3 d/week. Functional exercises include tandem and one-leg stands, squatting, chair stands, toe raises, and stepping over obstacles (WHO, 2020).

The 2018 ESC/ESH and 2020 ISH guidelines recommend at least 30 min of moderate-intensity dynamic aerobic exercise (i.e., walking, jogging, cycling, or swimming) on 5-7 d/week. Resistance exercise is also recommended 2 to 3 d/week (Unger et al., 2020; Williams et al., 2018). The 2017 guidelines of the ACC/AHA for patients with hypertension have except for aerobic exercise, both dynamic resistance (i.e., squats, climbing stairs, doing push-ups, or performing bicep curls) and isometric resistance exercise (i.e., wall sit, side plank, low squat) are recommended for patients suffering from hypertension or patients with elevated BP, as shown in **Table 16.4** (Whelton et al., 2018).

NUTRITION AND EXERCISE: COMBINED INTERVENTIONS

A lifestyle intervention including both diet and exercise is considered a more holistic intervention for reducing elevated BP.

In the ENCORE study, researchers compared the DASH diet alone, DASH diet combined with exercise and a weight management program, and a usual diet in 144 overweight or obese individuals with elevated BP (pre-hypertension or stage 1 hypertension) in a 16-week intervention program. A greater reduction in BP was observed in the group that received the DASH diet/exercise/weight management program compared to the DASH diet only group. Specifically, the reduction was 16.1 mm Hg in SBP and 9.9 mm Hg in DBP in the group with the triple intervention, compared to 11.2 and 7.5 mm Hg reductions

Table 16.4 Physical activity guidelines according to the American College of Cardiology/American Heart Association (2017).

Type of exercise	Duration	Rate	Detailed guidelines
Aerobic	90–150 min/week	65–75% heart rate reserve	-
Dynamic resistance	90–150 min/week	50–80% 1 rep maximum	6 exercises 3 sets/exercise 10 repetitions/set
Isometric resistance	3 sessions/week	30–40% maximum voluntary contraction	4 x 2 min (hand grip) 1 min rest between exercises

Source: (Adapted from Whelton et al., 2018).

Table 16.5 Dietary guidelines for the management of hypertension. ACC/AHA = American College of Cardiology/American Heart Association; ESC/ESH = European Society of Cardiology/European Society of Hypertension; ISH = International Society of Hypertension; BMI = body-mass index; DASH = Dietary Approach to Stop Hypertension; WC = waist circumference.

Dietary constituent	ACC/AHA, 2017 (Whelton et al., 2018)	ESC/ESH, 2018 (Williams et al., 2018)	ISH, 2020 (Unger et al., 2020)
Weight loss	• Ideal body weight • ↓ at least 1 kg for adults who are overweight	• Body-weight control; avoid obesity • Healthy BMI (20–25 kg/m²) and WC (<94 cm in men and <80 cm in women) should be achieved to reduce BP and CV risk.	Body-weight control; avoid obesity.
Healthy diet	Diet rich in fruits, vegetables, whole grains, and low-fat dairy products, and limit intake of saturated and trans-fat *(DASH diet)*	Healthy and balanced diet containing vegetables, fresh fruits, fish, nuts, and unsaturated fatty acids (olive oil), and low-fat dairy products, and have low consumption of red meat *(Mediterranean diet)*.	Diet rich in whole grains, fruits, vegetables, poly-unsaturated fats, and dairy products, and reducing food high in sugar, saturated fat and trans-fat *(DASH like)*.
Dietary sodium	• <1500 mg/d is optimal goal • at least 1,000 mg/d reduction in most adults	<2,000 mg/d	↓ salt added and high salt foods.
Dietary potassium	3500–5000 mg/d, mainly by adopting a diet rich in potassium	-	Foods and nutrients high in magnesium, calcium and potassium.
Alcohol	• Men: ≤2 drinks daily • Women: ≤1 drink daily	• Men: <14 units per week. • Women: <8 units per week.	• Men: ≤2 standard drinks daily • Women: ≤1.5 standard drink daily (10 g alcohol/ standard drink).
Physical activity	• Aerobic exercise 90–150 min/week • Dynamic resistance 90–150 min/week • Isometric resistance 3 sessions/week	Regular aerobic exercise at least 30 min of moderate dynamic exercise on 5–7 ds/week.	• Moderate-intensity aerobic exercise 30 min on 5–7 ds/ week or high-intensity interval training. • Resistance/strength exercises 2–3 ds/week.
Smoking cessation	-	✓	✓

Sources: (Whelton et al., 2018; Williams et al., 2018; Unger et al., 2020).

in the DASH diet only group (Blumenthal et al., 2010). These changes persisted for 8 months after the completion of the intervention, as shown by the 1-year follow up. Participants maintained diet modifications, but only 21% of those in the DASH diet/exercise/weight management group reported continuing to exercise. This finding suggests that even though lifestyle interventions for lowering BP may be effective for a short-term period, long-term adherence to the lifestyle is doubtful (Hinderliter et al., 2014).

The findings of the PREMIER clinical trial were also similar (Appel, 2003). In this study participants were randomly assigned to one of three groups; (i) an "established" group, e.g., a behavioral intervention based on current recommendations for lowering BP (weight loss, sodium reduction, increased physical activity, limited alcohol intake), (ii) an "established plus DASH diet" group, which additionally included the DASH diet, or (iii) an "advice only" control group (based on non-pharmacological factors that affect BP, such as weight, sodium intake, physical activity, and the DASH diet). Results showed greater improvements in BP for individuals who followed the established plus DASH diet group, achieving an optimal BP (<120 mm Hg SBP and <80 mm Hg DBP) to a greater extent, compared to individuals of the other groups (Appel, 2003).

In the EXERDIET-HTA study, 175 participants with overweight/obesity, sedentary lifestyle, and hypertension were randomly assigned into an attention control group or one of three supervised exercise groups [2 d/week: the high-volume moderate-intensity continuous training group (45 min), the high-volume high-intensity interval training group (45 min), or the low-volume high-intensity interval training group (20 min)] for 16 weeks. All participants received the same hypocaloric and controlled sodium diet (3–6 g/d). The diet was designed according to the DASH diet. The combination of the hypocaloric DASH diet with different supervised aerobic exercise programs 2 d/week improved BP, CRF, body composition, and pharmacological treatment (Gorostegi-Anduaga et al., 2018).

A meta-analysis of 17 RCTs, including 5014 participants, demonstrated that exercise and weight loss in combination with dietary changes, such as sodium reduction, had a significant reduction of 4.2/2.27 mm Hg in SBP/DBP (Ndanuko et al., 2016).

Taking all the above into consideration, a combination of diet and exercise could be more effective in patients with hypertension by helping them to reduce their BP **(Table 16.5)**.

OTHER STRATEGIES

The cessation of all products containing tobacco or nicotine, reducing stress, and inducing mindfulness as well as reducing exposure to air pollution and cold temperature are considered also important strategies for lowering BP (Unger et al., 2020).

KEY POINTS

- An SBP <140 mm Hg and DBP <90 mm Hg is considered normal BP. A chronic increase beyond these values in either SBP or DBP is considered hypertension.

- The risk of death from cardiovascular disease increases steadily as SBP or DBP increase. Thus, even small reductions in elevated BP result in a reduction of death from cardiovascular disease.

- In general, the available data support that the implementation of regular exercise alone, or combined with diet in patients with hypertension, can improve BP control at relatively lower doses of antihypertensive pharmacologic agents and reduced adverse events.

- Strong evidence supports the benefits of lifestyle modification for the prevention and management of hypertension. Adopting a healthy lifestyle (i.e., salt restriction, high consumption of vegetables and fruits, moderation of alcohol intake, weight reduction, maintaining an ideal body weight, regular physical activity, and smoking cessation) can prevent or delay the onset of hypertension as well as reduce the risk of cardiovascular disease.

- DASH and Mediterranean diets are the most effective diets for reducing BP based on the current available evidence.

- Lifestyle interventions including both diet and exercise interventions are more effective in lowering BP.

SELF-ASSESSMENT QUESTIONS

1. Define hypertension.
2. What are the most important risk factors for hypertension?
3. What are the most important cornerstones of the dietary intervention for hypertension?
4. Do you recommend dietary supplements such as magnesium and potassium for patients with hypertension? Why or why not?
5. What are the recommendations for exercise in patients with hypertension?
6. True or False: Regular aerobic exercise may be beneficial for both the prevention and treatment of hypertension, while resistance exercise is not recommended.
7. True or False: Body-weight control is recommended to avoid obesity.
8. True or False: People with hypertension should avoid the modest consumption of coffee, green and black tea.
9. True or False: The DASH diet is the only beneficial dietary pattern for the prevention and management of hypertension.
10. True or False: Smoking cessation, reducing stress, and inducing mindfulness as well as reducing exposure to air pollution and cold temperatures can help reduce BP.

Fill in the blank(s) to complete the following statements:

11. There is a(n) _____ association between alcohol consumption and the prevalence of hypertension.

12. Maintaining healthy body weight (BMI: _____ in individuals <60 years of age) and waist circumference (_____ for men and _____ for women) is recommended to prevent or treat hypertension.

13. Provision of _____ EPA+DHA reduces BP, especially in people with hypertension without antihypertension medications.

14. Both aerobic training and resistance training _____ SBP and DBP in older individuals.

15. Sodium reduction is _____ for individuals with hypertension. They should especially reduce _____ when preparing foods, and at _____, and avoid the consumption of _____ _____.

CASE SCENARIO

Mrs. KX is a 52-year-old woman with two children. She works as a teacher and describes feeling particularly anxious. She has had repeated measurements of SBP > 140 mm Hg despite receiving medication for hypertension for 2 years. Over the past 4 years, she has increased her body weight by 7 kg but, as she claims, has not changed anything in her diet. Her height is 1.53 m, body weight is 75 kg, and waist circumference is 104 cm. Her recent fasting biochemical evaluation revealed the following: total cholesterol of 185 mg/dl, LDL-cholesterol of 95 mg/dl, HDL-cholesterol of 65 mg/dl and glucose of 99 mg/, while her BP was 155/99 mm Hg. She is treated with Triacor.

Mrs. KX smokes between 6 and 10 cigarettes a day and is totally sedentary because her husband has been retired the last 2 years and drives her to and from work. In the afternoon, she stays at home because she feels too tired. However, she does all the housework. For breakfast, she usually consumes a cup of full-fat milk with cereal, two cheese pies, or a big piece of white cheese and one egg with two slices of bread. For lunch and dinner, she usually has red (pork) or white meat (chicken) 4 times/week (her typical portion size is approximately 250 g of cooked meat), fish 2 times/month, and pasta 2 times/week. In the afternoon, she usually consumes 1 cup of salted nuts. Also, she usually drinks 2 cups of coffee with sugar and milk per day as well as two sugar-sweetened beverages per week. She enjoys 4 to 5 glasses of wine with her family over Saturday and Sunday lunch. She does not have any food allergies, adds salt to cooking, sometimes also at the table, and reports difficulty consuming her food without salt.

Questions:

1. What patient problems/conditions may affect the dietary intervention?

2. What is the nutrition and dietetic diagnosis?

3. What are the aims of the dietary intervention?

4. Comment on the main sources of salt in Mrs. KX's diet.

5. What kind of advice would you give Mrs. KX regarding alcohol intake?

6. What kind of dietary pattern would you recommend to Mrs. KX and why?

7. What kind of exercise program would you recommend to Mrs. KX and why?

REFERENCES

Abdelhafiz, A. H., Marshall, R., Kavanagh, J., & El-Nahas, M. (2018). Management of hypertension in older people. *Expert Review of Endocrinology and Metabolism*, 13(4), 181–191. https://doi.org/10.1080/17446651.2018.1500893

Aburto, N. J., Ziolkovska, A., Hooper, L., Elliott, P., Cappuccio, F. P., & Meerpohl, J. J. (2013). Effect of lower sodium intake on health: Systematic review and meta-analyses. *BMJ (Online)*, 346(7903), 1–20. https://doi.org/10.1136/bmj.f1326

Agca, R., Heslinga, S. C., Rollefstad, S., Heslinga, M., McInnes, I. B., Peters, M. J. L., . . . Nurmohamed, M. T. (2016). EULAR recommendations for cardiovascular disease risk management in patients with rheumatoid arthritis and other forms of inflammatory joint disorders: 2015/2016 update. *Annals of the Rheumatic Diseases*, 76(1), 17–28. https://doi.org/10.1136/annrheumdis-2016-209775

Al Ghorani, H., Kulenthiran, S., Lauder, L., Böhm, M., & Mahfoud, F. (2021). Hypertension trials update. *Journal of Human Hypertension*, 35(5), 398–409. https://doi.org/10.1038/s41371-020-00477-1

Allen, T. S., Bhatia, H. S., Wood, A. C., Momin, S. R., & Allison, M. A. (2022). State-of-the-Art Review: Evidence on Red Meat Consumption and Hypertension Outcomes. *American Journal of Hypertension*, 35(8), 679–687. https://doi.org/10.1093/ajh/hpac064

Appel, L. J. (2003). Effects of Comprehensive Lifestyle Modification on Blood Pressure Control: Main Results of the PREMIER Clinical Trial. *Journal of the American Medical Association*, 289(16), 2083–2093. https://doi.org/10.1001/jama.289.16.2083

Appel, L. J. (2017). The Effects of Dietary Factors on Blood Pressure. *Cardiology Clinics*, 35(2), 197–212. https://doi.org/10.1016/j.ccl.2016.12.002

Appel, L. J., Moore, T. J., Obarzanek, E., Vollmer, W. M., Svetkey, L. P., Sacks, F. M., . . . Harsha, D. W. (1997). A Clinical Trial of the Effects of Dietary Patterns on Blood Pressure. *New England Journal of Medicine*, 336(16), 1117–1124. https://doi.org/10.1056/NEJM199704173361601

Bach-Faig, A., Berry, E. M., Lairon, D., Reguant, J., Trichopoulou, A., Dernini, S., . . . Padulosi, S. (2011). Mediterranean diet pyramid today. Science and cultural updates. *Public Health Nutrition*, Vol. 14, pp. 2274–2284. https://doi.org/10.1017/S1368980011002515

Bakker, E. A., Sui, X., Brellenthin, A. G., & Lee, D. C. (2018). Physical activity and fitness for the prevention of hypertension. *Current Opinion in Cardiology*, 33(4), 394–401. https://doi.org/10.1097/HCO.0000000000000526

Basu, A., Du, M., Leyva, M. J., Sanchez, K., Betts, N. M., Wu, M., ... Lyons, T. J. (2010). Blueberries decrease cardiovascular risk factors in obese men and women with metabolic syndrome. *Journal of Nutrition*, *140*(9), 1582–1587. https://doi.org/10.3945/jn.110.124701

Bercea, C. I., Cottrell, G. S., Tamagnini, F., & McNeish, A. J. (2021). Omega-3 polyunsaturated fatty acids and hypertension: a review of vasodilatory mechanisms of docosahexaenoic acid and eicosapentaenoic acid. *British Journal of Pharmacology*, *178*(4), 860–877. https://doi.org/10.1111/bph.15336

Blumenthal, J. A., Babyak, M. A., Hinderliter, A., Watkins, L. L., Craighead, L., Lin, P. H., ... Sherwood, A. (2010). Effects of the DASH diet alone and in combination with exercise and weight loss on blood pressure and cardiovascular biomarkers in men and women with high blood pressure: The ENCORE study. *Archives of Internal Medicine*, *170*(2), 126–135. https://doi.org/10.1001/archinternmed.2009.470

Borjesson, M., Onerup, A., Lundqvist, S., & Dahlof, B. (2016). Physical activity and exercise lower blood pressure in individuals with hypertension: Narrative review of 27 RCTs. *British Journal of Sports Medicine*, *50*(6), 356–361. https://doi.org/10.1136/bjsports-2015-095786

Bouchard, J., Valookaran, A. F., Aloud, B. M., Raj, P., Malunga, L. N., Thandapilly, S. J., & Netticadan, T. (2022). Impact of oats in the prevention/management of hypertension. *Food Chemistry*, *381*(July 2021), 132198. https://doi.org/10.1016/j.foodchem.2022.132198

Briasoulis, A., Agarwal, V., & Messerli, F. H. (2012). Alcohol Consumption and the Risk of Hypertension in Men and Women: A Systematic Review and Meta-Analysis. *Journal of Clinical Hypertension*, *14*(11), 792–798. https://doi.org/10.1111/jch.12008

Britton, A., & McKee, M. (2000). The relation between alcohol and cardiovascular disease in Eastern Europe: Explaining the paradox. *Journal of Epidemiology and Community Health*, *54*(5), 328–332. https://doi.org/10.1136/jech.54.5.328

Burnier, M. (2019). Should we eat more potassium to better control blood pressure in hypertension? *Nephrology Dialysis Transplantation*, *34*(2), 184–193. https://doi.org/10.1093/ndt/gfx340

Canale, M. P., Noce, A., Di Lauro, M., Marrone, G., Cantelmo, M., Cardillo, C., ... Tesauro, M. (2021). Gut dysbiosis and western diet in the pathogenesis of essential arterial hypertension: A narrative review. *Nutrients*, *13*(4). https://doi.org/10.3390/nu13041162

Carey, R. M., Muntner, P., Bosworth, H. B., & Whelton, P. K. (2018). Prevention and Control of Hypertension: JACC Health Promotion Series. *Journal of the American College of Cardiology*, *72*(11), 1278–1293. https://doi.org/10.1016/j.jacc.2018.07.008

Carpes, L., Costa, R., Schaarschmidt, B., Reichert, T., & Ferrari, R. (2022). High-intensity interval training reduces blood pressure in older adults: A systematic review and meta-analysis. *Experimental Gerontology*, *158*(October 2021), 111657. https://doi.org/10.1016/j.exger.2021.111657

Casonatto, J., Goessler, K. F., Cornelissen, V. A., Cardoso, J. R., & Polito, M. D. (2016). The blood pressure-lowering effect of a single bout of resistance exercise: A systematic review and meta-analysis of randomised controlled trials. *European Journal of Preventive Cardiology*, *23*(16), 1700–1714. https://doi.org/10.1177/2047487316664147

Chobanian, A. V., et al. (2003). The Seventh Report of the Joint National Committee on Prevention, Detection, Evaluation, and Treatment of High Blood Pressure: the JNC 7 report. *Jama*, *289*(19), 2560–2572.

Chow, C. K., Teo, K. K., Rangarajan, S., Islam, S., Gupta, R., Avezum, A., ... Yusuf, S. (2013). Prevalence, awareness, treatment, and control of hypertension in rural and urban communities in high-, middle-, and low-income countries. *JAMA - Journal of the American Medical Association*, *310*(9), 959–968. https://doi.org/10.1001/jama.2013.184182

Collins, R., et al. (1990). Blood pressure, stroke, and coronary heart disease. Part 2, Short-term reductions in blood pressure: overview of randomised drug trials in their epidemiological context. *Lancet*, *335*(8693), 827–838.

Colussi, G., Catena, C., Novello, M., Bertin, N., & Sechi, L. A. (2017). Impact of omega-3 polyunsaturated fatty acids on vascular function and blood pressure: Relevance for cardiovascular outcomes. *Nutrition, Metabolism and Cardiovascular Diseases*, *27*(3), 191–200. https://doi.org/10.1016/j.numecd.2016.07.011

Cormick, G., Ciapponi, A., Cafferata, M. L., Cormick, M. S., & Belizán, J. M. (2022). Calcium supplementation for prevention of primary hypertension. *Cochrane Database of Systematic Reviews*, *2022*(1). https://doi.org/10.1002/14651858.CD010037.pub4

Cornelissen, V. A., & Smart, N. A. (2013). Exercise training for blood pressure: a systematic review and meta-analysis. *Journal of the American Heart Association*, *2*(1), 1–9. https://doi.org/10.1161/JAHA.112.004473

Cowell, O. R., Mistry, N., Deighton, K., Matu, J., Griffiths, A., Minihane, A. M., ... Siervo, M. (2021). Effects of a Mediterranean diet on blood pressure: a systematic review and meta-analysis of randomized controlled trials and observational studies. *Journal of Hypertension*, *39*(4), 729–739. https://doi.org/10.1097/HJH.0000000000002667

D'Elia, L., La Fata, E., Galletti, F., Scalfi, L., & Strazzullo, P. (2019). Coffee consumption and risk of hypertension: a dose-response meta-analysis of prospective studies. *European Journal of Nutrition*, *58*(1), 271–280. https://doi.org/10.1007/s00394-017-1591-z

de Barcelos, G. T., Heberle, I., Coneglian, J. C., Vieira, B. A., Delevatti, R. S., & Gerage, A. M. (2022). Effects of Aerobic Training Progression on Blood Pressure in Individuals With Hypertension: A Systematic Review With Meta-Analysis and Meta-Regression. *Frontiers in Sports and Active Living*, *4*(February). https://doi.org/10.3389/fspor.2022.719063

De Giuseppe, R., Di Napoli, I., Granata, F., Mottolese, A., & Cena, H. (2019). Caffeine and blood pressure: A critical review perspective. *Nutrition Research Reviews*, *32*(2), 169–175. https://doi.org/10.1017/S0954422419000015

De Pergola, G., & D'alessandro, A. (2018). Influence of mediterranean diet on blood pressure. *Nutrients*, *10*(11), 2–7. https://doi.org/10.3390/nu10111700

DeMarco, V. G., Aroor, A. R., & Sowers, J. R. (2014). The pathophysiology of hypertension in patients with obesity. *Nature Reviews Endocrinology*, *10*(6), 364–376. https://doi.org/10.1038/nrendo.2014.44

Drawz, P. E., Alper, A. B., Anderson, A. H., Brecklin, C. S., Charleston, J., Chen, J., ... Ojo, A. (2016). Masked hypertension and elevated nighttime blood pressure in CKD: Prevalence and association with target organ damage. *Clinical Journal of the American Society of Nephrology*, *11*(4), 642–652. https://doi.org/10.2215/CJN.08530815

Egan, B. M., Li, J., Hutchison, F. N., & Ferdinand, K. C. (2014). Hypertension in the United States, 1999 to 2012: progress toward Healthy People 2020 goals. *Circulation*, *130*(19), 1692–1699. https://doi.org/10.1161/CIRCULATIONAHA.114.010676

Fernández-Solà, J. (2015). Cardiovascular risks and benefits of moderate and heavy alcohol consumption. *Nature Reviews Cardiology*, *12*(10), 576–587. https://doi.org/10.1038/nrcardio.2015.91

Filippou, C. D., Thomopoulos, C. G., Kouremeti, M. M., Sotiropoulou, L. I., Nihoyannopoulos, P. I., Tousoulis, D. M., & Tsioufis, C. P. (2021). Mediterranean diet and blood pressure reduction in adults with and without hypertension: A systematic review and meta-analysis of randomized controlled trials. *Clinical Nutrition*, *40*(5), 3191–3200. https://doi.org/10.1016/j.clnu.2021.01.030

Franklin, S. S., Larson, M. G., Khan, S. A., Wong, N. D., Leip, E. P., Kannel, W. B., & Levy, D. (2001). Does the relation of blood pressure to coronary heart disease risk change with aging?: The Framingham Heart Study. *Circulation*, *103*(9), 1245-1249. https://doi.org/10.1161/01.CIR.103.9.1245

Freis, E. D., et al. (1958). Treatment of essential hypertension with chlorothiazide (diuril); its use alone and combined with other antihypertensive agents. *J Am Med Assoc*, *166*(2), 137–140.

Freis, E. D. (1959). TREATMENT OF HYPERTENSION WITH CHLOROTHIAZIDE. *Journal of the American Medical Association*, *169*(2), 105–108.

Freis, E. D. (1959). Essential hypertension. *Heart Bull*, *8*(3):52–54.

Freis, E. D. (1969). The value of antihypertensive therapy. *Bull N Y Acad Med*, *45*(9), 951–962.

Freis, E. D, et al. (1974). The Veterans Administration Cooperative Study on Antihypertensive Agents. Implications for Stroke Prevention. *Stroke*, *5*(1), 76–77.

Freis, E. D. (1995). Hypertension: Pathophysiology, Diagnosis, and Management, Historical Development of Antihypertensive Treatment. *New York: Raven Press JHL Brenner*, 2nd ed.

Fu, J., Liu, Y., Zhang, L., Zhou, L., Li, D., Quan, H., . . . Zhao, Y. (2020). Non-pharmacologic interventions for reducing blood pressure in adults with prehypertension to established hypertension. *Journal of the American Heart Association*, *9*(19). https://doi.org/10.1161/JAHA.120.016804

Gibbs, J., Gaskin, E., Ji, C., Miller, M. A., & Cappuccio, F. P. (2021). The effect of plant-based dietary patterns on blood pressure: A systematic review and meta-analysis of controlled intervention trials. *Journal of Hypertension*, *39*(1), 23–37. https://doi.org/10.1097/HJH.0000000000002604

Gorostegi-Anduaga, I., Corres, P., MartinezAguirre-Betolaza, A., Pérez-Asenjo, J., Aispuru, G. R., Fryer, S. M., & Maldonado-Martín, S. (2018). Effects of different aerobic exercise programmes with nutritional intervention in sedentary adults with overweight/obesity and hypertension: EXERDIET-HTA study. *European Journal of Preventive Cardiology*, *25*(4), 343–353. https://doi.org/10.1177/2047487317749956

Grillo, A., Salvi, L., Coruzzi, P., Salvi, P., & Parati, G. (2019). Sodium intake and hypertension. *Nutrients*, *11*(9), 1–16. https://doi.org/10.3390/nu11091970

Guo, C., Zhou, Q., Zhang, D., Qin, P., Li, Q., Tian, G., . . . Hu, D. (2020). Association of total sedentary behaviour and television viewing with risk of overweight/obesity, type 2 diabetes and hypertension: A dose-response meta-analysis. *Diabetes, Obesity and Metabolism*, *22*(1), 79–90. https://doi.org/10.1111/dom.13867

Haber, S. L., & Gallus, K. (2012). Effects of dark chocolate on blood pressure in patients with hypertension. *American Journal of Health-System Pharmacy*, *69*(15), 1287–1293. https://doi.org/10.2146/ajhp110498

Hall, J. E. (2003). The kidney, hypertension, and obesity. *Hypertension*, *41*(3 II), 625–633. https://doi.org/10.1161/01.HYP.0000052314.95497.78

Hall, J. E., Do Carmo, J. M., Da Silva, A. A., Wang, Z., & Hall, M. E. (2015). Obesity-Induced Hypertension: Interaction of Neurohumoral and Renal Mechanisms. *Circulation Research*, *116*(6), 991–1006. https://doi.org/10.1161/CIRCRESAHA.116.305697

Hall, J. E., Granger, J. P., do Carmo, J. M., da Silva, A. A., Dubinion, J., George, E., . . . Hall, M. E. (2012). Hypertension: Physiology and pathophysiology. *Comprehensive Physiology*, *2*(4), 2393–2442. https://doi.org/10.1002/cphy.c110058

Hall, M. E., Cohen, J. B., Ard, J. D., Egan, B. M., Hall, J. E., Lavie, C. J., . . . Shimbo, D. (2021). Weight-Loss Strategies for Prevention and Treatment of Hypertension: A Scientific Statement from the American Heart Association. *Hypertension*, (November), E38–E50. https://doi.org/10.1161/HYP.0000000000000202

Han, H., Fang, X., Wei, X., Liu, Y., Jin, Z., Chen, Q., . . . Cao, Y. (2017). Dose-response relationship between dietary magnesium intake, serum magnesium concentration and risk of hypertension: A systematic review and meta-analysis of prospective cohort studies. *Nutrition Journal*, *16*(1), 1–12. https://doi.org/10.1186/s12937-017-0247-4

Hansford, H. J., Parmenter, B. J., McLeod, K. A., Wewege, M. A., Smart, N. A., Schutte, A. E., & Jones, M. D. (2021). The effectiveness and safety of isometric resistance training for adults with high blood pressure: a systematic review and meta-analysis. *Hypertension Research*, *44*(11), 1373–1384. https://doi.org/10.1038/s41440-021-00720-3

He, Q. Q. (2014). Association between alcohol consumption and risk of cardiovascular disease and all-cause mortality in patients with hypertension: a meta-analysis of prospective cohort studies. *Mayo Clinic Proceedings*, *89*(9), 1201–1210. https://doi.org/10.1016/j.mayocp.2014.05.014

Herrod, P. J. J., Doleman, B., Blackwell, J. E. M., O'Boyle, F., Williams, J. P., Lund, J. N., & Phillips, B. E. (2018). Exercise and other nonpharmacological strategies to reduce blood pressure in older adults: a systematic review and meta-analysis. *Journal of the American Society of Hypertension*, *12*(4), 248–267. https://doi.org/10.1016/j.jash.2018.01.008

Hinderliter, A. L., Sherwood, A., Craighead, L. W., Lin, P. H., Watkins, L., Babyak, M. A., & Blumenthal, J. A. (2014). The long-term effects of lifestyle change on blood pressure: One-year follow-up of the ENCORE study. *American Journal of Hypertension*, *27*(5), 734–741. https://doi.org/10.1093/ajh/hpt183

Ikdahl, E., Wibetoe, G., Rollefstad, S., Salberg, A., Bergsmark, K., Kvien, T. K., . . . Semb, A. G. (2019). Guideline recommended treatment to targets of cardiovascular risk is inadequate in patients with inflammatory joint diseases. *International Journal of Cardiology*, *274*, 311–318. https://doi.org/10.1016/j.ijcard.2018.06.111

Jafarnejad, S., Salek, M., & Clark, C. C. T. (2020). Cocoa Consumption and Blood Pressure in Middle-Aged and Elderly Subjects: a Meta-Analysis. *Current Hypertension Reports*, *22*(1). https://doi.org/10.1007/s11906-019-1005-0

Jama, H. A., Beale, A., Shihata, W. A., & Marques, F. Z. (2019). The effect of diet on hypertensive pathology: Is there a link via gut microbiota-driven immunometabolism? *Cardiovascular Research*, *115*(9), 1435–1447. https://doi.org/10.1093/cvr/cvz091

Jayedi, A., Rashidy-Pour, A., Khorshidi, M., & Shab-Bidar, S. (2018). Body mass index, abdominal adiposity, weight gain and risk of developing hypertension: a systematic review and dose-response meta-analysis of more than 2.3 million participants. *Obesity Reviews*, *19*(5), 654–667. https://doi.org/10.1111/obr.12656

Jayedi, Ahmad, & Zargar, M. S. (2019). Dietary calcium intake and hypertension risk: a dose response meta-analysis of prospective cohort studies. *European Journal of Clinical Nutrition*, *73*(7), 969–978. https://doi.org/10.1038/s41430-018-0275-y

Jordan, J., Kurschat, C., & Reuter, H. (2018). Arterial hypertension-diagnosis and treatment. *Deutsches Arzteblatt International*, *115*(33–34), 557–558. https://doi.org/10.3238/arztebl.2018.0557

Juraschek, S. P., Miller, E. R., Weaver, C. M., & Appel, L. J. (2017). Effects of Sodium Reduction and the DASH Diet in Relation to Baseline Blood Pressure. *Journal of the American College of Cardiology*, *70*(23), 2841–2848. https://doi.org/10.1016/j.jacc.2017.10.011

Kazeminia, M., Daneshkhah, A., Jalali, R., Vaisi-Raygani, A., Salari, N., & Mohammadi, M. (2020). The Effect of Exercise on the Older Adult's Blood Pressure Suffering Hypertension: Systematic Review and Meta-Analysis on Clinical Trial Studies. *International Journal of Hypertension*, *2020*. https://doi.org/10.1155/2020/2786120

Kearney, P. M., Whelton, M., Reynolds, K., Muntner, P., Whelton, P. K., & He, J. (2005). Global burden of hypertension: analysis of worldwide data. *The Lancet*, *365*(9455), 217–223. https://doi.org/10.1016/s0140-6736(05)17741-1

Kokkinos, P. (2014). Cardiorespiratory fitness, exercise, and blood pressure. *Hypertension*, *64*(6), 1160–1164. https://doi.org/10.1161/HYPERTENSIONAHA.114.03616

Lee, K. W., Loh, H. C., Ching, S. M., Devaraj, N. K., & Hoo, F. K. (2020). Effects of vegetarian diets on blood pressure lowering: A systematic review with meta-analysis and trial sequential analysis. *Nutrients*, *12*(6), 1–17. https://doi.org/10.3390/nu12061604

Lee, P. H., & Wong, F. K. Y. (2015). The Association Between Time Spent in Sedentary Behaviors and Blood Pressure: A Systematic Review and Meta-Analysis. *Sports Medicine*, *45*(6), 867–880. https://doi.org/10.1007/s40279-015-0322-y

Lelong, H., Blacher, J., Baudry, J., Adriouch, S., Galan, P., Fezeu, L., . . . Kesse-Guyot, E. (2017). Individual and combined effects of dietary factors on risk of incident hypertension prospective analysis from the nutrinet-santé cohort. *Hypertension*, *70*(4), 712–720. https://doi.org/10.1161/HYPERTENSIONAHA.117.09622

Lennon, S. L., DellaValle, D. M., Rodder, S. G., Prest, M., Sinley, R. C., Hoy, M. K., & Papoutsakis, C. (2017). 2015 Evidence Analysis Library Evidence-Based Nutrition Practice Guideline for the Management of Hypertension in Adults. *Journal of the Academy of Nutrition and Dietetics*, *117*(9), 1445–1458.e17. https://doi.org/10.1016/j.jand.2017.04.008

Liu, G., Mi, X. N., Zheng, X. X., Xu, Y. L., Lu, J., & Huang, X. H. (2014). Effects of tea intake on blood pressure: A meta-analysis of randomised controlled trials. *British Journal of Nutrition*, *112*(7), 1043–1054. https://doi.org/10.1017/S0007114514001731

Liu, X., Zhang, D., Liu, Y., Sun, X., Han, C., Wang, B., . . . Zhang, M. (2017). Dose-Response Association between Physical Activity and Incident Hypertension: A Systematic Review and Meta-Analysis of Cohort Studies. *Hypertension*, *69*(5), 813–820. https://doi.org/10.1161/HYPERTENSIONAHA.116.08994

Ma, C., Zheng, X., Yang, Y., & Bu, P. (2021). The effect of black tea supplementation on blood pressure: A systematic review and dose-response meta-analysis of randomized controlled trials. *Food and Function*, *12*(1), 41–56. https://doi.org/10.1039/d0fo02122a

MacDonald, H. V., Johnson, B. T., Huedo-Medina, T. B., Livingston, J., Forsyth, K. C., Kraemer, W. J., . . . Pescatello, L. S. (2016). Dynamic resistance training as stand-alone antihypertensive lifestyle therapy: A meta-analysis. *Journal of the American Heart Association*, *5*(10). https://doi.org/10.1161/JAHA.116.003231

MacMahon, S., et al. (1990). Blood pressure, stroke, and coronary heart disease. Part 1, Prolonged differences in blood pressure: prospective observational studies corrected for the regression dilution bias. *Lancet*, *335*(8692), 765–774.

Mahdavi-Roshan, M., Salari, A., Ghorbani, Z., & Ashouri, A. (2020). The effects of regular consumption of green or black tea beverage on blood pressure in those with elevated blood pressure or hypertension: A systematic review and meta-analysis. *Complementary Therapies in Medicine*, *51*(November 2019). https://doi.org/10.1016/j.ctim.2020.102430

Mahmood, S., Shah, K. U., Khan, T. M., Nawaz, S., Rashid, H., Baqar, S. W. A., & Kamran, S. (2019). Non-pharmacological management of hypertension: in the light of current research. *Irish Journal of Medical Science*, *188*(2), 437–452. https://doi.org/10.1007/s11845-018-1889-8

Medina, C., Janssen, I., Barquera, S., Bautista-Arredondo, S., González, M. E., & González, C. (2018). Occupational and leisure time physical inactivity and the risk of type II diabetes and hypertension among Mexican adults: A prospective cohort study. *Scientific Reports*, *8*(1), 4–10. https://doi.org/10.1038/s41598-018-23553-6

Miller, P. E., Van Elswyk, M., & Alexander, D. D. (2014). Long-chain Omega-3 fatty acids eicosapentaenoic acid and docosahexaenoic acid and blood pressure: A meta-analysis of randomized controlled trials. *American Journal of Hypertension*, *27*(7), 885–896. https://doi.org/10.1093/ajh/hpu024

Mills, K. T., Stefanescu, A., & He, J. (2020). The global epidemiology of hypertension. *Nature Reviews Nephrology*, *16*(4), 223–237. https://doi.org/10.1038/s41581-019-0244-2

Ndanuko, R. N., Tapsell, L. C., Charlton, K. E., Neale, E. P., & Batterham, M. J. (2016). Dietary patterns and blood pressure in adults: A systematic review and meta-analysis of randomized controlled trials. *Advances in Nutrition*, *7*(1), 76–89. https://doi.org/10.3945/an.115.009753

Neter, J. E., Stam, B. E., Kok, F. J., Grobbee, D. E., & Geleijnse, J. M. (2003). Influence of Weight Reduction on Blood Pressure: A Meta-Analysis of Randomized Controlled Trials. *Hypertension*, *42*(5), 878–884. https://doi.org/10.1161/01.HYP.0000094221.86888.AE

NICE guideline. (2019). Hypertension in adults: Diagnosis and management. *Https://Www.Nice.Org.Uk/Guidance/Ng136*, *49*(9).

Niu, Y., Cao, H., Zhou, H., Cao, J., & Wang, Z. (2022). Effects of a vegetarian diet combined with exercise on lipid profiles and blood pressure: A systematic review and meta-analysis. *Critical Reviews in Food Science and Nutrition*, *0*(0), 1–15. https://doi.org/10.1080/10408398.2022.2122923

O'Donnell, M. J., Denis, X., Liu, L., Zhang, H., Chin, S. L., Rao-Melacini, P., . . . Yusuf, S. (2010). Risk factors for ischaemic and intracerebral haemorrhagic stroke in 22 countries (the INTERSTROKE study): A case-control study. *The Lancet*, *376*(9735), 112–123. https://doi.org/10.1016/S0140-6736(10)60834-3

O'Donnell, M., Mente, A., & Yusuf, S. (2015). Sodium Intake and Cardiovascular Health. *Circulation Research*, *116*(6), 1046–1057. https://doi.org/10.1161/CIRCRESAHA.116.303771

Oliveros, E., Patel, H., Kyung, S., Fugar, S., Goldberg, A., Madan, N., & Williams, K. A. (2020). Hypertension in older adults: Assessment, management, and challenges. *Clinical Cardiology*, *43*(2), 99–107. https://doi.org/10.1002/clc.23303

Oparil, S., Acelajado, M. C., Bakris, G. L., Berlowitz, D. R., Cífková, R., Dominiczak, A. F., . . . Whelton, P. K. (2018). Hypertension. *Nature Reviews Disease Primers*, *4*. https://doi.org/10.1038/nrdp.2018.14

Organization World Health, & World Health Organization. (2012). Guideline: Sodium intake for adults and children. *World Health Organization*, 1–56. Retrieved from http://apps.who.int/iris/handle/10665/77985%5Cnhttp://www.ncbi.nlm.nih.gov/pubmed?term=Sodium%5BTitle%5D AND intake%5BTitle%5D AND adults%5BTitle%5D AND children%5BTitle%5D AND WHO%5BTitle%5D%5Cnhttp://www.ncbi.nlm.nih.gov/pubmed?term=Sodium%255BTitle%255

Panel, E., & Nda, A. (2015). Scientific Opinion on the safety of caffeine. *EFSA Journal*, *13*(5). https://doi.org/10.2903/j.efsa.2015.4102

Perumareddi, P. (2019). Prevention of Hypertension Related to Cardiovascular Disease. *Primary Care - Clinics in Office Practice*, *46*(1), 27–39. https://doi.org/10.1016/j.pop.2018.10.005

Pescatello, L. S., Buchner, D. M., Jakicic, J. M., Powell, K. E., Kraus, W. E., Bloodgood, B., . . . Piercy, K. L. (2019). Physical Activity to Prevent and Treat Hypertension: A Systematic Review. *Medicine and Science in Sports and Exercise*, *51*(6), 1314–1323. https://doi.org/10.1249/MSS.0000000000001943

Physical activity guidelines for Americans. (2008). *The Oklahoma Nurse*, *53*(4), 25. https://doi.org/10.1249/fit.0000000000000472

Piepoli, M. F., Hoes, A. W., Agewall, S., Albus, C., Brotons, C., Catapano, A. L., ... Verschuren, W. M. M. (2016). 2016 European Guidelines on cardiovascular disease prevention in clinical practice. *European Heart Journal, 37*(29), 2315–2381. https://doi.org/10.1093/eurheartj/ehw106

Poblete, P.F., et al. (1973). Effect of Treatment on Morbidity in Hypertension. Veterans Administration Cooperative Study on Antihypertensive Agents. *Circulation, 48*(3), 481–490.

Puddey, I. B., Mori, T. A., Barden, A. E., & Beilin, L. J. (2019). Alcohol and Hypertension—New Insights and Lingering Controversies. *Current Hypertension Reports, 21*(10). https://doi.org/10.1007/s11906-019-0984-1

Rees, K., Takeda, A., Martin, N., Ellis, L., Wijesekara, D., Vepa, A., ... Stranges, S. (2019). Mediterranean-style diet for the primary and secondary prevention of cardiovascular disease. *Cochrane Database of Systematic Reviews, 2019*(3). https://doi.org/10.1002/14651858.CD009825.pub3

Roccella, E. J. (1993). National High Blood Pressure Education Program Working Group Report on Primary Prevention of Hypertension. *Archives of Internal Medicine, 153*(2), 186–208. https://doi.org/10.1001/archinte.1993.00410020042003

Roerecke, M., Kaczorowski, J., Tobe, S. W., Gmel, G., Hasan, O. S. M., & Rehm, J. (2017). The effect of a reduction in alcohol consumption on blood pressure: a systematic review and meta-analysis. *The Lancet Public Health, 2*(2), e108–e120. https://doi.org/10.1016/S2468-2667(17)30003-8

Roerecke, M., Tobe, S. W., Kaczorowski, J., Bacon, S. L., Vafaei, A., Hasan, O. S. M., ... Rehm, J. (2018). Sex-specific associations between alcohol consumption and incidence of hypertension: A systematic review and meta-analysis of cohort studies. *Journal of the American Heart Association, 7*(13). https://doi.org/10.1161/JAHA.117.008202

Sacks, F. M., Svetkey, L. P., Vollmer, W. M., Appel, L. J., Bray, G. A., Harsha, D., ... Cutler, J. A. (2001). Effects on Blood Pressure of Reduced Dietary Sodium and the Dietary Approaches to Stop Hypertension (DASH) Diet. *New England Journal of Medicine, 344*(1), 3–10. https://doi.org/10.1056/NEJM200101043440101

Saco-Ledo, G., Valenzuela, P. L., Ramírez-Jiménez, M., Morales, J. S., Castillo-García, A., Blumenthal, J. A., ... Lucia, A. (2021). Acute Aerobic Exercise Induces Short-Term Reductions in Ambulatory Blood Pressure in Patients With Hypertension: A Systematic Review and Meta-Analysis. *Hypertension (Dallas, Tex. : 1979), 78*(6), 1844–1858. https://doi.org/10.1161/HYPERTENSIONAHA.121.18099

Samadian, F., Dalili, N., & Jamalian, A. (2016). Lifestyle modifications to prevent and control hypertension. *Iranian Journal of Kidney Diseases, 10*(5), 237–263.

Saneei, P., Salehi-Abargouei, A., Esmaillzadeh, A., & Azadbakht, L. (2014). Influence of Dietary Approaches to Stop Hypertension (DASH) diet on blood pressure: A systematic review and meta-analysis on randomized controlled trials. *Nutrition, Metabolism and Cardiovascular Diseases, 24*(12), 1253–1261. https://doi.org/10.1016/j.numecd.2014.06.008

Sardeli, A. V., Griffith, G. J., dos Santos, M. V. M. A., Ito, M. S. R., Nadruz, W., & Chacon-Mikahil, M. P. T. (2020). Do baseline blood pressure and type of exercise influence level of reduction induced by training in hypertensive older adults? A meta-analysis of controlled trials. *Experimental Gerontology, 140*(August). https://doi.org/10.1016/j.exger.2020.111052

Sardeli, A. V., Griffith, G. J., dos Santos, M. V. M. A., Ito, M. S. R., & Chacon-Mikahil, M. P. T. (2021). The effects of exercise training on hypertensive older adults: an umbrella meta-analysis. *Hypertension Research, 44*(11), 1434–1443. https://doi.org/10.1038/s41440-021-00715-0

Saydah, S., Bullard, K. M. K., Cheng, Y., Ali, M. K., Gregg, E. W., Geiss, L., & Imperatore, G. (2014). Trends in cardiovascular disease risk factors by obesity level in adults in the United States, NHANES 1999-2010. *Obesity, 22*(8), 1888–1895. https://doi.org/10.1002/oby.20761

Schwingshackl, L., Chaimani, A., Schwedhelm, C., Toledo, E., Pünsch, M., Hoffmann, G., & Boeing, H. (2019). Comparative effects of different dietary approaches on blood pressure in hypertensive and pre-hypertensive patients: A systematic review and network meta-analysis. *Critical Reviews in Food Science and Nutrition, 59*(16), 2674–2687. https://doi.org/10.1080/10408398.2018.1463967

Schwingshackl, L., Schwedhelm, C., Hoffmann, G., Knüppel, S., Iqbal, K., Andriolo, V., ... Boeing, H. (2017). Food groups and risk of hypertension: A systematic review and dose-response meta-analysis of prospective studies. *Advances in Nutrition, 8*(6), 793–803. https://doi.org/10.3945/an.117.017178

Shea, M. K., Nicklas, B. J., Houston, D. K., Miller, M. E., Davis, C. C., Kitzman, D. W., ... Kritchevsky, S. B. (2011). The effect of intentional weight loss on all-cause mortality in older adults: Results of a randomized controlled weight-loss trial. *American Journal of Clinical Nutrition, 94*(3), 839–846. https://doi.org/10.3945/ajcn.110.006379

Stamler, J., R. Stamler, and J. D. N. (1993). Blood pressure, systolic and diastolic, and cardiovascular risks. US population data. *Arch Intern Med, 153*(5), 598–615.

Stevens, V. J., Obarzanek, E., Cook, N. R., Lee, I. M., Appel, L. J., West, D. S., ... Cohen, J. (2001). Long-term weight loss and changes in blood pressure: Results of the trials of hypertension prevention, phase II. *Annals of Internal Medicine, 134*(1), 1–11. https://doi.org/10.7326/0003-4819-134-1-200101020-00007

The sixth report of the Joint National Committee on prevention, detection, evaluation, and treatment of high blood pressure. (1997). *Arch Intern Med, 157*(21), 2413–2446.

Travis D. Homan, Stephen Bordes, E. C. (2021). *Physiology*, Pulse Pressure.

Unger, T., Borghi, C., Charchar, F., Khan, N. A., Poulter, N. R., Prabhakaran, D., ... Schutte, A. E. (2020). 2020 International Society of Hypertension Global Hypertension Practice Guidelines. *Hypertension, 75*(6), 1334–1357. https://doi.org/10.1161/HYPERTENSIONAHA.120.15026

Valenzuela, P. L., Carrera-Bastos, P., Gálvez, B. G., Ruiz-Hurtado, G., Ordovas, J. M., Ruilope, L. M., & Lucia, A. (2021). Lifestyle interventions for the prevention and treatment of hypertension. *Nature Reviews Cardiology, 18*(4), 251–275. https://doi.org/10.1038/s41569-020-00437-9

van Mierlo, L. A. J., Arends, L. R., Streppel, M. T., Zeegers, M. P. A., Kok, F. J., Grobbee, D. E., & Geleijnse, J. M. (2006). Blood pressure response to calcium supplementation: a meta-analysis of randomized controlled trials. *Journal of Human Hypertension, 20*(8), 571–580. https://doi.org/10.1038/sj.jhh.1002038

Vasan, R.S., et al. (2001). Assessment of frequency of progression to hypertension in non-hypertensive participants in the Framingham Heart Study: a cohort study. *Lancet, 358*(9294), 1682–1686.

Veronese, N., Demurtas, J., Pesolillo, G., Celotto, S., Barnini, T., Calusi, G., ... Barbagallo, M. (2020). Magnesium and health outcomes: an umbrella review of systematic reviews and meta-analyses of observational and intervention studies. *European Journal of Nutrition, 59*(1), 263–272. https://doi.org/10.1007/s00394-019-01905-w

Wang, C. J., Shen, Y. X., & Liu, Y. (2016). Empirically Derived Dietary Patterns and Hypertension Likelihood: A Meta-Analysis. *Kidney and Blood Pressure Research, 41*(5), 570–581. https://doi.org/10.1159/000443456

Whelton, P. K., Appel, L. J., Espeland, M. A., Applegate, W. B., Ettinger, W. H., Kostis, J. B., ... Cutler, J. A. (1998). Sodium reduction and weight loss in the treatment of hypertension in older persons: A randomized controlled trial of nonpharmacologic interventions in the elderly (TONE).

Journal of the American Medical Association, 279(11), 839–846. https://doi.org/10.1001/jama.279.11.839

Whelton, P. K., Appel, L. J., Sacco, R. L., Anderson, C. A. M., Antman, E. M., Campbell, N., . . . Van Horn, L. V. (2012). Sodium, blood pressure, and cardiovascular disease: Further evidence supporting the American Heart Association sodium reduction recommendations. *Circulation, 126*(24), 2880–2889. https://doi.org/10.1161/CIR.0b013e318279acbf

Whelton, P. K., Carey, R. M., Aronow, W. S., Casey, D. E., Collins, K. J., Dennison Himmelfarb, C., . . . Wright, J. T. (2018). 2017 ACC/AHA/AAPA/ABC/ACPM/AGS/APhA/ASH/ASPC/NMA/PCNA Guideline for the Prevention, Detection, Evaluation, and Management of High Blood Pressure in Adults: Executive Summary: A Report of the American College of Cardiology/American Heart Association Task F. *Hypertension, 71*(6), 1269–1324. https://doi.org/10.1161/HYP.0000000000000066

Whelton, P. K., He, J., Cutler, J. A., Brancati, F. L., Appel, L. J., Follmann, D., . . . Pope, W. D. B. (1998). Effects of Oral Potassium on Blood Pressure. *Survey of Anesthesiology, 42*(2), 100. https://doi.org/10.1097/00132586-199804000-00041

WHO. (2016). WHO Guidelines on physical activity and sedentary behaviour. In *Routledge Handbook of Youth Sport*.

WHO. (2020). WHO Guidelines on physical activity and sedentary behaviour. In *Routledge Handbook of Youth Sport*.

Williams, B., Mancia, G., Spiering, W., Agabiti Rosei, E., Azizi, M., Burnier, M., . . . Brady, A. (2018). 2018 ESC/ESH Guidelines for the management of arterial hypertension. *European Heart Journal, 39*(33), 3021–3104. https://doi.org/10.1093/eurheartj/ehy339

Xu, R., Yang, K., Ding, J., & Chen, G. (2020). Effect of green tea supplementation on blood pressure. *Medicine, 99*(6), e19047. https://doi.org/10.1097/md.0000000000019047

Yokoyama, Y., Nishimura, K., Barnard, N. D., Takegami, M., Watanabe, M., Sekikawa, A., . . . Miyamoto, Y. (2014). Vegetarian diets and blood pressure. *JAMA Internal Medicine*, Vol. 174, pp. 577–587.

Zhou, B., Bentham, J., Di Cesare, M., Bixby, H., Danaei, G., Cowan, M. J., . . . Eggertsen, R. (2017). Worldwide trends in blood pressure from 1975 to 2015: a pooled analysis of 1479 population-based measurement studies with 19·1 million participants. *The Lancet, 389*(10064), 37–55. https://doi.org/10.1016/S0140-6736(16)31919-5

FURTHER READING

Bibliography

Bakker, E.A., Sui, X., Brellenthin, A.G., and Lee, D.C. (2018). Physical activity and fitness for the prevention of hypertension. *Current Opinions in Cardiology. 33*: 394–401.

Carey, R.M., Muntner, P., Bosworth, H.B., and Whelton, P.K. (2018). Prevention and control of hypertension: JACC health promotion series. *Journal of the American College of Cardiology 72*: 1278–1293.

Fu, J. et al. (2020). Nonpharmacologic interventions for reducing blood pressure in adults with prehypertension to established hypertension. *Journal of the American Heart Association. 9*.

Hall, M. E. et al. (2021). Weight-loss strategies for prevention and treatment of hypertension: A scientific statement from the American Heart Association. *Hypertension* E38–E50.

Jordan, J., Kurschat, C., and Reuter, H. (2018). Arterial hypertension-diagnosis and treatment. *Deutsches Ärzteblatt International. 115*: 557–558.

Kokkinos, P. (2014). Cardiorespiratory fitness, exercise, and blood pressure. *Hypertension 64*: 1160–1164.

Oparil, S. et al. (2018). Hypertension. *Nature Reviews Disease Primers 4*.

Samadian, F., Dalili, N., and Jamalian, A. (2016). Lifestyle modifications to prevent and control hypertension. *Iranian Journal of Kidney Diseases. 10*: 237–263.

Unger, T. et al. (2020). International Society of Hypertension global hypertension practice guidelines. *Hypertension 75*: 1334–1357.

Links

- https://www.heart.org/en/health-topics/high-blood-pressure
- https://www.ahajournals.org/journal/hyp
- https://www.bloodpressureuk.org/
- https://www.eshonline.org/
- https://www.who.int/health-topics/hypertension#tab=tab_1
- https://www.bhf.org.uk/informationsupport/risk-factors/high-blood-pressure
- https://www.kidney.org/atoz/atozTopic_HighBloodPressure
- https://www.heartfoundation.org.nz/wellbeing/managing-risk/managing-high-blood-pressure
- https://www.nice.org.uk/guidance/ng136

Dyslipidemia

CHAPTER 17

Introduction	259	Triglycerides	265
Epidemiology	259	Low-density Lipoprotein-cholesterol	266
Pathophysiology	260	High-density Lipoprotein-cholesterol	266
Risk Factors	260	Type of Exercise Training and Blood Lipids	267
Cardiovascular Disease Risk Assessment	261	Intensity of Training and Blood Lipids	267
Preventing ASCVD	261	Dyslipidemia in Older adults: The Role of Physical Activity and Diet	268
Management	262	Key Points	270
Diet	262	Self-assessment Questions	270
DASH Diet	264	Case Scenario	270
Mediterranean Diet	264	References	271
Physical Activity and Exercise Training Role on Blood Lipids	264	Further Reading	274
Physical-activity Recommendations	264	Bibliography	274
Total Cholesterol	265	Links	274

INTRODUCTION

Lipoproteins found in blood are chylomicrons, very low-density lipoprotein (VLDL), intermediate-density lipoprotein (IDL), low-density lipoprotein (LDL), and high-density lipoprotein (HDL) (Lee & Siddiqui, 2022). Chylomicrons, VLDL, IDL, and LDL are pro-atherogenic molecules, while HDL is an anti-atherogenic lipoprotein (Feingold, 2000a). (**Figure 17.1**).

Abnormal blood-lipid levels are a common health condition. High levels of total cholesterol, LDL-cholesterol, and/or triglycerides (TG) as well as low levels of HDL-cholesterol are defined as dyslipidemia or hyperlipidemia (Hill & Bordoni, 2022; Pirillo, Casula, Olmastroni, Norata, & Catapano, 2021). Guidelines on standard levels of blood lipids are shown in **Table 17.1** (NCEP, 2001).

Dyslipidemia may have a genetic background (primary or familial) or it may be acquired (secondary) (Hill & Bordoni, 2022). The most common causes of secondary dyslipidemia are diabetes mellitus, some rare endocrine disorders, nephrotic syndrome, renal failure, use of medications, hypothyroidism, alcohol consumption, and metabolic disorders (Nouh, Omar, & Younis, 2019). Most patients have both a family history of dyslipidemia and secondary factors, most commonly the use of medications (i.e., beta blockers, estrogens, thiazide diuretics, amiodarone, and glucocorticoids (Hill & Bordoni, 2022; Nouh et al., 2019)), hypothyroidism, uncontrolled diabetes, and/or an unhealthy lifestyle in terms of an unhealthy diet and physical inactivity.

EPIDEMIOLOGY

Dyslipidemia is a common health condition. Hypercholesterolemia – defined as an LDL-cholesterol level of ≥130 mg/dl [or ≥100 mg/dl in patients with Diabetes Mellitus (DM) or cardiovascular disease (CVD)] or the self-reported use of medication to control cholesterol – is considered a major risk factor for atherosclerotic cardiovascular disease (ASCVD) and mortality (Barquera et al., 2015).

Based on epidemiological data, in the 2003–2006 National Health and Nutrition Examination Survey (NHANES), 53%

Prevention and Management of Cardiovascular and Metabolic Disease: Diet, Physical Activity and Healthy Aging,
First Edition. Christina N. Katsagoni, Peter Kokkinos, and Labros S. Sidossis.
© 2023 John Wiley & Sons Ltd. Published 2023 by John Wiley & Sons Ltd.

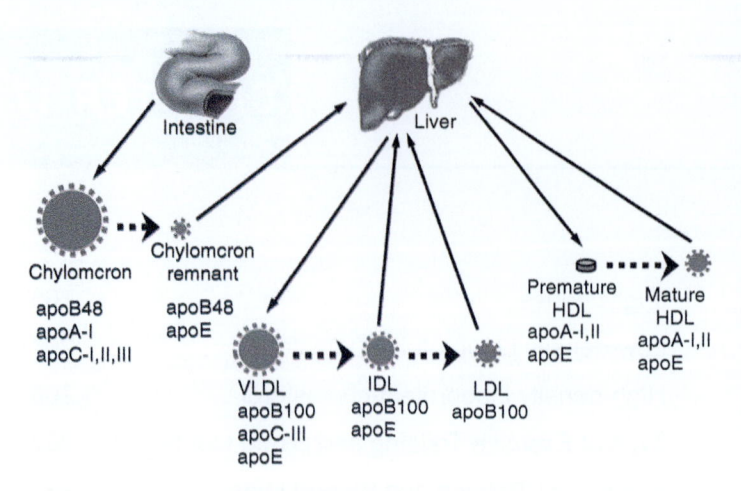

FIGURE 17.1 Overview of lipoprotein metabolism. Human lipoproteins are predominantly produced by the small intestine and the liver. Small intestine produces chylomicron, which contains apoB48, apoA-I, apoC-I, apoC-II, and apoC-III. The remnant particles, after use of lipids by the peripheral tissue, are taken up by the hepatocytes. The liver produces apoB-100-containing VLDL and premature HDL. VLDL is hydrolyzed in circulation and converted into IDL and LDL. Both IDL and LDL can be taken up by the hepatocytes. The discoidal shaped premature HDL becomes mature HDL in the circulation and serves an important role in reverse cholesterol transport. VLDL = very low-density lipoprotein; HDL = high-density lipoproteins; IDL = intermediate-density lipoprotein; LDL = low-density lipoprotein. Source: (Jiang, Robson, & Yao, 2013).

Table 17.1 Standard guidelines for blood-lipid levels.

Fasting triglycerides level	Normal: less than 150 mg/dL
	Mild hypertriglyceridemia: 150 to 499 mg/dL
	Moderate hypertriglyceridemia: 500 to 886 mg/dL
	Very high or severe hypertriglyceridemia: greater than 886 mg/dL
LDL-cholesterol level	Optimal: less than 100 mg/dL
	Near optimal/above optimal: 100 to 129 mg/dL
	Borderline high: 130 to 159 mg/dL
	High: 160 to 189 mg/dL
	Very high: greater than 190 mg/dL
HDL-cholesterol level	Low: less than 40
	High: greater than or equal to 60

Source: (NCEP, 2001).

(105.3 million) of US adults had lipid abnormalities, of which 27% had high LDL-cholesterol, 23% had low HDL-C, and 30% had high TG. Notably, 21% of US adults were found to have two lipid abnormalities at the same time, i.e., high LDL-cholesterol with either low HDL-cholesterol and/or high TG, while nearly 6% had all three lipid abnormalities (Tóth, Potter, & Ming, 2012). Based on the 2005–2008 NHANES survey, 33.5% (an estimated 71 million) of the US adults aged ≥20 years had high LDL-cholesterol (CDC, 2011). Moreover, according to the 2016 report from the American Heart Association, more than 100 million adults in the US over 20 years of age have total-cholesterol levels ≥200 mg/dL and almost 31 million have levels ≥240 mg/dL (Mozaffarian et al., 2016).

PATHOPHYSIOLOGY

Cholesterol may be synthesized in the liver or consumed through the diet. Cholesterol is needed by the body to synthesize steroid hormones, cell membranes, and bile acids, which are synthesized in the liver. It is also found in adipose tissue. Dyslipidemia occurs when pathway defects in lipoprotein synthesis, processing, and clearance can lead to accumulation of atherogenic lipids in plasma and endothelium formation (Nie & Luo, 2021; Nouh et al., 2019).

Elevated blood lipids - especially hypercholesterolemia - are associated with the development of atherosclerosis since they can change the cellular permeability of the arteries. This process causes inflammation. Briefly, monocytes from circulation adhere to the endothelial cells on the arterial walls. Selectins, special adhesion molecules expressed by endothelial cells, contribute to the migration of monocytes to the subendothelial. There, monocytes turn into foamy macrophages that are rich in cholesterol esters and free fatty acids and cause a thickening lesion on the arterial wall, called atherosclerotic plaque. Atherosclerotic plaque is prone to rupture that may form a clot able to block blood supply either to the heart, causing a heart attack, or to the brain, causing a stroke (Barquera et al., 2015).

RISK FACTORS

Several risk factors have been associated with the presence or risk for developing dyslipidemia. These risk factors may be non-modifiable or modifiable (Nouh et al., 2019). The non-modifiable risk factors include older age, sex (men are vulnerable at a younger age than women), and genetics.

However, it is possible to prevent or improve modifiable risk factors associated with dyslipidemia risk. Use of several medication (mentioned earlier in this chapter), unhealthy lifestyle, including high intake of saturated fatty acids (SFA) or trans fatty acids (TFA), high calorie intake leading to obesity, lack of physical activity, as well as smoking are common modifiable risk factors for dyslipidemia (Karr, 2017; Nouh et al., 2019).

Regarding the effects of SFA on lipid profile, in 2016, the WHO conducted a systematic review and meta-analysis of 84 clinical trials assessing the effects of SFA intake and its replacement with other nutrients in blood-lipid levels. Consumption of SFA was found to increase LDL-cholesterol levels (Mensink & World Health Organization, 2016). Moreover, replacing a mixture of SFA with cis-poly-unsaturated fatty acids (PUFA) (predominantly linoleic acid and α-linolenic acid) or cis-mono-unsaturated fatty acids (MUFA) (predominantly oleic acid) were more favorable than replacing SFA with a mixture of carbohydrates. Regarding total and LDL-cholesterol and TG the most favorable effects were observed for cis-PUFA.

A similar systematic review and meta-analysis was conducted by WHO for TFA, showing an increase in total cholesterol and LDL-cholesterol levels with the increase of TFA consumption (World Health Organization & Brouwer, 2016). Replacement of TFA from any source (industrial or ruminant TFA) by cis-PUFA was found to lessen total cholesterol, LDL-cholesterol, and ApoB for all TFA as well as improving HDL-cholesterol, and ratios of total cholesterol to HDL-cholesterol, and of LDL-cholesterol to HDL-cholesterol. These results highlight the connection of dietary factors with blood-lipid levels.

Abnormalities in lipid profile are very commonly observed in individuals with obesity (Feingold, 2000b). Up to 60% to 70% of subjects with obesity have dyslipidemia, which is known to further increase the risk for CVD (Bays et al., 2013). Obesity induced dyslipidemia recognized as "metabolic dyslipidemia" is driven by several pathophysiological factors including impaired production of adipokines and chronic low-grade inflammation in adipose tissue, which lead to insulin resistance, the main driving force in the development of metabolic dyslipidemia in obesity (Vekic, Zeljkovic, Stefanovic, Jelic-Ivanovic, & Spasojevic-Kalimanovska, 2019).

A sedentary lifestyle is also known to increase the risk for dyslipidemia. The association of sedentary behavior with abnormal blood-lipid levels have been observed in several studies indicating high total cholesterol, LDL-cholesterol and TG levels and low HDL-cholesterol levels in less active individuals (Crichton & Alkerwi, 2015; Pang et al., 2019; Park et al., 2018).

CARDIOVASCULAR DISEASE RISK ASSESSMENT

As dyslipidemia and especially hypercholesterolemia is highly correlated to atherosclerotic CVD (Hill & Bordoni, 2022; Pirillo et al., 2021), several tools exist for the assessment of CVD risk. CVD risk is defined as "the probability that an individual will experience an acute coronary or stroke event within a specific time period" (Zhao, Liu, Xie, & Qi, 2015).

These tools are of great importance for CVD prevention (Zhao et al., 2015). What is important is that the available tools differ according to the target population (i.e., American, European, Australian individuals etc.), the incorporated risk factors, and the predicted outcome. Most of these tools assess common risk factors for CVD, such as age, blood pressure, total-cholesterol or LDL-cholesterol levels, total cholesterol to HDL-cholesterol ratio, and smoking, while some models assess others, such as lipoprotein(a) level, C-reactive protein level, triglyceride level, family history of premature coronary heart disease (CHD), and obesity. Concerning the predicted outcome, some models are designed to predict total CVD risk, some may predict incidence of a CVD event, and some predict mortality.

Two of the most well-known CVD risk assessment tools are the American College of Cardiology/American Heart Association ASCVD risk estimator and the European SCORE. The 10-year ASCVD risk can be predicted for individuals aged 20 to 79 years using the American College of Cardiology/American Heart Association ASCVD risk estimator, by considering known risk factors, i.e., age, sex, race, SBP, DBP, total cholesterol, HDL-cholesterol, LDL-cholesterol, diabetes, smoking, treatment of hypertension, statin treatment, and aspirin treatment. $SCORE_2$ is a recently updated SCORE version aiming to estimate 10-year fatal and non-fatal CVD risk in individuals without previous CVD or diabetes aged 40 to 69 years in Europe (ESC, 2021). It incorporates known CVD risk factors, i.e., age, sex, SBP, non-HDL-cholesterol levels, and smoking, and it divides European regions into four CVD risk levels: low, moderate, high, and very high. Recently, an adjustment became available for older adults, over 70 years of age (ESC, 2021).

PREVENTING ASCVD

The prevention of dyslipidemia is eventually associated with the prevention of ASCVD. For the primary prevention of ASCVD it is important to identify the individuals who are at risk of dyslipidemia. Assessing the risk for ASCVD, monitoring blood-lipid levels, along with lifestyle modifications (Stone, Blumenthal, Lloyd-Jones, & Grundy, 2020) such as reduction in SFA intake, increase in physical activity, and weight control to lower cholesterol levels (NCEP, 2001) and pharmacological treatment, if needed, are the key messages in the 2020 guidelines for the primary prevention of dyslipidemia (Stone et al., 2020).

Secondary prevention refers to individuals with already confirmed clinical ASCVD (Virani, Smith, Stone, & Grundy, 2020). The 2020 guidelines for the secondary prevention of ASCVD highlight LDL-cholesterol as the primary treatment target, recommending a healthy lifestyle for all patients while giving emphasis on the management of blood-lipid levels (more about the management of dyslipidemia will be discussed later in this chapter).

Exercise is an important aspect of lifestyle that may contribute to the prevention and management of hypercholesterolemia and ASCVD. With regard to the dyslipidemia prevention, Bakker et al. (Bakker et al., 2018) examined the association of resistance exercise and the risk of developing hypercholesterolemia in men. Various characteristics of the participants, lifestyle factors (e.g., tobacco use or alcohol intake) and aerobic training were considered, but not diet or medication. The results showed that men who engaged in the suggested amount of resistance exercise (2 or more d/week) had a 13% lower risk of developing hypercholesterolemia, independent of the aerobic training. Individuals performing both aerobic and resistance training, according to the guidelines, had a 21% lower risk of developing hypercholesterolemia, compared to those who did not meet the recommendations for physical activity. In addition, one hour of resistance exercise was enough to lower the risk by 32%, while training 1 to 2 times/week was able to lower the risk by 31%, compared to a lack of resistance training. Notably, increasing the duration or frequency of exercise did not show any further benefit. Researchers concluded that combining resistance exercise with aerobic could be beneficial for preventing hypercholesterolemia in men (Bakker et al., 2018).

MANAGEMENT

Management of hyperlipidemia is essential for the prevention of atherosclerosis. This includes pharmacotherapy as well as lifestyle changes, i.e., diet, physical activity, and weight reduction (Fischer, Schatz, & Julius, 2015).

Concerning pharmacological treatment, statins are the first line of treatment for the management of hyperlipidemia (Fischer et al., 2015) and for primary and secondary prevention of ASCVD (Last, Ference, & Menzel, 2017). They work by reducing total cholesterol and LDL-cholesterol (Karr, 2017). Patients drinking grapefruit juice in large quantities, should be reminded of the potential for an interaction with statins. In case of statin intolerance, other lipid-lowering drugs may be used. These are bile-acid sequestrants, ezetimibe, fibric acids, niacin, cholesterol absorption and synthesis inhibitors, as well as the recently approved class, proprotein convertase subtilisin/kexin type 9 (PCSK9). Niacin, fibrates, and omega-3 fatty acids should not be routinely prescribed for primary or secondary prevention of ASCVD, as it seems that they do not affect patient-oriented outcomes (Karr, 2017; Last et al., 2017).

In the following paragraphs, the importance of diet and physical activity on the management of dyslipidemia will be discussed. The impact of several lifestyles changes on blood-lipid levels is shown on **Table 17.2** (ESC/EAS, 2019).

DIET

For the management of hyperlipidemia, fat quality and fat quantity are of great importance (E. A. Trautwein, Vermeer, Hiemstra, & Ras, 2018). The reduction of SFA and TFA is suggested in the case of dyslipidemia (Jacobson et al., 2015). According to the 2020 guidelines for the management of dyslipidemia, the reduction of SFA intake and their replacement with unsaturated fatty acids as well as the avoidance of TFA is suggested (Mach et al., 2020). As already mentioned, in order to reduce LDL-cholesterol, it is important to replace SFA with MUFA or PUFA, and this does not affect HDL-cholesterol or TG levels (Elke A. Trautwein & McKay, 2020). Evidence suggests that the replacement of SFA with PUFA has a greater reduction effect on LDL-cholesterol compared to MUFA (Mensink et al., 2016; Schwingshackl et al., 2018; Elke A. Trautwein & McKay, 2020). Moreover, the replacement of SFA with carbohydrates is not recommended as albeit the reduction in LDL-cholesterol, there is also a reduction in HDL-cholesterol and an increase in TG levels, which are both unfavorable outcomes (Mensink et al., 2016; Elke A. Trautwein & McKay, 2020).

Several studies exist assessing the effects of natural products, such as nutrients, specific foods or components of a plant-based diet on blood-lipid levels management (Bahmani et al., 2015; El-Tantawy & Temraz, 2019; Nie & Luo, 2021; Elke A. Trautwein & McKay, 2020). Evidence indicates that the consumption of β-glucans, a dietary fiber found in oat, has been shown to reduce total cholesterol and LDL-cholesterol (El-Tantawy & Temraz, 2019; Zhu et al., 2015). The hypocholesterolemic effect of β-glucans lies in their ability to increase bile-acid synthesis (El-Tantawy & Temraz, 2019).The ideal dose of β-glucans is still under investigation, but 3g/d may be an effective dosage (Nie & Luo, 2021). Phytosterols, plant sterols or stanols, are molecules that resemble cholesterol with cholesterol reduction action (Elke A. Trautwein & McKay, 2020). As far as food groups are concerned, all plant-based foods contain some amount of phytosterol. Good sources are vegetable oils, vegetable oil-based margarines, seeds, nuts, cereal grains, legumes, vegetables, and fruits as well as foods with added phytosterols (E. A. Trautwein et al., 2018). Phytosterols, because of their resemblance with cholesterol, can decrease intestinal absorption of cholesterol through the reduction of cholesterol content within the micelles, which subsequently decreases available

Table 17.2 Impact of specific lifestyle changes on lipid levels. The magnitude of the effect (+++ = >10%, ++ = 5–10%, + = <5%) and the level of evidence refer to the impact of each dietary modification on plasma levels of a specific lipoprotein class.

	Magnitude of the effect	Level
Lifestyle interventions to reduce TC and LDL-C levels		
Avoid dietary trans fats	++	A
Reduce dietary saturated fats	++	A
Increase dietary fibre	++	A
Use functional foods enriched with phytosterols	++	A
Use red yeast rice nutraceuticals	++	A
Reduce excessive body weight	++	A
Reduce dietary cholesterol	+	B
Increase habitual physical activity	+	B
Lifestyle interventions to reduce TG-rich lipoprotein levels		
Reduce excessive body weight	+	A
Reduce alcohol intake	+++	A
Increase habitual physical activity	++	A
Reduce total amount of dietary carbohydrates	++	A
Use supplements of n-3 polyunsaturated fats	++	A
Reduce intake of mono- and disaccharides	++	B
Replace saturated fats with mono- or polyunsaturated fats	+	B
Lifestyle interventions to increase HDL-C levels		
Avoid dietary trans fats	++	A
Increase habitual physical activity	+++	A
Reduce excessive body weight	++	A
Reduce dietary carbohydrates and replace them with unsaturated fats	++	A
Modest consumption in those who take alcohol may be continued	++	B
Quit smoking	+	B

Source: (ESC/EAS, 2019).

cholesterol for liver uptake. As a result, the expression of LDL-cholesterol receptors increases and the uptake of plasma LDL-cholesterol gets higher (El-Tantawy & Temraz, 2019). Recommended consumption of phytosterols is ≥2 g/d and can only be achieved through the consumption of enriched products.

Except for the use of single foods or nutrients for the management of dyslipidemia, research is focused on dietary patterns that may have beneficial effects. Some examples of dietary patterns researched for their benefits on the management of dyslipidemia are the Mediterranean diet (MD), Nordic diet, DASH diet, Portfolio diet, and vegetarian/vegan diet patterns (Elke A. Trautwein & McKay, 2020). More details about background and characteristics can be found in **Table 17.3**. What is common to all of them is the recommendation for a high consumption of plant-based foods, such as fruit, vegetables, legumes, whole grains, nuts, and seeds. However, long-standing literature including high quality evidence related to the management of dyslipidemia exist for both DASH diet and MD.

Table 17.3 Dietary patterns used for the management of dyslipidemia and their key characteristics.

Healthy Dietary Pattern	Background/Definition	Key Characteristics
Mediterranean (MED) diet	Traditionally based on dietary patterns typical of Crete, Greece, and Southern Italy in the early 1960s. No uniform definition of a MED diet, but MED dietary patterns emphasize plant-based foods and olive oil as main dietary fat source. Modified versions were studied in the PREDIMED trial[1].	Eating plenty of fruits, vegetables, legumes, (whole) grains, nuts; olive oils as main oil for daily use; moderate intake of fish; poultry and dairy foods like yogurt and cheese; eating less red meat, meat products and sweets; allows wine (in moderation) with meals. The MED diet is high in dietary fat and especially monounsaturated fatty acids but low in saturated fat.
Nordic diet	A dietary pattern comparable to the MED diet that emphasises traditional, locally grown, and seasonal foods of the Nordic countries. Developed as a diet to address health concerns such as obesity and taking local food culture, environmental aspects, and sustainability into account[2].	Emphasizes locally grown, seasonal foods; eating plenty of fruits, e.g., berries, vegetables, e.g., cabbage, legumes, potatoes, whole grains, e.g., oats and rye breads, nuts, seeds, fish and seafood, low-fat dairy, rapeseed oil, and, in moderation, game meats, free-range eggs, cheese, and yogurt; rarely eating red meats and animal fats; avoiding sugar-sweetened beverages, added sugars, processed meats. The Nordic diet is especially rich in dietary fiber and low in sugar and sodium.
Dietary approaches to stop hypertension (DASH) diet	A prescribed dietary pattern originally developed to lower blood pressure as studied in the DASH clinical trials[3].	Eating plenty of fruits, vegetables, legumes, whole grains; including fat-free or low-fat dairy products, fish, poultry, nuts, seeds, and vegetable oils; limiting fatty meats, tropical oils, sweets, sugar-sweetened beverages. The DASH diet is low in saturated fat, dietary cholesterol, salt (sodium), and high in dietary fiber, potassium, and calcium.
Portfolio diet	A predominately plant-based, vegan-type diet developed to further include a portfolio of foods/food components that are known to lower total and LDL-cholesterol[4].	Eating a diet low in fat (<30% of energy), especially saturated fat (<7% of energy), and high in fruits and vegetables with the addition of four plant-based, cholesterol-lowering foods: 50 g/day plant protein from various soy foods, legumes like beans, chickpeas, lentils; 45 g/day (about a handful) nuts such as peanuts, almonds; 20 g/day viscous soluble fiber from oats, barley, eggplant, okra, apples, berries, oranges, and psyllium; 2 g/day plant sterols from enriched foods such as spreads, dairy-type foods, or from supplements.
Vegetarian/vegan diet pattern	Dietary patterns of specific population groups that were adapted based on observational studies and randomized controlled trials.	Eating plenty of fruits, vegetables, legumes, whole grains, nuts and seeds, specific foods, e g., soy products and excluding meat and poultry and partly also dairy foods, eggs, and fish; lacto/ovo-vegetarians eat eggs and dairy products; lacto-vegetarians consume dairy products, ovo-vegetarians eat eggs, and pesco-vegetarians eat fish and seafood; vegans completely refrain of all animal-based foods including meat, poultry, eggs, dairy foods, and fish. Vegetarian/vegan diets are high in dietary fiber, and typically low in total and saturated fat, intake of n-3 fatty, acids, iron, and vitamin B_{12}.

Adapted in parts from Hemler and Hu, 2019; Zampelas and Magriplis, 2019; Magkos et al. 2020.
[1] Estruch et al., 2006;
[2] Bere and Brug;
[3] Appel et al., 1997;
[4] Jenkins et al.
Source: (Elke A. Trautwein & McKay, 2020).

DASH DIET

The DASH diet (Dietary Approaches to Stop Hypertension) is the commonly recommended diet for the reduction of CVD risk. It consists mostly of fruits, vegetables, and low-fat dairy products with reduced total and saturated fat (Appel et al., 1997). As described in **Chapter 16**, it was originally aiming to reduce blood pressure. However, it has also been proved to lower LDL-cholesterol, total cholesterol, and TG as well as HDL-cholesterol. Researchers tried a high-fat, low-carbohydrate alternative DASH diet in comparison to the standard DASH diet and a control diet. The results showed similar reductions in LDL-cholesterol between standard and alternative DASH diets, but the lower-fat DASH diet seemed to lower the HDL-cholesterol less, though this difference was not statistically significant (Chiu et al., 2016).

The OmniHeart trial examined the effects of three types of diet, a carbohydrate diet, very similar to the DASH diet, a high-protein diet, and a high-unsaturated fat diet (mostly MUFA), which followed both the main principles of DASH diet. Evidence showed that, compared to the carbohydrate diet, the protein diet decreased more total cholesterol, LDL, TG, and HDL. The high unsaturated-fat diet had the same effect on LDL-cholesterol as the carbohydrate diet had, but it decreased total cholesterol and TG more, while it increased HDL-cholesterol. The consumption of MUFA can, therefore, increase the serum levels of HDL (Appel et al., 2005).

MEDITERRANEAN DIET

MD is known for its beneficial effects on CVD. The MD, a plant-based dietary pattern (Bach-Faig et al., 2011) supplemented with extra virgin olive oil (high in MUFA) and the MD supplemented with nuts (high in MUFA and PUFA) were both evaluated for their effects on CVD, compared to a low-fat diet. Both of these MD versions were more beneficial for the blood-lipid profile than a typical low-fat diet, showing an increase in HDL-cholesterol serum levels and in the total cholesterol to HDL-cholesterol ratio (Estruch et al., 2006).

Combining the MD with weight loss and physical activity may have better results on the management of blood lipids than diet alone. The PREDIMED-plus trial included overweight and obese adults with metabolic syndrome and randomized them into an intervention group with intensive weight-loss lifestyle intervention, following an energy-restricted MD, physical activity, and behavioral support or a control group, in which participants were given information on the MD (Salas-Salvadó et al., 2018). After the 12-month intervention, the intervention group had a greater improvement in TG and HDL levels than the control group.

A recent randomized control-trial (RCT) investigated the effect of the MD on blood lipids, among other variables, in obese and overweight individuals (Meslier et al., 2020). Eighty-two adults participated in the 8-week trial and were randomized either to a MD group or to a habitual diet-control group. The energy intake of individuals in each group remained the same as baseline for each participant. Results showed that following a MD pattern leads to a decrease in total cholesterol, LDL-cholesterol, and HDL-cholesterol, independently of energy intake, and more importantly, the decrease in cholesterol was proportional to adherence rates of the dietary pattern.

According to a recent systematic review of clinical trials that assessed the use of olive oil compared with other types of oils, the consumption of olive oil was able to increase HDL-cholesterol by up to 7 mg/dL (Rondanelli et al., 2016). In summary, it appears that a diet rich in olive oil, especially virgin olive oil (Covas et al., 2006) such as the MD, is effective in raising HDL-cholesterol levels.

PHYSICAL ACTIVITY AND EXERCISE TRAINING ROLE ON BLOOD LIPIDS

Epidemiological and clinical data support a beneficial role of physical activity on the management of blood-lipid levels. Lin et al. conducted a meta-analysis including 160 RCTs published from 1965 to 2014, including 7487 participants in total. Researchers aimed to assess the relationship between any type of exercise training and blood-lipid levels (Lin et al., 2015). All RCTs had at least one intervention (exercise) group and a control group. Results showed that exercise training decreased TG levels and increased HDL-cholesterol levels, suggesting that exercise training may also affect cardiovascular health through other pathways, apart from modifying total cholesterol and LDL-cholesterol.

Physical activity may have a synergistic role with dietary fatty acids on altering lipid profile (Harris et al., 2018). In the study by Harris et al., the consumption of MUFA instead of carbohydrates was inversely associated with TG levels in both sexes, while the consumption of n-3 PUFA instead of carbohydrates was directly associated with HDL-cholesterol levels in women. However, these associations were mainly seen in participants with the lowest physical activity level or the highest time spent on sedentary activities (Harris et al., 2018), suggesting a cumulative effect of both dietary and physical activity alterations.

Several mechanisms by which physical activity improves the lipid profile have been suggested (He & Ye, 2020; Lin et al., 2015). One possible mechanism suggests that exercise may accelerate reverse cholesterol transport (Leaf, 2003; Lin et al., 2015). Reverse cholesterol transport is mediated by HDL-cholesterol. HDL-cholesterol is known for its anti-atherogenic effects, and its levels are increased after exercise training. HDL-cholesterol is able to mediate the transport of cholesterol from peripheral tissues to the liver in order to be excreted (Leaf, 2003). Another hypothesis is that lipoprotein lipase, which is the responsible enzyme for breaking down TG, is up-regulated by exercise, which results in a favorable lipid profile, i.e., decreased levels of TG and increased levels of HDL-cholesterol (Lin et al., 2015).

PHYSICAL-ACTIVITY RECOMMENDATIONS

According to the 2019 ACC/AHA guidelines for the primary prevention of CVD, adults should perform at least 150 min/week of moderate-intensity activity or 75 min/week of vigorous-activity

Table 17.4 Recommendations for exercise and physical activity for the primary prevention of CVD. ASCVD = atherosclerotic cardiovascular disease; COR = class (strength) of recommendation; LOE = level (quality) of evidence.

COR	LOE	Recommendations
I	B-R	1. Adults should be routinely counseled in healthcare visits to optimize a physically active lifestyle (S3.2-1,S3.2-2).
I	B-NR	2. Adults should engage in at least 150 minutes per week of accumulated moderate-intensity or 75 minutes per week of vigorous-intensity aerobic physical activity (or an equivalent combination of moderate and vigorous activity) to reduce ASCVD risk (S3.2-3-S3.2-8).
IIa	B-NR	3. For adults unable to meet the minimum physical activity recommendations (at least 150 minutes per week of accumulated moderate-intensity or 75 minutes per week of vigorous-intensity aerobic physical activity), engaging in some moderate- or vigorous-intensity physical activity, even if less than this recommended amount, can be beneficial to reduce ASCVD risk (S3.2-5,S3.2-6).
IIb	C-LD	4. Decreasing sedentary behavior in adults may be reasonable to reduce ASCVD risk (S3.2-3, S3.2-9-S3.2-11).

Source: (Arnett et al., 2019).

(Arnett et al., 2019) (**Table 17.4**). The 2021 guidelines from the European Society of Cardiology recommend even more; at least 150 to 300 min of moderate-intensity or 75 to 150 min of vigorous aerobic activity per week, or an equivalent combination of moderate- and vigorous-intensity exercise, in combination with resistance exercise, 2 times or more per week (Visseren et al., 2021). Guidelines also recommend that adults who are unable to reach the recommendation of 150 minutes of moderate-intensity exercise per week should stay as active as they are capable of.

As discussed thoroughly in **Unit 2**, exercise intensity can be estimated using several methods, such as: a) metabolic equivalent of task (MET-the energy cost of a given activity divided by resting energy expenditure); b) the percentage of measured or estimated maximum heart-rate (%HR_{max}); c) rating of perceived exertion—Borg scale score; or d) the talk test (Visseren et al., 2021). Examples of moderate-intensity exercise are walking at a moderate or brisk pace, slow cycling, vacuuming, gardening, ballroom dancing, or water aerobics, while examples of vigorous exercise could be race-walking, jogging, running, cycling, swimming, or tennis. Exercise may be classified as moderate when the MET is 3 to 5.9, %HR_{max} is 64 to 76, Borg scale score is 12 to 13, or when breathing is fast but the ability to speak full sentences remains (talk test), and as intense when MET is ≥6, %HR_{max} is 77 to 95, Borg scale score 14 to 17, or when breathing is very hard and the individual is not able to carry on a conversation comfortably (talk test).

TOTAL CHOLESTEROL

A lot of research has focused on the association of physical activity and total-cholesterol levels. A systematic review of meta-analyses of RCTs published between 1999 to 2019 examined the effect of exercise on blood lipids in individuals with or without disease and high levels of cholesterol (Palazón-Bru, Hernández-Lozano, & Gil-Guillén, 2021). Physical activity intervention was either aerobic exercise in many forms (i.e., walking, jogging, running, cycling, swimming, etc.), or a single type of exercise, aerobic, resistance, or other exercise such as yoga. From the 23 meta-analyses included in the review, 13 of them reported decreased total-cholesterol levels with exercise training, and a reduction was observed with all types of exercise.

When taking into account confounding factors such as changes in body composition and weight, exercise training has no significant effect on total-cholesterol concentrations, as it has been proven in early intervention studies (Gyntelberg et al., 1977; LaRosa et al., 1982; Thompson et al., 1988; P. D. Wood, Stefanick, Williams, & Haskell, 1991). In a recent review of meta-analyses of RCTs published between 1992 to 2020, researchers concluded that the observed increase in HDL-cholesterol and the observed decrease in LDL-cholesterol were comparable in exercise training and weight-loss interventions (Gaesser & Angadi, 2021). On the contrary, weight-loss interventions were more efficient in reducing TG than exercise training interventions.

Individuals with parallel co-morbidities and high cholesterol levels or dyslipidemia might benefit the most from physical-activity interventions. Results from a recent meta-analysis of 16 intervention studies suggested that, while no effects were seen in the overall sample, individuals with type 2 diabetes, hypertension, hyperlipidemia, or metabolic syndrome showed better improvements from exercise training, concerning their total-cholesterol levels, compared to healthy individuals (Lin et al., 2015).

Furthermore, the cholesterol levels of patients with insufficient physical activity might also benefit when getting more active. Evidence of an intervention study suggests that physical activity, instead of lowering total cholesterol, may counterbalance in increments that would happen by inactivity (Mann, Jimenez, Domone, & Beedie, 2016).

TRIGLYCERIDES

Triglyceride concentrations are known to be significantly reduced following exercise training (Barone Gibbs et al., 2021; Lin et al., 2015). The level of reduction in TG varies among studies. Kelly et al. in a meta-analysis of 13 clinical studies including only patients with overweight or obesity concluded that the reduction of TG may be as much as 11%, regardless of changes in body composition (Kelley, Kelley, & Vu Tran, 2005). Lin et al. in their meta-analysis of 160 RCTs, which investigated the effects of exercise training on blood-lipid levels, concluded that exercise training reduces TG levels by an average of 5.31 mg/dL (Lin et al., 2015).

Moreover, according to a recent scientific statement from the American Heart Association, aerobic training is able to reduce TG by 4 to 12 mg/dL (pooled average effects from meta-analyses) and resistance training by 8 mg/dL (Barone Gibbs et al., 2021). Overall, the consensus is that exercise training lowers blood TG concentration.

LOW-DENSITY LIPOPROTEIN-CHOLESTEROL

LDL is the lipoprotein responsible for carrying cholesterol (LDL-cholesterol) to the cells. It is the major carrier of cholesterol carrying approximately 60% to 80% of all blood cholesterol. Because the atherogenic properties of elevated LDL-cholesterol concentrations are well-documented (Brown & Goldstein, 1984; "The Lipid Research Clinics Coronary Primary Prevention Trial results. II. The relationship of reduction in incidence of coronary heart disease to cholesterol lowering," 1984), the interest in lowering LDL-cholesterol by increasing physical activity is elaborated in the literature, however results are not very consistent.

A recent meta-analysis of 160 RCTs, carried out from 1965 to 2014, evaluated the association between any type of exercise training and blood lipid, but failed to report any beneficial changes in LDL-cholesterol levels following exercise training (Lin et al., 2015). On the other hand, pooled results of two meta-analyses, one among men and one among women, presented in a scientific statement from American Heart Association yield a decrease of 3 to 4 mg/dL with aerobic exercise and 6mg/dL with resistance exercise (Barone Gibbs et al., 2021).

Co-morbidities may be a confounding factor. According to a recent meta-analysis, while physical activity had no overall effects on LDL-cholesterol, individuals with type 2 diabetes, hypertension, hyperlipidemia, or metabolic syndrome had a greater reduction of their LDL-cholesterol levels after intervention, compared to healthy individuals (Lin et al., 2015).

Additionally, the possible association of LDL-cholesterol levels and physical activity could be gender related. In the ARIC study, an increase of 180 MET-minutes per week from the baseline level of physical activity was associated with lower LDL-cholesterol levels only in women, especially African American women (Monda et al., 2009). On the other hand, results from a recent meta-analysis of 16 RCTs regarding the effects of physical activity on blood lipids showed that men had greater exercise-related improvement in LDL-cholesterol than women (Lin et al., 2015).

The efficacy and safety of statin treatment combined with physical activity has been also evaluated in many studies. A meta-analysis of a small number of trials (Gui et al., 2017), showed that exercise combined to statin monotherapy was safe and improved insulin sensitivity, inflammation, and peak oxygen uptake. However, there was no significant further improvement in total-cholesterol, LDL-cholesterol, HDL-cholesterol, or TG levels compared to statin treatment alone. From the lipid profile point of view, more research is needed on combination treatment and the numerous benefits of physical activity should not be disregarded.

HIGH-DENSITY LIPOPROTEIN-CHOLESTEROL

A lot of research exists on the relationship of physical activity and HDL-cholesterol. In a systematic review of meta-analyses of RCTs published from 1999 to 2019 researchers examined the effect of, mostly, aerobic exercise on HDL-cholesterol levels. All 23 meta-analyses concluded that physical activity raises HDL-cholesterol in both healthy and unhealthy participants (Palazón-Bru et al., 2021). The range of increment was 0.27 to 5.41 mg/dL. Moreover, data based on a pooled effect analysis of meta-analyses of the American Heart Association, yield similar results, that is, physical activity increases HDL-cholesterol by 1 to 2 mg/dL (Barone Gibbs et al., 2021).

Several factors may influence HDL-cholesterol increments with physical activity. Duration of physical activity, caloric expenditure, amount, and intensity of training have been proposed to affect the outcome.

According to Kokkinos et al., most changes in HDL-cholesterol occur when jogging (i.e., aerobic training) for approximately 101 to 124 min/week, at distances from 7 to 14 miles (Kokkinos et al., 1995). A meta-analysis of 25 RCTs published between 1966-2005 concluded to similar results. It was shown that at least 120 min/week of aerobic training are necessary for an increment in HDL-cholesterol levels, suggesting that the exercise duration was the most powerful predictor of this change. No information on the weekly distance was available since they included various types of aerobic training, not only running (Kodama et al., 2007).

Because caloric expenditure encompasses all three exercise components (intensity, duration, and frequency), it allows for more accurate comparisons among several studies. A caloric expenditure of 1000 to 1500 kcal/week has been defined as the threshold dose of exercise to favorably influence changes in HDL-cholesterol (Drygas, Jegler, & Kunski, 1988; Kokkinos et al., 1995). On the other hand, even lower energy expenditures, 900 kcal/week, has been reported to induce changes in HDL-cholesterol (Kodama et al., 2007).

Regarding the amount of exercise training required for optimal benefit, Kraus and co-investigators randomly assigned individuals to approximately 8 months in one of three exercise groups (Kraus et al., 2002): Group 1: Low-amount, moderate-intensity exercise, the equivalent of walking 12 miles per week at 40% to 55% of peak oxygen consumption; Group 2: Low-amount, high-intensity exercise, the equivalent of jogging 12 miles/week at 65% to 80% of peak oxygen consumption; Group 3: High-amount, high-intensity exercise, the caloric equivalent of jogging 20 miles/week at 65% to 80% of peak oxygen consumption; Group 4: The control group. The investigators reported favorable changes in a variety of lipid and lipoprotein variables in all exercise groups when compared to the control group. Higher amounts of exercise had the most beneficial effects when compared to individuals in the control group. In addition, the high amount of exercise resulted in greater improvements than did lower amounts of exercise. Researchers concluded that the improvements in lipid and lipoproteins were related to the amount of activity and not to the intensity of exercise or improvement in fitness (Kraus et al., 2002). Similar methodology has been used in the STRRIDE-PD study. Non-active, non-smoking overweight or obese adults were divided in four groups based on the amount and intensity of the physical activity: 1) Low-amount, moderate-intensity exercise (10 kcal/kg/week at 50% VO_2 reserve); 2) High-amount, moderate-intensity exercise (16 kcal/kg/week at 50% VO_2 reserve); 3) High-amount, vigorous-intensity exercise (16 kcal/kg/week at 75% VO$_2$ reserve); 4) Clinical lifestyle intervention, including both exercise and dietary intervention (10 kcal/kg/week at 50% VO$_2$ reserve and a weight-loss diet). Only those in the high-amount, vigorous-intensity exercise had a significant increase in HDL-cholesterol after 6 months of intervention (Sarzynski et al., 2018).

A dose-response relationship has also been observed as exercise duration increases. Kodama et al. propose that for every 10 more minutes of aerobic training, there is an increase of 1.4 mg/dl (0.036 mmol/L) in the HDL-cholesterol levels for training sessions that last between 23 and 74 minutes (Kodama et al., 2007). Thus, increasing the duration of each session, not the frequency of the exercise, may result in better changes to HDL-cholesterol.

TYPE OF EXERCISE TRAINING AND BLOOD LIPIDS

In contrast to the extensive research on the effects of aerobic training, relatively few studies have examined the effects of resistance training or strength training on lipoprotein-lipid profiles. Recently, more studies have addressed this topic, mostly in comparison with aerobic exercise.

Aerobic training is believed to have more favorable effects on blood lipids compared to resistance training and this point of view could be based on the characteristics of these two types of physical activity. For example, considering that the increase in HDL-cholesterol is positively associated with the volume of physical activity, it is easier to have long sessions of aerobic training rather than long sessions of resistance training. As a result, the two types of physical activity result in different energy expenditures, which could also influence the effect they both have on blood lipids (Gordon, Chen, & Durstine, 2014).

Early epidemiologic studies have indicated a low incidence of mortality from heart disease in men who are engaged in intense muscular activity (R. S. Paffenbarger & Hale, 1975; R. S. Paffenbarger, Jr., Laughlin, Gima, & Black, 1970). This led to a number of cross-sectional studies almost 40 years ago focusing on the association between resistance training and lipoprotein-lipid profiles (Berg, Keul, Ringwald, Deus, & Wybitul, 1980; Clarkson, Hintermister, Fillyaw, & Stylos, 1981; Cuppers, Erdmann, Schubert, Berchtold, & Berger, 1982; Farrell et al., 1982; Hurley et al., 1984; Yki-Jarvinen, Koivisto, Taskinen, & Nikkila, 1984). The results of these early studies yield mixed findings, mainly due to methodology issues. Since then, more research has been conducted evaluating the association of resistance physical activity and blood-lipid profile.

Resistance training can ameliorate blood-lipid profile. Several RCTs exist in the literature showing that resistance training have a positive effect on total cholesterol, (Kelley & Kelley, 2009), LDL-cholesterol (Kelley & Kelley, 2009; Tambalis, Panagiotakos, Kavouras, & Sidossis, 2009), TG and on the total-cholesterol to HDL-cholesterol ratio, but not on HDL-cholesterol alone (Kelley & Kelley, 2009).

Resistance training may be beneficial with respect to lipid profiles for specific populations such as older adults. The effects of aerobic or resistance training have been studied on elderly women. After 11 weeks of training, women in both groups, compared to the control group, had increased HDL-cholesterol and decreased levels of TG. Those who did resistance training also had lower LDL-cholesterol and total cholesterol than the control group. Those differences are the result of exercise alone since there was no change in diet or weight during those 11 weeks. The researchers concluded that, in the case of elderly women, high-intensity aerobic or resistance training are both able to improve the blood-lipid profile, independent of diet (Fahlman, Boardley, Lambert, & Flynn, 2002). James et. al randomly assigned older men into two groups, the control group in which participants were asked to walk for 30 min, 3 times per week, and the intervention group in which participants followed three hourly resistance trainings, for a period of 12 months (James et al., 2016). Participants in the intervention group had greater improvements in total-cholesterol and LDL-cholesterol levels compared with the control group, but no effects were observed in HDL-cholesterol concentrations.

A recent systematic review and meta-analysis aimed to assess the effects of aerobic, resistance or combined training on cardiovascular risk factors in adults with metabolic syndrome (Wewege, Thom, Rye, & Parmenter, 2018). Eleven clinical studies were included in the analysis, with 16 intervention groups (12 aerobic, 4 resistance). Aerobic training increased HDL-cholesterol and reduced TG, compared to the control group. No differences were observed concerning resistance training, but data were very limited.

Overall, based on the available evidence, resistance exercise has a positive effect on blood lipids and benefits have been proven also in certain populations or age groups. For these reasons, existing guidelines suggest that resistance training should be performed in combination with aerobic training (Visseren et al., 2021; Williams et al., 2007).

INTENSITY OF TRAINING AND BLOOD LIPIDS

The intensity of physical activity may influence the effect of training on blood-lipid levels. High-intensity interval training (HIIT) and moderate-intensity continuous training (MICT) are the two types of intensity of physical activity that are compared in most existing studies. HIIT, in most cases, refers to aerobic exercise at high intensity combined with active or passive recovery periods of lower intensity. On the other hand, MICT refers, in most cases, to medium intensity aerobic training.

In the systematic review and meta-analysis of 7 RCTs published by Ramos et al. (Ramos, Dalleck, Tjonna, Beetham, & Coombes, 2015), researchers examined the impact of HIIT compared to MICT on vascular function and traditional CVD risk factors, including lipid profile (Ramos et al., 2015). In total, 182 participants were included and the average duration of interventions was 12 to 16 weeks. HIIT was shown to be a better enhancer of vascular function than MICT, with a greater effect on cardiorespiratory fitness but, concerning lipid levels, no change in total cholesterol or TG was observed. In the case of HDL-cholesterol, HIIT increased HDL-cholesterol, but only in patients with metabolic syndrome or type 2 diabetes. Wood et. al evaluated the effect of HIIT and MICT on the blood lipids of healthy individuals (G. Wood, Murrell, van der Touw, & Smart, 2019). Twenty-six RCTs (823 participants in total), with intervention durations ≥4 weeks, were included in the meta-analysis. No difference was observed in total cholesterol, LDL-cholesterol, TG, or the total cholesterol to HDL-cholesterol ratio between the two groups. However, HIIT was shown to be superior to MICT in raising HDL-cholesterol (0.07 mmol/L (0.04–0.11), p <0.0001). A more recent systematic review and meta-analysis of RCTs (Mattioni Maturana, Martus, Zipfel, & Nieß, 2021), which included 1529 participants, compared effects of high-intensity interval exercise (HIIE, including HIIT and sprint interval training) and MICT on several cardio-metabolic risk factors, including blood lipids. Overall, no significant differences were observed between HIIE and MICT regarding total cholesterol, LDL-cholesterol, HDL-cholesterol, or TG.

The intensity of resistance training has been also evaluated in terms of lipid profile. Moro et. al examined the effect of high-intensity interval resistance training compared to traditional resistance training (RT) in blood lipids of individuals aged 60 to 80 years (Moro et al., 2017). Apolipoprotein A-1 and apolipoprotein B, total cholesterol, HDL-cholesterol, LDL-cholesterol, and TG were measured before and after the 4-month intervention period. Blood-lipid profiles improved in both groups, but individuals in the high-intensity interval resistance training group had a clinically significant improvement, i.e., 9% reduction in total cholesterol, 11% in LDL-cholesterol, and 18% in TG.

The impact of a 1-year combined HIIT with RT or a moderate continuous training with RT on lipid profile in individuals with type 2 diabetes was examined in a recent RCT, compared to a control group (Magalhães et al., 2020). According to the results, HIIT and RT combined improved total-cholesterol and LDL-cholesterol levels of individuals, while no effects were observed for TG and HDL-C.

Based on current evidence, the effects of intensity training on blood lipids are inconclusive. There is some evidence that HIIT favors HDL-cholesterol in healthy individuals or those with metabolic syndrome or type 2 diabetes. More research is needed to examine the factors that influence the association of exercise intensity with blood lipids.

DYSLIPIDEMIA IN OLDER ADULTS: THE ROLE OF PHYSICAL ACTIVITY AND DIET

Total-cholesterol, LDL-cholesterol, and TG levels increase as age increases and it is known that older adults are at risk of cardiovascular morbidity and mortality (Streja & Streja, 2020). More specifically, in men, cholesterol increases until 45 to 55 years and tends to stabilize at around 60 years of age, while in women, these procedures happen 10 years later (Félix-Redondo, Grau, & Fernández-Bergés, 2013; Noale, Limongi, & Maggi, 2020). The prevalence of hypercholesterolemia (total cholesterol >240 mg/dl) in older-adult individuals was found to be higher in Western countries, with up to 50% of older adults in Great Britain (Félix-Redondo et al., 2013).

In adults older than 70 years of age, LDL-cholesterol has been found to diminish (**Figure 17.2**) (Félix-Redondo et al., 2013). Various reasons could explain this observation. First of all, hyperlipidemic individuals may have died from a CVD event at a younger age; second, individuals born more recently may have been exposed to a less atherogenic diet with less SFAs; and finally, older adults may have reduced their fat intake knowing the consequences of a high-fat diet (Lind, Sundström, Ärnlöv, & Lampa, 2018). This reverse epidemiology of hypercholesterolemia, meaning a lower risk of death in hypercholesterolemic older adults, has been observed in the geriatric population, according to the results of several epidemiological studies, but evidence are not yet strong enough to suggest changes in the lipid-lowering treatment for older adults (Ahmadi et al., 2015).

In the 2019 ACC/AHA guidelines on the primary prevention of CVD, people ≥75 years old are referred as of advanced age. Concerning older-adult patients, no specific guidelines that may differ from those for younger individuals exist for the prevention or management of dyslipidemia with regards to diet and physical activity, however, older patients could benefit from a diet aiming to prevent and treat hypercholesterolemia (Félix-Redondo et al., 2013). Concerning lipid-lowering therapy in older-adult patients (i.e., statins and fibrates), treatment is indicated since older-adult individuals are at very high risk for morbidity and mortality from CVD events (Shanmugasundaram, Rough, & Alpert, 2010). Current guidelines for the management of blood cholesterol suggest that "in patients older than 75 years of age with clinical ASCVD, it is reasonable to initiate moderate- or high-intensity statin therapy after evaluation of the potential for ASCVD risk reduction, adverse effects, and drug–drug interactions as well as patient frailty and patient preferences" (Grundy et al., 2019).

Concerning physical activity in older-adult individuals, its prevalence decreases as age increases (**Figure 17.3**). Older-adult men have higher physical activity levels than older-adult women (Sun, Norman, & While, 2013). Nevertheless, physical activity is known to be beneficial for older adults, and it is inversely associated with blood-cholesterol levels (Noale et al., 2020). Yet, there is no ideal type or intensity of exercise training. What is worth to keep in mind is that older adults may not be capable of engaging in regular exercise training, mostly due to several health issues (Newson & Kemps, 2007) and thus tailored made physical activity programs are needed for this population.

Exercise and nutrition may have a synergistic role on lipid profiles of older adults with metabolic syndrome, based on evidence from a recent substudy of the PREDIMED trial (Sanllorente et al., 2021). Participants followed either an energy-restricted MD with physical activity or an energy-restricted MD without engaging in physical activity (control group) for a 6-month period. Results suggested that the energy-restricted MD with physical activity improved the metabolism of HDL-cholesterol, compared with the control group, even though levels of HDL-cholesterol did not differ between groups.

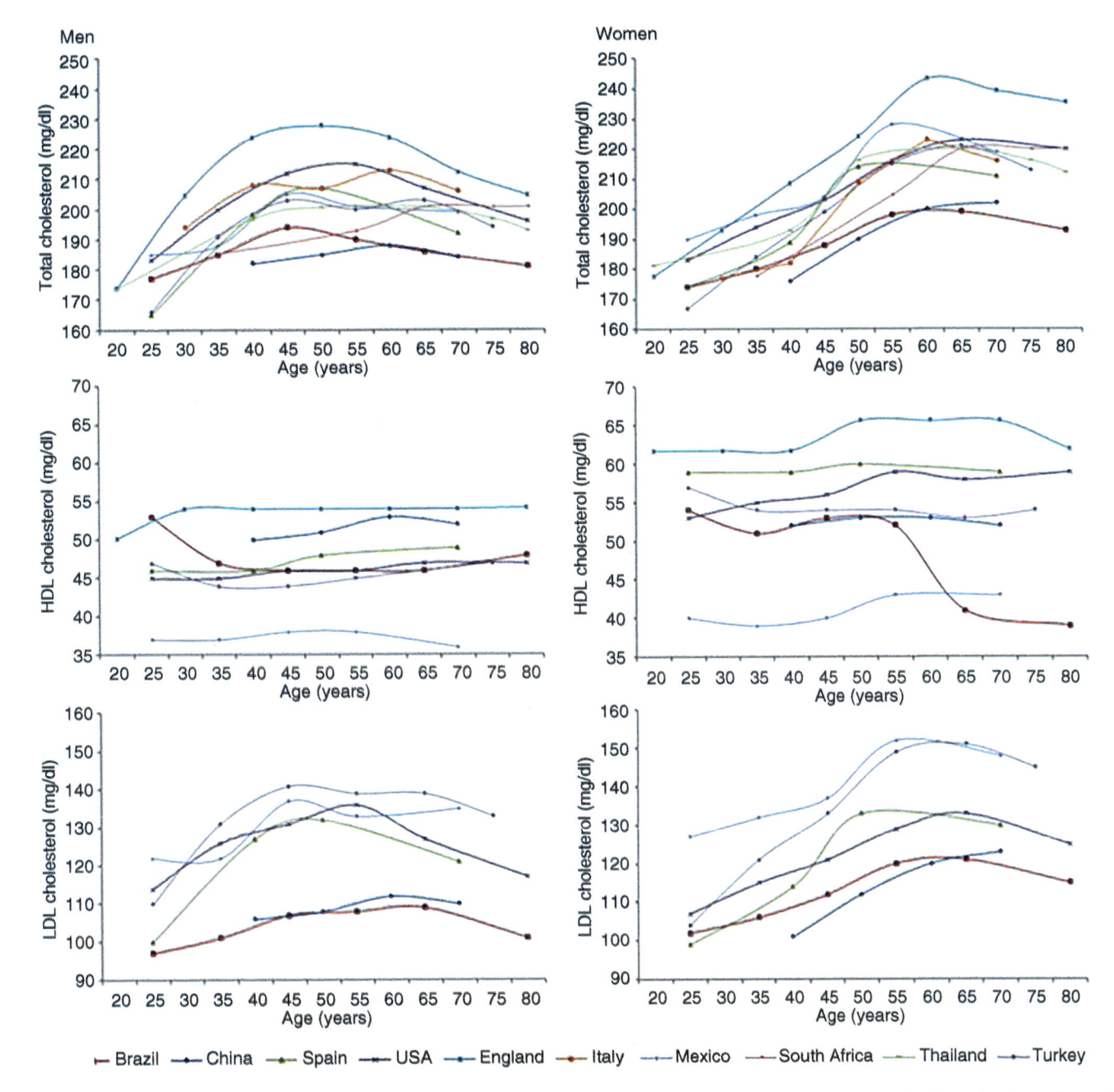

FIGURE 17.2 Total-cholesterol, HDL-cholesterol, and LDL-cholesterol levels by age, in men and women. Source: (Félix-Redondo et al., 2013).

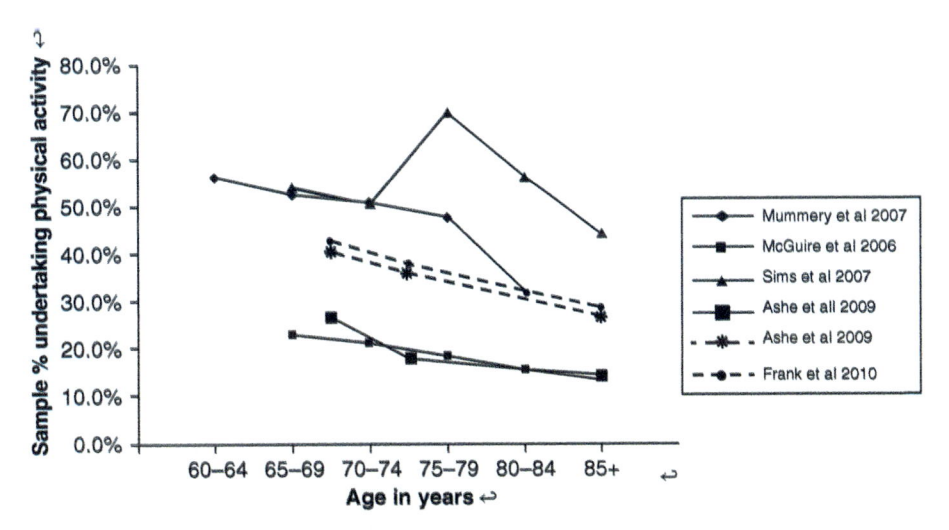

FIGURE 17.3 Physical-activity prevalence in elderly individuals. Source: (Sun et al., 2013 / Springer Nature / CC BY 2.0).

KEY POINTS

- A relationship exists between cholesterol and CHD. High blood concentrations of LDL-cholesterol are directly related to CHD. Conversely, high HDL-cholesterol concentrations are inversely related to CHD.
- Both prevention and management of dyslipidemia include physical activity and diet as basic elements.
- For the reduction of LDL-cholesterol, SFA need to be replaced by unsaturated fatty acids, preferably PUFA over MUFA.
- Exercise training or habitual physical activity favorably changes lipid- and lipoprotein-blood concentrations.
- The existing evidence suggests a possible association of physical activity with total cholesterol.
- Current evidence suggests that physical activity can decrease TG levels.
- There is consistent data indicating that physical activity increases HDL-cholesterol.
- Duration of training, caloric expenditure, and amount and intensity of physical activity may influence the increase of HDL-cholesterol after training.
- Aerobic physical activity is known to have positive effects on blood lipids, but recent evidence suggests that resistance physical activity may also be beneficial. Available evidence is not sufficient to support the idea of superiority of resistance over aerobic physical activity. Current guidelines suggest the combination of both aerobic and resistance training.
- Evidence cannot clearly support that HIIT is superior to MICT in terms of blood-lipid amelioration.
- A reverse epidemiology of hypercholesterolemia is observed in epidemiological studies of older adults. Further research is needed.
- No specific guidelines exist on diet and physical activity for older-adult individuals with hyperlipidemia. Drug lipid-lowering therapy should be individualized.

SELF-ASSESSMENT QUESTIONS

1. Define dyslipidemia.
2. True or False: Replacing SFA with PUFA will reduce LDL-cholesterol levels.
3. True or False: A low-fat, high-carbohydrate diet is the recommended diet pattern for a favorable blood-lipid profile.
4. Based on current evidence, briefly describe the effect of physical activity on blood lipids.
5. True or False: Aerobic physical activity is the only type of exercise with positive results on blood lipids.
6. True or False: The duration of physical activity can affect HDL-cholesterol after training.
7. True or False: Current guidelines suggest aerobic training, since this is the best form of physical activity for blood-lipid control.
8. True or False: Physical activity is not proposed by current guidelines to manage hyperlipidemia.

CASE SCENARIO

Mr. KI is 47 years old and a police officer. He has no significant previous medical history. In his annual standard audit, he received the following results:

Variable	Value	Reference range
TCHOL	270 mg/dL	<200 mg/dL
TG	180 mg/dL	<150 mg/dL
HDL	34 mg/dL	≥40 mg/dL
LDL	210 mg/dL	<130 mg/dL
ALT	40 IU/L	10–55 IU/L
AST	38 IU/L	10–40 IU/L
GGT	45 IU/L	5–40 IU/L

He immediately visited his family doctor for further evaluation of his condition. His doctor decided to start hypolipidemic treatment (statins) and referred him to you for a change in his lifestyle. The blood pressure was 124/82 mm Hg. According to the information you have collected:

His body weight is 145.6 kg and he is 187cm tall. He is married and has three children. He is not satisfied with his weight and has made various weight-loss efforts in the last year without many results. Mr. KI has a sedentary lifestyle, as he works in the office of his local police department. He does not perform any exercise. He has been a smoker since he was 22 years old.

Questions:

1. Calculate Mr. KI's cardiovascular risk using the ASCVD tool.
2. How do you find his lipid profile?
3. Please calculate his BMI.
4. What recommendations/advice would you give to the patient regarding his lifestyle?

REFERENCES

Ahmadi, S.-F., Streja, E., Zahmatkesh, G., Streja, D., Kashyap, M., Moradi, H., . . . Kalantar-Zadeh, K. (2015). Reverse Epidemiology of Traditional Cardiovascular Risk Factors in the Geriatric Population. *Journal of the American Medical Directors Association, 16*(11), 933-939. doi: https://doi.org/10.1016/j.jamda.2015.07.014

Appel, L. J., Moore, T. J., Obarzanek, E., Vollmer, W. M., Svetkey, L. P., Sacks, F. M., . . . Karanja, N. (1997). A clinical trial of the effects of dietary patterns on blood pressure. DASH Collaborative Research Group. *N Engl J Med, 336*(16), 1117-1124. doi: 10.1056/nejm199704173361601

Appel, L. J., Sacks, F. M., Carey, V. J., Obarzanek, E., Swain, J. F., Miller, E. R., 3rd, . . . Bishop, L. M. (2005). Effects of protein, monounsaturated fat, and carbohydrate intake on blood pressure and serum lipids: results of the OmniHeart randomized trial. *Jama, 294*(19), 2455-2464. doi: 10.1001/jama.294.19.2455

Arnett, D. K., Blumenthal, R. S., Albert, M. A., Buroker, A. B., Goldberger, Z. D., Hahn, E. J., . . . Ziaeian, B. (2019). 2019 ACC/AHA Guideline on the Primary Prevention of Cardiovascular Disease: A Report of the American College of Cardiology/American Heart Association Task Force on Clinical Practice Guidelines. *Circulation, 140*(11), e596-e646. doi: doi:10.1161/CIR.0000000000000678

Bach-Faig, A., Berry, E. M., Lairon, D., Reguant, J., Trichopoulou, A., Dernini, S., . . . Serra-Majem, L. (2011). Mediterranean diet pyramid today. Science and cultural updates. *Public Health Nutrition, 14*(12A), 2274-2284. doi: 10.1017/S1368980011002515

Bahmani, M., Mirhoseini, M., Shirzad, H., Sedighi, M., Shahinfard, N., & Rafieian-Kopaei, M. (2015). A Review on Promising Natural Agents Effective on Hyperlipidemia. *Journal of Evidence-Based Complementary & Alternative Medicine, 20*(3), 228-238. doi: 10.1177/2156587214568457

Bakker, E. A., Lee, D. C., Sui, X., Eijsvogels, T. M. H., Ortega, F. B., Lee, I. M., . . . Blair, S. N. (2018). Association of Resistance Exercise With the Incidence of Hypercholesterolemia in Men. *Mayo Clin Proc, 93*(4), 419-428. doi: 10.1016/j.mayocp.2017.11.024

Barone Gibbs, B., Hivert, M. F., Jerome, G. J., Kraus, W. E., Rosenkranz, S. K., Schorr, E. N., . . . Lobelo, F. (2021). Physical Activity as a Critical Component of First-Line Treatment for Elevated Blood Pressure or Cholesterol: Who, What, and How?: A Scientific Statement From the American Heart Association. *Hypertension, 78*(2), e26-e37. doi: 10.1161/hyp.0000000000000196

Barquera, S., Pedroza-Tobías, A., Medina, C., Hernández-Barrera, L., Bibbins-Domingo, K., Lozano, R., & Moran, A. E. (2015). Global Overview of the Epidemiology of Atherosclerotic Cardiovascular Disease. *Archives of Medical Research, 46*(5), 328-338. doi: https://doi.org/10.1016/j.arcmed.2015.06.006

Bays, H. E., Toth, P. P., Kris-Etherton, P. M., Abate, N., Aronne, L. J., Brown, W. V., . . . Samuel, V. T. (2013). Obesity, adiposity, and dyslipidemia: a consensus statement from the National Lipid Association. *J Clin Lipidol, 7*(4), 304-383. doi: 10.1016/j.jacl.2013.04.001

Berg, A., Keul, J., Ringwald, G., Deus, B., & Wybitul, K. (1980). Physical performance and serum cholesterol fractions in healthy young men. *Clinica Chimica Acta, 106*(3), 325-330. doi: https://doi.org/10.1016/0009-8981(80)90317-4

Brown, M. S., & Goldstein, J. L. (1984). How LDL receptors influence cholesterol and atherosclerosis. *Sci Am, 251*(5), 58-66. doi: 10.1038/scientificamerican1184-58

CDC. (2011). Vital signs: prevalence, treatment, and control of high levels of low-density lipoprotein cholesterol–United States, 1999-2002 and 2005-200. *MMWR Morb Mortal Wkly Rep, 60*(4), 109-114.

Chiu, S., Bergeron, N., Williams, P. T., Bray, G. A., Sutherland, B., & Krauss, R. M. (2016). Comparison of the DASH (Dietary Approaches to Stop Hypertension) diet and a higher-fat DASH diet on blood pressure and lipids and lipoproteins: a randomized controlled trial. *The American journal of clinical nutrition, 103*(2), 341-347. doi: 10.3945/ajcn.115.123281

Clarkson, P. M., Hintermister, R., Fillyaw, M., & Stylos, L. (1981). High density lipoprotein cholesterol in young adult weight lifters, runners and untrained subjects. *Hum Biol, 53*(2), 251-257.

Covas, M. I., Nyyssönen, K., Poulsen, H. E., Kaikkonen, J., Zunft, H. J., Kiesewetter, H., . . . Marrugat, J. (2006). The effect of polyphenols in olive oil on heart disease risk factors: a randomized trial. *Ann Intern Med, 145*(5), 333-341. doi: 10.7326/0003-4819-145-5-200609050-00006

Crichton, G. E., & Alkerwi, A. (2015). Physical activity, sedentary behavior time and lipid levels in the Observation of Cardiovascular Risk Factors in Luxembourg study. *Lipids Health Dis, 14*, 87. doi: 10.1186/s12944-015-0085-3

Cuppers, H. J., Erdmann, D., Schubert, H., Berchtold, P., & Berger, M. (1982). Glucose tolerance, serum insulin, and serum lipids in athletes. *Curr Probl Clin Biochem, 11*, 155-165.

Drygas, W., Jegler, A., & Kunski, H. (1988). Study on threshold dose of physical activity in coronary heart disease prevention. Part I. Relationship between leisure time physical activity and coronary risk factors. *Int J Sports Med, 9*(4), 275-278. doi: 10.1055/s-2007-1025021

El-Tantawy, W. H., & Temraz, A. (2019). Natural products for controlling hyperlipidemia: review. *Arch Physiol Biochem, 125*(2), 128-135. doi: 10.1080/13813455.2018.1441315

ESC. (2021). SCORE2 risk prediction algorithms: new models to estimate 10-year risk of cardiovascular disease in Europe. *European Heart Journal, 42*(25), 2439-2454. doi: 10.1093/eurheartj/ehab309

ESC/EAS. (2019). 2019 ESC/EAS guidelines for the management of dyslipidaemias: Lipid modification to reduce cardiovascular risk. *Atherosclerosis, 290*, 140-205. doi: 10.1016/j.atherosclerosis.2019.08.014

Estruch, R., Martinez-Gonzalez, M. A., Corella, D., Salas-Salvado, J., Ruiz-Gutierrez, V., Covas, M. I., . . . Ros, E. (2006). Effects of a Mediterranean-style diet on cardiovascular risk factors: a randomized trial. *Ann Intern Med, 145*(1), 1-11. doi: 10.7326/0003-4819-145-1-200607040-00004

Fahlman, M. M., Boardley, D., Lambert, C. P., & Flynn, M. G. (2002). Effects of Endurance Training and Resistance Training on Plasma Lipoprotein Profiles in Elderly Women. *The Journals of Gerontology: Series A, 57*(2), B54-B60. doi: 10.1093/gerona/57.2.B54

Farrell, P. A., Maksud, M. G., Pollock, M. L., Foster, C., Anholm, J., Hare, J., & Leon, A. S. (1982). A comparison of plasma cholesterol, triglycerides, and high density lipoprotein-cholesterol in speed skaters, weightlifters and non-athletes. *Eur J Appl Physiol Occup Physiol, 48*(1), 77-82. doi: 10.1007/bf00421167

Feingold, K. R. (2000a). Introduction to Lipids and Lipoproteins. In K. R. Feingold, B. Anawalt, A. Boyce, G. Chrousos, W. W. de Herder, K. Dhatariya, K. Dungan, J. M. Hershman, J. Hofland, S. Kalra, G. Kaltsas, C. Koch, P. Kopp, M. Korbonits, C. S. Kovacs, W. Kuohung, B. Laferrère, M. Levy, E. A. McGee, R. McLachlan, J. E. Morley, M. New, J. Purnell, R. Sahay, F. Singer, M. A. Sperling, C. A. Stratakis, D. L. Trence & D. P. Wilson (Eds.), *Endotext*. South Dartmouth (MA): MDText.com, Inc. Copyright © 2000-2022, MDText.com, Inc.

Feingold, K. R. (2000b). Obesity and Dyslipidemia. In K. R. Feingold, B. Anawalt, A. Boyce, G. Chrousos, W. W. de Herder, K. Dhatariya, K. Dungan, J. M. Hershman, J. Hofland, S. Kalra, G. Kaltsas, C. Koch, P. Kopp, M. Korbonits, C. S. Kovacs, W. Kuohung, B. Laferrère, M. Levy, E. A. McGee, R. McLachlan, J. E. Morley, M. New, J. Purnell, R. Sahay,

F. Singer, M. A. Sperling, C. A. Stratakis, D. L. Trence & D. P. Wilson (Eds.), *Endotext*. South Dartmouth (MA): MDText.com, Inc. Copyright © 2000-2022, MDText.com, Inc.

Félix-Redondo, F. J., Grau, M., & Fernández-Bergés, D. (2013). Cholesterol and cardiovascular disease in the elderly. Facts and gaps. *Aging and disease*, *4*(3), 154–169.

Fischer, S., Schatz, U., & Julius, U. (2015). Practical recommendations for the management of hyperlipidemia. *Atherosclerosis Supplements*, *18*, 194–198. doi: https://doi.org/10.1016/j.atherosclerosissup.2015.02.029

Gaesser, G. A., & Angadi, S. S. (2021). Obesity treatment: Weight loss versus increasing fitness and physical activity for reducing health risks. *iScience*, *24*(10), 102995-102995. doi: 10.1016/j.isci.2021.102995

Gordon, B., Chen, S., & Durstine, J. L. (2014). The effects of exercise training on the traditional lipid profile and beyond. *Curr Sports Med Rep*, *13*(4), 253–259. doi: 10.1249/jsr.0000000000000073

Grundy, S. M., Stone, N. J., Bailey, A. L., Beam, C., Birtcher, K. K., Blumenthal, R. S., . . . Yeboah, J. (2019). 2018 AHA/ACC/AACVPR/AAPA/ABC/ACPM/ADA/AGS/APhA/ASPC/NLA/PCNA Guideline on the Management of Blood Cholesterol: A Report of the American College of Cardiology/American Heart Association Task Force on Clinical Practice Guidelines. *Journal of the American College of Cardiology, 73*(24), e285–e350. doi: https://doi.org/10.1016/j.jacc.2018.11.003

Gui, Y. J., Liao, C. X., Liu, Q., Guo, Y., Yang, T., Chen, J. Y., . . . Xu, D. Y. (2017). Efficacy and safety of statins and exercise combination therapy compared to statin monotherapy in patients with dyslipidaemia: A systematic review and meta-analysis. *Eur J Prev Cardiol, 24*(9), 907–916. doi: 10.1177/2047487317691874

Gyntelberg, F., Brennan, R., Holloszy, J. O., Schonfeld, G., Rennie, M. J., & Weidman, S. W. (1977). Plasma triglyceride lowering by exercise despite increased food intake in patients with type IV hyperlipoproteinemia. *The American journal of clinical nutrition, 30*(5), 716–720. doi: 10.1093/ajcn/30.5.716

Harris, C. P., von Berg, A., Berdel, D., Bauer, C.-P., Schikowski, T., Koletzko, S., . . . Standl, M. (2018). Association of Dietary Fatty Acids with Blood Lipids is Modified by Physical Activity in Adolescents: Results from the GINIplus and LISA Birth Cohort Studies. *Nutrients, 10*(10), 1372. doi: 10.3390/nu10101372

He, N., & Ye, H. (2020). Exercise and Hyperlipidemia. In J. Xiao (Ed.), *Physical Exercise for Human Health* (pp. 79–90). Singapore: Springer Singapore.

Hill, M. F., & Bordoni, B. (2022). Hyperlipidemia *StatPearls*. Treasure Island (FL): StatPearls Publishing Copyright © 2022, StatPearls Publishing LLC.

Hurley, B. F., Seals, D. R., Hagberg, J. M., Goldberg, A. C., Ostrove, S. M., Holloszy, J. O., . . . Goldberg, A. P. (1984). High-density-lipoprotein cholesterol in bodybuilders v powerlifters. Negative effects of androgen use. *Jama, 252*(4), 507–513.

Jacobson, T. A., Maki, K. C., Orringer, C. E., Jones, P. H., Kris-Etherton, P., Sikand, G., . . . Underberg, J. A. (2015). National Lipid Association Recommendations for Patient-Centered Management of Dyslipidemia: Part 2. *J Clin Lipidol, 9*(6 Suppl), S1–122.e121. doi: 10.1016/j.jacl.2015.09.002

James, A. P., Whiteford, J., Ackland, T. R., Dhaliwal, S. S., Woodhouse, J. J., Prince, R. L., . . . Kerr, D. A. (2016). Effects of a 1-year randomised controlled trial of resistance training on blood lipid profile and chylomicron concentration in older men. *Eur J Appl Physiol, 116*(11-12), 2113–2123. doi: 10.1007/s00421-016-3465-0

Jiang, Z. G., Robson, S. C., & Yao, Z. (2013). Lipoprotein metabolism in nonalcoholic fatty liver disease. *Journal of biomedical research, 27*(1), 1–13. doi: 10.7555/JBR.27.20120077

Karr, S. (2017). Epidemiology and management of hyperlipidemia. *Am J Manag Care, 23*(9 Suppl), S139-s148.

Kelley, G. A., & Kelley, K. S. (2009). Impact of progressive resistance training on lipids and lipoproteins in adults: a meta-analysis of randomized controlled trials. *Prev Med, 48*(1), 9–19. doi: 10.1016/j.ypmed.2008.10.010

Kelley, G. A., Kelley, K. S., & Vu Tran, Z. (2005). Aerobic exercise, lipids and lipoproteins in overweight and obese adults: a meta-analysis of randomized controlled trials. *Int J Obes (Lond), 29*(8), 881–893. doi: 10.1038/sj.ijo.0802959

Kodama, S., Tanaka, S., Saito, K., Shu, M., Sone, Y., Onitake, F., . . . Sone, H. (2007). Effect of Aerobic Exercise Training on Serum Levels of High-Density Lipoprotein Cholesterol: A Meta-analysis. *JAMA Internal Medicine, 167*(10), 999–1008. doi: 10.1001/archinte.167.10.999

Kokkinos, P. F., Holland, J. C., Narayan, P., Colleran, J. A., Dotson, C. O., & Papademetriou, V. (1995). Miles run per week and high-density lipoprotein cholesterol levels in healthy, middle-aged men. A dose-response relationship. *Arch Intern Med, 155*(4), 415–420.

Kraus, W. E., Houmard, J. A., Duscha, B. D., Knetzger, K. J., Wharton, M. B., McCartney, J. S., . . . Slentz, C. A. (2002). Effects of the amount and intensity of exercise on plasma lipoproteins. *N Engl J Med, 347*(19), 1483–1492. doi: 10.1056/NEJMoa020194

LaRosa, J. C., Cleary, P., Muesing, R. A., Gorman, P., Hellerstein, H. K., & Naughton, J. (1982). Effect of Long-term Moderate Physical Exercise on Plasma Lipoproteins: The National Exercise and Heart Disease Project. *JAMA Internal Medicine, 142*(13), 2269–2274. doi: 10.1001/archinte.142.13.2269

Last, A. R., Ference, J. D., & Menzel, E. R. (2017). Hyperlipidemia: Drugs for Cardiovascular Risk Reduction in Adults. *Am Fam Physician, 95*(2), 78–87.

Leaf, D. A. (2003). The effect of physical exercise on reverse cholesterol transport. *Metabolism, 52*(8), 950–957. doi: 10.1016/s0026-0495(03)00147-1

Lee, Y., & Siddiqui, W. J. (2022). Cholesterol Levels *StatPearls*. Treasure Island (FL): StatPearls Publishing Copyright © 2022, StatPearls Publishing LLC.

Lin, X., Zhang, X., Guo, J., Roberts, C. K., McKenzie, S., Wu, W.-C., . . . Song, Y. (2015). Effects of Exercise Training on Cardiorespiratory Fitness and Biomarkers of Cardiometabolic Health: A Systematic Review and Meta-Analysis of Randomized Controlled Trials. *Journal of the American Heart Association, 4*(7), e002014. doi: 10.1161/JAHA.115.002014

Lind, L., Sundström, J., Ärnlöv, J., & Lampa, E. (2018). Impact of Aging on the Strength of Cardiovascular Risk Factors: A Longitudinal Study Over 40 Years. *Journal of the American Heart Association, 7*(1). doi: 10.1161/jaha.117.007061

The Lipid Research Clinics Coronary Primary Prevention Trial results. II. The relationship of reduction in incidence of coronary heart disease to cholesterol lowering. (1984). *Jama, 251*(3), 365–374.

Mach, F., Baigent, C., Catapano, A. L., Koskinas, K. C., Casula, M., Badimon, L., . . . Wiklund, O. (2020). 2019 ESC/EAS Guidelines for the management of dyslipidaemias: lipid modification to reduce cardiovascular risk. *Eur Heart J, 41*(1), 111–188. doi: 10.1093/eurheartj/ehz455

Magalhães, J. P., Santos, D. A., Correia, I. R., Hetherington-Rauth, M., Ribeiro, R., Raposo, J. F., . . . Sardinha, L. B. (2020). Impact of combined training with different exercise intensities on inflammatory and lipid markers in type 2 diabetes: a secondary analysis from a 1-year randomized controlled trial. *Cardiovascular diabetology, 19*(1), 169–169. doi: 10.1186/s12933-020-01136-y

Mann, S., Jimenez, A., Domone, S., & Beedie, C. (2016). Comparative effects of three 48-week community-based physical activity and exercise interventions on aerobic capacity, total cholesterol and mean arterial blood pressure. *BMJ open sport & exercise medicine, 2*(1), e000105-e000105. doi: 10.1136/bmjsem-2015-000105

Mattioni Maturana, F., Martus, P., Zipfel, S., & Nieß, A. M. (2021). Effectiveness of HIIE versus MICT in Improving Cardiometabolic Risk Factors in Health and Disease: A Meta-analysis. *Med Sci Sports Exerc*, 53(3), 559–573. doi: 10.1249/mss.0000000000002506

Mensink, R. P. & World Health Organization. (2016). *Effects of saturated fatty acids on serum lipids and lipoproteins: a systematic review and regression analysis*. Geneva: World Health Organization.

Meslier, V., Laiola, M., Roager, H. M., De Filippis, F., Roume, H., Quinquis, B., . . . Ercolini, D. (2020). Mediterranean diet intervention in overweight and obese subjects lowers plasma cholesterol and causes changes in the gut microbiome and metabolome independently of energy intake. *Gut*, 69(7), 1258–1268. doi: 10.1136/gutjnl-2019-320438

Moro, T., Tinsley, G., Bianco, A., Gottardi, A., Gottardi, G. B., Faggian, D., . . . Paoli, A. (2017). High intensity interval resistance training (HIIRT) in older adults: Effects on body composition, strength, anabolic hormones and blood lipids. *Exp Gerontol*, 98, 91–98. doi: 10.1016/j.exger.2017.08.015

Mozaffarian, D., Benjamin, E. J., Go, A. S., Arnett, D. K., Blaha, M. J., Cushman, M., . . . Turner, M. B. (2016). Heart Disease and Stroke Statistics—2016 Update. *Circulation*, 133(4), e38–e360. doi: doi:10.1161/CIR.0000000000000350

NCEP. (2001). Executive Summary of The Third Report of The National Cholesterol Education Program (NCEP) Expert Panel on Detection, Evaluation, And Treatment of High Blood Cholesterol In Adults (Adult Treatment Panel III). *Jama*, 285(19), 2486–2497. doi: 10.1001/jama.285.19.2486

Newson, R. S., & Kemps, E. B. (2007). Factors That Promote and Prevent Exercise Engagement in Older Adults. *Journal of Aging and Health*, 19(3), 470–481. doi: 10.1177/0898264307300169

Nie, Y., & Luo, F. (2021). Dietary Fiber: An Opportunity for a Global Control of Hyperlipidemia. *Oxidative Medicine and Cellular Longevity*, 2021, 5542342. doi: 10.1155/2021/5542342

Noale, M., Limongi, F., & Maggi, S. (2020). Epidemiology of Cardiovascular Diseases in the Elderly. In N. Veronese (Ed.), *Frailty and Cardiovascular Diseases: Research into an Elderly Population* (pp. 29–38). Cham: Springer International Publishing.

Nouh, F., Omar, M., & Younis, M. (2019). Risk Factors and Management of Hyperlipidemia (Review). 2, 1–10.

Paffenbarger, R. S., & Hale, W. E. (1975). Work activity and coronary heart mortality. *N Engl J Med*, 292(11), 545–550. doi: 10.1056/nejm197503132921101

Paffenbarger, R. S., Jr., Laughlin, M. E., Gima, A. S., & Black, R. A. (1970). Work activity of longshoremen as related to death from coronary heart disease and stroke. *N Engl J Med*, 282(20), 1109–1114. doi: 10.1056/nejm197005142822001

Palazón-Bru, A., Hernández-Lozano, D., & Gil-Guillén, V. F. (2021). Which Physical Exercise Interventions Increase HDL-Cholesterol Levels? A Systematic Review of Meta-analyses of Randomized Controlled Trials. *Sports Med*, 51(2), 243–253. doi: 10.1007/s40279-020-01364-y

Pang, Y., Kartsonaki, C., Du, H., Millwood, I. Y., Guo, Y., Chen, Y., . . . Chen, Z. (2019). Physical Activity, Sedentary Leisure Time, Circulating Metabolic Markers, and Risk of Major Vascular Diseases. *Circulation: Genomic and Precision Medicine*, 12(9), e002527. doi: doi:10.1161/CIRCGEN.118.002527

Park, J.-H., Joh, H.-K., Lee, G.-S., Je, S.-J., Cho, S.-H., Kim, S.-J., . . . Kwon, H.-T. (2018). Association between Sedentary Time and Cardiovascular Risk Factors in Korean Adults. *Korean J Fam Med*, 39(1), 29–36. doi: 10.4082/kjfm.2018.39.1.29

Pirillo, A., Casula, M., Olmastroni, E., Norata, G. D., & Catapano, A. L. (2021). Global epidemiology of dyslipidaemias. *Nature Reviews Cardiology*, 18(10), 689–700. doi: 10.1038/s41569-021-00541-4

Ramos, J. S., Dalleck, L. C., Tjonna, A. E., Beetham, K. S., & Coombes, J. S. (2015). The impact of high-intensity interval training versus moderate-intensity continuous training on vascular function: a systematic review and meta-analysis. *Sports Med*, 45(5), 679–692. doi: 10.1007/s40279-015-0321-z

Rondanelli, M., Giacosa, A., Morazzoni, P., Guido, D., Grassi, M., Morandi, G., . . . Perna, S. (2016). MediterrAsian Diet Products That Could Raise HDL-Cholesterol: A Systematic Review. *BioMed research international*, 2016, 2025687–2025687. doi: 10.1155/2016/2025687

Salas-Salvadó, J., Díaz-López, A., Ruiz-Canela, M., Basora, J., Fitó, M., Corella, D., . . . investigators, P.-P. (2018). Effect of a Lifestyle Intervention Program With Energy-Restricted Mediterranean Diet and Exercise on Weight Loss and Cardiovascular Risk Factors: One-Year Results of the PREDIMED-Plus Trial. *Diabetes Care*, 42(5), 777–788. doi: 10.2337/dc18-0836

Sanllorente, A., Soria-Florido, M. T., Castañer, O., Lassale, C., Salas-Salvadó, J., Martínez-González, M. Á., . . . Fitó, M. (2021). A lifestyle intervention with an energy-restricted Mediterranean diet and physical activity enhances HDL function: a substudy of the PREDIMED-Plus randomized controlled trial. *The American journal of clinical nutrition*, 114(5), 1666–1674. doi: 10.1093/ajcn/nqab246

Sarzynski, M. A., Ruiz-Ramie, J. J., Barber, J. L., Slentz, C. A., Apolzan, J. W., McGarrah, R. W., . . . Rohatgi, A. (2018). Effects of Increasing Exercise Intensity and Dose on Multiple Measures of HDL (High-Density Lipoprotein) Function. *Arteriosclerosis, thrombosis, and vascular biology*, 38(4), 943–952. doi: 10.1161/ATVBAHA.117.310307

Schwingshackl, L., Bogensberger, B., Benčič, A., Knüppel, S., Boeing, H., & Hoffmann, G. (2018). Effects of oils and solid fats on blood lipids: a systematic review and network meta-analysis. *J Lipid Res*, 59(9), 1771–1782. doi: 10.1194/jlr.P085522

Shanmugasundaram, M., Rough, S. J., & Alpert, J. S. (2010). Dyslipidemia in the Elderly: Should it Be Treated? *Clinical Cardiology*, 33(1), 4–9. doi: https://doi.org/10.1002/clc.20702

Stone, N. J., Blumenthal, R. S., Lloyd-Jones, D., & Grundy, S. M. (2020). Comparing Primary Prevention Recommendations. *Circulation*, 141(14), 1117–1120. doi: doi:10.1161/CIRCULATIONAHA.119.044562

Streja, E., & Streja, D. A. (2020). Management of Dyslipidemia in the Elderly. In K. R. Feingold, B. Anawalt, A. Boyce, G. Chrousos, W. W. de Herder, K. Dhatariya, K. Dungan, J. M. Hershman, J. Hofland, S. Kalra, G. Kaltsas, C. Koch, P. Kopp, M. Korbonits, C. S. Kovacs, W. Kuohung, B. Laferrère, M. Levy, E. A. McGee, R. McLachlan, J. E. Morley, M. New, J. Purnell, R. Sahay, F. Singer, M. A. Sperling, C. A. Stratakis, D. L. Trence & D. P. Wilson (Eds.), *Endotext*. South Dartmouth (MA): MDText.com, Inc. Copyright © 2000-2022, MDText.com, Inc.

Sun, F., Norman, I. J., & While, A. E. (2013). Physical activity in older people: a systematic review. *BMC Public Health*, 13(1), 449. doi: 10.1186/1471-2458-13-449

Tambalis, K., Panagiotakos, D. B., Kavouras, S. A., & Sidossis, L. S. (2009). Responses of blood lipids to aerobic, resistance, and combined aerobic with resistance exercise training: a systematic review of current evidence. *Angiology*, 60(5), 614–632. doi: 10.1177/0003319708324927

Thompson, P. D., Cullinane, E. M., Sady, S. P., Flynn, M. M., Bernier, D. N., Kantor, M. A., . . . Herbert, P. N. (1988). Modest changes in high-density lipoprotein concentration and metabolism with prolonged exercise training. *Circulation*, 78(1), 25–34. doi: 10.1161/01.cir.78.1.25

Tóth, P. P., Potter, D., & Ming, E. E. (2012). Prevalence of lipid abnormalities in the United States: The National Health and Nutrition Examination Survey 2003-2006. *Journal of Clinical Lipidology*, 6(4), 325–330. doi: https://doi.org/10.1016/j.jacl.2012.05.002

Trautwein, E. A., & McKay, S. (2020). The Role of Specific Components of a Plant-Based Diet in Management of Dyslipidemia and the Impact on Cardiovascular Risk. *Nutrients*, *12*(9), 2671.

Trautwein, E. A., Vermeer, M. A., Hiemstra, H., & Ras, R. T. (2018). LDL-Cholesterol Lowering of Plant Sterols and Stanols-Which Factors Influence Their Efficacy? *Nutrients*, *10*(9). doi: 10.3390/nu10091262

Vekic, J., Zeljkovic, A., Stefanovic, A., Jelic-Ivanovic, Z., & Spasojevic-Kalimanovska, V. (2019). Obesity and dyslipidemia. *Metabolism*, *92*, 71–81. doi: 10.1016/j.metabol.2018.11.005

Virani, S. S., Smith, S. C., Stone, N. J., & Grundy, S. M. (2020). Secondary Prevention for Atherosclerotic Cardiovascular Disease. *Circulation*, *141*(14), 1121–1123. doi: doi:10.1161/CIRCULATIONAHA.119.044282

Visseren, F. L. J., Mach, F., Smulders, Y. M., Carballo, D., Koskinas, K. C., Bäck, M., . . . Group, E. S. D. (2021). 2021 ESC Guidelines on cardiovascular disease prevention in clinical practice: Developed by the Task Force for cardiovascular disease prevention in clinical practice with representatives of the European Society of Cardiology and 12 medical societies With the special contribution of the European Association of Preventive Cardiology (EAPC). *European Heart Journal*, *42*(34), 3227–3337. doi: 10.1093/eurheartj/ehab484

Wewege, M. A., Thom, J. M., Rye, K. A., & Parmenter, B. J. (2018). Aerobic, resistance or combined training: A systematic review and meta-analysis of exercise to reduce cardiovascular risk in adults with metabolic syndrome. *Atherosclerosis*, *274*, 162–171. doi: 10.1016/j.atherosclerosis.2018.05.002

Williams, M. A., Haskell, W. L., Ades, P. A., Amsterdam, E. A., Bittner, V., Franklin, B. A., . . . Stewart, K. J. (2007). Resistance exercise in individuals with and without cardiovascular disease: 2007 update: a scientific statement from the American Heart Association Council on Clinical Cardiology and Council on Nutrition, Physical Activity, and Metabolism. *Circulation*, *116*(5), 572–584. doi: 10.1161/circulationaha.107.185214

Wood, G., Murrell, A., van der Touw, T., & Smart, N. (2019). HIIT is not superior to MICT in altering blood lipids: a systematic review and meta-analysis. *BMJ open sport & exercise medicine*, *5*(1), e000647. doi: 10.1136/bmjsem-2019-000647

Wood, P. D., Stefanick, M. L., Williams, P. T., & Haskell, W. L. (1991). The effects on plasma lipoproteins of a prudent weight-reducing diet, with or without exercise, in overweight men and women. *N Engl J Med*, *325*(7), 461–466. doi: 10.1056/nejm199108153250703

World Health Organization & Brouwer, I. A. (2016). *Effect of trans-fatty acid intake on blood lipids and lipoproteins: a systematic review and meta-regression analysis*. Geneva: World Health Organization.

Yki-Jarvinen, H., Koivisto, V. A., Taskinen, M. R., & Nikkila, E. (1984). Glucose tolerance, plasma lipoproteins and tissue lipoprotein lipase activities in body builders. *Eur J Appl Physiol Occup Physiol*, *53*(3), 253–259. doi: 10.1007/bf00776599

Zhao, D., Liu, J., Xie, W., & Qi, Y. (2015). Cardiovascular risk assessment: a global perspective. *Nature Reviews Cardiology*, *12*(5), 301–311. doi: 10.1038/nrcardio.2015.28

Zhu, X., Sun, X., Wang, M., Zhang, C., Cao, Y., Mo, G., . . . Zhu, S. (2015). Quantitative assessment of the effects of beta-glucan consumption on serum lipid profile and glucose level in hypercholesterolemic subjects. *Nutr Metab Cardiovasc Dis*, *25*(8), 714–723. doi: 10.1016/j.numecd.2015.04.008

FURTHER READING

Bibliography

Arnett, D. K., Blumenthal, R. S., Albert, M. A., Buroker, A. B., Goldberger, Z. D., Hahn, E. J., . . . Ziaeian, B. (2019). 2019 ACC/AHA Guideline on the Primary Prevention of Cardiovascular Disease: A Report of the American College of Cardiology/American Heart Association Task Force on Clinical Practice Guidelines. *Circulation*, *140*(11), e596–e646. doi: 10.1161/cir.0000000000000678

Grundy, S. M., Stone, N. J., Bailey, A. L., Beam, C., Birtcher, K. K., Blumenthal, R. S., . . . Yeboah, J. (2019). 2018 AHA/ACC/AACVPR/AAPA/ABC/ACPM/ADA/AGS/APhA/ASPC/NLA/PCNA Guideline on the Management of Blood Cholesterol: Executive Summary: A Report of the American College of Cardiology/American Heart Association Task Force on Clinical Practice Guidelines. *J Am Coll Cardiol*, *73*(24), 3168–3209. doi: 10.1016/j.jacc.2018.11.002

Stewart, J., Addy, K., Campbell, S., & Wilkinson, P. (2020). Primary prevention of cardiovascular disease: Updated review of contemporary guidance and literature. *JRSM Cardiovasc Dis*, *9*, 2048004020949326. doi: 10.1177/2048004020949326

Streja, E., & Streja, D. A. (2000). Management of Dyslipidemia in the Elderly. In K. R. Feingold, B. Anawalt, A. Boyce, G. Chrousos, W. W. de Herder, K. Dhatariya, K. Dungan, J. M. Hershman, J. Hofland, S. Kalra, G. Kaltsas, C. Koch, P. Kopp, M. Korbonits, C. S. Kovacs, W. Kuohung, B. Laferrère, M. Levy, E. A. McGee, R. McLachlan, J. E. Morley, M. New, J. Purnell, R. Sahay, F. Singer, M. A. Sperling, C. A. Stratakis, D. L. Trence & D. P. Wilson (Eds.), Endotext. South Dartmouth (MA): MDText.com, Inc.

Visseren, F. L. J., Mach, F., Smulders, Y. M., Carballo, D., Koskinas, K. C., Bäck, M., . . . Williams, B. (2021). 2021 ESC Guidelines on cardiovascular disease prevention in clinical practice. *Eur Heart J*, *42*(34), 3227–3337. doi: 10.1093/eurheartj/ehab484

Links

- https://www.heart.org/
- https://www.acc.org/
- https://www.escardio.org/
- https://www.escardio.org/static-file/Escardio/Subspecialty/EACPR/Documents/score-charts.pdf
- https://www.escardio.org/Education/Practice-Tools/CVD-prevention-toolbox/SCORE-Risk-Charts
- https://tools.acc.org/ldl/ascvd_risk_estimator/index.html#!/calulate/estimator/

Obesity and Metabolic Syndrome

CHAPTER 18

Introduction	275
Definition, Assessment, and Classification of Obesity	275
Epidemiology of Obesity	276
Pathogenesis of Obesity	277
Complications and Co-morbidities of Obesity	277
Obesity Paradox	278
Metabolically Healthy Obesity	279
Prevention of Obesity	279
Early Strategies	279
Healthy Weight	280
Dietary Sugar	280
Dietary Patterns	280
Physical Activity	281
Treatment of Obesity	281
Goals	281
Who Needs Weight Loss?	281
Dietary Strategies	281
Physical Activity and Obesity	284
Nutrition and Exercise: Combined Interventions	285
Pharmacotherapy and Bariatric Surgery	286
Lifestyle Modifications During Weight-loss Maintenance	286
Introduction to Metabolic Syndrome	287
Epidemiology of Metabolic Syndrome	288
Diagnosis of Metabolic Syndrome	288
Lifestyle and Risk of Metabolic Syndrome	288
Diet	288
Physical Activity	289
Management of Metabolic Syndrome	289
Diet	289
Physical Activity	290
Exercise and Nutrition: Combined Intervention	290
Recommendations	290
Key Points	291
Self-assessment Questions	291
Case Scenario	291
References	292
Further Reading	297
Bibliography	297
Links	297

INTRODUCTION

The rates of overweight and obesity are increasing worldwide and, in parallel, an increasing prevalence of metabolic syndrome is observed. These conditions are strongly associated with several adverse effects, including impaired quality of life and a higher risk of morbidity and mortality. Hence, there is a need for prevention strategies as well as optimal interventions to manage and reduce the incidence of these conditions as well as their co-morbidities.

DEFINITION, ASSESSMENT, AND CLASSIFICATION OF OBESITY

According to the World Health Organization (WHO), overweight and obesity are defined as abnormal or excessive fat accumulation that causes negative health consequences (World Health Organization, 2021). The classification of overweight and obesity in adults most commonly uses the body-mass index (BMI), which is a simple index of weight-for-height. It is

Prevention and Management of Cardiovascular and Metabolic Disease: Diet, Physical Activity and Healthy Aging,
First Edition. Christina N. Katsagoni, Peter Kokkinos, and Labros S. Sidossis.
© 2023 John Wiley & Sons Ltd. Published 2023 by John Wiley & Sons Ltd.

Table 18.1 Adult BMI and waist circumference cutoff points in white people.

	Obesity class	BMI (kg/m^2)	Waist circumference	Associated health risk
Underweight		<18.5		
Normal		18.5–24.9		Average
Overweight		25.0–29.9	Men: ≥94 cm Women: ≥80 cm	Increased
Obesity	I	30.0–34.9	Men: ≥102 cm Women: ≥88 cm	Moderate
Moderate obesity	II	35.0–39.9		High
Severe obesity	III	≥40		Very high

Source: (NICE clinical guideline 189, 2014).

calculated as a person's weight in kilograms divided by the square of height in meters (kg/m^2). The classification of overweight and obesity is presented in **Table 18.1** (World Health Organization, 2021). The main drawback of BMI is that it does not take into account body composition and thus only provides a rough estimation of obesity and undernutrition.

Overweight is defined as a BMI between 25 and 29.9 kg/m^2 and obesity as a BMI >30 kg/m^2 (World Health Organization, 2021). This cutoff value is not valid for non-Caucasian ethnicities, people with increased muscle mass, such as bodybuilders, as well as children and adolescents (Durrer Schutz et al., 2019; Jensen, Ryan, Donato, et al., 2014; NICE clinical guideline 189, 2014). BMI represents the sum of fat-mass index (FMI) and fat-free mass index (FFMI), with the latter accounting for skeletal muscle mass, bone, and organs and FMI consisting of the peripheral and visceral adipose tissues. These components of BMI contribute differently to health status, and BMI changes are not related to a proportional and linear modification of body compartments (Donini, Pinto, Giusti, Lenzi, & Poggiogalle, 2020; Dulloo, Jacquet, Solinas, Montani, & Schutz, 2010; Rothman, 2008). Consequently, the BMI classification should be used with caution for older adults as the progressive "natural" weight gain that occurs between 20 and 65 years, could "hide" the fat-free mass loss that happens through aging. Indeed, central/visceral fat and relative loss of fat-free mass may become relatively more important than BMI for the assessment of obesity-related health risks in the elderly. In association with the rapid increase of life expectancy and the rising prevalence of obesity, the so called "obesity paradox" in the elderly has been explored by many studies (more in **Unit 3**) (Bosello & Vanzo, 2021; Durrer Schutz et al., 2019; Flicker et al., 2010). Except for older adults, the obesity paradox also refers to evidence showing that obesity in patients with chronic diseases may be protective and associated with decreased mortality (more later in this chapter).

Waist circumference is a good measure for the assessment of the visceral fat and a good predictor of cardiovascular diseases. "Normal" waist circumference references are <80 cm for women and <94 cm for men. Cutoff points indicating higher cardio-metabolic risk are >88 cm for women and >102 cm for men (**Table 18.1**) (Lean, Han, & Morrison, 1995; Manolopoulos, Karpe, & Frayn, 2010; Zhu et al., 2002).

Assessing body fat is not a simple task. As direct assessment of body fat is not practical, several indirect techniques and technologies have been developed over the years to assess body composition, including bioimpedance analysis (BIA), dual-energy X-ray absorptiometry (DXA), air-displacement plethysmography (BodPod), and body scanning procedures (Cornier et al., 2011; Silver, E. Brian Welch, Malcolm J. Avison, & Kevin D. Niswender, 2010). The assessment of body composition (fat mass and fat-free mass) is not a routine procedure for the management of obesity in clinical practice but may be a useful tool before and during treatment or in specific category of patients such as in older adults. However, body composition measurements are recommended for research purposes (Durrer Schutz et al., 2019; Yumuk et al., 2015).

EPIDEMIOLOGY OF OBESITY

Despite growing recognition of the problem, the prevalence of overweight and obesity in the US and around the world continues to rise. In US, according to 2015–2016 data, the prevalence of overweight and obesity in men was 74.7% and 38% respectively, while the corresponding prevalence in women was 68.9% and 41.5%, respectively. It is estimated that by 2030 most American adults will suffer either from overweight or obesity, with central obesity estimated to reach 55.6% in men and 80.0% in women (Y. Wang et al., 2021). According to the WHO, the prevalence of obesity worldwide in 2016 was almost three times higher than that in 1975 (World Health Organization, 2021). **Figure 18.1** shows the estimated global prevalence and numbers of adults living with obesity from 2010 to 2030.

Adult obesity prevalence	2010		2025		2030	
	% adults	number	% adults	number	% adults	number
Obesity (Class I, II and III) BMI ≥30 kg/m^2	11.4%	511m	16.1%	892m	17.5%	1,025m
of which, severe obesity (Class II and III) BMI ≥35 kg/m^2	3.2%%	143m	5.1%	284m	5.7%	333m
and of these, severe obesity (Class III) BMI ≥40 kg/m^2	0.9%	42m	1.7%	93m	1.9%	111m

FIGURE 18.1 Estimated global prevalence and numbers of adults living with obesity in 2010–2030. Source: (WHO, 2022 / with permission of Elsevier).

PATHOGENESIS OF OBESITY

The causes of obesity are complex and multifactorial. The complex interaction between genetic, epigenetic, behavioral, social, and environmental factors is likely to contribute to obesity. Specifically, obesity is the result of a chronic imbalance between caloric intake and caloric expenditure. A net deficit in energy balance, either through a reduction in energy intake or an increase in energy expenditure, leads to weight reduction. Conversely, a net excess in energy balance due to a reduction in energy expenditure or an increase in energy intake, leads to weight gain (Gjermeni et al., 2021; X. Lin & Li, 2021).

Peripheral signals from various body organs are integrated to control energy homeostasis. Therefore, small changes in one of these determinants can bring over time substantial changes in body weight. A host of hormones, including insulin, leptin, adiponectin, and ghrelin, communicate with the hypothalamus to control a person's energy intake and body weight. Moreover, the heritability of obesity is estimated at between 40% and 70%, with evidence involving mutations and variations in several genes (Waalen, 2014). Obesity has been also associated with changes in the composition of the intestinal microbiota (Gjermeni et al., 2021; X. Lin & Li, 2021). Intestinal flora has been found to regulate a variety of host physiological functions, such as energy absorption, intestinal barrier permeability, secondary synthesis of bile acids, and intestinal hormone release. When metabolites of the intestinal flora enter the circulation, they can affect appetite and adipose tissue synthesis, decomposition, thermogenesis, and browning. Moreover, increased intestinal permeability is also associated with systemic chronic inflammation, which is a further factor leading to insulin resistance (K. Lin, Zhu, & Yang, 2022).

Lifestyle is a major contributor to the development of overweight and obesity. A high-energy density diet, increased portion size, lack of exercise, and a sedentary lifestyle are important risk factors for the development of obesity (X. Lin & Li, 2021). The dietary fat model of obesity postulates that high intake of fat and sugars leads to increased overall energy intake. Moreover, an increase in physical inactivity due to adopting a sedentary lifestyle, or due to the sedentary nature of many forms of work, increasing urbanization, and changing modes of transportation, all contribute to the development of obesity (World Health Organization, 2021).

COMPLICATIONS AND CO-MORBIDITIES OF OBESITY

Obesity is a chronic systematic disease that affects almost every organ and system of the body, including the endocrine, gastrointestinal, cardiovascular, and central nervous systems (**Figure 18.2**) (Bischoff et al., 2017). Obesity can progressively cause and/or exacerbate a wide spectrum of co-morbidities, including cardiovascular diseases (CVD), type 2 diabetes, hypertension, dyslipidemia, liver dysfunction, musculoskeletal disorders (especially osteoarthritis), asthma, sleep apnea syndrome, psychosocial problems, cognition, and certain types of cancer, such as colorectal, kidney, and breast cancers (Bischoff et al., 2017; Fruh, 2017; World Health Organization, 2021). The different co-morbidities associated with obesity are shown in **Figure 18.3**.

Consequently, the excess adiposity is a well-established risk factor for all-cause mortality, which is mediated through its effects on this wide range of chronic diseases. Indeed, in an early systematic review and meta-analysis of 97 prospective, observational cohort studies, including more than 2.88 million individuals, researchers aimed to examine the effect of body weight on all-cause mortality. They showed that those suffering from obesity (all grates) or grade II and grade III obesity, compared to normal weight, had higher risk of all-cause mortality by 18% and

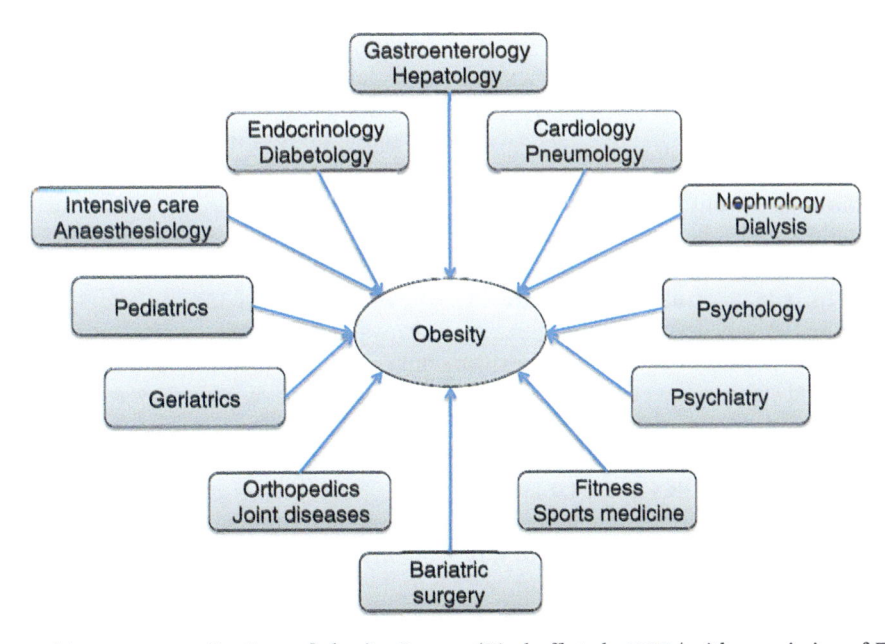

FIGURE 18.2 Multiorgan, multi-system complications of obesity. Source: (Bischoff et al., 2017 / with permission of Elsevier).

Obesity and co-morbidities

Pulmonary disease
Abnormal function
Obstructive sleep apnea
Hypoventilation syndrome

Nonalcoholic fatty liver disease
Steatosis
Steatohepatitis
Cirrhosis

Gall bladder disease

Gynaecologic abnormalities
Abnormal menses
Infertility
Polycystic ovarian syndrome

Osteoarthritis

Skin

Idiopathic intracranial hypertension

Stroke

Cataracts

Coronary heart disease
← Diabetes
← Dyslipidaemia
← Hypertension

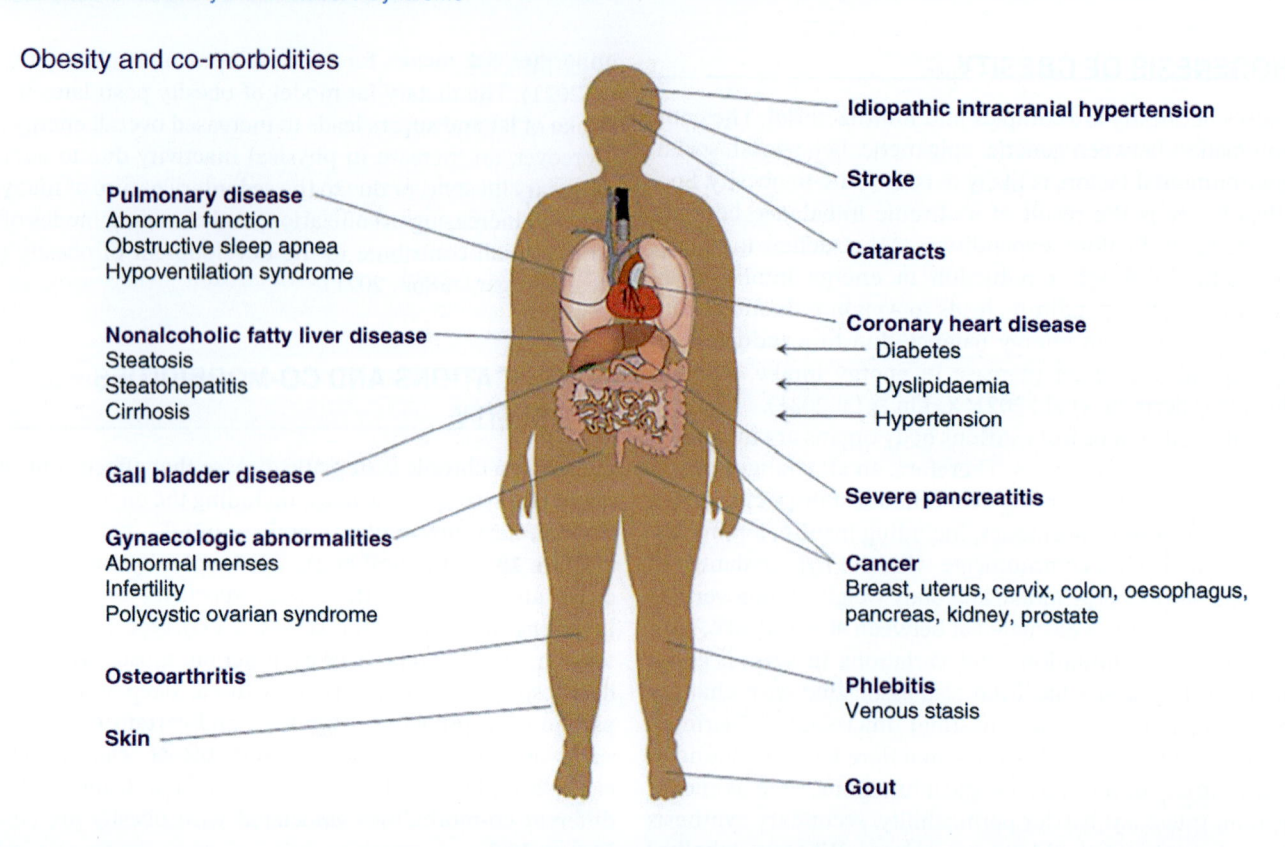

Severe pancreatitis

Cancer
Breast, uterus, cervix, colon, oesophagus, pancreas, kidney, prostate

Phlebitis
Venous stasis

Gout

FIGURE 18.3 Obesity and its co-morbidities affecting many systems, organs, and tissues. Source: (Durrer Schutz et al., 2019 / with permission of Karger Publishers).

29%, respectively, while grade I obesity was not correlated with higher or lower mortality. On the contrary, overweight correlated with lower mortality risk by 6% compared to normal weight (Flegal, Kit, Orpana, & Graubard, 2013).

OBESITY PARADOX

Numerous studies have indicated that obesity offers a survival advantage among older adults and in patients with several chronic diseases.

Indeed, although obesity is positively associated with CVD risk, it paradoxically leads to a more favorable prognosis in individuals with chronic heart failure and other cardiovascular diseases such as coronary heart disease, hypertension, and atrial fibrillation (Lavie et al., 2016; Oktay et al., 2017) (more in **Chapter 12**), a phenomenon commonly defined as the "obesity paradox" (S. Wang & Ren, 2018). Kokkinos et al. observed this paradox in African American and Caucasian veterans with type 2 diabetes. The cohort consisted of 4156 men with a mean age of 60 years who were followed for 7.5 years. Researchers found that individuals with a normal BMI (between 18.5 and 24.9 kg/m^2) had a significantly increased risk of mortality compared to those with obesity (hazard ratio 1.70 [95% CI 1.36-2.1]). The risk was even greater for African American, compared to Caucasian veterans. They also highlighted the important role of exercise on mortality in the same population. Those with increased exercise capacity had a lower mortality risk, independent of their weight status (Kokkinos et al., 2012). In a cohort study published two years later, in 2014, some authors of the previous study concluded to similar results; lower values of BMI (18,5-23,9 kg/m^2) compared to a BMI of 24.0 to 27.9 kg/m^2 were associated with higher mortality risk in male veterans. Researchers also further examined the cardio-respiratory fitness of the individuals and its association with BMI and mortality. The association was not present in high-fit individuals, but only in moderate-fit and low-fit individuals, suggesting that the increased mortality rate in lower values of BMIs could be due to considerable weight loss accompanied by a reduction in muscle mass (Kokkinos et al., 2014).

Obesity paradox is even more pronounced in older adults. A meta-analysis of 32 population-based cohort studies, including 197,940 participants, with an average follow up of 12 years, demonstrated that being overweight was not associated with an increased risk of mortality while the optimal BMI for people aged ≥65 years was 28 kg/m^2 (**Figure 18.4**) (Winter, MacInnis, Wattanapenpaiboon, & Nowson, 2014).

Nevertheless, according to a narrative review published in 2020, which summarized the evidence underlying the concept of obesity paradox researchers found great discrepancies between studies. The attributed causes of these discrepancies were the use of BMI in the definition of obesity, instead of excess body fat and the different adjustments for potential confounders in the studies

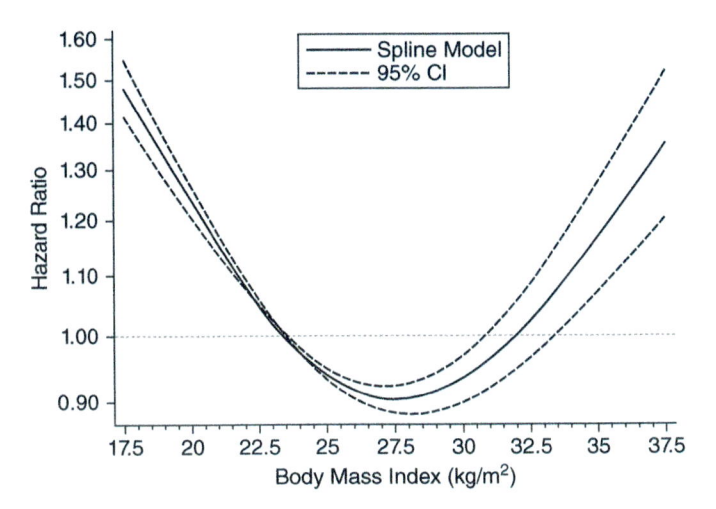

FIGURE 18.4 Hazard ratio of all-cause mortality according to BMI for men and women aged ≥65 year. Source: (Winter et al., 2014 / with permission of Oxford University Press).

(e.g., stage and grade of diseases, body composition etc) that could scale down the protective role of obesity in terms of mortality. However, they acknowledged a few biases among studies (e.g., reverse causation, attrition bias, selection bias of healthy obese subjects or resilient survivors) that could affect the trajectories of mortality in a number of diseases (Donini et al., 2020).

METABOLICALLY HEALTHY OBESITY

Metabolically healthy obesity is defined as obesity in the absence of a clearly defined cardio-metabolic disorder, such as MetS, insulin resistance, hypertension, diabetes, or dyslipidemia. Identifying individuals with metabolically healthy obesity may potentially help avoid wasting time, effort, and resources on people who may not benefit—or benefit less—from weight-loss management. However, the term "metabolically" is often misinterpreted as meaning without any sort of complications whatsoever and, consequently, without the need for treatment. Besides cardio-metabolic diseases, obesity may be associated with orthopedic problems, reproductive disorders, depression, asthma, sleep apnea, renal disease, back pain, skin infections, cognitive decline, social stigma, and overall reduced quality of life (Magkos, 2019) and thus individuals with metabolically healthy obesity will seek assistance from a healthcare professional at some point in their life.

However, meta-analyses of prospective studies have demonstrated that metabolically healthy individuals with obesity have approximately half the risk of developing type 2 diabetes and CVD compared with metabolically unhealthy individuals with obesity (Bell, Kivimaki, & Hamer, 2014; N. Eckel, Meidtner, Kalle-Uhlmann, Stefan, & Schulze, 2016). Nevertheless, the cardio-metabolic disease risk is still significantly elevated by 50% to 300% compared with metabolically healthy lean individuals. Therefore, there is an obvious need to deal with both phenotypes of obesity, both unhealthy and healthy (Magkos, 2019).

PREVENTION OF OBESITY

EARLY STRATEGIES

Factors that contribute to obesity in life are already present from the time of gestation. The first months of life seem to play a crucial role in the development of obesity later in life. Preventing overweight or obesity from the early stages of life could be an important strategy (M. et al., 2013). A position paper from the Academy of Nutrition and Dietetics published in 2013 proposed interventions for the prevention of excess body weight in children and treatment of children with overweight or obesity (**Table 18.2**) (Hoelscher, Kirk, Ritchie, & Cunningham-Sabo, 2013).

Breastfeeding has been associated with a modest reduction in the risk of developing overweight or obesity later in life by inducing lower plasma insulin levels, thereby

Table 18.2 Summary of recommendations from the review of child obesity primary prevention literature.

1. **Integrate education with supportive environmental change.** In school and childcare settings, the most successful interventions at achieving behavior change coupled educational messages with institutional change, so that children are taught about healthy eating and physical activity while provided healthy foods and more opportunities for physical activity.
2. **Include both nutrition education and physical education.** The most successful interventions were those that included both nutrition and physical activity as integral parts of the intervention. Targeting obesity prevention through physical activity alone does not seem to be as effective without incorporating nutrition education. Younger children appear to learn best when exposed to behaviorally based or hands-on (rather than didactic) activities including ample opportunities for tasting, touching, and working with food. Providers, caregivers, and parents should be reminded that repeated exposure is typically required to promote acceptance of new foods by children.
3. **Build in parent engagement for younger children.** Interventions that aimed to involve parents were generally more successful than those that did not, especially among preschool and elementary school-age children. Efforts to include parents are most effective when the parent not only receives information that reflects what the child is learning but is also given guidance and at-home activities to aid in the progression of healthier lifestyle changes for the child at home.
4. **Promote community engagement in schools and childcare.** School and childcare based interventions show better results when coupled with community efforts that reinforce healthy eating and activity as well as consistent messaging, both in and out of school and childcare.
5. **Policies that limit food availability show promise.** Policies that limit food availability, especially in schools, seem to be associated with lower BMI.
6. **Dose and continuity is important.** Children are inundated with messages promoting the consumption of high-energy foods, so it is important to intensify and sustain the dose of nutrition education. More intensive interventions show better results. Although including health education in curricula is important, more innovative and "out of the box" messaging and other strategies should be explored, such as role model stories or novels, social media, and the incorporation of health outcomes and consequences into all facets of society.

Source: (Hoelscher et al., 2013).

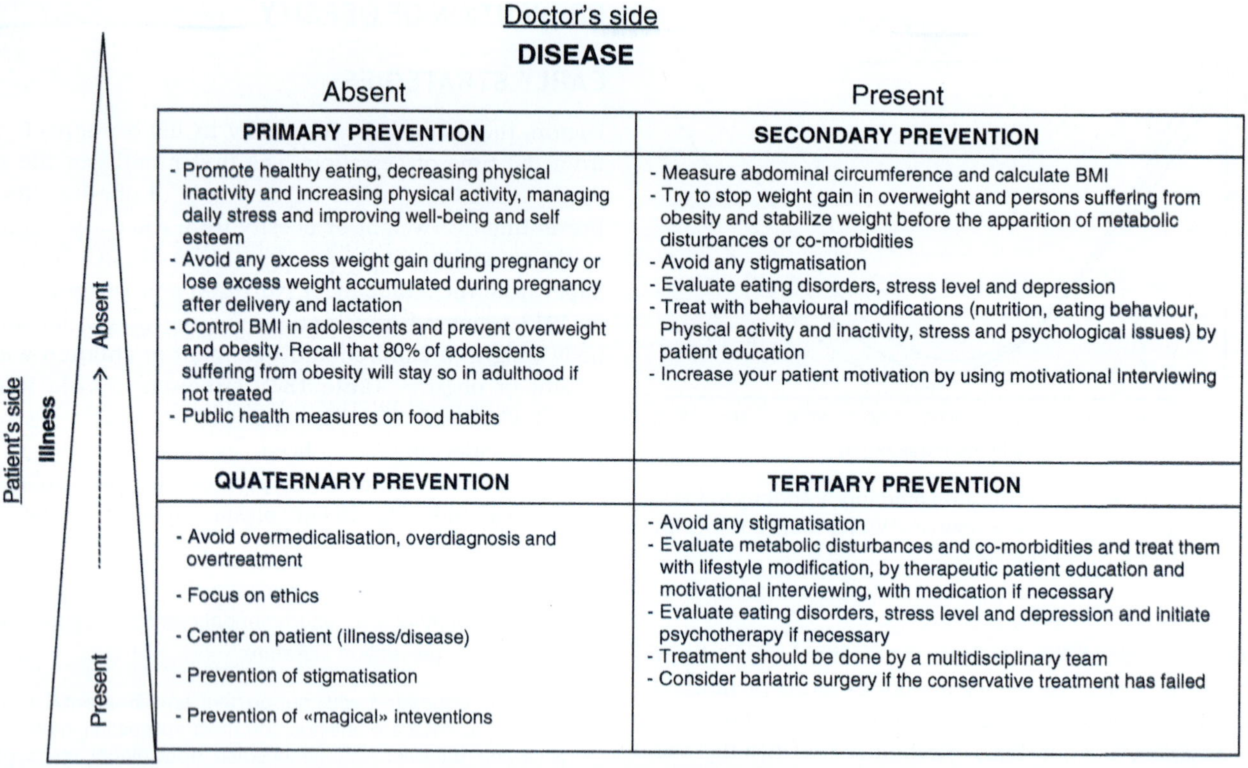

	Doctor's side	
	DISEASE	
	Absent	Present
Patient's side Illness — Absent	**PRIMARY PREVENTION** - Promote healthy eating, decreasing physical inactivity and increasing physical activity, managing daily stress and improving well-being and self esteem - Avoid any excess weight gain during pregnancy or lose excess weight accumulated during pregnancy after delivery and lactation - Control BMI in adolescents and prevent overweight and obesity. Recall that 80% of adolescents suffering from obesity will stay so in adulthood if not treated - Public health measures on food habits	**SECONDARY PREVENTION** - Measure abdominal circumference and calculate BMI - Try to stop weight gain in overweight and persons suffering from obesity and stabilize weight before the apparition of metabolic disturbances or co-morbidities - Avoid any stigmatisation - Evaluate eating disorders, stress level and depression - Treat with behavioural modifications (nutrition, eating behaviour, Physical activity and inactivity, stress and psychological issues) by patient education - Increase your patient motivation by using motivational interviewing
Patient's side Illness — Present	**QUATERNARY PREVENTION** - Avoid overmedicalisation, overdiagnosis and overtreatment - Focus on ethics - Center on patient (illness/disease) - Prevention of stigmatisation - Prevention of «magical» inteventions	**TERTIARY PREVENTION** - Avoid any stigmatisation - Evaluate metabolic disturbances and co-morbidities and treat them with lifestyle modification, by therapeutic patient education and motivational interviewing, with medication if necessary - Evaluate eating disorders, stress level and depression and initiate psychotherapy if necessary - Treatment should be done by a multidisciplinary team - Consider bariatric surgery if the conservative treatment has failed

FIGURE 18.5 Primary, secondary, tertiary, and quaternary preventions with their respective explanations. Source: (Durrer Schutz et al., 2019 / with permissions of Karger Publishers).

decreasing fat storage and preventing excessive early adipocyte development. The higher protein content of artificial infant milk compared to the lower-protein content in breast milk is responsible for the increased growth rate and adiposity, promoting growth acceleration, whereas breastfeeding has been shown to promote slower growth. Therefore, enhancing breastfeeding can be suggested to reduce the risk of obesity (Wendy H Oddy, 2012).

HEALTHY WEIGHT

Although the development of overweight and obesity is multifactorial, the decline in energy expenditure is considered as one of the most important determinants of excessive body weight. Body weight increases because of a positive energy balance when energy intake exceeds energy expenditure. So, aiming to or maintaining a healthy weight, which is achieved when energy intake is adjusted to energy expenditure is considered the main goal for preventing overweight/obesity (Lavie et al., 2018). Four categories of prevention—primary, secondary, tertiary, and fourth (quaternary prevention)—are shown in **Figure 18.5** (Durrer Schutz et al., 2019).

DIETARY SUGAR

Counseling people to reduce the intake of sugar and the consumption of sugar-sweetened beverages (SSBs) is important for controlling body weight and therefore the risk for obesity-related chronic diseases (Ebbeling, 2014). A meta-analysis of 30 randomized controlled trials (RCTs) and 38 prospective cohort studies showed that intake of sugar or SSBs is a determinant of body weight among free-living people involving *ad libitum* diets (Morenga, Mallard, & Mann, 2013). Moreover, high intake of SSBs has been linked to higher risk of type 2 diabetes, CVD, and some types of cancers. SSBs are believed to promote weight gain through incomplete compensation for liquid calories at subsequent meals (Malik & Hu, 2019).

DIETARY PATTERNS

A low-calorie healthy food pattern either based on the components of a vegetarian or a Mediterranean dietary pattern may offer a possible solution to the ongoing challenges to prevent and manage obesity and CVDs.

A meta-analysis of 12 cross-sectional studies and one case-control study, including 26,974 and 174 participants, respectively, demonstrated that *a posteriori* healthy dietary patterns characterized as high in fruits, vegetables, and whole grains decrease the risk of central obesity (Rezagholizadeh, Djafarian, Khosravi, & Shab-Bidar, 2017). Moreover, in a meta-analysis of six prospective cohort studies, including a total of 244,678 participants, higher adherence to the Mediterranean diet (MD) was associated with a 9% lower risk of suffering from overweight and/or obesity, while closer adherence to the MD, as assessed by the MD score was inversely associated with weight gain over 5 years (Lotfi, Saneei, Hajhashemy, & Esmaillzadeh, 2022).

PHYSICAL ACTIVITY

The role of physical activity in the prevention of excessive body weight is well-documented. As mentioned in previous chapters, the World Health Organization in the 2020 guidelines provides age-appropriate recommendations for PA for children, adults and older adults (WHO, 2020). In brief, adults (from 18 to 64 years old) should undertake 150–300 min of moderate-intensity physical activity, or 75–150 min of vigorous-intensity physical activity, or some equivalent combination of moderate-intensity and vigorous-intensity aerobic physical activity, per week. Among children and adolescents, an average of 60 min/day of moderate-to-vigorous intensity aerobic physical activity across the week provides health benefits.

Older adults should also participate in varied multi-component physical activity emphasizing functional balance and strength training (i.e., circuit training) at moderate or greater intensity, 3 or more days a week. Functional exercises include tandem and one-leg stands, squatting, chair stands, toe raises, and stepping over obstacles (WHO, 2020).

TREATMENT OF OBESITY

GOALS

According to 2019 European guidelines for adults with obesity (Durrer Schutz et al., 2019), the main goals of obesity treatment are to prevent complications, to prevent or treat co-morbidities if they are present, to reduce stigmatization, and to induce well-being, positive body image, and self-esteem. Body weight *per se* is not a priority, while obesity treatment cannot focus only on weight reduction. The goals can focus more on lifestyle changes, reducing waist circumference, and body composition than weight loss. Modest weight loss (i.e., 5–10% of the initial body weight) within 6 months may lead to significant clinical benefits, and 5–15% of weight loss can be feasible depending on the pathology (Durrer Schutz et al., 2019; Yumuk et al., 2015).

WHO NEEDS WEIGHT LOSS?

Individuals suffering from overweight or obesity, in most cases, require weight loss. However, there are patients that are not eligible or prepared for this kind of intervention. The main goal is to assess every individual and provide tailor-made advice and customized intervention based on a person's needs.

According to the 2013 American Heart Association/American College of Cardiology task force on practice guidelines and The Obesity Society (AHA/ACC/TOS) guideline for the management of overweight and obesity in adults, a weight-loss intervention should be performed in individuals with obesity or overweight, who additionally have one indicator of increased cardiovascular risk or any obesity-related comorbidity. Risk factors indicating increased cardiovascular risk are diabetes or prediabetes, hypertension, dyslipidaemia, and elevated waist circumference. It is possible, though, that some of these patients who need weight loss might reject the intervention. In this case, a patient's intention in losing weight should be frequently assessed and they should be advised to avoid further weight gain.

Individuals with a normal body weight or individuals with overweight without cardiovascular disease risk factors or co-morbidities linked to obesity should not be advised to lose weight, but to avoid additional weight gain. Furthermore, generally healthy individuals with overweight or currently normal weight individuals who used to suffer from overweight or obesity should be advised to measure their body weight, alter their energy intake, when appropriate, and engage with physical activity to avoid weight gain (Jensen, Ryan, Donato, et al., 2014).

In older adults with overweight, weight-reducing diets may be avoided so as to prevent loss of muscle mass and functional decline, whereas in older adults with obesity, weight-reducing diets may only be considered after weighing the benefits and risks (Volkert et al., 2019).

DIETARY STRATEGIES

Over the past decades, a considerable number of diets have been used to induce weight loss in people living with overweight or obesity (examples in **Table 18.3**). Even though there are a lot of differences between them, all of them aim at the same thing, caloric restriction. What varies is the way of achieving this. The question is, which is the most effective?

A low-calorie diet (LCD) usually ranges from 1200 to 1600 kcal/d with the use of a meal plan, in which all food choices and portion sizes for all meals and snacks are provided. The use of meal replacements, usually liquid shakes and bars, containing a known amount of energy and macronutrient content, is also appropriate. These methods enhance adherence to a LCD by reducing problematic food choices and decreasing any challenges in making healthy choices (Raynor & Champagne, 2016). A meta-analysis of six RCTs showed that an LCD composed of conventional foods or meal replacements led to a 2.54 kg and 2.43 kg greater weight loss in the partial meal-replacement group for the 3-month and 1-year follow ups, respectively (Heymsfield, Van Mierlo, Van Der Knaap, Heo, & Frier, 2003).

A very low-calorie diet (VLCD) provides ≤800 kcal per day and are usually consumed as liquid shakes. Specifically, a VLCD is usually appropriate only for individuals with a BMI ≥30 kg/m^2 and is used before bariatric surgery to reduce overall surgical risk in individuals with severe obesity. A meta-analysis of six RCTs showed that VLCDs produce significantly greater weight loss in the short-term compared to LCD, whereas there was no difference in weight loss between the diets in long-term follow up (>1 year) (Tsai & Wadden, 2006).

Although calorie intake seems to play a crucial role for the management of overweight or obesity, current evidence indicates that different diets with different macronutrient content (low-carbohydrate diets- low CHO, carbohydrate intake ≤ 40% vs. low-fat diets-LFD, fat intake < 30%), may promote similar percentages of weight loss while it is the adherence to each diet that will predict their success. According to a systematic review and meta-analysis comparing low CHO diets with isoenergetic

Table 18.3 Common weight-loss diets.

Diet name	Composition	Need for prescribed energy restriction
Low-calorie	Not specific	Prescribed energy restriction.
Higher protein	• 25% energy from protein • 30% energy from fat • 45% energy from carbohydrate	Choice of foods that lead to an energy deficit.
Higher protein Zone™-type	5 meals/d, each with: • 40% energy from carbohydrate • 30% energy from protein • 30% energy from fat	Without prescribed energy restriction. Automatically leads to energy deficit.
Lacto–ovo–vegetarian–style	Typical diet composition	Prescribed energy restriction.
European Association for the Study of Diabetes Guidelines	Focuses on targeting food groups and achieving an energy deficit.	Without prescribed energy restriction.
Low-carbohydrate	<20 g/d carbohydrate	Without prescribed energy restriction. Automatically leads to energy deficit.
Low-fat vegan-style	• 10–25% energy from fat • Vegan food choices	Without prescribed energy restriction. Automatically leads to energy deficit.
Low-fat	20% energy from fat	Without prescribed energy restriction. Automatically leads to energy deficit.
Low–glycemic load	Food choices with low–glycemic load	With or without prescribed energy restriction but leading to energy deficit either way.
Lower-fat, high-dairy diets with or without increased fiber and/or low–glycemic index (low–glycemic load)	• ≤30% energy from fat • 4 servings/d dairy	Prescribed energy restriction.
Macronutrient-targeted	• 15–25% energy from protein • 20–40% energy from fat • 35%, 45%, 55%, or 65% energy from carbohydrate	Prescribed energy restriction.
Mediterranean-style	Typical MD food choices	Prescribed energy restriction.
Moderate-protein	• 12% energy from protein • 58% energy from carbohydrate • 30% energy from fat	Choice of foods that lead to an energy deficit.
High-glycemic or low–glycemic load	Based on food glycemic load	Prescribed energy restriction.
The AHA-style Step 1 diet	• <30% energy from fat • <10% energy from saturated fat	Prescribed energy restriction of 1500 to 1800 kcal/d.

Source: (Jensen, Ryan, Apovian, et al., 2014)

balanced weight-loss diets in adults with overweight or obesity, there is little or no difference in weight loss or cardiovascular risk factors when comparing low CHO diets with balanced diets as long as they are isoenergetic. Results are similar either assesing the individuals in the short (3–6 months) or in the long term (up to two years of follow-up). (Naude et al., 2014). Another research team resulted in a similar finding. When they compared a LFD with low CHO diets or higher-fat diets, they inferred that it is the intensity of the intervention that most strongly affect the final weight loss and not the macronutrient intake (Mansoor, Vinknes, Veierod, & Retterstol, 2016).

Nevertheless, in a meta-analysis of 11 RCTs of, at least, a 6-month duration, individuals with obesity followed a low CHO diet and compared to those who followed an LFD. The low CHO diet showed a greater decrease in body weight (mean difference ~2.2 kg) and in triglycerides as well as a greater increase in high-density lipoprotein-cholesterol (HDL-cholesterol) and in low-density lipoprotein-cholesterol (LDL-cholesterol) compared to the LFD (Mansoor et al., 2016). This last consequence should be taken into consideration based on patient's medical history and risk factors to assess the pros and cons of losing weight but also increasing LDL. Another meta-analysis of 13 RCTs, with durations of 12 months or more, compared a very low CHO-ketogenic diet with a typical LFD with energy restriction. The low CHO diet resulted in a greater weight loss (mean difference 0.9 kg), (Mansoor et al., 2016), while an amelioration in diastolic blood pressure was also observed (Bueno, De Melo, De Oliveira, & Da Rocha Ataide, 2013).

These results indicate that health care providers may choose among different dietary options to manage individuals with overweight or obesity and that there is not an optimally effective diet for all individuals to lose weight. Moreover, a higher level of adherence to a dietary weight-loss approach, regardless of the type of the diet will determine its success (Freire, 2020). Higher adherence to a diet is significantly correlated with the amount of weight loss and lower weight regain compared to less or no weight loss observed in individuals with difficulties in adhering to a weight-loss dietary program (Freire, 2020).

High-protein diets (at least 20% of energy derived from protein) for weight loss have also been thoroughly studied, mainly as a means to maintain lean mass. A meta-analysis of 37 RCTs demonstrated that people with increased protein intake (ranging from 18–59% of energy requirements) reduced body weight by 1.6 kg compared to controls (digestible carbohydrate, fiber, fat, or no supplementation [no placebo used]). The same study concluded that people with prediabetes may benefit more from a diet high in protein compared to people with normoglycemia (Hansen, Astrup, & Sjödin, 2021). Another meta-analysis of 20 RCTs, including 1174 participants, showed that older adults aged ≥50 years retained more lean mass while losing body fat mass during weight loss when they consumed energy-restricted higher protein (≥25 energy percentage) rather than normal protein diets (<25 energy percentage) (Kim, O'Connor, Sands, Slebodnik, & Campbell, 2016). Regarding CVD factors, meta-analyses have concluded that a high-protein diet is not superior to a standard diet during weight loss on changes in serum triglycerides, HDL, and LDL-cholesterol compared to a standard diet during weight loss (Santesso et al., 2012; Wycherley, Moran, Clifton, Noakes, & Brinkworth, 2012). Finally, diets high in protein have not been found to beneficially affect hunger and the desire to eat, food cravings, or overall well-being (Li, Armstrong, & Campbell, 2016; Nerylee A. Watson et al., 2018; Nerylee Ann Watson et al., 2018).

Whatever the intervention is for the management of overweight or obesity, it is important to refer each individual who is willing to lose weight to a qualified registered dietitian that can evaluate which type of diet will be more effective for the patient. The aim is to achieve the greatest adherence to the weight-loss diet, so that the patient can benefit as much as possible. The summary findings of these studies on dietary modifications for weight loss in individuals with overweight or obesity are shown in **Table 18.4** (Yannakoulia, Poulimeneas, Mamalaki, & Anastasiou, 2019).

However, there is a great number of individuals who choose to follow, without any supervision, the so called "fad diets" for weight loss. Fad diets are popular in promising easy and quick weight loss. Typical examples of such diets are shown in **Table 18.5** (Mattson, Longo, & Harvie, 2017). These diets may have a positive impact on health as they are based on extreme caloric restriction, leading to rapid weight loss. What is concerning is the safety of these methods and the tendency for individuals to regain weight once they start consuming a normal diet again (Obert, Pearlman, Obert, & Chapin, 2017).

As nutrition research and epidemiology have focused on the relationship between health/disease and dietary patterns—rather than single nutrients, the role of specific dietary patterns in the management of overweight and obesity has been evaluated.

The MD dietary pattern is the most extensively studied pattern for a variety of health outcomes, including obesity and weight treatment. The PREDIMED study is a large study, with two MD intervention arms, one supplemented with olive oil and the other supplemented with nuts, and a low-fat diet as the control group. All diets were provided without an energy restriction. The results of this trial did not reveal a difference between the three arms regarding body weight over 5 years. In contrast, waist circumference increased less in the MD plus nuts group compared with the control group (Estruch et al., 2019). Moreover, another meta-analysis of nine RCTs, including 1178 diabetic individuals, demonstrated that a MD improved outcomes of glycemic control, weight loss, and CVD risk factors (Huo et al., 2015).

Table 18.4 Summary findings of the studies on dietary modifications for weight loss in people with overweight and obesity, published beyond the 2013 AHA/ACC/TOC guidelines.

Dietary intervention	Summary of findings
Very low-carbohydrate diets	• Greater weight loss compared to a moderately energy-restricted, and/or a low-fat diet.
Low-carbohydrate diets	• Equal weight loss compared to an isocaloric diet with higher carbohydrate content.
High-protein diets	• No consistent evidence for a beneficial effect for weight loss and body composition of a high-protein intake.
Intermittent fasting/severe energy restriction	• No additional benefit on weight loss, compared to the continuous energy restriction.
Meal replacements	• Greater weight loss, compared to conventional dietary plans.
Diets promoting specific food groups	• Without a definite energy restriction, only minimal weight loss. • Evidence for improvements in the quality of the diet and other health-enhancing benefits.
Diets close to the MD	• Benefits for weight reduction only in the context of a hypocaloric diet • Evidence for other health-enhancing benefits.
Diets with varying energy distribution throughout the day	• Greater weight loss when an early eating pattern is used.

Source: (Yannakoulia et al., 2019 / with permission of Elsevier).

Table 18.5 Common fad diets.

Diet Name	Composition
Juicing or detoxification	All meals are replaced with juices Sometimes they contain supplements Duration: 2–21 days
Paleo (Paleolithic)	Includes only food that existed in the Stone Age Foods included: fresh vegetables, fruit, lean meats, poultry, fish, eggs, tofu, nuts, seeds Foods prohibited: cereals, grains, legumes, and dairy
Intermittent fasting	Fasting for an extended period (16–48 h) with little or no calorie intake, followed by periods of normal eating

Source: (Adapted from Mattson et al., 2017).

Table 18.6 General nutritional and behavioral advice given to individuals with obesity.

1. Decrease energy density of food; increase vegetables and eat 2 portions of fruit per day; decrease fatty foods, especially saturated fat; decrease refined carbohydrates, sugar, and sweetened beverages; decrease portion size, use a smaller plate, and eat only one portion per meal
2. Avoid snacking and skipping meals (breakfast, for example: if you are not hungry early in the morning, you can eat your breakfast later, when you will feel hungrier)
3. Eat only in response to your sensation of hunger and stop when you feel a sensation of satiety; avoid eating if you are not hungry and avoid finishing your food if you feel full before the end of your meal
4. Eat slowly; a sensation of satiety will appear about 20 min after the beginning of the meal
5. Eat mindfully
    a. Take a moment to relax, listen to your favorite music, and try to anticipate the meal to come
    b. Sit down at a table (no standing or walking) to eat without doing anything else (television, smartphone, tablet, radio, reading, etc.)
    c. Be aware of how the intensity of your hunger decreases throughout the meal
    d. Eat slowly and enjoy it, paying attention to the tastes, flavors, textures, and temperature of the food; put down your knife and fork between bites
    e. Observe your emotions while eating
    f. Stop eating when you feel full and the pleasure of eating decreases
6. Keep a diary so you become aware of your eating behavior (snacking, volume of meals, etc.) and to identify the triggers for eating when you are not hungry (watching television, using a smartphone or tablet, walking past a bakery, feeling bored or frustrated, etc.)

Source: (Durrer Schutz et al., 2019).

In an RCT including participants with central obesity, the Nordic diet (high in fruits, vegetables, whole grains, and fish) provided *ad libitum*, resulted in ~3.5 kg larger weight loss compared to a group receiving an average Danish diet (Poulsen et al., 2014). Moreover, a meta-analysis of 12 RCTs, including 1151 participants, concluded that vegetarian diets had significant benefits on weight reduction compared to non-vegetarian diets (Huang, Huang, Hu, & Chavarro, 2016).

To sum up, several dietary manipulations may lead to weight loss as long as they cause changes in energy intake leading to negative energy balance, apart from the other health benefits they may have (Yannakoulia et al., 2019).

Most people with obesity do not recognize the physiological sensations of hunger and satiety that determine food intake. They usually eat for emotional compensation or because it is time to eat. Therefore, it is important to perceive the act of eating through all person's senses. There are practical tips for people with obesity, which are presented in **Table 18.6** (Durrer Schutz et al., 2019).

PHYSICAL ACTIVITY AND OBESITY

Regular physical activity, with and without weight loss, can improve many cardio-metabolic risk factors (i.e., hyperglycemia, insulin sensitivity, high blood pressure, dyslipidemia), health-related quality of life, mood disorders (i.e., depression, anxiety) as well as body image in people with overweight or obesity (AbouAssi et al., 2015; Baillot et al., 2018; Baker, Sirois-Leclerc, & Tulloch, 2016; Kuhle, Steffen, Anderson, & Murad, 2014; Lemes, Turi-Lynch, Cavero-Redondo, Linares, & Monteiro, 2018).

It is generally believed that physical activity programs aim mainly at weight loss, but in some cases, body composition might be equally important to body weight. Individuals with obesity may achieve health improvements by adopting a lifestyle that includes exercise and a balanced diet with minimal, or no, weight loss. This could be due to the reduction in visceral fat accumulation and central obesity (Ross & Bradshaw, 2009). Researchers in a meta-analysis of 115 intervention studies compared the effects of exercise programs versus hypocaloric diets for treating obesity. Hypocaloric diet interventions resulted in a greater weight loss, when compared to exercise, while exercise resulted in a greater reduction in visceral adiposity tissue, even if there was no reduction in body weight (Verheggen et al., 2016).

Regarding the type of exercise, several studies have randomly assigned individuals with obesity to either resistance or aerobic exercise. A meta-analysis of 45 RCTs, including 3566 participants, demonstrated that combining high-intensity aerobic and high-load resistance training has beneficial effects that are superior to any other exercise modality at reducing abdominal adiposity, improving lean body mass, and increasing cardio-respiratory fitness (O'Donoghue, Blake, Cunningham, Lennon, & Perrotta, 2021). Another meta-analysis of 18 RCTs, including 3964 participants, showed that all training types (aerobic, resistance, combined aerobic plus resistance, and high-intensity interval training) can improve cardio-respiratory fitness as measured by maximal oxygen consumption per kg body weight in people with overweight or obesity. Specifically, high-intensity interval training and aerobic training were the most effective. Regarding muscle strength benefits, resistance training and combined aerobic and resistance training increased muscle strength (van Baak et al., 2021).

With regard to the intensity of training, high-intensity training improves cardiopulmonary fitness and reduced the percentage of body fat in people with obesity compared to traditional forms of exercise (Türk et al., 2017), but at this time there is no clear evidence that high-intensity training causes more body fat reduction compared to moderate exercise (Keating, Johnson, Mielke, & Coombes, 2017; M. Wewege, van den Berg, Ward, & Keech, 2017).

Therefore, aerobic physical activity, especially 30 to 60 min of moderate-to-vigorous intensity most days of the week (corresponding to approximately 225 to 300 mins/week of moderate-intensity physical activity or lesser amounts of vigorous physical activity), can be proposed for people who want to achieve small amounts of weight and fat loss, as it favors the maintenance of fat-free mass during weight loss, while increasing cardiovascular fitness and mobility (Hwang, Wu, & Chou, 2011; Johnston et al., 2014; Mabire, Mani, Liu, Mulligan, & Baxter, 2017; Washburn et al., 2014). Moreover, resistance training, at least 2 d/week as well as

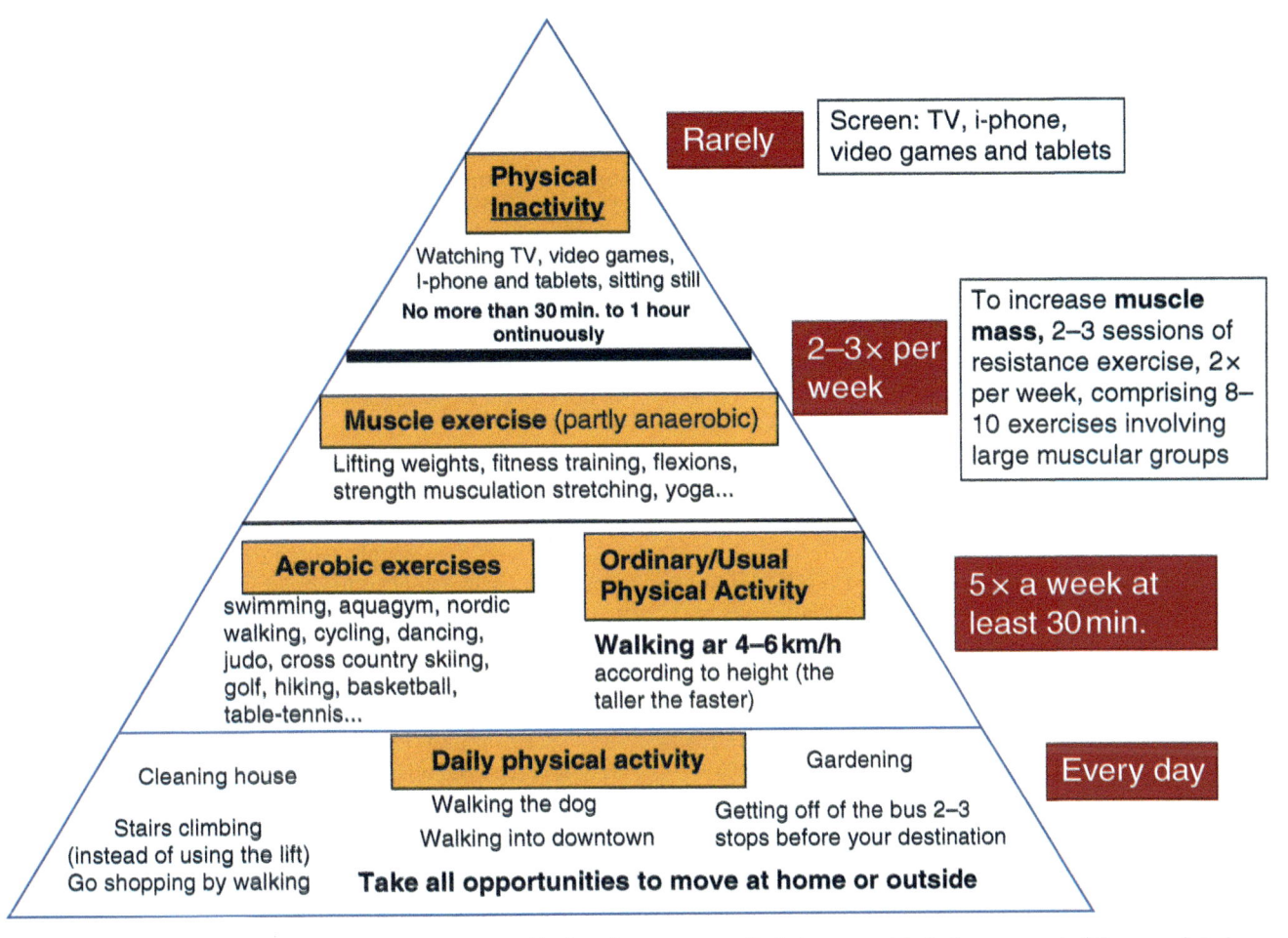

FIGURE 18.6 The principle of the physical-activity pyramid is that the more you climb the pyramid, the less amount of time needs to be dedicated to the activity. Source: (Durrer Schutz et al., 2019 / with permission of Karger Publishers).

reducing the amount of daily sedentary time, can promote weight maintenance, modest increases in muscle mass, or fat-free mass and mobility in individuals with overweight or obesity (Mann et al., 2018). Increasing exercise intensity, including high-intensity interval training, can also lead to greater increases in cardiovascular fitness and achieve benefits sooner than lower intensity exercise (Hwang et al., 2011; Ross, Stotz, & Lam, 2015). Some examples of appropriate sports for people with obesity are swimming, aqua gymnastics, cycling, dancing, judo, skiing, golf, hiking, table tennis, muscle strengthening, and cardio training under supervision (Durrer Schutz et al., 2019). A schematic diagram is shown in **Figure 18.6**.

NUTRITION AND EXERCISE: COMBINED INTERVENTIONS

Both dietary and exercise interventions are effective in reducing body weight and altering body composition. Taking this fact into consideration, it is expected that individuals with overweight or obesity, willing to lose weight benefit more from a lifestyle intervention program that includes a combination of diet and exercise modifications (Hassan et al., 2016).

Indeed, a systematic review and meta-analysis examined the effects of lifestyle interventions, either diet or exercise alone, or their combination, on weight loss in peri- and post-menopausal women. Eleven studies, eight RCTs, and three prospective longitudinal studies, were included in the meta-analysis, and all of them compared the intervention with a control group. Mean weight loss from dietary intervention alone was ~6.6 kg and from exercise alone ~3.5 kg. Women who engaged in both exercise and dietary interventions, experienced greater weight loss, 1.2 kg more, than those who only reduced their caloric intake (Cheng, Hsu, & Liu, 2018). Moreover, a meta-analysis of 56 intervention studies showed that lifestyle changes incorporating apart from diet and a physical activity component (supervised or semi-supervised exercise session, non-supervised exercise program or physical activity recommendations) can improve weight and cardio-metabolic factors (i.e., blood pressure, total cholesterol, LDL-C, triglycerides, and fasting insulin) in people with obesity (Baillot et al., 2015). Findings like this support the hypotheses that a lifestyle intervention, including both diet and exercise, can have favorable effects on weight loss in obesity.

A combination of dietary and exercise interventions is preferred in older adults >60 years old with obesity as well. This is because it can moderate the muscle and bone mass loss compared with interventions that include only nutritional aspects (Batsis et al., 2017). Therefore, according to the 2019 clinical nutrition and hydration guidelines in geriatrics from the European Society for Clinical Nutrition and Metabolism (ESPEN) dietary interventions may be combined with physical activity whenever possible in older adults with obesity in order to preserve muscle mass (Volkert et al., 2019).

PHARMACOTHERAPY AND BARIATRIC SURGERY

Although lifestyle interventions are recommended to all patients with overweight or obesity, in some cases they have been shown to be unsuccessful. Therefore, pharmacotherapy may be considered as an adjunctive therapy (Wharton et al., 2020). Anti-obesity drugs should not be used as a monotherapy. Over the past decades they have been shown to be modestly effective, although newer drugs, such as glucagon-like peptide-1 (GLP-1) agonists seem to be promising for obesity treatment (Stehouwer, 2021). Furthermore, bariatric surgery has been shown to be the most effective therapy for patients with severe obesity, and it has been associated with relative weight loss of 20% to 40%, while the majority of multimodal interventions have been associated with up to 10% of weight loss (Sjöström, 2013).

The costs of pharmacotherapy and bariatric surgery as well as the invasiveness of the latter, make these options suitable for some but not all patients. More specifically, anti-obesity drugs may be given to patients with a BMI >30 kg/m^2 or >27 kg/m^2 with adiposity-related co-morbidities. On the other hand, bariatric surgery may be considered when other treatments are not successful over a certain period of time and whether the patients have a BMI ≥40 kg/m^2 or >35 kg/m^2 with at least one adiposity-related disease (Durrer Schutz et al., 2019; Wharton et al., 2020).

LIFESTYLE MODIFICATIONS DURING WEIGHT-LOSS MAINTENANCE

To treat individuals with overweight or obesity appropriately and to evaluate the treatment options correctly, a phase-dependent therapy is required (**Figure 18.7**) (Bischoff & Schweinlin, 2020). This means that the indication for treatment depends on BMI and the type of treatment varies according to the phase of the disease. If the goal is primary prevention or secondary prevention (weight maintenance), healthy food according to individual requirements, behavioral training, and lifestyle modification are needed. If the goal is weight reduction, a negative energy balance is needed (Bischoff & Schweinlin, 2020). People who achieved any weight loss face new challenges related to weight-loss maintenance. The challenge resides in maintaining weight loss or a significant body weight reduction over time since evidence suggests that 95% of body weight-loss strategies are followed by weight regain. This weight regain might be even greater than the weight initially lost (Bédard & Richard, 2019). Health care providers should recognize the behavioral and/or clinical characteristics of successful weight-loss maintainers in order to provide specific dietary advice for weight-loss maintenance, but sufficient dietary interventions in this area are still lacking.

Regarding the characteristics of the optimal diet for weight maintenance, the adoption of a lacto-vegetarian dietary pattern characterized by a high intake of fruits, vegetables, dairy, and high-fiber foods may lead to lower excess weight rates, or weight maintenance. Moreover, individuals may maintain their weight over time, even if they occasionally consume high-fat or high-sugar foods (fast food, butter, processed meat, sweets, traditional desserts, and high-fat dairy) and at the same time continue to consume adequate portions of fruits, vegetables, and high-fiber foods (Koutras, Chrysostomou, Poulimeneas, & Yannakoulia, 2022). Additionally, the MedWeight study, a large cohort of maintainers and regainers of weight loss, concluded that higher

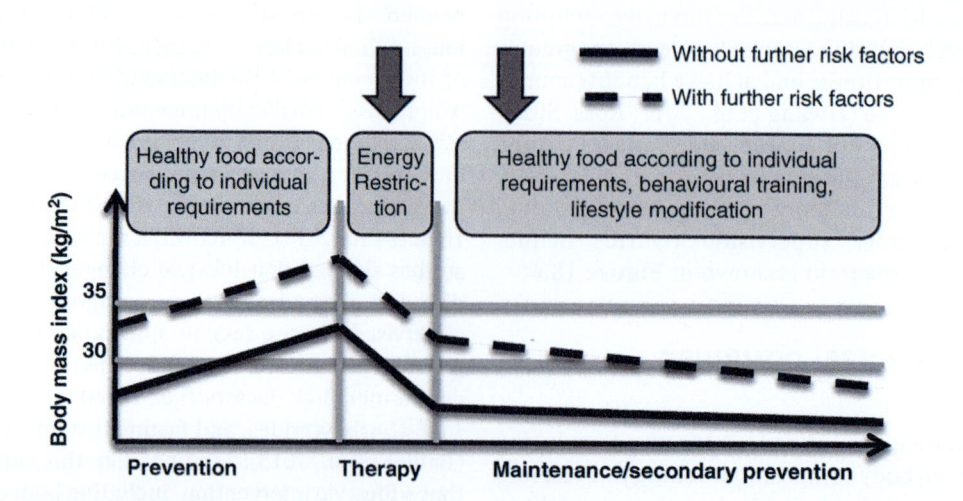

FIGURE 18.7 Phase-dependent therapy. This means that the indication for treatment depends on BMI and the type of treatment varies according to the phase of the disease. If the goal is primary prevention or secondary prevention (weight maintenance), healthy food according to individual requirements, behavioral training, and lifestyle modification are needed. If the goal is weight reduction, a negative energy balance is needed. Source: (Bischoff & Schweinlin, 2020 / with permission of Elsevier).

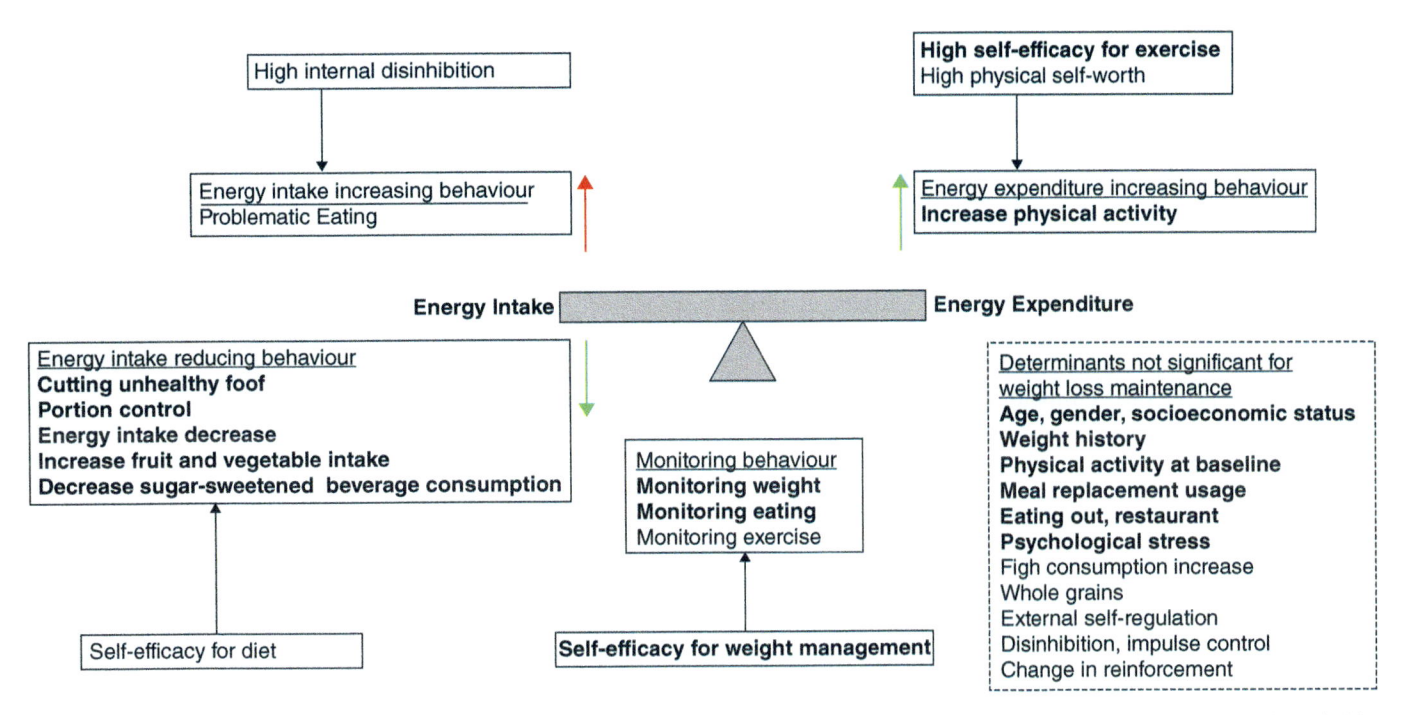

FIGURE 18.8 Determinants of weight-loss maintenance. Determinants in bold have a strong level of evidence, whereas others without bold have a moderate level of evidence. The green arrows indicate positive factors for weight-loss maintenance. The red arrow indicates negative determinants in weight-loss maintenance. Source: (Varkevisser et al., 2019 / with permission of John Wiley & Sons).

adherence to the MD was associated with a 2-fold increased likelihood of weight-loss maintenance (Poulimeneas et al., 2020).

The MedWeight study also showed that breakfast, the first eating episode of the day, when consumed at home, may influence weight-loss maintenance and be protective against weight regaining (Brikou, Zannidi, Karfopoulou, Anastasiou, & Yannakoulia, 2016). Additional behaviors associated with maintenance were eating at home, involvement in meal preparation, higher eating frequency, and slower eating rate (Karfopoulou et al., 2017). A meta-analysis of eight RCTs also demonstrated that an intensive approach (weight-maintenance intervention at fixed follow up, 12 months) after weight loss may be important to ensure greater success in the maintenance phase in addition to a behavioral approach that seems to play a crucial role (Flore et al., 2022).

Weight-loss maintenance is not entirely dependent on the demographics of the individual but on the behavioral determinants involved in the energy balance and the determinants that promote it (**Figure 18.8**). Current literature on psychological/cognitive, social, physical, and macro-environmental determinants is scarce or ambiguous. Weight-loss maintenance programs may focus on changing behavior to reduce energy intake through avoiding unhealthy foods, portion control, reducing sugar-sweetened beverage consumption, and fat intake, increasing vegetable and fruit consumption, and adhering to a diet. Moreover, increased energy expenditure should be promoted through increasing physical activity. The monitoring of this balance through self-monitoring should be regarded as part of the intervention (Paixão et al., 2020; Varkevisser, van Stralen, Kroeze, Ket, & Steenhuis, 2019). Indeed, a meta-analysis of 45 RCTs, including 7788 participants, demonstrated that behavioral interventions focusing on both diet and physical activity resulted in small but significant benefits for weight-loss maintenance for up to 24 months (Dombrowski, Knittle, Avenell, Araújo-Soares, & Sniehotta, 2014).

According to 2019 AHA/ACC/TOS guidelines, participation in a long-term (≥1 year) comprehensive weight-loss maintenance programs, with monthly or more frequent contact, face-to-face or by the telephone, can improve successful weight maintenance. Moreover, people should be advised to consume a reduced-calorie diet (needed to maintain lower body weight), to adopt higher levels of physical activity, approximately 200 to 300 min/week of moderate- intensity physical activity, and to monitor body weight regularly (i.e., weekly or more frequently) for weight-loss maintenance (Jensen, Ryan, Apovian, et al., 2014).

INTRODUCTION TO METABOLIC SYNDROME

Metabolic syndrome (MetS) refers to a cluster of specific CVD and type 2 diabetes risk factors that usually occur simultaneously, instead of separately. These risk factors include elevated blood pressure, dyslipidemia (high levels of triglycerides, low levels of HDL-cholesterol), impaired fasting glucose levels, and central obesity (Alberti et al., 2009).

Regarding its pathophysiology, MetS seem to be the result of various complex interactions between genetic factors and the environment, which can modulate the two main proposed pathogenetic factors, namely insulin resistance and central obesity (Kahn et al., 2005). Notably, it is estimated that approximately 10% of the variance of MetS may be associated with genes, while the remaining 90% seems to be explained by environmental factors (Chen et al., 2008; Lusis, Attie, & Reue, 2008).

EPIDEMIOLOGY OF METABOLIC SYNDROME

The prevalence of MetS is increasing worldwide in parallel to the growing incidence of obesity and diabetes mellitus in the last decades. According to 2003 to 2012 NHANES (National Health and Nutrition Examination Survey) data, the overall prevalence of MetS in US adults (≥20 years) was 33%. The prevalence was higher in women than men, 35.6% compared to 30.3%. Considering the race/ethnicity, Hispanic people have the highest prevalence of the syndrome, followed by non-Hispanic white and African-American individuals (Aguilar, Bhuket, Torres, Liu, & Wong, 2015). The prevalence appears to increase with increasing age, from 19.5% in adults aged 20-39 years to 48,6% in older adults (Hirode & Wong, 2020). It is expected that the incidence of MetS will reach 53% in 2035 (Gierach, Gierach, Ewertowska, Arndt, & Junik, 2014).

DIAGNOSIS OF METABOLIC SYNDROME

A lot of disagreement existed regarding the diagnosis of MetS over the past few years between the various organizations. This has led to a variety of possible diagnoses and confusion among the physicians. In 2009, there was a consensus by the International Diabetes Federation (IDF), the American Heart Association, and the National Heart, Lung, and Blood Institute (AHA/NHLBI). According to this joint statement, MetS is identified by the presence of at least three components as shown in **Table 18.7** (Fahed et al., 2022). According to these criteria, most patients with type 2 diabetes mellitus also have MetS (Alberti et al., 2009).

LIFESTYLE AND RISK OF METABOLIC SYNDROME

The increasing prevalence of MetS and its complications, sets a significant public health challenge that should be primarily prevented and addressed (Engin, 2017). It is associated with a 2-fold increased risk of coronary heart disease, 5-fold higher risk of diabetes, 2.5-fold higher cardiovascular mortality, and 1.5-fold increased risk of all-cause mortality. Current literature demonstrates a favorable effect of modifiable lifestyle factors, such as diet and physical activity, on the incidence and prevention of MetS.

DIET

Little evidence exists regarding the association of specific nutrients or food groups on the likelihood or risk of

Table 18.7 Diagnostic criteria for metabolic syndrome throughout the years. AHA = American Heart Association; ATPIII = National Cholesterol Education Program Adult Treatment Panel III; BP = blood pressure; dx = diagnosis; EGIR = European group for study of insulin resistance; Glc = glucose; HDL = high-density lipoprotein; HTN = hypertension; IR = insulin resistance; IDF = International Diabetes Federation; IGT = impaired glucose tolerance; IFG = impaired fasting glucose; NHLBI = National Heart, Lung, and Blood Institute; TG = triglyceride; txt = treatment; WC = waist circumference; WHO = World Health Organization.

Clinical measure	Criteria					Diagnosis
	Central obesity	**Blood glucose**	**High TG**	**Low HDL**	**High BP**	
AHA/NHLBI (2009) (Grundy et al., 2005)	WC >40" (men) or >35" (women)	• IFG or • on high blood Glc txt or • T2DM dx	• 150 mg/dL or • on TG txt	• <40 mg/dL (men) or • <50 mg/dL (women) or • on HDL txt	• ≥130 mm Hg systolic and/or • ≥85 mm Hg diastolic or • on HTN txt	≥3 criteria
IDF (2005) (Eckel, 2010; McCracken, 2018)	• WC >37" (men) or >32" (women) or • BMI >30 kg/m²					≥3 criteria one of which should be central obesity
ATPIII (2001) (Cleeman, 2001)	WC >40" (men) or >35" (women)		• ≥150 mg/dL	• <40 mg/dL (men) or • <50 mg/dL (women)	• ≥130 mm Hg systolic and ≥85 mm Hg diastolic or • on HTN txt	≥3 criteria
EGIR (1999) (Balkau & Charles, 1999)	WC >37" (men) or >32" (women)	• IFG or • IGT		• <39 mg/dL (men and women)	• ≥140 mm Hg systolic and ≥90 mm Hg diastolic or • on HTN txt	≥3 criteria one of which should be IR[1]
WHO (1998) (Reaven, 1988)	• Waist/hip ratio >0.9 (men) or >0.85 (women) or • BMI >30 kg/m²	• IFG or x • IIGT or • T2DM dx		• <35 mg/dL (men) or • <39 mg/dL (women)	• ≥140 mm Hg systolic and ≥90 mm Hg diastolic	≥3 criteria one of which should be IR[2]

Source: (Fahed et al., 2022 / MDPI / CC BY 4.0).

IFG is defined as ≥110 mg/dL in 2001, but this was modified in 2004 to be ≥100 mg/dL, IGT is defined as 2-h glucose >140 mg/dL.

[1] EGIR IR is defined as plasma insulin levels >75th percentile.

[2] WHO IR is defined as presence of IR or IFG or IGT.

developing MetS. Dietary fiber found in plant foods, including fruits, vegetables, whole grains, nuts, seeds, beans, and legumes, is consistently inversely associated with a lower risk of MetS (Shay et al., 2012). In terms of foods and food groups, a meta-analysis of 16 observational studies, 3 cohort studies and 13 cross-sectional studies, showed that fruit or/and vegetable consumption may be inversely associated with the likelihood or risk of MetS (Tian, Su, Wang, Duan, & Jiang, 2018).

With regard to dietary patterns, two main *posteriori* dietary patterns, a healthy/prudent and an unhealthy/Western dietary pattern have been inversely and positively associated with the risk of developing MetS, respectively. Indeed, a meta-analysis of 28 cross-sectional studies and three cohort studies demonstrated that a healthy/prudent dietary pattern, rich in fresh fruits, vegetables, whole grains, and fish, was associated with a lower prevalence of MetS. On the contrary, an unhealthy/Western dietary pattern, which is composed of red meat, processed meat, refined grains, sweets, French fries, desserts, eggs, and high-fat dairy products, was associated with an increased likelihood of having MetS in cross-sectional studies but not in cohort studies (Rodríguez-Monforte, Sánchez, Barrio, Costa, & Flores-Mateo, 2017). Another two meta-analyses, one including 19 cross-sectional studies and the other 40 observation studies, 4 cohort studies, 1 case-control study, and 35 cross-sectional, showed similar results; a greater adherence to a healthy/prudent dietary pattern was associated with a lower risk of MetS, while an unhealthy/Western dietary pattern was associated with an increased risk of MetS (Fabiani, Naldini, & Chiavarini, 2019; Shab-Bidar, Golzarand, Hajimohammadi, & Mansouri, 2018).

Regarding *a priori* dietary patterns, the most well-studied is MD. The MD is an effective dietary pattern for both the primary and the secondary prevention of MetS. According to a meta-analysis of 50 studies (32 clinical trials, 2 prospective and 13 cross-sectional), adherence to the MD was associated with 31% reduced risk of MetS compared to lower compliance or a control diet (low-fat diet or usual care). (Kastorini et al., 2011). The protective effect of the MD on the MetS risk ranges from 19% to 31%. In a meta-analysis of eight cross-sectional and four prospective studies, including 33,847 individuals and 6324 cases of MetS, high adherence to the MD was associated with a 19% lower risk of MetS compared to the lowest adherence (Godos et al., 2017). Moreover, the MD seems to provide a positive effect not only on the risk of MetS but on its components as well. In the meta-analysis of Kastorini et al., results from both clinical trials and epidemiological studies showed that the MD has a protective effect on several components of MetS, like glucose, triglycerides and HDL-cholesterol levels, diastolic blood pressure as well as on waist circumference. Moreover, in a more updated meta-analysis including 57 clinical trials with 36,983 participants, the MD resulted in greater beneficial changes on all components and most risk factors of MetS, in addition to CVD and stroke incidence (Papadaki, Nolen-Doerr, & Mantzoros, 2020).

PHYSICAL ACTIVITY

Most individuals with MetS follow mainly a sedentary lifestyle. According to a cross-sectional analysis from the PREDIMED-PLUS RCT, including approximately 6000 individuals with MetS and overweight or obesity, participants with the highest MetS severity score had more sedentary time and lower moderate- and vigorous-intensity leisure-time physical activity (Gallardo-Alfaro et al., 2020). Therefore, there is a need for strategies to raise the awareness of these patients regarding the benefits of physical activity.

Current evidence regarding the association between physical activity and the incidence of MetS derives from epidemiological studies. These demonstrate that being physically active can lower both the risk of developing MetS and the risk of its components. For instance, in a 2017 meta-analysis of cohort studies a negative linear association between leisure-time physical activity and the risk of MetS has been shown. A further dose-response analysis reported a 8% reduction in the risk of MetS for each 10 METs increase per week (Zhang et al., 2017). Moreover, in the TROMSO study, in which ~11,000 individuals were studied for approximately seven years, there was a dose-response relationship between higher levels of physical activity and improved BMI and lipid levels (Thune, Njølstad, Løchen, & Førde, 1998). Furthermore, in the same study, an improvement in metabolic profiles was observed in individuals who increased their leisure-time activity and a negative impact in those that decreased leisure time. Although there is inconclusive data regarding the exact duration, current evidence support that meeting the minimum recommendation of 150 min/week of moderate-intensity activity or 75 min/week of vigorous physical activity is associated with reduced prevalence of the MetS (Nylén, Gandhi, & Lakshman, 2019).

Physical activity can protect individuals from developing MetS through various mechanisms, including improved insulin sensitivity and glucose metabolism as well as reduced blood pressure (Golbidi, Mesdaghinia, & Laher, 2012). Moreover, a contribution to the maintenance of a healthy weight and the prevention of excessive body weight gain has been proposed, as previously reported in this chapter.

MANAGEMENT OF METABOLIC SYNDROME

DIET

The initial and most important step to address MetS is lifestyle modification with changes in physical activity levels and dietary habits.

Most intervention studies targeted at weight loss seem to be associated with improvements in all MetS parameters. Notably, even moderate weight reduction (i.e., approximately 7%) is related to significant improvements in glucose, triglycerides, and total cholesterol levels as well as in blood pressure (Case, Jones, Nelson, O'Brian Smith, & Ballantyne, 2002; Phelan et al., 2007).

Diet plays an important role in the management of MetS, yet little is known about the optimal composition of the diet or the ideal dietary intervention for patients with MetS. Among the various dietary patterns that have been suggested for individuals with MetS, the most well studied is the MD, followed by the dietary approaches to stop hypertension (DASH diet) (Pérez-Martínez et al., 2017). Both MD and DASH diet are plant-based diets, high in fruits, vegetables, fibers and generally foods that have shown beneficial effects for dyslipidemia, blood pressure, glucose and insulin abnormalities. Furthermore, individuals who follow the MD or DASH diet are less prone to being overweight and obesity (Akhlaghi, 2020).

Adherence to the MD has been shown to be an effective dietary strategy, even in the absence of weight loss, because it exerts many beneficial effects on various components of MetS, as well as on inflammatory and oxidative states that often found in patients with MetS. These recognized effects make MD a very useful alternative to weight-loss intervention, especially for patients with MetS who hardly achieve or sustain weight-loss.

The DASH diet has also been associated with favorable effects on each component of MetS, especially blood pressure and excess body weight (Castro-Barquero, Ruiz-León, Sierra-Pérez, Estruch, & Casas, 2020). There is also some data demonstrating the effectiveness of different types of DASH-like diets. For instance, results from the OmniHeart study comparing three types of DASH-like diets, high in carbohydrates, high in protein, or high in mono- and poly-unsaturated fats, (21% and 10% respectively vs 13% and 8% in other diets) suggested that all of them are beneficial for MetS components, especially those high in protein or high in mono-and poly-unsaturated fat (Root & Dawson, 2014).

PHYSICAL ACTIVITY

There is growing evidence that physical activity improves each one of the MetS components as well as the syndrome itself (Pedersen & Saltin, 2015). A systematic review and meta-analysis of 11 RCTs (with interventions of at least 4 weeks duration) examined the effects of aerobic, resistance exercise or their combination on risk factors for CVD among patients with MetS without diabetes (M. A. Wewege, Thom, Rye, & Parmenter, 2018). Aerobic exercise was significantly associated with improvements in all MetS components, while resistance training had no significant effect, though there were limited data regarding the latter. Moreover, in a meta-analysis of 16 intervention studies in patients with MetS (approximately 800 exercising participants with an intervention duration ranging from 8 weeks to 1 year), both aerobic exercise and combined aerobic and resistance exercise were correlated with significant improvements in all MetS components (Ostman et al., 2017).

Current research data suggests that individuals with MetS follow the general recommendations for physical activity for adults. Although the evidence is strong, mainly for aerobic activities, it is plausible that physical activity should combine aerobic exercise and strength training to prevent adiposity-related complications and to improve cardio-respiratory fitness. Notably, some patients with MetS have elevated blood pressure, hence recommendations should be tailored and increased gradually (Pedersen & Saltin, 2015).

EXERCISE AND NUTRITION: COMBINED INTERVENTION

There is solid evidence that the combination of dietary therapy and physical activity is associated with the improvement of MetS (Pedersen & Saltin, 2015). Moreover, combining diet with exercise and behavioral support may have favorable results in the treatment of individuals with MetS. In the PREDIMED-PLUS RCT, individuals who followed an energy-reduced MD in combination with physical activity and behavioral support, compared to the control group who followed the MD without caloric restriction, exercise, or behavioral intervention, had better adherence to the diet at 12 months and improvement in common cardiovascular risk factors (Sayón-Orea et al., 2019).

RECOMMENDATIONS

As obesity is considered the key etiological condition that predisposes to the development of MetS and central obesity itself, weight loss constitutes the first line of intervention for the management of the MetS (Bédard & Richard, 2019).

According to an international panel recommendation, lifestyle recommendations for the management of MetS are shown in **Table 18.8**. People with overweight/obesity and MetS should achieve 5% weight loss through calorie restriction and increased physical activity, 30 to 60 min/d. Regarding the dietary approach to treatment over the last decade, research in nutrition epidemiology has moved from the single food approach to the dietary pattern strategy, which better reflects the complexity of interacting effects of several nutrients on health status. The MD, with or without energy restriction, can be recommended for all individuals with MetS as an effective component of the treatment strategy. Moreover, it is recommended to reduce the intake of salt, limit saturated and trans fats, and the consumption of SSBs while increasing the intake of dietary fiber (Pérez-Martínez et al., 2017).

Table 18.8 Lifestyle recommendations for management of MetS.

- Smoking cessation
- 30–60 min of daily physical activity
- For patients with overweight/obese and MetS: healthy diet designed to achieve 5% weight loss
- Plant-based MD, with or without energy restriction, Dietary Approaches to Stop Hypertension diet, or vegetarian diet as a component of the treatment strategy
- Specific dietary recommendations include:
  - Limit saturated and trans fats
  - Increase dietary fiber
  - Reduce intake of SSBs
  - Moderate alcohol intake
  - Restrict salt intake

Source: (Pérez-Martínez et al., 2017).

KEY POINTS

- "Overweight and obesity are defined as abnormal or excessive fat accumulation that presents a risk to health" (WHO).
- For weight loss, the chosen diet should always be adjusted to the needs of each individual to achieve better adherence to the intervention.
- A balanced hypocaloric diet, regardless of the type of the diet, containing at least the recommended protein intake, is considered appropriate for weight loss in individuals with overweight or obesity.
- Lifestyle interventions that include both diet and exercise have better results in weight loss and overall health.
- For weight loss, 30 to 60 min of moderate-to-vigorous intensity most days of the week (corresponding to approximately 225 to 300 mins/week of moderate-intensity physical activity or lesser amounts of vigorous physical activity) and resistance activity at least 2 d/week, as well as reduction of daily sedentary time are recommended.
- Every successful weight loss requires a subsequent weight-maintenance strategy.
- For weight-loss maintenance, a reduced-calorie diet, high levels of physical activity, approximately 200 to 300 min/week, and monitoring body weight regularly (i.e., weekly, or more frequently) are recommended.
- The prevalence of MetS is increasing worldwide in parallel to the growing incidence of overweight, obesity, and diabetes.
- Lifestyle modification is the first-line approach for the treatment of MetS, including physical activity, weight loss, and a healthy dietary pattern (i.e., the MD, DASH).

SELF-ASSESSMENT QUESTIONS

1. Define overweight and obesity.
2. What the is the optimal treatment for weight loss?
3. Define metabolically healthy obesity.
4. What are the recommendations for exercise in weight-loss maintenance?
5. What are the most important cornerstones of the dietary intervention for MetS?
6. What are the 2009 diagnostic criteria for MetS?
7. True or False: Body weight per se is a priority in the treatment for obesity.
8. True or False: For weight maintenance, people should adopt aerobic exercise, at least 150 min/week, and resistance exercise, two times per week.
9. True or False: The MD is an effective dietary pattern for the primary and secondary prevention of the MetS.
10. True or False: A low-carbohydrate diet is the preferable diet for inducing weight loss in participants living with overweight or obesity.
11. True or False: Combining diet, physical activity, and behavioral strategies leads to greater weight loss than an intervention that uses these same components singularly for the management of obesity.

Fill in the blank(s) to complete the following statements:

12. In older people who are _____, weight-reducing diets may be _____ to prevent the loss of _____ and functional decline, whereas in older adults with _____, weight-reducing diets may only be considered after weighing the benefits and risks.
13. The main goals in obesity management are to prevent _____, to prevent or treat _____ if they are present, to reduce _____, and to induce _____, a _____ body image and self-esteem.
14. For weight-loss maintenance, people should be advised to consume a _____ diet, to adopt _____ levels of physical activity, approximately _____ min/week, and to _____ body weight regularly (i.e., _____ or _____ frequently).
15. MD, with or without _____, can be _____ for all individuals with _____ as an effective component of the treatment strategy.

CASE SCENARIO

HS is a 53-year-old man. He is an accountant working for approximately 9 h/d, who gets to work by car and follows a sedentary lifestyle. He weighs 105 kg, his height is 187 cm, and his waist circumference 106 cm. Recent blood test showed fasting glucose levels of 116 mg/dL, triglyceride levels of 170 mg/dL, and HDL-cholesterol levels of 55 mg/dL. His blood pressure was 140/81 mm Hg. These results made him anxious, and he started following a hypocaloric, low-fat diet (<20% of total energy) to lose weight, but his adherence is low.

Questions:

1. Does HS have metabolic syndrome according to the 2009 diagnostic criteria?
2. What is the goal of weight loss to observe benefits in biochemical indices?
3. Is there any specific dietary pattern that can be recommended?
4. He claims that he does not have enough free time to participate in a supervised exercise program. What physical activity can be recommended?

REFERENCES

AbouAssi, H., Slentz, C. A., Mikus, C. R., Tanner, C. J., Bateman, L. A., Willis, L. H., ... Kraus, W. E. (2015). The effects of aerobic, resistance, and combination training on insulin sensitivity and secretion in overweight adults from STRRIDE AT/RT: A randomized trial. *Journal of Applied Physiology*, 118(12), 1474–1482. https://doi.org/10.1152/japplphysiol.00509.2014

Aguilar, M., Bhuket, T., Torres, S., Liu, B., & Wong, R. J. (2015). Prevalence of the metabolic syndrome in the United States, 2003-2012. *Jama*, 313(19), 1973–1974. https://doi.org/10.1001/jama.2015.4260

Akhlaghi, M. (2020). Dietary Approaches to Stop Hypertension (DASH): Potential mechanisms of action against risk factors of the metabolic syndrome. *Nutrition Research Reviews*, 33(1), 1–18. https://doi.org/10.1017/S0954422419000155

Alberti, K. G. M. M., Eckel, R. H., Grundy, S. M., Zimmet, P. Z., Cleeman, J. I., Donato, K. A., ... Smith, S. C. (2009). Harmonizing the metabolic syndrome: A joint interim statement of the international diabetes federation task force on epidemiology and prevention; National heart, lung, and blood institute; American heart association; World heart federation; International. *Circulation*, 120(16), 1640–1645. https://doi.org/10.1161/CIRCULATIONAHA.109.192644

Baillot, A., Romain, A. J., Boisvert-Vigneault, K., Audet, M., Baillargeon, J. P., Dionne, I. J., ... Langlois, M. F. (2015). Effects of lifestyle interventions that include a physical activity component in class II and III obese individuals: A systematic review. *PLoS ONE*, 10(4), 1–32. https://doi.org/10.1371/journal.pone.0119017

Baillot, A., Saunders, S., Brunet, J., Romain, A. J., Trottier, A., & Bernard, P. (2018). A systematic review and meta-analysis of the effect of exercise on psychosocial outcomes in adults with obesity: A call for more research. *Mental Health and Physical Activity*, 14, 1–10. https://doi.org/10.1016/j.mhpa.2017.12.004

Baker, A., Sirois-Leclerc, H., & Tulloch, H. (2016). The Impact of Long-Term Physical Activity Interventions for Overweight/Obese Postmenopausal Women on Adiposity Indicators, Physical Capacity, and Mental Health Outcomes: A Systematic Review. *Journal of Obesity*, 2016(Ci). https://doi.org/10.1155/2016/6169890

Balkau, B., & Charles, M. A. (1999). Comment on the provisional report from the WHO consultation. *Diabetic Medicine*, 16(5), 442–443. https://doi.org/10.1046/j.1464-5491.1999.00059.x

Batsis, J. A., Gill, L. E., Masutani, R. K., Adachi-Mejia, A. M., Blunt, H. B., Bagley, P. J., ... Bartels, S. J. (2017). Weight Loss Interventions in Older Adults with Obesity: A Systematic Review of Randomized Controlled Trials Since 2005. *Journal of the American Geriatrics Society*, 65(2), 257–268. https://doi.org/10.1111/jgs.14514

Bédard, A., & Richard, C. (2019). The Mediterranean Diet for an Effective Management of Metabolic Syndrome in Both Men and Women. *Bioactive Food as Dietary Interventions for Diabetes*, 317–333. https://doi.org/10.1016/b978-0-12-813822-9.00021-7

Bell, J. A., Kivimaki, M., & Hamer, M. (2014). Metabolically healthy obesity and risk of incident type 2 diabetes: A meta-analysis of prospective cohort studies. *Obesity Reviews*, 15(6), 504–515. https://doi.org/10.1111/obr.12157

Bischoff, S. C., Boirie, Y., Cederholm, T., Chourdakis, M., Cuerda, C., Delzenne, N. M., ... Barazzoni, R. (2017). Towards a multidisciplinary approach to understand and manage obesity and related diseases. *Clinical Nutrition*, 36(4), 917–938. https://doi.org/10.1016/j.clnu.2016.11.007

Bischoff, S. C., & Schweinlin, A. (2020). Obesity therapy. *Clinical Nutrition ESPEN*, 38(2020), 9–18. https://doi.org/10.1016/j.clnesp.2020.04.013

Bosello, O., & Vanzo, A. (2021). Obesity paradox and aging. *Eating and Weight Disorders*, 26(1), 27–35. https://doi.org/10.1007/s40519-019-00815-4

Brikou, D., Zannidi, D., Karfopoulou, E., Anastasiou, C. A., & Yannakoulia, M. (2016). Breakfast consumption and weight-loss maintenance: Results from the MedWeight study. *British Journal of Nutrition*, 115(12), 2246–2251. https://doi.org/10.1017/S0007114516001550

Bueno, N. B., De Melo, I. S. V., De Oliveira, S. L., & Da Rocha Ataide, T. (2013). Very-low-carbohydrate ketogenic diet v. low-fat diet for long-term weight loss: A meta-analysis of Randomised controlled trials. *British Journal of Nutrition*, 110(7), 1178–1187. https://doi.org/10.1017/S0007114513000548

Case, C. C., Jones, P. H., Nelson, K., O'Brian Smith, E., & Ballantyne, C. M. (2002). Impact of weight loss on the metabolic syndrome. *Diabetes, Obesity and Metabolism*, 4(6), 407–414. https://doi.org/10.1046/j.1463-1326.2002.00236.x

Castro-Barquero, S., Ruiz-León, A. M., Sierra-Pérez, M., Estruch, R., & Casas, R. (2020). Dietary strategies for metabolic syndrome: A comprehensive review. *Nutrients*, 12(10), 1–21. https://doi.org/10.3390/nu12102983

Chen, Y., Zhu, J., Lum, P. Y., Yang, X., Pinto, S., MacNeil, D. J., ... Schadt, E. E. (2008). Variations in DNA elucidate molecular networks that cause disease. *Nature*, 452(7186), 429–435. https://doi.org/10.1038/nature06757

Cheng, C. C., Hsu, C. Y., & Liu, J. F. (2018). Effects of dietary and exercise intervention on weight loss and body composition in obese postmenopausal women: A systematic review and meta-analysis. *Menopause*, 25(7), 772–782. https://doi.org/10.1097/GME.0000000000001085

Cleeman, J. I. (2001). Executive summary of the third report of the National Cholesterol Education Program (NCEP) expert panel on detection, evaluation, and treatment of high blood cholesterol in adults (adult treatment panel III). *Journal of the American Medical Association*, 285(19), 2486–2497. https://doi.org/10.1001/jama.285.19.2486

Cornier, M. A., Després, J. P., Davis, N., Grossniklaus, D. A., Klein, S., Lamarche, B., ... Poirier, P. (2011). Assessing adiposity: A scientific statement from the american heart association. *Circulation*, 124(18), 1996–2019. https://doi.org/10.1161/CIR.0b013e318233bc6a

Dombrowski, S. U., Knittle, K., Avenell, A., Araújo-Soares, V., & Sniehotta, F. F. (2014). Long term maintenance of weight loss with non-surgical interventions in obese adults: Systematic review and meta-analyses of randomised controlled trials. *BMJ (Online)*, 348(May), 1–12. https://doi.org/10.1136/bmj.g2646

Donini, L. M., Pinto, A., Giusti, A. M., Lenzi, A., & Poggiogalle, E. (2020). Obesity or BMI Paradox? Beneath the Tip of the Iceberg. *Frontiers in Nutrition*, 7(May), 1–6. https://doi.org/10.3389/fnut.2020.00053

Dulloo, A. G., Jacquet, J., Solinas, G., Montani, J. P., & Schutz, Y. (2010). Body composition phenotypes in pathways to obesity and the metabolic syndrome. *International Journal of Obesity*, 34(S2), S4–S17. https://doi.org/10.1038/ijo.2010.234

Durrer Schutz, D., Busetto, L., Dicker, D., Farpour-Lambert, N., Pryke, R., Toplak, H., ... Schutz, Y. (2019). European Practical and Patient-Centred Guidelines for Adult Obesity Management in Primary Care. *Obesity Facts*, 12(1), 40–66. https://doi.org/10.1159/000496183

Ebbeling, C. B. (2014). Sugar-sweetened beverages and body weight. *Current Opinion in Lipidology*, 25(1), 1–7. https://doi.org/10.1097/MOL.0000000000000035

Eckel, N., Meidtner, K., Kalle-Uhlmann, T., Stefan, N., & Schulze, M. B. (2016). Metabolically healthy obesity and cardiovascular events: A systematic review and meta-analysis. *European Journal of Preventive Cardiology*, 23(9), 956–966. https://doi.org/10.1177/2047487315623884

Eckel, R. H., Alberti, K. G. M. M., Grundy, S. M., & Zimmet, P. Z. (2010). The metabolic syndrome. *The Lancet*, *375*(9710), 181–183. https://doi.org/10.1016/S0140-6736(09)61794-3

Engin, A. (2017). *The Definition and Prevalence of Obesity and Metabolic Syndrome*. https://doi.org/10.1007/978-3-319-48382-5_1

Estruch, R., Martínez-González, M. A., Corella, D., Salas-Salvadó, J., Fitó, M., Chiva-Blanch, G., ... Ros, E. (2019). Effect of a high-fat Mediterranean diet on bodyweight and waist circumference: a prespecified secondary outcomes analysis of the PREDIMED randomised controlled trial. *The Lancet Diabetes and Endocrinology*, *7*(5), e6–e17. https://doi.org/10.1016/S2213-8587(19)30074-9

Fabiani, R., Naldini, G., & Chiavarini, M. (2019). Dietary patterns and metabolic syndrome in adult subjects: A systematic review and meta-analysis. *Nutrients*, *11*(9), 1–36. https://doi.org/10.3390/nu11092056

Fahed, G., Aoun, L., Zerdan, M. B., Allam, S., Zerdan, M. B., Bouferraa, Y., & Assi, H. I. (2022). Metabolic Syndrome: Updates on Pathophysiology and Management in 2021. *International Journal of Molecular Sciences*, *23*(2). https://doi.org/10.3390/ijms23020786

Flegal, K. M., Kit, B. K., Orpana, H., & Graubard, B. I. (2013). Association of All-Cause Mortality With Overweight and Obesity Using Standard Body Mass Index Categories. *JAMA*, *309*(1), 71. https://doi.org/10.1001/jama.2012.113905

Flicker, L., McCaul, K. A., Hankey, G. J., Jamrozik, K., Brown, W. J., Byles, J. E., & Almeida, O. P. (2010). Body mass index and survival in men and women aged 70 to 75. *Journal of the American Geriatrics Society*, *58*(2), 234–241. https://doi.org/10.1111/j.1532-5415.2009.02677.x

Flore, G., Preti, A., Carta, M. G., Deledda, A., Fosci, M., Nardi, A. E., ... Velluzzi, F. (2022). Weight Maintenance after Dietary Weight Loss: Systematic Review and Meta-Analysis on the Effectiveness of Behavioural Intensive Intervention. *Nutrients*, *14*(6). https://doi.org/10.3390/nu14061259

Freire, R. (2020). Scientific evidence of diets for weight loss: Different macronutrient composition, intermittent fasting, and popular diets. *Nutrition*, *69*. https://doi.org/10.1016/j.nut.2019.07.001

Fruh, S. M. (2017). Obesity: Risk factors, complications, and strategies for sustainable long-term weight management. *Journal of the American Association of Nurse Practitioners*, *29*, S3–S14. https://doi.org/10.1002/2327-6924.12510

Gallardo-Alfaro, L., Bibiloni, M. del M., Mascaró, C. M., Montemayor, S., Ruiz-Canela, M., Salas-Salvadó, J., ... Tur, J. A. (2020). Leisure-Time Physical Activity, Sedentary Behaviour and Diet Quality are Associated with Metabolic Syndrome Severity: The PREDIMED-Plus Study. *Nutrients*, *12*(4), 1013. https://doi.org/10.3390/nu12041013

Gierach, M., Gierach, J., Ewertowska, M., Arndt, A., & Junik, R. (2014). Correlation between Body Mass Index and Waist Circumference in Patients with Metabolic Syndrome. *ISRN Endocrinology*, *2014*, 1–6. https://doi.org/10.1155/2014/514589

Gjermeni, E., Kirstein, A. S., Kolbig, F., Kirchhof, M., Bundalian, L., Katzmann, J. L., ... Le Duc, D. (2021). Obesity–an update on the basic pathophysiology and review of recent therapeutic advances. *Biomolecules*, *11*(10). https://doi.org/10.3390/biom11101426

Godos, J., Zappalà, G., Bernardini, S., Giambini, I., Bes-Rastrollo, M., & Martínez-González, M. (2017). Adherence to the Mediterranean diet is inversely associated with metabolic syndrome occurrence: a meta-analysis of observational studies. *International Journal of Food Sciences and Nutrition*, *68*(2), 138–148. https://doi.org/10.1080/09637486.2016.1221900

Golbidi, S., Mesdaghinia, A., & Laher, I. (2012). Exercise in the Metabolic Syndrome. *Oxidative Medicine and Cellular Longevity*, *2012*, 1–13. https://doi.org/10.1155/2012/349710

Grube, M., Bergmann, S., Keitel, A., Herfurth-Majstorovic, K., Wendt, V., von Klitzing, K., & Klein, A. M. (2013). Obese parents – obese children? Psychological-psychiatric risk factors of parental behavior and experience for the development of obesity in children aged 0 – 3: study protocol. *BMC Public Health*, *13*(1), 1193. https://doi.org/10.1186/1471-2458-13-1193

Grundy, S. M., Cleeman, J. I., Daniels, S. R., Donato, K. A., Eckel, R. H., Franklin, B. A., ... Costa, F. (2005). Diagnosis and management of the metabolic syndrome: An American Heart Association/National Heart, Lung, and Blood Institute scientific statement. *Circulation*, *112*(17), 2735–2752. https://doi.org/10.1161/CIRCULATIONAHA.105.169404

Hansen, T. T., Astrup, A., & Sjödin, A. (2021). Are dietary proteins the key to successful body weight management? A systematic review and meta-analysis of studies assessing body weight outcomes after interventions with increased dietary protein. *Nutrients*, *13*(9). https://doi.org/10.3390/nu13093193

Hassan, Y., Head, V., Jacob, D., Bachmann, M. O., Diu, S., & Ford, J. (2016). Lifestyle interventions for weight loss in adults with severe obesity: a systematic review. *Clinical Obesity*, *6*(6), 395–403. https://doi.org/10.1111/cob.12161

Heymsfield, S. B., Van Mierlo, C. A. J., Van Der Knaap, H. C. M., Heo, M., & Frier, H. I. (2003). Weight management using a meal replacement strategy: Meta and pooling analysis from six studies. *International Journal of Obesity*, *27*(5), 537–549. https://doi.org/10.1038/sj.ijo.0802258

Hirode, G., & Wong, R. J. (2020). Trends in the Prevalence of Metabolic Syndrome in the United States, 2011-2016. *JAMA*, *323*(24), 2526. https://doi.org/10.1001/jama.2020.4501

Hoelscher, D. M., Kirk, S., Ritchie, L., & Cunningham-Sabo, L. (2013). Position of the Academy of Nutrition and Dietetics: Interventions for the Prevention and Treatment of Pediatric Overweight and Obesity. *Journal of the Academy of Nutrition and Dietetics*, *113*(10), 1375–1394. https://doi.org/10.1016/j.jand.2013.08.004

Huang, R. Y., Huang, C. C., Hu, F. B., & Chavarro, J. E. (2016). Vegetarian Diets and Weight Reduction: a Meta-Analysis of Randomized Controlled Trials. *Journal of General Internal Medicine*, *31*(1), 109–116. https://doi.org/10.1007/s11606-015-3390-7

Huo, R., Du, T., Xu, Y., Xu, W., Chen, X., Sun, K., & Yu, X. (2015). Effects of Mediterranean-style diet on glycemic control, weight loss and cardiovascular risk factors among type 2 diabetes individuals: A meta-analysis. *European Journal of Clinical Nutrition*, *69*(11), 1200–1208. https://doi.org/10.1038/ejcn.2014.243

Hwang, C. L., Wu, Y. T., & Chou, C. H. (2011). Effect of aerobic interval training on exercise capacity and metabolic risk factors in people with cardiometabolic disorders: a meta-analysis. *Journal of Cardiopulmonary Rehabilitation and Prevention*, *31*(6), 378–385. https://doi.org/10.1097/HCR.0b013e31822f16cb

Jensen, M. D., Ryan, D. H., Apovian, C. M., Ard, J. D., Comuzzie, A. G., Donato, K. A., ... Yanovski, S. Z. (2014). 2013 AHA/ACC/TOS Guideline for the Management of Overweight and Obesity in Adults. *Circulation*, *129*(25 suppl 2), S102–S138. https://doi.org/10.1161/01.cir.0000437739.71477.ee

Jensen, M. D., Ryan, D. H., Donato, K. A., Apovian, C. M., Ard, J. D., Comuzzie, A. G., ... Yanovski, S. Z. (2014). Executive summary: Guidelines (2013) for the management of overweight and obesity in adults: A Report of the American College of Cardiology/American Heart Association Task Force on Practice Guidelines and the Obesity Society Published by the Obesity Socie. *Obesity*, *22*(SUPPL. 2). https://doi.org/10.1002/oby.20821

Johnston, B. C., Kanters, S., Bandayrel, K., Wu, P., Naji, F., Siemieniuk, R. A., ... Mills, E. J. (2014). Comparison of weight loss among named diet programs in overweight and obese adults: A meta-analysis. *JAMA -*

Journal of the American Medical Association, 312(9), 923–933. https://doi.org/10.1001/jama.2014.10397

Kahn, R., Buse, J., Ferrannini, E., & Stern, M. (2005). The Metabolic Syndrome: Time for a Critical Appraisal. *Diabetes Care, 28*(9), 2289–2304. https://doi.org/10.2337/diacare.28.9.2289

Karfopoulou, E., Brikou, D., Mamalaki, E., Bersimis, F., Anastasiou, C. A., Hill, J. O., & Yannakoulia, M. (2017). Dietary patterns in weight loss maintenance: results from the MedWeight study. *European Journal of Nutrition, 56*(3), 991–1002. https://doi.org/10.1007/s00394-015-1147-z

Kastorini, C. M., Milionis, H. J., Esposito, K., Giugliano, D., Goudevenos, J. A., & Panagiotakos, D. B. (2011). The effect of mediterranean diet on metabolic syndrome and its components: A meta-analysis of 50 studies and 534,906 individuals. *Journal of the American College of Cardiology, 57*(11), 1299–1313. https://doi.org/10.1016/j.jacc.2010.09.073

Keating, S. E., Johnson, N. A., Mielke, G. I., & Coombes, J. S. (2017). A systematic review and meta-analysis of interval training versus moderate-intensity continuous training on body adiposity. *Obesity Reviews, 18*(8), 943–964. https://doi.org/10.1111/obr.12536

Kim, J. E., O'Connor, L. E., Sands, L. P., Slebodnik, M. B., & Campbell, W. W. (2016). Effects of dietary protein intake on body composition changes after weight loss in older adults: a systematic review and meta-analysis. *Nutrition Reviews, 74*(3), 210–224. https://doi.org/10.1093/nutrit/nuv065

Kokkinos, P., Faselis, C., Myers, J., Pittaras, A., Sui, X., Zhang, J., . . . Kokkinos, J. P. (2014). Cardiorespiratory fitness and the paradoxical BMI-mortality risk association in male veterans. *Mayo Clinic Proceedings, 89*(6), 754–762. https://doi.org/10.1016/j.mayocp.2014.01.029

Kokkinos, P., Myers, J., Faselis, C., Doumas, M., Kheirbek, R., & Nylén, E. (2012). BMI-mortality paradox and fitness in African American and Caucasian men with type 2 diabetes. *Diabetes Care, 35*(5), 1021–1027. https://doi.org/10.2337/dc11-2407

Koutras, Y., Chrysostomou, S., Poulimeneas, D., & Yannakoulia, M. (2022). Examining the associations between a posteriori dietary patterns and obesity indexes: Systematic review of observational studies. *Nutrition and Health, 28*(2), 149–162. https://doi.org/10.1177/02601060211020975

Kuhle, C. L., Steffen, M. W., Anderson, P. J., & Murad, M. H. (2014). Effect of exercise on anthropometric measures and serum lipids in older individuals: A systematic review and meta-analysis. *BMJ Open, 4*(6). https://doi.org/10.1136/bmjopen-2014-005283

Lavie, C. J., De Schutter, A., Parto, P., Jahangir, E., Kokkinos, P., Ortega, F. B., . . . Milani, R. V. (2016). Obesity and Prevalence of Cardiovascular Diseases and Prognosis-The Obesity Paradox Updated. *Progress in Cardiovascular Diseases, 58*(5), 537–547. https://doi.org/10.1016/j.pcad.2016.01.008

Lavie, C. J., Laddu, D., Arena, R., Ortega, F. B., Alpert, M. A., & Kushner, R. F. (2018). Healthy Weight and Obesity Prevention: JACC Health Promotion Series. *Journal of the American College of Cardiology, 72*(13), 1506–1531. https://doi.org/10.1016/j.jacc.2018.08.1037

Lean, M. E. J., Han, T. S., & Morrison, C. E. (1995). Waist circumference as a measure for indicating need for weight management. *Bmj, 311*(6998), 158. https://doi.org/10.1136/bmj.311.6998.158

Lemes, Í. R., Turi-Lynch, B. C., Cavero-Redondo, I., Linares, S. N., & Monteiro, H. L. (2018). Aerobic training reduces blood pressure and waist circumference and increases HDL-c in metabolic syndrome: a systematic review and meta-analysis of randomized controlled trials. *Journal of the American Society of Hypertension, 12*(8), 580–588. https://doi.org/10.1016/j.jash.2018.06.007

Li, J., Armstrong, C., & Campbell, W. (2016). Effects of Dietary Protein Source and Quantity during Weight Loss on Appetite, Energy Expenditure, and Cardio-Metabolic Responses. *Nutrients, 8*(2), 63. https://doi.org/10.3390/nu8020063

Lin, K., Zhu, L., & Yang, L. (2022). Gut and obesity/metabolic disease: Focus on microbiota metabolites. *MedComm, 3*(3), 1–21. https://doi.org/10.1002/mco2.171

Lin, X., & Li, H. (2021). Obesity: Epidemiology, Pathophysiology, and Therapeutics. *Frontiers in Endocrinology, 12*(September), 1–9. https://doi.org/10.3389/fendo.2021.706978

Lotfi, K., Saneei, P., Hajhashemy, Z., & Esmaillzadeh, A. (2022). Adherence to the Mediterranean Diet, Five-Year Weight Change, and Risk of Overweight and Obesity: A Systematic Review and Dose-Response Meta-Analysis of Prospective Cohort Studies. *Advances in Nutrition, 13*(1), 152–166. https://doi.org/10.1093/advances/nmab092

Lusis, A. J., Attie, A. D., & Reue, K. (2008). Metabolic syndrome: from epidemiology to systems biology. *Nature Reviews Genetics, 9*(11), 819–830. https://doi.org/10.1038/nrg2468

Mabire, L., Mani, R., Liu, L., Mulligan, H., & Baxter, D. (2017). The Influence of Age, Sex and Body Mass Index on the Effectiveness of Brisk Walking for Obesity Management in Adults: A Systematic Review and Meta-Analysis. *Journal of Physical Activity and Health, 14*(5), 389–407. https://doi.org/10.1123/jpah.2016-0064

Magkos, F. (2019). Metabolically healthy obesity: What's in a name? *American Journal of Clinical Nutrition, 110*(3), 533–537. https://doi.org/10.1093/ajcn/nqz133

Malik, V. S., & Hu, F. B. (2019). Sugar-Sweetened Beverages and Cardiometabolic Health: An Update of the Evidence. *Nutrients, 11*(8), 1840. https://doi.org/10.3390/nu11081840

Mann, S., Jimenez, A., Steele, J., Domone, S., Wade, M., & Beedie, C. (2018). Programming and supervision of resistance training leads to positive effects on strength and body composition: Results from two randomised trials of community fitness programmes. *BMC Public Health, 18*(1), 1–11. https://doi.org/10.1186/s12889-018-5289-9

Manolopoulos, K. N., Karpe, F., & Frayn, K. N. (2010). Gluteofemoral body fat as a determinant of metabolic health. *International Journal of Obesity, 34*(6), 949–959. https://doi.org/10.1038/ijo.2009.286

Mansoor, N., Vinknes, K. J., Veierod, M. B., & Retterstol, K. (2016). Effects of low-carbohydrate diets v. low-fat diets on body weight and cardiovascular risk factors a meta-analysis of randomised controlled trials. *British Journal of Nutrition, 115*(3), 466–479. https://doi.org/10.1017/S0007114515004699

Mattson, M. P., Longo, V. D., & Harvie, M. (2017). Impact of intermittent fasting on health and disease processes. *Ageing Research Reviews, 39*, 46–58. https://doi.org/10.1016/j.arr.2016.10.005

McCracken, E., Monaghan, M., & Sreenivasan, S. (2018). Pathophysiology of the metabolic syndrome. *Clinics in Dermatology, 36*(1), 14–20. https://doi.org/10.1016/j.clindermatol.2017.09.004

Morenga, L. Te, Mallard, S., & Mann, J. (2013). Dietary sugars and body weight: Systematic review and meta-analyses of randomised controlled trials and cohort studies. *BMJ (Online), 345*(7891), 1–25. https://doi.org/10.1136/bmj.e7492

Naude, C. E., Schoonees, A., Senekal, M., Young, T., Garner, P., & Volmink, J. (2014). Low carbohydrate versus isoenergetic balanced diets for reducing weight and cardiovascular risk: A systematic review and meta-analysis. *PLoS ONE, 9*(7). https://doi.org/10.1371/journal.pone.0100652

NICE clinical guideline 189. (2014). *Obesity : identification, assessment and management of overweight and obesity in children, young people and adults.*

Nylén, E. S., Gandhi, S. M., & Lakshman, R. (2019). Cardiorespiratory Fitness, Physical Activity, and Metabolic Syndrome. *Cardiorespiratory Fitness in Cardiometabolic Diseases: Prevention and Management in Clinical Practice*, 207–215. https://doi.org/10.1007/978-3-030-04816-7_12

O'Donoghue, G., Blake, C., Cunningham, C., Lennon, O., & Perrotta, C. (2021). What exercise prescription is optimal to improve body composition and cardiorespiratory fitness in adults living with obesity? A network meta-analysis. *Obesity Reviews*, *22*(2), 1–19. https://doi.org/10.1111/obr.13137

Obert, J., Pearlman, M., Obert, L., & Chapin, S. (2017). Popular Weight Loss Strategies: a Review of Four Weight Loss Techniques. *Current Gastroenterology Reports*, *19*(12), 17–20. https://doi.org/10.1007/s11894-017-0603-8

Oktay, A. A., Lavie, C. J., Kokkinos, P. F., Parto, P., Pandey, A., & Ventura, H. O. (2017). The Interaction of Cardiorespiratory Fitness With Obesity and the Obesity Paradox in Cardiovascular Disease. *Progress in Cardiovascular Diseases*, *60*(1), 30–44. https://doi.org/10.1016/j.pcad.2017.05.005

Ostman, C., Smart, N. A., Morcos, D., Duller, A., Ridley, W., & Jewiss, D. (2017). The effect of exercise training on clinical outcomes in patients with the metabolic syndrome: a systematic review and meta-analysis. *Cardiovascular Diabetology*, *16*(1), 110. https://doi.org/10.1186/s12933-017-0590-y

Paixão, C., Dias, C. M., Jorge, R., Carraça, E. V., Yannakoulia, M., de Zwaan, M., . . . Santos, I. (2020). Successful weight loss maintenance: A systematic review of weight control registries. *Obesity Reviews*, *21*(5), 1–15. https://doi.org/10.1111/obr.13003

Papadaki, A., Nolen-Doerr, E., & Mantzoros, C. S. (2020). The effect of the mediterranean diet on metabolic health: A systematic review and meta-analysis of controlled trials in adults. *Nutrients*, *12*(11), 1–21. https://doi.org/10.3390/nu12113342

Pedersen, B. K., & Saltin, B. (2015). Exercise as medicine - evidence for prescribing exercise as therapy in 26 different chronic diseases. *Scandinavian Journal of Medicine & Science in Sports*, *25*, 1–72. https://doi.org/10.1111/sms.12581

Pérez-Martínez, P., Mikhailidis, D. P., Athyros, V. G., Bulló, M., Couture, P., Covas, M. I., . . . López-Miranda, J. (2017). Lifestyle recommendations for the prevention and management of metabolic syndrome: An international panel recommendation. *Nutrition Reviews*, *75*(5), 307–326. https://doi.org/10.1093/nutrit/nux014

Phelan, S., Wadden, T. A., Berkowitz, R. I., Sarwer, D. B., Womble, L. G., Cato, R. K., & Rothman, R. (2007). Impact of weight loss on the metabolic syndrome. *International Journal of Obesity*, *31*(9), 1442–1448. https://doi.org/10.1038/sj.ijo.0803606

Poulimeneas, D., Anastasiou, C. A., Santos, I., Hill, J. O., Panagiotakos, D. B., & Yannakoulia, M. (2020). Exploring the relationship between the Mediterranean diet and weight loss maintenance: The MedWeight study. *British Journal of Nutrition*, *124*(8), 874–880. https://doi.org/10.1017/S0007114520001798

Poulsen, S. K., Due, A., Jordy, A. B., Kiens, B., Stark, K. D., Stender, S., . . . Larsen, T. M. (2014). Health effect of the new nordic diet in adults with increased waist circumference: A 6-mo randomized controlled trial. *American Journal of Clinical Nutrition*, *99*(1), 35–45. https://doi.org/10.3945/ajcn.113.069393

Raynor, H. A., & Champagne, C. M. (2016). Position of the Academy of Nutrition and Dietetics: Interventions for the Treatment of Overweight and Obesity in Adults. *Journal of the Academy of Nutrition and Dietetics*, *116*(1), 129–147. https://doi.org/10.1016/j.jand.2015.10.031

Reaven, G. M. (1988). Role of Insulin Resistance in Human Disease. *Diabetes*, *37*(12), 1595–1607. https://doi.org/10.2337/diab.37.12.1595

Rezagholizadeh, F., Djafarian, K., Khosravi, S., & Shab-Bidar, S. (2017). A posteriori healthy dietary patterns may decrease the risk of central obesity: findings from a systematic review and meta-analysis. *Nutrition Research*, *41*, 1–13. https://doi.org/10.1016/j.nutres.2017.01.006

Rodríguez-Monforte, M., Sánchez, E., Barrio, F., Costa, B., & Flores-Mateo, G. (2017). Metabolic syndrome and dietary patterns: a systematic review and meta-analysis of observational studies. *European Journal of Nutrition*, *56*(3), 925–947. https://doi.org/10.1007/s00394-016-1305-y

Root, M. M., & Dawson, H. R. (2014). DASH-like diets high in protein or monounsaturated fats improve metabolic syndrome and calculated vascular risk. *International Journal for Vitamin and Nutrition Research*, *83*(4), 224–231. https://doi.org/10.1024/0300-9831/a000164

Ross, R., & Bradshaw, A. J. (2009). The future of obesity reduction: Beyond weight loss. *Nature Reviews Endocrinology*, *5*(6), 319–326. https://doi.org/10.1038/nrendo.2009.78

Ross, R., Stotz, P. J., & Lam, M. (2015). Effects of exercise amount and intensity on abdominal obesity and glucose tolerance in obese adults: A randomized trial. *Annals of Internal Medicine*, *162*(5), 325–334. https://doi.org/10.7326/M14-1189

Rothman, K. J. (2008). BMI-related errors in the measurement of obesity. *International Journal of Obesity*, *32*, S56–S59. https://doi.org/10.1038/ijo.2008.87

Santesso, N., Akl, E. A., Bianchi, M., Mente, A., Mustafa, R., Heels-Ansdell, D., & Schünemann, H. J. (2012). Effects of higher- versus lower-protein diets on health outcomes: a systematic review and meta-analysis. *European Journal of Clinical Nutrition*, *66*(7), 780–788. https://doi.org/10.1038/ejcn.2012.37

Sayón-Orea, C., Razquin, C., Bulló, M., Corella, D., Fitó, M., Romaguera, D., . . . Martínez-González, M. A. (2019). Effect of a Nutritional and Behavioral Intervention on Energy-Reduced Mediterranean Diet Adherence Among Patients With Metabolic Syndrome. *JAMA*, *322*(15), 1486. https://doi.org/10.1001/jama.2019.14630

Shab-Bidar, S., Golzarand, M., Hajimohammadi, M., & Mansouri, S. (2018). A posteriori dietary patterns and metabolic syndrome in adults: A systematic review and meta-analysis of observational studies. *Public Health Nutrition*, *21*(9), 1681–1692. https://doi.org/10.1017/S1368980018000216

Shay, C. M., Van Horn, L., Stamler, J., Dyer, A. R., Brown, I. J., Chan, Q., . . . Elliott, P. (2012). Food and nutrient intakes and their associations with lower BMI in middle-aged US adults: the International Study of Macro-/Micronutrients and Blood Pressure (INTERMAP). *The American Journal of Clinical Nutrition*, *96*(3), 483–491. https://doi.org/10.3945/ajcn.111.025056

Silver, H. J., E. Brian Welch, Malcolm J. Avison, & Kevin D. Niswender. (2010). Imaging body composition in obesity and weight loss: challenges and opportunities. *Diabetes, Metabolic Syndrome and Obesity: Targets and Therapy*, 337. https://doi.org/10.2147/dmsott.s9454

Sjöström, L. (2013). Review of the key results from the Swedish Obese Subjects (SOS) trial - a prospective controlled intervention study of bariatric surgery. *Journal of Internal Medicine*, *273*(3), 219–234. https://doi.org/10.1111/joim.12012

Stehouwer, C. D. A. (2021). Treating Obesity: Lifestyle, New Options in Pharmacotherapy, and the Obesogenic Environment. *Journal of Endocrinology and Metabolism*, *11*(2), 33–34. https://doi.org/10.14740/jem737

Thune, I., Njølstad, I., Løchen, M.-L., & Førde, O. H. (1998). Physical Activity Improves the Metabolic Risk Profiles in Men and Women. *Archives of Internal Medicine, 158*(15), 1633. https://doi.org/10.1001/archinte.158.15.1633

Tian, Y., Su, L., Wang, J., Duan, X., & Jiang, X. (2018). Fruit and vegetable consumption and risk of the metabolic syndrome: a meta-analysis. *Public Health Nutrition, 21*(4), 756–765. https://doi.org/10.1017/S136898001700310X

Tsai, A. G., & Wadden, T. A. (2006). The evolution of very-low-calorie diets: An update and meta-analysis. *Obesity, 14*(8), 1283–1293. https://doi.org/10.1038/oby.2006.146

Türk, Y., Theel, W., Kasteleyn, M. J., Franssen, F. M. E., Hiemstra, P. S., Rudolphus, A., . . . Braunstahl, G. J. (2017). High intensity training in obesity: a Meta-analysis. *Obesity Science and Practice, 3*(3), 258–271. https://doi.org/10.1002/osp4.109

van Baak, M. A., Pramono, A., Battista, F., Beaulieu, K., Blundell, J. E., Busetto, L., . . . Oppert, J. M. (2021). Effect of different types of regular exercise on physical fitness in adults with overweight or obesity: Systematic review and meta-analyses. *Obesity Reviews, 22*(S4), 1–11. https://doi.org/10.1111/obr.13239

Varkevisser, R. D. M., van Stralen, M. M., Kroeze, W., Ket, J. C. F., & Steenhuis, I. H. M. (2019). Determinants of weight loss maintenance: a systematic review. In *Obesity Reviews* (Vol. 20). https://doi.org/10.1111/obr.12772

Verheggen, R. J. H. M., Maessen, M. F. H., Green, D. J., Hermus, A. R. M. M., Hopman, M. T. E., & Thijssen, D. H. T. (2016). A systematic review and meta-analysis on the effects of exercise training versus hypocaloric diet: distinct effects on body weight and visceral adipose tissue. *Obesity Reviews, 17*(8), 664–690. https://doi.org/10.1111/obr.12406

Volkert, D., Beck, A. M., Cederholm, T., Cruz-Jentoft, A., Goisser, S., Hooper, L., . . . Bischoff, S. C. (2019). ESPEN guideline on clinical nutrition and hydration in geriatrics. *Clinical Nutrition, 38*(1), 10–47. https://doi.org/10.1016/j.clnu.2018.05.024

Waalen, J. (2014). The genetics of human obesity. *Translational Research, 164*(4), 293–301. https://doi.org/10.1016/j.trsl.2014.05.010

Wang, S., & Ren, J. (2018). Obesity Paradox in Aging: From Prevalence to Pathophysiology. *Progress in Cardiovascular Diseases, 61*(2), 182–189. https://doi.org/10.1016/j.pcad.2018.07.011

Wang, Y., Beydoun, M. A., Min, J., Xue, H., Kaminsky, L. A., & Cheskin, L. J. (2021). Has the prevalence of overweight, obesity and central obesity levelled off in the United States? Trends, patterns, disparities, and future projections for the obesity epidemic. *International Journal of Epidemiology, 49*(3), 810–823. https://doi.org/10.1093/IJE/DYZ273

Washburn, R. A., Szabo, A. N., Lambourne, K., Willis, E. A., Ptomey, L. T., Honas, J. J., . . . Donnelly, J. E. (2014). Does the method of weight loss effect long-term changes in weight, body composition or chronic disease risk factors in overweight or obese adults? A systematic review. *PLoS ONE, 9*(10). https://doi.org/10.1371/journal.pone.0109849

Watson, Nerylee A., Dyer, K. A., Buckley, J. D., Brinkworth, G. D., Coates, A. M., Parfitt, G., . . . Murphy, K. J. (2018). Reductions in food cravings are similar with low-fat weight loss diets differing in protein and carbohydrate in overweight and obese adults with type 2 diabetes: A randomized clinical trial. *Nutrition Research, 57*, 56–66. https://doi.org/10.1016/j.nutres.2018.05.005

Watson, Nerylee Ann, Dyer, K. A., Buckley, J. D., Brinkworth, G. D., Coates, A. M., Parfitt, G., . . . Murphy, K. J. (2018). Comparison of two low-fat diets, differing in protein and carbohydrate, on psychological wellbeing in adults with obesity and type 2 diabetes: a randomised clinical trial. *Nutrition Journal, 17*(1), 62. https://doi.org/10.1186/s12937-018-0367-5

Wendy H Oddy. (2012). Infant feeding and obesity risk in the child. *Breastfeed Rev, 20*(2), 7–12.

Wewege, M. A., Thom, J. M., Rye, K.-A., & Parmenter, B. J. (2018). Aerobic, resistance or combined training: A systematic review and meta-analysis of exercise to reduce cardiovascular risk in adults with metabolic syndrome. *Atherosclerosis, 274*, 162–171. https://doi.org/10.1016/j.atherosclerosis.2018.05.002

Wewege, M., van den Berg, R., Ward, R. E., & Keech, A. (2017). The effects of high-intensity interval training vs. moderate-intensity continuous training on body composition in overweight and obese adults: a systematic review and meta-analysis. *Obesity Reviews, 18*(6), 635–646. https://doi.org/10.1111/obr.12532

Wharton, S., Lau, D. C. W., Vallis, M., Sharma, A. M., Biertho, L., Campbell-Scherer, D., . . . Wicklum, S. (2020). Obesity in adults: A clinical practice guideline. *Cmaj, 192*(31), E875–E891. https://doi.org/10.1503/cmaj.191707

WHO. (2016). WHO Guidelines on physical activity and sedentary behaviour. In *Routledge Handbook of Youth Sport*.

WHO. (2022). *World Obesity Atlas 2022*. (March), 289.

Winter, J. E., MacInnis, R. J., Wattanapenpaiboon, N., & Nowson, C. A. (2014). BMI and all-cause mortality in older adults: A meta-analysis. *American Journal of Clinical Nutrition, 99*(4), 875–890. https://doi.org/10.3945/ajcn.113.068122

World Health Organization. (2021). Obesity and overweight. https://doi.org/https://www.who.int/news-room/fact-sheets/detail/obesity-and-overweight

Wycherley, T. P., Moran, L. J., Clifton, P. M., Noakes, M., & Brinkworth, G. D. (2012). Effects of energy-restricted high-protein, low-fat compared with standard-protein, low-fat diets: a meta-analysis of randomized controlled trials. *The American Journal of Clinical Nutrition, 96*(6), 1281–1298. https://doi.org/10.3945/ajcn.112.044321

Yannakoulia, M., Poulimeneas, D., Mamalaki, E., & Anastasiou, C. A. (2019, March). Dietary modifications for weight loss and weight loss maintenance. *Metabolism: Clinical and Experimental*, Vol. 92, pp. 153–162. https://doi.org/10.1016/j.metabol.2019.01.001

Yumuk, V., Tsigos, C., Fried, M., Schindler, K., Busetto, L., Micic, D., & Toplak, H. (2015). European Guidelines for Obesity Management in Adults. *Obesity Facts, 8*(6), 402–424. https://doi.org/10.1159/000442721

Zhang, D., Liu, X., Liu, Y., Sun, X., Wang, B., Ren, Y., . . . Hu, D. (2017). Leisure-time physical activity and incident metabolic syndrome: a systematic review and dose-response meta-analysis of cohort studies. *Metabolism: Clinical and Experimental, 75*, 36–44. https://doi.org/10.1016/j.metabol.2017.08.001

Zhu, S. K., Wang, Z. M., Heshka, S., Heo, M., Faith, M. S., & Heymsfield, S. B. (2002). Waist circumference and obesity-associated risk factors among whites in the third National Health and Nutrition Examination Survey: Clinical action thresholds. *American Journal of Clinical Nutrition, 76*(4), 743–749. https://doi.org/10.1093/ajcn/76.4.743

FURTHER READING

Bibliography

Bischoff, S. C., and Schweinlin, A. (2020). Obesity therapy. *Clinical Nutrition ESPEN*, *38*: 9–18. doi: 10.1016/j.clnesp.2020.04.013

Jensen, M. D., et al. (2014). 2013 AHA/ACC/TOS guideline for the management of overweight and obesity in adults. *Circulation*, *129*(25 suppl 2): S102–S138.

Pérez-Martínez, P., Mikhailidis, D. P., Athyros, V. G., et. al., (2017). Lifestyle recommendations for the prevention and management of metabolic syndrome: An international panel recommendation. *Nutrition Reviews*, *75*(5): 307–326. doi: 10.1093/nutrit/nux014

Raynor, H. A., and Champagne, C. M. (2016). Position of the Academy of Nutrition and Dietetics: Interventions for the treatment of overweight and obesity in adults. *Journal of the Academy of Nutrition and Dietetics*, *116*(1): 129–147. doi: 10.1016/j.jand.2015.10.031

Varkevisser, R. D. M., van Stralen, M. M., Kroeze, W., Ket, J. C. F., and Steenhuis, I. H. M. (2019). Determinants of weight loss maintenance: A systematic review. *Obesity Reviews*, *20*. doi: 10.1111/obr.12772

Yannakoulia, M., Poulimeneas, D., Mamalaki, E., and Anastasiou, C. A. (2019). Dietary modifications for weight loss and weight loss maintenance. *Metabolism: Clinical and Experimental*, *92*: 153–162. doi: 10.1016/j.metabol.2019.01.001

Links

- https://www.obesity.org/
- https://www.worldobesity.org/
- https://www.americanobesity.org/
- https://www.who.int/news-room/fact-sheets/detail/obesity-and-overweight
- https://www.nhlbi.nih.gov/health/overweight-and-obesity
- https://www.heart.org/en/health-topics/metabolic-syndrome/about-metabolic-syndrome
- https://www.heartuk.org.uk/genetic-conditions/metabolic-syndrome

Obstructive Sleep Apnea

CHAPTER 19

Introduction	299	Physical Activity, Fitness, and Obstructive Sleep Apnea	311
Diagnosis	300	Exercise Training and Obstructive Sleep Apnea Management	312
Prevalence	302	Key Points	314
Pathophysiology and Risk Factors	303	Self-assessment Questions	315
Complications	305	Case Scenario	316
Management	307	References	317
Nutrition in Obstructive Sleep Apnea	308	Further Reading	324
Diet as a Risk Factor for Obstructive Sleep Apnea Development and Progression	308	Bibliography	324
Dietary Modifications for Obstructive Sleep Apnea Management	308	Links	325
Role of the Mediterranean Diet/Lifestyle in Obstructive Sleep Apnea	310		

INTRODUCTION

According to the *International Classification of Sleep Disorders* by the American Academy of Sleep Medicine, obstructive sleep apnea (OSA) belongs to a group of sleep-related breathing disorders, along with central sleep apnea, sleep-related hypoventilation, and sleep-related hypoxemia disorder (*International Classification of Sleep Disorders*, 2014). It is a chronic pathological condition characterized by recurrent pauses of breathing during sleep due to obstruction of the upper airways, which leads to sleep disruption (Eckert & Malhotra, 2008; Jordan, McSharry, & Malhotra, 2014) (**Figure 19.1**). Specifically, in the context of OSA, narrowing or complete obstructions of the upper airways are observed in the pharyngeal region during sleep, when the tone of upper-airway dilator muscles decreases normally and leads to temporary partial or complete cessation of breathing (respiratory events) despite respiratory effort. Breathing pauses are accompanied by a decrease in blood oxygen saturation (hypoxemia) and carbon dioxide retention (hypercapnia) that lead to sleep disruption (awakening) to restore the tone of the upper-airway dilator muscles and normal airflow. However, after sleep restoration, upper-airway obstructions reoccur and repetitive awakenings end up disrupting sleep architecture, duration, and quality (Eckert & Malhotra, 2008; Jordan et al., 2014).

The clinical presentation of OSA includes symptoms that occur during both sleep and daytime. During sleep, OSA is characterized by a distinct pattern of snoring, which involves intervals of loud noises and respiratory efforts that alternate with intervals of silence due to complete breathing cessations. In most patients, snoring symptoms are usually present for many years, but the decision to undergo a sleep diagnostic procedure is usually made due to the aggravation of snoring frequency and/or intensity as reported by patients' bedpartners. This aggravation is usually reported when alcohol has been consumed before bedtime or as a result of recent weight gain (Lurie, 2011; Stansbury & Strollo, 2015). Patients' respiratory events can vary in severity, and in the case of severe OSA, they are maintained for several seconds before respiratory movements are observed and cause cyanosis due to hypoxemia. The end of respiratory events is usually accompanied by intense snoring and sounds that resemble "groans" or "squeals", while awakenings are often accompanied by whole-body movements, which can be sharp or even violent. The majority of patients are not fully aware of the breathing pauses and repetitive awakenings that occur during

---

Prevention and Management of Cardiovascular and Metabolic Disease: Diet, Physical Activity and Healthy Aging,
First Edition. Christina N. Katsagoni, Peter Kokkinos, and Labros S. Sidossis.
© 2023 John Wiley & Sons Ltd. Published 2023 by John Wiley & Sons Ltd.

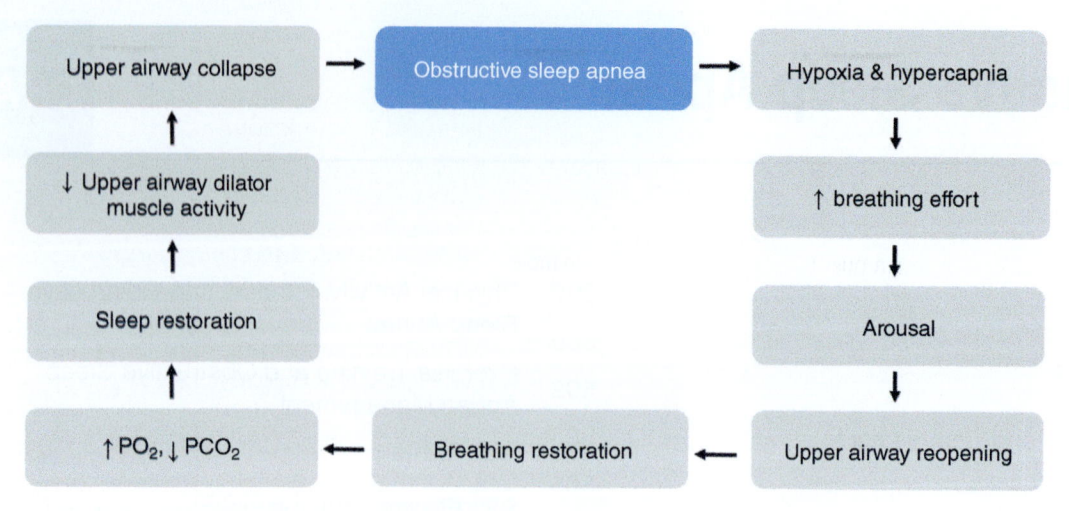

FIGURE 19.1 Schematic representation of the typical pathophysiological sequence that occurs in OSA. PCO_2 = partial pressure of carbon dioxide; PO_2 = partial pressure of oxygen.

sleep but usually report insomnia symptoms and a sense of "restless" sleep (Lurie, 2011; Stansbury & Strollo, 2015). Nocturnal symptoms of the disease also include heavy sweating and nocturia, while early daytime symptoms manifest as fatigue, decreased rejuvenation, disorientation, mental sluggishness, lack of coordination, and headaches that often require analgesics (Lurie, 2011; Stansbury & Strollo, 2015).

DIAGNOSIS

Polysomnography (PSG) is the gold-standard method for OSA diagnosis (Epstein et al., 2009; Kapur et al., 2017; Qaseem et al., 2014). PSG is non-invasive and consists of a simultaneous recording of multiple physiologic parameters related to sleep and wakefulness. The procedure is usually performed during night sleep in a laboratory (e.g., a sleep center) under the supervision of specialized medical personnel (sleep technologists and somnologists). In the context of the PSG, brain activity via electroencephalography, eye movements via electrooculography, muscle activity via electromyography, heart rate via electrocardiography, respiratory airflow via pressure transducers, respiratory effort via abdominal movement sensors, and blood oxygen levels via pulse oximetry are assessed during real sleep conditions, and all data are simultaneously recorded on a multi-channel digital system (**Figure 19.2**) (Epstein et al., 2009; Kapur et al., 2017; Qaseem et al., 2014). After the procedure is completed, all recorded data are scored and analyzed according to the American Academy of Sleep Medicine guidelines (*The AASM Manual for the Scoring of Sleep and Associated Events: Rules, Terminology and Technical Specifications*, 2015), providing a detailed assessment of the patient's sleep architecture and cardio-respiratory function.

With regard to sleep architecture, PSG analyses provide data on wake time, and time spent in non-rapid eye movement (NREM) sleep, which consists of stage 1 (N1), stage 2 (N2), and stage 3 (N3) sleep as well as rapid eye movement (REM) sleep; for each sleep stage, the relative contribution to total sleep period is calculated as ([(time spent in sleep stage [min] ÷ total sleep period [min]) × 100]). **Table 19.1** presents an overview of adult sleep staging and disturbances observed in OSA patients (Jordan et al., 2014). In general, human sleep consists of distinct sleep circles, each starting from a period of non-REM sleep (N1 to N3) that is followed by a shorter period of REM sleep, which are repeated several times along with some arousals until the final

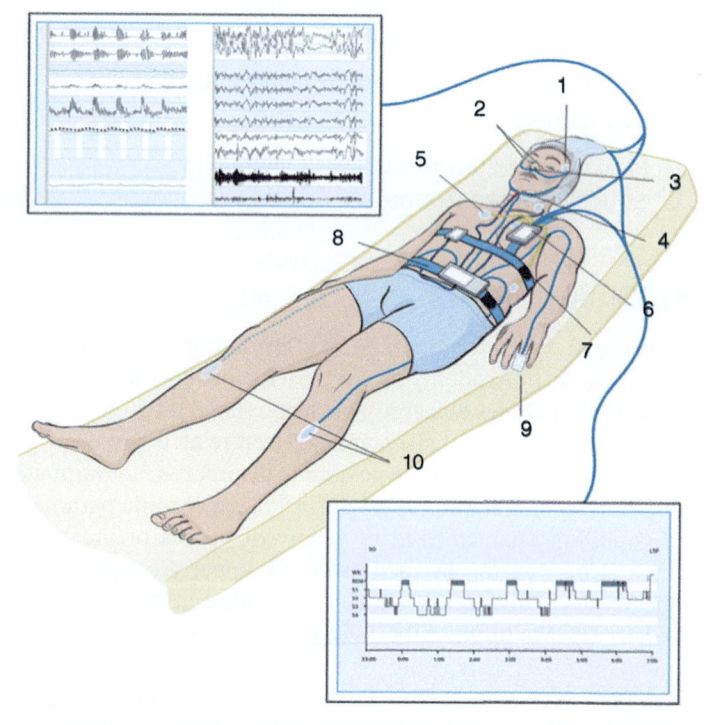

FIGURE 19.2 Schematic illustration of polysomnography. During the procedure, the following assessments are simultaneously performed: (1) electroencephalography, (2) electrooculography, (3) assessment of respiratory airflow, (4) mandible electromyography, (5) electrocardiography (heart rate), (6) assessment of body position, (7) assessment of respiratory effort (thoracic movements), (8) assessment of abdominal movements, (9) pulse oximetry (blood oxygen), and (10) lower limb electromyography. Source: (Sadek, Siyanbade, Abdulrazak, 2023)

Table 19.1 Adult sleep staging and arousal scoring. REM = rapid eye movement; OSA = obstructive sleep apnea; EEG = electroencephalogram; EMG = electromyogram.

	EEG characteristics	Relevance to OSA	Normal amounts
Wake	Low voltage, mixed frequency when eyes are open or alert; α activity (8–13 Hz) while relaxed with eyes closed	Typically increased	15–20% of time in bed
N1	Predominantly low amplitude and relatively fast θ activity (3–7 Hz) accompanied by slow rolling-type eye movements	Typically increased	4–6%, more in older patients
N2	Sleep spindles (12–14 Hz bursts lasting >0·5 s) and K complexes (large negative EEG wave followed immediately by a slower positive wave) on a background of low voltage, mixed frequency EEG	Typically increased	50–65%, more in older patients
N3	Slow (<2 Hz), high amplitude (> 75 μV) EEG waves for more than half the epoch	Often absent or reduced; associated with improved severity or absence of OSA when present	15–20%, less in older patients
REM	Low voltage, mixed frequency EEG with periodic runs of sawtooth waves accompanied by irregular movements of both eyes and low muscle tone	Often absent or reduced; often accompanied by worsening of respiratory events and more pronounced desaturation than the non-REM stages	15–20%
Arousals	3–15 s return of waking or faster activity in the EEG; concurrent increase in EMG must be recorded in REM sleep	Commonly occur at the end of respiratory events, but also occur spontaneously or because of other stimuli (e.g., leg movements)	20 per h of sleep

Source: (Jordan et al., 2014).

awakening. Most patients with OSA spend more time awake, in N1, and N2 sleep and less time in N3 and REM sleep due to repetitive airway obstructions that lead to awakenings, disrupt normal sleep architecture, and prevent deeper sleep stages. Sleep latency (min), i.e., time from lights out to sleep onset, is also recorded, and sleep efficiency (%) is calculated as [(sleep time [min] ÷ time in bed [min]) × 100].

Respiratory events are classified as apneas (obstructive, central, or mixed) and hypopneas (*The AASM Manual for the Scoring of Sleep and Associated Events: Rules, Terminology and Technical Specifications*, 2015), depending on the severity of airflow reduction (**Table 19.2**). Based on the assessment of respiratory events, the apnea index (AI), the hypopnea index (HI), and the apnea-hypopnea index (AHI) (total, non-REM, and REM) are calculated as the number of corresponding respiratory events per hour of sleep [respiratory events (total number) ÷ sleep period (h)].

The respiratory disturbance index (RDI) can also be calculated; it is based on the number of apneas and hypopneas just like the AHI but also includes respiratory effort-related arousals and usually receives slightly higher values compared to the AHI. Oximetry indices, such as average and minimum oxygen saturation (SaO_2) are also recorded during PSG, and respiratory events accompanied by a decrease in SaO_2 equal or greater than 4% during sleep, compared to SaO_2 during wake period, are recorded to calculate the oxygen desaturation index (ODI) as [oxygen desaturation events (total number) ÷ sleep period (h)]. Electromyography of the anterior tibialis is also often performed to assess limb movements that might alter sleep stage or respiration and body position is monitored because of the position-specific nature of OSA in many patients. Other parameters, such as

Table 19.2 Adult respiratory event scoring.

	Definition
Apnea	Airflow reduced to less than 10% of baseline for more than 10 s; obstructive if respiratory effort is present, central if no respiratory effort is present
Hypopnea (recommended definition)	Airflow reduced to less than 30% of baseline for more than 10 s, in association with a 4% oxygen desaturation
Hypopnea (alternative definition)	Airflow reduced to less than 50% of baseline for more than 10 s, in association with a 3% oxygen desaturation or an arousal from sleep
Respiratory effort-related arousal	Sequence of breaths lasting more than 10 s that do not meet the standard hypopnea definition but are characterized by high upper-airway resistance (snoring and flattened inspiratory nasal pressure signal) and terminate in arousal from sleep

Source: (Jordan et al., 2014).

average and highest heart rate, including episodes of bradycardia, asystole, tachycardia, atrial fibrillation, snoring, and any unusual or atypical behavioral events occurring during sleep and/or wakefulness are also recorded during PSG. **Figure 19.3** provides an example of the signals recorded during an overnight PSG.

According to the American Academy of Sleep Medicine *International Classification of Sleep Disorders* (*International Classification of Sleep Disorders*, 2014), the diagnosis of OSA requires the presence of signs-symptoms (e.g., arousals accompanied by breathing difficulty or choking, snoring or witness of apneas during sleep, and daytime sleepiness) or co-morbidities (e.g., hypertension, coronary heart disease, atrial fibrillation,

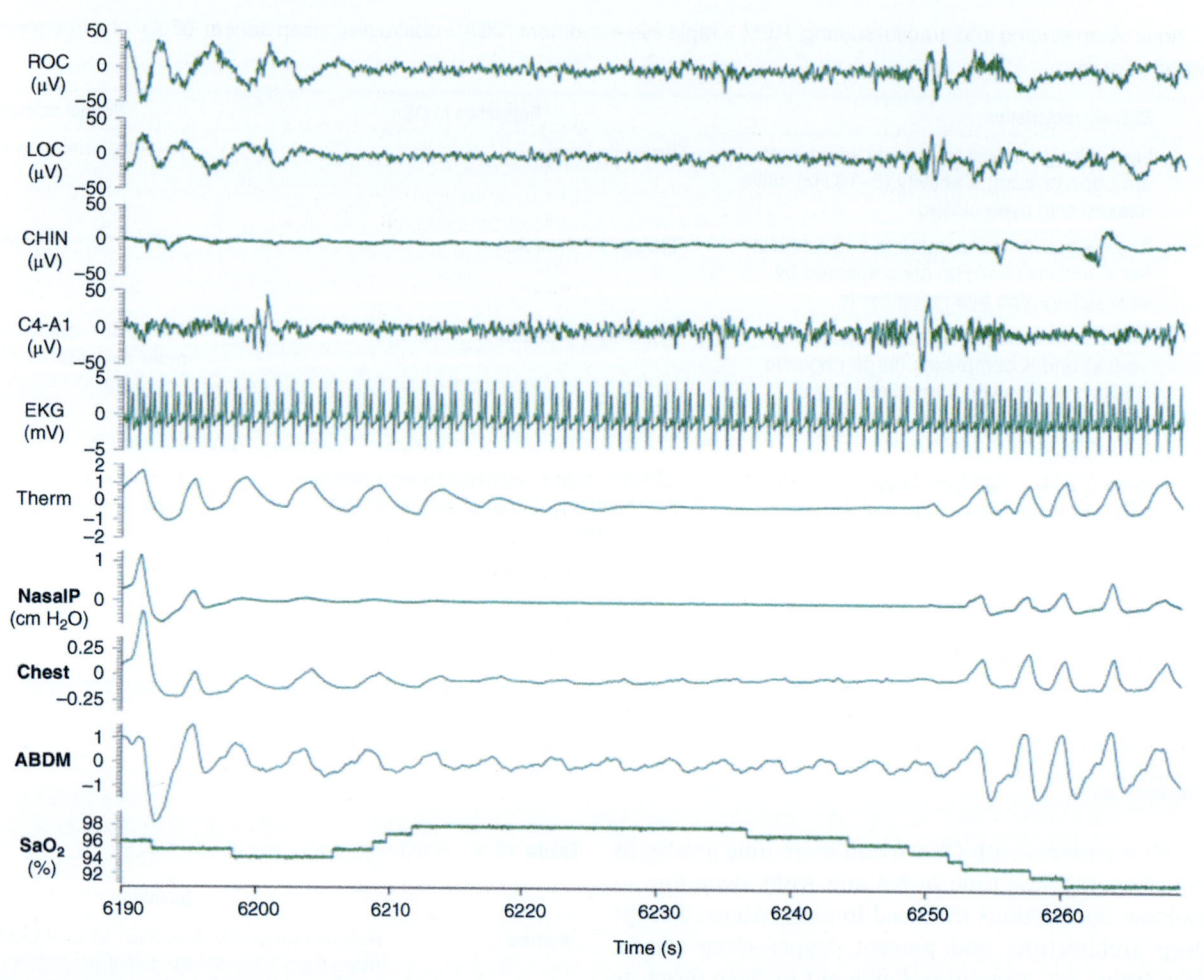

FIGURE 19.3 An example of the signals recorded during overnight polysomnography. The polysomnogram shows an obstructive apnea with cessation of airflow for more than 10 s despite persistent respiratory efforts shown on the chest and abdominal respiratory bands. The apnea is associated with arterial oxygen desaturation and is terminated by arousal from sleep. C4-A1 = electroencephalogram; LOC = left electro-oculogram; ROC = right electro-oculogram; CHIN = chin electromyogram; CHEST = respiratory inductance plethysmography bands placed around the thorax; ABDM = respiratory inductance plethysmography bands placed around the abdomen; PNasal = airflow monitoring by nasal air pressure; Therm = airflow monitoring by thermal air sensor; SaO_2 = arterial oxygen saturation; EKG = electrocardiogram; ABDM = abdomen. Source: (Jordan, McSharry, & Malhotra, 2014)

congestive heart failure, stroke, diabetes mellitus, cognitive impairment, or psychiatric disorder), in combination with more than five, mainly obstructive, respiratory episodes per hour of sleep during a sleep study. Alternatively, OSA can be diagnosed in the presence of ≥15 respiratory events per hour of sleep even in the absence of associated signs-symptoms or co-morbidities. In clinical practice, the AHI, i.e., the number of apneas and hypopneas per hour of sleep, is the most important PSG measure, based on which OSA diagnosis and severity is evaluated (Sateia, 2014). An OSA diagnosis is established when the AHI receives values ≥5 events/h and the disease is further classified as mild (5–14 events/h), moderate (15–29 events/h) or severe OSA (≥30 events/h). OSA severity evaluation based on ODI and RDI values is similar to AHI classification, but these indexes are not widely used for OSA diagnosis and severity assessment in clinical practice.

Although an overnight attended PSG is the gold-standard method for OSA diagnosis and provides definitive results, the procedure is expensive, time consuming, burdensome for most patients, and requires specialized personnel and equipment. Simplified home sleep studies using portable devices also provide basic information on sleep architecture and respiratory events and can alternatively be used for OSA diagnosis. Available evidence suggests that a home-based diagnosis, if properly performed, is not inferior to a laboratory diagnosis and can be of great value for individuals with mobility problems who have difficulty accessing a sleep center or when an attended PSG is not available (Masa et al., 2011; Mulgrew, Fox, Ayas, & Ryan, 2007; Rosen et al., 2012).

PREVALENCE

Even though the first reports of OSA date back to antiquity (Kryger, 1985), epidemiological data on the prevalence of the disease were not available until the early 1990s. The Wisconsin sleep cohort study, a prospective epidemiological study initiated in 1988 with the aim of investigating the prevalence and natural history of sleep-related breathing disorders, is a landmark for the epidemiology of OSA (T. Young et al., 1993). According to analyses of

602 US men and women aged 30 to 60, the prevalence of OSA—defined as the presence of ≥5 apneas-hypopneas/h based on PSG combined with increased daytime sleepiness—was 4% in men and 2% in women. Subsequent epidemiological studies in the USA, Europe, Australia, and Asia (Franklin & Lindberg, 2015; Punjabi, 2008; Senaratna et al., 2017) have shown that the prevalence of OSA in the general population, defined as AHI/ODI ≥5 events/h, ranges from 9% to 36%; disease rates are higher in men (from 13% to 33%) compared to women (from 6% to 19%) and increase with age, reaching 90% and 80% in older men and women, respectively. According to a comprehensive review of epidemiological studies examining global estimates of OSA prevalence published in 2019 (Benjafield et al., 2019), 936 million adults aged 30 to 69 years have mild-to-severe OSA and 425 million have moderate-to-severe disease; the number of affected individuals was highest in China, followed by the USA, Brazil, and India.

It is worth mentioning, however, that despite the widespread recognition of OSA as a major public health problem, available estimates of its prevalence probably underestimate its true extent, given that a large part of the general population (approximately 20%) experiences the respiratory manifestations of the disease in the absence of accompanying symptoms or co-morbidities that usually lead to diagnostic sleep testing. Moreover, a large proportion of patients, even those with symptoms or those at increased risk for co-morbidities, remain undiagnosed due to the practical difficulties of PSG.

PATHOPHYSIOLOGY AND RISK FACTORS

OSA has been traditionally considered a disease of abnormal upper-airway anatomy and neuromuscular pathology, in which abnormal craniofacial structure or excess body fat decreases the size of the pharyngeal airway lumen and, combined with upper-airway muscle dysfunction, leads to an increased likelihood of pharyngeal collapse during sleep (Eckert & Malhotra, 2008; Horner, 2008; Patil, Schneider, Schwartz, & Smith, 2007). The pharynx is a common organ for the respiratory system and the gastrointestinal tract, and it is involved in many vital body functions, such as swallowing, speaking, and breathing. It is unsupported by bones or cartilaginous tissue, but it contains several groups of muscles and soft tissues, along with a section that can be closed, which extends from the hard palate to the larynx (Ayappa & Rapoport, 2003). This ability of the pharynx to close is essential for speech and swallowing while awake, but it also provides the grounds for an undesirable obstruction under certain conditions during sleep.

During wakefulness, the upper airway is held open by the high activity of the numerous upper-airway dilator muscles. After the onset of sleep, when muscle activity is normally reduced, the airway is susceptible to obstruction, especially in the presence of a detrimental upper-airway anatomy. The size of the upper airways in the pharyngeal region depends on many factors, as the pharyngeal lumen is surrounded lengthwise by bones, such as the nasal bones, jaw bones, and the hyoid bone, as well as soft tissues, such as the tongue, the soft palate, the tonsils, the epiglottis, fat particles, and blood vessels. In general, a disproportionately high proportion of soft tissue mass, relative to the space available from the skeletal structures surrounding the pharynx, favors its obstruction (C. M. Ryan & Bradley, 2005). Patients with OSA often present with disorders of the skeletal structures surrounding the pharyngeal cavity, such as hypoplasia and/or dislocation of the jaws and displacement of the hyoid bone as well as enlargement of the soft tissues surrounding the pharynx, such as the thickening of the lateral walls of the pharynx (secondary to the accumulation of fat in the area, swelling of the pharyngeal mucosa due to vascular congestion or inflammation, or swelling of the veins in the area in the presence of fluid accumulation due to heart failure or chronic kidney disease) or the swelling of the soft palate and the tonsils (Eckert & Malhotra, 2008; Horner, 2008; Patil et al., 2007). In addition to this detrimental upper-airway anatomy, compared to healthy subjects, patients with OSA also experience a greater reduction in genioglossus muscle activity, the most important upper-airway dilator muscle, and its response to local stimuli during sleep. Upper-airway muscle fatigue is also thought to be involved in OSA pathogenesis, caused by chronic muscle trauma and inflammation due to continuous low-frequency vibrations of snoring and recurrent hypoxia (Eckert & Malhotra, 2008; Horner, 2008; Patil et al., 2007). Therefore, although healthy individuals experience only a small degree of respiratory instability at the onset of sleep, a person with a detrimental upper respiratory tract anatomy who relies more on muscle tone to support respiration is particularly prone to developing OSA when the function of the upper-airway dilator muscles is compromised.

Although upper-airway anatomy and muscle function are crucial for the development of OSA, accumulated research over the last decades has also identified several non-anatomical and non-neuromuscular factors that contribute to OSA pathophysiology in patients with apparently normal upper-airway anatomy and very responsive upper-airway dilator muscles. These factors include the instability of the central respiratory control system, increased tendency to wake up (low arousal threshold), and low lung volume (Eckert & Malhotra, 2008; Horner, 2008; Patil et al., 2007). In addition, the close relationship between OSA and cardio-metabolic diseases has led the scientific community to reconsider its traditional view as merely an anatomical disease of the upper respiratory system and investigate cardio-metabolic factors as potential pathogenetic mechanisms. In this context, the landmark theory of Vgontzas et al. (Vgontzas, Bixler, & Chrousos, 2003, 2005; Vgontzas, Gaines, Ryan, & McNicholas, 2016) suggests that cardio-metabolic disorders in the context of the metabolic syndrome, i.e., central obesity, insulin resistance, dyslipidemia, and hypertension are implicated in OSA pathogenesis. In particular, while the majority of researchers argue that inflammation and oxidative stress resulting from intermittent hypoxia in the context of OSA lead to cardio-metabolic morbidity, Vgontas et al. (Vgontzas et al., 2003, 2005; Vgontzas et al., 2016) suggest that the pathophysiology of the metabolic syndrome actually precedes the onset of OSA, with central fat deposition triggering upper-airway dysfunction through insulin resistance, inflammation and oxidative stress, and that OSA should be essentially be considered as the manifestation of the metabolic syndrome in the respiratory system of obese individuals. This hypothesis is based on evidence that: i) obesity, and diseases in which insulin resistance and inflammation play a central role, such as diabetes mellitus, are associated with symptoms of OSA (e.g., daytime sleepiness) in the absence of a formal OSA diagnosis; ii) treatment of OSA-related respiratory disorders is not accompanied by benefits in glucose metabolism, inflammation, and oxidative stress, suggesting that these disorders precede OSA rather than manifest as a result of the disease; iii) exercise can reduce OSA severity through improvements in inflammation and insulin resistance in the absence of weight loss; iv) the presence of the metabolic syndrome is associated with sarcopenia and skeletal muscle dysfunction and may consequently contribute to upper-airway dilator muscle dysfunction; v) elevated leptin levels, a key feature of obesity, can disrupt central respiratory control; vi) the prevalence of OSA and the metabolic syndrome has a similar age distribution in the general population, reaching a maximum in middle age, a fact that supports their causal relationship; and vii) inflammation is present in patients with OSA regardless of the presence of obesity (Vgontzas et al., 2003, 2005; Vgontzas et al., 2016).

Risk factors for developing OSA resemble those of cardiovascular diseases and include increased age, obesity, male gender, smoking, and heavy alcohol consumption (Gharibeh & Mehra, 2010; Punjabi, 2008). OSA also exhibits a hereditary pattern, with up to 35% of the variation in disease severity being attributed to genetic factors regardless of age and body-weight status (Gharibeh & Mehra, 2010; Punjabi, 2008).

Among modifiable risk factors, obesity has emerged as the most important factor leading to sleep-disordered breathing and the progression of OSA. Epidemiological studies suggest that being overweight occurs in approximately 60% of patients undergoing diagnostic sleep testing. The Wisconsin sleep cohort study was the first large-scale prospective study to test longitudinal associations between weight change and OSA indices (Peppard, Young, Palta, Dempsey, & Skatrud, 2000). In a sample of 690 participants from Wisconsin, USA who were followed for 4 years, compared to weight-stable conditions, a 5%, 10%, and 20% weight gain predicted a 15%, 32%, and 70% increase in the AHI, respectively, while weight loss was associated with analogous decreases in the AHI (Peppard et al., 2000). Similar observations were subsequently reported by the sleep heart health study among 2968 middle-aged men and women from several US communities during a 5-year follow-up period, compared to weight-stable individuals; those who gained weight experienced increases in the RDI in a dose-response manner and vice versa (Newman et al., 2005). Several case-control studies have also revealed a significant positive association between the presence of overweight/obesity and odds of OSA both in children and adults (Dong et al., 2020). Results of available interventional studies reinforce the epidemiological observations, as weight loss has been shown to improve the severity of OSA in most patients (these data are discussed below in detail). The involvement of obesity in the pathophysiology of OSA can be explained through several mechanisms, including: i) central fat accumulation, mainly in abdominal viscera and around the neck, which leads to increased mechanical load on upper airways; ii) increased leptin resistance, which can impair central respiratory control and lead to abnormal hypercapnic ventilatory response; iii) expression of pro-inflammatory cytokines, which negatively impact upper-airway neuromuscular control; and iv) a state of increased oxidative stress, which reduces the force-generating capacity of upper-airway muscles (**Figure 19.4**) (Dobrosielski, Papandreou, Patil, & Salas-Salvado, 2017). It is also worth noting that, regardless of total body mass, an

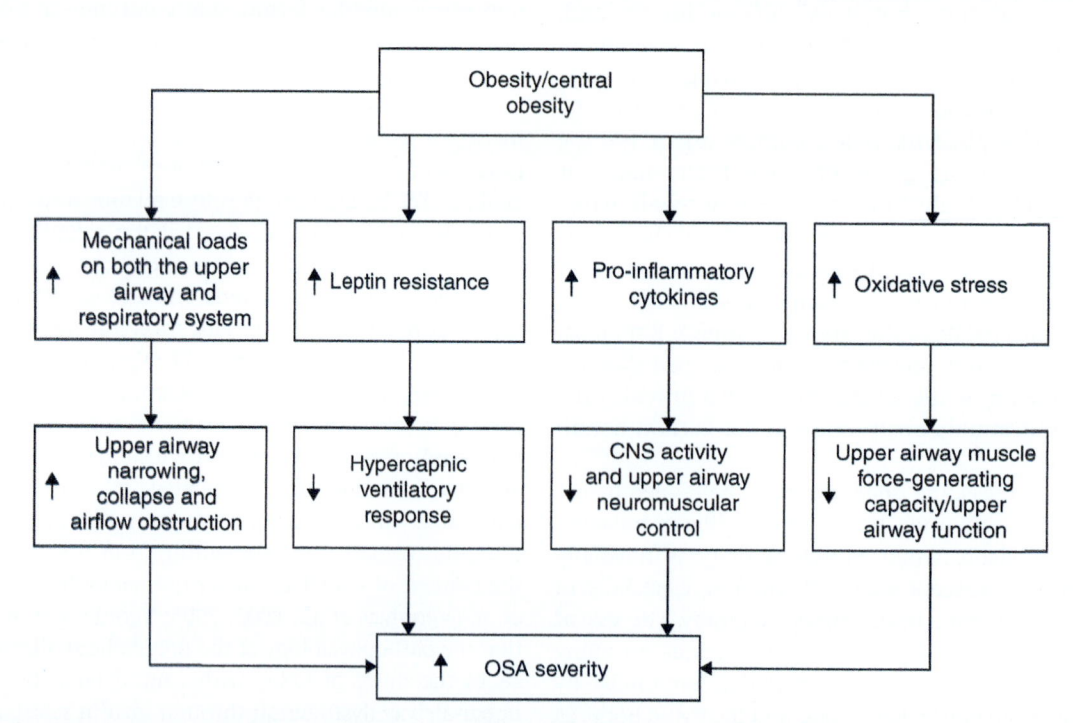

FIGURE 19.4 Schematic diagram indicating the possible mechanisms linking obesity/central obesity with OSA development. CNS = central nervous system; OSA = obstructive sleep apnea. Source: (Dobrosielski et al., 2017).

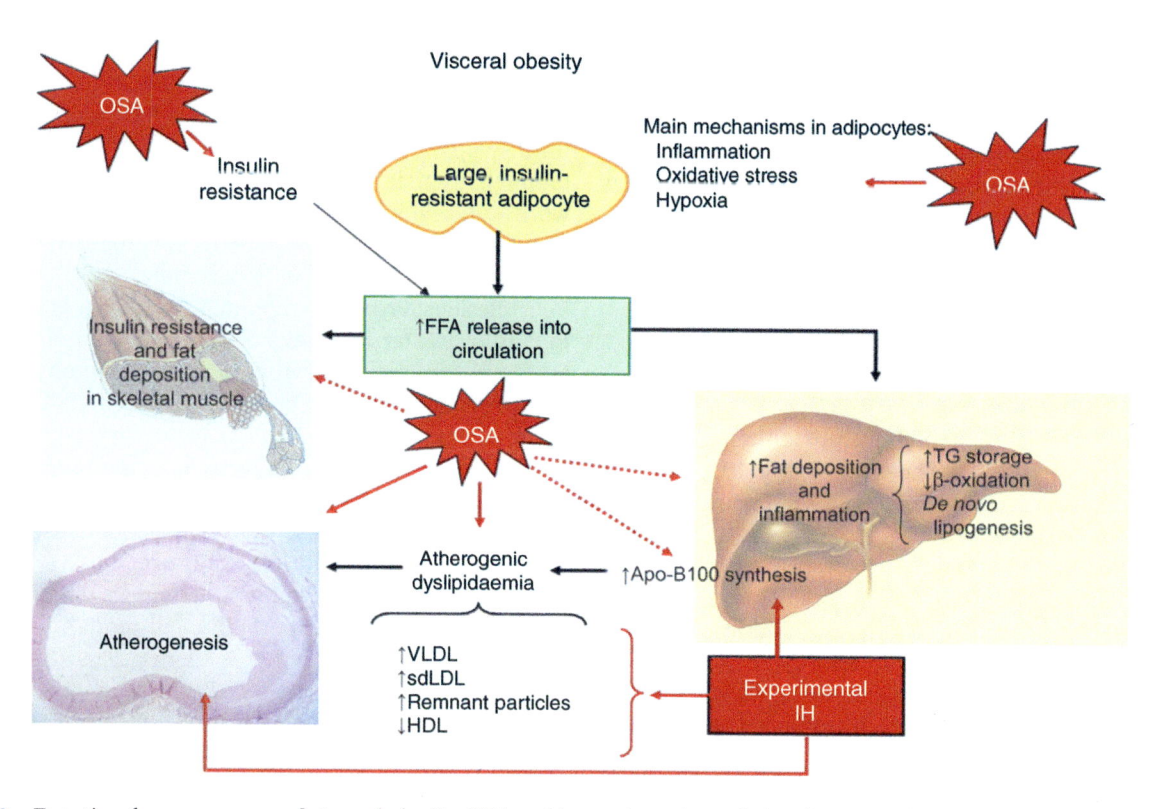

FIGURE 19.6 Functional consequences of visceral obesity, OSA and intermittent hypoxia in adipocytes, skeletal muscle, the liver, and the vessel wall. TG = triglycerides; FFA = free fatty acid; Apo = apolipoprotein; VLDL = very low-density lipoproteins; sdLDL = small dense low-density lipoproteins; HDL = high-density lipoproteins; IH = intermittent hypoxia; OSA = obstructive sleep apnea. Source: (Bonsignore et al., 2012).

subsequent awakenings in the context of OSA cause an abnormal increase in sympathetic activity during sleep, which is followed by an increase in catecholamine levels. Hyperactivity of the sympathetic nervous system is accompanied by an increase in blood pressure, a disorder that often persists during the day and, in the long term can lead to the establishment of hypertension. This increase in blood pressure levels, combined with the fluctuating intrathoracic pressure due to respiratory effort and the reduction of oxygen supply to body tissues due to hypoxemia, significantly impairs myocardial and vascular function and increases the risk of cardiac arrhythmias, heart failure, and ischemic stroke (Bonsignore et al., 2012; Bradley & Floras, 2009). In addition, recurrent episodes of oxygen desaturation and re-oxygenation within OSA lead to the production of oxygen free radicals and the establishment of an environment of increased oxidative stress, which in turn results in macromolecular peroxidation, changes in cellular homeostasis, and increased expression of inflammatory genes controlled by the nuclear factor κB. This change in the expression of inflammatory genes results in an increased production of inflammatory markers, mainly tumor necrosis factor-α, C-reactive protein, interleukin-6, and interleukin-8 as well as a decreased production of anti-inflammatory markers, such as adiponectin. The combination of sympathetic nervous system hyperactivation, oxidative stress, and chronic subclinical inflammation leads to long-term endothelial dysfunction and arterial stiffness, factors that play a central role in the establishment and development of atherosclerosis, the background of cardiovascular disease (Bonsignore et al., 2012; Bradley & Floras, 2009). Finally, chronic sleep deprivation or poor sleep quality, combined with oxidative stress and chronic inflammation, also adversely affect the body's metabolic homeostasis, triggering insulin resistance. Insulin resistance, combined with obesity, which is present in the majority of patients with OSA, lead to increased adipose tissue lipolysis and increased availability of free fatty acids to the circulation, which are stored ectopically in the liver and lead to hepatic steatosis, increased *de novo* lipogenesis, and eventually to atherogenic dyslipidemia, which manifests as elevated triglycerides (TG), total cholesterol (TC), low-density lipoprotein cholesterol (LDL-cholesterol), and very low-density lipoprotein cholesterol (VLDL-cholesterol), and low levels of high-density lipoprotein cholesterol (HDL-cholesterol) (Bonsignore et al., 2012; Bradley & Floras, 2009).

The hemodynamic, oxidative, inflammatory, and metabolic complications of OSA lead to an overall increased cardio-metabolic risk. This hypothesis is supported by numerous cross-sectional epidemiological studies showing an increased prevalence of cardiovascular diseases in patients with OSA and vice versa (Floras, 2018; Sarkar, Mukherjee, Chai-Coetzer, & McEvoy, 2018) as well as prospective epidemiological studies that reveal a strong positive relationship between the presence and severity of OSA and the risk of hypertension, diabetes mellitus, arrhythmias, coronary heart disease, heart failure, stroke, cardiovascular, and total mortality (Hou et al., 2018; Wang, Bi, Zhang, & Pan, 2013; Xie, Zhu, Tian, & Wang, 2017).

increasing number of studies highlight the potential aggravating role of upper body fat deposition in the development of OSA, in particular visceral adipose tissue (Kritikou et al., 2013; Vgontzas et al., 2000), a metabolic active tissue associated with cardio-metabolic disorders, and the adipose tissue that accumulates in the area of the upper airways (Mortimore, Marshall, Wraith, Sellar, & Douglas, 1998; Pahkala, Seppa, Ikonen, Smirnov, & Tuomilehto, 2014), which, as mentioned above, contributes to the thickening of the lateral walls of the pharynx.

COMPLICATIONS

Disruption of the normal sleep architecture is the main short-term complication of OSA. As shown in **Table 19.1**, sleep is divided into NREM and REM sleep, while NREM sleep is further subdivided into three stages (N1 to N3), which represent the successive transition from lighter to deeper sleep (Kales, Rechtschaffen, University of California, Brain Information, & Network, 1968). Under normal conditions, in adults, N1 sleep accounts for 5%, N2 sleep for 50% to 65%, N3 sleep for 15% to 20%, and REM sleep for 15% to 20% of total sleep (Karacan, 1970). In OSA, these patterns are significantly disturbed, with the duration of N1 and N2 sleep being increased, and the duration of N3 (slow-wave sleep) and REM sleep being significantly reduced (Jordan et al., 2014) due to repeated interruptions of breathing leading to awakenings. Given the significant disruption of normal sleep architecture, OSA is typically characterized by a wide variety of daytime symptoms, including sleepiness, fatigue, low vitality, inability to concentrate, impaired reflexes, and memory deficits (Bucks, Olaithe, & Eastwood, 2013; Wallace & Bucks, 2013). The most prevalent daytime symptom is sleepiness, which is evident in most patients when at a relaxed state, e.g., after lunch, when reading, or watching TV, and in severe OSA manifests as involuntary sleep episodes during social circumstances (e.g., theater or cinema), work environment (e.g., meetings), and driving (Black, 2003; Pagel, 2008). OSA daytime symptoms collectively lead to reduced functionality and productivity that can negatively affect personal relationships or work efficiency and contribute to psychological disorders (Brown, 2005), while most patients are prone to self-injuries and accidents (Ellen et al., 2006; Rodenstein, 2009).

Besides daytime symptomatology, OSA is strongly linked to cardiovascular morbidity. This association is partly because OSA and cardiovascular disease share common risk factors, as discussed earlier in this chapter. However, OSA has also been suggested as an independent risk factor for cardiovascular disorders, a theory based on its adverse effects on the cardiovascular system, which is exposed to a vicious cycle of hemodynamic, oxidative, inflammatory, and metabolic disorders during sleep-disordered breathing (**Figure 19.5**) (Bradley & Floras, 2009). Overall, the literature agrees that OSA is a major cause of cardiovascular morbidity and mortality and not just a respiratory disorder (Bradley & Floras, 2009; Kasai, Floras, & Bradley, 2012; Sanchez-de-la-Torre, Campos-Rodriguez, & Barbe, 2013). Several health organizations, such as the European and the American Heart Association, recognize OSA as a modifiable risk factor for cardiovascular disease (Piepoli et al., 2016; Somers et al., 2008).

Intermittent hypoxia plays a central role in the pathogenesis of cardio-metabolic complications of OSA, due to its effects on the central nervous system and its various oxidative, inflammatory, and metabolic consequences (**Figure 19.6**) (Bonsignore, McNicholas, Montserrat, & Eckel, 2012; Bradley & Floras, 2009). During normal sleep, the parasympathetic activity of the central nervous system outweighs the sympathetic one; however, intermittent hypoxemia and the

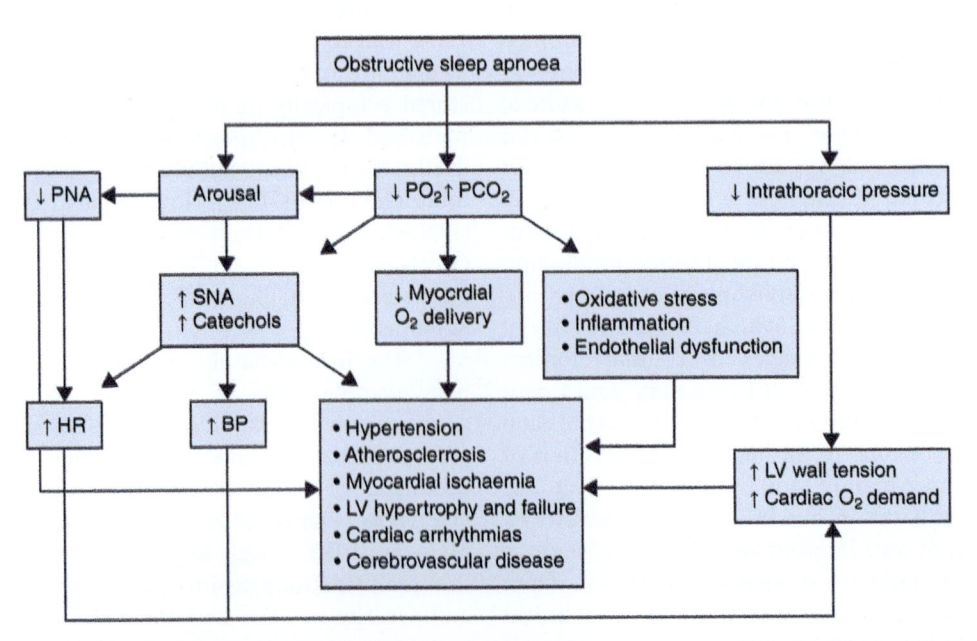

FIGURE 19.5 Pathophysiological effects of OSA on the cardiovascular system. PNA = parasympathetic nervous system activity; PO_2 = partial pressure of oxygen; PCO_2 = partial pressure of carbon dioxide; SNA = sympathetic nervous system activity; HR = heart rate; BP = blood pressure; LV = left ventricle. Source: (Bradley & Floras, 2009).

MANAGEMENT

Treatment modalities for OSA aim to reverse the underlying pathology, i.e., to prevent the obstruction of the upper airways during sleep, and include: i) the administration of positive airway pressure (PAP), which is currently the first-line treatment for all OSA patients; ii) weight loss in overweight/obese patients (a detailed overview of data on weight loss and OSA management is presented later in this chapter); and iii) the use of oral devices or surgical procedures in patients with severe upper respiratory tract anatomical disorders (Gaisl, Haile, Thiel, Osswald, & Kohler, 2019; Patil et al., 2019; Veasey et al., 2006). Positional therapy, i.e., avoidance of sleeping in the supine position in which the upper airway becomes more susceptible to obstruction due to gravity, and sleep hygiene techniques (e.g., maintaining a regular bedtime schedule, avoidance of sleeping pills, avoidance of alcohol, caffeine, or other stimulants before sleep, consumption of a light dinner to prevent gastrointestinal symptoms that can further disrupt sleep, etc.) are also used as secondary measures for OSA management (Gaisl et al., 2019; Patil et al., 2019; Veasey et al., 2006). Regarding pharmacotherapy, to date, there is no established pharmacological treatment for OSA, and specific medications are individually prescribed to patients in the presence of co-morbidities (e.g., hypolipidemic agents in case of dyslipidemia).

CPAP was introduced as a therapeutic approach for OSA in 1981 (Sullivan, Issa, Berthon-Jones, & Eves, 1981) and ever since has been recommended as the first-line treatment for the disease (Epstein et al., 2009; Qaseem et al., 2013). It is a form of PAP ventilation in which a constant level of pressure greater than atmospheric is continuously applied to the upper respiratory tract of a patient during sleep, to prevent upper airway collapse and respiratory events (**Figure 19.7**). CPAP is currently prescribed as long-life standard care to most patients with OSA in clinical practice and has been found efficient in minimizing the frequency of sleep-disordered breathing, reducing OSA symptoms (e.g., daytime sleepiness), and improving patient quality of life compared to control therapies. However, it is also characterized by several limitations. Low adherence to CPAP, typically defined as use for <70% of nights and <4 h/night, has been documented in up to 80% of patients with OSA (Bakker, Weaver, Parthasarathy, & Aloia, 2019; Giles, 2015; Rotenberg, Murariu, & Pang, 2016; Sawyer et al., 2011), while in some cases its discontinuation even for one night leads to the recurrence of OSA manifestations, i.e., respiratory events and daytime symptoms (Kribbs et al., 1993; Rossi, Schwarz, Bloch, Stradling, & Kohler, 2014; Sforza & Lugaresi, 1995; L. R. Young et al., 2013). Moreover, evidence of the cardio-metabolic benefits of CPAP is currently lacking. According to meta-analyses of the available well-designed randomized controlled clinical trials, CPAP therapy does not seem to improve glucose metabolism indices, lipidemic profile, low-grade inflammation biomarkers, or cardiovascular morbidity and mortality (Feng, Zhang, & Dong, 2015; Jullian-Desayes et al., 2015; Yu et al., 2017), a fact that significantly limits its value as the sole treatment for most high cardiovascular risk OSA patients. Finally, CPAP has been shown to promote a modest but significant increase in body weight (possibly due to reversing chronic hypoxemia, which has been associated with increases in resting energy expenditure), further aggravating overweight/obesity in patients with OSA initiated on CPAP therapy (Drager et al., 2015; Hoyos et al., 2019). These limitations challenge the value of CPAP as the sole treatment for OSA and highlight the importance of novel therapies for the disease management. In this context, behavioral interventions toward weight loss through beneficial changes in dietary and physical habits that do not require sophisticated equipment and can be feasible in all healthcare services can constitute a realistic and efficient plan for the management of OSA in clinical practice (Hudgel et al., 2018), as presented in detail later in this chapter.

The use of oral devices and surgical procedures are alternative treatments for some patients with OSA, especially those with a detrimental upper-airway anatomy. Oral appliances aim to move the lower jaw forward or to restore the correct position of the tongue, with the ultimate goal of maintaining the accessibility of the upper airways during sleep through a geometrically favorable air flow geometry (A. T. Ng, Gotsopoulos, Qian, & Cistulli, 2003; C. F. Ryan, Love, Peat, Fleetham, & Lowe, 1999). Most clinical trials to date suggest that these devices can improvement the severity of the OSA and its symptoms, albeit to a lesser extent than that achieved by application of CPAP therapy (Lim, Lasserson, Fleetham, & Wright, 2006; Sharples et al., 2016). Possible side effects include pain in face

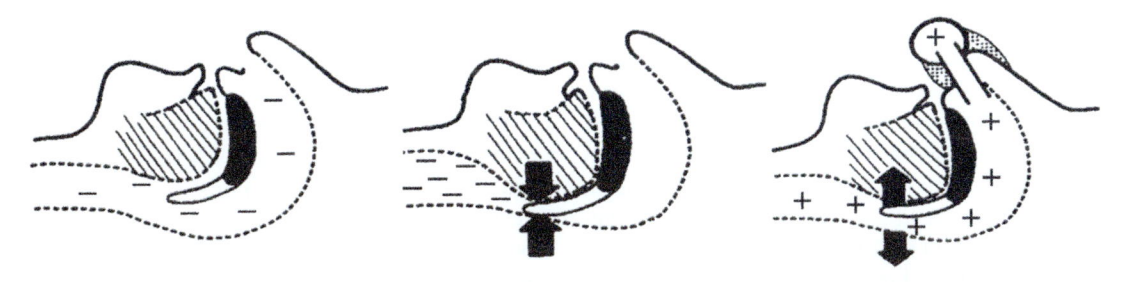

FIGURE 19.7 Mechanism of upper-airway occlusion and its prevention by CPAP. When the patient is awake (left), muscle tone prevents collapse of the airway during inspiration. During sleep, the tongue and soft palate are sucked against the posterior oropharyngeal wall (middle). CPAP with low pressure provides a pneumatic splint and keeps the airway open (right). CPAP = continuous positive airway pressure.
Source: (Sullivan et al., 1981).

muscles, temporomandibular joints and teeth, excessive salivation, xerostomia (dry mouth), and gum irritation (Ferguson, Cartwright, Rogers, & Schmidt-Nowara, 2006). The surgical treatment of OSA aims to increase the cross-sectional area of the upper airways by correcting the aggravated anatomy of the upper respiratory tract, either by removing unnecessary/enlarged parts of the soft tissues of the pharynx or by correcting the skeletal structures that surround it. Various surgical procedures have been investigated in the context of OSA management, the main one being uvulopalatopharyngoplasty, i.e., the removal of the tonsils, the uvula, and part of the soft palate, which was first applied in 1981 (Fujita, Conway, Zorick, & Roth, 1981); other techniques have also been developed over time and include functional rhinoplasty, septoplasty, turbinoplasty, palatal surgery, and orthognathic surgery (Tanna et al., 2016). Overall, the implementation of surgery to treat OSA has been shown to lead to moderate improvements in disease severity, especially in patients with severe structural abnormalities of the upper respiratory tract; however, these improvements are not greater than those resulting from CPAP treatment, while improvements in daytime sleepiness and patients' quality of life has not been confirmed by all available studies (Back et al., 2009; Ceylan et al., 2009; Ferguson, Heighway, & Ruby, 2003; Larrosa et al., 2004; Li, Wang, Lee, Chen, & Fang, 2006; Stuck, Sauter, Hormann, Verse, & Maurer, 2005; Woodson, Steward, Weaver, & Javaheri, 2003).

NUTRITION IN OBSTRUCTIVE SLEEP APNEA

DIET AS A RISK FACTOR FOR OBSTRUCTIVE SLEEP APNEA DEVELOPMENT AND PROGRESSION

Data on the association between long-term dietary habits and the presence or severity of OSA are so far scarce, and most studies have focused on specific dietary nutrients. Available epidemiological case-control studies have reported a higher intake of saturated fatty acids and a lower intake of carbohydrates, dietary fiber, thiamine, folic acid, vitamin E, and potassium among patients with OSA and/or other sleep disorders (e.g., chronic insomnia) compared to healthy controls (Stelmach-Mardas, Mardas, Iqbal, Kostrzewska, & Piorunek, 2017; Tan et al., 2015). In addition, epidemiological cross-sectional studies among OSA patients with varying degrees of disease severity have revealed higher intakes of protein, total fat, cholesterol, and saturated fatty acids in patients with severe OSA compared to those with mild or moderate disease (Vasquez, Goodwin, Drescher, Smith, & Quan, 2008). The levels of docosahexaenoic acid (DHA) in red blood cell membranes have also been negatively correlated with OSA severity after adjustment for habitual fish consumption and the use of omega-3 fatty acid supplements (Ladesich, Pottala, Romaker, & Harris, 2011); although there are no data linking dietary omega-3 fatty acid intake to the presence and/or severity of OSA, it is possible that omega-3 fatty acids can alleviate OSA severity due to their strong anti-inflammatory properties and contribute to a more favorable cardio-metabolic profile, a hypothesis that remains to be confirmed (Scorza et al., 2013). Besides individual nutrients, OSA severity has been positively correlated to the consumption of red meat, meat products, and refined grains and negatively correlated to the consumption of whole grains and total dietary quality assessed through the alternative healthy eating index (Kechribari et al., 2020; Kechribari et al., 2021; Reid et al., 2019).

Although the aforementioned data come from epidemiological studies, which cannot establish causal relationships, it is possible that adherence to prudent dietary patterns characterized by a high consumption of fruits, vegetables, whole grains, legumes, nuts, vegetable oils (e.g., olive oil), and fish, and a low consumption of animal-based products, such as red meat, cold cuts, butter, and processed foods, can offer protection against the development and progression of OSA and should be encouraged as a strategy for preventing sleep-disordered breathing in the general population. Beyond its potential impact on respiratory events, the adoption of a heathy dietary pattern can also act toward cardio protection and the prevention of OSA-related cardio-metabolic morbidity.

DIETARY MODIFICATIONS FOR OBSTRUCTIVE SLEEP APNEA MANAGEMENT

Despite the lack of evidence on the role of long-term dietary habits as a risk factor for OSA, nutrition has an important role in the management of sleep-disordered breathing. Given the close relationship between OSA and obesity, dietary modifications toward weight loss have long been considered essential for most patients with OSA and are currently advocated as an ancillary treatment for the disease. Randomized controlled clinical trials (Foster et al., 2009; Johansson et al., 2011; Johansson et al., 2009; Kemppainen et al., 2008; Kuna et al., 2013; Nerfeldt, Nilsson, Udden, Rossner, & Friberg, 2008; S. S. Ng et al., 2015; Sahlman et al., 2012; Schwartz et al., 1991; Smith, Gold, Meyers, Haponik, & Bleecker, 1985; H. Tuomilehto et al., 2010; H. Tuomilehto et al., 2013; H. P. Tuomilehto et al., 2009) comparing the effects of an intensive weight-loss intervention (usually a prescription of very low- or low-calorie diets combined with lifestyle counseling or counseling toward reduction in energy intake in individual or group sessions without a standard dietary plan) versus standard care (simple dietary/lifestyle advice or no active intervention) on OSA management have consistently highlighted the benefits of weight loss in improving disease severity (e.g., decline in the AHI) and symptomatology (e.g., alleviation of daytime sleepiness). Meta-analyses of these studies reveal that an intensive weight-loss intervention can lower the AHI by approximately 15 events/h compared to standard care (Anandam, Akinnusi, Kufel, Porhomayon, & El-Solh, 2013; Mitchell et al., 2014), which is considered a clinically meaningful reduction especially for patients with mild-to-moderate OSA. Uncontrolled clinical trials (Aubert-Tulkens, Culee, & Rodenstein, 1989; Barnes, Goldsworthy, Cary, & Hill, 2009; Dobrosielski, Patil, Schwartz, Bandeen-Roche, & Stewart, 2015; Fujii, Miyamoto, Miyamoto, & Muto, 2010; Hakala, Maasilta, & Sovijarvi, 2000; Hakala, Mustajoki, Aittomaki, & Sovijarvi, 1995; Hernandez et al., 2009; Kajaste, Telakivi, Mustajoki, Pihl, & Partinen, 1994; Kansanen et al., 1998; Kiselak, Clark, Pera,

Rosenberg, & Redline, 1993; Kulkas et al., 2015; Lojander, Mustajoki, Ronka, Mecklin, & Maasilta, 1998; Nahmias, Kirschner, & Karetzky, 1993; Nerfeldt, Nilsson, Mayor, Udden, & Friberg, 2010; Nerfeldt, Nilsson, Mayor, et al., 2008; Noseda, Kempenaers, Kerkhofs, Houben, & Linkowski, 1996; Papandreou, Hatzis, & Fragkiadakis, 2015; Papandreou, Schiza, Bouloukaki, et al., 2012; Papandreou, Schiza, Tzatzarakis, et al., 2012; Pasquali et al., 1990; Rajala et al., 1991; Sampol et al., 1998; Suratt, McTier, Findley, Pohl, & Wilhoit, 1987; H. P. Tuomilehto et al., 2009) have also shown that weight loss can promote significant improvements in respiratory events, oximetry indices, sleep architecture, and quality of life among overweight and obese OSA patients with varying degrees of disease severity. In most studies, baseline OSA severity and the degree of weight loss were the strongest predictors of improvement.

Although the dose-response relationship between the magnitude of weight loss and OSA management requires further investigation, most clinical trials have revealed that the greater the weight loss, the greater the improvements in OSA severity, with patients achieving a ≥5% to 10% weight loss exhibiting the greatest benefits (Georgoulis et al., 2022; Kulkas et al., 2015; Papandreou et al., 2015; H. P. Tuomilehto et al., 2009). This is in line with current guidelines for obesity management that suggest a 5% to 10% weight loss over 6 months as a realistic goal sufficient to produce health benefits in most overweight/obese individuals; an even greater degree of weight loss of ≥10% may be suitable for patients with higher degrees of obesity, however, even a mild weight loss of 3% to 5% is considered beneficial for health, especially for obese patients at high risk of, or with, established obesity-related chronic diseases and could constitute an initial goal for OSA patients who struggle with long-term weight regulation (Jensen et al., 2014; Stegenga, Haines, Jones, Wilding, & Guideline Development, 2014; Yumuk et al., 2015). A similar dose-response pattern has been reported for weight loss and improvements in cardio-metabolic disorders, with which OSA frequently co-occurs or shares a common pathogenetic background, such as type 2 diabetes mellitus, dyslipidemia, hypertension, and non-alcoholic fatty liver disease (D. H. Ryan & Yockey, 2017). However, not all scientific data support this dose-response relationship. For example, Dixon et al. (Dixon et al., 2012) reported that laparoscopic adjustable gastric banding did not result in a statistically greater reduction in 2-year AHI levels compared to conventional weight-loss therapy through dietary modification, despite an almost 6-fold greater weight loss among 60 obese participants with a baseline AHI of ≥20 events/h. They also observed a strong positive correlation between weight loss and AHI decline in the conventional weight-loss group but not in the bariatric surgery group. The authors concluded that there was a non-linear link between weight loss and OSA severity with considerable individual effect variability as well as a complex, rather than pure mechanical load, pathogenesis of OSA in obese individuals (Dixon et al., 2012). It is therefore possible that although mild-to-moderate weight loss (5-15%) is associated with proportional improvements in the AHI, the dose-response relationship eventually reaches a plateau with limited additional benefit from further weight loss.

Whether lifestyle-induced weight loss and CPAP treatment are similarly effective for OSA management has so far been investigated in a small number of studies. A randomized clinical trial (Chakravorty, Cayton, & Szczepura, 2002) comparing a non-intensive lifestyle modification program (sleep hygiene, smoking cessation, stress management, avoidance of alcohol, and simple advice on weight loss and physical activity) with CPAP treatment revealed benefits from both interventions in sleep architecture and daytime sleepiness; the lifestyle intervention resulted in greater weight loss, while CPAP therapy led to greater improvements in the AHI, oxygen saturation, and quality of life. A few more randomized clinical trials (Ballester et al., 1999; Lam et al., 2007; Monasterio et al., 2001) have compared the combination of a weight-loss intervention with CPAP versus a weight-loss intervention alone in OSA and showed the superiority of the combination therapy in reducing OSA severity and symptoms; however, the weight-loss intervention used in these studies involved a generalized, non-intensive lifestyle program that included simple sleep hygiene tips and weight-loss recommendations, which served as a control treatment and probably had little effect on OSA. More recent data from well-designed, randomized controlled clinical trials (Georgoulis, Yiannakouris, Kechribari, et al., 2021; Helena, Margareta, Eva, & Pernilla, 2014; Igelstrom, Asenlof, Emtner, & Lindberg, 2018) have shown that, compared to CPAP alone, its combination with an intensive weight-loss intervention (counseling sessions targeting weight loss, prudent dietary habits, and adequate physical activity) is superior in improving anthropometric indices, lifestyle habits, and OSA severity and symptomatology, which highlights the necessity of weight loss on top of CPAP prescription for overweight/obese patients with OSA.

Besides improvements in respiratory lesions, recent research has also focused on the cardio-metabolic benefits of weight loss in OSA. In the clinical trial of Chirinos et al. (Chirinos et al., 2014) published in 2014, 181 patients with AHI ≥15 events/h were randomly allocated to three interventions, i.e., CPAP treatment, weight loss (hypocaloric diet), or a combination of both, for 24 weeks. The study revealed benefits in arterial pressure in all three study groups, but only patients receiving the weight-loss regimen exhibited improvements in lipidemic profile indices, triglycerides, LDL-cholesterol, and C-reactive protein as well as an increase in insulin sensitivity as assessed through an oral glucose tolerance test, compared to baseline (Chirinos et al., 2014). In addition, the combination therapy led to a greater improvement in triglycerides and insulin sensitivity compared to CPAP alone, but not compared to weight loss alone (Chirinos et al., 2014). In another randomized controlled clinical trial by Georgoulis et al. (Georgoulis et al., 2020; Georgoulis, Yiannakouris, Tenta, et al., 2021), 180 moderate-to-severe OSA patients were randomized to a standard care group, a Mediterranean diet group, or a Mediterranean lifestyle group. All groups were prescribed CPAP, while intervention arms also participated in a 6-month behavioral weight-loss intervention based on the Mediterranean diet/lifestyle. The study revealed improvements in glucose metabolism indices, blood lipids, liver enzymes, blood pressure, plasma high-sensitivity C-reactive protein, and urinary isoprostanes (a marker of lipid peroxidation) only in patients allocated in the weight-loss behavioral intervention, while at the end of the 6-month study the relative risk of metabolic syndrome was significantly lower in intervention arms compared to the standard care group (Georgoulis et al., 2020; Georgoulis, Yiannakouris, Tenta, et al., 2021). A study by Tuomilehto et al. (Sahlman et al., 2012; H. Tuomilehto et al., 2010; H. P. Tuomilehto et al., 2009) is also of interest, as it explored the long-term cardio-metabolic benefits of weight loss in patients with OSA. The study included 81 patients with mild OSA (AHI: 5-15 events/h) who were randomized to either an intensive weight-loss intervention (3 months of a very low-calorie diet and then monthly individual counseling sessions to improve lifestyle habits) or to a control group (3 individual lifestyle counseling sessions), for 1 year. In the annual follow-up, compared with the control arm, the intervention arm group showed a greater reduction in insulin and triglyceride levels, while no significant differences were observed in fasting glucose, high-density lipoprotein cholesterl, blood pressure, and various inflammatory markers such as CRP and interleukin-6 (Sahlman et al., 2012; H. P. Tuomilehto et al., 2009). However, at the 2-year follow-up, the aforementioned cardiovascular improvements of the intervention arm faded, possibly due to partial weight regain (approximately 3%) relative to the 1-year follow-up, and the differences between the two groups were no longer statistically significant (H. Tuomilehto et al., 2010). A few more uncontrolled clinical trials have also highlighted the cardio-metabolic benefits of weight loss (improvements in glycemic control indices, lipid profile, liver enzymes, and blood pressure) in patients with OSA (Barnes et al., 2009; Nerfeldt et al., 2010). Combined, these data suggest that CPAP alone, despite being the first-line therapy for OSA, is insufficient for managing its cardio-metabolic manifestations and that weight loss through lifestyle modifications is equally important in the context of a comprehensive OSA management.

Although the above findings highlight the importance of weight loss for OSA management, it is worth noting that in most studies, weight loss was achieved through strict dietary protocols, mainly through the administration of very low-calorie diets. Very low-calorie diets are 800 kcal diet regimens that are usually applied for ≤12 weeks by completely replacing conventional foods with special low-calorie solid or liquid products/formulas and have been used since the 1970s for rapid weight loss (Tsai & Wadden, 2006; "Very low-calorie diets. National Task Force on the Prevention and Treatment of Obesity, National Institutes of Health," 1993). These diets lead to an average loss of 1.5 to 2.5 kg/week and in the short term seem to be more effective than low-calorie diets (800-1500 kcal), which lead to an average loss of 0.4 to 0.5 kg/week. However, the long-term effectiveness of the two types of diets is almost the same, which suggests that a large proportion of the weight lost is regained after very low-calorie diets are discontinued. Weight regain, along with their difficult application, which requires medical/dietary monitoring and their possible side effects (e.g., fatigue, menstrual disorders in women, cholelithiasis, fatty liver, nutritional deficiencies, and significant loss of lean mass if adequate protein intake is not achieved), limit the use of very low-calorie diets only in individuals with morbid obesity when rapid weight loss is necessary (e.g., pre-op) (Tsai & Wadden, 2006; "Very low-calorie diets. National Task Force on the Prevention and Treatment of Obesity, National Institutes of Health," 1993). In this context, future research should focus more on the application of weight-loss interventions through diet regimens that meet the principles of a life-long prudent diet, combined with cognitive-behavioral techniques to facilitate behavior change, for a long-term weight-loss maintenance and successful management of OSA.

Finally, it should be noted that despite evidence of the beneficial effect of weight loss on OSA, it is not clear whether lifestyle interventions alone are sufficient to cure the disease and completely normalize breathing during sleep in the whole OSA population. For example, according to the results of three randomized controlled clinical trials (Foster et al., 2009; Johansson et al., 2009; H. P. Tuomilehto et al., 2009) and three uncontrolled clinical trials (Barnes et al., 2009; Nerfeldt et al., 2010; Pasquali et al., 1990), a 10% to 15% weight loss seems to lead to a 20% to 50% reduction in the AHI; this reduction is clinically significant, but may not be sufficient to treat OSA in patients with severe disease (AHI ≥30 events/h). In addition, out of all the available weight-loss interventional studies in patients with OSA, only a few (Johansson et al., 2009; H. P. Tuomilehto et al., 2009) have so far provided data on complete disease resolution, showing success only in patients with mild OSA. Although the available literature is not sufficient to establish weight-loss interventions as the sole treatment for OSA, they have an important role for its management as an adjunct to patient standard care in clinical practice (CPAP prescription).

ROLE OF THE MEDITERRANEAN DIET/LIFESTYLE IN OBSTRUCTIVE SLEEP APNEA

The Mediterranean diet is one of the most studied dietary patterns worldwide, and its health benefits are well-established in the fields of nutritional epidemiology and clinical dietetics. The term Mediterranean diet was first conceived in the 1950s and 1960s by Ancel Keys, a US physiologist, based on his observations of the dietary habits of the Mediterranean populations in a landmark study called the "seven countries study". These unique dietary habits were considered to be the main reason for the low incidence of cardiovascular and neoplastic diseases observed in some Mediterranean countries, such as Greece and Italy, compared to other countries, such as the USA (Keys et al., 1986). In rough terms, the Mediterranean diet can be described as a dietary pattern characterized by high consumption of olive oil (as the main source of dietary fat), fruits, vegetables, legumes, whole-grain cereals, nuts, and seeds, moderate consumption of white meat, fish-seafood, and dairy products, low consumption of red meat products, and moderate consumption of wine with main meals (Sofi, 2009). According to numerous prospective and interventional studies, a high adherence to the Mediterranean diet has been shown to reduce mortality from all causes, cardiovascular disease, and cancer; to protect against the development of neurodegenerative diseases and diabetes mellitus; and to negatively associate with the presence of various other diseases, such as hypertension, dyslipidemia, the metabolic syndrome, non-alcoholic fatty liver disease, rheumatoid arthritis, and asthma

(Georgoulis, Kontogianni, & Yiannakouris, 2014; Kastorini et al., 2011; Sofi, 2009; Sofi & Casini, 2014; Sofi, Macchi, Abbate, Gensini, & Casini, 2010, 2013, 2014; Trichopoulou, Bamia, & Trichopoulos, 2009; Yannakoulia, Kontogianni, & Scarmeas, 2015). The beneficial effects of the Mediterranean diet have been mainly attributed to its strong anti-inflammatory and antioxidant properties and its negative correlation to insulin resistance, which arises as a result of the synergistic effects of the various nutrients present in typical Mediterranean foods (Bullo, Lamuela-Raventos, & Salas-Salvado, 2011; Estruch, 2010; Kontogianni, Zampelas, & Tsigos, 2006). In addition, the Mediterranean diet has been proposed as a highly palatable dietary pattern, even when combined with energy restriction, given that it encourages the consumption of a wide variety of foods and does not pose strict dietary restrictions (Sofi et al., 2014). This might explain its negative association with the likelihood of obesity observed in epidemiological studies and its superiority in obesity management compared to other diets (mainly low-fat diets) in interventional studies, especially when combined with adequate physical activity or when adopted in the long term (Buckland, Bach, & Serra-Majem, 2008; Esposito, Kastorini, Panagiotakos, & Giugliano, 2011). Besides the Mediterranean diet, other lifestyle habits observed in the Mediterranean region, such as consumption of seasonal and eco-friendly food products, regular exercise as part of family and social activities, adequate rest during the day and traditional culinary activities, have also been identified as beneficial for health, and along with the Mediterranean diet form what is known as the Mediterranean lifestyle (Bach-Faig et al., 2011; Estruch & Bach-Faig, 2019; Serra-Majem et al., 2020).

Given the health benefits of the Mediterranean diet and the close link between OSA, obesity, and cardio-metabolic morbidity, one could speculate that the Mediterranean diet is probably a highly beneficial dietary model for most patients with OSA. Although this theory has not been systematically explored, there is some preliminary evidence of the beneficial role of the Mediterranean diet in OSA patients. In 2012, Papandreou et al. (Papandreou, Schiza, Bouloukaki, et al., 2012; Papandreou, Schiza, Tzatzarakis, et al., 2012) randomized 40 obese patients with moderate-to-severe OSA treated with CPAP to either a Mediterranean-style diet (emphasis on high consumption of fruits, vegetables, legumes, nuts, whole-grain cereals, and fish, moderate amounts of red wine, and low consumption of red meat) or a prudent (healthy) diet, both being calorie-restricted (1200-1500 kcal/d for women and 1500-1800 kcal/d for men), along with instructions to increase daily physical activity. According to the results of the study, compared to the prudent diet, the Mediterranean-style diet resulted in a greater reduction in AHI during REM sleep, a fact that was attributed to a parallel greater improvement in anthropometric indices; however, no difference was observed between the two dietary patterns in other sleep parameters. As the authors concluded, "further studies in larger samples are needed in order to clarify the role of the Mediterranean in the therapeutic plan of patients with OSA, and to address the potential mechanisms of its protective effects" (Papandreou, Schiza, Bouloukaki, et al., 2012; Papandreou, Schiza, Tzatzarakis, et al., 2012). In a subsequent randomized controlled clinical trial, compared to CPAP alone, its combination with a behavioral intervention based on the Mediterranean diet/lifestyle was found superior at reducing respiratory events, OSA daytime symptomatology, and the prevalence of cardio-metabolic disorders associated with the metabolic syndrome, regardless of weight loss (Georgoulis et al., 2020; Georgoulis, Yiannakouris, Kechribari, et al., 2021; Georgoulis, Yiannakouris, Tenta, et al., 2021); this suggests that qualitative features of the Mediterranean lifestyle can also have a positive impact on sleep-disordered breathing and should be encouraged in OSA patients on top of weight loss. Most importantly, the intervention based on the Mediterranean lifestyle, combining the Mediterranean diet, physical activity, and optimal sleep habits, was superior in improving sleep architecture, daytime sleepiness, and various cardio-metabolic indices (e.g., insulin resistance and HDLC levels) compared to the intervention based solely on the Mediterranean diet, highlighting the positive synergistic effect or various healthy lifestyle habits on OSA management (Georgoulis et al., 2020; Georgoulis, Yiannakouris, Kechribari, et al., 2021; Georgoulis, Yiannakouris, Tenta, et al., 2021). Although the relevant literature is currently insufficient, the Mediterranean diet/lifestyle could be the first-line dietary/lifestyle choice for OSA, given its strong anti-inflammatory and antioxidant properties and its beneficial effects on body composition, which can improve upper-airway neuromuscular control and prevent respiratory disturbances during sleep (**Figure 19.8**) (Dobrosielski et al., 2017).

PHYSICAL ACTIVITY, FITNESS, AND OBSTRUCTIVE SLEEP APNEA

Although the protective role of physical activity against other chronic diseases, especially those of the cardio-metabolic nature, has been extensively explored, little is known about its association with the development and progression of OSA. Available data come from either cross-sectional or case-control studies and collectively reveal a negative association between physical activity level and the presence or severity of OSA (Hong & Dimsdale, 2003; Igelstrom, Emtner, Lindberg, & Asenlof, 2013; Kline, Krafty, Mulukutla, & Hall, 2017; Murillo et al., 2016; Peppard & Young, 2004; Quan et al., 2007; Simpson et al., 2015; Verwimp, Ameye, & Bruyneel, 2013; Vivodtzev et al., 2017). For instance, according to data published in 2007 from 4275 participants of the sleep heart health study, engaging in ≥3 h/week of high-intensity exercise was associated with approximately 30% lower likelihood of at least moderate OSA (RDI ≥15 events/h), after adjusting for obesity, obstructed spirometry, self-reported cardiovascular disease, hypertension, gender, marital status, age, education, and sleepiness (Quan et al., 2007). In a study by Simpson et al. (Simpson et al., 2015), of 2430 patients with OSA and 1931 healthy controls, participants categorized as very physically active had approximately 40% lower odds of moderate OSA, whereas individuals classified as mildly active or inactive had 1.6 and 2.7 higher odds, respectively, compared to moderately physically active individuals (Simpson et al., 2015). In another multi-center population-based study among 14,087 self-identified Hispanic/Latinos patients aged 18 to 74 years, meeting the recommended time (≥150 min/week) of moderate-to-vigorous

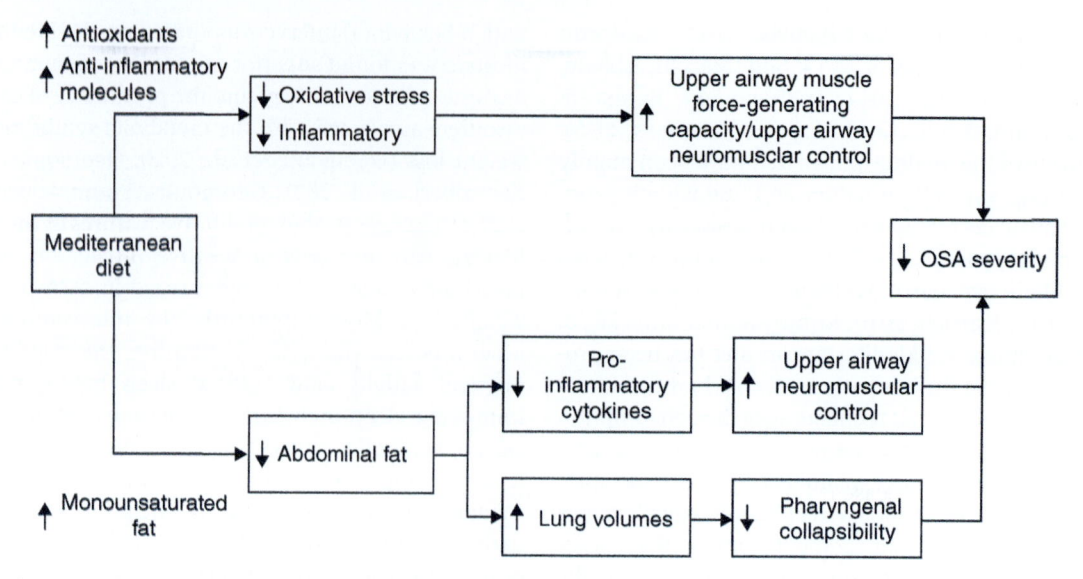

FIGURE 19.8 Schematic diagram indicating the possible mechanisms through which the Mediterranean diet may improve the severity of OSA, independent of weight loss. OSA = obstructive sleep apnea. Source: (Dobrosielski et al., 2017).

physical activity was associated with 30% lower odds of mild OSA and 25% lower odds of moderate-to-severe OSA, after adjusting for sociodemographics, smoking, and body-mass index; engaging in medium or high levels of transportation activity was also associated with 15% lower odds of mild OSA, while performing some recreational moderate-to-vigorous physical activity was associated with an 18% lower likelihood of mild and 21% lower likelihood of moderate-to-severe OSA (Murillo et al., 2016).

Although the aforementioned data support a negative correlation between physical activity and OSA severity, given their cross-sectional nature they could also reflect patients' inability to adopt a physically active lifestyle or their low cardiorespiratory fitness (Beitler et al., 2014). In fact, sleep apnea itself is a possible causal factor for physical inactivity due to daytime sleepiness and fatigue and can greatly influence patient's energy balance and exercise capacity. Several studies have demonstrated that aerobic capacity is significantly impaired in OSA patients compared to healthy controls (Beitler et al., 2014). Moreover, a positive correlation has been observed between OSA severity and exercise intolerance, as supported by data showing that the AHI is a significant independent predictor of aerobic exercise capacity, even after adjusting for possible confounders including body-weight status; for example, approximately 16% of the variability observed in percent predicted VO_2max can be explained by the AHI (Ucok et al., 2009). OSA patients also have a low physical condition and an inappropriate hemodynamic response to exercise, which is related to OSA severity (Przybylowski et al., 2007). During peak exercise and recovery, OSA patients exhibit increased blood pressure and heart rate, decreased stroke volume, and delayed heart rate recovery compared to healthy individuals (Alameri, Al-Kabab, & BaHammam, 2010; Beitler et al., 2014); increased blood pressure is predicted to be a limiting factor for aerobic exercise capacity in 20% of patients (Przybylowski et al., 2007). The exaggerated cardiopulmonary response is caused by an increase in autonomic sympathetic activity and arterial vasoconstriction (Alameri et al., 2010; Quadri et al., 2017). Impaired skeletal muscle energy metabolism, indicating abnormal oxidative and glycolytic metabolism of exercising muscles, has also been observed in OSA patients (Alameri et al., 2010). Altogether, these data suggest that patients with OSA have an impaired aerobic exercise capacity and a poor hemodynamic response to exercise; these factors constitute not only cardiovascular risk factors but also significant barriers for physical activity and should be considered before exercise prescription.

EXERCISE TRAINING AND OBSTRUCTIVE SLEEP APNEA MANAGEMENT

Starting from the early 2000s, the importance of exercise as part of the management of sleep-disordered breathing gradually began to spread in the scientific community along with the recognition of OSA as a disease of cardio-metabolic nature, and study protocols implementing supervised exercise interventions in the OSA population gradually emerged in the literature. So far, research has mainly focused on supervised aerobic exercise programs, either alone or in combination with other types of exercise (mainly resistance), which appear to lead to significant improvements in the severity and symptoms of OSA, sleep quality, and architecture as well as patient fitness level and physical functioning (Ackel-D'Elia et al., 2012; Cavagnolli et al., 2014; Desplan et al., 2014; Guimaraes, Drager, Genta, Marcondes, & Lorenzi-Filho, 2009; Karlsen et al., 2016; Kline et al., 2011, 2013; Kline et al., 2012; Mendelson et al., 2016; Norman, Von Essen, Fuchs, & McElligott, 2000; Schutz et al., 2013; Sengul, Ozalevli, Oztura, Itil, & Baklan, 2011; Servantes et al., 2018; Servantes et al., 2012; Ueno et al., 2009; Yang, Liu, Zheng, Liu, & Mei, 2018). According to meta-analyses of available clinical trials, when compared to control interventions, exercise interventions lead to a greater decline in the AHI by approximately 5 to 10 events/h

(Aiello et al., 2016; Iftikhar, Kline, & Youngstedt, 2014; Mendelson et al., 2018). Although the effect of exercise on respiratory events is moderate, improvements in the AHI following exercise protocols are observed in the absence of significant changes in anthropometric indices; this observation highlights the weight-loss independent benefits of physical activity for the management of OSA and the importance of integrating exercise as part of multi-component strategies for disease management.

It is worth noting that, to date, there are no data on the optimal type of exercise for patients with OSA. A study by Servantes et al. (Servantes et al., 2012) is the only randomized controlled clinical trial that compared the effect of the combination of aerobic and resistance exercise with that of aerobic exercise alone on the management of the disease. According to the results of the study, compared to the control group (no active intervention), both exercise groups showed significantly greater improvements in the AHI, the severity of OSA (decline from severe to moderate disease), the number of awakenings, sleep efficiency, quality of life, and cardio-respiratory endurance while the only difference between intervention arms was a greater improvement in isokinetic muscle strength and endurance tests in the group that underwent the combined aerobic and resistance exercise program (Servantes et al., 2012).

The comparison of the effectiveness of exercise interventions and CPAP treatment has also been investigated in a few clinical trials (Ackel-D'Elia et al., 2012; Schutz et al., 2013; Servantes et al., 2018), which show that both regimens are efficient in improving OSA severity (AHI and oxygen saturation) and symptomatology (daytime sleepiness) as well as patient quality of life. However, each type of intervention seems to be superior in terms of improving specific endpoints; exercise interventions lead to greater improvements in quality of life, drowsiness, fitness, and cardio-metabolic profile indices, while CPAP treatment is superior in reducing respiratory events (Ackel-D'Elia et al., 2012; Schutz et al., 2013; Servantes et al., 2018).

The beneficial effect of exercise on OSA management can be explained through several mechanisms, including: i) improvements in body composition (i.e., decline in body fat mass and preservation/enhancement of fat free mass), which helps reduce the mechanical load on the upper airways; ii) improvement of upper-airway airflow by reducing nasal congestion; iii) prevention of fluid movement in the upper body (neck region) during sleep, which can add to upper-airway mechanical load and contribute to obstruction; iv) upper-airway muscle strengthening (muscles of the pharynx, tongue, and lungs) allowing for a better breathing control; and v) improvements in metabolic disturbances (e.g., enhancement of insulin sensitivity and reduction of systemic inflammation and oxidative stress), which can further aggravate upper-airway dysfunction (**Figure 19.9**) (Mendelson et al., 2018).

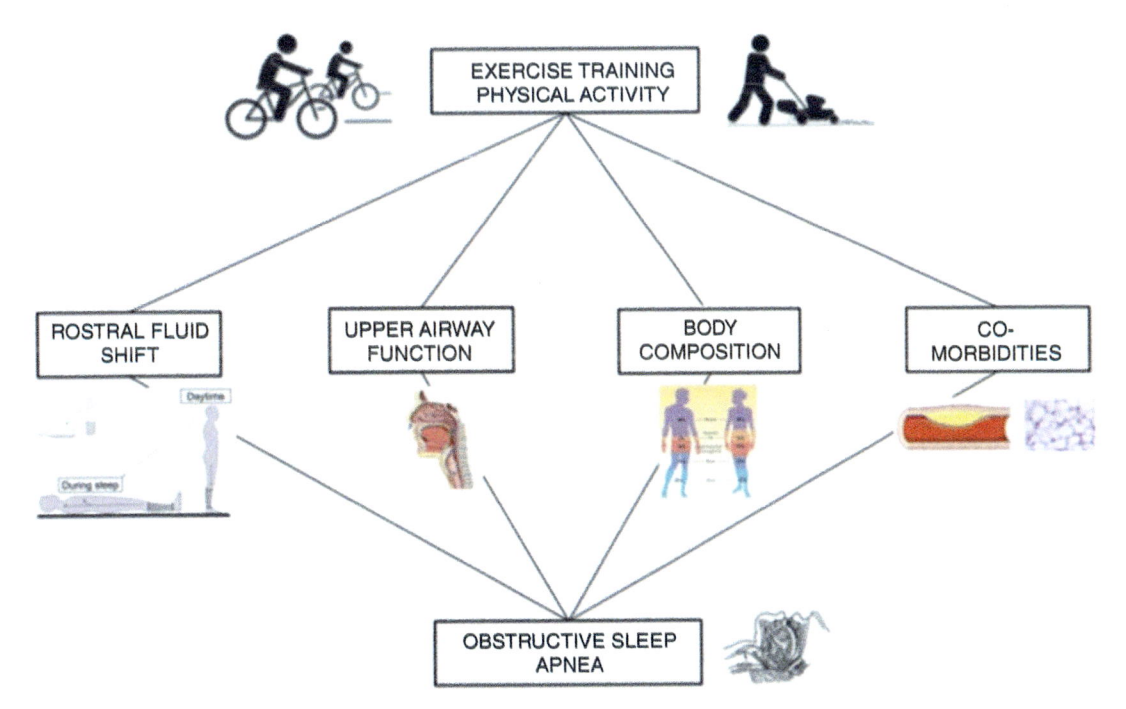

FIGURE 19.9 Hypothetical relationship between exercise training/physical activity and obstructive sleep apnea (OSA). The rostral fluid shift contributes to the pathogenesis of OSA and its attenuation via physical activity and exercise training has been shown to alleviate OSA. The strength and fatigability of the upper-airway dilators have been shown to be altered in patients with OSA. Specific exercise training modalities may improve upper-airway function in OSA patients and thus contribute to decrease OSA severity. An elevated body-mass index (BMI) is a key risk factor for the development of OSA while sleep disturbances can influence body composition. Exercise training has been shown to favorably modify body composition (increase lean mass, decrease fat mass) and reduce BMI, therefore potentially alleviating the severity of OSA. OSA is often accompanied by cardiovascular and metabolic co-morbidities, which can impair exercise tolerance. Exercise training has been shown to be beneficial for the improvement of a number of these co-morbidities (hypertension, dyslipidemia, type 2 diabetes, etc.). Source: (Mendelson et al., 2018).

Although, to date, there are no specific exercise guidelines for patients with OSA, the 2020 World Health Organization guidelines on physical activity and sedentary behavior (2020) are probably suitable for the OSA population, as they provide evidence-based public health recommendations for the amount of physical activity (frequency, intensity, and duration) required to offer significant health benefits and mitigate health risks. According to these guidelines, all adults should do at least 150 to 300 min of moderate-intensity aerobic physical activity, or at least 75 to 150 min of vigorous-intensity aerobic physical activity, or an equivalent combination of moderate- and vigorous-intensity activity throughout the week for substantial health benefits (2020). For additional health benefits, increasing aerobic physical activity to more than 300 min/week of moderate intensity, more than 150 min/week of vigorous-intensity, or an equivalent combination of both as well as undertaking muscle-strengthening activities at moderate or greater intensity that involve all major muscle groups on 2 or more days a week and limiting sedentary behavior to a minimum, is also recommended (2020). Given that most patients with OSA are sedentary and characterized by increased body weight, they should start by doing small amounts of physical activity and gradually increase the frequency, intensity, and duration over time. Older patients with OSA and co-morbidities should be as physically active as their functional ability allows and adjust their level of physical effort to their level of fitness.

> **KEY POINTS**

- According to the *International Classification of Sleep Disorders* of the American Academy of Sleep Medicine, OSA belongs to the group of sleep-related breathing disorders and is a chronic disease characterized by recurrent pauses of breathing during sleep, due to obstruction of the upper airways, which leads to sleep disruption.

- Although traditionally viewed as an anatomical disease of the upper respiratory tract, OSA is currently recognized as a complex disease of cardio-metabolic nature.

- Novel theories suggest that the pathophysiology of the metabolic syndrome precedes the onset of OSA, with central fat deposition triggering upper-airway dysfunction through insulin resistance, inflammation, and oxidative stress; OSA can be viewed as the respiratory manifestation of the metabolic syndrome in obese individuals.

- CPAP is currently the first-line treatment for OSA and is prescribed as long-life care to most OSA patients in clinical practice to minimize respiratory events during sleep.

- CPAP is characterized by several limitations, most importantly patients' low adherence and its doubtable efficiency in improving cardio-metabolic indices, which limit its value as the sole treatment option for OSA.

- Patients with OSA have impaired aerobic exercise capacity and a poor hemodynamic response to exercise; these factors constitute cardiovascular risk factors and barriers for physical activity and should be considered before exercise prescription.

- Supervised aerobic exercise programs, either alone or in combination with resistance exercise, appear to lead to significant improvements in the severity and symptoms of OSA as well as patient sleep quality, fitness level, and physical functioning.

- Improvements in the AHI following exercise interventions are observed in the absence of significant changes in patients' anthropometric indices, a fact that highlights the weight-loss independent benefits of physical activity for OSA.

- Patents with OSA should be advised to follow the international guidelines for physical activity by the World Health Organization. These suggest at least 150 to 300 min of moderate-intensity aerobic physical activity, at least 75 to 150 min of vigorous-intensity aerobic physical activity, or an equivalent combination of moderate- and vigorous-intensity activity throughout the week. For additional health benefits, increasing aerobic physical activity, undertaking muscle-strengthening activities, and limiting sedentary behavior to a minimum are also recommended.

- Given that most patients with OSA are sedentary and characterized by increased body weight, they should start by doing small amounts of physical activity and gradually increase the frequency, intensity, and duration over time.

- Older patients with OSA and co-morbidities should be as physically active as their functional ability allows and adjust their level of physical effort to their level of fitness.

- Adherence to prudent dietary patterns characterized by a high consumption of fruits, vegetables, whole grains, legumes, nuts, vegetable oils, and fish as well as prudent consumption of animal-based products and processed foods, can offer protection against the development and progression of OSA and related cardio-metabolic diseases.

- Weight loss is essential for most patients with OSA and is advocated as an ancillary treatment for the disease. Weight-loss interventions can improve OSA severity (e.g., decline in the AHI), symptoms (e.g., alleviation of daytime sleepiness), sleep architecture, and quality of life and lead to significant cardio-metabolic benefits.

- Mild-to-moderate weight loss (5-15%) is associated with proportional improvements in the AHI. However, the dose-response relationship eventually seems to reach a plateau with limited additional benefit from further weight loss.

- Despite evidence of the beneficial effect of weight loss on OSA, it is not clear whether lifestyle interventions alone are sufficient to cure the disease and completely normalize breathing during sleep, especially in patients with severe disease.

- Although available data are insufficient, the Mediterranean diet/lifestyle could be a beneficial choice for OSA, given its strong anti-inflammatory and antioxidant properties as well as its beneficial effects on body composition, which can improve upper-airway neuromuscular control and prevent respiratory disturbances during sleep.

SELF-ASSESSMENT QUESTIONS

1. Define OSA and describe its main pathophysiological sequence.

2. Briefly discuss the link between OSA and cardio-metabolic morbidity.

3. True or False: The AHI represents the number of apneas, hypopneas, and respiratory-effort related arousals per hour of sleep.

4. True or False: OSA is recognized as a modifiable risk factor for cardiovascular disease by health organizations, such as the European and the American Heart Association.

5. True or False: Improvements in the AHI following exercise interventions are attributed to weight loss because of increased energy expenditure.

6. True or False: During normal sleep, the sympathetic activity of the central nervous system outweighs the parasympathetic one.

7. True or False: Home-based diagnosis of OSA, if properly performed, is not inferior to laboratory diagnosis and can be of great value for individuals with mobility problems who have difficulty accessing a sleep center or when attended PSG is not available.

8. True or False: The Mediterranean diet is a dietary pattern characterized by high consumption of fruits, vegetables, legumes, nuts, seeds, white meat, and dairy products, moderate consumption of fish/seafood, low consumption of vegetable oils and red meat products, and a moderate consumption of alcohol with main meals.

9. True or False: Although CPAP is the first-line treatment for OSA, its effectiveness in improving patients' cardio-metabolic status remains controversial.

10. True or False: This ability of the pharynx to close is essential for speech and swallowing while awake, but it also provides the grounds for an undesirable obstruction under certain conditions during sleep.

11. True or False: OSA is a disease attributed solely to abnormal upper-airway anatomy and neuromuscular pathology.

12. Describe CPAP and discuss its benefits and limitations for OSA management.

13. Provide an overview of the benefits of exercise in OSA.

Fill in the blank(s) to complete the following statements:

14. Given the significant disruption of normal sleep architecture, OSA is typically characterized by a wide variety of daytime symptoms, including _____.

15. Various surgical procedures have been investigated in the context of OSA management, the main one being _____, i.e., the removal of _____.

16. While most researchers argue that inflammation and oxidative stress resulting from _____ in the context of OSA lead to cardio-metabolic morbidity, novel theories suggest that the _____ actually precedes the onset of OSA, with central fat deposition triggering upper-airway dysfunction through _____, _____.

17. Very low-calorie diets lead to an average loss of _____ kg/week, and in the short term seem to be _____ effective than low-calorie diets.

18. Recurrent episodes of oxygen desaturation and re-oxygenation within OSA lead to the production of _____ and the establishment of an environment of increased _____, which in turn results in macromolecular peroxidation, changes in cellular homeostasis, and increased expression of inflammatory genes.

19. Positional therapy in OSA suggests avoidance of sleeping in the _____ position, in which the upper airway becomes more susceptible to obstruction due to _____.

20. Besides the Mediterranean diet, other lifestyle habits observed in the Mediterranean region, such as _____ _____ _____, are also beneficial for health and combined, form the _____.

21. During wakefulness, the upper airway is held open by the high activity of _____ _____. After the onset of sleep, when muscle activity is normally reduced, the airway is susceptible to obstruction, especially in the presence of a _____ _____.

22. According to the World Health Organization guidelines, all adults should do at least _____ min of moderate-intensity aerobic physical activity, at least _____ min of vigorous-intensity aerobic physical activity, or an equivalent combination of moderate- and vigorous-intensity activity throughout the week.

23. Hyperactivity of the sympathetic nervous system is accompanied by an increase in _____, a disorder that often persists during the day and in the long term can lead to the establishment of _____.

24. A _____ weight loss seems to lead to a _____ reduction in the AHI; this reduction is clinically significant but may not be sufficient to treat OSA in _____ _____.

25. Insulin resistance leads to _____ adipose tissue lipolysis and availability of free fatty acids to the circulation, which are stored ectopically in the liver and lead to increased _____ and eventually to atherogenic _____.

26. Under normal conditions, in adults, N1 sleep accounts for _____, N2 sleep for _____, N3 sleep for _____, and REM sleep for _____ of total sleep. In OSA these patterns are significantly disturbed, with the duration of _____ sleep being increased and the duration of _____ sleep being significantly reduced due to repeated awakenings.

27. On a food-group level, OSA severity has been positively correlated to the consumption of_____, and negatively correlated to the consumption of _____.

28. How can OSA affect exercise capacity?

29. Make a brief review of the available data on the role of diet quality in OSA.

30. True or False: Cardio-metabolic disorders in the context of the metabolic syndrome, e.g., central obesity, insulin resistance, dyslipidemia, hypertension, subclinical inflammation, and oxidative stress are implicated in OSA pathogenesis.

31. True or False: Adipose tissue accumulating around the upper airways (e.g., the neck) contributes to the thickening of the lateral walls of the pharynx and is a risk factor for OSA development.

32. True or False: Sleep is divided into NREM sleep and REM sleep, while REM sleep is further subdivided into five stages (N1 to N5), which represent the successive transition from lighter to deeper sleep.

33. True or False: Chronic sleep deprivation or poor sleep quality, combined with oxidative stress and chronic inflammation, can enhance insulin sensitivity.

34. True or False: The use of oral devices is the first-line treatment for all OSA patients, while CPAP use is advised only for patients with severe disease (AHI ≥30 events/h).

35. True or False: Very low-calorie diets are 800–1500 kcal nutritionally complete diet regimens that can be used as a life-long approach of obesity management and produce a similar weight loss compared to low-calorie diets in the long term.

36. True or False: The Mediterranean lifestyle, combining the Mediterranean diet, adequate physical activity, and optimal sleep habits (duration and quality), can lead to greater health benefits for patients with OSA compared to the Mediterranean diet alone.

37. True or False: An AHI value of 20 events/h is indicative of moderate-severity OSA.

38. True or False: Hypolipidemic agents, metformin, and laxatives are the only established and efficient pharmacological treatments for OSA.

39. Describe the Mediterranean diet and the mechanisms through which it can contribute to OSA management.

CASE SCENARIO

Mr. LG is a 45-year-old white man who recently visited a sleep center as part of his annual health check-up. His wife has been complaining about his loud snoring for several years but recently witnessed him experience breathing pauses and choking episodes during his sleep and convinced him to undergo sleep testing. The results of an attended overnight PSG revealed an AHI of 68 events/h, and Mr. LG was diagnosed with severe OSA. The medical team of the sleep center prescribed CPAP treatment and suggested weight loss. Mr. LG's height is 1.82 m and current body weight is 128 kg. His medical history includes a 5-year diagnosis of hypertension and a 3-year diagnosis of dyslipidemia for which he receives appropriate medication, i.e., Norvasc (antihypertensive) and Lipitor (hypolipidemic). His recent fasting biochemical evaluation revealed the following (numbers in parentheses indicate normal values): fasting glucose 102 of mg/dL (65–110 mg/dL), TC of 235 mg/dL (<200 mg/dL), triglycerides of 168 mg/dl (<150 mg/dL), HDL-cholesterol of 38 (>50 mg/dL), and CRP of 8.8 (<3 mg/L).

Mr. LG is a police officer and lives with his wife and two teenage children. He has a rotating shift schedule at work with alternating morning and night shifts throughout a typical working week. Given his difficult work schedule, he only consumes one meal (either lunch or dinner) at home, and all other meals and snacks are fast-food choices, such as pizza, burger, or sandwiches. Mr. LG loves food and his wife always tries to cook whatever he wants to please him. He particularly likes all kinds of red meat, which he consumes almost daily, and after his meal he always has a sweet dessert. He does not eat fish and legumes, he is allergic to nuts, and drinks an average of 3 cups of coffee daily, each with added cream and sugar. Mr. LG used to play soccer as a youth, from the age of 10 until the age of 21. Since then, he has never exercised systematically, and his job involves many sedentary hours, due to office work. Although his work is sedentary, he usually feels sleepy and tired, a fact that he used to attribute to night shifts and stress until his OSA diagnosis. He always uses his car for transportation to/from work and all other daily activities.

Questions:

1. Evaluate the patient's body weight in relation to his height. Please use the body-mass index calculator and the instructions for categorizing its values on the following link: https://www.nhlbi.nih.gov/health/educational/lose_wt/BMI/bmicalc.htm.

2. Review the patient's biochemical profile and medical history. How is his overall health status related to OSA pathophysiology? Do you have any evidence to suspect that Mr. LG fulfils the criteria for the presence of metabolic syndrome?

3. Mr. LG was recently prescribed CPAP for OSA management. What kind of information would you give him on CPAP use? Would you leave Mr. LG thinking that CPAP alone is enough to optimize his health? Justify your answer.

4. What kind of exercise program would you recommend to Mr. LG and why? Outline the main points of your counseling about the benefits of exercise in OSA.

5. Based on his dietary habits, what kind of advice would you give to Mr. LG toward the adoption of a healthier diet? Would you recommend weight loss to Mr. LG? If so, what would be a realistic and efficient weight-loss goal for this patient?

REFERENCES

(2020). In *WHO Guidelines on Physical Activity and Sedentary Behaviour*. Geneva.

The AASM Manual for the Scoring of Sleep and Associated Events: Rules, Terminology and Technical Specifications. (2015). Retrieved from Darien, IL:

Ackel-D'Elia, C., da Silva, A. C., Silva, R. S., Truksinas, E., Sousa, B. S., Tufik, S., . . . Bittencourt, L. R. (2012). Effects of exercise training associated with continuous positive airway pressure treatment in patients with obstructive sleep apnea syndrome. *Sleep Breath, 16*(3), 723-735. doi:10.1007/s11325-011-0567-0

Aiello, K. D., Caughey, W. G., Nelluri, B., Sharma, A., Mookadam, F., & Mookadam, M. (2016). Effect of exercise training on sleep apnea: A systematic review and meta-analysis. *Respir Med, 116*, 85-92. doi:10.1016/j.rmed.2016.05.015

Alameri, H., Al-Kabab, Y., & BaHammam, A. (2010). Submaximal exercise in patients with severe obstructive sleep apnea. *Sleep Breath, 14*(2), 145-151. doi:10.1007/s11325-009-0300-4

Anandam, A., Akinnusi, M., Kufel, T., Porhomayon, J., & El-Solh, A. A. (2013). Effects of dietary weight loss on obstructive sleep apnea: a meta-analysis. *Sleep Breath, 17*(1), 227-234. doi:10.1007/s11325-012-0677-3

Aubert-Tulkens, G., Culee, C., & Rodenstein, D. O. (1989). Cure of sleep apnea syndrome after long-term nasal continuous positive airway pressure therapy and weight loss. *Sleep, 12*(3), 216-222. Retrieved from http://www.ncbi.nlm.nih.gov/pubmed/2662343

Ayappa, I., & Rapoport, D. M. (2003). The upper airway in sleep: physiology of the pharynx. *Sleep Med Rev, 7*(1), 9-33. doi:10.1053/smrv.2002.0238

Bach-Faig, A., Berry, E. M., Lairon, D., Reguant, J., Trichopoulou, A., Dernini, S., . . . Mediterranean Diet Foundation Expert, G. (2011). Mediterranean diet pyramid today. Science and cultural updates. *Public Health Nutr, 14*(12A), 2274-2284. doi:10.1017/S1368980011002515

Back, L. J., Liukko, T., Rantanen, I., Peltola, J. S., Partinen, M., Ylikoski, J., & Makitie, A. A. (2009). Radiofrequency surgery of the soft palate in the treatment of mild obstructive sleep apnea is not effective as a single-stage procedure: A randomized single-blinded placebo-controlled trial. *Laryngoscope, 119*(8), 1621-1627. doi:10.1002/lary.20562

Bakker, J. P., Weaver, T. E., Parthasarathy, S., & Aloia, M. S. (2019). Adherence to CPAP: What Should We Be Aiming For, and How Can We Get There? *Chest, 155*(6), 1272-1287. doi:10.1016/j.chest.2019.01.012

Ballester, E., Badia, J. R., Hernandez, L., Carrasco, E., de Pablo, J., Fornas, C., . . . Montserrat, J. M. (1999). Evidence of the effectiveness of continuous positive airway pressure in the treatment of sleep apnea/hypopnea syndrome. *Am J Respir Crit Care Med, 159*(2), 495-501. doi:10.1164/ajrccm.159.2.9804061

Barnes, M., Goldsworthy, U. R., Cary, B. A., & Hill, C. J. (2009). A diet and exercise program to improve clinical outcomes in patients with obstructive sleep apnea--a feasibility study. *J Clin Sleep Med, 5*(5), 409-415. Retrieved from http://www.ncbi.nlm.nih.gov/pubmed/19961023

Beitler, J. R., Awad, K. M., Bakker, J. P., Edwards, B. A., DeYoung, P., Djonlagic, I., . . . Malhotra, A. (2014). Obstructive sleep apnea is associated with impaired exercise capacity: a cross-sectional study. *J Clin Sleep Med, 10*(11), 1199-1204. doi:10.5664/jcsm.4200

Benjafield, A. V., Ayas, N. T., Eastwood, P. R., Heinzer, R., Ip, M. S. M., Morrell, M. J., . . . Malhotra, A. (2019). Estimation of the global prevalence and burden of obstructive sleep apnoea: a literature-based analysis. *Lancet Respir Med, 7*(8), 687-698. doi:10.1016/S2213-2600(19)30198-5

Black, J. (2003). Sleepiness and residual sleepiness in adults with obstructive sleep apnea. *Respir Physiol Neurobiol, 136*(2-3), 211-220. Retrieved from http://www.ncbi.nlm.nih.gov/pubmed/12853012

Bonsignore, M. R., McNicholas, W. T., Montserrat, J. M., & Eckel, J. (2012). Adipose tissue in obesity and obstructive sleep apnoea. *Eur Respir J, 39*(3), 746-767. doi:10.1183/09031936.00047010

Bradley, T. D., & Floras, J. S. (2009). Obstructive sleep apnoea and its cardiovascular consequences. *Lancet, 373*(9657), 82-93. doi:10.1016/S0140-6736(08)61622-0

Brown, W. D. (2005). The psychosocial aspects of obstructive sleep apnea. *Semin Respir Crit Care Med, 26*(1), 33-43. doi:10.1055/s-2005-864199

Buckland, G., Bach, A., & Serra-Majem, L. (2008). Obesity and the Mediterranean diet: a systematic review of observational and intervention studies. *Obes Rev, 9*(6), 582-593. doi:10.1111/j.1467-789X.2008.00503.x

Bucks, R. S., Olaithe, M., & Eastwood, P. (2013). Neurocognitive function in obstructive sleep apnoea: a meta-review. *Respirology, 18*(1), 61-70. doi:10.1111/j.1440-1843.2012.02255.x

Bullo, M., Lamuela-Raventos, R., & Salas-Salvado, J. (2011). Mediterranean diet and oxidation: nuts and olive oil as important sources of fat and antioxidants. *Curr Top Med Chem, 11*(14), 1797-1810. Retrieved from http://www.ncbi.nlm.nih.gov/pubmed/21506929

Cavagnolli, D. A., Esteves, A. M., Ackel-D'Elia, C., Maeda, M. Y., de Faria, A. P., Tufik, S., & de Mello, M. T. (2014). Aerobic exercise does not change C-reactive protein levels in non-obese patients with obstructive sleep apnoea. *Eur J Sport Sci, 14* Suppl 1, S142-147. doi:10.1080/17461391.2012.663412

Ceylan, K., Emir, H., Kizilkaya, Z., Tastan, E., Yavanoglu, A., Uzunkulaoglu, H., . . . Felek, S. A. (2009). First-choice treatment in mild to moderate obstructive sleep apnea: single-stage, multilevel, temperature-controlled radiofrequency tissue volume reduction or nasal continuous positive airway pressure. *Arch Otolaryngol Head Neck Surg, 135*(9), 915-919. doi:10.1001/archoto.2009.117

Chakravorty, I., Cayton, R. M., & Szczepura, A. (2002). Health utilities in evaluating intervention in the sleep apnoea/hypopnoea syndrome. *Eur Respir J, 20*(5), 1233-1238. Retrieved from http://www.ncbi.nlm.nih.gov/pubmed/12449179

Chirinos, J. A., Gurubhagavatula, I., Teff, K., Rader, D. J., Wadden, T. A., Townsend, R., . . . Pack, A. I. (2014). CPAP, Weight Loss, or Both for Obstructive Sleep Apnea. *N Engl J Med, 370*(24), 2265-2275. Retrieved from http://www.ncbi.nlm.nih.gov/entrez/query.fcgi?cmd=Retrieve&db=PubMed&dopt=Citation&list_uids=24918371

Desplan, M., Mercier, J., Sabate, M., Ninot, G., Prefaut, C., & Dauvilliers, Y. (2014). A comprehensive rehabilitation program improves disease severity in patients with obstructive sleep apnea syndrome: a pilot randomized controlled study. *Sleep Med, 15*(8), 906-912. doi:10.1016/j.sleep.2013.09.023

Dixon, J. B., Schachter, L. M., O'Brien, P. E., Jones, K., Grima, M., Lambert, G., . . . Naughton, M. T. (2012). Surgical vs conventional therapy for weight loss treatment of obstructive sleep apnea: a randomized controlled trial. *JAMA, 308*(11), 1142-1149. doi:10.1001/2012.jama.11580

Dobrosielski, D. A., Papandreou, C., Patil, S. P., & Salas-Salvado, J. (2017). Diet and exercise in the management of obstructive sleep apnoea and cardiovascular disease risk. *Eur Respir Rev, 26*(144). doi:10.1183/16000617.0110-2016

Dobrosielski, D. A., Patil, S., Schwartz, A. R., Bandeen-Roche, K., & Stewart, K. J. (2015). Effects of exercise and weight loss in older adults with obstructive sleep apnea. *Med Sci Sports Exerc, 47*(1), 20–26. doi:10.1249/MSS.0000000000000387

Dong, Z., Xu, X., Wang, C., Cartledge, S., Maddison, R., & Shariful Islam, S. M. (2020). Association of overweight and obesity with obstructive sleep apnoea: A systematic review and meta-analysis. *Obesity Medicine, 17*, 100185. doi:https://doi.org/10.1016/j.obmed.2020.100185

Drager, L. F., Brunoni, A. R., Jenner, R., Lorenzi-Filho, G., Bensenor, I. M., & Lotufo, P. A. (2015). Effects of CPAP on body weight in patients with obstructive sleep apnoea: a meta-analysis of randomised trials. *Thorax, 70*(3), 258–264. doi:10.1136/thoraxjnl-2014-205361

Eckert, D. J., & Malhotra, A. (2008). Pathophysiology of adult obstructive sleep apnea. *Proc Am Thorac Soc, 5*(2), 144–153. doi:10.1513/pats.200707-114MG

Ellen, R. L., Marshall, S. C., Palayew, M., Molnar, F. J., Wilson, K. G., & Man-Son-Hing, M. (2006). Systematic review of motor vehicle crash risk in persons with sleep apnea. *J Clin Sleep Med, 2*(2), 193–200. Retrieved from http://www.ncbi.nlm.nih.gov/pubmed/17557495

Epstein, L. J., Kristo, D., Strollo, P. J., Jr., Friedman, N., Malhotra, A., Patil, S. P., . . . Adult Obstructive Sleep Apnea Task Force of the American Academy of Sleep, M. (2009). Clinical guideline for the evaluation, management and long-term care of obstructive sleep apnea in adults. *J Clin Sleep Med, 5*(3), 263–276. Retrieved from http://www.ncbi.nlm.nih.gov/pubmed/19960649

Esposito, K., Kastorini, C. M., Panagiotakos, D. B., & Giugliano, D. (2011). Mediterranean diet and weight loss: meta-analysis of randomized controlled trials. *Metab Syndr Relat Disord, 9*(1), 1–12. doi:10.1089/met.2010.0031

Estruch, R. (2010). Anti-inflammatory effects of the Mediterranean diet: the experience of the PREDIMED study. *Proc Nutr Soc, 69*(3), 333–340. doi:10.1017/S0029665110001539

Estruch, R., & Bach-Faig, A. (2019). Mediterranean diet as a lifestyle and dynamic food pattern. *Eur J Clin Nutr, 72*(Suppl 1), 1–3. doi:10.1038/s41430-018-0302-z

Feng, Y., Zhang, Z., & Dong, Z. Z. (2015). Effects of continuous positive airway pressure therapy on glycaemic control, insulin sensitivity and body mass index in patients with obstructive sleep apnoea and type 2 diabetes: a systematic review and meta-analysis. *NPJ Prim Care Respir Med, 25*, 15005. doi:10.1038/npjpcrm.2015.5

Ferguson, K. A., Cartwright, R., Rogers, R., & Schmidt-Nowara, W. (2006). Oral appliances for snoring and obstructive sleep apnea: a review. *Sleep, 29*(2), 244–262. Retrieved from http://www.ncbi.nlm.nih.gov/pubmed/16494093

Ferguson, K. A., Heighway, K., & Ruby, R. R. (2003). A randomized trial of laser-assisted uvulopalatoplasty in the treatment of mild obstructive sleep apnea. *Am J Respir Crit Care Med, 167*(1), 15–19. doi:10.1164/rccm.2108050

Floras, J. S. (2018). Sleep Apnea and Cardiovascular Disease: An Enigmatic Risk Factor. *Circ Res, 122*(12), 1741–1764. doi:10.1161/CIRCRESAHA.118.310783

Foster, G. D., Borradaile, K. E., Sanders, M. H., Millman, R., Zammit, G., Newman, A. B., . . . Sleep, A. R. G. o. L. A. R. G. (2009). A randomized study on the effect of weight loss on obstructive sleep apnea among obese patients with type 2 diabetes: the Sleep AHEAD study. *Arch Intern Med, 169*(17), 1619–1626. doi:10.1001/archinternmed.2009.266

Franklin, K. A., & Lindberg, E. (2015). Obstructive sleep apnea is a common disorder in the population-a review on the epidemiology of sleep apnea. *J Thorac Dis, 7*(8), 1311–1322. doi:10.3978/j.issn.2072-1439.2015.06.11

Fujii, H., Miyamoto, M., Miyamoto, T., & Muto, T. (2010). Weight loss approach during routine follow-up is effective for obstructive sleep apnea hypopnea syndrome subjects receiving nasal continuous positive airway pressure treatment. *Ind Health, 48*(4), 511–516. Retrieved from http://www.ncbi.nlm.nih.gov/pubmed/20720344

Fujita, S., Conway, W., Zorick, F., & Roth, T. (1981). Surgical correction of anatomic azbnormalities in obstructive sleep apnea syndrome: uvulopalatopharyngoplasty. *Otolaryngol Head Neck Surg, 89*(6), 923–934. Retrieved from http://www.ncbi.nlm.nih.gov/pubmed/6801592

Gaisl, T., Haile, S. R., Thiel, S., Osswald, M., & Kohler, M. (2019). Efficacy of pharmacotherapy for OSA in adults: A systematic review and network meta-analysis. *Sleep Med Rev, 46*, 74–86. doi:10.1016/j.smrv.2019.04.009

Georgoulis, M., Kontogianni, M. D., & Yiannakouris, N. (2014). Mediterranean diet and diabetes: prevention and treatment. *Nutrients, 6*(4), 1406–1423. doi:10.3390/nu6041406

Georgoulis, M., Yiannakouris, N., Kechribari, I., Lamprou, K., Perraki, E., Vagiakis, E., & Kontogianni, M. D. (2020). Cardiometabolic Benefits of a Weight-Loss Mediterranean Diet/Lifestyle Intervention in Patients with Obstructive Sleep Apnea: The "MIMOSA" Randomized Clinical Trial. *Nutrients, 12*(6). doi:10.3390/nu12061570

Georgoulis, M., Yiannakouris, N., Kechribari, I., Lamprou, K., Perraki, E., Vagiakis, E., & Kontogianni, M. D. (2021). The effectiveness of a weight-loss Mediterranean diet/lifestyle intervention in the management of obstructive sleep apnea: Results of the "MIMOSA" randomized clinical trial. *Clin Nutr, 40*(3), 850–859. doi:10.1016/j.clnu.2020.08.037

Georgoulis, M., Yiannakouris, N., Kechribari, I., Lamprou, K., Perraki, E., Vagiakis, E., & Kontogianni, M. D. (2022). Dose-response relationship between weight loss and improvements in obstructive sleep apnea severity after a diet/lifestyle interventions: secondary analyses of the "MIMOSA" randomized clinical trial. *J Clin Sleep Med, 18*(5), 1251–1261. doi:10.5664/jcsm.9834

Georgoulis, M., Yiannakouris, N., Tenta, R., Fragopoulou, E., Kechribari, I., Lamprou, K., . . . Kontogianni, M. D. (2021). A weight-loss Mediterranean diet/lifestyle intervention ameliorates inflammation and oxidative stress in patients with obstructive sleep apnea: results of the "MIMOSA" randomized clinical trial. *Eur J Nutr*. doi:10.1007/s00394-021-02552-w

Gharibeh, T., & Mehra, R. (2010). Obstructive sleep apnea syndrome: natural history, diagnosis, and emerging treatment options. *Nat Sci Sleep, 2*, 233–255. doi:10.2147/NSS.S6844

Giles, K. (2015). Adherence to CPAP in obstructive sleep apnoea. *Nurs Times, 111*(7), 23. Retrieved from http://www.ncbi.nlm.nih.gov/pubmed/26477183

Guimaraes, K. C., Drager, L. F., Genta, P. R., Marcondes, B. F., & Lorenzi-Filho, G. (2009). Effects of oropharyngeal exercises on patients with moderate obstructive sleep apnea syndrome. *Am J Respir Crit Care Med, 179*(10), 962–966. doi:10.1164/rccm.200806-981OC

Hakala, K., Maasilta, P., & Sovijarvi, A. R. (2000). Upright body position and weight loss improve respiratory mechanics and daytime oxygenation in obese patients with obstructive sleep apnoea. *Clin Physiol, 20*(1), 50–55. Retrieved from http://www.ncbi.nlm.nih.gov/pubmed/10651792

Hakala, K., Mustajoki, P., Aittomaki, J., & Sovijarvi, A. R. (1995). Effect of weight loss and body position on pulmonary function and gas exchange abnormalities in morbid obesity. *Int J Obes Relat Metab Disord, 19*(5), 343-346. Retrieved from http://www.ncbi.nlm.nih.gov/pubmed/7647827

Helena, I., Margareta, E., Eva, L., & Pernilla, A. (2014). Tailored behavioral medicine intervention for enhanced physical activity and healthy eating in patients with obstructive sleep apnea syndrome and overweight. *Sleep Breath, 18*(3), 655-668. doi:10.1007/s11325-013-0929-x

Hernandez, T. L., Ballard, R. D., Weil, K. M., Shepard, T. Y., Scherzinger, A. L., Stamm, E. R., . . . Eckel, R. H. (2009). Effects of maintained weight loss on sleep dynamics and neck morphology in severely obese adults. *Obesity (Silver Spring), 17*(1), 84-91. doi:10.1038/oby.2008.485

Hong, S., & Dimsdale, J. E. (2003). Physical activity and perception of energy and fatigue in obstructive sleep apnea. *Med Sci Sports Exerc, 35*(7), 1088-1092. doi:10.1249/01.MSS.0000074566.94791.24

Horner, R. L. (2008). Pathophysiology of obstructive sleep apnea. *J Cardiopulm Rehabil Prev, 28*(5), 289-298. doi:10.1097/01.HCR.0000336138.71569.a2

Hou, H., Zhao, Y., Yu, W., Dong, H., Xue, X., Ding, J., . . . Wang, W. (2018). Association of obstructive sleep apnea with hypertension: A systematic review and meta-analysis. *J Glob Health, 8*(1), 010405. doi:10.7189/jogh.08.010405

Hoyos, C. M., Murugan, S. M., Melehan, K. L., Yee, B. J., Phillips, C. L., Killick, R., . . . Marshall, N. S. (2019). Dose-dependent effects of continuous positive airway pressure for sleep apnea on weight or metabolic function: Individual patient-level clinical trial meta-analysis. *J Sleep Res, 28*(5), e12788. doi:10.1111/jsr.12788

Hudgel, D. W., Patel, S. R., Ahasic, A. M., Bartlett, S. J., Bessesen, D. H., Coaker, M. A., . . . Respiratory, N. (2018). The Role of Weight Management in the Treatment of Adult Obstructive Sleep Apnea. An Official American Thoracic Society Clinical Practice Guideline. *Am J Respir Crit Care Med, 198*(6), e70-e87. doi:10.1164/rccm.201807-1326ST

Iftikhar, I. H., Kline, C. E., & Youngstedt, S. D. (2014). Effects of exercise training on sleep apnea: a meta-analysis. *Lung, 192*(1), 175-184. doi:10.1007/s00408-013-9511-3

Igelstrom, H., Asenlof, P., Emtner, M., & Lindberg, E. (2018). Improvement in obstructive sleep apnea after a tailored behavioural sleep medicine intervention targeting healthy eating and physical activity: a randomised controlled trial. *Sleep Breath, 22*(3), 653-661. doi:10.1007/s11325-017-1597-z

Igelstrom, H., Emtner, M., Lindberg, E., & Asenlof, P. (2013). Physical activity and sedentary time in persons with obstructive sleep apnea and overweight enrolled in a randomized controlled trial for enhanced physical activity and healthy eating. *Sleep Breath, 17*(4), 1257-1266. doi:10.1007/s11325-013-0831-6

International Classification of Sleep Disorders. (2014). Retrieved from Darien, IL:

Jensen, M. D., Ryan, D. H., Apovian, C. M., Ard, J. D., Comuzzie, A. G., Donato, K. A., . . . Obesity, S. (2014). 2013 AHA/ACC/TOS guideline for the management of overweight and obesity in adults: a report of the American College of Cardiology/American Heart Association Task Force on Practice Guidelines and The Obesity Society. *Circulation, 129*(25 Suppl 2), S102-138. doi:10.1161/01.cir.0000437739.71477.ee

Johansson, K., Hemmingsson, E., Harlid, R., Trolle Lagerros, Y., Granath, F., Rossner, S., & Neovius, M. (2011). Longer term effects of very low energy diet on obstructive sleep apnoea in cohort derived from randomised controlled trial: prospective observational follow-up study. *BMJ, 342*, d3017. doi:10.1136/bmj.d3017

Johansson, K., Neovius, M., Lagerros, Y. T., Harlid, R., Rossner, S., Granath, F., & Hemmingsson, E. (2009). Effect of a very low energy diet on moderate and severe obstructive sleep apnoea in obese men: a randomised controlled trial. *BMJ, 339*, b4609. doi:10.1136/bmj.b4609

Jordan, A. S., McSharry, D. G., & Malhotra, A. (2014). Adult obstructive sleep apnoea. *Lancet, 383*(9918), 736-747. doi:10.1016/S0140-6736(13)60734-5

Jullian-Desayes, I., Joyeux-Faure, M., Tamisier, R., Launois, S., Borel, A. L., Levy, P., & Pepin, J. L. (2015). Impact of obstructive sleep apnea treatment by continuous positive airway pressure on cardiometabolic biomarkers: a systematic review from sham CPAP randomized controlled trials. *Sleep Med Rev, 21*, 23-38. doi:10.1016/j.smrv.2014.07.004

Kajaste, S., Telakivi, T., Mustajoki, P., Pihl, S., & Partinen, M. (1994). Effects of a cognitive-behavioural weight loss programme on overweight obstructive sleep apnoea patients. *J Sleep Res, 3*(4), 245-249. Retrieved from http://www.ncbi.nlm.nih.gov/pubmed/10607132

Kales, A., Rechtschaffen, A., University of California, L. A., Brain Information, S., & Network, N. N. I. (1968). *A manual of standardized terminology, techniques and scoring system for sleep stages of human subjects.* Allan Rechtschaffen *and* Anthony Kales*, editors*. Bethesda, Md.: US National Institute of Neurological Diseases and Blindness, Neurological Information Network.

Kansanen, M., Vanninen, E., Tuunainen, A., Pesonen, P., Tuononen, V., Hartikainen, J., . . . Uusitupa, M. (1998). The effect of a very low-calorie diet-induced weight loss on the severity of obstructive sleep apnoea and autonomic nervous function in obese patients with obstructive sleep apnoea syndrome. *Clin Physiol, 18*(4), 377-385. Retrieved from http://www.ncbi.nlm.nih.gov/pubmed/9715765

Kapur, V. K., Auckley, D. H., Chowdhuri, S., Kuhlmann, D. C., Mehra, R., Ramar, K., & Harrod, C. G. (2017). Clinical Practice Guideline for Diagnostic Testing for Adult Obstructive Sleep Apnea: An American Academy of Sleep Medicine Clinical Practice Guideline. *J Clin Sleep Med, 13*(3), 479-504. doi:10.5664/jcsm.6506

Karacan, I. (1970). Sleep: Physiology and pathology. *JAMA, 211*(9), 1547-1547. doi:10.1001/jama.1970.03170090063022

Karlsen, T., Nes, B. M., Tjonna, A. E., Engstrom, M., Stoylen, A., & Steinshamn, S. (2016). High-intensity interval training improves obstructive sleep apnoea. *BMJ Open Sport Exerc Med, 2*(1). doi:10.1136/bmjsem-2016-000155 bmjsem-2016-000155 [pii]

Kasai, T., Floras, J. S., & Bradley, T. D. (2012). Sleep apnea and cardiovascular disease: a bidirectional relationship. *Circulation, 126*(12), 1495-1510. doi:10.1161/CIRCULATIONAHA.111.070813

Kastorini, C. M., Milionis, H. J., Esposito, K., Giugliano, D., Goudevenos, J. A., & Panagiotakos, D. B. (2011). The effect of Mediterranean diet on metabolic syndrome and its components: a meta-analysis of 50 studies and 534,906 individuals. *J Am Coll Cardiol, 57*(11), 1299-1313. doi:10.1016/j.jacc.2010.09.073

Kechribari, I., Kontogianni, M. D., Georgoulis, M., Lamprou, K., Mourati, I., Vagiakis, E., & Yiannakouris, N. (2020). Associations between Red Meat Intake and Sleep Parameters in Patients with Obstructive Sleep Apnea. *J Acad Nutr Diet, 120*(6), 1042-1053. doi:10.1016/j.jand.2019.10.016

Kechribari, I., Kontogianni, M. D., Georgoulis, M., Lamprou, K., Vagiakis, E., & Yiannakouris, N. (2021). Higher refined cereal grain intake is positively associated with apnoea-hypopnoea index in patients with obstructive sleep apnoea. *J Hum Nutr Diet.* doi:10.1111/jhn.12933

Kemppainen, T., Ruoppi, P., Seppa, J., Sahlman, J., Peltonen, M., Tukiainen, H., . . . Tuomilehto, H. (2008). Effect of weight reduction on rhinometric measurements in overweight patients with obstructive sleep apnea. *Am J Rhinol, 22*(4), 410–415. doi:10.2500/ajr.2008.22.3203

Keys, A., Menotti, A., Karvonen, M. J., Aravanis, C., Blackburn, H., Buzina, R., . . . et al. (1986). The diet and 15-year death rate in the seven countries study. *Am J Epidemiol, 124*(6), 903–915. Retrieved from http://www.ncbi.nlm.nih.gov/pubmed/3776973

Kiselak, J., Clark, M., Pera, V., Rosenberg, C., & Redline, S. (1993). The association between hypertension and sleep apnea in obese patients. *Chest, 104*(3), 775–780. Retrieved from http://www.ncbi.nlm.nih.gov/pubmed/8365288

Kline, C. E., Crowley, E. P., Ewing, G. B., Burch, J. B., Blair, S. N., Durstine, J. L., . . . Youngstedt, S. D. (2011). The effect of exercise training on obstructive sleep apnea and sleep quality: a randomized controlled trial. *Sleep, 34*(12), 1631–1640. doi:10.5665/sleep.1422

Kline, C. E., Crowley, E. P., Ewing, G. B., Burch, J. B., Blair, S. N., Durstine, J. L., . . . Youngstedt, S. D. (2013). Blunted heart rate recovery is improved following exercise training in overweight adults with obstructive sleep apnea. *Int J Cardiol, 167*(4), 1610–1615. doi:10.1016/j.ijcard.2012.04.108

Kline, C. E., Ewing, G. B., Burch, J. B., Blair, S. N., Durstine, J. L., Davis, J. M., & Youngstedt, S. D. (2012). Exercise training improves selected aspects of daytime functioning in adults with obstructive sleep apnea. *J Clin Sleep Med, 8*(4), 357–365. doi:10.5664/jcsm.2022

Kline, C. E., Krafty, R. T., Mulukutla, S., & Hall, M. H. (2017). Associations of sedentary time and moderate-vigorous physical activity with sleep-disordered breathing and polysomnographic sleep in community-dwelling adults. *Sleep Breath, 21*(2), 427–434. doi:10.1007/s11325-016-1434-9

Kontogianni, M. D., Zampelas, A., & Tsigos, C. (2006). Nutrition and inflammatory load. *Ann N Y Acad Sci, 1083*, 214–238. doi:10.1196/annals.1367.015

Kribbs, N. B., Pack, A. I., Kline, L. R., Getsy, J. E., Schuett, J. S., Henry, J. N., . . . Dinges, D. F. (1993). Effects of one night without nasal CPAP treatment on sleep and sleepiness in patients with obstructive sleep apnea. *Am Rev Respir Dis, 147*(5), 1162–1168. doi:10.1164/ajrccm/147.5.1162

Kritikou, I., Basta, M., Tappouni, R., Pejovic, S., Fernandez-Mendoza, J., Nazir, R., . . . Vgontzas, A. N. (2013). Sleep apnoea and visceral adiposity in middle-aged male and female subjects. *Eur Respir J, 41*(3), 601–609. doi:10.1183/09031936.00183411

Kryger, M. H. (1985). Fat, sleep, and Charles Dickens: literary and medical contributions to the understanding of sleep apnea. *Clin Chest Med, 6*(4), 555–562. Retrieved from http://www.ncbi.nlm.nih.gov/pubmed/3910333

Kulkas, A., Leppanen, T., Sahlman, J., Tiihonen, P., Mervaala, E., Kokkarinen, J., . . . Tuomilehto, H. (2015). Amount of weight loss or gain influences the severity of respiratory events in sleep apnea. *Med Biol Eng Comput, 53*(10), 975–988. doi:10.1007/s11517-015-1290-y

Kuna, S. T., Reboussin, D. M., Borradaile, K. E., Sanders, M. H., Millman, R. P., Zammit, G., . . . Sleep, A. R. G. o. t. L. A. R. G. (2013). Long-term effect of weight loss on obstructive sleep apnea severity in obese patients with type 2 diabetes. *Sleep, 36*(5), 641–649A. doi:10.5665/sleep.2618

Ladesich, J. B., Pottala, J. V., Romaker, A., & Harris, W. S. (2011). Membrane level of omega-3 docosahexaenoic acid is associated with severity of obstructive sleep apnea. *J Clin Sleep Med, 7*(4), 391–396. doi:10.5664/JCSM.1198

Lam, B., Sam, K., Mok, W. Y., Cheung, M. T., Fong, D. Y., Lam, J. C., . . . Ip, M. S. (2007). Randomised study of three non-surgical treatments in mild to moderate obstructive sleep apnoea. *Thorax, 62*(4), 354–359. doi:10.1136/thx.2006.063644

Larrosa, F., Hernandez, L., Morello, A., Ballester, E., Quinto, L., & Montserrat, J. M. (2004). Laser-assisted uvulopalatoplasty for snoring: does it meet the expectations? *Eur Respir J, 24*(1), 66–70. Retrieved from http://www.ncbi.nlm.nih.gov/pubmed/15293606

Li, H. Y., Wang, P. C., Lee, L. A., Chen, N. H., & Fang, T. J. (2006). Prediction of uvulopalatopharyngoplasty outcome: anatomy-based staging system versus severity-based staging system. *Sleep, 29*(12), 1537–1541. Retrieved from http://www.ncbi.nlm.nih.gov/pubmed/17252884

Lim, J., Lasserson, T. J., Fleetham, J., & Wright, J. (2006). Oral appliances for obstructive sleep apnoea. *Cochrane Database Syst Rev(1)*, CD004435. doi:10.1002/14651858.CD004435.pub3

Lojander, J., Mustajoki, P., Ronka, S., Mecklin, P., & Maasilta, P. (1998). A nurse-managed weight reduction programme for obstructive sleep apnoea syndrome. *J Intern Med, 244*(3), 251–255. Retrieved from http://www.ncbi.nlm.nih.gov/pubmed/9747748

Lurie, A. (2011). Obstructive sleep apnea in adults: epidemiology, clinical presentation, and treatment options. *Adv Cardiol, 46*, 1–42. doi:10.1159/000327660

Masa, J. F., Corral, J., Pereira, R., Duran-Cantolla, J., Cabello, M., Hernandez-Blasco, L., . . . Montserrat, J. M. (2011). Effectiveness of home respiratory polygraphy for the diagnosis of sleep apnoea and hypopnoea syndrome. *Thorax, 66*(7), 567–573. doi:10.1136/thx.2010.152272

Mendelson, M., Bailly, S., Marillier, M., Flore, P., Borel, J. C., Vivodtzev, I., . . . Pepin, J. L. (2018). Obstructive Sleep Apnea Syndrome, Objectively Measured Physical Activity and Exercise Training Interventions: A Systematic Review and Meta-Analysis. *Front Neurol, 9*, 73. doi:10.3389/fneur.2018.00073

Mendelson, M., Lyons, O. D., Yadollahi, A., Inami, T., Oh, P., & Bradley, T. D. (2016). Effects of exercise training on sleep apnoea in patients with coronary artery disease: a randomised trial. *Eur Respir J, 48*(1), 142–150. doi: 10.1183/13993003.01897-2015

Mitchell, L. J., Davidson, Z. E., Bonham, M., O'Driscoll, D. M., Hamilton, G. S., & Truby, H. (2014). Weight loss from lifestyle interventions and severity of sleep apnoea: a systematic review and meta-analysis. *Sleep Med, 15*(10), 1173–1183. doi:10.1016/j.sleep.2014.05.012

Monasterio, C., Vidal, S., Duran, J., Ferrer, M., Carmona, C., Barbe, F., . . . Montserrat, J. M. (2001). Effectiveness of continuous positive airway pressure in mild sleep apnea-hypopnea syndrome. *Am J Respir Crit Care Med, 164*(6), 939–943. doi:10.1164/ajrccm.164.6.2008010

Mortimore, I. L., Marshall, I., Wraith, P. K., Sellar, R. J., & Douglas, N. J. (1998). Neck and total body fat deposition in nonobese and obese patients with sleep apnea compared with that in control subjects. *Am J Respir Crit Care Med, 157*(1), 280–283. doi:10.1164/ajrccm.157.1.9703018

Mulgrew, A. T., Fox, N., Ayas, N. T., & Ryan, C. F. (2007). Diagnosis and initial management of obstructive sleep apnea without polysomnography: a randomized validation study. *Ann Intern Med, 146*(3), 157–166. doi:10.7326/0003-4819-146-3-200702060-00004

Murillo, R., Reid, K. J., Arredondo, E. M., Cai, J., Gellman, M. D., Gotman, N. M., . . . Daviglus, M. L. (2016). Association of self-reported physical activity with obstructive sleep apnea: Results from the Hispanic Community Health Study/Study of Latinos (HCHS/SOL). *Prev Med, 93*, 183–188. doi:10.1016/j.ypmed.2016.10.009

Nahmias, J., Kirschner, M., & Karetzky, M. S. (1993). Weight loss and OSA and pulmonary function in obesity. *N J Med, 90*(1), 48–53. Retrieved from http://www.ncbi.nlm.nih.gov/pubmed/8419857

Nerfeldt, P., Nilsson, B. Y., Mayor, L., Udden, J., & Friberg, D. (2010). A two-year weight reduction program in obese sleep apnea patients. *J Clin Sleep Med*, *6*(5), 479-486. Retrieved from http://www.ncbi.nlm.nih.gov/pubmed/20957850

Nerfeldt, P., Nilsson, B. Y., Mayor, L., Udden, J., Rossner, S., & Friberg, D. (2008). Weight reduction improves sleep, sleepiness and metabolic status in obese sleep apnoea patients. *Obes Res Clin Pract*, *2*(4), I-II. doi:10.1016/j.orcp.2008.08.001

Nerfeldt, P., Nilsson, B. Y., Udden, J., Rossner, S., & Friberg, D. (2008). Weight reduction improves nocturnal respiration in obese sleep apnoea patients-A randomized controlled pilot study. *Obes Res Clin Pract*, *2*(2), 71-142. doi:10.1016/j.orcp.2008.03.002

Newman, A. B., Foster, G., Givelber, R., Nieto, F. J., Redline, S., & Young, T. (2005). Progression and regression of sleep-disordered breathing with changes in weight: the Sleep Heart Health Study. *Arch Intern Med*, *165*(20), 2408-2413. doi:10.1001/archinte.165.20.2408

Ng, A. T., Gotsopoulos, H., Qian, J., & Cistulli, P. A. (2003). Effect of oral appliance therapy on upper airway collapsibility in obstructive sleep apnea. *Am J Respir Crit Care Med*, *168*(2), 238-241. doi:10.1164/rccm.200211-1275OC

Ng, S. S., Chan, R. S., Woo, J., Chan, T. O., Cheung, B. H., Sea, M. M., . . . Hui, D. S. (2015). A Randomized Controlled Study to Examine the Effect of a Lifestyle Modification Program in OSA. *Chest*, *148*(5), 1193-1203. doi:10.1378/chest.14-3016

Norman, J. F., Von Essen, S. G., Fuchs, R. H., & McElligott, M. (2000). Exercise training effect on obstructive sleep apnea syndrome. *Sleep Res Online*, *3*(3), 121-129. Retrieved from http://www.ncbi.nlm.nih.gov/pubmed/11382910

Noseda, A., Kempenaers, C., Kerkhofs, M., Houben, J. J., & Linkowski, P. (1996). Sleep apnea after 1 year domiciliary nasal-continuous positive airway pressure and attempted weight reduction. Potential for weaning from continuous positive airway pressure. *Chest*, *109*(1), 138-143. Retrieved from http://www.ncbi.nlm.nih.gov/pubmed/8549176

Pagel, J. F. (2008). The burden of obstructive sleep apnea and associated excessive sleepiness. *J Fam Pract*, *57*(8 Suppl), S3-8. Retrieved from http://www.ncbi.nlm.nih.gov/pubmed/18687237

Pahkala, R., Seppa, J., Ikonen, A., Smirnov, G., & Tuomilehto, H. (2014). The impact of pharyngeal fat tissue on the pathogenesis of obstructive sleep apnea. *Sleep Breath*, *18*(2), 275-282. doi:10.1007/s11325-013-0878-4

Papandreou, C., Hatzis, C. M., & Fragkiadakis, G. A. (2015). Effects of different weight loss percentages on moderate to severe obstructive sleep apnoea syndrome. *Chron Respir Dis*, *12*(3), 276-278. doi:10.1177/1479972315587516

Papandreou, C., Schiza, S. E., Bouloukaki, I., Hatzis, C. M., Kafatos, A. G., Siafakas, N. M., & Tzanakis, N. E. (2012). Effect of Mediterranean diet versus prudent diet combined with physical activity on OSAS: a randomised trial. *Eur Respir J*, *39*(6), 1398-1404. doi:10.1183/09031936.00103411

Papandreou, C., Schiza, S. E., Tzatzarakis, M. N., Kavalakis, M., Hatzis, C. M., Tsatsakis, A. M., . . . Tzanakis, N. E. (2012). Effect of Mediterranean diet on lipid peroxidation marker TBARS in obese patients with OSAHS under CPAP treatment: a randomised trial. *Sleep Breath*, *16*(3), 873-879. doi:10.1007/s11325-011-0589-7

Pasquali, R., Colella, P., Cirignotta, F., Mondini, S., Gerardi, R., Buratti, P., . . . et al. (1990). Treatment of obese patients with obstructive sleep apnea syndrome (OSAS): effect of weight loss and interference of otorhinolaryngoiatric pathology. *Int J Obes*, *14*(3), 207-217. Retrieved from http://www.ncbi.nlm.nih.gov/pubmed/2341227

Patil, S. P., Ayappa, I. A., Caples, S. M., Kimoff, R. J., Patel, S. R., & Harrod, C. G. (2019). Treatment of Adult Obstructive Sleep Apnea With Positive Airway Pressure: An American Academy of Sleep Medicine Systematic Review, Meta-Analysis, and GRADE Assessment. *J Clin Sleep Med*, *15*(2), 301-334. doi:10.5664/jcsm.7638

Patil, S. P., Schneider, H., Schwartz, A. R., & Smith, P. L. (2007). Adult obstructive sleep apnea: pathophysiology and diagnosis. *Chest*, *132*(1), 325-337. doi:10.1378/chest.07-0040

Peppard, P. E., & Young, T. (2004). Exercise and sleep-disordered breathing: an association independent of body habitus. *Sleep*, *27*(3), 480-484. doi:10.1093/sleep/27.3.480

Peppard, P. E., Young, T., Palta, M., Dempsey, J., & Skatrud, J. (2000). Longitudinal study of moderate weight change and sleep-disordered breathing. *JAMA*, *284*(23), 3015-3021. doi:10.1001/jama.284.23.3015

Piepoli, M. F., Hoes, A. W., Agewall, S., Albus, C., Brotons, C., Catapano, A. L., . . . Group, E. S. C. S. D. (2016). 2016 European Guidelines on cardiovascular disease prevention in clinical practice: The Sixth Joint Task Force of the European Society of Cardiology and Other Societies on Cardiovascular Disease Prevention in Clinical Practice (constituted by representatives of 10 societies and by invited experts)Developed with the special contribution of the European Association for Cardiovascular Prevention & Rehabilitation (EACPR). *Eur Heart J*, *37*(29), 2315-2381. doi:10.1093/eurheartj/ehw106

Przybylowski, T., Bielicki, P., Kumor, M., Hildebrand, K., Maskey-Warzechowska, M., Korczynski, P., & Chazan, R. (2007). Exercise capacity in patients with obstructive sleep apnea syndrome. *J Physiol Pharmacol*, *58 Suppl 5(Pt 2)*, 563-574. Retrieved from http://www.ncbi.nlm.nih.gov/pubmed/18204170

Punjabi, N. M. (2008). The epidemiology of adult obstructive sleep apnea. *Proc Am Thorac Soc*, *5*(2), 136-143. doi:10.1513/pats.200709-155MG

Qaseem, A., Dallas, P., Owens, D. K., Starkey, M., Holty, J. E., Shekelle, P., & Clinical Guidelines Committee of the American College of, P. (2014). Diagnosis of obstructive sleep apnea in adults: a clinical practice guideline from theAmerican College of Physicians. *Ann Intern Med*, *161*(3), 210-220. doi:10.7326/M12-3187

Qaseem, A., Holty, J. E., Owens, D. K., Dallas, P., Starkey, M., Shekelle, P., & Clinical Guidelines Committee of the American College of, P. (2013). Management of obstructive sleep apnea in adults: A clinical practice guideline from the American College of Physicians. *Ann Intern Med*, *159*(7), 471-483. doi:10.7326/0003-4819-159-7-201310010-00704

Quadri, F., Boni, E., Pini, L., Bottone, D., Venturoli, N., Corda, L., & Tantucci, C. (2017). Exercise tolerance in obstructive sleep apnea-hypopnea (OSAH), before and after CPAP treatment: Effects of autonomic dysfunction improvement. *Respir Physiol Neurobiol*, *236*, 51-56. doi:10.1016/j.resp.2016.11.004

Quan, S. F., O'Connor, G. T., Quan, J. S., Redline, S., Resnick, H. E., Shahar, E., . . . Sherrill, D. L. (2007). Association of physical activity with sleep-disordered breathing. *Sleep Breath*, *11*(3), 149-157. doi:10.1007/s11325-006-0095-5

Rajala, R., Partinen, M., Sane, T., Pelkonen, R., Huikuri, K., & Seppalainen, A. M. (1991). Obstructive sleep apnoea syndrome in morbidly obese patients. *J Intern Med*, *230*(2), 125-129. Retrieved from http://www.ncbi.nlm.nih.gov/pubmed/1865163

Reid, M., Maras, J. E., Shea, S., Wood, A. C., Castro-Diehl, C., Johnson, D. A., . . . Redline, S. (2019). Association between diet quality and sleep apnea in the Multi-Ethnic Study of Atherosclerosis. *Sleep*, *42*(1). doi:10.1093/sleep/zsy194

Rodenstein, D. (2009). Sleep apnea: traffic and occupational accidents--individual risks, socioeconomic and legal implications. *Respiration*, *78*(3), 241–248. doi:10.1159/000222811

Rosen, C. L., Auckley, D., Benca, R., Foldvary-Schaefer, N., Iber, C., Kapur, V., . . . Redline, S. (2012). A multisite randomized trial of portable sleep studies and positive airway pressure autotitration versus laboratory-based polysomnography for the diagnosis and treatment of obstructive sleep apnea: the HomePAP study. *Sleep*, *35*(6), 757–767. doi:10.5665/sleep.1870

Rossi, V. A., Schwarz, E. I., Bloch, K. E., Stradling, J. R., & Kohler, M. (2014). Is continuous positive airway pressure necessarily an everyday therapy in patients with obstructive sleep apnoea? *Eur Respir J*, *43*(5), 1387–1393. doi:10.1183/09031936.00180213

Rotenberg, B. W., Murariu, D., & Pang, K. P. (2016). Trends in CPAP adherence over twenty years of data collection: a flattened curve. *J Otolaryngol Head Neck Surg*, *45*(1), 43. doi:10.1186/s40463-016-0156-0

Ryan, C. F., Love, L. L., Peat, D., Fleetham, J. A., & Lowe, A. A. (1999). Mandibular advancement oral appliance therapy for obstructive sleep apnoea: effect on awake calibre of the velopharynx. *Thorax*, *54*(11), 972–977. Retrieved from http://www.ncbi.nlm.nih.gov/pubmed/10525554

Ryan, C. M., & Bradley, T. D. (2005). Pathogenesis of obstructive sleep apnea. *J Appl Physiol (1985)*, *99*(6), 2440–2450. doi:10.1152/japplphysiol.00772.2005

Ryan, D. H., & Yockey, S. R. (2017). Weight Loss and Improvement in Comorbidity: Differences at 5%, 10%, 15%, and Over. *Curr Obes Rep*, *6*(2), 187–194. doi:10.1007/s13679-017-0262-y

Sahlman, J., Seppa, J., Herder, C., Peltonen, M., Peuhkurinen, K., Gylling, H., . . . Tuomilehto, H. (2012). Effect of weight loss on inflammation in patients with mild obstructive sleep apnea. *Nutr Metab Cardiovasc Dis*, *22*(7), 583–590. doi:10.1016/j.numecd.2010.10.007

Sampol, G., Munoz, X., Sagales, M. T., Marti, S., Roca, A., Dolors de la Calzada, M., . . . Morell, F. (1998). Long-term efficacy of dietary weight loss in sleep apnoea/hypopnoea syndrome. *Eur Respir J*, *12*(5), 1156–1159. Retrieved from http://www.ncbi.nlm.nih.gov/pubmed/9864013

Sanchez-de-la-Torre, M., Campos-Rodriguez, F., & Barbe, F. (2013). Obstructive sleep apnoea and cardiovascular disease. *Lancet Respir Med*, *1*(1), 61–72. doi:10.1016/S2213-2600(12)70051-6

Sarkar, P., Mukherjee, S., Chai-Coetzer, C. L., & McEvoy, R. D. (2018). The epidemiology of obstructive sleep apnoea and cardiovascular disease. *J Thorac Dis*, *10*(Suppl 34), S4189–S4200. doi:10.21037/jtd.2018.12.56

Sateia, M. J. (2014). International classification of sleep disorders-third edition: highlights and modifications. *Chest*, *146*(5), 1387–1394. doi:10.1378/chest.14-0970

Sawyer, A. M., Gooneratne, N. S., Marcus, C. L., Ofer, D., Richards, K. C., & Weaver, T. E. (2011). A systematic review of CPAP adherence across age groups: clinical and empiric insights for developing CPAP adherence interventions. *Sleep Med Rev*, *15*(6), 343–356. doi:10.1016/j.smrv.2011.01.003

Schutz, T. C., Cunha, T. C., Moura-Guimaraes, T., Luz, G. P., Ackel-D'Elia, C., Alves Eda, S., . . . Bittencourt, L. (2013). Comparison of the effects of continuous positive airway pressure, oral appliance and exercise training in obstructive sleep apnea syndrome. *Clinics (Sao Paulo)*, *68*(8), 1168–1174. doi:10.6061/clinics/2013(08)17

Schwartz, A. R., Gold, A. R., Schubert, N., Stryzak, A., Wise, R. A., Permutt, S., & Smith, P. L. (1991). Effect of weight loss on upper airway collapsibility in obstructive sleep apnea. *Am Rev Respir Dis*, *144*(3 Pt 1), 494–498. doi:10.1164/ajrccm/144.3_Pt_1.494

Scorza, F. A., Cavalheiro, E. A., Scorza, C. A., Galduroz, J. C., Tufik, S., & Andersen, M. L. (2013). Omega-3 intake in people with obstructive sleep apnea: beauty sleep for the heart. *Epilepsy Behav*, *29*(2), 424–426. doi:10.1016/j.yebeh.2013.07.029

Senaratna, C. V., Perret, J. L., Lodge, C. J., Lowe, A. J., Campbell, B. E., Matheson, M. C., . . . Dharmage, S. C. (2017). Prevalence of obstructive sleep apnea in the general population: A systematic review. *Sleep Med Rev*, *34*, 70–81. doi:10.1016/j.smrv.2016.07.002

Sengul, Y. S., Ozalevli, S., Oztura, I., Itil, O., & Baklan, B. (2011). The effect of exercise on obstructive sleep apnea: a randomized and controlled trial. *Sleep Breath*, *15*(1), 49–56. doi:10.1007/s11325-009-0311-1

Serra-Majem, L., Tomaino, L., Dernini, S., Berry, E. M., Lairon, D., Ngo de la Cruz, J., . . . Trichopoulou, A. (2020). Updating the Mediterranean Diet Pyramid towards Sustainability: Focus on Environmental Concerns. *Int J Environ Res Public Health*, *17*(23). doi:10.3390/ijerph17238758

Servantes, D. M., Javaheri, S., Kravchychyn, A. C. P., Storti, L. J., Almeida, D. R., de Mello, M. T., . . . Bittencourt, L. (2018). Effects of Exercise Training and CPAP in Patients With Heart Failure and OSA: A Preliminary Study. *Chest*, *154*(4), 808–817. doi:10.1016/j.chest.2018.05.011

Servantes, D. M., Pelcerman, A., Salvetti, X. M., Salles, A. F., de Albuquerque, P. F., de Salles, F. C., . . . Filho, J. A. (2012). Effects of home-based exercise training for patients with chronic heart failure and sleep apnoea: a randomized comparison of two different programmes. *Clin Rehabil*, *26*(1), 45–57. doi:10.1177/0269215511403941

Sforza, E., & Lugaresi, E. (1995). Daytime sleepiness and nasal continuous positive airway pressure therapy in obstructive sleep apnea syndrome patients: effects of chronic treatment and 1-night therapy withdrawal. *Sleep*, *18*(3), 195–201. Retrieved from http://www.ncbi.nlm.nih.gov/pubmed/7610316

Sharples, L. D., Clutterbuck-James, A. L., Glover, M. J., Bennett, M. S., Chadwick, R., Pittman, M. A., & Quinnell, T. G. (2016). Meta-analysis of randomised controlled trials of oral mandibular advancement devices and continuous positive airway pressure for obstructive sleep apnoea-hypopnoea. *Sleep Med Rev*, *27*, 108–124. doi:10.1016/j.smrv.2015.05.003

Simpson, L., McArdle, N., Eastwood, P. R., Ward, K. L., Cooper, M. N., Wilson, A. C., . . . Mukherjee, S. (2015). Physical Inactivity Is Associated with Moderate-Severe Obstructive Sleep Apnea. *J Clin Sleep Med*, *11*(10), 1091–1099. doi:10.5664/jcsm.5078

Smith, P. L., Gold, A. R., Meyers, D. A., Haponik, E. F., & Bleecker, E. R. (1985). Weight loss in mildly to moderately obese patients with obstructive sleep apnea. *Ann Intern Med*, *103*(6 Pt 1), 850–855. Retrieved from http://www.ncbi.nlm.nih.gov/pubmed/3933396

Sofi, F. (2009). The Mediterranean diet revisited: evidence of its effectiveness grows. *Curr Opin Cardiol*, *24*(5), 442–446. doi:10.1097/HCO.0b013e32832f056e

Sofi, F., & Casini, A. (2014). Mediterranean diet and non-alcoholic fatty liver disease: new therapeutic option around the corner? *World J Gastroenterol*, *20*(23), 7339–7346. doi:10.3748/wjg.v20.i23.7339

Sofi, F., Macchi, C., Abbate, R., Gensini, G. F., & Casini, A. (2010). Effectiveness of the Mediterranean diet: can it help delay or prevent Alzheimer's disease? *J Alzheimers Dis*, *20*(3), 795–801. doi:10.3233/JAD-2010-1418

Sofi, F., Macchi, C., Abbate, R., Gensini, G. F., & Casini, A. (2013). Mediterranean diet and health. *Biofactors*, *39*(4), 335–342. doi:10.1002/biof.1096

Sofi, F., Macchi, C., Abbate, R., Gensini, G. F., & Casini, A. (2014). Mediterranean diet and health status: an updated meta-analysis and a proposal for a literature-based adherence score. *Public Health Nutr*, *17*(12), 2769–2782. doi:10.1017/S1368980013003169

Somers, V. K., White, D. P., Amin, R., Abraham, W. T., Costa, F., Culebras, A., . . . American College of Cardiology, F. (2008). Sleep apnea and cardiovascular disease: an American Heart Association/american College Of Cardiology Foundation Scientific Statement from the American Heart Association Council for High Blood Pressure Research Professional Education Committee, Council on Clinical Cardiology, Stroke Council, and Council On Cardiovascular Nursing. In collaboration with the National Heart, Lung, and Blood Institute National Center on Sleep Disorders Research (National Institutes of Health). *Circulation*, *118*(10), 1080–1111. doi:10.1161/CIRCULATIONAHA.107.189375

Stansbury, R. C., & Strollo, P. J. (2015). Clinical manifestations of sleep apnea. *J Thorac Dis*, *7*(9), E298–310. doi:10.3978/j.issn.2072-1439.2015.09.13

Stegenga, H., Haines, A., Jones, K., Wilding, J., & Guideline Development, G. (2014). Identification, assessment, and management of overweight and obesity: summary of updated NICE guidance. *BMJ*, *349*, g6608. doi:10.1136/bmj.g6608

Stelmach-Mardas, M., Mardas, M., Iqbal, K., Kostrzewska, M., & Piorunek, T. (2017). Dietary and cardio-metabolic risk factors in patients with Obstructive Sleep Apnea: cross-sectional study. *PeerJ*, *5*, e3259. doi:10.7717/peerj.3259

Stuck, B. A., Sauter, A., Hormann, K., Verse, T., & Maurer, J. T. (2005). Radiofrequency surgery of the soft palate in the treatment of snoring. A placebo-controlled trial. *Sleep*, *28*(7), 847–850. Retrieved from http://www.ncbi.nlm.nih.gov/pubmed/16124664

Sullivan, C. E., Issa, F. G., Berthon-Jones, M., & Eves, L. (1981). Reversal of obstructive sleep apnoea by continuous positive airway pressure applied through the nares. *Lancet*, *1*(8225), 862–865. doi:10.1016/s0140-6736(81)92140-1

Suratt, P. M., McTier, R. F., Findley, L. J., Pohl, S. L., & Wilhoit, S. C. (1987). Changes in breathing and the pharynx after weight loss in obstructive sleep apnea. *Chest*, *92*(4), 631–637. Retrieved from http://www.ncbi.nlm.nih.gov/pubmed/3652748

Tan, X., Alen, M., Cheng, S. M., Mikkola, T. M., Tenhunen, J., Lyytikainen, A., . . . Cheng, S. (2015). Associations of disordered sleep with body fat distribution, physical activity and diet among overweight middle-aged men. *J Sleep Res*, *24*(4), 414–424. doi:10.1111/jsr.12283

Tanna, N., Smith, B. D., Zapanta, P. E., Karanetz, I., Andrews, B. T., Urata, M. M., & Bradley, J. P. (2016). Surgical Management of Obstructive Sleep Apnea. *Plast Reconstr Surg*, *137*(4), 1263–1272. doi:10.1097/PRS.0000000000002017

Trichopoulou, A., Bamia, C., & Trichopoulos, D. (2009). Anatomy of health effects of Mediterranean diet: Greek EPIC prospective cohort study. *BMJ*, *338*, b2337. doi:10.1136/bmj.b2337

Tsai, A. G., & Wadden, T. A. (2006). The evolution of very-low-calorie diets: an update and meta-analysis. *Obesity (Silver Spring)*, *14*(8), 1283–1293. doi:10.1038/oby.2006.146

Tuomilehto, H., Gylling, H., Peltonen, M., Martikainen, T., Sahlman, J., Kokkarinen, J., . . . Kuopio Sleep Apnea, G. (2010). Sustained improvement in mild obstructive sleep apnea after a diet- and physical activity-based lifestyle intervention: postinterventional follow-up. *Am J Clin Nutr*, *92*(4), 688–696. doi:10.3945/ajcn.2010.29485

Tuomilehto, H., Seppa, J., Uusitupa, M., Tuomilehto, J., Gylling, H., & Kuopio Sleep Apnea, G. (2013). Weight reduction and increased physical activity to prevent the progression of obstructive sleep apnea: A 4-year observational postintervention follow-up of a randomized clinical trial. [corrected]. *JAMA Intern Med*, *173*(10), 929–930. doi:10.1001/jamainternmed.2013.389

Tuomilehto, H. P., Seppa, J. M., Partinen, M. M., Peltonen, M., Gylling, H., Tuomilehto, J. O., . . . Kuopio Sleep Apnea, G. (2009). Lifestyle intervention with weight reduction: first-line treatment in mild obstructive sleep apnea. *Am J Respir Crit Care Med*, *179*(4), 320–327. doi:10.1164/rccm.200805-669OC

Ucok, K., Aycicek, A., Sezer, M., Genc, A., Akkaya, M., Caglar, V., . . . Unlu, M. (2009). Aerobic and anaerobic exercise capacities in obstructive sleep apnea and associations with subcutaneous fat distributions. *Lung*, *187*(1), 29–36. doi:10.1007/s00408-008-9128-0

Ueno, L. M., Drager, L. F., Rodrigues, A. C., Rondon, M. U., Braga, A. M., Mathias, W., Jr., . . . Negrao, C. E. (2009). Effects of exercise training in patients with chronic heart failure and sleep apnea. *Sleep*, *32*(5), 637–647. Retrieved from http://www.ncbi.nlm.nih.gov/pubmed/19480231

Vasquez, M. M., Goodwin, J. L., Drescher, A. A., Smith, T. W., & Quan, S. F. (2008). Associations of dietary intake and physical activity with sleep disordered breathing in the Apnea Positive Pressure Long-Term Efficacy Study (APPLES). *J Clin Sleep Med*, *4*(5), 411–418. Retrieved from http://www.ncbi.nlm.nih.gov/pubmed/18853696

Veasey, S. C., Guilleminault, C., Strohl, K. P., Sanders, M. H., Ballard, R. D., & Magalang, U. J. (2006). Medical therapy for obstructive sleep apnea: a review by the Medical Therapy for Obstructive Sleep Apnea Task Force of the Standards of Practice Committee of the American Academy of Sleep Medicine. *Sleep*, *29*(8), 1036–1044. Retrieved from http://www.ncbi.nlm.nih.gov/pubmed/16944672

Verwimp, J., Ameye, L., & Bruyneel, M. (2013). Correlation between sleep parameters, physical activity and quality of life in somnolent moderate to severe obstructive sleep apnea adult patients. *Sleep Breath*, *17*(3), 1039–1046. doi:10.1007/s11325-012-0796-x

Very low-calorie diets. National Task Force on the Prevention and Treatment of Obesity, National Institutes of Health. (1993). *JAMA*, *270*(8), 967–974. Retrieved from http://www.ncbi.nlm.nih.gov/pubmed/8345648

Vgontzas, A. N., Bixler, E. O., & Chrousos, G. P. (2003). Metabolic disturbances in obesity versus sleep apnoea: the importance of visceral obesity and insulin resistance. *J Intern Med*, *254*(1), 32–44. Retrieved from http://www.ncbi.nlm.nih.gov/pubmed/12823641

Vgontzas, A. N., Bixler, E. O., & Chrousos, G. P. (2005). Sleep apnea is a manifestation of the metabolic syndrome. *Sleep Med Rev*, *9*(3), 211–224. doi:10.1016/j.smrv.2005.01.006

Vgontzas, A. N., Gaines, J., Ryan, S., & McNicholas, W. T. (2016). Cross-Talk proposal: Metabolic syndrome causes sleep apnoea. *J Physiol*. doi:10.1113/JP272114

Vgontzas, A. N., Papanicolaou, D. A., Bixler, E. O., Hopper, K., Lotsikas, A., Lin, H. M., . . . Chrousos, G. P. (2000). Sleep apnea and daytime sleepiness and fatigue: relation to visceral obesity, insulin resistance, and hypercytokinemia. *J Clin Endocrinol Metab*, *85*(3), 1151–1158. doi:10.1210/jcem.85.3.6484

Vivodtzev, I., Mendelson, M., Croteau, M., Gorain, S., Wuyam, B., Tamisier, R., . . . Pepin, J. L. (2017). Physiological correlates to spontaneous physical activity variability in obese patients with already treated sleep apnea syndrome. *Sleep Breath*, *21*(1), 61–68. doi:10.1007/s11325-016-1368-2

Wallace, A., & Bucks, R. S. (2013). Memory and obstructive sleep apnea: a meta-analysis. *Sleep*, *36*(2), 203–220. doi:10.5665/sleep.2374

Wang, X., Bi, Y., Zhang, Q., & Pan, F. (2013). Obstructive sleep apnoea and the risk of type 2 diabetes: a meta-analysis of prospective cohort studies. *Respirology*, *18*(1), 140–146. doi:10.1111/j.1440-1843.2012.02267.x

Woodson, B. T., Steward, D. L., Weaver, E. M., & Javaheri, S. (2003). A randomized trial of temperature-controlled radiofrequency, continuous positive airway pressure, and placebo for obstructive sleep apnea syndrome. *Otolaryngol Head Neck Surg, 128*(6), 848-861. Retrieved from http://www.ncbi.nlm.nih.gov/pubmed/12825037

Xie, C., Zhu, R., Tian, Y., & Wang, K. (2017). Association of obstructive sleep apnoea with the risk of vascular outcomes and all-cause mortality: a meta-analysis. *BMJ Open, 7*(12), e013983. doi:10.1136/bmjopen-2016-013983

Yang, H., Liu, Y., Zheng, H., Liu, G., & Mei, A. (2018). Effects of 12 weeks of regular aerobic exercises on autonomic nervous system in obstructive sleep apnea syndrome patients. *Sleep Breath, 22*(4), 1189-1195. doi:10.1007/s11325-018-1736-110.1007/s11325-018-1736-1 [pii]

Yannakoulia, M., Kontogianni, M., & Scarmeas, N. (2015). Cognitive health and Mediterranean diet: just diet or lifestyle pattern? *Ageing Res Rev, 20*, 74-78. doi:10.1016/j.arr.2014.10.003

Young, L. R., Taxin, Z. H., Norman, R. G., Walsleben, J. A., Rapoport, D. M., & Ayappa, I. (2013). Response to CPAP withdrawal in patients with mild versus severe obstructive sleep apnea/hypopnea syndrome. *Sleep, 36*(3), 405-412. doi:10.5665/sleep.2460

Young, T., Palta, M., Dempsey, J., Skatrud, J., Weber, S., & Badr, S. (1993). The occurrence of sleep-disordered breathing among middle-aged adults. *N Engl J Med, 328*(17), 1230-1235. doi:10.1056/NEJM199304293281704

Yu, J., Zhou, Z., McEvoy, R. D., Anderson, C. S., Rodgers, A., Perkovic, V., & Neal, B. (2017). Association of Positive Airway Pressure With Cardiovascular Events and Death in Adults With Sleep Apnea: A Systematic Review and Meta-analysis. *JAMA, 318*(2), 156-166. doi:10.1001/jama.2017.7967

Yumuk, V., Tsigos, C., Fried, M., Schindler, K., Busetto, L., Micic, D., . . . Obesity Management Task Force of the European Association for the Study of, O. (2015). European Guidelines for Obesity Management in Adults. *Obes Facts, 8*(6), 402-424. doi:10.1159/000442721

FURTHER READING

Bibliography

Aiello, K.D., Caughey, W.G., Nelluri, B., et al. (2016). Effect of exercise training on sleep apnea: A systematic review and meta-analysis. *Respiratory Medicine. 116*: 85-92.

Bach-Faig, A., Berry, E.M., Lairon, D., et al. (2011). Mediterranean diet pyramid today. Science and cultural updates. *Public Health Nutrition. 14*(12A): 2274-2284.

Benjafield, A.V., Ayas, N.T., Eastwood, P.R., et al. (2019). Estimation of the global prevalence and burden of obstructive sleep apnoea: a literature-based analysis. *The Lancet Respiratory Medicine. 7*(8) :687-98.

Bradley, T.D., Floras, J.S. (2009). Obstructive sleep apnoea and its cardiovascular consequences. *Lancet. 373*(9657): 82-93.

Chirinos, J.A., Gurubhagavatula, I., Teff, K., et al. (2014). CPAP, weight loss, or both for obstructive sleep apnea. *The New England Journal of Medicine. 370*(24) :2265-2275.

Dobrosielski, D.A., Papandreou, C., Patil, S.P., Salas-Salvado, J. (2017). Diet and exercise in the management of obstructive sleep apnoea and cardiovascular disease risk. *European Respiratory Review. 26*(144).

Dong, Z., Xu, X., Wang, C., Cartledge, S., Maddison, R., Shariful Islam, S.M. (2020). Association of overweight and obesity with obstructive sleep apnoea: A systematic review and meta-analysis. *Obesity Medicine. 17*: 100185.

Eckert, D.J., Malhotra, A. (2008). Pathophysiology of adult obstructive sleep apnea. *Proceedings of the American Thoracic Society. 5*(2): 144-153.

Georgoulis, M., Yiannakouris, N., Kechribari, I., et al. (2021). The effectiveness of a weight-loss Mediterranean diet/lifestyle intervention in the management of obstructive sleep apnea: Results of the "MIMOSA" randomized clinical trial. *Clinical Nutrition. 40*(3): 850-859.

Hudgel, D.W., Patel, S.R., Ahasic, A.M., et al. (2018). The role of weight management in the treatment of adult obstructive sleep apnea: An official American Thoracic Society clinical practice guideline. *American Journal of Respiratory and Critical Care Medicine. 198*(6): e70-e87.

Jordan, A.S., McSharry, D.G., Malhotra, A. (2014). Adult obstructive sleep apnoea. *Lancet. 383*(9918): 736-747.

Kapur, V.K., Auckley, D.H., Chowdhuri, S., et al. (2017). Clinical practice guideline for diagnostic testing for adult obstructive sleep apnea: An American Academy of Sleep Medicine clinical practice guideline. *Journal of Clinical Sleep Medicine. 13*(3): 479-504.

Kasai, T., Floras, J.S., Bradley, T.D. (2012). Sleep apnea and cardiovascular disease: a bidirectional relationship. *Circulation. 126*(12):1495-1510.

Mendelson, M., Bailly, S., Marillier, M., et al. (2018). Obstructive sleep apnea syndrome objectively measured physical activity and exercise training interventions: A systematic review and meta-analysis. *Frontiers in Neurology. 9*: 73.

Mitchell, L.J., Davidson, Z.E., Bonham, M., O'Driscoll, D.M., Hamilton, G.S., Truby, H. (2014). Weight loss from lifestyle interventions and severity of sleep apnoea: a systematic review and meta-analysis. *Sleep Medicine. 15*(10): 1173-1183.

Patil, S.P., Ayappa, I.A., Caples, S.M., Kimoff, R.J., Patel, S.R., Harrod, C.G. (2019). Treatment of adult obstructive sleep apnea with positive airway pressure: An American Academy of Sleep Medicine systematic review, meta-analysis, and GRADE assessment. *Journal of Clinical Sleep Medicine. 15*(2): 301-334.

Sadek, I., Siyanbade, J., & Abdulrazak, B. Unobtrusive Monitoring of Sleep Cycles. Encyclopedia. https://encyclopedia.pub/entry/21218 (accessed on 28 February 2023).

Sofi, F., Macchi, C., Abbate, R., Gensini, G.F., Casini, A. (2014). Mediterranean diet and health status: an updated meta-analysis and a proposal for a literature-based adherence score. *Public Health Nutrition. 17*(12): 2769-2782.

The AASM Manual for the Scoring of Sleep and Associated Events: Rules, Terminology and Technical Specifications. (2015). Darien, IL: American Academy of Sleep Medicine.

Vgontzas, A.N., Bixler, E.O., Chrousos, G.P. (2005). Sleep apnea is a manifestation of the metabolic syndrome. *Sleep Medicine Reviews. 9*(3): 211-224.

Vgontzas, A.N., Gaines, J., Ryan, S., McNicholas, W.T. (2016). CrossTalk proposal: Metabolic syndrome causes sleep apnoea. *The Journal of Physiology. 594*(17): 4687-4690.

Links

- https://www.ersnet.org
- https://esrs.eu
- https://www.aarc.org
- https://aasm.org
- https://www.sleepfoundation.org
- https://worldsleepsociety.org
- https://www.behavioralsleep.org
- https://www.sleepsociety.org.uk
- https://www.sleepapnea.org
- https://www.sleepassociation.org
- https://sleep-apnoea-trust.org

Chronic Kidney Disease

CHAPTER 20

Introduction	327
Definition	328
Prevalence	328
Etiology	329
Complications	329
Management	330
Nutrition in Chronic Kidney Disease	330
Physical Activity, Fitness, and Chronic Kidney Disease	333
Physical Activity and Fitness Status of Chronic Kidney Disease Patients	333
Physical Activity, Fitness, and Risk of Chronic Kidney Disease	334
Physical Activity, Fitness, and Mortality Risk in Chronic Kidney Disease	335
Exercise Training and Chronic Kidney Disease Management	336
Physical Function	336
Disease Progression	337
Cardiovascular Risk	337
Physical Activity Recommendations	338
Key Points	341
Self-assessment Questions	341
Case Scenario	342
References	342
Further Reading	345
Bibliography	345
Links	346

INTRODUCTION

The urinary system, also known as the renal system or urinary tract, consists of the kidneys, ureters, bladder, and the urethra, and its main function in the human body is the production, storage, and eventual removal of urine, the fluid waste excreted by the kidneys. The kidneys are complex organs of the urinary system considered vital in maintaining body physiology. A human being's survival depends, to a large degree, on the crucial functions and processes performed by the kidneys, which aim at maintaining a stable internal environment (homeostasis) for optimal cell and tissue metabolism. These include: i) the regulation of plasma osmolarity by modulating the amount of water and electrolytes (e.g., sodium, potassium, phosphates) in the blood; ii) the removal of metabolic waste products (e.g., nitrogenous substances) and foreign substances (e.g., drugs) from the body through urine; iii) the regulation of long-term acid-base balance by modulating the excretion of hydrogen ions and the reabsorption of bicarbonate; iv) the production of several important hormones, such as erythropoietin, which stimulates the production of red blood cells and renin, which is involved in blood-pressure regulation; and v) the conversion of vitamin D to its active form, which is crucial for intestinal calcium absorption (Ogobuiro & Tuma, 2020).

Kidney disorders can develop suddenly (acute) or over a long period (chronic). Acute kidney injury (AKI) is the sudden loss of kidney function over a period of hours or days. It is usually caused by an event that leads to kidney malfunction, such as severe dehydration, blood loss from major surgery or injury, or improper use of potentially nephrotoxic medication. It is considered reversible given that a prompt workup of the underlying cause is pursued and proper care is implemented (e.g., optimization of volume status and avoidance of nephrotoxic substances) (Moore, Hsu, & Liu, 2018). On the other hand, chronic kidney disease (CKD) is the gradual loss of kidney function over a period of years or even decades, usually caused by a long-term medical condition and aggravated by risk factors. CKD encompasses a wide spectrum of renal dysfunction that ranges from a mild loss of kidney function to renal failure, also called end-stage renal disease (ESRD), which represents the most common form

---

Prevention and Management of Cardiovascular and Metabolic Disease: Diet, Physical Activity and Healthy Aging,
First Edition. Christina N. Katsagoni, Peter Kokkinos, and Labros S. Sidossis.
© 2023 John Wiley & Sons Ltd. Published 2023 by John Wiley & Sons Ltd.

of kidney disease. CKD is now recognized as a major cause of morbidity and mortality, and its efficient management remains a challenge for the medical community (Bikbov, Perico, Remuzzi, & on behalf of the, 2018).

DEFINITION

CKD refers to the progressive and irreversible decline in renal function and is defined as the presence of either chronic impaired renal clearance capacity or chronic kidney damage (National Kidney, 2002; Stevens, Levin, & Kidney Disease: Improving Global Outcomes Chronic Kidney Disease Guideline Development Work Group, 2013). Renal clearance capacity refers to the rate at which kidneys filter blood, while kidney damage refers to either functional abnormalities of the kidneys (such as proteinuria or abnormalities of the urinary sediment, such as dysmorphic red cells) or structural abnormalities of the kidneys as noted on imaging studies (National Kidney, 2002; Stevens et al., 2013).

In clinical practice, the ability of the kidneys to clear blood from waste products and to reserve proteins are combined to determine CKD presence, severity, and risk of progression (Vart & Grams, 2016). The clearance capacity of the kidneys is typically expressed through the glomerular filtration rate (GFR), a measure of how much blood (in mL) is "cleaned" by the kidneys per minute. In the absence of methods to directly measure the number of nephrons and single-nephron GFR, overall GFR is estimated indirectly from the clearance rate of exogenous markers, such as inulin, or endogenous markers, such as creatinine and cystatin C, using appropriate equations that take body size into account, assuming that the average adult body size is 1.73 m². Estimated GFR is expressed as mL/min/1.73 m² and low values are indicative of impaired renal clearance efficiency (Vart & Grams, 2016). The protein reservation capacity of kidneys is typically estimated through the degree of proteinuria, a condition in which protein abnormally leaks into urine. Given that albumin is the most abundant high molecular-weight protein in plasma, the albumin:creatinine ratio (ACR) is the dominant marker of the abnormal leakage of albumin into urine (albuminuria). ACR is expressed in mg/g or mg/mmol, and high values are indicative of a pathologic alteration of the glomerular filtration barrier and an impaired kidney protein reabsorption function (Vart & Grams, 2016).

In general, CKD is defined as the presence of decreased kidney function with GFR <60 mL/min/1.73 m² or kidney damage with an ACR ≥30 mg/g or ≥3 mg/mmol for 3 or more months (National Kidney, 2002; Stevens et al., 2013). The diagnosis, staging, and progression risk assessment of CKD based on the categorization of GFR and ACR values is summarized in **Table 20.1** (Levey et al., 2011).

PREVALENCE

CKD is a global health burden with a high economic cost to health systems. According to the available epidemiological studies, the mean global CKD prevalence is estimated as high as 13.4% (11.7–15.1%), of which 3.5% (2.8–4.2%) corresponds to stage 1 (GFR > 90 mL/min/1.73 m² + ACR > 30 mg/g), 3.9% (2.7–5.3%) corresponds to stage 2 (GFR 60–89 mL/min/1.73 m² + ACR > 30 mg/g), 7.6% (6.4–8.9%) corresponds to stage 3 (GFR 30–59 mL/min/1.73 m²), 0.4% (0.3–0.5%) corresponds to stage 4 (GFR 29-15 mL/min/1.73 m²), and 0.1% (0.1–0.1%) corresponds to stage 5 CKD (GFR < 15 mL/min/1.73 m²) (Hill et al., 2016). In 2016, the global number of individuals with CKD reached

Table 20.1 Diagnosis and prognosis of CKD based on the criteria of kidney disease improving global outcomes (KDIGO). ACR = albumin:creatitine ratio; GFR = glomerular filtration rate.

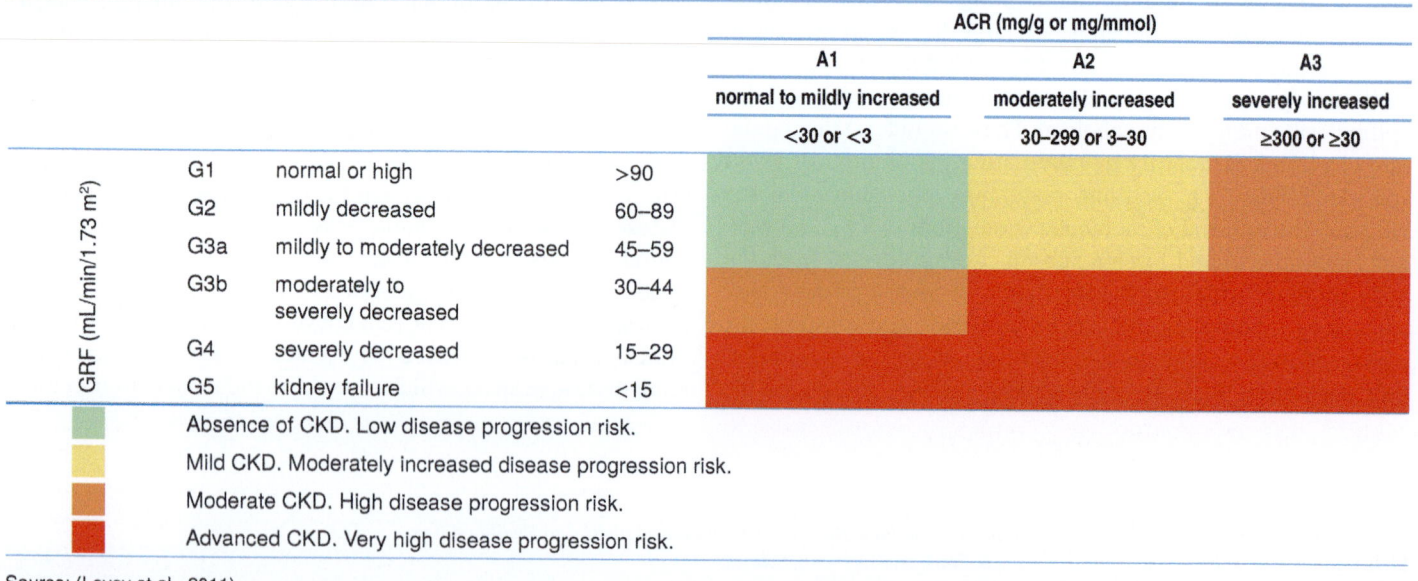

GFR (mL/min/1.73 m²)				ACR (mg/g or mg/mmol)		
				A1 normal to mildly increased <30 or <3	A2 moderately increased 30–299 or 3–30	A3 severely increased ≥300 or ≥30
	G1	normal or high	>90			
	G2	mildly decreased	60–89			
	G3a	mildly to moderately decreased	45–59			
	G3b	moderately to severely decreased	30–44			
	G4	severely decreased	15–29			
	G5	kidney failure	<15			

- Absence of CKD. Low disease progression risk.
- Mild CKD. Moderately increased disease progression risk.
- Moderate CKD. High disease progression risk.
- Advanced CKD. Very high disease progression risk.

Source: (Levey et al., 2011).

752.7 million, of which 417.0 million were women and 335.7 million were men, while the most prevalent form of CKD in both genders is albuminuria (ACR > 30 mg/g) with preserved GFR (Bikbov et al., 2018).

ETIOLOGY

The most common causes of CKD are diabetes mellitus and hypertension, which are responsible for up to two-thirds of the cases (Drawz & Rahman, 2015). Other risk factors for CKD include autoimmune diseases, systemic infections, urinary tract infections, nephrolithiasis, lower urinary tract obstruction, hyperuricemia, AKI, and a family history of CKD as well as sociodemographic and lifestyle factors, such as smoking, heavy alcohol consumption, being an older adult, Black, and/or overweight/obese as well as the use of nonsteroidal anti-inflammatory drugs (Drawz & Rahman, 2015).

Diabetes mellitus is a group of metabolic diseases characterized by hyperglycemia resulting from defects in insulin production, insulin action, or both ("2. Classification and Diagnosis of Diabetes: Standards of Medical Care in Diabetes-2019," 2019). It is a well-established risk factor for kidney injury that can eventually lead to the development of diabetic kidney disease (DKD) through mechanisms that include hyperaminoacidemia, a promoter of glomerular hyperfiltration, and hyperperfusion as well as hyperglycemia, which induces chronic inflammation and oxidative stress through an increased production of advanced glycosylation end products, reactive oxygen species, and inflammatory cytokines (Alicic, Rooney, & Tuttle, 2017). DKD develops in approximately 40% of patients who are diabetic and is the leading cause of CKD worldwide. If poorly treated, DKD can eventually lead to ESRD, however, the majority of DKD patients die from cardiovascular diseases and infections related to diabetes before reaching ESRD. Therefore, optimal glycemic control is crucial for all DKD patients to reduce the progression of CKD, the incidence of ESRD, and mortality risk (Alicic et al., 2017).

Hypertension (systolic/diastolic pressure ≥140/90 mm Hg) and CKD are closely interlinked, given that sustained hypertension can lead to the deterioration of kidney function and that a decline in kidney function can conversely lead to poor blood-pressure control (Hamrahian, 2017; Ku, Lee, Wei, & Weir, 2019). It is well established that hypertension is the second leading cause of CKD worldwide after diabetes mellitus and accounts for approximately 30% of all ESRD patients. The leading theory explaining this relationship is that systemic hypertension is transmitted to intraglomerular capillary pressure, which leads to glomerulosclerosis and gradual loss of kidney function. However, the pathophysiology of hypertension in CKD is complex and is a sequela of multiple factors, including reduced nephron mass, increased sodium retention and extracellular volume expansion, sympathetic nervous system overactivity, activation of the renin-angiotensin-aldosterone system, and endothelial dysfunction. Regardless of the cause-effect relationship of the two entities, hypertension is highly prevalent in CKD patients and its efficient management is of high importance, as it can help toward both slowing CKD progression and reducing cardiovascular risk (Hamrahian, 2017; Ku et al., 2019).

COMPLICATIONS

Mild CKD (estimated GFR >60 mL/min/1.73 m^2) is usually an asymptomatic disorder with no physical findings specific to decreased kidney function. On the contrary, advanced CKD is associated with serious complications, including cardiovascular disorders, cachexia, cognitive dysfunction, and metabolic abnormalities such as anemia, dyslipidemia, renal osteodystrophy, secondary hyperparathyroidism, and electrolyte disturbances (Thomas, Kanso, & Sedor, 2008). Most importantly, advanced CKD is recognized as a major cause of mortality. As shown in **Figure 20.1**, according to a 2010 collaborative meta-analysis of 14 general population cohorts with 105,872 participants (Matsushita et al., 2010), a GFR <60 ml/min/1.73 m^2 and ACR ≥10 mg/g were highlighted as independent predictors of mortality risk in the general population. Notably, this increased risk for all-cause mortality is largely driven by cardiovascular deaths, which constitute approximately 60% of the deaths in CKD patients (Tonelli et al., 2006).

Cardiovascular disorders in CKD include: (a) atherosclerosis, which predisposes the patient to ischemic cardiac events (myocardial infarction/angina), cerebrovascular events (strokes, transient ischemic attacks), and peripheral vascular events (gangrene, amputation); (b) arteriosclerosis, which predisposes the patient to left ventricular hypertrophy and ischemic heart disease; (c) cardiomyopathy is associated with disorders of cardiac structure (concentric and eccentric hypertrophy) and function (diastolic and systolic dysfunction), which predispose the patient to pulmonary edema; (d) arrhythmogenic disorders resulting in atrial fibrillation and sudden cardiac death; and (e) cardiac valvular disorders, particularly affecting the aortic and mitral valves (Parfrey & Barrett, 2015). The close relationship between CKD and cardiovascular diseases can be explained by both traditional and non-traditional cardiovascular risk factors that are present in most CKD patients. Traditional risk factors include smoking, sedentariness, obesity, hypertension, dyslipidemia, and diabetes mellitus, while non-traditional risk factors are mainly related to uremia, i.e., high levels of urea in the blood due to insufficient excretion in urine and include low levels of hemoglobin, albuminuria, and related malnutrition (loss of lean body mass) as well as abnormal bone and mineral metabolism (Alani, Tamimi, & Tamimi, 2014). Interestingly, it has been shown that the heart and the kidneys are closely linked, with the disease of one organ causing dysfunction of the other, and ultimately leading to the failure of both, a condition known as cardio-renal syndrome. Cardiovascular involvement in CKD is known as type-4 cardio-renal syndrome or chronic reno-cardiac syndrome, a condition characterized by the hemodynamic cross-talk between failing kidneys and the heart as well as by significant alterations in neurohormonal markers and inflammatory molecular signatures that derive from the pathophysiology of CKD and result in a highly increased cardiovascular risk (**Figure 20.2**) (Ronco, Haapio, House, Anavekar, & Bellomo, 2008).

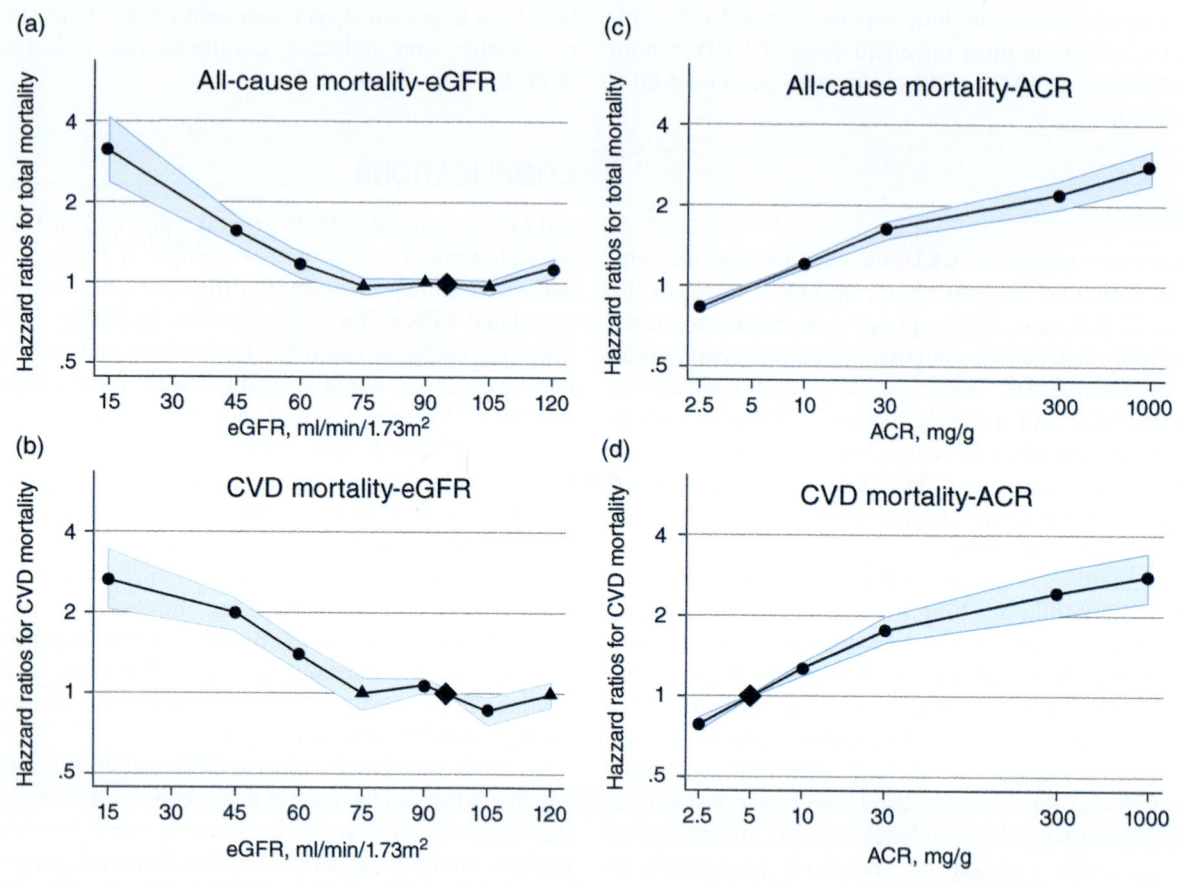

FIGURE 20.1 All-cause and cardiovascular mortality according to eGFR and ACR adjusted for each other, age, gender, race, cardiovascular history, systolic blood pressure, diabetes, smoking, and total cholesterol levels. The reference categories are GFR 95 ml/min/1.73 m² and ACR 5 mg/g (0.6 mg/mmol). Dots and triangles represent statistically significant and non-significant differences compared to reference categories, respectively. ACR = albumin:creatinine ratio; CVD = cardiovascular disease; eGFR = estimated glomerular filtration rate. Source: (Matsushita et al., 2010).

MANAGEMENT

Given the complex nature and complications of CKD, optimal disease management is best accomplished through a collaboration between different medical specialties in the context of a multidisciplinary team. In the early stages of CKD, the main goals of treatment include slowing the decline in kidney function and the likelihood of reaching ESRD, preventing the establishment of cardiovascular diseases, and treating CKD metabolic complications. To accomplish these goals, dietary protein intake should be <1.0g/kg/d, blood pressure should be closely monitored and kept within normal range in patients with hypertension, and glycemia should be controlled in patients with diabetes mellitus using available therapies (Drawz & Rahman, 2015).

In ESRD, treatment should facilitate a transition to renal replacement therapy, usually advised to start once the estimated GFR is <15 mL/min/1.73 m² and the patient is symptomatic. Common indications to initiate renal replacement therapy are volume overload unresponsive to diuretics, pericarditis, uremic encephalopathy, major bleeding secondary to uremic platelets, and hypertension that does not respond to treatment. Hyperkalemia and metabolic acidosis that cannot be managed medically and progressive "uremic" symptoms, such as fatigue, nausea and vomiting, loss of appetite, and evidence of malnutrition, are also indications for renal replacement therapy. Renal replacement therapy options include dialysis, i.e., the process of removing excess water, solutes, and toxins from the blood in the form of hemodialysis, peritoneal dialysis, hemofiltration, hemodiafiltration, or intestinal dialysis as well as renal transplantation (Hakim & Lazarus, 1995).

NUTRITION IN CHRONIC KIDNEY DISEASE

Nutritional therapy in CKD is of high importance. As already mentioned, CKD is progressive, irreversible, and affects various metabolic pathways. Altered energy homeostasis, abnormal protein catabolism, and acid-base derangements are typical manifestations of the disease. As CKD progresses, nutritional status deteriorates and protein-energy wasting occurs, a condition that requires dietary adjustments. Reasons for the establishment of

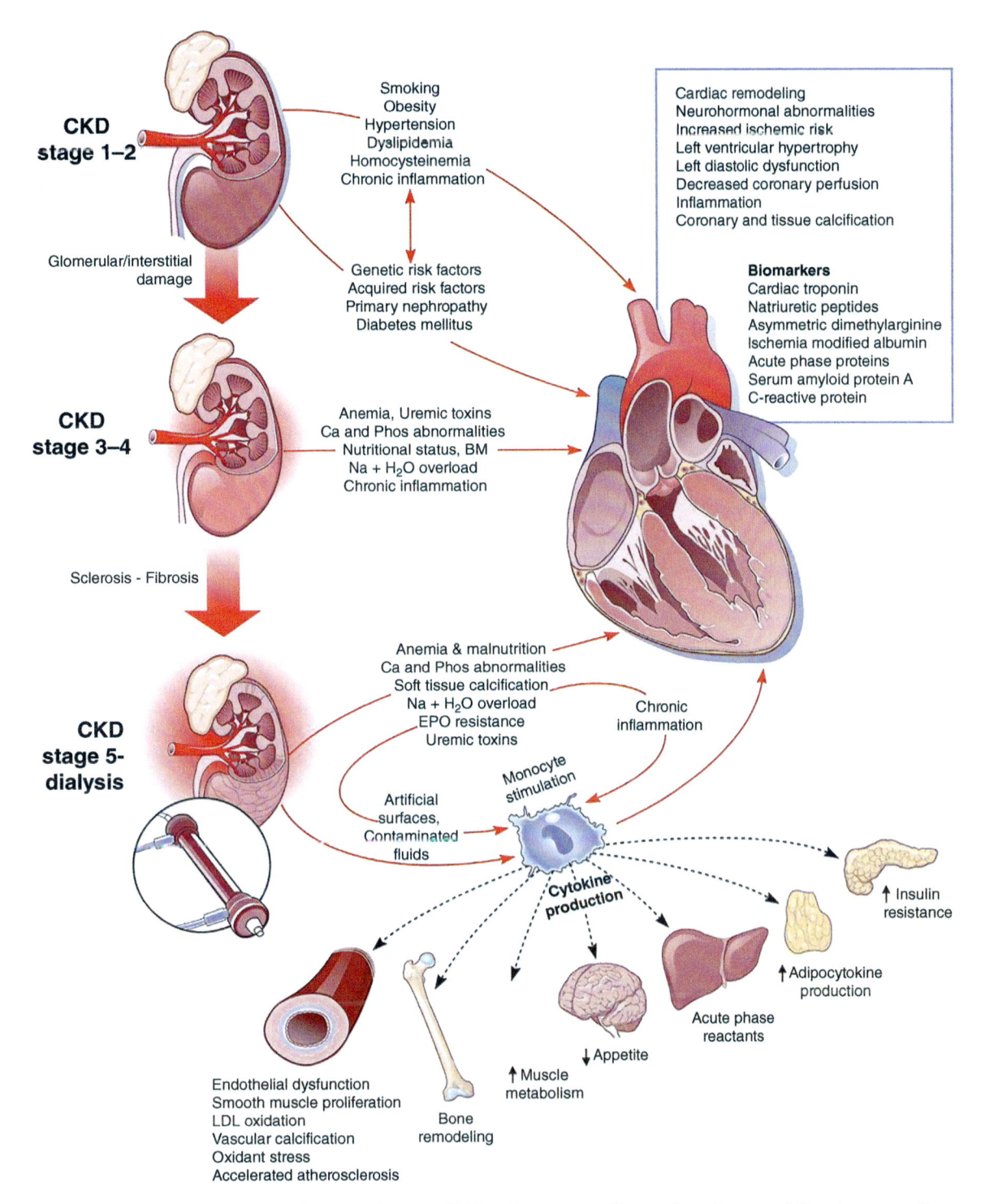

FIGURE 20.2 Pathophysiological interactions between heart and kidney in type 4 cardio-renal syndrome or "chronic renocardiac syndrome". BMI = body-mass index; CKD = chronic kidney disease; EPO = erythropoietin; LDL = low-density lipoprotein. Source: (Ronco et al., 2008).

protein-energy wasting in the CKD population include: the accumulation of nitrogen-containing products from dietary and intrinsic protein catabolism in the body that may distort taste and smell and blunt patients' appetite, which results in insufficient energy intake; coexisting medical conditions, and frailty, particularly in elderly patients who account for a large proportion of those who are affected by CKD; abnormal gastrointestinal nutrient absorption due to uremia, which affects the microbiome and disrupts intestinal epithelia.

However, beyond dietary adjustments to prevent or manage malnutrition, nutritional therapy may also help manage uremia and other CKD complications, such as electrolyte imbalances, water and salt retention, and bone disorders. Given the high prevalence of CKD and considering the

Table 20.2 Dietary guidelines for the management of CKD. BMI = body-mass index; CKD = chronic kidney disease; EAA = essential amino acids; GFR = glomerular filtration rate; HBV = high biologic value; KA = ketoacids; LPD = low-protein diet; PEW = protein-energy wasting.

Dietary constituent	Normal kidney function with increased CKD risk	Mild-to-moderate CKD	Advanced CKD	Ongoing dialysis or any stage with PEW
Energy (kcal/kg/d)	30–35; adjust to target weight reduction if BMI>30 kg/m^2	30–35; increase proportion with LPD	30–35; increase proportion with LPD	30–35; target higher intake if PEW present or imminent
Protein (g/kg/d)	<1.0; increase proportion of plant-based proteins	<1.0 (consider 0.6–0.8 if GFR<45 ml/min/1.73 m^2 or rapid progression)	0.6–0.8, including 50% HBV protein, or <0.6 with addition of EAA or KA	1.2–1.4; may require >1.5 if hypercatabolic state develops
Sodium (g/d)	<4 (<3 in patients with hypertension)	<4; avoid intake of <1.5 if hyponatremia likely	<3; avoid intake of <1.5 if hyponatremia likely	<3
Potassium (g/d)	4.7 (same as recommended for general population)	4.7 unless frequent or severe hyperkalemia excursions likely	<3 if hyperkalemia occurs frequently during high-fiber intake	<3; target high-fiber intake
Phosphorus (mg/d)	<1000; minimize added inorganic phosphorus in preservatives and processed foods	<800; minimize added inorganic phosphorus and encourage consumption of more plant-based foods	<800; minimize added inorganic phosphorus and encourage consumption of more plant-based foods	<800; minimize added inorganic phosphorus; add phosphorus binder as needed
Calcium (mg/d)	1000–1300 (adjusted for age)	800–1000	800–1000	<800
Dietary fibers (g/d)	25–30; target higher proportion (>50%) of plant-based foods	25–30 or more; higher proportion (>50%) of plant-based foods	25–30 or more; consider >70% plant-based foods	25–30 or more; suggest avoiding strict vegan diet

Source: (Kalantar-Zadeh & Fouque, 2017).

exceptionally high costs and burden of maintenance dialysis therapy and kidney transplantation, dietary interventions are increasingly chosen as a conservative management strategy for the disease. Nutritional management of CKD is generally focused on dietary protein, sodium, potassium, and phosphorus and aims at both managing CKD complications and achieving an optimal nutritional status. A synopsis of the dietary guidelines for the management of CKD is presented in **Table 20.2** (Kalantar-Zadeh & Fouque, 2017).

The optimal protein intake for patients with CKD is probably one of the most debated and challenging issues in disease management, given that the quantity and quality of ingested protein has been proposed as a risk factor for CKD. On the one hand, experimental evidence suggests that long-term dietary protein intake exceeding 1.5 g/kg/d may cause glomerular hyperfiltration and proinflammatory gene expression (Hostetter, Meyer, Rennke, & Brenner, 1986; Tovar-Palacio et al., 2011), which are known risk factors for CKD. On the other hand, a very low-protein intake can aggravate muscle wasting and contribute to both uremia, due to increased intrinsic protein catabolism, and severe malnutrition, given that CKD patients often suffer from cachexia (Wright, Southcott, MacLaughlin, & Wineberg, 2019). Altogether, the current evidence suggests that the ideal protein intake for CKD patients can vary from 0.6 to 0.8 g/kg/d for adults with moderate-to-advanced CKD (GFR <45 ml/min/1.73 m^2) and those with substantial proteinuria (urinary protein excretion > 0.3 g/d) to 1.2 to 1.4 g/kg/d for CKD patients on dialysis or with malnutrition aiming at preventing or correcting protein-energy wasting. In either case, about half of the protein ingested should be of "high biologic value" (e.g., from dairy products and lean meat) and adequate energy (30–35 kcal/kg/d) along with ongoing nutritional education should be provided to preserve muscle mass (Kalantar-Zadeh & Fouque, 2017).

Dietary sodium restriction is also an integral part of CKD nutritional management to control fluid retention, hypertension, and to improve patients' cardiovascular risk profile. Observations in the general population suggest a J-shaped association between sodium intake and cardiovascular risk, with an intake of >5 g/d or <3 g/d being associated with an increased risk of cardiovascular disease and death (Stolarz-Skrzypek et al., 2011). Although a daily dietary allowance <2.3 g of sodium (<100 mmol) is often recommended for patients with cardiovascular disease, there is no evidence that patients with CKD will benefit from this strict sodium restriction, given the risk of hyponatremia, worsening of nutritional status due to an unpalatable diet, and adverse cardiovascular outcomes. Therefore, a daily dietary sodium intake of <4 g (<174 mmol) is recommended for the overall management of CKD and its associated risks, and a sodium intake <3 g (<131 mmol) is recommended for CKD patients with symptomatic fluid retention, severe hypertension, or proteinuria (Kalantar-Zadeh & Fouque, 2017). A sodium restriction <3-4 g/d is translated into a diet characterized by a minimum consumption of packaged products (e.g., salty snacks and pastries), processed foods (e.g., cold cuts), or pre-cooked meals, a modest consumption of dairy products, grains, and meat, and allows for the addition of approximately 1 teaspoon of salt during cooking daily.

Dietary potassium is also an important target of the nutritional management of CKD, given that hyperkaliemia frequently occurs in patients with advanced disease and can be lethal. A modest dietary potassium restriction is therefore beneficial for most CKD patients. However, a very low dietary potassium intake can expose patients to unintended side-effects, such as an unhealthy atherogenic diet, given that many potassium-rich foods (e.g. fresh fruits and vegetables) are high in dietary fibers and vitamins and generally considered an integral part of a cardio-protective diet, and constipation, which may actually result in higher gut potassium absorption (Khoueiry et al., 2011; St-Jules, Goldfarb, & Sevick, 2016). Given the aforementioned, patients with mild-to-moderate CKD should aim for a potassium intake similar to that of the general population (4.7 g/d), while in patients with a tendency toward hyperkalemia (>5.5 mmol/L), a dietary potassium intake of <3 g/d (<77 mmol/d) is recommended, with the condition that a balanced intake of fresh fruits and vegetables with high fiber is not compromised (Kalantar-Zadeh & Fouque, 2017). To achieve this goal, CKD patients must be educated on the dietary sources of potassium, techniques to lower the natural potassium content of foods (e.g., peeling, cutting in smaller pieces, and changing water during cooking), and how to balance high- and low-potassium foods in their meals when they design their daily dietary plan.

Regarding phosphorus, hyperphosphatemia is also common in kidney failure, however a modest protein intake (0.8 g/kg/d) is generally equivalent to a diet with a modest phosphorus content, given that most high-protein foods, such as dairy and meat products, are also rich in phosphorus. Restricting dietary phosphorus intake to <800 mg/d (26 mmol/d) is recommended for patients with moderate-to-advanced CKD, this requires a modest fish consumption (no more than 1 serving/week) and the limitation of processed foods, in which food additives include readily absorbable inorganic phosphorus that can lead to a high phosphorus burden (Kalantar-Zadeh & Fouque, 2017). It should be noted that in dialysis, for patients who are at increased risk for protein-energy malnutrition, a strict reduction of protein intake to control hyperphosphatemia may be associated with poor outcomes and is therefore contraindicated (Lynch, Lynch, Curhan, & Brunelli, 2011). In this case, an individualized approach that incorporates the optimal use of phosphorus binders with meals that contain phosphorus (usually main meals, i.e., breakfast, lunch, and dinner), and the avoidance of phosphorus-rich snacks throughout the day is crucial for the optimal management of CKD (Tonelli, Pannu, & Manns, 2010).

Other important aspects of the nutritional management of CKD include an appropriate calcium intake, which in advanced CKD, is lower than that recommended for the general population (increased calcium release from bones in hyperactive renal bone disease is can cause a positive calcium balance that may worsen vascular calcification), an adequate vitamin D intake to manage renal osteodystrophy, an adequate intake of unrefined carbohydrates from plant-based foods to prevent constipation and promote a more favorable microbiome, a healthy dietary lipid profile with emphasis on mono- and poly-unsaturated fatty acids over saturated fatty acids, a reduced protein intake with a greater proportion of diet from plant-based foods to correct acidosis as well as the assessment and individualized correction of micronutrient deficiencies (e.g., iron, zinc, copper, folate, vitamin K, and vitamin D) through supplementation (Kalantar-Zadeh & Fouque, 2017).

PHYSICAL ACTIVITY, FITNESS, AND CHRONIC KIDNEY DISEASE

PHYSICAL ACTIVITY AND FITNESS STATUS OF CHRONIC KIDNEY DISEASE PATIENTS

CKD patients are characterized by low levels of physical activity and markedly poor exercise capacity. Decreased physical activity and fitness in CKD patients represent the beginning of a vicious cycle of declining physical function and disability, which, if left uncontrolled, continues to escalate progressively and negatively affects all aspects of the disease, including kidney failure, cardiovascular risk, and mortality (**Figure 20.3**) (P. Painter & Roshanravan, 2013).

Regarding physical activity, CKD patients can be characterized as a highly sedentary population. Most available data refer to dialysis patients, who have been shown to fail to meet physical activity guidelines and norms of the general population (Avesani et al., 2012; Johansen et al., 2010) and to report a significantly lower level of physical activity, assessed through accelerometers or pedometers, compared with gender- and age-matched healthy controls (Baria et al., 2011; Johansen et al., 2000; Zamojska, Szklarek, Niewodniczy, & Nowicki, 2006). It is worth mentioning that although data are insufficient for pre-dialysis patients, Agarwal et al. (Agarwal & Light, 2011) showed that actimetry-assessed physical activity level decreases as CKD progresses, with dialysis patients being the most sedentary, followed by pre-dialysis patients, and healthy controls. Although the etiology of inadequate physical activity in CKD has not been fully elucidated, possible explanations include: (a) the metabolic and nutritional consequences of the disease, such as fluid and electrolyte imbalances, uremia, anemia, bone disease, and malnutrition that combined lead to impaired muscle function and fatigue; (b) the presence of co-morbidities, such as obesity, hypertension, diabetes mellitus, and cardiovascular diseases that can contribute to reduced exercise capacity; (c) renal replacement therapy for ESRD patients, possibly due to the period of inactivity for the dialysis procedure itself (typically includes three 4-hour sessions per week), and to the post-dialysis fatigue syndrome often observed in ESRD patients; and (d) fear of injury or aggravating the disease, lack of guidance from healthcare professionals, and lack of local exercise facilities, which are reported by patients as barriers to exercise (Clarke et al., 2015; Roshanravan, Gamboa, & Wilund, 2017).

Regarding physical fitness, several cross-sectional studies clearly demonstrate that peak oxygen consumption (VO_2max) is significantly lower in CKD patients compared with population norms or with healthy control groups, averaging 50% to 80% of healthy levels (Johansen & Painter, 2012). This low VO_2max level suggests that most patients with CKD do not have the exercise capacity to sustain even simple lifestyle activities, such as housework and shopping, and that most of them meet criteria for cardiovascular disability. Besides VO_2max, performance in several other fitness tests, including hand-grip strength, leg extension strength, symptom-limited test, sit-to-stand test, timed up-and-go test, 400-m walk, and comfortable and maximal

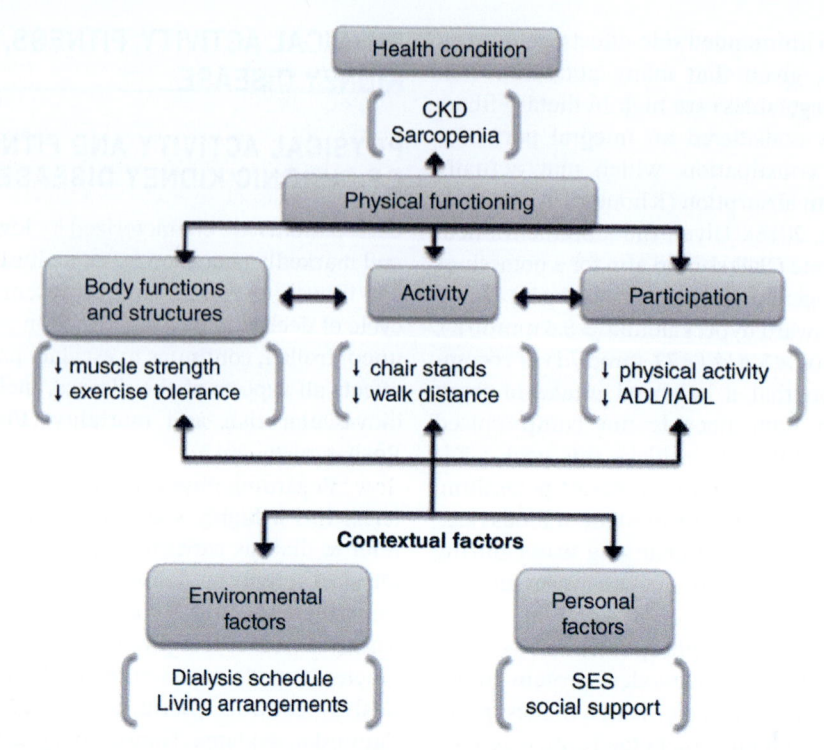

FIGURE 20.3 The impact of CKD on the components of functioning as described in the *International Classification of Function Framework*. The health condition and co-morbidities associated with CKD, such as sarcopenia, vascular dysfunction, inflammation, and malnutrition affect the three components of functioning: body functions and structures (at the level of body or specific organs and functioning of those systems); activity (the individual level—ability to ambulate, perform physical tasks); and participation (the whole person in their environment—participation in physical activity, ability to participate in life activities). Contextual factors of environment and personal factors affect both activity and participation components. ADL = activities of daily living; CKD = chronic kidney disease; IADL = instrumental activities of daily living; SES = socio-economic status. Source: (P. Painter & Roshanravan, 2013).

6-min-walking test, has been found significantly reduced in CKD patients compared to population norms, indicating that the CKD population is characterized by low muscle mass and strength and poor physical functioning (Brodin, Ljungman, & Sunnerhagen, 2008; Clyne, Jogestrand, Lins, & Pehrsson, 1994; Odden et al., 2006; Padilla et al., 2008). In addition, the few available prospective studies provide evidence of a gradual decrease in fitness indices, such as VO_2max, gait speed, and muscle area and density as CKD severity advances (Leikis et al., 2006; Liu et al., 2014; Roshanravan et al., 2015). Several CKD-related factors, such as uremic toxins, vitamin D deficiency, hyperparathyroidism, metabolic acidosis, and anemia have been proposed as causes of muscle wasting, altered neuromuscular function, and poor fitness in the CKD population, however, advanced age, the presence of co-morbidities, and low physical inactivity level are also possible mediators (Johansen & Painter, 2012).

PHYSICAL ACTIVITY, FITNESS, AND RISK OF CHRONIC KIDNEY DISEASE

Although the protective role of physical activity against other chronic diseases has been described extensively, little is known about its association with the development and progression of CKD. The findings of the available large-scale cross-sectional epidemiological studies suggest that a high physical activity level is positively associated with kidney function, i.e., higher values of GFR, and inversely associated with the prevalence of CKD both in the general population (Finkelstein, Joshi, & Hise, 2006; Hallan et al., 2006; Hawkins et al., 2011) and in diabetic patients (Kriska, LaPorte, Patrick, Kuller, & Orchard, 1991; Waden et al., 2008). However, given the cross-sectional design of these studies, it is not possible to distinguish whether low physical activity predisposes the patient to the development of renal dysfunction, reflects the poor exercise capacity of individuals with established CKD, or both.

Longitudinal studies on the association between physical activity and CKD are scarce, however, available data provide some evidence of the beneficial role of physical activity in CKD development and progression. The earliest report is dated in 1999, when results from the atherosclerosis risk in communities study of 1434 middle-aged diabetic adults revealed that a one unit increase in a leisure-time physical activity score (range 1 to 5; higher values indicate higher physical activity level) was associated with a 50% lower risk of early renal function decline, defined as a 0.4 mg/dL increase in serum creatinine levels, during 3 years of follow up (Krop et al., 1999). In a 2003 analysis of combined data from the national health and nutrition examination survey and the Medicare ESRD registry with a total sample of 9082 individuals who were followed for a 12- to 16-year period, Stengel et al. (Stengel, Tarver-Carr, Powe, Eberhardt,

& Brancati, 2003) showed that those who reported being inactive had approximately twice the risk of CKD, defined as either treatment of ESRD due to any cause or death related to CKD, compared to those who reported being very active, after adjusting for several confounders, including age, gender, race, body-mass index, alcohol, smoking, presence of cardio-metabolic diseases, and baseline GFR. Results from the Tromso study in Norway also support that among 4441 individuals without signs of CKD at baseline who were followed for 7 years, high self-reported physical activity (>1 hour of vigorous activity and/or >3 hours of light activity per week) predicted a significant increase (0.30 mL/min/1.73 m^2 per year) in GFR in women, although a similar trend was not observed in men. Moreover, in 2009, Robinson-Cohen et al. (Robinson-Cohen et al., 2009) analyzed self-reported physical activity and GFR data from 4011 men and women ≥65 years old who participated in the cardiovascular health study. A composite physical activity score was constructed based on leisure-time activities and walking pace (range 2–8; higher values indicate higher physical activity level) and, during a 7-year median follow up, participants with medium (4–6) and high values (7–8) had 15% and 30% lower risk of rapid kidney function decline, defined as the loss of GFR >3.0 mL/min/1.73 m^2 per year, compared to those with the lowest values (2–3), after adjusting for demographics, clinical, and subclinical disease characteristics. A few years later (2014) the same research team conducted the Seattle kidney study of 256 stage 3–4 CKD patients and showed that during a median 3.7-year follow up, participants who reported >150 minutes of physical activity per week had the lowest rate of GFR loss (−6.2% per year) compared with inactive participants (−9.6% per year); in adjusted analyses, each 60-min increment in weekly physical activity duration was associated with a 0.5% slower annual decline in GFR (Robinson-Cohen et al., 2014).

Besides physical activity, exercise capacity has also been inversely associated with the risk of CKD development. In a report from the Veterans Affairs Medical Center, Washington, DC (Kokkinos et al., 2015), exercise capacity was assessed in 5812 male veterans without CKD at baseline using a standard treadmill test; peak exercise capacity was estimated using standardized equations and was further categorized on the basis of age-stratified quartiles of peak metabolic equivalents achieved. According to the results of the study, during a median follow-up period of 7.9 years, the risk of CKD was approximately 20% lower for every one metabolic equivalent increase in exercise capacity. Moreover, compared with the least-fit individuals, low-fit, moderate-fit, and high-fit patients had approximately 15%, 35%, and 60% lower risk of CKD, respectively, after adjusting for several confounders (**Figure 20.4**).

PHYSICAL ACTIVITY, FITNESS, AND MORTALITY RISK IN CHRONIC KIDNEY DISEASE

Besides CKD development and progression, it is well established that physical inactivity and low levels of physical functioning are also associated with other clinical outcomes, and most importantly mortality, among CKD patients. As early as 2003, analysis of the United States renal data system dialysis morbidity and mortality study wave II data of approximately 2500 patients at

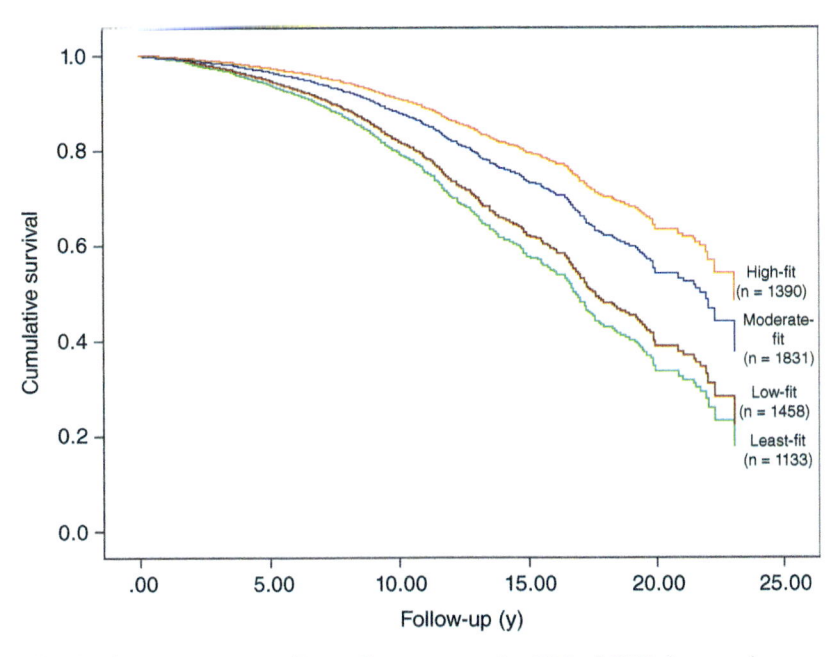

FIGURE 20.4 Cumulative risk for developing CKD according to fitness categories. Risk of CKD decreased progressively as fitness status increased. When compared with the least-fit individuals (reference group), the hazard ratios for the fully adjusted model (confounders: age, race, baseline GFR, body-mass index, cardiovascular diseases, cardiovascular risk factors, including hypertension, diabetes mellitus, dyslipidemia, sleep apnea, history of alcohol abuse, history of smoking, cardiac/hypertension medications, and lipid-lowering and hypoglycemic agents) were 0.87 (95% CI, 0.74–1.03) for low-fit, 0.55 (95% CI, 0.47–0.66) for moderate-fit, and 0.42 (95% CI, 0.33–0.52) for high-fit individuals. Source: (Kokkinos et al., 2015).

the time of initiation of dialysis showed that those who were sedentary (reported to exercise never or almost never) had a 60% greater risk for mortality than the non-sedentary ones during a 1-year follow-up period, after adjusting for co-morbidities and several other factors associated with mortality (O'Hare, Tawney, Bacchetti, & Johansen, 2003). A few years later, results of the same study revealed that mortality risk was significantly increased by 70% and 50% for patients who reported severe limitations in moderate and vigorous physical activities, respectively, compared with those reporting minimal or no limitations, during a median follow up of 4 years (Stack, Molony, Rives, Tyson, & Murthy, 2005). The beneficial effect of physical activity on health parameters of ESRD is also supported by the dialysis outcomes and practice patterns study (Tentori et al., 2010). Among a sample of 20,920 randomly selected hemodialysis patients from 12 countries who responded to a single question of exercise frequency, a 25% lower mortality risk was observed in patients reporting ≥1 time per week of exercise, compared to <1 time per week or never, after adjusting for demographics, co-morbidities, and socio-economic indicators. In addition, higher exercise frequency was also associated with higher scores in self-reported mental and physical health scales, less body pain, better appetite, better sleep, more positive affect, and less depression symptoms.

The national health and nutrition examination survey III is, to date, the only study that aimed to evaluate the association between physical activity and mortality in pre-dialysis CKD patients (Beddhu, Baird, Zitterkoph, Neilson, & Greene, 2009). In this study, 6% of the 15,368 participants had reduced renal function as indicated by a GFR<60 ml/min/1.73 m^2 and physical activity was assessed through self-reported data on frequency of leisure-time participation in moderate or vigorous activity, based upon which participants were categorized as inactive, insufficiently active, or active. As referenced to the inactive group, the risk of death was lower in both the insufficiently active group (−40%) and the active group (−55%); however, no difference in the risk of mortality was observed between the insufficiently active and active groups.

It is also worth mentioning that physical activity is associated with lower mortality risk in renal transplant recipients. In 2011, Zelle et al. (Zelle et al., 2011) reported that higher self-reported physical activity was associated with a significantly reduced risk of both cardiovascular and all-cause mortality as well as with a lower prevalence of metabolic syndrome and a higher creatinine clearance among 540 renal transplant recipients who were at least 1-year post-transplantation and followed for an average of 5.4 years. Another study in a sample of 507 kidney transplant patients showed that a higher physical activity level at the time of transplantation was associated with significantly reduced all-cause mortality and death with a functioning graft during a 8.4-year follow-up period (Rosas et al., 2012).

Besides physical activity, fitness level has also emerged as a strong predictor of mortality in the CKD population. In a 2013 report of 385 ambulatory, stroke-free participants with stage 2–4 CKD enrolled in clinic-based cohorts at the University of Washington, University of Maryland, and Veterans Affairs Maryland healthcare systems (Roshanravan et al., 2013), lower performance in hand-grip strength, usual gait speed, timed-up-and-go-test, and 6-minute walking distance measures was associated with significantly higher mortality among CKD patients during a median 3-year follow-up period. In adjusted analyses for age, gender, race, education, study site, smoking, body-mass index, GFR, hemoglobin, C-reactive protein, diabetes, and prevalent coronary artery disease, each 0.1-m/s decrease in gait speed was associated with a 25% higher risk for death, and each 1-s longer timed-up-and-go-test was associated with a 10% higher risk for death. Notably, gait speed and the timed-up-and-go-test more strongly predicted 3-year mortality than individual markers of kidney function or commonly measured serum biomarkers, i.e., GFR, serum bicarbonate, hemoglobin, C-reactive protein, albumin, and phosphate.

EXERCISE TRAINING AND CHRONIC KIDNEY DISEASE MANAGEMENT

Over the last several decades, numerous data have documented a broad range of important health benefits associated with exercise and these observations have served as the basis for the incorporation of exercise interventions as an integral part of disease prevention and health promotion (Kokkinos & Myers, 2010). However, CKD is a chronic condition that is still largely overlooked as a potential target for exercise therapy, in which the delivery of rehabilitation programs and exercise advice falls far behind that of pulmonary and cardiac services.

PHYSICAL FUNCTION

The effect of exercise on improving physical function is well established in CKD patients. Most data refer to dialysis patients, in whom aerobic exercise training has repeatedly been shown to improve physical functioning, which leads to improvements in VO_2max with an average increase of 20%, as well as in physical performance measures (gait speed, 6-minute walk and sit-to-stand test) and self-reported physical functioning (Cheema & Singh, 2005; Parsons & King-Vanvlack, 2009). In pre-dialysis patients, aerobic exercise has also been shown to significantly increase VO_2max (Aoike et al., 2012; Boyce et al., 1997; Eidemak, Haaber, Feldt-Rasmussen, Kanstrup, & Strandgaard, 1997; Mustata et al., 2011), exercise tolerance (Clyne, Ekholm, Jogestrand, Lins, & Pehrsson, 1991; Kosmadakis et al., 2012; Leehey et al., 2009; Pechter et al., 2003), and anaerobic threshold (Toyama, Sugiyama, Oka, Sumida, & Ogawa, 2010) with concomitant improvements in physical functioning measures and physical and overall quality of life (Aoike et al., 2012; Kosmadakis et al., 2012; Mustata et al., 2011). Although most studies in the CKD population have focused on the effects of aerobic training on physical function, evidence exists that resistance training can help increase muscular strength in pre-dialysis (Bohm et al., 2014; Heiwe, Tollback, & Clyne, 2001; Rossi, Burris, Lucas, Crocker, & Wasserman, 2014; Watson et al., 2015), dialysis (Baggetta et al., 2018) and post-transplant (P. L. Painter et al., 2002) patients. This is of high importance, given that one of the main causes for reduced exercise capacity in CKD is muscle weakness and that most CKD patients suffer from cachexia, a condition causing ongoing muscle loss that cannot be entirely reversed with nutritional supplementation. The beneficial effect of exercise on physical function is also supported by meta-analyses of the literature, suggesting that exercise interventions regardless of type, duration, or intensity, result in significant improvements in aerobic capacity, walking capacity and muscle strength (Heiwe & Jacobson, 2011, 2014). All in all, data so far suggest that all forms of exercise are effective at improving exercise and functional capacity in CKD patients, but more research is required to identify the optimal training methods. Physical activities that use large muscle groups and can be maintained continuously, such as walking, are most effective, although resistance training should be combined to improve muscular mass and strength, which can consequently improve functional capacity (e.g., walking) (Wilkinson, Shur, & Smith, 2016).

DISEASE PROGRESSION

A key aim in the treatment of CKD is slowing disease progression, and ultimately preventing the need for renal replacement therapy. While higher levels of physical activity have been associated with slower declines in kidney function, evidence regarding the effect of exercise-based interventions on improving kidney function or slowing CKD progression is little and controversial. Some interventional studies have failed to show beneficial effects on the GFR following exercise interventions (Boyce et al., 1997; Clyne et al., 1991; Leehey et al., 2009; Pechter et al., 2003), while others have reported statistically significant, albeit modestly clinically significant, increases in GFR (Baria et al., 2014; Castaneda et al., 2001; Toyama et al., 2010) indicative of exercise-induced improvements in the kidney function of pre-dialysis CKD patients that need to be further explored.

For instance, as early as 2001, Castaneda et al. (Castaneda et al., 2001) conducted a randomized controlled clinical trial among 26 CKD patients ≥50 years old and reported a significant increase in GFR levels (+1.18 ml/min/1.73 m^2) in patients who were subjected to a 12-week resistance exercise program (3 sessions/week, each involving 3 sets of 8 repetitions in chest and leg press, latissimus pull-down, knee extension, and knee flexion for about 45 minutes under the supervision of an exercise physiologist), versus a decline of -1.62 ml/min/1.73 m^2 observed in the control group. In another prospective open-labeled clinical trial by Toyama et al. (Toyama et al., 2010) among 19 CKD patients with established cardiovascular disease, a weekly in-hospital aerobic exercise (half-an-hour bicycle ergometer) plus home exercise (half-an-hour daily walking) intervention for 12 weeks significantly improved GFR (from 47.0 ± 13.7 to 55.2 ± 16.9 ml/min/1.73 m^2), with a significant difference compared to the control group, in which a trend for decreased GFR was observed (from 47.9 ± 9.5 to 44.6 ± 8.2 ml/min/1.73 m^2). Moreover, in 2014, Baria et al. (Baria et al., 2014) randomized 27 sedentary overweight CKD stage 3–4 men to a center-based supervised exercise group (n = 10; aerobic training on a treadmill 3 times/week for 12 weeks under supervision of an exercise physiologist), a home-based unsupervised exercise group (n = 8; aerobic training at locations nearby their home, backyard, park or street 3 times/week for 12 weeks according to the instructions), or a control group (n = 9; no intervention); a significant increase in GFR (+3.6 ± 4.6 mL/min) was only observed in the center-based supervised exercise group, with a significant group-by-time interaction versus the control group, suggesting that a more intense supervised exercise program is necessary for promoting renal function in CKD patients.

Although it remains inconclusive as to whether exercise impacts progression of CKD, the lack of consensus is mainly due to the lack of large-scale, long-term, well-designed randomized controlled trials with disease progression as the primary outcome. Despite the challenging nature of these trials, the primary aim of treatment in early CKD is preventing or slowing disease progression, therefore such research is well indicated and needed.

CARDIOVASCULAR RISK

To date, evidence of the effect of exercise on cardiovascular outcomes, i.e., cardiovascular morbidity and mortality, in CKD is scarce. However, a few studies have examined the effects of exercise on potential mediators of cardiovascular risk, such as blood pressure, arterial stiffness, and markers of inflammation and oxidative stress in the CKD population all point toward the cardio-protective effects of exercise.

With regards to blood pressure, Headley et al. (Headley et al., 2008) studied the acute effects of aerobic exercise (40 min of moderate walking at 50–60% VO$_2$max) on blood pressure in 24 pre-dialysis CKD patients taking antihypertensive medication and showed significant decreases for up to 60 min following exercise. Boyce et al. (Boyce et al., 1997) explored the effects of 4 months of aerobic exercise (supervised walking and cycling performed 3 times/week at a target intensity of 70% heart rate reserve for up to 60 min) on blood pressure in eight pre-dialysis patients with hypertension and reported significant reductions in systolic and diastolic blood pressure, which returned to baseline values following 2 months of detraining. Moreover, Kosmadakis et al. (Kosmadakis et al., 2012) investigated the benefits of walking exercise (30 min walking at a rate of perceived exertion of 12–14 performed 5 times/week) in 20 hypertensive CKD patients at stages 4–5 not on dialysis, compared to 20 CKD patients who served as a control group, and reported no significant changes in blood-pressure levels of exercising subjects; however, a reduction in the number of antihypertensives required to maintain good blood-pressure control was observed, along with stable values for stroke volume, heart rate, and cardiac output in the exercise group, compared to the usual-activity control group, which had an increase in antihypertensive prescriptions and reductions in stroke volume, heart rate, and cardiac output. Similar improvements in blood pressure have also been noticed in dialysis CKD patients following exercise interventions (Toussaint, Polkinghorne, & Kerr, 2008; Tsuyuki et al., 2003).

Exercise has also been shown to improve both arterial stiffness, i.e., the thickening of the arterial walls, and arterial compliance, i.e., the elasticity of arteries, in the CKD population. Mustata et al. (Mustata et al., 2011) performed a randomized controlled trial, in which 20 medically stable sedentary patients with stage 3–4 CKD were randomized either to 12 months of exercise (supervised training including twice-weekly in-center sessions with the choice of treadmill, stationary cycle, or elliptical trainer at a target intensity of 40% to 60% of VO_2max for 5–20 minutes, combined with home-based exercise of walking 3 d/week) or to standard care, and reported a significantly lower augmentation index, derived from pulse wave analysis of the radial artery indicative of arterial stiffness in the exercise arm compared to the standard care group (−11.7%). In addition, Toussaint et al. (Toussaint et al., 2008) designed a prospective crossover trial in 19 dialysis patients who were subjected either to an intradialytic exercise program (use of a bicycle ergometer for a minimum 30 min at each dialysis session) for 3 months or a 3-month period without exercise, with a 1-month wash-out period in-between. The exercise intervention resulted in improvements in pulse wave velocity compared with no exercise, suggesting that regular exercise in CKD may be associated with improvements in arterial compliance and a reduction in CVD risk.

Besides traditional CVD risk factors, CKD is also associated with increased inflammation and oxidative stress and although relevant data are limited, exercise interventions have been shown to be efficient at reducing both inflammation and oxidative stress markers in the CKD population. Castaneda et al. (Castaneda et al., 2004) performed a 12-week randomized controlled study of resistance exercise training 3 times/week among 26 patients with CKD on a low-protein diet (0.6 g/kg/d) and found that inflammatory markers, i.e., C-reactive protein and interleukin-6, were reduced following exercise compared to the control group (C-reactive protein: −1.7 mg/L in the exercise group vs. +1.5 mg/L in the control group; interleukin-6: −4.2 pg/mL in the exercise group vs. +2.3 pg/mL in the control group). In addition, Viana et al. (Viana et al., 2014) investigated the effect of acute and regular moderate-intensity aerobic exercise on neutrophil degranulation, activation of T lymphocytes and monocytes, and several plasma inflammatory markers (interleukin-6, interleukin-10, soluble tumor necrosis factor receptors, and C-reactive protein) in patients with pre-dialysis CKD. A single 30-min (acute) bout of walking induced a normal pattern of leukocyte mobilization and had no effect on T-lymphocyte and monocyte activation but improved neutrophil responsiveness to a bacterial challenge in the post-exercise period. Furthermore, acute exercise induced a systemic anti-inflammatory environment, evidenced by a marked increase in plasma interleukin-10 levels (peaked at 1-h post-exercise), that was most likely mediated by increased plasma interleukin-6 levels (peaked immediately post-exercise). Six months of regular walking exercise (30 min/d for 5 times/week) also exerted anti-inflammatory effects (reduction in the ratio of plasma interleukin-6 to interleukin-10 levels) and a downregulation of T-lymphocyte and monocyte activation, but it had no effect on circulating immune cell numbers or neutrophil degranulation responses. These findings provide evidence that walking exercise is safe regarding immune and inflammatory responses and has the potential to be an effective anti-inflammatory therapy in pre-dialysis CKD. Finally, in a 12-week study of a water-based exercise intervention in 17 CKD patients, Pechter et al. (Pechter et al., 2003) reported a reduction in oxidative stress, indicated by a decrease in products of lipid peroxidation and an increase in reduced glutathione.

PHYSICAL ACTIVITY RECOMMENDATIONS

Although evidence of the beneficial role of exercise in CKD is constantly emerging, targeted exercise recommendations for this population have not yet been produced, as opposed to other chronic diseases, such as diabetes mellitus and cardiovascular diseases, for which exercise guidelines have long been available to guide clinical practice. The lack of exercise recommendations for CKD patients can be largely attributed to the methodological discrepancies of the available interventional studies, which make the identification of the optimal exercise training program for this population difficult.

For instance, most available interventional exercise studies have been designed in dialysis patients, while data are limited for patients with CKD stages 2–5 and patients who have undergone kidney transplantation, therefore limiting the generalization of the effects of exercise in the whole CKD population. In addition, although aerobic training has been sufficiently studied, resistance training and its combination with aerobic exercise have been used only in a limited number of clinical trials in CKD patients. Regarding exercise intensity, frequency, and duration, available studies have mostly used moderate- to high-intensity exercise protocols, with varying frequency from 2 to 7 times/week (usually 3–5 times/week), varying exercise bout duration from 20 to 110 min (usually 30–60 min/week) per session, and varying total intervention duration from 2 to 12 months (usually 3–6 months). Although at this time, data are insufficient to identify the optimal training program for CKD, patients with impaired kidney function should be encouraged to avoid sedentariness and exercise should be used as an adjunct treatment to help improve many of the CKD-related morbidities, such as poor functional capacity, elevated cardiovascular risk, and cachexia (Heiwe & Jacobson, 2014), provided that consideration of potential risks associated with exercise and CKD-related contradictions are taken into account.

The most important consideration for exercise in CKD is related to patients' cardiovascular health. So far, no cardiac events have been reported in any of the published exercise training studies in CKD patients. In addition, the few available studies in which CKD patients were subjected to symptom-limited exercise testing reported some exercise-induced adverse outcomes, such as positive stress tests, hypertensive/hypotensive responses, or ventricular ectopy, only in a small number of patients with established cardiac disease (Leehey et al., 2009; Padilla et al., 2008). Beyond these data, the risks associated with exercise in the CKD population have not been studied, leaving the medical community to weigh the risks of exercise and physical inactivity based on what is known in other populations. It is well established that although physically active individuals have a lower risk of cardiovascular events both during activity and inactivity compared to inactive individuals, all individuals, even those who are regularly active, have greater risk of sudden adverse cardiac events while engaged in vigorous physical activity than when they are less active (Thompson et al., 2007). This risk is significantly lower for light and moderate-intensity activities compared to vigorous-intensity activities, and also greater for those who persist with a sedentary lifestyle than those who gradually increase their regular levels of physical activity (Thompson et al., 2007). With a view of preventing acute cardiovascular events during intense exercise, current guidelines for exercise prescription advise exercise testing prior to exercise training for individuals with diabetes mellitus or known cardiovascular disease and additionally state that exercise testing should also be considered in individuals who appear to be at a greater risk of having underlying coronary artery disease before engaging in a vigorous (>6 METs or >60% of peak heart rate) exercise training program (Gibbons et al., 2002; Thompson, Arena, Riebe, Pescatello, & American College of Sports, 2013). Regarding light- and moderate-intensity exercise training, a requirement for exercise testing would constitute a substantial barrier to participation for many individuals and could contribute to the increased risk associated with remaining sedentary. Furthermore, given that exercise testing is a symptom-limited or near maximal effort, its risks are probably greater than those of increasing participation in light or moderate-intensity activity.

Besides the potential cardiovascular risks of vigorous-intensity exercise, other important parameters that need to be considered before prescribing exercise to patients with CKD are the presence of hypertension, the risk of musculoskeletal injuries, and whether the patient is on renal replacement therapy. As previously mentioned, hypertension is highly common in CKD and consists of the main causes of the disease. Hypertension should be controlled before exercise, and the American College of Sports Medicine recommends not exercising if resting systolic blood pressure exceeds 200 mm Hg and/or diastolic blood pressure exceeds 110 mm Hg (Thompson et al., 2007). Musculoskeletal risk may also be increased in CKD patients due to renal bone disease, and fragility fractures and spontaneous quadriceps tendon ruptures have been reported in the CKD population. Additional special considerations need to be given to dialysis patients who may experience frequent fluid and electrolyte balance shifts. While exercise may be safer on non-dialysis days, studies have shown that exercise is also safe and effective on dialysis days and does not exacerbate systemic inflammation or immune dysfunction. In this context, intradialytic exercise, generally using a specially designed cycle ergometer, is available in some renal units and offers a valuable opportunity for supervised exercise (Smith & Burton, 2012). Patients can exercise their fistula arm but should not apply weight to that area.

Based on these data, it can be concluded that CKD patients should be encouraged to participate in light- and moderate-intensity physical activity to reduce the health risks associated with sedentariness. Risk assessment and preparticipation screening should be done on an individual basis as CKD patients are likely to be at a higher risk of exercise-induced death than the general population but also stand to benefit more from increasing physical activity. Potential risks from exercise can be reduced with appropriate education of the patients about abnormal responses, symptoms, and when to reduce intensity of exercise, defer exercise on a given day, stop exercise, and contact the physician; prudent recommendations for starting and progressing with the program; and regular assessment of participation and responses to the program. Given that the prevalence of CKD rises dramatically with age, with the majority of patients being >60 years old, and that several co-morbidities and some degree of functional disability often coexist with CKD, 2 sets of existing physical activity guidelines seem to be suitable for CKD patients: i) the physical activity guidelines published in 2018 by the US Department of Health and Human Services with emphasis on recommendations for older adults and those with chronic health conditions and disabilities (**Table 20.3**) (Piercy et al., 2018) and ii) the World Health Organization recommendations on physical activity and sedentary behavior published in 2020, with emphasis on recommendations for older adults, which are also relevant to individuals with chronic non-communicable diseases or disabilities (**Table 20.4**) (World Health Organization, 2020).

According to both sets of guidelines, to promote and maintain health older adults are encouraged to participate in moderate-intensity aerobic physical activity for a minimum of 150 min/week, i.e., a minimum of 30 min on 5 d/week (World Health Organization, 2020; Piercy et al., 2018). An equivalent amount of intense aerobic physical activity (60–75 min/week) or a combination of both moderate- and high-intensity exercise is also recommended, however, both guidelines emphasize that one should start with small amounts of physical activity and gradually increase duration, frequency, and intensity over time to the extent that their abilities and conditions allow (World Health Organization, 2020; Piercy et al., 2018). Moderate and vigorous activity corresponds to a level of effort relative to an individual's aerobic fitness, and the guidelines state that given the heterogeneity of fitness levels in older adults, for some a moderate intensity is a slow walk, and for others it is a brisk walk. On top of aerobic training, muscle-strengthening exercises as well as flexibility and balance exercises, also tailored to an individual's exercise capacity and progressed gradually, are also recommended with the aim to preserving and/or enhancing muscle strength and improving motor control (World Health Organization, 2020; Piercy et al., 2018). Until targeted recommendations for CKD patients are available, these guidelines can serve as a reference point for exercise prescription in the CKD population in clinical practice. Whenever possible, referral to a trained health care professional who is qualified to work with patients with chronic disease, such as physical/occupational therapists, cardiac rehabilitation specialists, or clinical exercise physiologists, is highly recommended.

Table 20.3 Physical activity recommendations for older adults and adults with chronic health conditions and disabilities by the US Department of Health and Human Services.

Key recommendations for adults (including older adults and those with chronic health conditions and disabilities).

- In general, adults should be as physically active as possible and limit sedentariness, since some physical activity is better than none and any amount of physical activity can lead to significant health benefits.
- Adults should do at least 150–300 min (equivalent to 2.5–5 h) per week of moderate-intensity, or 75–150 min (equivalent to 1.25–2.5 h) per week of vigorous-intensity aerobic physical activity, or an equivalent combination of both types of activity, to achieve health benefits. The column of aerobic activity should preferably be spread throughout the week.
- Additional health benefits can be gained by more than 300 min (5 h) of moderate-intensity aerobic physical activity per week.
- On top of aerobic activity, muscle-strengthening activities of moderate or greater intensity that involve all major muscle groups should be performed on 2 or more days a week, as these activities provide additional health benefits.

Additional recommendations specific for older adults

- Older adults can benefit from a multi-component physical activity regimen that includes balance training, aerobic, and muscle-strengthening activities.
- Older adults should determine and adjust their level of effort for physical activity based on their level of physical fitness.
- Older adults with chronic health conditions should understand whether and how their medical status affects their ability to perform physical activity safely.
- When older adults are not able to meet physical activity recommendations due to chronic health conditions, they should be as physically active as their abilities and conditions allow.

Additional recommendations specific for adults with health conditions and disabilities

- When adults with chronic conditions or disabilities are not able to meet physical activity recommendations for the general adult population, they should avoid inactivity and engage in as much activity their health status permits.
- Adults with chronic conditions or disabilities should be under the care of a health professional and consult a physical activity specialist about the type, amount, and intensity of physical activity appropriate for their health status.

Source: (Piercy et al., 2018).

Table 20.4 Recommendations on physical activity and sedentary behavior for adults aged 65 and above by the World Health Organization.

- All older adults should undertake regular physical activity.
- Older adults should do at least 150–300 min of moderate-intensity aerobic physical activity; at least 75–150 min of vigorous-intensity aerobic physical activity; or an equivalent combination of moderate- and vigorous-intensity activity throughout the week, for substantial health benefits.
- Older adults should also do muscle-strengthening activities at moderate or greater intensity that involve all major muscle groups on 2 or more days a week, as these provide additional health benefits.
- As part of their weekly physical activity, older adults should do varied multi-component physical activity that emphasizes functional balance and strength training at moderate or greater intensity, on 3 or more days a week, to enhance functional capacity and to prevent falls.
- Older adults may increase moderate-intensity aerobic physical activity to more than 300 min; do more than 150 min of vigorous-intensity aerobic physical activity; or an equivalent combination of moderate- and vigorous-intensity activity throughout the week, for additional health benefits.
- Older adults should limit the amount of time spent being sedentary. Replacing sedentary time with physical activity of any intensity (including light intensity) provides health benefits.
- To help reduce the detrimental effects of high levels of sedentary behavior on health, older adults should aim to do more than the recommended levels of moderate-to-vigorous-intensity physical activity.

Notes:

- For adults of this age group, physical activity can be undertaken as part of recreation and leisure (play, games, sports, or planned exercise), transportation (wheeling, walking, and cycling), work, or household chores, in the context of daily occupational, educational, home or community settings.
- Doing some physical activity is better than doing none.
- If older adults are not meeting the recommendations, doing some physical activity will bring benefits to health.
- Older adults should start by doing small amounts of physical activity, and gradually increase the frequency, intensity, and duration over time.
- Older adults should be as physically active as their functional ability allows and adjust their level of effort for physical activity relative to their level of fitness.

Source: (World Health Organization, 2020).

KEY POINTS

- CKD refers to a progressive and irreversible decline in renal function and is a major cause of mortality, mainly of cardiovascular etiology.
- CKD leads to metabolic abnormalities and nutritional deficiencies.
- Nutrition care in CKD aims to manage the complications of the disease, such as uremia and electrolyte imbalances, and preventing/managing malnutrition.
- Nutritional management of CKD involves an individualized protein, sodium, potassium, and phosphorus intake based on CKD stage and the patients' characteristics, along with ongoing nutritional education, support, and surveillance.
- CKD patients are sedentary and have markedly poor exercise capacity.
- A high physical activity level is positively associated with kidney function and inversely associated with the risk of CKD and mortality risk in CKD patients.
- In CKD patients, exercise can slow the disease progression, enhance physical functioning, and improve cardiovascular health.
- Exercise risk assessment and preparticipation screening in CKD should be done on an individual basis, however, light-to-moderate intensity exercise is considered safe for most CKD patients and should be recommended.
- The optimal exercise regimen for CKD patients has not yet been determined. Patients should generally be advised to avoid sedentariness and participate in moderate-intensity aerobic physical activity for a minimum of 150 min/week, with a gradual increase in physical activity according to their capabilities. Resistance training can additionally enhance muscular mass and strength as well as improve functional capacity.

SELF-ASSESSMENT QUESTIONS

1. What is the role of kidneys in human body metabolism and homeostasis?
2. Define CKD.
3. Briefly describe the link between CKD and cardiovascular diseases.
4. Provide an overview of the benefits of exercise in CKD.
5. Which are the most important risk considerations for exercise in CKD?
6. Why is optimal nutrition important for patients with CKD?
7. True or False: Exercise testing is a near maximal effort, and its risks are probably greater than those of undertaking light- or moderate-intensity activity in CKD.
8. True or False: Physical activities that utilize large muscle groups, such as walking, is the preferable type of exercise for CKD patients to enhance physical functioning, while resistance training has little additional value and is not recommended.
9. True or False: Patients with hyperkalemia (>5.5 mmol/L) should aim for a dietary potassium intake of <3 g/d through a minimal intake of fresh fruits and vegetables.
10. True or False: A modest protein intake, i.e., 0.8 g/kg/d, is generally equivalent to a diet with a modest phosphorus content.
11. True or False: Recommended calcium intake in CKD is higher than that recommended for the general population, due to increased risk of osteopenia and osteoporosis.

Fill in the blank(s) to complete the following statements:

12. Renal replacement therapy is advised once the estimated GFR is _____.
13. A high physical activity level is _____ associated with kidney function, i.e., _____ values of GFR, and _____ associated with the prevalence of CKD.
14. Exercise can improve both arterial stiffness, i.e., _____, and arterial compliance, i.e., _____, in the CKD population.
15. Current evidence suggests that the ideal protein intake for CKD patients can vary from _____ for adults with moderate-to-advanced CKD and substantial proteinuria to _____ for CKD patients on dialysis or with malnutrition.
16. A sodium restriction of <3–4 g/d is translated into a diet characterized by a minimum consumption of _____ _____, _____, and allows for the addition of approximately _____ of salt during cooking daily.

CASE SCENARIO

Mrs. MJ is a 58-year-old African-American woman who has been visiting the outpatient nephrology clinic of a public hospital due to a decline in her kidney function for 4 years. Her height is 1.60 m, body weight is 78 kg, and current urine production is 1200 to 1500 ml/day. Her medical history includes a 10-year diagnosis of hypertension, which has not always been adequately treated by medication. Her recent fasting biochemical evaluation revealed the following (numbers in parentheses indicate normal values): hematocrit at 36% (38–54%), glucose at 88 mg/dL (65–110 mg/dL), total cholesterol of 245 mg/dL (<200 mg/dL), triglycerides of 142 mg/dL (<150 mg/dL), creatinine of 2.5 mg/dL (0.6–1.3 mg/dL), urea of 105 mg/dL (17–55 mg/dL), uric acid at 8.7 mg/dL (2–7 mg/dL), sodium at 138 mmol/L (136–145 mmol/L), potassium at 5.3 mmol/L (3.5–5.1 mmol/L), and phosphorus at 5.0 mg/dL (2.7–4.5 mg/dL). She is currently treated with the following medications: Norvasc (antihypertensive), Tenormin (antihypertensive), tritralac (phosphorous binder), and Zyloric (antihyperuricemic).

Mrs. MJ is retired and lives with her younger sister who helps her in food supply and cooking. For lunch and dinner, she usually has red (pork) or white meat (chicken) 5 times/week (her typical portion size is approximately 250 g of cooked meat), fish once a week, and pasta once a week. She is particularly fond of dairy products, which she consumes daily, such as a cup of full-fat milk with cereals for breakfast, yogurt with fruit, or a big piece of white cheese with two slices of bread as a snack. She usually drinks 2 cups of coffee with sugar and milk per day and avoids sugar-sweetened beverages. She does not have any food allergies, drinks alcohol rarely during social occasions, and reports difficulty consuming her food without salt. Mrs. MJ recognizes the benefits of exercise and used to participate in organized group dancing and aerobic classes during her early adulthood. At the time of your evaluation, she is completely sedentary because she usually feels too tired to even walk for recreation, and the only type of physical activity she performs is light housework 1 to 2 times/week.

Questions:

1. Estimate the patient's GFR and assess her CKD stage (on-line GFR calculator: https://www.kidney.org/professionals/kdoqi/gfr_calculator).

2. Evaluate the patient's biochemical profile and medical history. Do you have any evidence to suspect that Mrs. MJ is at increased cardiovascular risk?

3. What kind of exercise program would you recommend to Mrs. MJ and why? Would you advise exercise testing prior to the initiation of the program? Which variables/endpoints would you want to assess in the long-term to evaluate the effects of exercise on her kidney function and overall health?

4. What kind of advice would you give Mrs. MJ regarding dietary protein, sodium, potassium, and phosphorous intake? Justify your recommendations based on current guidelines for the dietary management of CKD and her medication.

REFERENCES

Agarwal, R., & Light, R. P. (2011). Sleep and activity in chronic kidney disease: a longitudinal study. *Clin J Am Soc Nephrol, 6*(6), 1258–1265. doi:10.2215/CJN.10581110

Alani, H., Tamimi, A., & Tamimi, N. (2014). Cardiovascular co-morbidity in chronic kidney disease: Current knowledge and future research needs. *World J Nephrol, 3*(4), 156–168. doi:10.5527/wjn.v3.i4.156

Alicic, R. Z., Rooney, M. T., & Tuttle, K. R. (2017). Diabetic Kidney Disease: Challenges, Progress, and Possibilities. *Clin J Am Soc Nephrol, 12*(12), 2032–2045. doi:10.2215/CJN.11491116

Aoike, D. T., Baria, F., Rocha, M. L., Kamimura, M. A., Mello, M. T., Tufik, S., . . . Cuppari, L. (2012). Impact of training at ventilatory threshold on cardiopulmonary and functional capacity in overweight patients with chronic kidney disease. *J Bras Nefrol, 34*(2), 139–147. doi:10.1590/s0101-28002012000200006

Avesani, C. M., Trolonge, S., Deleaval, P., Baria, F., Mafra, D., Faxen-Irving, G., . . . Fouque, D. (2012). Physical activity and energy expenditure in haemodialysis patients: an international survey. *Nephrol Dial Transplant, 27*(6), 2430–2434. doi:10.1093/ndt/gfr692

Baggetta, R., D'Arrigo, G., Torino, C., ElHafeez, S. A., Manfredini, F., Mallamaci, F., . . . group, E. W. (2018). Effect of a home based, low intensity, physical exercise program in older adults dialysis patients: a secondary analysis of the EXCITE trial. *BMC Geriatr, 18*(1), 248. doi:10.1186/s12877-018-0938-5

Baria, F., Kamimura, M. A., Aoike, D. T., Ammirati, A., Rocha, M. L., de Mello, M. T., & Cuppari, L. (2014). Randomized controlled trial to evaluate the impact of aerobic exercise on visceral fat in overweight chronic kidney disease patients. *Nephrol Dial Transplant, 29*(4), 857–864. doi:10.1093/ndt/gft529

Baria, F., Kamimura, M. A., Avesani, C. M., Lindholm, B., Stenvinkel, P., Draibe, S. A., & Cuppari, L. (2011). Activity-related energy expenditure of patients undergoing hemodialysis. *J Ren Nutr, 21*(3), 226–234. doi:10.1053/j.jrn.2010.06.022

Beddhu, S., Baird, B. C., Zitterkoph, J., Neilson, J., & Greene, T. (2009). Physical activity and mortality in chronic kidney disease (NHANES III). *Clin J Am Soc Nephrol, 4*(12), 1901–1906. doi:10.2215/CJN.01970309

Bikbov, B., Perico, N., Remuzzi, G., & on behalf of the, G. B. D. G. D. E. G. (2018). Disparities in Chronic Kidney Disease Prevalence among Males and Females in 195 Countries: Analysis of the Global Burden of Disease 2016 Study. *Nephron, 139*(4), 313–318. doi:10.1159/000489897

Bohm, C., Stewart, K., Onyskie-Marcus, J., Esliger, D., Kriellaars, D., & Rigatto, C. (2014). Effects of intradialytic cycling compared with pedometry on physical function in chronic outpatient hemodialysis: a prospective randomized trial. *Nephrol Dial Transplant, 29*(10), 1947–1955. doi:10.1093/ndt/gfu248

Boyce, M. L., Robergs, R. A., Avasthi, P. S., Roldan, C., Foster, A., Montner, P., . . . Nelson, C. (1997). Exercise training by individuals with predialysis renal failure: cardiorespiratory endurance, hypertension, and renal function. *Am J Kidney Dis, 30*(2), 180–192. doi:10.1016/s0272-6386(97)90051-2

Brodin, E., Ljungman, S., & Sunnerhagen, K. S. (2008). Rising from a chair: a simple screening test for physical function in predialysis patients. *Scand J Urol Nephrol, 42*(3), 293-300. doi:10.1080/00365590701797556

Castaneda, C., Gordon, P. L., Parker, R. C., Uhlin, K. L., Roubenoff, R., & Levey, A. S. (2004). Resistance training to reduce the malnutrition inflammation complex syndrome of chronic kidney disease. *Am J Kidney Dis, 43*(4), 607-616. doi:10.1053/j.ajkd.2003.12.025

Castaneda, C., Gordon, P. L., Uhlin, K. L., Levey, A. S., Kehayias, J. J., Dwyer, J. T., . . . Singh, M. F. (2001). Resistance training to counteract the catabolism of a low-protein diet in patients with chronic renal insufficiency. A randomized, controlled trial. *Ann Intern Med, 135*(11), 965-976. doi:10.7326/0003-4819-135-11-200112040-00008

Cheema, B. S., & Singh, M. A. (2005). Exercise training in patients receiving maintenance hemodialysis: a systematic review of clinical trials. *Am J Nephrol, 25*(4), 352-364. doi:10.1159/000087184

Clarke, A. L., Young, H. M., Hull, K. L., Hudson, N., Burton, J. O., & Smith, A. C. (2015). Motivations and barriers to exercise in chronic kidney disease: a qualitative study. *Nephrol Dial Transplant, 30*(11), 1885-1892. doi:10.1093/ndt/gfv208

Classification and Diagnosis of Diabetes: Standards of Medical Care in Diabetes-2019. (2019). *Diabetes Care, 42*(Suppl 1), S13-s28. doi:10.2337/dc19-S002

Clyne, N., Ekholm, J., Jogestrand, T., Lins, L. E., & Pehrsson, S. K. (1991). Effects of exercise training in predialytic uremic patients. *Nephron, 59*(1), 84-89. doi:10.1159/000186524

Clyne, N., Jogestrand, T., Lins, L. E., & Pehrsson, S. K. (1994). Progressive decline in renal function induces a gradual decrease in total hemoglobin and exercise capacity. *Nephron, 67*(3), 322-326. doi:10.1159/000187987

Drawz, P., & Rahman, M. (2015). Chronic kidney disease. *Ann Intern Med, 162*(11), ITC1-16. doi:10.7326/AITC201506020

Eidemak, I., Haaber, A. B., Feldt-Rasmussen, B., Kanstrup, I. L., & Strandgaard, S. (1997). Exercise training and the progression of chronic renal failure. *Nephron, 75*(1), 36-40. doi:10.1159/000189497

Finkelstein, J., Joshi, A., & Hise, M. K. (2006). Association of physical activity and renal function in subjects with and without metabolic syndrome: a review of the Third National Health and Nutrition Examination Survey (NHANES III). *Am J Kidney Dis, 48*(3), 372-382. doi:10.1053/j.ajkd.2006.05.013

Gibbons, R. J., Balady, G. J., Bricker, J. T., Chaitman, B. R., Fletcher, G. F., Froelicher, V. F., . . . American College of Cardiology/American Heart Association Task Force on Practice, G. (2002). ACC/AHA 2002 guideline update for exercise testing: summary article: a report of the American College of Cardiology/American Heart Association Task Force on Practice Guidelines (Committee to Update the 1997 Exercise Testing Guidelines). *Circulation, 106*(14), 1883-1892. doi:10.1161/01.cir.0000034670.06526.15

Hakim, R. M., & Lazarus, J. M. (1995). Initiation of dialysis. *J Am Soc Nephrol, 6*(5), 1319-1328. Retrieved from http://www.ncbi.nlm.nih.gov/pubmed/8589305

Hallan, S., de Mutsert, R., Carlsen, S., Dekker, F. W., Aasarod, K., & Holmen, J. (2006). Obesity, smoking, and physical inactivity as risk factors for CKD: are men more vulnerable? *Am J Kidney Dis, 47*(3), 396-405. doi:10.1053/j.ajkd.2005.11.027

Hamrahian, S. M. (2017). Management of Hypertension in Patients with Chronic Kidney Disease. *Curr Hypertens Rep, 19*(5), 43. doi:10.1007/s11906-017-0739-9

Hawkins, M. S., Sevick, M. A., Richardson, C. R., Fried, L. F., Arena, V. C., & Kriska, A. M. (2011). Association between physical activity and kidney function: National Health and Nutrition Examination Survey. *Med Sci Sports Exerc, 43*(8), 1457-1464. doi:10.1249/MSS.0b013e31820c0130

Headley, S. A., Germain, M. J., Milch, C. M., Buchholz, M. P., Coughlin, M. A., & Pescatello, L. S. (2008). Immediate blood pressure-lowering effects of aerobic exercise among patients with chronic kidney disease. *Nephrology (Carlton), 13*(7), 601-606. doi:10.1111/j.1440-1797.2008.01030.x

Heiwe, S., & Jacobson, S. H. (2011). Exercise training for adults with chronic kidney disease. *Cochrane Database Syst Rev*(10), CD003236. doi:10.1002/14651858.CD003236.pub2

Heiwe, S., & Jacobson, S. H. (2014). Exercise training in adults with CKD: a systematic review and meta-analysis. *Am J Kidney Dis, 64*(3), 383-393. doi:10.1053/j.ajkd.2014.03.020

Heiwe, S., Tollback, A., & Clyne, N. (2001). Twelve weeks of exercise training increases muscle function and walking capacity in elderly predialysis patients and healthy subjects. *Nephron, 88*(1), 48-56. doi:10.1159/000045959

Hill, N. R., Fatoba, S. T., Oke, J. L., Hirst, J. A., O'Callaghan, C. A., Lasserson, D. S., & Hobbs, F. D. (2016). Global Prevalence of Chronic Kidney Disease - A Systematic Review and Meta-Analysis. *PLoS One, 11*(7), e0158765. doi:10.1371/journal.pone.0158765

Hostetter, T. H., Meyer, T. W., Rennke, H. G., & Brenner, B. M. (1986). Chronic effects of dietary protein in the rat with intact and reduced renal mass. *Kidney Int, 30*(4), 509-517. doi:10.1038/ki.1986.215

Johansen, K. L., Chertow, G. M., Kutner, N. G., Dalrymple, L. S., Grimes, B. A., & Kaysen, G. A. (2010). Low level of self-reported physical activity in ambulatory patients new to dialysis. *Kidney Int, 78*(11), 1164-1170. doi:10.1038/ki.2010.312

Johansen, K. L., Chertow, G. M., Ng, A. V., Mulligan, K., Carey, S., Schoenfeld, P. Y., & Kent-Braun, J. A. (2000). Physical activity levels in patients on hemodialysis and healthy sedentary controls. *Kidney Int, 57*(6), 2564-2570. doi:10.1046/j.1523-1755.2000.00116.x

Johansen, K. L., & Painter, P. (2012). Exercise in individuals with CKD. *Am J Kidney Dis, 59*(1), 126-134. doi:10.1053/j.ajkd.2011.10.008

Kalantar-Zadeh, K., & Fouque, D. (2017). Nutritional Management of Chronic Kidney Disease. *N Engl J Med, 377*(18), 1765-1776. doi:10.1056/NEJMra1700312

Khoueiry, G., Waked, A., Goldman, M., El-Charabaty, E., Dunne, E., Smith, M., . . . El-Sayegh, S. (2011). Dietary intake in hemodialysis patients does not reflect a heart healthy diet. *J Ren Nutr, 21*(6), 438-447. doi:10.1053/j.jrn.2010.09.001

Kokkinos, P., Faselis, C., Myers, J., Sui, X., Zhang, J., Tsimploulis, A., . . . Palant, C. (2015). Exercise capacity and risk of chronic kidney disease in US veterans: a cohort study. *Mayo Clin Proc, 90*(4), 461-468. doi:10.1016/j.mayocp.2015.01.013

Kokkinos, P., & Myers, J. (2010). Exercise and physical activity: clinical outcomes and applications. *Circulation, 122*(16), 1637-1648. doi:10.1161/CIRCULATIONAHA.110.948349

Kosmadakis, G. C., John, S. G., Clapp, E. L., Viana, J. L., Smith, A. C., Bishop, N. C., . . . Feehally, J. (2012). Benefits of regular walking exercise in advanced pre-dialysis chronic kidney disease. *Nephrol Dial Transplant, 27*(3), 997-1004. doi:10.1093/ndt/gfr364

Kriska, A. M., LaPorte, R. E., Patrick, S. L., Kuller, L. H., & Orchard, T. J. (1991). The association of physical activity and diabetic complications in individuals with insulin-dependent diabetes mellitus: the Epidemiology of Diabetes Complications Study-VII. *J Clin Epidemiol, 44*(11), 1207-1214. doi:10.1016/0895-4356(91)90153-z

Krop, J. S., Coresh, J., Chambless, L. E., Shahar, E., Watson, R. L., Szklo, M., & Brancati, F. L. (1999). A community-based study of explanatory factors for the excess risk for early renal function decline in blacks vs whites with diabetes: the Atherosclerosis Risk in Communities study. *Arch Intern Med*, *159*(15), 1777–1783. doi:10.1001/archinte.159.15.1777

Ku, E., Lee, B. J., Wei, J., & Weir, M. R. (2019). Hypertension in CKD: Core Curriculum 2019. *Am J Kidney Dis*, *74*(1), 120–131. doi:10.1053/j.ajkd.2018.12.044

Leehey, D. J., Moinuddin, I., Bast, J. P., Qureshi, S., Jelinek, C. S., Cooper, C., ... Collins, E. G. (2009). Aerobic exercise in obese diabetic patients with chronic kidney disease: a randomized and controlled pilot study. *Cardiovasc Diabetol*, *8*, 62. doi:10.1186/1475-2840-8-62

Leikis, M. J., McKenna, M. J., Petersen, A. C., Kent, A. B., Murphy, K. T., Leppik, J. A., ... McMahon, L. P. (2006). Exercise performance falls over time in patients with chronic kidney disease despite maintenance of hemoglobin concentration. *Clin J Am Soc Nephrol*, *1*(3), 488–495. doi:10.2215/CJN.01501005

Levey, A. S., de Jong, P. E., Coresh, J., El Nahas, M., Astor, B. C., Matsushita, K., ... Eckardt, K. U. (2011). The definition, classification, and prognosis of chronic kidney disease: a KDIGO Controversies Conference report. *Kidney Int*, *80*(1), 17–28. doi:10.1038/ki.2010.483

Liu, C. K., Lyass, A., Massaro, J. M., D'Agostino, R. B., Sr., Fox, C. S., & Murabito, J. M. (2014). Chronic kidney disease defined by cystatin C predicts mobility disability and changes in gait speed: the Framingham Offspring Study. *J Gerontol A Biol Sci Med Sci*, *69*(3), 301–307. doi:10.1093/gerona/glt096

Lynch, K. E., Lynch, R., Curhan, G. C., & Brunelli, S. M. (2011). Prescribed dietary phosphate restriction and survival among hemodialysis patients. *Clin J Am Soc Nephrol*, *6*(3), 620–629. doi:10.2215/CJN.04620510

Matsushita, K., van der Velde, M., Astor, B. C., Woodward, M., Levey, A. S., de Jong, P. E., ... Gansevoort, R. T. (2010). Association of estimated glomerular filtration rate and albuminuria with all-cause and cardiovascular mortality in general population cohorts: a collaborative meta-analysis. *Lancet*, *375*(9731), 2073–2081. doi:10.1016/S0140-6736(10)60674-5

Moore, P. K., Hsu, R. K., & Liu, K. D. (2018). Management of Acute Kidney Injury: Core Curriculum 2018. *Am J Kidney Dis*, *72*(1), 136–148. doi:10.1053/j.ajkd.2017.11.021

Mustata, S., Groeneveld, S., Davidson, W., Ford, G., Kiland, K., & Manns, B. (2011). Effects of exercise training on physical impairment, arterial stiffness and health-related quality of life in patients with chronic kidney disease: a pilot study. *Int Urol Nephrol*, *43*(4), 1133–1141. doi:10.1007/s11255-010-9823-7

National Kidney, F. (2002). K/DOQI clinical practice guidelines for chronic kidney disease: evaluation, classification, and stratification. *Am J Kidney Dis*, *39*(2 Suppl 1), S1–266. Retrieved from http://www.ncbi.nlm.nih.gov/pubmed/11904577

O'Hare, A. M., Tawney, K., Bacchetti, P., & Johansen, K. L. (2003). Decreased survival among sedentary patients undergoing dialysis: results from the dialysis morbidity and mortality study wave 2. *Am J Kidney Dis*, *41*(2), 447–454. doi:10.1053/ajkd.2003.50055

Odden, M. C., Chertow, G. M., Fried, L. F., Newman, A. B., Connelly, S., Angleman, S., ... Study, H. (2006). Cystatin C and measures of physical function in elderly adults: the Health, Aging, and Body Composition (HABC) Study. *Am J Epidemiol*, *164*(12), 1180–1189. doi:10.1093/aje/kwj333

Ogobuiro, I., & Tuma, F. (2020). Physiology, Renal. In *StatPearls*. Treasure Island (FL).

Padilla, J., Krasnoff, J., Da Silva, M., Hsu, C. Y., Frassetto, L., Johansen, K. L., & Painter, P. (2008). Physical functioning in patients with chronic kidney disease. *J Nephrol*, *21*(4), 550–559. Retrieved from http://www.ncbi.nlm.nih.gov/pubmed/18651545

Painter, P., & Roshanravan, B. (2013). The association of physical activity and physical function with clinical outcomes in adults with chronic kidney disease. *Curr Opin Nephrol Hypertens*, *22*(6), 615–623. doi:10.1097/MNH.0b013e328365b43a

Painter, P. L., Hector, L., Ray, K., Lynes, L., Dibble, S., Paul, S. M., ... Ascher, N. L. (2002). A randomized trial of exercise training after renal transplantation. *Transplantation*, *74*(1), 42–48. doi:10.1097/00007890-200207150-00008

Parfrey, P. S., & Barrett, B. J. (2015). Chapter 16 - Cardiovascular Disease and Chronic Kidney Disease. In P. L. Kimmel & M. E. Rosenberg (Eds.), *Chronic Renal Disease* (pp. 181–198). San Diego: Academic Press.

Parsons, T. L., & King-Vanvlack, C. E. (2009). Exercise and end-stage kidney disease: functional exercise capacity and cardiovascular outcomes. *Adv Chronic Kidney Dis*, *16*(6), 459–481. doi:10.1053/j.ackd.2009.08.009

Pechter, U., Ots, M., Mesikepp, S., Zilmer, K., Kullissaar, T., Vihalemm, T., ... Maaroos, J. (2003). Beneficial effects of water-based exercise in patients with chronic kidney disease. *Int J Rehabil Res*, *26*(2), 153–156. doi:10.1097/00004356-200306000-00013

Piercy, K. L., Troiano, R. P., Ballard, R. M., Carlson, S. A., Fulton, J. E., Galuska, D. A., ... Olson, R. D. (2018). The Physical Activity Guidelines for Americans. *JAMA*, *320*(19), 2020–2028. doi:10.1001/jama.2018.14854

Robinson-Cohen, C., Katz, R., Mozaffarian, D., Dalrymple, L. S., de Boer, I., Sarnak, M., ... Kestenbaum, B. (2009). Physical activity and rapid decline in kidney function among older adults. *Arch Intern Med*, *169*(22), 2116–2123. doi:10.1001/archinternmed.2009.438

Robinson-Cohen, C., Littman, A. J., Duncan, G. E., Weiss, N. S., Sachs, M. C., Ruzinski, J., ... Kestenbaum, B. R. (2014). Physical activity and change in estimated GFR among persons with CKD. *J Am Soc Nephrol*, *25*(2), 399–406. doi:10.1681/ASN.2013040392

Ronco, C., Haapio, M., House, A. A., Anavekar, N., & Bellomo, R. (2008). Cardiorenal syndrome. *J Am Coll Cardiol*, *52*(19), 1527–1539. doi:10.1016/j.jacc.2008.07.051

Rosas, S. E., Reese, P. P., Huan, Y., Doria, C., Cochetti, P. T., & Doyle, A. (2012). Pretransplant physical activity predicts all-cause mortality in kidney transplant recipients. *Am J Nephrol*, *35*(1), 17–23. doi:10.1159/000334732

Roshanravan, B., Gamboa, J., & Wilund, K. (2017). Exercise and CKD: Skeletal Muscle Dysfunction and Practical Application of Exercise to Prevent and Treat Physical Impairments in CKD. *Am J Kidney Dis*, *69*(6), 837–852. doi:10.1053/j.ajkd.2017.01.051

Roshanravan, B., Patel, K. V., Robinson-Cohen, C., de Boer, I. H., O'Hare, A. M., Ferrucci, L., ... Kestenbaum, B. (2015). Creatinine clearance, walking speed, and muscle atrophy: a cohort study. *Am J Kidney Dis*, *65*(5), 737–747. doi:10.1053/j.ajkd.2014.10.016

Roshanravan, B., Robinson-Cohen, C., Patel, K. V., Ayers, E., Littman, A. J., de Boer, I. H., ... Seliger, S. (2013). Association between physical performance and all-cause mortality in CKD. *J Am Soc Nephrol*, *24*(5), 822–830. doi:10.1681/ASN.2012070702

Rossi, A. P., Burris, D. D., Lucas, F. L., Crocker, G. A., & Wasserman, J. C. (2014). Effects of a renal rehabilitation exercise program in patients with CKD: a randomized, controlled trial. *Clin J Am Soc Nephrol*, *9*(12), 2052–2058. doi:10.2215/CJN.11791113

Smith, A. C., & Burton, J. O. (2012). Exercise in kidney disease and diabetes: time for action. *J Ren Care*, *38* Suppl 1, 52–58. doi:10.1111/j.1755-6686.2012.00279.x

St-Jules, D. E., Goldfarb, D. S., & Sevick, M. A. (2016). Nutrient Non-equivalence: Does Restricting High-Potassium Plant Foods Help to

Prevent Hyperkalemia in Hemodialysis Patients? *J Ren Nutr*, *26*(5), 282–287. doi:10.1053/j.jrn.2016.02.005

Stack, A. G., Molony, D. A., Rives, T., Tyson, J., & Murthy, B. V. (2005). Association of physical activity with mortality in the US dialysis population. *Am J Kidney Dis*, *45*(4), 690–701. doi:10.1053/j.ajkd.2004.12.013

Stengel, B., Tarver-Carr, M. E., Powe, N. R., Eberhardt, M. S., & Brancati, F. L. (2003). Lifestyle factors, obesity and the risk of chronic kidney disease. *Epidemiology*, *14*(4), 479–487. doi:10.1097/01.EDE.0000071413.55296.c4

Stevens, P. E., Levin, A., & Kidney Disease: Improving Global Outcomes Chronic Kidney Disease Guideline Development Work Group, M. (2013). Evaluation and management of chronic kidney disease: synopsis of the kidney disease: improving global outcomes 2012 clinical practice guideline. *Ann Intern Med*, *158*(11), 825–830. doi:10.7326/0003-4819-158-11-201306040-00007

Stolarz-Skrzypek, K., Kuznetsova, T., Thijs, L., Tikhonoff, V., Seidlerova, J., Richart, T., . . . European Project on Genes in Hypertension, I. (2011). Fatal and nonfatal outcomes, incidence of hypertension, and blood pressure changes in relation to urinary sodium excretion. *JAMA*, *305*(17), 1777–1785. doi:10.1001/jama.2011.574

Tentori, F., Elder, S. J., Thumma, J., Pisoni, R. L., Bommer, J., Fissell, R. B., . . . Robinson, B. M. (2010). Physical exercise among participants in the Dialysis Outcomes and Practice Patterns Study (DOPPS): correlates and associated outcomes. *Nephrol Dial Transplant*, *25*(9), 3050–3062. doi:10.1093/ndt/gfq138

Thomas, R., Kanso, A., & Sedor, J. R. (2008). Chronic kidney disease and its complications. *Prim Care*, *35*(2), 329–344, vii. doi:10.1016/j.pop.2008.01.008

Thompson, P. D., Arena, R., Riebe, D., Pescatello, L. S., & American College of Sports, M. (2013). ACSM's new preparticipation health screening recommendations from ACSM's guidelines for exercise testing and prescription, ninth edition. *Curr Sports Med Rep*, *12*(4), 215–217. doi:10.1249/JSR.0b013e31829a68cf

Thompson, P. D., Franklin, B. A., Balady, G. J., Blair, S. N., Corrado, D., Estes, N. A., 3rd, . . . American College of Sports, M. (2007). Exercise and acute cardiovascular events placing the risks into perspective: a scientific statement from the American Heart Association Council on Nutrition, Physical Activity, and Metabolism and the Council on Clinical Cardiology. *Circulation*, *115*(17), 2358–2368. doi:10.1161/CIRCULATIONAHA.107.181485

Tonelli, M., Pannu, N., & Manns, B. (2010). Oral phosphate binders in patients with kidney failure. *N Engl J Med*, *362*(14), 1312–1324. doi:10.1056/NEJMra0912522

Tonelli, M., Wiebe, N., Culleton, B., House, A., Rabbat, C., Fok, M., . . . Garg, A. X. (2006). Chronic kidney disease and mortality risk: a systematic review. *J Am Soc Nephrol*, *17*(7), 2034–2047. doi:10.1681/ASN.2005101085

Toussaint, N. D., Polkinghorne, K. R., & Kerr, P. G. (2008). Impact of intradialytic exercise on arterial compliance and B-type natriuretic peptide levels in hemodialysis patients. *Hemodial Int*, *12*(2), 254–263. doi:10.1111/j.1542-4758.2008.00262.x

Tovar-Palacio, C., Tovar, A. R., Torres, N., Cruz, C., Hernandez-Pando, R., Salas-Garrido, G., . . . Correa-Rotter, R. (2011). Proinflammatory gene expression and renal lipogenesis are modulated by dietary protein content in obese Zucker fa/fa rats. *Am J Physiol Renal Physiol*, *300*(1), F263–271. doi:10.1152/ajprenal.00171.2010

Toyama, K., Sugiyama, S., Oka, H., Sumida, H., & Ogawa, H. (2010). Exercise therapy correlates with improving renal function through modifying lipid metabolism in patients with cardiovascular disease and chronic kidney disease. *J Cardiol*, *56*(2), 142–146. doi:10.1016/j.jjcc.2010.06.007

Tsuyuki, K., Kimura, Y., Chiashi, K., Matsushita, C., Ninomiya, K., Choh, K., . . . Dohi, S. (2003). Oxygen uptake efficiency slope as monitoring tool for physical training in chronic hemodialysis patients. *Ther Apher Dial*, *7*(4), 461–467. doi:10.1046/j.1526-0968.2003.00084.x

Vart, P., & Grams, M. E. (2016). Measuring and Assessing Kidney Function. *Semin Nephrol*, *36*(4), 262–272. doi:10.1016/j.semnephrol.2016.05.003

Viana, J. L., Kosmadakis, G. C., Watson, E. L., Bevington, A., Feehally, J., Bishop, N. C., & Smith, A. C. (2014). Evidence for anti-inflammatory effects of exercise in CKD. *J Am Soc Nephrol*, *25*(9), 2121–2130. doi:10.1681/ASN.2013070702

Waden, J., Forsblom, C., Thorn, L. M., Saraheimo, M., Rosengard-Barlund, M., Heikkila, O., . . . FinnDiane Study, G. (2008). Physical activity and diabetes complications in patients with type 1 diabetes: the Finnish Diabetic Nephropathy (FinnDiane) Study. *Diabetes Care*, *31*(2), 230–232. doi:10.2337/dc07-1238

Watson, E. L., Greening, N. J., Viana, J. L., Aulakh, J., Bodicoat, D. H., Barratt, J., . . . Smith, A. C. (2015). Progressive Resistance Exercise Training in CKD: A Feasibility Study. *Am J Kidney Dis*, *66*(2), 249–257. doi:10.1053/j.ajkd.2014.10.019

Wilkinson, T. J., Shur, N. F., & Smith, A. C. (2016). "Exercise as medicine" in chronic kidney disease. *Scand J Med Sci Sports*, *26*(8), 985–988. doi:10.1111/sms.12714

World Health Organization. (2020). In *WHO Guidelines on Physical Activity and Sedentary Behaviour*. Geneva.

Wright, M., Southcott, E., MacLaughlin, H., & Wineberg, S. (2019). Clinical practice guideline on undernutrition in chronic kidney disease. *BMC Nephrol*, *20*(1), 370. doi:10.1186/s12882-019-1530-8

Zamojska, S., Szklarek, M., Niewodniczy, M., & Nowicki, M. (2006). Correlates of habitual physical activity in chronic haemodialysis patients. *Nephrol Dial Transplant*, *21*(5), 1323–1327. doi:10.1093/ndt/gfi323

Zelle, D. M., Corpeleijn, E., Stolk, R. P., de Greef, M. H., Gans, R. O., van der Heide, J. J., . . . Bakker, S. J. (2011). Low physical activity and risk of cardiovascular and all-cause mortality in renal transplant recipients. *Clin J Am Soc Nephrol*, *6*(4), 898–905. doi:10.2215/CJN.03340410

FURTHER READING

Bibliography

Drawz, P., and Rahman, M. (2015). Chronic kidney disease. *Annals of Internal Medicine*. *162*(11): ITC1-16.

Heiwe, S., and Jacobson, S.H. (2014). Exercise training in adults with CKD: a systematic review and meta-analysis. *American Journal of Kidney Disease*. *64*(3): 383–393.

Johansen, K.L., and Painter, P. (2012). Exercise in individuals with CKD. *American Journal of Kidney Disease.* *59*(1): 126–134.

Kalantar-Zadeh, K., and Fouque, D. (2017). Nutritional management of chronic kidney disease. New England Journal of Medicine. *377*(18): 1765–1776.

Painter, P., and Roshanravan, B. (2013). The association of physical activity and physical function with clinical outcomes in adults with chronic kidney disease. *Current Opinion in Nephrology and Hypertension*, *22*(6): 615–623.

Smith, A.C., and Burton, J.O. (2012). Exercise in kidney disease and diabetes: Time for action. *Journal of Renal Care.* *38*(Suppl 1): 52–58.

Stevens, P.E., Levin, A., and M. (2013). Kidney disease: Improving global outcomes chronic kidney disease guideline development work group, evaluation, and management of chronic kidney disease: synopsis of the kidney disease: improving global outcomes 2012 clinical practice guideline. *Annals of Internal Medicine.* *158*(11): 825–830.

Vart, P., and Grams, M.E. (2016). Measuring and assessing kidney function. *Seminars in Nephrology.* *36*(4): 262–272.

Wilkinson, T.J., Shur, N.F., and Smith, A.C. (2016). "Exercise as medicine" in chronic kidney disease. *Scandinavian Journal of Medicine & Science in Sports.* *26*(8): 985–988.

Links

- https://www.kidney.org
- https://www.kidney.org.uk
- https://nccd.cdc.gov/ckd
- https://www.theisn.org
- https://www.asn-online.org
- https://www.era-edta.org
- https://www.niddk.nih.gov/health-information/kidney-disease
- https://www.kidney.org/professionals/kdoqi/gfr_calculator

Cancer

CHAPTER 21

Introduction	347	Nutrition and Physical Activity in Patients Living With or Beyond Cancer	356
Risk Factors	347	Body Weight, Body Composition, and Physical Activity during Therapy	357
Excess Body Fat	348	Role of Nutrition and Physical Activity during Therapy	358
Alcohol	350	Role in Prehabilitation for Surgery	358
Red and Processed Meat	350	Role in Long-term Survivorship	359
Dietary Fiber, Whole Grains, Fruits, and Vegetables	351	Key Points	360
Calcium and Dairy Products	352	Self-assessment Questions	361
Sugar-Sweetened Drinks, Fast and Ultra-processed Foods	352	Case Scenario	361
Dietary Patterns	352	References	362
Dietary Supplements	353	Further Reading	366
Sedentary Behavior	353	Bibliography	366
Physical Activity	353	Links	366
Diet and Physical Activity Recommendations for Prevention	354		

INTRODUCTION

Cancer is one of the leading causes of death worldwide, ranking first or second after cardiovascular disease, in most countries. Worldwide in 2020, it was estimated, that 19.3 million new cancer cases and 10 million cancer deaths occurred (Sung et al., 2021). Almost one-quarter of total cancer cases as well as 19.6% and 14.2% of global cancer deaths were observed in Europe and America, respectively. Regarding cancer cases, female breast cancer was the most commonly diagnosed, while lung cancer was the leading cause of cancer death worldwide. Concerning gender, lung cancer was the most commonly diagnosed among men, while breast cancer was among women. The same was observed for cancer deaths (Sung et al., 2021).

These numbers are expected to rise, as 23.6 million new cancer cases will be diagnosed annually by 2040 due to aging and growth of the population (Jemal A et al., 2019). Therefore, optimal primary prevention and management actions should be taken to address this public health issue.

RISK FACTORS

Cancer research has expanded in the last decades, increasing our understanding in the molecular pathways that lead to cancer development. Cancer development is associated with a disruption of molecular pathways and the function of specific genes that control normal cell proliferation, growth, and apoptosis through genetic and epigenetic changes. Despite the fact that there are numerous relevant molecular events, the main characteristics of most cancers are known as the "hallmarks of cancer" and are summarized in the 2018 expert report of the World Cancer Research Fund (WCRF) and the American Institute for Cancer Research (AICR) (**Figure 21.1**) (WCRF/AICR, 2018).

The process of cancer development typically lasts many years. During these years, lots of different environmental factors, including diet and physical activity may interact with host factors and, as a consequence, can protect from or increase the susceptibility to cancer development (**Figure 21.2**) (WCRF/AICR, 2018).

Prevention and Management of Cardiovascular and Metabolic Disease: Diet, Physical Activity and Healthy Aging,
First Edition. Christina N. Katsagoni, Peter Kokkinos, and Labros S. Sidossis.
© 2023 John Wiley & Sons Ltd. Published 2023 by John Wiley & Sons Ltd.

Our first knowledge of the effects of environmental exposures on the risk of developing cancer dates back to the 1960s, when individuals, who moved from countries with low risk of some cancers to high risk countries were reported to have an increase in cancer rates at equal levels, or even higher, compared to the host population (Shimizu H. et al., 1987). Since then, there is abundant evidence, mainly from observational studies that have shown the importance of environmental factors, which account for 90% to 95% of cancer cases, while the remaining 5% to 10% are due to genes (Anand et al., 2008).

According to the WHO, between 30% and 50% of all cancer cases worldwide are estimated to be prevented though lower exposure to tobacco, infectious agents, and occupational carcinogens as well as through alterations in lifestyle factors, such as adherence to a healthy diet, preventing or managing overweight or obesity, and engaging with physical activity (WHO, 2019). Considering current estimates about lifestyle, diet is attributable to 20% to 25% of cancer burden. This range seems to include a 10% to 15%, which encompasses excess body weight and physical inactivity, approximately 5% is attributed to alcohol and the remaining 5% to dietary factors (Giovannucci, 2018). Therefore, understanding the magnitude of these factors is of major importance to potentially prevent several cancer cases through lifestyle modifications.

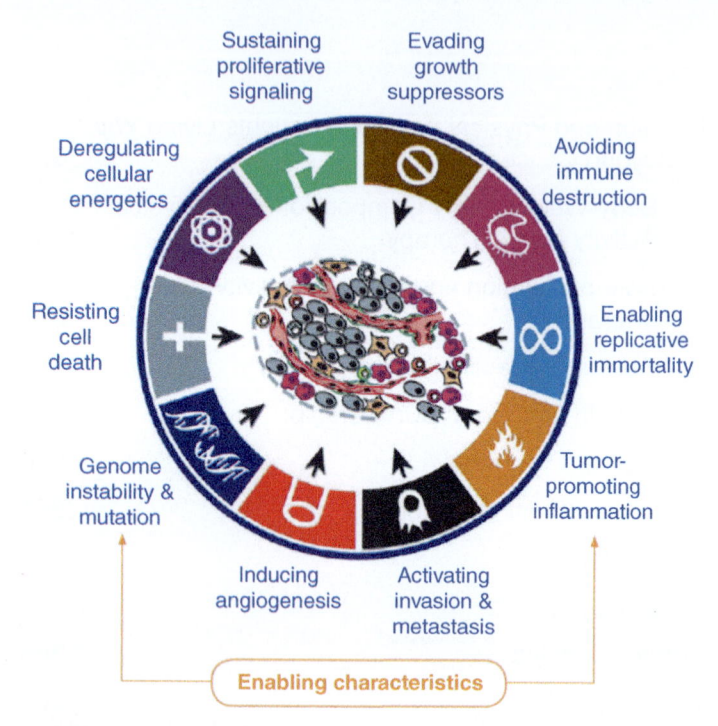

FIGURE 21.1 Hallmarks of cancer and two enabling characteristics. Source: (WCRF/AICR, 2018).

EXCESS BODY FAT

Overweight and obesity are collectively characterized by abnormal, and excess, fat accumulation associated with the incidence of several different disease entities. Data by the WHO have shown that 1.9 billion adults and 340 million children and adolescents were living with excess body weight in 2016, and it is estimated that these numbers will be increased (WHO, 2020).

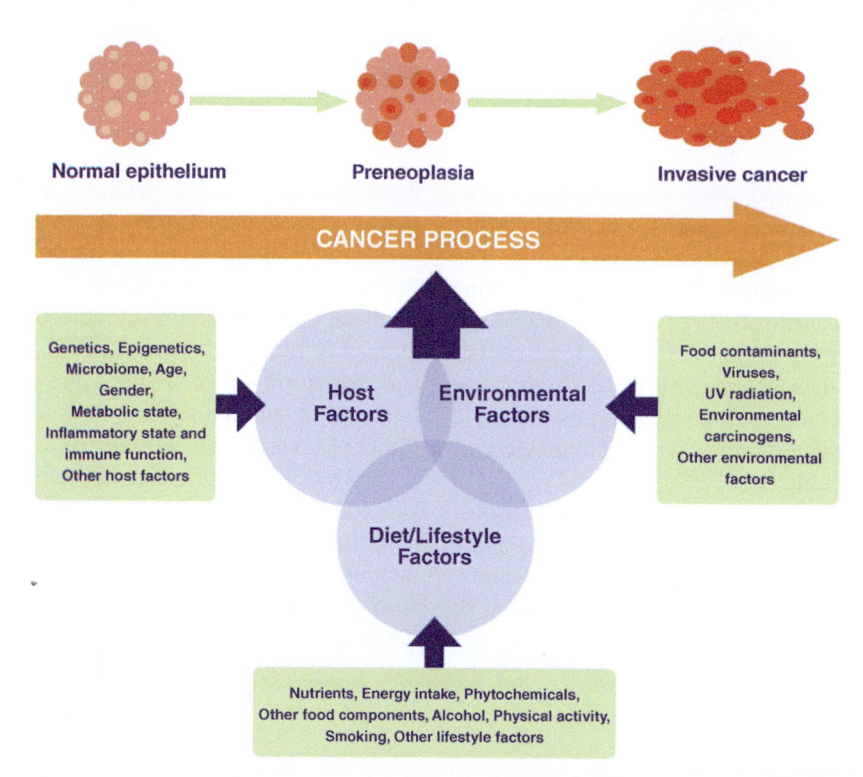

FIGURE 21.2 Diet, nutrition, physical activity, other environmental exposures, and host factors interact to affect the cancer process. Source: (WCRF/AICR, 2018).

Worldwide, considering lifestyle factors, obesity is ranked as the second leading preventable cause after smoking and, in general, is considered the third risk factor for cancer incidence after smoking and infections. Should obesity trends continue to rise over the next years, it is projected to lead, in the USA, to at least 500,000 additional cases annually and will be the leading modifiable risk factor of cancer, exceeding smoking. At a global level, approximately 3.9% of all types of cancers in 2012 were attributable to overweight and obesity levels in 2002 (Arnold et al., 2015), with the proportions across countries varying widely, ranging from 0.4% to 8.2%.

There is consistent data over the last several decades that support the association between overweight, obesity, and cancer risk. The 2018 WCRF/AICR expert report concluded that being overweight or obesity in adulthood increases the risk of some types of cancers, including colorectum, post-menopausal breast, kidney, endometrium, adenocarcinoma of esophagus, liver, pancreas, advanced prostate, gastric cardia, oral, oropharyngeal, and larynx, while weight gain in adults is strongly associated with a high risk of post-menopausal cancer (WCRF/AICR, 2018).

Endometrial cancer has one of the strongest associations with obesity, with each 5 kg/m² increase in body-mass index (BMI) related to a 54% higher risk of cancer (D. Aune et al., 2015). Moreover, the *International Agency for Research on Cancer (IARC) Handbook* reported evidence that excess body weight is further associated with a high risk of thyroid cancer, meningioma, and multiple myeloma (Lauby-Secretan et al., 2016). On the other hand, it seems that being overweight or obesity in young adulthood (i.e.,18–30 years) protects against both pro- and post-menopausal breast cancer, although the higher risk of post-menopausal breast cancer later in life outweighs any potential benefit (WCRF/AICR, 2018).

Given the burden of overweight and obesity, there were interesting data from recent observational studies regarding weight management and the risk of developing cancer. A pooled analysis of prospective studies with regard to diet and cancer (Teras et al., 2020) including approximately 180,000 women aged ≥50 years, reported that women who sustained weight loss (more than 2 kg between baseline and the first follow up, that was not regained after a 10-year final follow up) had a lower risk of breast cancer compared with women whose weight was stable. In general, this study demonstrated that the greater the weight loss, the lower the risk of breast cancer. In the same context, the UK women's cohort study (Moy et al., 2018) concluded that women who lost weight had a lower risk of post-menopausal breast cancer compared to women who gained weight or had a stable weight. Moreover, the women's health initiative study demonstrated lower risks of both endometrial and breast cancers' incidence in women with weight loss compared with those whose weight remained stable (Chlebowski et al., 2019; Luo et al., 2017).

Moreover, data from the Look AHEAD trial demonstrated, that individuals with overweight or obesity and type 2 diabetes, who successfully achieved weight loss by reducing energy intake and increasing physical activity, had a 16% lower risk of cancers related to obesity (Yeh et al., 2020). There are, also, few data regarding the beneficial effects of bariatric surgery in cancer risk. According to a 2019 systematic review and meta-analysis of eight population-based cohort studies that included 635,642 patients (114,020 patients who have undergone bariatric surgery and 521,622 controls), bariatric surgery was significantly associated with a 45% lower incidence of obesity-associated tumor types (Wiggins et al., 2019).

Multiple mechanisms have been proposed to explain the link between excess body weight and cancer incidence (**Figure 21.3**). In obesity, hypoxia of the adipose tissue contributes to a chronic low grade inflammatory state, which leads to changes in its structural and functional damage, such as abnormal adipokines secretion, e.g., adiponectin and leptin. Increased leptin levels, as observed in obesity, have been shown to trigger tumor initiation and further metastasis in several types of cancer, including liver, lung, breast, colorectal, kidney, and prostate cancers (Ghasemi et al., 2019; Sánchez-Jiménez et al., 2019).

Furthermore, hyperinsulinemia, insulin resistance, and abnormalities in the insulin-like growth factor-1 (IGF-1) axis

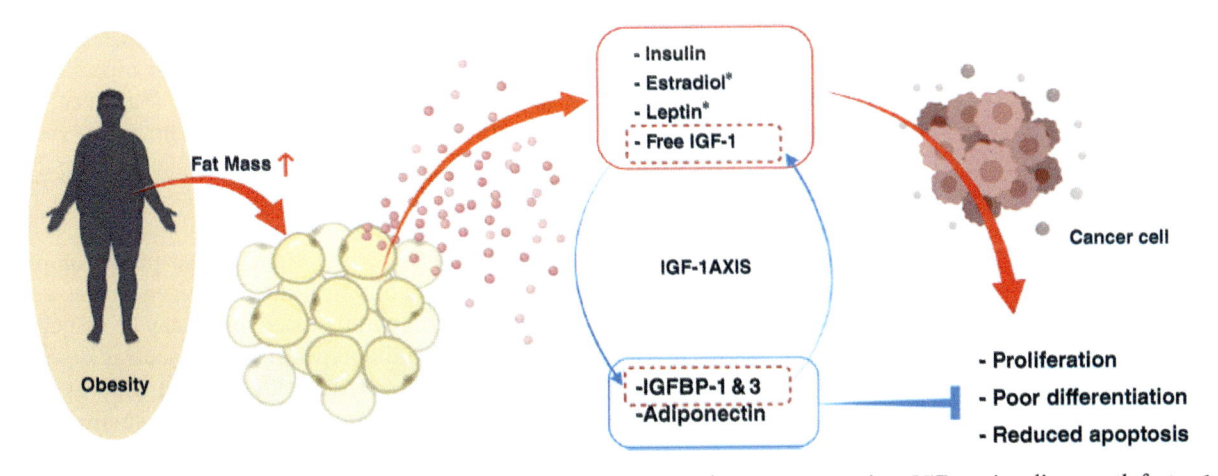

FIGURE 21.3 Proposed mechanisms for the association between body fatness and cancer progression. IGF-1 = insulin growth factor-1; IGFBP1 & 3 = insulin growth factor binding proteins-1 & 3. Source: (Wilson et al., 2022).

have been proposed as important mechanisms. Insulin can promote carcinogenesis through direct and indirect stimulation of cells. It can increase the circulation levels of the IGF-1 through a reduction in the circulating levels of its binding proteins. IGF-1 and insulin can activate mechanisms related to proliferation, angiogenesis, and inhibition of apoptosis, all of which are associated with tumorigenesis (Hopkins et al., 2020; Jiramongkol & Lam, 2020). It is well-established that both insulin resistance and hyperinsulinemia are common in obesity, and as a result they can increase cancer risk in obese individuals.

Finally, in the context of obesity, higher levels of estrogens are observed due to the higher activity of the enzyme aromatase in adipose tissue. Consequently, higher conversion rates of androgens to estradiol are observed. Elevated levels of estrogens can promote carcinogenesis and have been shown to increase breast cancer risk (Fortner et al., 2016) as well as endometrial cancer (Shaw et al., 2016).

ALCOHOL

Alcoholic beverages have been classified as carcinogenic to humans since 1988 (IARC, 1988). Only in 2012 was it estimated that 5.5% of new cancer cases was attributed to alcohol consumption (Praud et al., 2016). Recently, both the updated IARC monographs and the 2018 WCRF/AIRC report concluded that there is sufficient evidence that alcohol consumption increases the risk of several types of cancer, including cancers of upper aerodigestive tract, e.g., mouth, larynx, pharynx, esophagus (squamous cell carcinoma), and cancers of the liver, colorectum, stomach, and female breast (WCRF/AICR, 2018; Wild CP, 2020). According to the 2018 WCRF/AICR report, there is probable evidence that alcoholic drinks consumption is associated with a higher risk of cancers of the pancreas, lung, and skin (basal cell carcinoma and malignant melanoma), although, this relationship may be confounded by other lifestyle factors, such as smoking. On the other hand, the same report concluded that there is probable evidence showing an inverse association between moderate alcohol consumption (up to 2 alcoholic drinks per day) and risk of kidney cancer (WCRF/AICR, 2018).

Both the amount of alcohol consumed and the type of cancer may affect the magnitude of the increase of cancer risk. The greater risks are observed in heavy (namely ≥3 drinks per day or ≥8 drinks per week for women; ≥4 drinks per day or ≥15 drinks per week for men) and moderate (defined as ≤1 drink per day for women and ≤2 drinks per day for men) alcohol consumption categories (LoConte et al., 2018). However, the risk for some types of cancer is present even at low levels of consumption, as reported in a meta-analysis of observational studies of approximately 92,000 light drinkers (up to 1 drink/d), in which drinking no more than one alcoholic beverage per day was associated with a higher risk of oropharyngeal cancer, female breast cancer, and esophageal cancer (squamous cell carcinoma) (Bagnardi et al., 2013).

Alcohol contains a plethora of substances. Some of them, such as resveratrol, a phytochemical found in red wine, have been shown in laboratory studies to associate with anticarcinogenic properties (Dybkowska E. et al., 2018). However, human studies have not reported benefits from drinking red wine regarding cancer prevention. The 2018 WCRF/AIRC report concluded that the devastating effects of alcoholic beverages in cancer risk have been observed consistently, regardless of the type of alcoholic drink.

There is an emerging body of research showing that despite the presence of several carcinogenic compounds, the major cause of the relationship between alcohol consumption and cancer development is ethanol. Its metabolite, acetaldehyde, is characterized as human carcinogen that can rapidly bind to DNA and cause mutations (Liu et al., 2015). Furthermore, through its metabolism, reactive oxygen species are generated and as a consequence, DNA damage is observed. Moreover, it is considered that ethanol can act as a solvent that enhances the penetration of carcinogenic compounds into cells. People exposed to the concurrent use of alcohol and tobacco have higher risks of cancers of the respiratory tract and upper digestive area. A further mechanism that may explain the higher risk of breast cancer and hormone sensitive cancers in general, is the increase of estrogen circulating levels and the higher proliferation of estrogen receptors (Liu et al., 2015).

RED AND PROCESSED MEAT

Unprocessed meat, such as beef, lamp, pork, mutton, goat, and veal meat are referred to as red meat. The term "processed meat" includes meat that has been processed through smoking, curing, salting, and fermentation as well as procedures used to preserve foods or enhance flavor. This can include bacon, ham, salami, and sausages, except for fresh sausages that may not always be included as processed meat (Bouvard et al., 2015).

In 2015, IARC experts reported that processed meat was classified as a Group 1 carcinogen (strong evidence that it causes cancer), whereas red meat as a Group 2A carcinogen (it probably causes cancer), based on sufficient data with regard to colorectal cancer (IARC, 2015). A meta-analysis published in 2011 included 10 cohort studies and concluded that there was a significant 17% increased risk of colorectal cancer per 100 g/d of red meat, and an 18% increased risk per 50 g/d of processed red meat (Chan et al., 2011). Similarly, the 2018 WCRF/AICR report demonstrated that there is strong evidence that processed meat "convincingly" increases colorectal cancer incidence, whereas red meat is "probably" associated with an increased risk of colorectal cancer. The analysis of the available data reported that per 100 g/d of red meat, the risk of colorectal cancer increases by 12%, whereas per 50 g/d of processed red meat, it increases by 16% (WCRF/AICR, 2018). Notably, except for colorectal cancer, there is growing, but still limited evidence that a higher consumption of red and processed meat may be associated with an increased risk of other types of cancer, such as stomach, prostate and breast cancers (IARC, 2015; Inoue-Choi et al., 2016; Wu et al., 2016). In a systematic review and meta-analysis of 148 prospective studies, the high intake of total red and processed meat further increased the risk of lung and renal cancers by approximately 20% and 19%, respectively (Farvid et al., 2021).

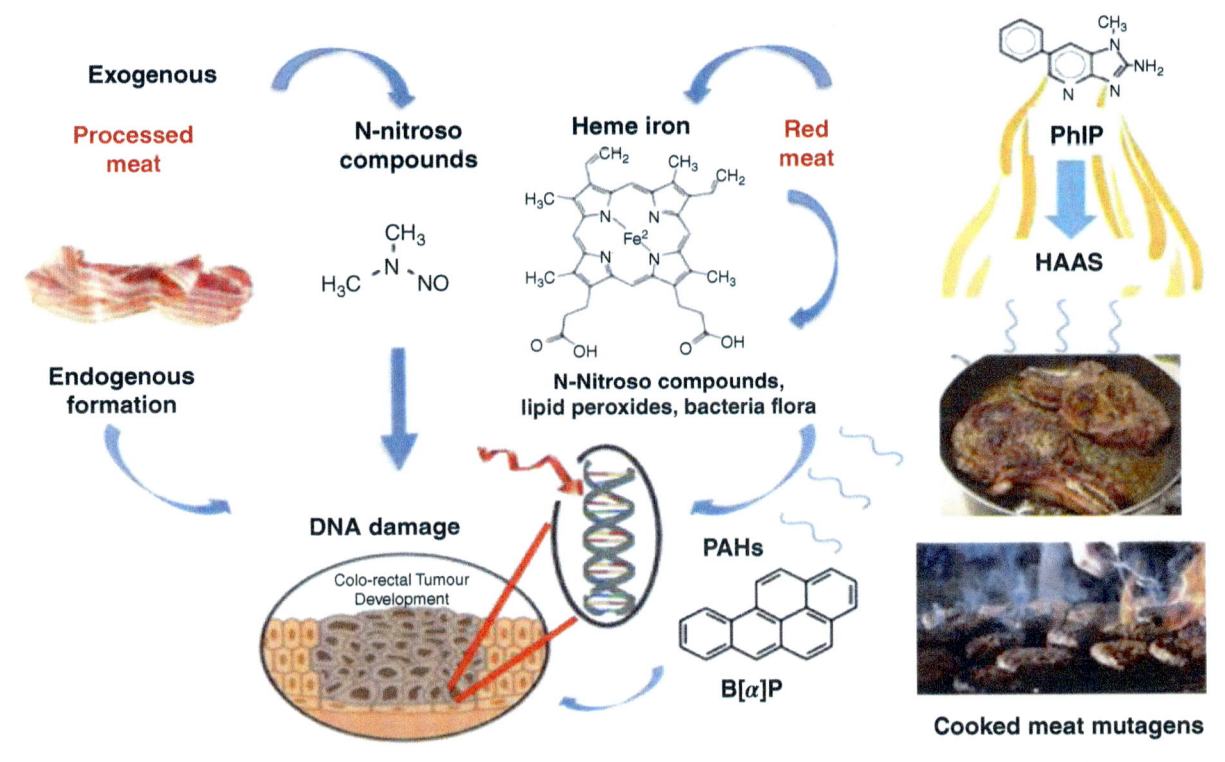

FIGURE 21.4 Proposed mechanisms linking processed and red meat to colorectal cancer development. PAHs = polycyclic aromatic hydrocarbons; HAAs = heterocyclic aromatic amines. Source: (Turesky, 2018 / with permission of Swiss Chemical Society).

There is mounting evidence for the potential biological mechanisms that explain these associations (**Figure 21.4**). Processing meat, for example during smoking and curing, produces several carcinogens, including polycyclic aromatic hydrocarbons and N-nitroso compounds, while cooking meat at high temperature, such as grilling or barbecuing, leads further to the formation of heterocyclic amines. Besides, it is suggested that the heme iron, which is present at high levels in red and processed meat, can promote carcinogenesis through lipid peroxidation and the formation of DNA adducts and N-nitroso compounds (Joosen et al., 2009; Sinha et al., 1998).

DIETARY FIBER, WHOLE GRAINS, FRUITS, AND VEGETABLES

Dietary fiber, which could be defined briefly as the constituents of the plant walls that are not digested in the small intestine, is found mainly in plant foods, such as whole-grain products, fruits, vegetables, nuts, seeds, and legumes. Their intake is considered probably related to a reduced risk of colorectal cancer, with an increase of 10 g/d of dietary fiber associated with a 9% reduced risk of colorectal cancer (WCRF/AICR, 2018).

Their intake through the consumption of whole plant foods has been also associated with a reduced likelihood of gaining weight and overweight or obesity, which results in a lower risk of obesity-related types of cancers (WCRF/AICR, 2018). Dietary fiber reduces gastrointestinal transit time, dilutes carcinogens in the colon, and reduces their absorption and contact with the epithelial cells. Furthermore, fiber promotes the avoidance of gut microbial dysbiosis as well as the fermentation of intestinal bacteria and the increase of production of short-chain fatty acids, like butyrate, which has been shown to inhibit cell proliferation and promote apoptosis (Baena & Salinas, 2015; de Vries, 2015; Romaneiro & Parekh, 2012).

Whole grains, according to the American Association of Cereal Chemists (AACC), are defined as consisting of the "intact, ground, cracked, or flaked caryopsis, whose principal anatomical components, including the starchy endosperm, germ, and bran are present in the same relative proportions as they exist in the intact caryopsis" (AACC, 2000). Retaining the original kernel makes whole grains rich in several substances and dietary factors, such as vitamins, dietary fibers, and phytochemicals and is one of the reasons why their consumption has been consistently associated with lower cancer risk, with the strongest evidence for colorectal, pancreatic, gastric, and esophageal cancers based on a systematic review of meta-analyses of observational studies (Gaesser, 2020). The 2018 WCRF/AIRC report states that the consumption of whole grains is strongly associated with a lower risk only of colorectal cancer. Each 90 g/d increase in the consumption of whole grains has been reported to reduce the risk of colorectal cancer by 17% (WCRF/AICR, 2018). In the same context, in a meta-analysis of nine prospective studies, the risk of colorectal cancer was reduced by 5% for each 30 g/d increase in intake (Schwingshackl et al., 2018).

Nutrients, substances, and bioactive compounds of whole grains have been demonstrated to have potential anticarcinogenic properties, reduce oxidative stress, and ameliorate levels of insulin and proinflammatory cytokines (Fardet, 2010; Slavin, 2003; Song et al., 2015). In addition, whole-grain intake is associated with lower excess body weight and as a result they could have a beneficial role in lowering the risk of adiposity-related type of cancers (Harland & Garton, 2008).

Considering fruits and vegetables, older studies demonstrated strong and convincing evidence between their consumption and reduced cancer risk. However, the results of long-term studies in the last decade weaken this association. Therefore, the 2018 WCRF/AIRC report concluded that the greater consumption of whole fruits and/or non-starchy vegetables was "probably" associated with a lower incidence of aerodigestive cancers, such as mouth, pharynx, larynx, nasopharynx, and esophagus as well as stomach and lung cancers (WCRF/AICR, 2018). There are, also, some promising results on specific-tumor subtypes, as demonstrated in a systematic review and meta-analysis of prospective studies published in 2021, in which total fruits and vegetables consumption was associated with a 9% lower overall breast cancer risk, but also with 11% and 26% lower risk of estrogen-receptor and progesterone-receptor positive and negative breast cancer, respectively (Farvid, Barnett, et al., 2021).

As plant-based foods, fruits and vegetables contain numerous nutrients and bioactive compounds that have been reported to protect against cancer development. Furthermore, they are low energy-dense foods, high in dietary fiber, and their consumption has been shown to likely increase satiety and reduce the likelihood of weight gain, overweight, and obesity (WCRF/AICR, 2018).

Although the intake of whole grains, vegetables, and legumes seems to be beneficial, it should be noted that there are some factors to be considered. For example, grains and legumes can be contaminated by aflatoxins, that are produced by some molds, and it is observed mainly in low and middle income countries (Wild et al., 2020). Aflatoxin is classified as carcinogenic to humans according to the IARC and has been shown to strongly increase the incidence of liver cancer (WCRF/AICR, 2018; Wild et al., 2020). Except for aflatoxin, the positive effects of the consumption of these plant foods may be disrupted by the consumption of preserved non-starchy vegetables. The 2018 WCRF/AIRC report demonstrated, that higher intake of foods preserved by salting, including preserved vegetables, such as those, which are pickled or salted can probably increase the risk of developing stomach cancer (WCRF/AICR, 2018). Hence, given these results, individuals should be aware of the safety and quality of the plant foods they consume to be protected against cancer.

CALCIUM AND DAIRY PRODUCTS

The association between dairy products, calcium and cancer risk is complicated, because there are several data indicating reduced risk of some cancers and increased risk of others. Indeed, the 2018 WCRF/AICR report supports an inverse association between intake of dairy and the risk of colorectal cancer risk (WCRF/AICR, 2018). Regarding dairy consumption, for each 400 g the risk was reduced by approximately 13%. Moreover, it reported that diets high in calcium may reduce breast cancer risk, although the evidence is considered as limited/suggestive. On the other hand, there is limited evidence that diets high in dairy products and calcium may increase the risk of prostate cancer. For each 400 g of dairy consumption, prostate cancer risk was estimated to increase by 7%. However, it should be noted that the more pronounced positive associations with calcium are observed in higher intakes (approximately more than 1500 mg per day) compared to the Recommended Dietary Allowance (1000–1200 mg) and even higher doses (> 2000 mg) has been associated with advanced prostate cancer (Aune et al., 2015; Wilson et al., 2015).

Dairy products may lead to a reduced risk of colorectal cancer mainly due to their calcium concentration. The main mechanisms include the binding of calcium to the potentially toxic free fatty acids and secondary bile acids, the preservation of integrity of epithelial cells and the reduction of intestinal inflammation (Norat & Riboli, 2003; Song et al., 2015). In contrast, considering prostate cancer, the principal mechanism involves the increase in IGF-1 levels, although it is not completely understood. There is some evidence demonstrating that milk intake may increase IGF-1 levels and as a consequence the risk of prostate cancer (Harrison et al., 2017). The other suggested mechanism includes the downregulation of the 1,25-dihydroxyvitamin D formation, which is the active form of vitamin D (Abu el Maaty & Wölfl, 2017). In this regard, cellular proliferation in the prostate is increased.

SUGAR-SWEETENED DRINKS, FAST AND ULTRAPROCESSED FOODS

Both sugar-sweetened drinks, which include liquids with added sugars, such as sodas, energy, and sports drinks, as well as fast foods tend to be high energy-dense and have a low impact on satiety. Their consumption has been associated with higher risk of long-term weight gain, overweight and obesity, and as a consequence indirectly may be a cause of cancer development (WCRF/AICR, 2018). However, data from PREDIMED study demonstrated a significant positive association between simple sugars in liquid form and cancer risk, regardless of BMI and energy intake, which should be further researched in the future (Laguna et al., 2021). Moreover, there are interesting data from the Nutrinet-Santé prospective cohort study (approximately 105,000 adults were assessed) with regard to ultra-processed foods (e.g., cookies, cakes, soft drinks, salty snacks) demonstrating that a 10% increase in the intake of those foods has been associated with a 12% greater risk in overall cancer risk (Fiolet et al., 2018).

DIETARY PATTERNS

Examining the effects of single nutrients or food groups in cancer risk is a proposed reason why some relevant studies have failed to show consistent results. Therefore, in the last several decades there is a shift in nutrition research to more holistic dietary patterns, which can take into consideration all the interactions between food components. To this context, there is some data demonstrating that *a priori* dietary patterns and numerous dietary indices have been associated with either reduced or higher risk of various cancer types. The strongest evidence has been shown with regard to colorectal and breast cancer, with the healthy eating index (HEI-2005 or HEI-2010), Mediterranean diet score and dietary approaches to stop hypertension (DASH) associated with a reduced risk (Steck & Murphy, 2020). Furthermore, there are numerous prospective and case-control studies that have assessed the effects of *a posteriori* dietary patterns in cancer incidence. Two main patterns were found, including "healthy" or "prudent" and "unhealthy" or "Western" patterns. The former has been associated with a lower risk of colorectal, breast, and lung cancers and the latter has been consistently related to an increased risk of colorectal cancer, while there are inconsistent results regarding breast, pancreatic, and prostate cancers. Hence, case-control studies have reported a positive association while prospective studies have demonstrated no consistent results (Steck & Murphy, 2020). Considering single nutrients and foods, healthy patterns include mainly fruits and vegetables, whole grains, legumes, nuts/seeds, fish, and polyunsaturated fats, while they are characterized by low amounts of red and processed meat, added sugars, saturated and trans fats. On the other hand, unhealthy patterns are characterized by the opposite features (Grosso et al., 2017).

Notably, while the evidence regarding the direct association of Mediterranean diet (MD) and Western diet with lower and higher cancer risk, respectively, is inconclusive, the 2018 WCRF/AIRC report suggest that MD is "convincingly" associated with a reduced risk of weight gain, overweight, or obesity. On the other hand, a Western dietary pattern is "probably" associated with an increased risk of being overweight or obese. Therefore, these patterns may, also, indirectly have a huge impact on cancer development. Furthermore, the same report concluded that diets with high glycemic load are "probably" associated with a higher risk of endometrial cancer, with one unit increment to be related with a 15% higher risk. Considering the relevant mechanisms, a diet higher in glycemic load can increase the postprandial glucose and insulin levels in the short-term, while in the long-term it may be associated with a higher risk of obesity and diabetes, which may further increase the risk of endometrial cancer (WCRF/AICR, 2018).

DIETARY SUPPLEMENTS

Although there is evidence that a high intake of plant-based foods, including fruits and vegetables may lower the cancer risk, the evidence regarding the use of vitamin supplements for cancer prevention is limited. Notably, despite the limited evidence in terms of higher plasma levels of vitamin D and lower colorectal cancer risk, the results of its supplementation are inconsistent (Dimitrakopoulou et al., 2017; Manson et al., 2019; WCRF/AICR, 2018). Consequently, to date, there is no recommendation to assess vitamin D levels and provide supplementation, in case of deficiency, to prevent cancer incidence. Furthermore, there is strong evidence that high-doses of beta carotene can "convincingly" increase the risk of lung cancer in individuals who smoke or used to smoke as well as that high-doses of vitamin E may increase prostate cancer incidence (WCRF/AICR, 2018). For these reasons, no dietary supplement is recommended for cancer prevention, instead individuals should obtain nutrients and these compounds from foods that provide the potential for synergistic effects against cancer (Rock et al., 2020; WCRF/AICR, 2018).

SEDENTARY BEHAVIOR

Sedentary behavior is defined as "any waking behavior that characterized by an energy expenditure less than or equal to 1.5 Metabolic Equivalents of Task (METs) while in a sitting or reclining posture" (Sedentary Behaviour Research Network, 2012). In the last several decades, sedentary behavior has been evaluated with regard to cancer risk and now it seems to be a further important modifiable risk factor, especially given that some data demonstrate that physical inactivity is attributable to approximately 2.9% of all cancer cases in the United States (Islami et al., 2018).

In a meta-analysis that includes 14 observational studies, a 24% higher risk of cancer has been shown when high levels of time were spent sitting compared to low, after adjusting for physical activity (Biswas et al., 2015). Considering the types of cancer, the strongest evidence has been demonstrated for colon, breast, and endometrial cancers. In a meta-analysis of 43 observational studies, each increase of 2 h/d sitting time was associated with 8% and 10% greater risk of colon and endometrial cancer, respectively (Schmid & Leitzmann, 2014).

The 2018 WCRF/AIRC report concluded that sedentary behavior increases the risk only of endometrial cancer and graded the evidence as "limited-suggestive" (WCRF/AICR, 2018). The 2018 physical activity guidelines advisory committee (PAGAC) report demonstrated that there is moderate evidence for a significant association between increased levels of sedentary behavior and a greater risk of colon, endometrial, and lung cancer (PAGAC, 2018).

The relevant mechanisms are not fully understood. Although, there are inconsistent data, sedentary behavior may increase the risk of weight gain, overweight, or obesity that may lead to cancer development.

PHYSICAL ACTIVITY

Research about physical activity and cancer has emerged in the past decade and, to date, evidence was derived mainly from multiple observational epidemiological studies showing that higher levels of physical activity are consistently associated with a lower risk of several cancers. Almost all the available data in the literature focused on aerobic physical activity, and they are summarized and evaluated by the 2018 PAGAC and 2018 WCRF/AIRC expert reports (PAGAC, 2018; WCRF/AICR, 2018). After thorough evaluation, they concluded that there is some evidence demonstrating a reduced risk of 13 types of cancer, when comparing the individuals in the highest category of physical activity to those in the lowest. More specifically, the PAGAC concluded that there is strong evidence that being physically active reduces the risk of breast, bladder, endometrial, colon, esophageal adenocarcinoma, gastric cardia, and renal cancers. It is also

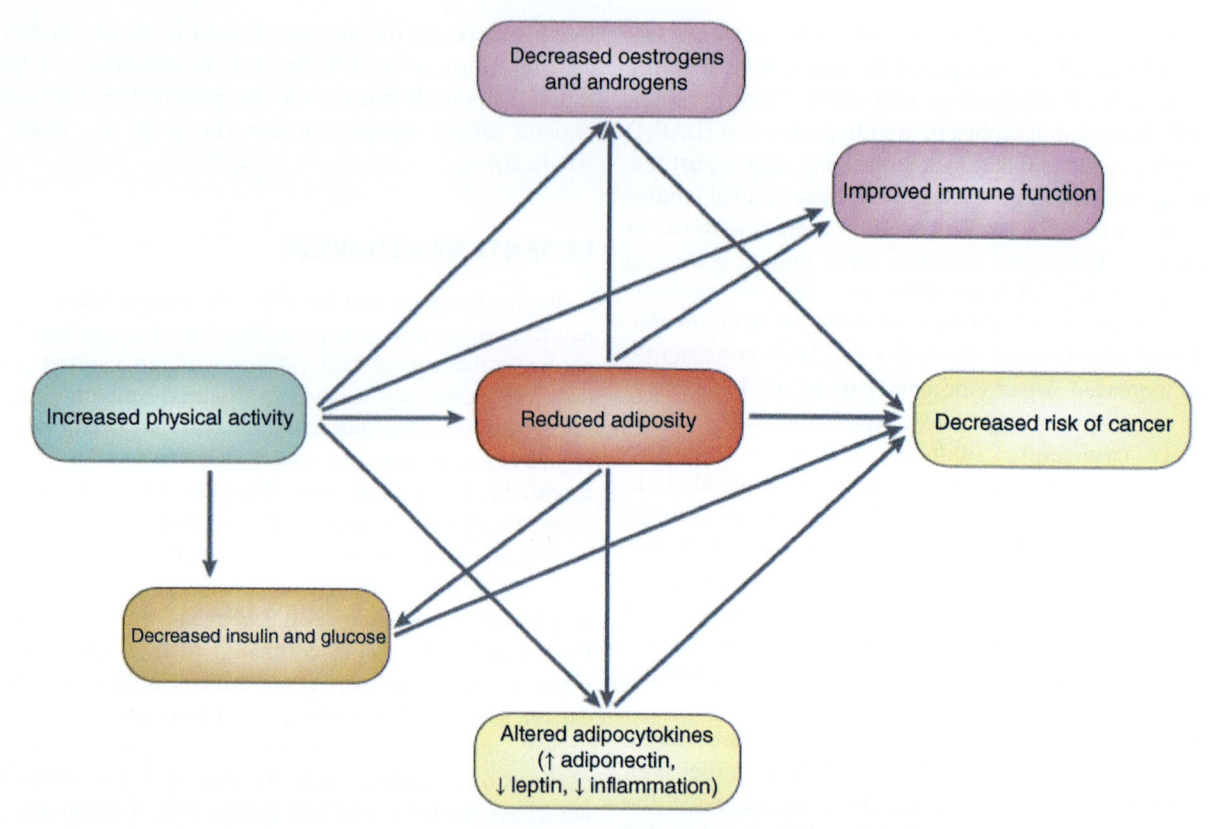

FIGURE 21.5 Mechanisms linking physical activity to decreased cancer risk. Source: (McTiernan, 2008).

demonstrated moderate evidence for lung cancer, although smoking may be an important confounder, and limited for hematologic, ovary, head and neck, pancreas and prostate cancers (PAGAC, 2018). Given the different criteria for grading, the 2018 WCRF/AICR report found strong evidence regarding a "convincing" association between physical activity and a reduced risk of colon cancer as well as a "probable" association with a lower risk of endometrial and post-menopausal breast cancers. In a meta-analysis of the available cohort studies published by WCRF/AICR, researchers found that when comparing the highest levels of total physical activity with the lowest, risk was reduced by 20% and 13% in colon cancer and post-menopausal breast cancer, respectively (WCRF/AICR, 2018). Moreover, in the same report, the association between physical activity and decreased risk of esophagus, liver, post-menopausal breast, and lung cancers was graded as "limited". In 2019, the American College of Sports Medicine (ACSM) published an expert review demonstrating similar conclusions compared with the 2018 PAGAC report, except for an additional protective role of physical activity against liver cancer incidence. The magnitude of the reductions in relative risks for most cancer types ranges from approximately 10% to 20% (Patel et al., 2019).

Furthermore, regarding the intensity and the type of physical activity, and given the different methods reported in the literature for measuring its levels, it is difficult to determine the precise levels and type of exercise training that can reduce the risk of most cancer types. However, in this context, and according to the 2018 WCRF/AICR report, there is strong evidence that vigorous (>6 METs or >60% of peak heart rate) physical activity is "probably" associated with 21% and 10% lower risk of premenopausal and post-menopausal breast cancer risk, respectively, when comparing the highest and lowest levels (WCRF/AICR, 2018).

An emerging body of research suggests a variety of mechanisms though which physical activity can have a beneficial role in developing cancer (**Figure 21.5**). Exercise training may have direct effects on minimizing chronic inflammation and improving function of the immune system. Moreover, it may indirectly prevent weight gain as well as being overweight or obese through the management of body weight and the maintenance of healthy body fat levels. It may, also, be associated with the reduction of bioavailable sex-hormones levels, the improvement of insulin sensitivity, and the consequent reduction of insulin levels. Furthermore, considering the risk of colon cancer, exercise may lead to a decreasing transit time and, as a result, a reduced exposure of intestinal epithelial cells to carcinogens (Hojman et al., 2018).

DIET AND PHYSICAL ACTIVITY RECOMMENDATIONS FOR PREVENTION

Regarding diet, nutrition, and cancer prevention, the available recommendations are the updated 2018 WCRF/AIRC recommendations and the 2020 American Cancer Society (ACS) guidelines on nutrition and physical activity (**Tables 21.1** and **21.2**, respectively). Briefly, they promote a body weight within the

Table 21.1 The 2018 WCRF/AICR recommendations for cancer prevention. AICR = American Institute for Cancer Research; BMI = body-mass index; WCRF = World Cancer Research Fund; WHO = World Health Organization.

Recommendations	Details	Goals
Be a healthy weight	Keep your weight within the healthy range and avoid weight gain in adult life.	• Ensure that body weight during childhood and adolescence projects toward the lower end of the healthy adult BMI range. • Keep your weight as low as you can within the healthy range throughout life. • Avoid weight gain (measured as body weight or waist circumference) throughout adulthood.
Be physically active	Be physically active as part of everyday life and life—walk more and sit less.	• Be at least moderately physically active and follow or exceed national guidelines. • Limit sedentary habits.
Eat a diet rich in wholegrains, vegetables, fruit, and beans	Make wholegrains, vegetables, fruit, and pulses (legumes) such as beans and lentils a major part of your usual diet.	• Consume a diet that provides at least 30 g/day of fiber from food sources. • Include in more meals foods containing wholegrains, non-starchy vegetables, fruit, and pulses (legumes) such as beans and lentils. • Eat a diet high in all types of plant foods including at least five portions or servings (at least 400 g or 15 oz in total) of a variety of non-starchy vegetables and fruit every day. • If you eat starchy roots and tubers as staple foods, eat non-starchy vegetables, fruit, and pulses (legumes) regularly too if possible.
Limit consumption of "fast foods" and other processed foods high in fat, starches, or sugars	Limiting these foods helps control calorie intake and maintain a healthy weight.	Limit consumption of processed foods high in fat, starches or sugars—including "fast foods", many pre-pared dishes, snacks, bakery foods and desserts; and confectionery (candy).
Limit consumption of red and processed meat	Eat no more than moderate amounts of red meat, such as beef, pork, and lamb. Eat little, if any, processed meat.	If you eat red meat, limit consumption to no more than about three portions per week. Three portions are equivalent to about 350 to 500 g (about 12 to 18 oz) cooked weight of red meat. Consume very little, if any, processed meat.
Limit consumption of sugar-sweetened drinks	Drink mostly water and unsweetened drinks.	Do not consume sugar-sweetened drinks.
Limit alcohol consumption	For cancer prevention, it is best not to drink alcohol.	For cancer prevention, it is best not to drink alcohol.
Do not use supplements for cancer prevention	Aim to meet nutritional needs through diet alone.	High-dose dietary supplements are not recommended for cancer prevention—aim to meet nutritional needs through diet alone.
For mothers: breastfeed your baby if you can	Breastfeeding is good for both mother and baby.	This recommendation aligns with the advice of the WHO, which recommends infants are exclusively breastfed for 6 months, and then up to 2 years of age or beyond alongside appropriate complementary foods.
After a cancer diagnosis: follow our recommendations if you can	Check with your health professional what is right for you.	• All cancer survivors should receive nutritional care and guidance on physical activity from trained professionals • Unless otherwise advised, and if you can, all cancer survivors are advised to follow the cancer prevention recommendations as far as possible after the acute stage of treatment.

Source: (WCRF/AICR, 2018).

Table 21.2 2020 American Cancer Society guideline on diet and physical activity for cancer prevention.

Recommendations for individuals

1. Achieve and maintain a healthy body weight throughout life.
   - Keep body weight within the healthy range and avoid weight gain in adult life.
2. Be physically active.
   - Adults should engage in 150–300 min/week of moderate-intensity physical activity, or 75–150 min/week of vigorous-intensity physical activity, or an equivalent combination; achieving or exceeding the upper limit of 300 min/week is optimal.
   - Children and adolescents should engage in at least 1 h/d of moderate- or vigorous-intensity activity.
   - Limit sedentary behavior, such as sitting, lying down, watching television, and other forms of screen-based entertainment.
3. Follow a healthy eating pattern at all ages.
   - A healthy eating pattern includes:
     - Foods that are high in nutrients in amounts that help achieve and maintain a healthy body weight;
     - A variety of vegetables—dark green, red, and orange, fiber-rich legumes (beans and peas), and others;
     - Fruits, especially whole fruits with a variety of colors; and
     - Whole grains.
   - A healthy eating pattern limits or does not include:
     - Red and processed meats;
     - Sugar-sweetened beverages; or
     - Highly processed foods and refined grain products.
4. It is best not to drink alcohol.
   - People who do choose to drink alcohol should limit their consumption to no more than 1 drink per day for women and 2 drinks per day for men.

Source: (Rock et al., 2020).

healthy range and a healthy dietary pattern rich in vegetables, fruits, whole grains, and beans, while suggesting the limitation of red and processed meat, sugar-sweetened drinks, processed foods, fast foods, and refined grains consumption. They also recommend against the use of supplements for cancer prevention. Furthermore, regarding alcohol consumption, both recommend individuals limit their consumption to national guidelines (e.g., in the United States: 1 drink per day for women, 2 drinks for men), although the WCRF/AIRC suggests even to avoid drinking. Moreover, the 2018 WCRF/AIRC recommendations suggest specific quantities of some foods and nutrients, as at least 30 g/d of fiber and 400 g/d of non-starchy vegetables and fruits as well as consumption of red meat with no more than three portions (350–500 g) per week (Rock et al., 2020; WCRF/AICR, 2018).

Regarding the available recommendations for physical activity, the ACS recommends adults get at least 150 min of moderate-intensity physical activity or 75 min of vigorous-intensity physical activity weekly. In this context, the WCRF/AICR suggests following the recommendations and trying to be physically active daily. Moreover, the ACSM recommend at least 30 min of moderate to vigorous aerobic physical activity five times weekly as well as the implementation of activities that support muscle strengthening at least 2 d/week (Patel et al., 2019). Although, not specifically referring to cancer prevention, the 2020 physical activity guidelines for Americans are consistent with others, as they recommend moderate aerobic for at least 150 to 300 min, 75 to 150 min of vigorous aerobic physical activity per week, or a combination of them (Piercy et al., 2018). In general, as the available data show that the more active an individual is, the lower the risk of cancer, these guidelines can be increased for greater cancer prevention.

Interestingly, there are some data regarding the association of the adherence to recommendations, mainly of WCRF/AIRC and the risk of cancer. To this context, a standardized scoring system was developed in 2019 by the experts of WCRF and other organizations to examine the adherence to the WCRF/AIRC recommendations. This score gives a full point for meeting a recommendation and points for lower adherence and total score ranges from 0 to 7 (Shams-White et al., 2019). Consequently, in a 2021 study, in which data from prospective cohort studies were assessed, individuals in the highest category of the score had a 12% lower risk of cancer compared to those in the lowest category. Moreover, it was shown that each 1-point increment in adherence to the score was significantly associated with a 3% lower risk of cancer. This study also highlighted the lack of or intermediate adherence to the majority of recommendations as well as the need to inform and educate individuals regarding the importance of lifestyle factors for cancer prevention (Kaluza et al., 2020). Furthermore, a 2016 systematic review assessed the effects of adherence to the 2007 WCRF/AICR recommendations and the 2012 ACS guidelines and reported that a higher adherence to these guidelines was significantly associated with reduced incidence of overall cancer as well as a lower risk of colorectal, breast, and endometrial cancers when compared to lower adherence (Kohler et al., 2016).

NUTRITION AND PHYSICAL ACTIVITY IN PATIENTS LIVING WITH OR BEYOND CANCER

The improvements in cancer treatments as well as early detection through screening programs and the increased aging population have already led to an increased number of patients living with and beyond cancer worldwide. It is estimated that in 2016 approximately 15.5 million Americans were living with a diagnosis of cancer, and this number is projected to reach 20.3 million by 2026 (Miller et al., 2016). Although, patients living with or beyond cancer are often characterized in the literature with the term "cancer survivors", there is a controversy regarding its definition. According to the US National Cancer Institute, the term "cancer survivors" refers to those individuals who have been diagnosed with cancer, throughout the whole journey, including the time before, during, and after treatment (Marzorati et al., 2017). In the same context, the ACS refers to anyone who has been diagnosed with cancer, regardless of the course of the disease. However, the European society of enteral and parenteral nutrition (ESPEN) uses this term for patients cured of their cancer (Arends et al., 2017). In this chapter, to avoid misunderstanding, when the term "cancer survivors" is used, it will be referred to people living beyond cancer who have completed active anti-cancer treatments.

BODY WEIGHT, BODY COMPOSITION, AND PHYSICAL ACTIVITY DURING THERAPY

Body weight, body composition, and the ability of patients with cancer to exercise during active treatments may be adversely affected due to multiple factors. The anatomical location of the tumor, especially in patients with esophageal or head and neck cancers, may lead to dysphagia and swallowing problems and hence to the restriction of dietary intake. Moreover, the cancer cachexia syndrome can result in significant weight loss, malnutrition, and changes in body composition. It is defined as "a multi-factorial syndrome characterized by ongoing loss of muscle mass (with or without loss of fat mass), which cannot be completely reversed by conventional nutritional support and eventually leads to progressive functional impairments" (Fearon et al., 2011).

Its main mechanisms include a variety of different factors, involving overproduction of proinflammatory mediators and cytokines as well as altered hormonal signals resulting to anorexia, systemic inflammation, insulin resistance and increased energy expenditure. The prevalence of cancer cachexia varies among types of cancer and patients with lung, head and neck, pancreatic and gastro-esophageal cancers are more likely to develop cachexia rather than patients with prostate or breast cancer (Baracos et al., 2018).

Other factors, like the presence of co-morbidities and aging may contribute to changes in body composition, difficulties around weight management, and malnutrition. The median age of patients with cancer is approximately 66-years old, therefore problems associated with aging itself may have already adversely affected the nutritional status as well as the physical performance of patients. Notably, sarcopenia associated with aging may be present, defined by low physical function, low muscle mass, and potential low performance status (Cruz-Jentoft et al., 2019).

Sarcopenia may also be developed secondarily due to anti-cancer treatments. There are data showing that certain drugs, such as steroids, commonly used in patients with cancer, and targeted therapies may directly affect myocytes and lead progressively to muscle loss (Egerman & Glass, 2014). Interestingly, some therapies, such as the androgen-deprivation therapy (ADT) used in prostate cancer, can progressively lead to so called sarcopenic obesity, namely loss of lean body mass along with an increase in fat mass and a reduction in both muscle strength and endurance, which is associated with a number of adverse outcomes (**Figure 21.6**) (Donini et al., 2022). The loss of lean body mass in prostate cancer patients undergoing ADT has been estimated to be 1% after 12 months and 2.4% after 36 months (Smith et al., 2012). Furthermore, a range of symptoms and side effects related to treatments, like symptoms from the gastrointestinal tract (nausea, vomiting, taste alterations, diarrhea, constipation, mucositis), anorexia, and fatigue can adversely affect dietary intake leading to unintentional weight loss, malnutrition, and sarcopenia.

In some cases, weight gain may also be observed. Notably, 30% to 60% of early breast cancer patients receiving chemotherapy seem to significantly increase their body weight (Vance et al., 2011). Sometimes, this may be over 5% of the starting body weight within the first 12 months after diagnosis and is often the result of a positive energy balance, especially due to lower physical activity (Gandhi et al., 2019).

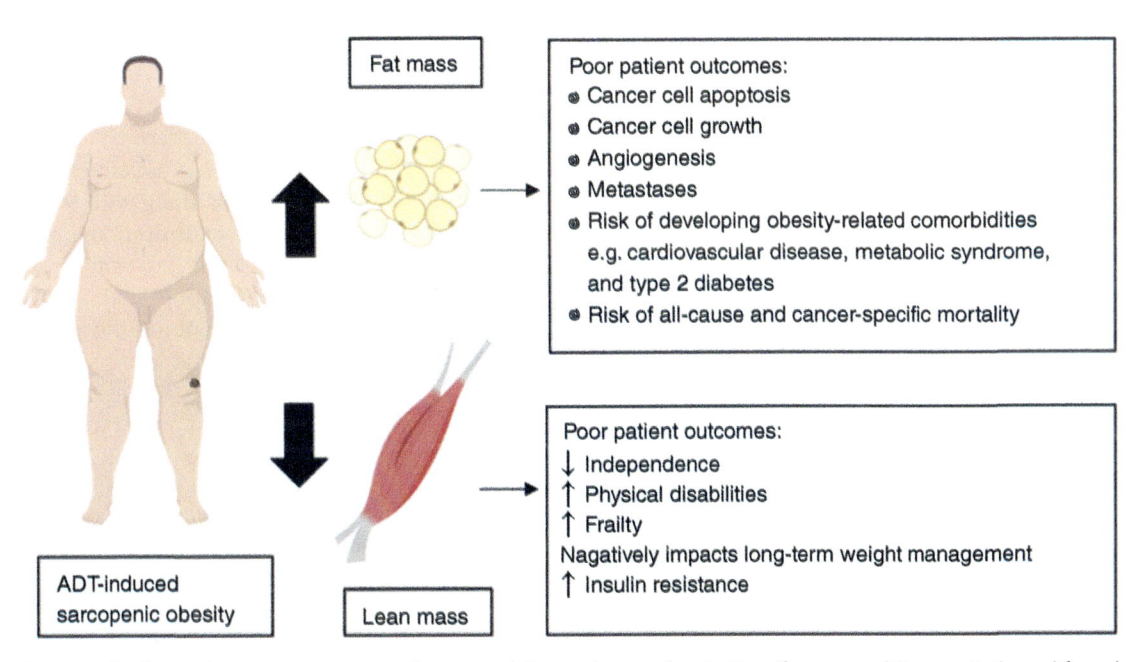

FIGURE 21.6 Sarcopenic obesity in prostate cancer patients receiving androgen-deprivation therapy and its association with various outcomes. ADT = androgen-deprivation therapy. Source: (Wilson et al., 2021).

The latter is frequent among patients with cancer during treatments and is related to several factors like the side effects of treatment, especially fatigue and pain, the emotional stress during the cancer journey, and cachexia. It has been estimated that patients with cachexia take approximately 4,000 steps daily, and they spend only a few hours walking or standing (Ferriolli et al., 2012). Physical inactivity and all the other aforementioned factors related to the tumor itself and anti-cancer treatments can lead to a well-established reduction of cardio-respiratory fitness, which refers to the ability for oxygen to be delivered to the skeletal muscles for the production of energy (Jones et al., 2008).

ROLE OF NUTRITION AND PHYSICAL ACTIVITY DURING THERAPY

Malnutrition, sarcopenia, and sarcopenic obesity (the loss of lean body mass along with an increase in fat mass) as well as cachexia are consistently associated with adverse outcomes among patients with cancer, resulting in increased treatment toxicities, reduced physical activity, impaired quality of life (QOL) and decreased overall survival (Arends et al., 2017). Weight gain, obesity, and excess body fat that are observed in some cases, like in breast cancer, have been associated with higher risk of impaired QOL, treatment-related toxicities and all-cause mortality (Anderson et al., 2021). Given the global burden of overweight and obesity, many patients already have excess body weight upon diagnosis, which often leads to masking these features. Therefore, patients with cancer should get an appropriate nutritional assessment followed by optimal nutrition and physical activity interventions to prevent or manage them, despite the lack of solid and robust evidence about the effectiveness of dietary interventions (Laviano, 2021).

The main goals of nutrition interventions during cancer therapy are to cover energy and protein demands, manage nutrition-related problems, maintain, or target normal body composition, and improve QOL.

To date, the available research data about specific dietary patterns or foods that could be recommended during treatments to improve cancer outcomes, are insufficient. According to the guidelines of the American Society of Clinical Oncology (ASCO) published in 2022, dietary interventions like low-fat diets, ketogenic or low carbohydrates diets, fasting, or diets high in functional foods cannot be recommended to improve QOL, treatment-related toxicities, and in general, cancer management (**Table 21.3** summarizes the ASCO guidelines) (Ligibel et al., 2022). Though, dietary interventions should aim to cover energy requirements, providing 25 to 30 kcal/kg/d as well as protein needs, providing at least 1 g/kg/d (if possible, up to 1.5 g/kg/d) (Arends et al., 2017). Furthermore, a 2021 expert report suggests that protein intake should be at least 1.2 g/kg/d to achieve muscle maintenance and support (Ford et al., 2022). It also states the importance of taking into consideration the source of protein. Given several different characteristics based on the protein source, such as amino acid composition, animal protein seems to provide a higher anabolic potential than plant-based protein and result in a more positive impact on muscles. Therefore, unlike cancer prevention recommendations that focus primarily on plant-based foods, patients with cancer during active treatments may benefit from a combination of protein sources with an emphasis on animal protein (at least 65%) to support muscle mass and avoid malnutrition, while the initiation of a vegetarian or vegan diet is not recommended at this stage (Ford et al., 2022).

Besides nutritional care, physical activity programs should be further provided so as to minimize side effects related to treatments and functional decline, by supporting muscle mass, physical function, and metabolic pattern (Schmitz et al., 2019). Combined nutrition and physical therapy is recommended for the optimal management of patients with cancer during therapies (Arends et al., 2017).

Therefore, regarding physical activity prescription, there is strong evidence that it is safe and well-tolerated during anti-cancer treatment, even among patients with advanced cancer. The guidelines suggest that patients with cancer should avoid physical inactivity and get at least 150 min/week of moderate physical activity and at least 2 d/week of muscle strengthening activities (Rock et al., 2022). However, given the complexity of cancer treatments and the presence of possible co-morbidities, any physical exercise prescription should consider several factors, including, but not limited to, peripheral neuropathy, presence of central catheters, lymphedema, stomas, surgical wounds, low levels of white blood-cell count, and anemia. Medical screening and thorough monitoring are necessary to make physical activity feasible and to keep all patients safe. There is evidence that physical activity is associated with reduced fatigue, decreased muscle catabolism, improvements in physical function and cardio-respiratory fitness, reduced emotional stress, and in general, a better QOL (Schmitz et al., 2019).

It should be noted that nutrition and physical activity interventions should be provided considering the type and stage of cancer and the patients' characteristics, including the assessment of body composition. Therefore, the goal in terms of weight management may be different among patients with various types of cancer. As previously mentioned, weight loss during active treatment may negatively affect outcomes in certain cancers. However, in some cases intentional weight loss, involving loss of excess body fat along with the maintenance of lean body mass may be desirable. Indeed, the 2022 ASCO guidelines states that intentional weight loss may be feasible in breast and possibly prostate cancers (Ligibel et al., 2022). Nevertheless, to date, it is unclear if interventions aiming at reducing body fatness during active treatment would lead to significant improvement of outcomes (WCRF/AICR, 2018). Notably, even among breast cancer patients, there may be exceptions, such as in patients with triple-negative metastatic breast cancer, who commonly have a rapid progression of their disease.

ROLE IN PREHABILITATION FOR SURGERY

Prehabilitation seems to be promising for patients with cancer waiting for a surgery. Its aim is to improve physical and/or psychological factors of patients with cancer and prepare them

Table 21.3 Exercise, diet, and weight management during cancer treatment: ASCO guideline.

Questions	Recommendations
Does exercise during cancer treatment safely improve outcomes related to QOL, treatment toxicity, or cancer control?	**Recommendation 1.1** Oncology providers should recommend aerobic and resistance exercise during active treatment with curative intent to mitigate side effects of cancer treatment (Type: evidence based; benefits outweigh harms; Evidence quality: moderate to low; Strength of recommendation: strong).
	Recommendation 1.2 Oncology providers may recommend preoperative exercise for patients undergoing surgery for lung cancer to reduce length of hospital stay and postoperative complications (Type: evidence based, benefits outweigh harms; Evidence quality: low; Strength of recommendation: weak).
Does consuming a particular dietary pattern or food(s) during cancer treatment safely improve outcomes related to QOL, treatment toxicity, or cancer control?	**Recommendation 2.1.** There is currently insufficient evidence to recommend for or against dietary interventions such as ketogenic or low-carbohydrate diets, low-fat diets, functional foods, or fasting to improve outcomes related to QOL, treatment toxicity, or cancer control.
	Recommendation 2.2. Neutropenic diets (specifically diets that exclude raw fruits and vegetables) are not recommended to prevent infection in patients with cancer during active treatment (Type: evidence based, harms likely to outweigh benefits; Evidence quality: low; Strength of recommendation: weak).
Do interventions to promote intentional weight loss or avoidance of weight gain during cancer treatment safely improve outcomes related to QOL, treatment toxicity, or cancer control?	There is currently insufficient evidence to recommend for or against intentional weight loss or prevention of weight gain interventions during active treatment to improve outcomes related to QOL, treatment toxicity, or cancer control.

Notes
- Exercise interventions during active treatment reduce fatigue; preserve cardiorespiratory fitness, physical functioning, and strength; and in some populations, improve QOL and reduce anxiety and depression. In addition, exercise interventions during treatment have a low risk of adverse events. Evidence was not sufficient to recommend for or against exercise during treatment to improve cancer control outcomes (recurrence or survival) or treatment completion rates.
- The Expert Panel felt strongly that the current lack of evidence regarding diet and weight management interventions during cancer treatment should be a call to conduct more research in these critical areas. Diet and weight management strategies that provide health benefits to the general population could also provide important benefits to people who are undergoing cancer treatment. The Expert Panel is not discouraging clinicians from discussing healthy diet and weight with their patients, but did refrain from making specific recommendations, given gaps in the evidence.

Source: (Ligibel et al., 2022).

for cancer treatment. It is a multimodal approach, in which exercise and nutritional interventions combined with possible psychological interventions are the main core (Davis et al., 2022). More specifically, they may include a combination of aerobic, anaerobic, and balance training, nutritional interventions aiming to minimize catabolism and support anabolism, and interventions aiming to reduce stress levels and implement healthy habits. They are usually provided for 2 to 6 weeks prior to cancer treatment and may be continued during treatment. There is some evidence that these interventions are associated with improvement in cardio-respiratory fitness, nutritional, and neuro-cognitive status. Furthermore, they may lead to a reduction in length of hospital stay and better recovery after cancer treatments (Faithfull et al., 2019).

In addition, with regard to achieving better outcomes perioperatively, the ESPEN recommends the implementation of the Enhanced Recovery After Surgery (ERAS) program (Arends et al., 2017). Nutritional care is a fundamental part of this, aiming to support patients by avoiding fasting, providing them with fluids and carbohydrates preoperatively, and re-establishing oral nutrition as soon as possible postoperatively. The main goals of the ERAS program are to maintain nutritional status, minimize perioperative stress, lower the risk of postoperative complications, and optimize recovery rates (Pędziwiatr et al., 2018). Especially, the early detection of patients with cancer, who are at risk of malnutrition or are already malnourished, is essential for both pre- and postoperative management.

ROLE IN LONG-TERM SURVIVORSHIP

After the completion of active treatments, the main goals of lifestyle interventions are to reduce the risk of recurrence and other chronic diseases, such as coronary heart disease, diabetes, and osteoporosis as well as to lower the risk of morbidity and mortality (Rock et al., 2022). According to the 2018 WCRF/AIRC report, in this phase and due to the absence of strong evidence regarding the association between diet, and the long-term survivorship, cancer survivors should follow recommendations for cancer prevention, namely to maintain a body weight within a healthy range, avoid weight gain, and follow a diet rich in plant-based foods while restricting alcohol, processed foods, and meats and limiting red meat consumption (WCRF/AICR, 2018). However, it should be noted that the first weeks or months after the completion of active treatments may be challenging for many cancer survivors due to the presence of potential persistent or late nutrition-related symptoms and treatment side effects. Therefore, a further goal of nutrition care during this period should be the recovery of nutritional status along with minimizing these problems.

Most of the existing studies regarding the long-term data of cancer survivors have been conducted mainly in breast as well as in colorectal and prostate cancer survivors. Diets characterized by better overall quality, as assessed using a variety of diet indices, have consistently shown an improvement in overall survival in breast and colorectal cancer survivors (Castro-Espin & Agudo, 2022). Moreover, individuals living beyond colorectal or prostate cancers, who had a higher adherence to the MD, had a lower risk of mortality compared to those who reported a low adherence, as assessed by the MD score (Castro-Espin & Agudo, 2022). In a meta-analysis of prospective cohort studies with regard to breast cancer survivors, a higher diet quality, compared to lower diet quality, was associated with a 23% lower risk of overall mortality (Castro-Espin & Agudo, 2022).

Besides epidemiological data, two large randomized clinical trials assessed the association between dietary patterns and outcomes in breast cancer survivors. The women's intervention nutrition study (WINS) randomized approximately 2400 women with early-stage breast cancer to follow either a low-fat or a standard diet (Chlebowski et al., 2006). After 5 years, the intervention group had a significantly reduced risk of recurrence by 24% compared to the control group. The women's healthy eating and living study (WHEL) studied about 3000 breast cancer patients and randomized them to follow either a low-fat diet high in fruits, vegetables, and dietary fiber or a standard diet (Pierce et al., 2007). After 7 years, there was no difference regarding a recurrence between the groups. Therefore, to date, it is unknown whether a specific dietary pattern can positively impact cancer recurrence.

It seems that aerobic exercise (e.g., cycling, walking) and weight training can have a variety of benefits for cancer survivors after active treatment. According to the 2018 WCRF/AIRC report, there is good evidence that physical activity is associated with an improvement in fatigue, depression, and aerobic fitness, whereas there is limited evidence with regard to cancer-specific and overall survival (WCRF/AICR, 2018). However, reviews by the ACSM conclude that there is "substantial evidence" that exercise is related to lower risk of cancer-specific survival for colon, breast, and prostate cancer (Schmitz et al., 2019). Post-treatment exercise programs should aim to optimize recovery of physical function and physical performance of individuals. The expected benefits for individuals who participate in exercise training programs, as summarized by the ACSM in 2019, are shown in **Table 21.4** (Campbell et al., 2019). The ACSM suggests that anxiety, fatigue, depressive symptoms, QOL, and physical function could be improved by "doing thrice-weekly aerobic activity for 30 minutes and that there is also evidence of a benefit for most of those same outcomes from twice-weekly resistance exercise: one exercise per major muscle group, 8 to 15 repetitions per set, 2 sets per exercise, progressing with small increments" (Schmitz et al., 2019).

Adherence to the 2012 ACS recommendations for cancer survivors has been shown to improve health-related QOL (Koh et al., 2019). Moreover, a high adherence to the 2018 WCRF/AIRC recommendations, as assessed by the WCRF score, has been shown to be associated with better QOL and lower levels of fatigue 2 to 10 years after diagnosis in 150 colorectal cancer survivors (Kenkhuis et al., 2021).

Table 21.4 Expected patient benefits from exercise training by mode. QOL = quality of life.

Aerobic	Resistance	Aerobic plus Resistance
Reduced anxiety	Less fatigue	Reduced anxiety
Fewer depressive symptoms	Better QOL	Fewer depressive symptoms
Less fatigue	No risk of exacerbating lymphedema	Less fatigue
Better QOL	Improved perceived physical function	Better QOL
Improved perceived physical function		Improved perceived physical function

Source: (Patel et al., 2019).

> [!NOTE] KEY POINTS
> - Cancer is the second leading cause of death worldwide.
> - 30% to 50% of cancer cases could be prevented through lifestyle modifications.
> - Excess body weight is ranked as a second leading preventable cause of cancer after smoking.
> - Several dietary factors (e.g., alcohol, processed meat, whole grains) may negatively or positively affect susceptibility to cancer development.
> - Physical inactivity and a sedentary lifestyle may increase the risk of cancer, whereas higher levels of physical activity are consistently associated with a lower risk of several cancers.
> - Nutrition care in patients with cancer aims to cover energy and protein demands; maintain or target normal body composition; prevent or manage malnutrition, sarcopenia, cachexia, nutrition-related problems; and improve QOL.
> - Exercise regimens aim to minimize side effects related to treatments as well as functional decline by supporting muscle mass, physical function, and metabolic patterns in patients with cancer.
> - Combined nutrition and exercise interventions are recommended for the optimal management of patients with cancer during anticancer treatments.
> - After the completion of active cancer treatment, individuals should follow, if possible, recommendations for cancer prevention to reduce the risk of recurrence, other chronic diseases, morbidity, and mortality.

SELF-ASSESSMENT QUESTIONS

1. Briefly describe the main mechanisms linking excess body fatness to cancer development.
2. According to the PAGAC, which types of cancer have been shown to associated with physical activity?
3. Provide the definition of cancer cachexia according to Fearon et al.
4. What are the goals of following nutrition and physical activity recommendations for cancer survivors after active treatment?
5. True or False: Moderate consumption of alcohol is not associated with any type of cancer.
6. True or False: The available data have shown that obesity is associated with a higher risk of cancer, regardless of menopausal status.
7. True or False: According to the WCRF/AIRC report, the risk of colorectal cancer increases by 16% per 50 g of processed red meat consumed per day.
8. True or False: In any case, a vitamin D supplementation should be prescribed for cancer prevention.
9. True or False: Excess body weight is ranked as a second leading preventable cause of cancer after smoking.
10. True or False: Energy intake for all patients with cancer should be at least 35 kcal/d.
11. True or False: Exercise is not safe for most patients with cancer during anti-cancer treatments.
12. True or False: During long-term survivorship, individuals should increase unprocessed red meat to increase their protein intake.

Fill in the blank(s) to complete the following statements:

13. The term "processed meat" includes meat that has been processed through _____ _____.
14. Energy and protein intake for patients with cancer should be ____ kcal/kg/d, at least ____ g/kg/d, and if possible, up to ____ g/kg/d.
15. Sedentary behavior is defined as _____.
16. Prehabilitation is a multimodal approach, including _____ interventions.

CASE SCENARIO

Mrs. TH is a 66-year-old woman who recently diagnosed with early-stage breast cancer (estrogen-receptor and progesterone-receptor positive, HER/2 neu negative) after a referral due to an abnormal mammogram. She has undergone a breast-conserving surgery and now she has completed two cycles of adjuvant chemotherapy. At the time of evaluation, she is 5 feet 3 inches tall, weighs 165 pounds, and reports an increase in body weight by 3 pounds after diagnosis and treatment-related symptoms, including constipation and fatigue. She also has a history of osteoporosis and hypertension. She feels "very tired", and she believes that any exercise program would aggravate this feeling. Therefore, she is doing light housework activities. At present, she is taking a high-dose multivitamin supplement that also contains ginseng and guarana to mainly address the symptom of fatigue.

Questions:

1. Estimate the patient's BMI. Do you need other anthropometric or body composition indices?
2. Is there evidence linking physical activity to worsened fatigue? What physical activity recommendations would you give the patient? How would you assess the long-term effects of the physical activity program?
3. What dietary recommendations would you suggest and why? Is weight loss an evidence-based approach in this patient? In this context, what variables should you assess in the long-term?
4. Should Mrs. TH continue to take the multivitamin supplement?

After the completion of chemotherapy, a hormonal therapy (letrozole) is planned for at least 5 years to further reduce the risk of recurrence. Anticipated side effects include, among others, hypercholesterolemia and osteoporosis.

5. What kind of dietary and physical activity advice would you give Mrs. TH on this stage of survivorship and why?

REFERENCES

AACC. (2000). American Association of Cereal Chemists Committee to Define Whole Grain. AACC members agree on definition of whole grain. *Cereal Foods World, 45,* 79.

Abu el Maaty, M., & Wölfl, S. (2017). Vitamin D as a Novel Regulator of Tumor Metabolism: Insights on Potential Mechanisms and Implications for Anti-Cancer Therapy. *International Journal of Molecular Sciences, 18*(10), 2184. https://doi.org/10.3390/ijms18102184

Anand, P., Kunnumakara, A. B., Sundaram, C., Harikumar, K. B., Tharakan, S. T., Lai, O. S., Sung, B., & Aggarwal, B. B. (2008). Cancer is a Preventable Disease that Requires Major Lifestyle Changes. *Pharmaceutical Research, 25*(9), 2097–2116. https://doi.org/10.1007/s11095-008-9661-9

Anderson, A. S., Martin, R. M., Renehan, A. G., Cade, J., Copson, E. R., Cross, A. J., Grimmett, C., Keaver, L., King, A., Riboli, E., Shaw, C., Saxton, J. M., Anderson, A., Beeken, R., Cade, J., Cross, A., King, A., Martin, R., Mitrou, G., ... Renehan, A. (2021). Cancer survivorship, excess body fatness and weight-loss intervention—where are we in 2020? *British Journal of Cancer, 124*(6), 1057–1065. https://doi.org/10.1038/s41416-020-01155-2

Arends, J., Baracos, V., Bertz, H., Bozzetti, F., Calder, P. C., Deutz, N. E. P., Erickson, N., Laviano, A., Lisanti, M. P., Lobo, D. N., McMillan, D. C., Muscaritoli, M., Ockenga, J., Pirlich, M., Strasser, F., de de van der Schueren, M., Van Gossum, A., Vaupel, P., & Weimann, A. (2017). ESPEN expert group recommendations for action against cancer-related malnutrition. *Clinical Nutrition, 36*(5), 1187–1196. https://doi.org/10.1016/j.clnu.2017.06.017

Arends, Jann, Bachmann, P., Baracos, V., Barthelemy, N., Bertz, H., Bozzetti, F., Fearon, K., Hütterer, E., Isenring, E., Kaasa, S., Krznaric, Z., Laird, B., Larsson, M., Laviano, A., Mühlebach, S., Muscaritoli, M., Oldervoll, L., Ravasco, P., Solheim, T., ... Preiser, J. C. (2017). ESPEN guidelines on nutrition in cancer patients. *Clinical Nutrition, 36*(1), 11–48. https://doi.org/10.1016/j.clnu.2016.07.015

Arnold, M., Pandeya, N., Byrnes, G., Renehan, A. G., Stevens, G. A., Ezzati, M., Ferlay, J., Miranda, J. J., Romieu, I., Dikshit, R., Forman, D., & Soerjomataram, I. (2015). Global burden of cancer attributable to high body-mass index in 2012: a population-based study. *The Lancet Oncology, 16*(1), 36–46. https://doi.org/10.1016/S1470-2045(14)71123-4

Aune, D., Navarro Rosenblatt, D. A., Chan, D. S. M., Vingeliene, S., Abar, L., Vieira, A. R., Greenwood, D. C., Bandera, E. V., & Norat, T. (2015). Anthropometric factors and endometrial cancer risk: a systematic review and dose–response meta-analysis of prospective studies. *Annals of Oncology, 26*(8), 1635–1648. https://doi.org/10.1093/annonc/mdv142

Aune, Dagfinn, Navarro Rosenblatt, D. A., Chan, D. S., Vieira, A. R., Vieira, R., Greenwood, D. C., Vatten, L. J., & Norat, T. (2015). Dairy products, calcium, and prostate cancer risk: a systematic review and meta-analysis of cohort studies. *The American Journal of Clinical Nutrition, 101*(1), 87–117. https://doi.org/10.3945/ajcn.113.067157

Baena, R., & Salinas, P. (2015). Diet and colorectal cancer. *Maturitas, 80*(3), 258–264. https://doi.org/10.1016/j.maturitas.2014.12.017

Bagnardi, V., Rota, M., Botteri, E., Tramacere, I., Islami, F., Fedirko, V., Scotti, L., Jenab, M., Turati, F., Pasquali, E., Pelucchi, C., Bellocco, R., Negri, E., Corrao, G., Rehm, J., Boffetta, P., & La Vecchia, C. (2013). Light alcohol drinking and cancer: a meta-analysis. *Annals of Oncology, 24*(2), 301–308. https://doi.org/10.1093/annonc/mds337

Baracos, V. E., Martin, L., Korc, M., Guttridge, D. C., & Fearon, K. C. H. (2018). Cancer-associated cachexia. *Nature Reviews Disease Primers, 4*(January). https://doi.org/10.1038/nrdp.2017.105

Biswas, A., Oh, P. I., Faulkner, G. E., Bajaj, R. R., Silver, M. A., Mitchell, M. S., & Alter, D. A. (2015). Sedentary Time and Its Association With Risk for Disease Incidence, Mortality, and Hospitalization in Adults. *Annals of Internal Medicine, 162*(2), 123–132. https://doi.org/10.7326/M14-1651

Bouvard, V., Loomis, D., Guyton, K. Z., Grosse, Y., Ghissassi, F. El, Benbrahim-Tallaa, L., Guha, N., Mattock, H., & Straif, K. (2015). Carcinogenicity of consumption of red and processed meat. *The Lancet Oncology, 16*(16), 1599–1600. https://doi.org/10.1016/S1470-2045(15)00444-1

Campbell, K. L., Winters-Stone, K. M., Wiskemann, J., May, A. M., Schwartz, A. L., Courneya, K. S., Zucker, D. S., Matthews, C. E., Ligibel, J. A., Gerber, I. H., Morris, G. S., Patel, A. V., Hue, T. F., Perna, F. M., & Schmitz, K. H. (2019). Exercise Guidelines for Cancer Survivors: Consensus Statement from International Multidisciplinary Roundtable. *Medicine & Science in Sports & Exercise, 51*(11), 2375–2390. https://doi.org/10.1249/MSS.0000000000002116

Castro-Espin, C., & Agudo, A. (2022). The Role of Diet in Prognosis among Cancer Survivors: A Systematic Review and Meta-Analysis of Dietary Patterns and Diet Interventions. *Nutrients, 14*(2), 348. https://doi.org/10.3390/nu14020348

Chan, D. S. M., Lau, R., Aune, D., Vieira, R., Greenwood, D. C., Kampman, E., & Norat, T. (2011). Red and Processed Meat and Colorectal Cancer Incidence: Meta-Analysis of Prospective Studies. *PLoS ONE, 6*(6), e20456. https://doi.org/10.1371/journal.pone.0020456

Chlebowski, R. T., Blackburn, G. L., Thomson, C. A., Nixon, D. W., Shapiro, A., Hoy, M. K., Goodman, M. T., Giuliano, A. E., Karanja, N., McAndrew, P., Hudis, C., Butler, J., Merkel, D., Kristal, A., Caan, B., Michaelson, R., Vinciguerra, V., Del Prete, S., Winkler, M., ... Elashoff, R. M. (2006). Dietary Fat Reduction and Breast Cancer Outcome: Interim Efficacy Results From the Women's Intervention Nutrition Study. *JNCI: Journal of the National Cancer Institute, 98*(24), 1767–1776. https://doi.org/10.1093/jnci/djj494

Chlebowski, R. T., Luo, J., Anderson, G. L., Barrington, W., Reding, K., Simon, M. S., Manson, J. E., Rohan, T. E., Wactawski-Wende, J., Lane, D., Strickler, H., Mosaver-Rahmani, Y., Freudenheim, J. L., Saquib, N., & Stefanick, M. L. (2019). Weight loss and breast cancer incidence in postmenopausal women. *Cancer, 125*(2), 205–212. https://doi.org/10.1002/cncr.31687

Cruz-Jentoft, A. J., Bahat, G., Bauer, J., Boirie, Y., Bruyère, O., Cederholm, T., Cooper, C., Landi, F., Rolland, Y., Sayer, A. A., Schneider, S. M., Sieber, C. C., Topinkova, E., Vandewoude, M., Visser, M., Zamboni, M., Bautmans, I., Baeyens, J. P., Cesari, M., ... Schols, J. (2019). Sarcopenia: Revised European consensus on definition and diagnosis. *Age and Ageing, 48*(1), 16–31. https://doi.org/10.1093/ageing/afy169

Davis, J. F., van Rooijen, S. J., Grimmett, C., West, M. A., Campbell, A. M., Awasthi, R., Slooter, G. D., Grocott, M. P., Carli, F., & Jack, S. (2022). From Theory to Practice: An International Approach to Establishing Prehabilitation Programmes. *Current Anesthesiology Reports, 12*(1), 129–137. https://doi.org/10.1007/s40140-022-00516-2

de Vries, J. (2015). Effects of cereal fiber on bowel function: A systematic review of intervention trials. *World Journal of Gastroenterology, 21*(29), 8952. https://doi.org/10.3748/wjg.v21.i29.8952

Dimitrakopoulou, V. I., Tsilidis, K. K., Haycock, P. C., Dimou, N. L., Al-Dabhani, K., Martin, R. M., Lewis, S. J., Gunter, M. J., Mondul, A., Shui, I. M., Theodoratou, E., Nimptsch, K., Lindström, S., Albanes, D., Kühn, T., Key, T. J., Travis, R. C., Vimaleswaran, K. S., Kraft, P., ... Schildkraut, J. M. (2017). Circulating vitamin D concentration and risk of seven cancers: Mendelian randomisation study. *BMJ, j4761.* https://doi.org/10.1136/bmj.j4761

Donini, L. M., Busetto, L., Bischoff, S. C., Cederholm, T., Ballesteros-Pomar, M. D., Batsis, J. A., Bauer, J. M., Boirie, Y., Cruz-Jentoft, A. J., Dicker, D., Frara, S., Frühbeck, G., Genton, L., Gepner, Y., Giustina, A., Gonzalez, M. C., Han, H.-S., Heymsfield, S. B., Higashiguchi, T., . . . Barazzoni, R. (2022). Definition and diagnostic criteria for sarcopenic obesity: ESPEN and EASO consensus statement. *Clinical Nutrition*, *41*(4), 990–1000. https://doi.org/10.1016/j.clnu.2021.11.014

Dybkowska E., Sadowska A., Świderski F., Rakowska R., W. K. (2018). The occurrence of resveratrol in foodstuffs and its potential for supporting cancer prevention and treatment. A review. *Rocz Panstw Zakl Hig*, *69*(1), 5–14.

Egerman, M. A., & Glass, D. J. (2014). Signaling pathways controlling skeletal muscle mass. *Critical Reviews in Biochemistry and Molecular Biology*, *49*(1), 59–68. https://doi.org/10.3109/10409238.2013.857291

Faithfull, S., Turner, L., Poole, K., Joy, M., Manders, R., Weprin, J., Winters-Stone, K., & Saxton, J. (2019). Prehabilitation for adults diagnosed with cancer: A systematic review of long-term physical function, nutrition and patient-reported outcomes. *European Journal of Cancer Care*, *28*(4). https://doi.org/10.1111/ecc.13023

Fardet, A. (2010). New hypotheses for the health-protective mechanisms of whole-grain cereals: what is beyond fibre? *Nutrition Research Reviews*, *23*(1), 65–134. https://doi.org/10.1017/S0954422410000041

Farvid, M. S., Barnett, J. B., & Spence, N. D. (2021). Fruit and vegetable consumption and incident breast cancer: a systematic review and meta-analysis of prospective studies. *British Journal of Cancer*, *125*(2), 284–298. https://doi.org/10.1038/s41416-021-01373-2

Farvid, M. S., Sidahmed, E., Spence, N. D., Mante Angua, K., Rosner, B. A., & Barnett, J. B. (2021). Consumption of red meat and processed meat and cancer incidence: a systematic review and meta-analysis of prospective studies. *European Journal of Epidemiology*, *36*(9), 937–951. https://doi.org/10.1007/s10654-021-00741-9

Fearon, K., Strasser, F., Anker, S. D., Bosaeus, I., Bruera, E., Fainsinger, R. L., Jatoi, A., Loprinzi, C., MacDonald, N., Mantovani, G., Davis, M., Muscaritoli, M., Ottery, F., Radbruch, L., Ravasco, P., Walsh, D., Wilcock, A., Kaasa, S., & Baracos, V. E. (2011). Definition and classification of cancer cachexia: An international consensus. *The Lancet Oncology*, *12*(5), 489–495. https://doi.org/10.1016/S1470-2045(10)70218-7

Ferriolli, E., Skipworth, R. J. E., Hendry, P., Scott, A., Stensteth, J., Dahele, M., Wall, L., Greig, C., Fallon, M., Strasser, F., Preston, T., & Fearon, K. C. H. (2012). Physical activity monitoring: A responsive and meaningful patient-centered outcome for surgery, chemotherapy, or radiotherapy? *Journal of Pain and Symptom Management*, *43*(6), 1025–1035. https://doi.org/10.1016/j.jpainsymman.2011.06.013

Fiolet, T., Srour, B., Sellem, L., Kesse-Guyot, E., Allès, B., Méjean, C., Deschasaux, M., Fassier, P., Latino-Martel, P., Beslay, M., Hercberg, S., Lavalette, C., Monteiro, C. A., Julia, C., & Touvier, M. (2018). Consumption of ultra-processed foods and cancer risk: results from NutriNet-Santé prospective cohort. *BMJ*, *k322*. https://doi.org/10.1136/bmj.k322

Ford, K. L., Arends, J., Atherton, P. J., Engelen, M. P. K. J., Gonçalves, T. J. M., Laviano, A., Lobo, D. N., Phillips, S. M., Ravasco, P., Deutz, N. E. P., & Prado, C. M. (2022). The importance of protein sources to support muscle anabolism in cancer: An expert group opinion. *Clinical Nutrition*, *41*(1), 192–201. https://doi.org/10.1016/j.clnu.2021.11.032

Fortner, R. T., Katzke, V., Kühn, T., & Kaaks, R. (2016). *Obesity and Breast Cancer* (pp. 43–65). https://doi.org/10.1007/978-3-319-42542-9_3

Gaesser, G. A. (2020). Whole Grains, Refined Grains, and Cancer Risk: A Systematic Review of Meta-Analyses of Observational Studies. *Nutrients*, *12*(12), 3756. https://doi.org/10.3390/nu12123756

Gandhi, A., Copson, E., Eccles, D., Durcan, L., Howell, A., Morris, J., Howell, S., McDiarmid, S., Sellers, K., Gareth Evans, D., & Harvie, M. (2019). Predictors of weight gain in a cohort of premenopausal early breast cancer patients receiving chemotherapy. *The Breast*, *45*, 1–6. https://doi.org/10.1016/j.breast.2019.02.006

Ghasemi, A., Saeidi, J., Azimi-Nejad, M., & Hashemy, S. I. (2019). Leptin-induced signaling pathways in cancer cell migration and invasion. *Cellular Oncology*, *42*(3), 243–260. https://doi.org/10.1007/s13402-019-00428-0

Giovannucci, E. (2018). Nutritional epidemiology and cancer: A Tale of Two Cities. *Cancer Causes & Control*, *29*(11), 1007–1014. https://doi.org/10.1007/s10552-018-1088-y

Grosso, G., Bella, F., Godos, J., Sciacca, S., Del Rio, D., Ray, S., Galvano, F., & Giovannucci, E. L. (2017). Possible role of diet in cancer: systematic review and multiple meta-analyses of dietary patterns, lifestyle factors, and cancer risk. *Nutrition Reviews*, *75*(6), 405–419. https://doi.org/10.1093/nutrit/nux012

Harland, J. I., & Garton, L. E. (2008). Whole-grain intake as a marker of healthy body weight and adiposity. *Public Health Nutrition*, *11*(6), 554–563. https://doi.org/10.1017/S1368980007001279

Harrison, S., Lennon, R., Holly, J., Higgins, J. P. T., Gardner, M., Perks, C., Gaunt, T., Tan, V., Borwick, C., Emmet, P., Jeffreys, M., Northstone, K., Rinaldi, S., Thomas, S., Turner, S. D., Pease, A., Vilenchick, V., Martin, R. M., & Lewis, S. J. (2017). Does milk intake promote prostate cancer initiation or progression via effects on insulin-like growth factors (IGFs)? A systematic review and meta-analysis. *Cancer Causes & Control*, *28*(6), 497–528. https://doi.org/10.1007/s10552-017-0883-1

Hojman, P., Gehl, J., Christensen, J. F., & Pedersen, B. K. (2018). Molecular Mechanisms Linking Exercise to Cancer Prevention and Treatment. *Cell Metabolism*, *27*(1), 10–21. https://doi.org/10.1016/j.cmet.2017.09.015

Hopkins, B. D., Gonçalves, M. D., & Cantley, L. C. (2020). Insulin–PI3K signalling: an evolutionarily insulated metabolic driver of cancer. *Nature Reviews Endocrinology*, *16*(5), 276–283. https://doi.org/10.1038/s41574-020-0329-9

IARC. (1988). Alcohol drinking. *IARC Monogr Eval Carcinog Risks Hum*, *44*, 1–378.

IARC. (2015). *International Agency for Research on Cancer (IARC). Consumption of red meat and processed meat. IARC Working Group. Lyon*. 114.

Inoue-Choi, M., Sinha, R., Gierach, G. L., & Ward, M. H. (2016). Red and processed meat, nitrite, and heme iron intakes and postmenopausal breast cancer risk in the NIH-AARP Diet and Health Study. *International Journal of Cancer*, *138*(7), 1609–1618. https://doi.org/10.1002/ijc.29901

Islami, F., Goding Sauer, A., Miller, K. D., Siegel, R. L., Fedewa, S. A., Jacobs, E. J., McCullough, M. L., Patel, A. V., Ma, J., Soerjomataram, I., Flanders, W. D., Brawley, O. W., Gapstur, S. M., & Jemal, A. (2018). Proportion and number of cancer cases and deaths attributable to potentially modifiable risk factors in the United States. *CA: A Cancer Journal for Clinicians*, *68*(1), 31–54. https://doi.org/10.3322/caac.21440

Jemal A, Torre L, Soerjomataram I, B. F. (Eds.). (2019). The Cancer Atlas. Third Ed. Atlanta, GA: American Cancer Society. Also Available at: Www.Cancer.Org/Canceratlas.

Jiramongkol, Y., & Lam, E. W.-F. (2020). *Multifaceted Oncogenic Role of Adipocytes in the Tumour Microenvironment* (pp. 125–142). https://doi.org/10.1007/978-3-030-34025-4_7

Jones, L. W., Eves, N. D., Haykowsky, M., Joy, A. A., & Douglas, P. S. (2008). Cardiorespiratory exercise testing in clinical oncology research: systematic review and practice recommendations. *The Lancet Oncology*, *9*(8), 757–765. https://doi.org/10.1016/S1470-2045(08)70195-5

Joosen, A. M. C. P., Kuhnle, G. G. C., Aspinall, S. M., Barrow, T. M., Lecommandeur, E., Azqueta, A., Collins, A. R., & Bingham, S. A. (2009). Effect of processed and red meat on endogenous nitrosation and DNA damage. *Carcinogenesis*, *30*(8), 1402–1407. https://doi.org/10.1093/carcin/bgp130

Kaluza, J., Harris, H. R., Håkansson, N., & Wolk, A. (2020). Adherence to the WCRF/AICR 2018 recommendations for cancer prevention and risk of cancer: prospective cohort studies of men and women. *British Journal of Cancer*, *122*(10), 1562–1570. https://doi.org/10.1038/s41416-020-0806-x

Kenkhuis, M.-F., van der Linden, B. W. A., Breedveld-Peters, J. J. L., Koole, J. L., van Roekel, E. H., Breukink, S. O., Mols, F., Weijenberg, M. P., & Bours, M. J. L. (2021). Associations of the dietary World Cancer Research Fund/American Institute for Cancer Research (WCRF/AICR) recommendations with patient-reported outcomes in colorectal cancer survivors 2–10 years post-diagnosis: a cross-sectional analysis. *British Journal of Nutrition*, *125*(10), 1188–1200. https://doi.org/10.1017/S0007114520003487

Koh, D., Song, S., Moon, S.-E., Jung, S.-Y., Lee, E. S., Kim, Z., Youn, H. J., Cho, J., Yoo, Y. B., Lee, S. K., Lee, J. E., Nam, S. J., & Lee, J. E. (2019). Adherence to the American Cancer Society Guidelines for Cancer Survivors and Health-Related Quality of Life among Breast Cancer Survivors. *Nutrients*, *11*(12), 2924. https://doi.org/10.3390/nu11122924

Kohler, L. N., Garcia, D. O., Harris, R. B., Oren, E., Roe, D. J., & Jacobs, E. T. (2016). Adherence to Diet and Physical Activity Cancer Prevention Guidelines and Cancer Outcomes: A Systematic Review. *Cancer Epidemiology Biomarkers & Prevention*, *25*(7), 1018–1028. https://doi.org/10.1158/1055-9965.EPI-16-0121

Laguna, J. C., Alegret, M., Cofán, M., Sánchez-Tainta, A., Díaz-López, A., Martínez-González, M. A., Sorlí, J. V., Salas-Salvadó, J., Fitó, M., Alonso-Gómez, Á. M., Serra-Majem, L., Lapetra, J., Fiol, M., Gómez-Gracia, E., Pintó, X., Muñoz, M. A., Castañer, O., Ramírez-Sabio, J. B., Portu, J. J., ... Ros, E. (2021). Simple sugar intake and cancer incidence, cancer mortality and all-cause mortality: A cohort study from the PREDIMED trial. *Clinical Nutrition*, *40*(10), 5269–5277. https://doi.org/10.1016/j.clnu.2021.07.031

Lauby-Secretan, B., Scoccianti, C., Loomis, D., Grosse, Y., Bianchini, F., & Straif, K. (2016). Body Fatness and Cancer — Viewpoint of the IARC Working Group. *New England Journal of Medicine*, *375*(8), 794–798. https://doi.org/10.1056/NEJMsr1606602

Laviano, A. (2021). Current guidelines for nutrition therapy in cancer: The arrival of a long journey or the starting point? *Journal of Parenteral and Enteral Nutrition*, *45*(S2). https://doi.org/10.1002/jpen.2288

Ligibel, J. A., Bohlke, K., May, A. M., Clinton, S. K., Demark-Wahnefried, W., Gilchrist, S. C., Irwin, M. L., Late, M., Mansfield, S., Marshall, T. F., Meyerhardt, J. A., Thomson, C. A., Wood, W. A., & Alfano, C. M. (2022). Exercise, Diet, and Weight Management During Cancer Treatment: ASCO Guideline. *Journal of Clinical Oncology*. https://doi.org/10.1200/JCO.22.00687

Liu, Y., Nguyen, N., & Colditz, G. A. (2015). Links between Alcohol Consumption and Breast Cancer: A Look at the Evidence. *Women's Health*, *11*(1), 65–77. https://doi.org/10.2217/WHE.14.62

LoConte, N. K., Brewster, A. M., Kaur, J. S., Merrill, J. K., & Alberg, A. J. (2018). Alcohol and Cancer: A Statement of the American Society of Clinical Oncology. *Journal of Clinical Oncology*, *36*(1), 83–93. https://doi.org/10.1200/JCO.2017.76.1155

Luo, J., Chlebowski, R. T., Hendryx, M., Rohan, T., Wactawski-Wende, J., Thomson, C. A., Felix, A. S., Chen, C., Barrington, W., Coday, M., Stefanick, M., LeBlanc, E., & Margolis, K. L. (2017). Intentional Weight Loss and Endometrial Cancer Risk. *Journal of Clinical Oncology*, *35*(11), 1189–1193. https://doi.org/10.1200/JCO.2016.70.5822

Manson, J. E., Cook, N. R., Lee, I.-M., Christen, W., Bassuk, S. S., Mora, S., Gibson, H., Gordon, D., Copeland, T., D'Agostino, D., Friedenberg, G., Ridge, C., Bubes, V., Giovannucci, E. L., Willett, W. C., & Buring, J. E. (2019). Vitamin D Supplements and Prevention of Cancer and Cardiovascular Disease. *New England Journal of Medicine*, *380*(1), 33–44. https://doi.org/10.1056/NEJMoa1809944

Marzorati, C., Riva, S., & Pravettoni, G. (2017). Who Is a Cancer Survivor? A Systematic Review of Published Definitions. *Journal of Cancer Education*, *32*(2), 228–237. https://doi.org/10.1007/s13187-016-0997-2

McTiernan, A. (2008). Mechanisms linking physical activity with cancer. *Nature Reviews Cancer*, *8*(3), 205–211. https://doi.org/10.1038/nrc2325

Miller, K. D., Siegel, R. L., Lin, C. C., Mariotto, A. B., Kramer, J. L., Rowland, J. H., Stein, K. D., Alteri, R., & Jemal, A. (2016). Cancer treatment and survivorship statistics, 2016. *CA: A Cancer Journal for Clinicians*, *66*(4), 271–289. https://doi.org/10.3322/caac.21349

Moy, F. M., Greenwood, D. C., & Cade, J. E. (2018). Associations of clothing size, adiposity and weight change with risk of postmenopausal breast cancer in the UK Women's Cohort Study (UKWCS). *BMJ Open*, *8*(9), e022599. https://doi.org/10.1136/bmjopen-2018-022599

Norat, T., & Riboli, E. (2003). Dairy products and colorectal cancer. A review of possible mechanisms and epidemiological evidence. *European Journal of Clinical Nutrition*, *57*(1), 1–17. https://doi.org/10.1038/sj.ejcn.1601522

PAGAC. (2018). *2018 Physical Activity Guidelines Advisory Committee. 2018 Physical Activity Guidelines Advisory Committee Scientific Report*. Washington, DC: US Department of Health and Human Services.

Patel, A. V., Friedenreich, C. M., Moore, S. C., Hayes, S. C., Silver, J. K., Campbell, K. L., Winters-Stone, K., Gerber, I. H., George, S. M., Fulton, J. E., Denlinger, C., Morris, G. S., Hue, T., Schmitz, K. H., & Matthews, C. E. (2019). American College of Sports Medicine Roundtable Report on Physical Activity, Sedentary Behavior, and Cancer Prevention and Control. *Medicine & Science in Sports & Exercise*, *51*(11), 2391–2402. https://doi.org/10.1249/MSS.0000000000002117

Pędziwiatr, M., Mavrikis, J., Witowski, J., Adamos, A., Major, P., Nowakowski, M., & Budzyński, A. (2018). Current status of enhanced recovery after surgery (ERAS) protocol in gastrointestinal surgery. *Medical Oncology*, *35*(6), 95. https://doi.org/10.1007/s12032-018-1153-0

Pierce, J. P., Natarajan, L., Caan, B. J., Parker, B. A., Greenberg, E. R., Flatt, S. W., Rock, C. L., Kealey, S., Al-Delaimy, W. K., Bardwell, W. A., Carlson, R. W., Emond, J. A., Faerber, S., Gold, E. B., Hajek, R. A., Hollenbach, K., Jones, L. A., Karanja, N., Madlensky, L., ... Stefanick, M. L. (2007). Influence of a Diet Very High in Vegetables, Fruit, and Fiber and Low in Fat on Prognosis Following Treatment for Breast Cancer. *JAMA*, *298*(3), 289. https://doi.org/10.1001/jama.298.3.289

Piercy, K. L., Troiano, R. P., Ballard, R. M., Carlson, S. A., Fulton, J. E., Galuska, D. A., George, S. M., & Olson, R. D. (2018). The Physical Activity Guidelines for Americans. *JAMA*, *320*(19), 2020. https://doi.org/10.1001/jama.2018.14854

Praud, D., Rota, M., Rehm, J., Shield, K., Zatoński, W., Hashibe, M., La Vecchia, C., & Boffetta, P. (2016). Cancer incidence and mortality attributable to alcohol consumption. *International Journal of Cancer*, *138*(6), 1380–1387. https://doi.org/10.1002/ijc.29890

Rock, C. L., Thomson, C. A., Sullivan, K. R., Howe, C. L., Kushi, L. H., Caan, B. J., Neuhouser, M. L., Bandera, E. V., Wang, Y., Robien, K., Basen-Engquist, K. M., Brown, J. C., Courneya, K. S., Crane, T. E., Garcia, D. O., Grant, B. L., Hamilton, K. K., Hartman, S. J., Kenfield, S. A., ... McCullough, M. L. (2022). American Cancer Society nutrition and physical activity guideline for cancer survivors. *CA: A Cancer Journal for Clinicians*, *72*(3), 230–262. https://doi.org/10.3322/caac.21719

Rock, C. L., Thomson, C., Gansler, T., Gapstur, S. M., McCullough, M. L., Patel, A. V., Andrews, K. S., Bandera, E. V., Spees, C. K., Robien, K., Hartman, S., Sullivan, K., Grant, B. L., Hamilton, K. K., Kushi, L. H., Caan, B. J., Kibbe, D., Black, J. D., Wiedt, T. L., ... Doyle, C. (2020). American Cancer Society guideline for diet and physical activity for cancer prevention. *CA: A Cancer Journal for Clinicians*, 70(4), 245–271. https://doi.org/10.3322/caac.21591

Romaneiro, S., & Parekh, N. (2012). Dietary Fiber Intake and Colorectal Cancer Risk. *Topics in Clinical Nutrition*, 27(1), 41–47. https://doi.org/10.1097/TIN.0b013e3182461dd4

Sánchez-Jiménez, F., Pérez-Pérez, A., de la Cruz-Merino, L., & Sánchez-Margalet, V. (2019). Obesity and Breast Cancer: Role of Leptin. *Frontiers in Oncology*, 9. https://doi.org/10.3389/fonc.2019.00596

Schmid, D., & Leitzmann, M. F. (2014). Television Viewing and Time Spent Sedentary in Relation to Cancer Risk: A Meta-Analysis. *JNCI: Journal of the National Cancer Institute*, 106(7). https://doi.org/10.1093/jnci/dju098

Schmitz, K. H., Campbell, A. M., Stuiver, M. M., Pintó, B. M., Schwartz, A. L., Morris, G. S., Ligibel, J. A., Cheville, A., Galvão, D. A., Alfano, C. M., Patel, A. V., Hue, T., Gerber, L. H., Sallis, R., Gusani, N. J., Stout, N. L., Chan, L., Flowers, F., Doyle, C., ... Matthews, C. E. (2019). Exercise is medicine in oncology: Engaging clinicians to help patients move through cancer. *CA: A Cancer Journal for Clinicians*, 69(6), 468–484. https://doi.org/10.3322/caac.21579

Schwingshackl, L., Schwedhelm, C., Hoffmann, G., Knüppel, S., Laure Preterre, A., Iqbal, K., Bechthold, A., De Henauw, S., Michels, N., Devleesschauwer, B., Boeing, H., & Schlesinger, S. (2018). Food groups and risk of colorectal cancer. *International Journal of Cancer*, 142(9), 1748–1758. https://doi.org/10.1002/ijc.31198

Sedentary Behaviour Research Network. (2012). Letter to the Editor: Standardized use of the terms "sedentary" and "sedentary behaviours." *Applied Physiology, Nutrition, and Metabolism*, 37(3), 540–542. https://doi.org/10.1139/h2012-024

Shams-White, M. M., Brockton, N. T., Mitrou, P., Romaguera, D., Brown, S., Bender, A., Kahle, L. L., & Reedy, J. (2019). Operationalizing the 2018 World Cancer Research Fund/American Institute for Cancer Research (WCRF/AICR) Cancer Prevention Recommendations: A Standardized Scoring System. *Nutrients*, 11(7), 1572. https://doi.org/10.3390/nu11071572

Shaw, E., Farris, M., McNeil, J., & Friedenreich, C. (2016). *Obesity and Endometrial Cancer* (pp. 107–136). https://doi.org/10.1007/978-3-319-42542-9_7

Shimizu H, Mack TM, Ross RK, H. B. (1987). Cancer of the gastrointestinal tract among Japanese and white immigrants in Los Angeles County. *J Natl Cancer Inst*, 78(2), 223–228.

Sinha, R., Rothman, N., Salmon, C. P., Knize, M. G., Brown, E. D., Swanson, C. A., Rhodes, D., Rossi, S., Felton, J. S., & Levander, O. A. (1998). Heterocyclic amine content in beef cooked by different methods to varying degrees of doneness and gravy made from meat drippings. *Food and Chemical Toxicology*, 36(4), 279–287. https://doi.org/10.1016/S0278-6915(97)00162-2

Slavin, J. (2003). Why whole grains are protective: biological mechanisms. *Proceedings of the Nutrition Society*, 62(1), 129–134. https://doi.org/10.1079/PNS2002221

Smith, M. R., Saad, F., Egerdie, B., Sieber, P. R., Tammela, T. L. J., Ke, C., Leder, B. Z., & Goessl, C. (2012). Sarcopenia during androgen-deprivation therapy for prostate cancer. *Journal of Clinical Oncology*, 30(26), 3271–3276. https://doi.org/10.1200/JCO.2011.38.8850

Song, M., Garrett, W. S., & Chan, A. T. (2015). Nutrients, Foods, and Colorectal Cancer Prevention. *Gastroenterology*, 148(6), 1244–1260.e16. https://doi.org/10.1053/j.gastro.2014.12.035

Steck, S. E., & Murphy, E. A. (2020). Dietary patterns and cancer risk. *Nature Reviews Cancer*, 20(2), 125–138. https://doi.org/10.1038/s41568-019-0227-4

Sung, H., Ferlay, J., Siegel, R. L., Laversanne, M., Soerjomataram, I., Jemal, A., & Bray, F. (2021). Global Cancer Statistics 2020: GLOBOCAN Estimates of Incidence and Mortality Worldwide for 36 Cancers in 185 Countries. *CA: A Cancer Journal for Clinicians*, 71(3), 209–249. https://doi.org/10.3322/caac.21660

Teras, L. R., Patel, A. V, Wang, M., Yaun, S.-S., Anderson, K., Brathwaite, R., Caan, B. J., Chen, Y., Connor, A. E., Eliassen, A. H., Gapstur, S. M., Gaudet, M. M., Genkinger, J. M., Giles, G. G., Lee, I.-M., Milne, R. L., Robien, K., Sawada, N., Sesso, H. D., ... Smith-Warner, S. A. (2020). Sustained Weight Loss and Risk of Breast Cancer in Women 50 Years and Older: A Pooled Analysis of Prospective Data. *JNCI: Journal of the National Cancer Institute*, 112(9), 929–937. https://doi.org/10.1093/jnci/djz226

Turesky, R. J. (2018). Mechanistic Evidence for Red Meat and Processed Meat Intake and Cancer Risk: A Follow-up on the International Agency for Research on Cancer Evaluation of 2015. *CHIMIA*, 72(10), 718. https://doi.org/10.2533/chimia.2018.718

Vance, V., Mourtzakis, M., McCargar, L., & Hanning, R. (2011). Weight gain in breast cancer survivors: prevalence, pattern and health consequences. *Obesity Reviews*, 12(4), 282–294. https://doi.org/10.1111/j.1467-789X.2010.00805.x

WCRF/AICR. (2018). *Diet, nutrition, physical activity and cancer: a global perspective. Continuous Update Project Expert Report 2018*. World Cancer Research Fund/American Institute for Cancer Research. Available from: https://www.wcrf.org/dietandcancer

WHO. (2019). *Cancer prevention*. Http://Www.Who.Int/Cancer/Prevention/En/. Accessed March 19, 2022.

WHO. (2020). *Obesity Estimates*. Geneva: *World Health Organisation*. https://www.who.int/news-room/fact-sheets/detail/obesity-and-overweight

Wiggins, T., Antonowicz, S. S., & Markar, S. R. (2019). Cancer Risk Following Bariatric Surgery—Systematic Review and Meta-analysis of National Population-Based Cohort Studies. *Obesity Surgery*, 29(3), 1031–1039. https://doi.org/10.1007/s11695-018-3501-8

Wild CP, Weiderpass E, Stewart BW, E. (2020). *World Cancer Report: Cancer Research for Cancer Prevention*. Lyon, France: International Agency for Research on Cancer. Available from: http://publications.iarc.fr/586.

Wilson, K. M., Shui, I. M., Mucci, L. A., & Giovannucci, E. (2015). Calcium and phosphorus intake and prostate cancer risk: a 24-y follow-up study. *The American Journal of Clinical Nutrition*, 101(1), 173–183. https://doi.org/10.3945/ajcn.114.088716

Wilson, R. L., Taaffe, D. R., Newton, R. U., Hart, N. H., Lyons-Wall, P., & Galvão, D. A. (2021). Using Exercise and Nutrition to Alter Fat and Lean Mass in Men with Prostate Cancer Receiving Androgen Deprivation Therapy: A Narrative Review. *Nutrients*, 13(5), 1664. https://doi.org/10.3390/nu13051664

Wilson, R. L., Taaffe, D. R., Newton, R. U., Hart, N. H., Lyons-Wall, P., & Galvão, D. A. (2022). Obesity and prostate cancer: A narrative review. *Critical Reviews in Oncology/Hematology*, 169, 103543. https://doi.org/10.1016/j.critrevonc.2021.103543

Wu, K., Spiegelman, D., Hou, T., Albanes, D., Allen, N. E., Berndt, S. I., van den Brandt, P. A., Giles, G. G., Giovannucci, E., Alexandra Goldbohm, R., Goodman, G. G., Goodman, P. J., Håkansson, N., Inoue, M., Key, T. J., Kolonel, L. N., Männistö, S., McCullough, M. L., Neuhouser, M. L., ... Smith-Warner, S. A. (2016). Associations between unprocessed red and processed meat, poultry, seafood and egg intake and the risk of prostate cancer: A pooled analysis of 15 prospective cohort studies. *International Journal of Cancer, 138*(10), 2368–2382. https://doi.org/10.1002/ijc.29973

Yeh, H., Bantle, J. P., Cassidy-Begay, M., Blackburn, G., Bray, G. A., Byers, T., Clark, J. M., Coday, M., Egan, C., Espeland, M. A., Foreyt, J. P., Garcia, K., Goldman, V., Gregg, E. W., Hazuda, H. P., Hesson, L., Hill, J. O., Horton, E. S., Jakicic, J. M., . . . Yanovski, S. Z. (2020). Intensive Weight Loss Intervention and Cancer Risk in Adults with Type 2 Diabetes: Analysis of the Look AHEAD Randomized Clinical Trial. *Obesity, 28*(9), 1678–1686. https://doi.org/10.1002/oby.22936

FURTHER READING

Bibliography

2018 Physical Activity Guidelines Advisory Committee. (2018). 2018 Physical Activity Guidelines Advisory Committee Scientific Report. Washington, DC: US Department of Health and Human Services.

Arends, J. *et al.* (2017). ESPEN guidelines on nutrition in cancer patients. *Clinical Nutrition. 36*: 11–48.

Campbell, K. L. *et al.* (2019). Exercise guidelines for cancer survivors: Consensus statement from international multidisciplinary roundtable. *Medicine & Science in Sports & Exercise. 51*: 2375–2390.

International Agency for Research on Cancer. (2015). Consumption of red meat and processed meat. IARC Working Group. Lyon. 114.

Lauby-Secretan, B. et al. (2016). Body fatness and cancer—Viewpoint of the IARC working group. *New England Journal of Medicine. 375*: 794–798.

Ligibel, J. A. et al. (2022). Exercise, diet, and weight management during cancer treatment: ASCO guideline. *Journal of Clinical Oncology.*

LoConte, N.K., Brewster, A.M., Kaur, J.S., Merrill, J.K., and Alberg, A.J. (2018). Alcohol and cancer: A statement of the American Society of Clinical Oncology. *Journal of Clinical Oncology. 36*: 83–93.

Rock, C. L. et al. (2020). American Cancer Society guideline for diet and physical activity for cancer prevention. *CA: A Cancer Journal for Clinicians. 70*: 245–271.

Rock, C. L. et al. (2022). American Cancer Society nutrition and physical activity guideline for cancer survivors. *CA: A Cancer Journal for Clinicians. 72*: 230–262.

WCRF/AICR. (2018). Diet, nutrition, physical activity, and cancer: a global perspective. Continuous update project expert report 2018. World Cancer Research Fund/American Institute for Cancer Research. Available from: https://www.wcrf.org/dietandcancer.

Wild, C.P., Weiderpass, E., and Stewart, B.W., editors. (2020). World cancer report: Cancer research for cancer prevention. Lyon, France: International Agency for Research on Cancer. Available from: http://publications.iarc.fr/586.

Links

- https://www.wcrf.org/
- https://www.cancer.org/
- https://beta.asco.org/
- https://www.iarc.who.int/
- https://www.who.int/activities/preventing-cancer
- https://www.who.int/news-room/fact-sheets/detail/obesity-and-overweight
- https://www.acsm.org/education-resources/trending-topics-resources/resource-library/detail?id=d081604d-aff3-4961-bbe8-4e4220193c54

Answers to Self-assessment Questions

APPENDIX

Chapter 1	367	Chapter 12	373
Chapter 2	368	Chapter 13	374
Chapter 3	368	Chapter 14	374
Chapter 4	369	Chapter 15	375
Chapter 5	369	Chapter 16	375
Chapter 6	369	Chapter 17	376
Chapter 7	370	Chapter 18	376
Chapter 8	370	Chapter 19	376
Chapter 9	370	Chapter 20	378
Chapter 10	371	Chapter 21	379
Chapter 11	372		

CHAPTER 1:

1.
   (a) True
   (b) False
   (c) False
   (d) False

2.
   (a) >2 g /day; 5 g salt/day
   (b) Viscosity; Fermentation
   (c) 10% or less
   (d) Five portions; 400 g
   (e) 5–10% of total energy intake
   (f) Total fat; Animal proteins; Added sugars; Fiber

3. Trans fatty acids might promote inflammation and endoplasmic reticulum stress as well as fat storage in the liver at the expense of adipose tissue compared to cis-unsaturated fatty acids and SFAs.

4. The WHO defines added/free sugar as "monosaccharides and disaccharides added to foods and beverages by the manufacturer, cook or consumer, and sugars naturally present in honey, syrups, fruit juices and fruit juice concentrates".

5. Physical inactivity is defined by an individual's inability to follow their current age group recommendations regarding weekly levels of physical activity.

6. b

7. For adults, recommendations suggest at least 150 minutes of moderate-intensity aerobic physical activity per week, or at least 75 minutes of vigorous-intensity aerobic physical activity throughout the week, or an equivalent combination of moderate- and vigorous-intensity activity.

8. An unhealthy pattern is not always synonymous with developing CVD. Those patterns do not necessarily represent food choices that pose the highest CVD risk rather than a mix of food choices including those with a protective role.

9. The pathophysiology behind high amounts of sugar via SSBs and ultra-processed foods is that the latter may lead to the production of high reactive oxygen-carbons, which further increase the possibility of atherosclerosis, hypertension,

Prevention and Management of Cardiovascular and Metabolic Disease: Diet, Physical Activity and Healthy Aging,
First Edition. Christina N. Katsagoni, Peter Kokkinos, and Labros S. Sidossis.
© 2023 John Wiley & Sons Ltd. Published 2023 by John Wiley & Sons Ltd.

peripheral vascular disease, coronary artery disease, cardiomyopathy, heart failure, and cardiac arrhythmias.

10.
   (a) Hypertension; Cardiovascular disease
   (b) 2300 mg/day
   (c) Salt
   (d) Processed foods; Ready-to-eat meals; Salt added in food preparation; Cooking; Table salt.
   (e) Blood pressure in both hypertensive and normotensive individuals

CHAPTER 2:

1. True. Epigenetic changes can be inherited by offspring and the following generations.

2. d

3. Over the last several decades, considerable scientific data suggests that the *in utero* environment can affect the phenotype of the fetus, leaving epigenetic imprints on genes that can modify the health status of the offspring. Maternal overnutrition, through excessive energy and fat consumption, alter the genome of the fetus, making the child more prone to develop metabolic abnormalities, obesity, impaired glucose tolerance, and hyperlipidemia, throughout its life.

4. Excessive body weight and weight gain during pregnancy favors the increase of adipose content in the fetus and newborn (macrosomia), and predisposes to childhood and adolescent obesity. It has been hypothesized that high maternal glucose, free fatty acid, and amino acid concentrations result in permanent changes in appetite control, neuroendocrine functioning and/or energy metabolism in the developing fetus, thus increasing the risk of adiposity, metabolic and cardiovascular disease in later life.

5. d

6. False. Both oocyte and sperm possess their own unique epigenomes. Maternal as well as paternal lifestyle, including physical activity, nutrition, and exposure to hazardous substances can alter the epigenome and affect the health of their children.

7. Emerging data indicate that air pollution exposure modulates the epigenetic mark, DNA methylation, and that these changes might in turn influence inflammation and disease development. In vitro and in vivo models have established that epigenetic modifications caused by *in utero* exposure to environmental toxicants can induce alterations in gene expression that may persist throughout life.

8. While genetic mutations tend to be irreversible, epigenetic changes are inherently reversible and potentially preventable. The overall disease risk can be decreased through preventive health care, including screenings; eating a low-fat, high fiber diet; getting regular exercise; maintaining an appropriate weight; and managing stress.

9. The epigenetic diet is a diet regimen that can be used therapeutically for health or preventive purposes. This term was introduced to indicate the consumption of foods such as soy, cruciferous vegetables, and green tea, which influence epigenetic mechanisms capable of protecting against cancer and the aging process.

10. a and c

CHAPTER 3:

1. According to the 2020–2025 Dietary Guidelines for Americans, a healthy dietary pattern should represent all foods and beverages consumed, include foods and beverages across all food groups in nutrient-dense forms, in recommended amounts and within calorie limits; individuals should have more than one way to achieve a healthy dietary pattern.

2. b

3. Olive oil induces cardio-protective effects due to the presence of polyphenolic compounds. Several mechanistic studies demonstrated that olive oil polyphenols increase the HDL level, prevent damage from oxidative stress, reduce thrombogenicity, endothelial dysfunction, BP, and inflammation, and alter gene expression responsible for atherosclerosis process.

4. Please complete the phrase:
   (a) 6% of energy; 27% of daily calorie intake; 150 mg/d approximately
   (b) from 1500 to 2300 mg/day
   (c) >30 g/day.
   (d) prevent and treat hypertension.

5. A notable difference between the ND and MedDiet is the use of rapeseed (canola) oil instead of olive oil.

6. The first type is the vegan diet, in which all animal products are avoided (such as meat, poultry, fish, seafood, eggs, dairy products). The second type is vegetarian, in which all meats are avoided but may include eggs (ovo-vegetarian), dairy products (lacto-vegetarian), eggs and dairy products (acto-ovo-vegetarian) or eggs, dairy products, and fish and/or shellfish (pescetarian).

7. a non-strict vegetarian diet in which individuals may occasionally eat meat or fish.

8. A well-structured vegetarian diet can provide adequate nutrient intake throughout their life; it can be a helpful therapeutic approach for some chronic diseases. However, some vegetarian diets, e.g. the vegan diet, may be low in certain nutrients, such as calcium, vitamins B-12 and D, omega-3 fatty acids, iodine, iron, and zinc. Individuals following such a dietary pattern need appropriate planning and are encouraged to habitually consume good sources of those micronutrients to avoid becoming deficient.

9. The 2021 AHA guidance to improve cardiovascular health emphasizes the important role of the US-style (USDA), healthy Mediterranean-style, DASH, and healthy vegetarian eating patterns as heart-healthy dietary patterns.

10.
   (a) True
   (b) False
   (c) False
   (d) True

CHAPTER 4:

1. The use of oxygen to extract energy is referred to as aerobic metabolism (from the Greek "aerobiosis", which means air-dependent living). Conversely, extracting energy without using oxygen is anaerobic (air-independent living) metabolism.

2. Cardiorespiratory fitness is the ability to perform dynamic exercise using large muscles for prolonged periods, at specific intensities, and frequencies.

3. The fat-free mass, which includes the skeleton, muscles and body water, and the fat mass in human bodies.

4. The maximal force a muscle or group of muscles can exert is assessed by tests that require maximum effort against the greatest resistance that one can move through the full range of motion once; this is known as the 1-repetition maximum (1-RM).

5. The joint range of motion is generally affected by age, sex, obesity, and physical activity.

CHAPTER 5:

1. Structured physical activity or exercise is a planned, structured program designed to beneficially promote health and physical fitness.

2. PA and exercise can be quantified based on (1) the mode or type of the activity, i.e. specific activity performed; (2) the frequency of the activity; (3) the duration of the activity; and (4) the intensity of the performing activity.

3. There are several methods for quantifying PA intensity. Three of those methods are: metabolic equivalents (METs), oxygen consumption (VO_2), and heart rate (HR).

4. AEE kcal/day = 0.9 × TEE kcal/day − REE kcal/day =
   = 0.9 × 2380 kcal/day − 1450 kcal/day =
   = 692 kcal/day

5. PAL = TEE/BMR = 2220/ 1350 = 1.64 (sedentary lifestyle or light activity lifestyle)

6. Borg Scale = 9 = very light physical activity. Examples: folding clothes, making the bed, washing dishes, playing billiard.

7. d & e.

8. HR_{max} = 220 − Age = 220 − 52 = 168 bpm/min.

9. According to 2020 WHO physical activity recommendations, moderate-intensity aerobic exercise is recommended in any duration, highlighting the value of total physical activity volume, irrespective of bout length, which differs from the the previous WHO 2010 guidelines that require bouts of at least 10 min.

10. Exercise volume is the byproduct of all exercise components. That is, exercise volume is the outcome of exercise intensity, exercise duration, and frequency.

CHAPTER 6:

1. The definition of physical inactivity has changed through the years, from failing to meet previous recommendations of 30 min of moderate-intensity physical activity on at least 5 days per week, or 20 min of vigorous physical activity on at least 3 days per week, or a combination of walking, moderate-intensity or vigorous-intensity activities for a total of 600 MET minutes per week to current recommendations of at least 150 min of moderate-to-vigorous-intensity physical activity per week regardless of how many days the activity is accumulated.

2. 6% of the global burden of coronary heart disease (CHD); 7% of type 2 diabetes mellitus (T2DM); 10% of breast cancer

3. Sedentary behavior is defined as any behavior with an energy expenditure of ≤1.5 METs, which typically refers to sitting, lying, and reclining behaviors during waking hours rather than an absence of MVPA.

4. Any physical activity other than none is beneficial for all-cause mortality, which will help those struggling to follow the guidelines to engage more with physical activity.

5. Routine physical activity is an effective method for the primary and secondary prevention of more than 25 chronic medical conditions including CVD/CAD, hypertension, stroke, osteoporosis, and T2DM.

6. (a) False
   (b) True
   (c) False
   (d) True

7. (i) improvements in cardiorespiratory and health-related physical fitness, (ii) better exercise toleration and functional status, (iii) improvements in body composition (e.g., strategies against obesity, reduced central obesity, weight management).

8. Adults should perform at least 150 to 300 minutes of MVPA per week and muscle strengthening activities at least 2 days a week.

9. Such remote and device-based interventions have a strong, short-term efficacy in both adult and older adult

CHAPTER 7:

1. The rate of aging is controlled, to some extent, by genetic pathways and biochemical processes. Furthermore, it is associated with the physical and social environment (external factors: ethnicity, culture, religion, security, social inequities, and scientific/technological advances), as well as personal characteristics – such as sex, ethnicity, or socioeconomic status.

2. Rowe and Kahn stated that successful aging involved three main factors: (1) being free of disability or disease, (2) having high cognitive and physical abilities, and (3) interacting with others in meaningful ways.

3. c

4. Healthy and successful aging are used interchangeably, nevertheless they represent different values. Successful aging is related to the Western view of success, which encompasses failure, a term that promotes ageism.

5. Healthy aging consists of five key components: physical capability, cognition, metabolic and physiological health, psychological well-being, and social well-being.

6. True

7. False

8. The older we get the happier we are. As we get old, we compensate for the declines that aging brings and establish new criteria for well-being; our overall mental health, including mood, sense of well-being, and ability to handle stress improves up until the very end of life.

9. True. Early life exposures, even *in utero*, can significantly affect healthy aging.

10. False. Health status, per se, does not reflect healthy aging. There is not an agreed standard measure, given the complexity of the aging process and the lack of consensus about how to define healthy aging. Overall, healthy aging reflects physical capability, cognition, metabolic and physiological health, psychological well-being, and social well-being.

CHAPTER 8:

1. Lifespan and health span seem to be strongly related, and individuals who live longer tend to be healthier throughout their life. Centenarians are generally considered a healthy aging model. They have reduced mortality rates and are less prone to the diseases that accompany aging. Centenarians seem to postpone critical disease into their later years of life, and the diseases and morbidities that centenarians suffer may be less severe or influence them to a lesser extent.

2. To live to 100, one must inherit the right genetic variants from parents or acquire epigenetic variants through the environment. Longevity and healthy aging are highly inherited traits.

3. Longevity clusters within families suggest a strong genetic predisposition that is expressed later in life. It exerts its effect for survival to ages beyond the age of 90.

4. False. Centenarians do not appear to lack common complex disease risk alleles. Instead, they have some protective genetic variants that buffer the risk alleles, allowing them to remain healthy. This genetic predisposition might make individuals less prone or more resistant to aging-related diseases.

5. Lifestyle factors that favor an increased health and life span, include eating in moderation, regular exercise, purposeful living, and strong social support systems.

6. False. Diet is an important, but not the sole, factor that affects the lifespan of people living in blue zones. It seems that longevity is not solely attributed to what they eat but also to how they live. Daily exercise from manual labor and rural living. The midday rest, even a short nap, protects and improves cardiac function. Emotional attachments to others, including strong family and social ties. The relaxed pace of daily life, without anxiety and stress, and living lives full of optimism, also contributes to longevity.

7. a and b

8. Complete the following statements:

    (a) ... living longer does not necessarily entail living healthier.

    (b) ... why some individuals live a longer and healthier life, without suffering from the diseases that most people come to confront much earlier in their lives.

    (c) ... women suffer from more illness and chronic health problems than do men but die at lower rates from all the major causes of death.

9. True

10. False

CHAPTER 9:

1. From a cardiovascular perspective, aging intensifies the influence of stress hormones due to their elevated levels, which deteriorates vascular stiffness due to excessive fibrosis and calcification and decreases the responsiveness to b-adrenergic stimulation. These conditions, along with

the presence of atherosclerotic mechanisms, result in impaired cardiac output and functionality, which in the long term can accelerate the development of age-related cardiovascular pathology such as hypertension, congestive heart failure, atrioventricular block, and aortic stenosis.

2. From a respiratory perspective, aging processes reduce: the available surface for gas exchange, tissue elasticity, chest-wall compliance, and diffusion capacity. When combined with a diminished central drive to the respiratory muscles, decreased pulmonary muscle strength, and reduced efficacy of mucociliary clearance, there is a higher risk of hypoxemia, hypercapnia, augmented mechanical load, and/or infectious diseases.

3. Infamm-aging is the age-related, chronic, low-grade production of pro-inflammatory cytokines such as the nuclear factor kappa-light-chain-enhancer of activated B cells (NF-κb) transcription factor and tumor necrosis factor (TNF)-α. The aging and chronically hyper-activated immune system cannot respond efficiently to chronic or acute stressors that can occur in later stages of life: thus, older people are more prone to infectious, malignant, autoimmune, neurodegenerative, and/or wasting diseases.

4. Sarcopenia and frailty are common geriatric syndromes that entail a loss of muscle mass, strength, and functionality. More specifically, sarcopenia and frailty are mediated by increased inflammation levels, which in the long-term impair the ability to ambulate and independently execute daily activities. Sarcopenia and frailty negatively affect the quality of life of elderly citizens, as they become more susceptible to falls and fractures, cardiac and respiratory disease, and cognitive deterioration. Both conditions are clinically recognized as pathological entities that need systematic detection and management, so as to meet the WHO goals to ensure adequate levels of good health and well-being.

5. The timed "Up & Go" test (TUG) is a single physical performance test recommended by the CDC to assess the risk of falls and balance impairments in the elderly. Balance assessments are essential in these age groups, since the timely diagnosis of potential balance impairments can significantly lessen the risk of falls and maintain ambulatory capabilities.

   The TUG test reliably assesses the functional mobility of the elderly. After requesting the participant to sit on a chair (height of 46 cm and with arms rest height of 65 cm) placed against a wall. They are next asked to stand and walk at their normal pace until they cover a straight distance of 3 m. At the 3 m point, they should turn around and return to the chair along the same path. The time is recorded in seconds (s) and the test is completed when the patient's buttocks touch the chair. The procedure is repeated three times with adequate time to rest between each session. The mean of the three scores is the TUG score.

6. c
7. a
8. b
9. b
10. False
11. True
12. True
13. False
14. True

CHAPTER 10:

1. Plant-based diets are food patterns that emphasize the consumption of food that is mainly plant-derived while minimizing, or even excluding the consumption of animal products. Most plant-based food patterns consist of low-processed fruits, vegetables, whole grains, legumes, nuts, seeds, herbs, spices. Vegetarian diets are a subgroup of plant-based diets that may exclude the consumption of some or all forms of animal foods and products. Vegan diet patterns are the strictest forms of plant-based diets; they completely omit all animal products, including meat, dairy, fish, eggs, and (usually) honey. Instead, they base their daily caloric and nutrient intake on vegetable, fruit, nut, seed, legume, and plant-derived oils. Less strict forms of vegetarian diets can include to some extent the consumption of eggs, dairy products, poultry, and fish, or a combination of them. The raw vegan diet, which does not cook at temperatures above 48 °C, is considered the last type of plant-based diets

2. Older adults have higher protein needs because of the anabolic resistance phenomenon, which describes the reduced stimulation of muscle protein synthesis to a given dose of protein/amino acids and contributes to a decline in skeletal muscle mass. Anabolic resistance causes older individuals to have higher protein needs, especially when combined with other chronic or acute conditions characterized by high inflammatory loads. A reduced appetite, sensory degradation, poor oral health, physical pain, and painful medical conditions are among the most common reasons for lower energy, and therefore, protein intake, which makes muscle maintenance even more difficult for the elderly.

3. Chronically high blood-glucose levels are partially responsible for most degenerative diseases, including hypertension, heart failure, kidney dysfunction, dementia, and cataracts. In human cells, the presence of a high glucose content produces negative effects of aging on endothelial progenitor cells (EPCs) and fibroblasts. It also enhances various aging-related phenotypes through the activation of the p38 mitogen-activated protein kinase (MAPK) and induces downregulation of sirtuins, which result in reducing FOXO activity and accelerated cellular senescence. Lastly, glucose-rich conditions exacerbate inflammation by increasing ROS and AGE (Advanced

Glycation End) production, which lead to tissue stiffening and reduced enzyme functionality.

4. b – 1.0–1.2 g/kg body weight
5. a Leucine
6. b 67 base pairs
7. b 20–30g/day
8. a 250–500mg/day
9. False
10. True
11. False
12. True
13. False
14. False
15. i = a, c; ii = b, f; iii = d; iv = e, g
16. The MD is a dietary pattern that focuses on plant-derived foods that are locally and seasonally produced along with the intake of animal products in controlled quantities. More specifically, it is mainly plant-based, with a focus on seasonal vegetables, fresh fruits as a dessert, nuts, legumes, whole grains, and seeds on an everyday basis. This pattern also includes the moderate consumption of fish (2–3 times per week), regular intake of dairy in limited quantities, infrequent consumption of sweets (a few times per week), rare consumption of red or processed meat in very small quantities, and moderate use of eggs (3–4 per week). Olive oil is the first and foremost source of (unsaturated) fat, while the intake of saturated fats remains extremely low. According to the MD, water is the main beverage and drinking wine is permitted occasionally and in moderation, especially during social gatherings accompanied by food. For extra taste, seasonal and local herbs and spices are preferred to salt. In addition to the dietary recommendations, the MD also includes an adequate amount of everyday rest and social interactions, regular connection with nature, and moderate physical activity daily.

    Adherence to the MD during midlife is correlated with a 36% to 46% greater likelihood of healthy aging. Chronic consumption of these nutrients, which act synergistically by various biological and molecular mechanisms, lessen the overall risk of NCDs. Studies conducted in European older adults indicate that adherence to the MD, even at this late stage of life, can reduce the risk for all-cause mortality, independent aging indices, frailty, and cognitive deterioration.

17. The staple components of the ND are berries, apples, pears, and Nordic fruits in general, fatty fish (Baltic herring, mackerel, and salmon), lean fish, vegetables (cabbage, tomatoes, lettuce, cucumbers, legumes, and roots–except for potatoes) and whole-grain cereals (barley, oats, and rye). Nordic vegetables and fruits are located at the bottom of the pyramid due to their crucial role in health preservation and promotion. Whole-grain products rich in fiber are found in the intermediate levels of the pyramid before fish, low-fat or fat-free milk products, and oils used for cooking. A notable point of difference between the ND and MD is the use of rapeseed (canola) oil instead of olive oil. Milk and sour milk are the only drinks illustrated in the pyramid because of its important role in Nordic nutrition. Water and tea are preferred to address thirst, while light to moderate alcohol drinking is tolerated. Foods like processed meat, butter, sweets, chocolate, and sweet bakery products are located at the top of the pyramid, implying the need for very considerate or minimal consumption.

18. True
19. False
20. True
21. True
22. Okinawan dietary patterns are characterized by a high consumption of vegetables and legumes (mostly soy-derived); moderate consumption of fish products; low intake of meat, dairy, and meat products; and moderate alcohol consumption. Consequently, the traditional Okinawan diet includes a very low-fat intake, especially saturated fat, versus a very high intake of unrefined carbohydrates through the consumption of orange-yellow root vegetables, such as sweet potatoes, green leafy vegetables, and seaweeds. Spices such as bitter greens, peppers, and turmeric are preferred instead of salt, which along with their rich antioxidant phytonutrient content and low glycemic load, explain the significant cardioprotective effects of the Okinawan diet.

    The Okinawan diet pattern is characterized as low in calories yet nutritionally dense, particularly in vitamins, minerals, and phytonutrients. Additionally, the Okinawa diet pattern differs from the MD pattern as it is rich in high quality carbohydrates and extra low in fat; in the MD, carbohydrates and fats provide up to 42% and 45% of daily energy intake, respectively. They have more commonalities, however, than discrepancies and include a high intake of unrefined carbohydrates and phytonutrients, mostly from vegetables; moderate to high legume consumption; an emphasis on fish and/or lean meats; and a healthy fat profile (increased n-3 and monounsaturated fat intake with a low saturated fat intake). The resemblances in these nutrient and food patterns are considered the key that leads to decreased rates of CVD, certain cancers, and diabetes mainly through mechanisms involved in oxidative stress.

CHAPTER 11:

1. According to the WHO, a person is considered physically inactive when they do not meet the relative (to their age) recommendations regarding weekly levels of physical activity.

2. Physical inactivity is an actual cause of the numerous abnormal physiological values (physiological dysfunctions) that in turn cause (usually) permanent pathological changes. Over time, these changes lead to overt, diagnosed chronic diseases that culminate as contributors to premature mortality. Conversely, physical activity produces primary and tertiary preventive health benefits for the same chronic diseases, using different pathways. Chronically inactive individuals tend to express a different kind and number of genes, which in the long term predispose them to a higher risk of developing cardiovascular disease, type 2 diabetes, obesity, and several types of cancer. Furthermore, the time needed for exercise to show its protective effects is often longer than the respective time that a more sedentary lifestyle adoptions need to negatively impact molecular and tissue functionality. Physical inactivity deteriorates endothelial function by immediate, negative remodeling of the vessels and increased levels of inflammation.

3. Regular physical activity influences, in a direct or indirect manner, the most common risk factors for most non-communicable chronic diseases as well as the mechanisms that govern the aging process. A lack of physical activity can decrease the CRF and consequently deteriorate glycaemia, lipid and lipoprotein profile, body composition, blood pressure, and levels of systematic inflammation, which are all risk factors for all-causes morbidity. From an immunological perspective, regular exercise contributes to better oxidative-stress management through a decrease in inflammation levels, better antioxidant capacity, and therefore, prolonged cellular life and normal function. Moreover, many programs that implement physical activity in the everyday routine of older adults to manage geriatric syndromes like sarcopenia and frailty, grant a higher quality of everyday living through better musculoskeletal functionality and therefore, better functional, balance, and ambulatory capacity. Finally, physical activity has neuroprotective effects by promoting structural and functional brain-plasticity, which consequently has a positive effect on cognition, memory, and mental health as well as sustains an older individual's autonomy and self-respect.

4. When it comes to wasting syndromes like sarcopenia and frailty, physical activity can be used as a treatment and a prevention strategy. Physical activity, in the form of multicomponent programs that address resistance, endurance, balance, and flexibility, can improve physical performance, upper- and lower-body strength, and muscle strength in general. Implementing systematic physical exercise in an older person's weekly routine reduces muscle-quality deterioration due to aging, the risk of sarcopenia and frailty, and consequently, the risk of falls, fractures, and a lower overall functional capacity.

5. b

6. a

7. a

8. c

9. b

10. False

11. False

12. False

13. True

14. False

CHAPTER 12:

1. Heart failure is a "complex clinical syndrome that can result from any structural or functional cardiac disorder that impairs the ability of the ventricle to fill or eject blood." HF is a set of complex and heterogeneous condition with underlying variability in etiology, pathophysiology, metabolic, and other individual factors. HF constitutes an end stage of several cardiovascular disorders, coronary heart disease (CHD), and hypertension being the most common in high-income countries. The diagnosis of heart failure as a clinical syndrome rests on three cornerstones: typical symptoms (including shortness of breath, ankle swelling, orthopnea, lower limb swelling, and chronic fatigue); signs (jugular vein stasis, pulmonary crackles, and pitting edema); and findings from supporting diagnostic tests (e.g., electrocardiogram, transthoracic echocardiography, serum natriuretic peptides) that can all be attributed to cardiac dysfunction, often caused by a structural and/or functional cardiac abnormality resulting in reduced cardiac output and/or elevated intracardiac pressures.

2. The classification of heart failure is based on different etiologies and associated mechanistic disturbances of cardiac function. One classification is based on left ventricular ejection fraction (LVEF), which is estimated by an echocardiographic estimate of left ventricular systolic function, since LVEF is a strong marker for underlying pathophysiology, as well as a marker for sensitivity to pharmacotherapy. The classification depends on the level of LVEF, thus for LVEF < 40%, there is a heart failure with reduced ejection fraction (HFrEF), whereas for LVEF > 50%, there is a preserved Heart failure with preserved ejection fraction (HFpEF). Furthermore, heart failure is classified according to the state, if it is a chronic state then the definition is chronic heart failure, and if the disease has a rapid onset with new or worsening signs and symptoms, it is called acute heart failure (AHF).

3. There is growing evidence that nutrition is a critical factor in the incidence and progression of HF. Patients diagnosed with HF have a poor prognosis that is also linked to poor nutritional status. Related features to HF are obesity, sarcopenia, and in combination (sarcopenic & obesity), or weight loss (both lean and fat mass, even tissue loss, i.e., cachexia). Furthermore, HF is related to hypertension, type 2 diabetes mellitus (T2D), chronic inflammation,

and coronary artery disease. It is important to study possible nutrition recommendations regarding HF prevention and therapy to improve clinical outcomes.

4. DASH and MD dietary patterns, micronutrient deficiencies, and recommendations for sodium and fluid. However, there is a lack of dietary therapies that have demonstrated a relative role. HF patients should adhere to a healthy dietary pattern and recommendations should be individualized.

5. Physical activity is linked to various health effects, including reduced total and cardiovascular morbidity, mortality, and risk factors. PA has a positive effect on many of the risk factors for CHD and HF, such as hypertension, and is related to the risk of HF. Exercise also plays an important role in the three stages of HF. It affects the presentation of HF and seems to have a protective role by positively affecting HF in secondary prevention and influencing the prognosis of HF in the future for HF patients. Multiple studies indicate that exercise training can be considered a highly effective therapy for patients with HF as well as safe, feasible, and beneficial. It increases functional capacity, resting heart rate, ventilatory efficiency, ejection fraction, and quality of life as well as reducing the incidence of major cardiovascular events, hospitalizations, cardiac mortality, and the rate of new-onset atrial arrhythmias, but not ventricular arrhythmias, in patients with HF. However, as highlighted in the recent ESC Guidelines on Sports Cardiology, exercise should be individually tailored, and sporting activities may be restricted in some patients.

6. True
7. False
8. True
9. education groups; diaries; goal settings
10. a
11. c
12. a
13. a
14. c
15. c

CHAPTER 13:

1. Atrial fibrillation is one of the most common types of cardiac arrhythmias, i.e., irregular heartbeats, which increase the risk of stroke, heart failure, and other cardiovascular-related complications.

2. Atrial fibrillation is a multifactorial condition. Four risk factors associated with atrial fibrillation include: (i) increased age, (ii) hypertension, (iii) coronary artery disease, and (iv) congenital heart diseases.

3. There are three mechanisms for the initiation and progression of atrial fibrillation: (i) autonomous nervous system, (ii) electrophysiology of the pulmonary veins, and (iii) substrate abnormalities.

4. The Atrial Fibrillation Better Care (ABC) pathway is an integrated approach for atrial fibrillation management across all healthcare levels and among different specialties. In the ABC pathway, "A" stands for "Anticoagulation/Avoid stroke", "B" for "Better symptom management", and "C" for "Comorbidity optimization".

5. The Mediterranean diet (emphasizing olive oil, nuts, fresh fruits, vegetables, fish, legumes, white meat, and moderate consumption of wine with meals) supplemented with either olive oil or nuts was superior at reducing cardiovascular disease risk compared to a low-fat diet; the Mediterranean diet can therefore be recommended as a prudent dietary pattern for the prevention and management of atrial fibrillation.

6. The dose-response relationship between physical activity and atrial fibrillation risk shows a U-shaped pattern, meaning that both inactivity and a very high level of physical activity are associated with an increased risk of atrial fibrillation compared to the intermediate category, i.e., a low-to-moderate physical activity level.

CHAPTER 14:

1. The epithelium is one of the five main types of animal tissues, and it serves as a covering or lining of various bodily surfaces and cavities. The other four are nerve tissue, connective tissue, muscle tissue, and vascular tissue.

2. The endothelium is a special type of epithelium that lines the blood and lymphatic vessels. It consists of a single layer of smooth thin cells that form an interface between circulating blood or lymph in the lumen and the rest of the vessel wall.

3. Endothelial dysfunction, i.e., the loss of normal endothelial function, is a hallmark of vascular diseases and is recognized as a key early event in the development of atherosclerosis.

4. Despite its prominent role in cardiovascular health, endothelial function is not easy to assess. This is because i) few symptoms are directly referable or specific to the endothelium; ii) the endothelium is hidden from view and not amenable to traditional physical diagnostic procedures; and iii) the endothelium is not spatially confined and therefore difficult to image using anatomic imaging methodologies.

5. favorable

6. For people that are overweight or obese, the available clinical trials are highly encouraging and indicate that endothelial dysfunction is at least partially reversible by weight loss. Moreover, dietary fat appears to affect endothelial function in a complex way.

A diet rich in foods with unsaturated fat, such as vegetable oils, nuts, and fish is beneficial for the endothelium compared to foods rich in saturated and trans fat, such as red and processed meat, butter, stick margarine, and high-processed foods. Some micronutrients, such as folic acid and vitamin C, can also have beneficial properties for the endothelium.

Given that obesity, inflammation, and oxidative stress are implicated in the pathogenesis of endothelial dysfunction, the Mediterranean diet could be a first-line dietary pattern for enhancing endothelial function.

7. Although the effect of exercise on the endothelium is less well-studied, the available evidence suggests that exercise can improve endothelial function and result in a favorable vascular remodeling through several mechanisms, including vasodilation, a favorable effect on the oxidative balance of the endothelium, the promotion of fibrinolysis and angiogenesis, and a chronic anti-inflammatory effect.

CHAPTER 15:

1. Diabetes mellitus is a group of metabolic disorders characterized by chronic hyperglycemia (i.e., high concentrations of blood glucose) that results from defects in insulin production, insulin action, or both and is associated with disturbances in glucose, lipid, and protein metabolism

2. Type 1 and Type 2 diabetes

3. The diagnosis of diabetes is based on blood-glucose levels. The fasting plasma glucose (FPG) or the plasma glucose (PG) after a 2-hour, 75-g oral glucose tolerance test (OGTT) or the A1C criteria are used to determine the diagnosis, with equal effectiveness for type 2 diabetes.

4. heart disease and stroke; high blood pressure; kidney disease; complications in pregnancy.

5. Sedentary behavior (defined as waking behavior of ≤1.5 Metabolic Equivalent of Task [MET]) as well as physical inactivity (i.e., not meeting specified physical activity guidelines) increases the risk of T2DM onset and other chronic diseases.

6. Resistance training decreases blood glucose during training with smaller changes after the training session. This may diminish patients' fear of hypoglycemia during or after exercise in patients with diabetes type 1.

7. An ideal percentage of calories from carbohydrates, protein, and lipids does not exist for all patients with diabetes.

8. According to the latest guidelines of the American Diabetes Association, adults with diabetes, type 1 or 2, or prediabetes should perform aerobic exercise for 150 minutes or more on a weekly basis, at a moderate-to-vigorous intensity, at least three times a week and once in two days. For younger and more physically active individuals, 75 minutes per week of vigorous exercise or interval training might be enough. Adult patients should, also engage in resistance training for 2 to 3 times per week, but not for consecutive days.

CHAPTER 16:

1. In accordance with most major guidelines, hypertension is diagnosed when the SBP is ≥140 mm Hg and/or DBP is ≥90 mm Hg. According to the ACC/AHA recommendation, hypertension is defined as a SBP >130 mm Hg or DBP >80 mm Hg.

2. Primary hypertension originates from a combination of genetic and environmental factors, including the aging process of kidney function and peripheral resistance, vascular inflammation, genetic expression, and environmental influences, such as overweight/obesity, an unhealthy diet, excessive dietary sodium, inadequate dietary potassium, insufficient physical activity, and consumption of alcohol. The most important modifiable environmental factors are an unhealthy diet and insufficient physical activity.

3. According to the ESC/ESH and the ISH recommendations, people with hypertension should do at least 30 minutes of moderate-intensity dynamic aerobic exercise (i.e., walking, jogging, cycling, or swimming) 5 to 7 days per week and resistance exercise 2 to 3 days per week. According to the ACC/AHA recommendations, individuals with hypertension should complete 90 to 150 min per week of aerobic exercise, 90 to 150 min per week of dynamic resistance exercise, and three sessions per week of isometric resistance exercise.

4. Weight-loss interventions in patients with obesity and hypertension are effective treatments of hypertension. Patients with hypertension should adopt a diet that is rich in whole grains, fruits, vegetables, poly-unsaturated fats, and dairy products with a low consumption of food high in sugar, saturated fat, and trans fats, such as the DASH diet and the Mediterranean diet. Moreover, sodium reduction is highly recommended for individuals with hypertension. They should reduce salt added when preparing foods and at the table as well as avoid consumption of high salt foods (i.e., fast foods, soy sauce, nuts, chips, processed food). Moreover, moderate consumption of coffee, green and black tea is proposed. Finally, alcohol, if consumed, should be ingested with moderation, whereas binge drinking should be avoided.

5. Dietary supplements of calcium, magnesium, or potassium are recommended for people with hypertension who are unable to meet the DRI with a food source and diet alone. Individuals with hypertension should consume adequate amounts of dietary calcium, magnesium, or potassium through food sources high in these micronutrients.

6. False

7. True

8. False
9. False
10. True
11. positive
12. 20–25 kg/m²; <94 cm; <80 cm
13. ≥2 g per day
14. reduced
15. recommended; salt added; the table; high salt foods (i.e., fast foods, soy sauce, processed food)

CHAPTER 17:

1. High levels of total cholesterol, LDL-cholesterol, triglycerides, or low levels, in the case of HDL-cholesterol, are defined as dyslipidemia.
2. True
3. False
4. There is some evidence that exercise training may decrease total cholesterol, but confounding factors may influence this association. Concerning blood triglycerides, exercise training is known to lower their levels. The observed, in some studies, decrease in LDL-cholesterol could be because of concurrent weight loss, comorbidity, or sex-related differences. There are consistent data indicating that exercise training increases HDL-cholesterol, but several factors may influence the increase.
5. False
6. True
7. False
8. False

CHAPTER 18:

1. Regarding the WHO, overweight and obesity are defined as abnormal or excessive fat accumulation that presents a risk to health.
2. Obesity treatment should consist of a dietary prescription with an energy deficit of at least 500 kcal per day, a physical prescription of at least 150 minutes of moderate- to vigorous-intensity physical activity per week and structured behavior-change intervention. A balanced hypocaloric diet containing at least the recommended protein intake, irrespective of food sources, is adequate for weight loss. Moreover, food-focused dietary approaches or specific dietary patterns may also lead to weight loss if they cause changes in dietary intake and thus decrease total energy and/or negative energy balance, apart from the other health benefits they may have.
3. Metabolically healthy obesity is defined as obesity in the absence of a clearly defined cardiometabolic disorder, such as metabolic syndrome, insulin resistance, hypertension, diabetes, or dyslipidemia. Identifying individuals with metabolically healthy obesity may prevent wasting time, effort, and resources on people who may not benefit—or benefit less—from weight-loss management.
4. For weight-loss maintenance, people should adopt higher levels of physical activity, approximately 200 to 300 min per week.
5. Individuals with overweight/obesity and MetS should lose approximately 5% of their initial body weight. They should also adopt a healthy dietary pattern, such as the Mediterranean diet or DASH diet. A Mediterranean diet, with or without energy restriction, can especially be recommended for all individuals with MetS an effective component of the treatment strategy. Moreover, reducing the intake of salt and limiting saturated and trans fats as well as the consumption of sugar-sweetened beverages, while increasing the intake of dietary fiber are also recommended.
6. MetS is identified by the presence of at least three components:
   - Waist circumference >40 cm for men or >35 for women
   - Impaired fasting glucose, high blood glucose, or type 2 diabetes
   - High triglyceride ≥150 mg/dL or on triglyceride treatment
   - Low HDL <40 mg/dL for men, <50 mg/dL for women, or HDL treatment.
   - High blood pressure ≥130 mmHg systolic and/or ≥85 mmHg diastolic or upon hypertension treatment.
7. False
8. False
9. True
10. False
11. True
12. overweight; avoided; muscle mass; obesity
13. complications; co-morbidities; stigmatization; well-being; positive
14. reduced-calorie; higher; 200–300; monitor; weekly; more
15. energy restriction; recommended; MetS

CHAPTER 19:

1. According to the International Classification of Sleep Disorders of the American Academy of Sleep Medicine, OSA belongs to the group of sleep-related breathing disorders. It is a chronic and complex pathological

condition, characterized by recurrent pauses of breathing during sleep due to obstruction of the upper airways, which leads to sleep disruption. In the context of OSA, narrowing or complete obstructions of the upper airways are observed in the pharyngeal region during sleep, when the tone of upper airway dilator muscles decreases normally, which leads to temporary cessation of breathing despite respiratory effort. Breathing pauses are accompanied by hypoxemia and hypercapnia, and lead to sleep disruption, which restores the tone of the upper airway dilator muscles and normal airflow. However, after sleep restoration, upper airway obstructions reoccur, and repetitive awakenings eventually lead to sleep fragmentation.

2. In the context of OSA, the cardiovascular system is exposed to a vicious cycle of hemodynamic, oxidative, inflammatory, and metabolic disorders. Intermittent hypoxemia and the subsequent awakenings in the context of OSA cause an abnormal increase in sympathetic activity during sleep, which can lead to the establishment of hypertension in the long term. Hypertension, combined with fluctuations in intrathoracic pressure and hypoxemia can impair myocardial and vascular function. Intermittent hypoxemia also leads to increased oxidative stress, which triggers inflammation, long-term endothelial dysfunction, and arterial stiffness, all major factors predisposing to atherosclerosis. Chronic sleep deprivation or poor sleep quality, combined with oxidative stress and chronic inflammation, can disrupt the body's metabolic homeostasis, triggering insulin resistance, fatty liver, and atherogenic dyslipidemia. All these hemodynamic, oxidative, inflammatory, and metabolic complications increase the risk for diabetes mellitus, coronary heart disease, heart failure, stroke, cardiovascular, and total mortality.

3. False
4. True
5. False
6. False
7. True
8. False
9. True
10. True
11. False
12. CPAP is a form of positive airway pressure ventilation in which a constant level of pressure, greater than atmospheric, is continuously applied to the upper respiratory tract of a patient during sleep to prevent upper airway collapse and respiratory events. CPAP is currently the first-line treatment for OSA, it is prescribed as long-life care to most OSA patients in clinical practice and is efficient in minimizing respiratory events, ameliorating OSA symptoms (e.g., daytime sleepiness), and improving patients' quality of life compared to control therapies. However, it is also characterized by a number of limitations, including: i) low adherence (documented in up to 80% of patients), and the recurrence of OSA manifestations after its discontinuation even for one night, ii) doubtable efficiency in improving patients' cardiometabolic health (e.g., glucose metabolism indices, lipidemic profile, low-grade inflammation, or cardiovascular morbidity and mortality) and iii) a modest but significant increase in body weight after its initiation, which can further aggravate overweight/obesity in patients with OSA.

13. The importance of exercise as part of the management of sleep-disordered breathing has been consistently shown in studies implementing supervised exercise interventions in the OSA population. Research so far has shown that supervised aerobic exercise programs, either alone or in combination with resistance exercise, lead to significant improvements in the severity and symptoms of OSA, sleep quality, and architecture as well as patients' fitness level, physical functioning, and cardiometabolic profile. Although the effect of exercise on respiratory events is moderate (decline in the AHI by approximately 5 to 10 events/h compared to control interventions), improvements in the AHI following exercise are observed in the absence of significant changes in anthropometric indices, highlighting the weight-loss independent benefits of physical activity for OSA. The beneficial effect of exercise on OSA can be explained through: i) improvements in body composition which helps reduce the mechanical load on the upper airways; ii) improvement of upper airway airflow by reducing nasal congestion; iii) prevention of fluid movement in the upper body during sleep that can add to upper airway mechanical load and contribute to obstruction; iv) upper airway muscle strengthening, allowing for a better breathing control; and v) improvements in metabolic disturbances that can aggravate upper airway dysfunction.

14. sleepiness, fatigue, low vitality, inability to concentrate, impaired reflexes, and memory deficits

15. uvulopalatopharyngoplasty; the tonsils, the uvula and part of the soft palate

16. intermittent hypoxia; metabolic syndrome; insulin resistance, inflammation, and oxidative stress.

17. 1.5 to 2.5; more

18. oxygen free radicals; oxidative stress

19. supine; gravity

20. consumption of seasonal and eco-friendly food products, regular exercise as part of family and social activities, adequate rest during the day and traditional culinary activities; Mediterranean lifestyle

21. upper airway dilator muscles; detrimental upper airway anatomy.
22. 150–300; 75–150
23. blood pressure; hypertension
24. 10–15%; 20–50%; patients with severe disease (AHI ≥30 events/h)
25. increased; de novo lipogenesis; dyslipidemia.
26. 5%; 50–65%; 15–20%; 15–20%; N1 and N2; N3 (slow-wave sleep) and REM
27. red meat and refined grains; whole grains
28. Sleep apnea can lead to physical inactivity due to symptoms of daytime sleepiness and fatigue and can greatly influence a patient's energy balance and exercise capacity. Several studies have demonstrated that aerobic capacity is significantly impaired in OSA patients compared to healthy controls. Moreover, a positive correlation has been observed between OSA severity and exercise intolerance, as supported by data showing that the AHI is a significant independent predictor of aerobic exercise capacity, even after adjusting for possible confounders including body weight status; for example, approximately 16% of the variability observed in percent predicted VO_2 max can be explained by the AHI. OSA patients also have a low physical condition and an inappropriate hemodynamic response to exercise, which is related to OSA severity. During peak exercise and recovery, OSA patients exhibit increased blood pressure and heart rate, decreased stroke volume, and delayed heart rate recovery compared to healthy individuals. Additionally, OSA patients have impaired skeletal muscle energy metabolism, indicating abnormal oxidative and glycolytic metabolism of exercising muscles. Altogether, OSA have an impaired aerobic exercise capacity and a poor hemodynamic response to exercise, which is important to consider since these factors constitute not only cardiovascular risk factors but also significant barriers for physical activity.
29. Data on the association between diet quality and the presence or severity of OSA are so far scarce. Available epidemiological studies have shown that the intake of certain nutrients, such as total fat, cholesterol, and saturated fatty acids might be detrimental for OSA development, while the intake of dietary fiber, thiamine, folic acid, vitamin E, and potassium might protect against the disease. Besides individual nutrients, OSA severity was positively correlated with the consumption of red meat, meat products, and refined grains, and negatively correlated to the consumption of whole grains. Although available data come from epidemiological studies, which cannot establish causality, it is possible that adherence to prudent dietary patterns that emphasize high amounts of a variety of plant-based foods, and prudent consumption of animal-based products and processed foods, can offer protection against the development and progression of OSA and act toward the prevention of OSA-related cardiometabolic morbidity.
30. True
31. True
32. False
33. False
34. False
35. False
36. True
37. True
38. False
39. The Mediterranean diet is one of the most studied dietary patterns worldwide, and its health benefits are well-established in the fields of nutritional epidemiology and clinical dietetics. In rough terms, the Mediterranean diet can be defined as the collection of dietary habits adopted by populations bordering the Mediterranean Sea in the 1950s and 60s. In its modern version, it is a dietary pattern characterized by high consumption of olive oil (as the main source of dietary fat), fruits, vegetables, legumes, whole-grain cereals, nuts, and seeds; a moderate consumption of white meat, fish/seafood, and dairy products; a low consumption of red meat products; and a moderate consumption of wine with main meals. According to numerous prospective and interventional studies, a high adherence to the Mediterranean diet has been shown to reduce mortality from all causes, cardiovascular disease, and cancer; to protect against the development of neurodegenerative diseases and diabetes mellitus; to negatively associate with the presence of various other diseases; and to be a highly palatable diet that is able to produce weight loss and contribute to the management of obesity. Given the well-established cardiometabolic benefits of the Mediterranean diet and the close link between OSA, obesity, and cardiometabolic morbidity, this unique dietary pattern is probably a highly beneficial dietary model for most patients with OSA. Although this theory has not been systematically explored, there is some preliminary clinical evidence of the benefits of the Mediterranean diet in OSA patients; these benefits can probably be explained through the strong anti-inflammatory and antioxidant properties of the Mediterranean diet and its beneficial effects on body composition, which can improve upper airway neuromuscular control and therefore prevent respiratory disturbances during sleep.

CHAPTER 20:

1. The kidneys are complex organs of the urinary system and are considered vital in maintaining body physiology and homeostasis. Their fundamental functions include

the regulation of plasma osmolarity by modulating the amount of water and electrolytes in the blood, the removal of metabolic waste products and foreign substances from the body through urine, the regulation of long-term acid-base balance by modulating the excretion of hydrogen ions and the reabsorption of bicarbonate, the production of several important hormones, such as erythropoietin and renin, as well as the conversion of vitamin D to its active form, which is crucial for intestinal calcium absorption and bone health.

2. CKD refers to the progressive and irreversible decline in renal function and is defined as the presence of either chronic, impaired renal clearance capacity or chronic kidney damage. Renal clearance capacity refers to the rate at which kidneys filter blood, while kidney damage refers to either functional or structural abnormalities of the kidneys.

3. Cardiovascular disorders are the most frequent and life-threatening complications of CKD and include atherosclerosis, ischemic heart disease, cerebrovascular events, peripheral vascular events, left ventricular hypertrophy, cardiomyopathy, and arrhythmogenic disorders. The close relationship between CKD and cardiovascular diseases can be explained by both traditional (e.g., smoking, obesity, hypertension, diabetes mellitus) and non-traditional cardiovascular risk factors (e.g., low levels of hemoglobin, albuminuria, malnutrition) that are present in most CKD patients. Current theories in CKD pathophysiology suggest that the heart and the kidneys are closely linked, with the disease of one organ causing dysfunction of the other, which ultimately leads to the failure of both, a condition known as cardiorenal syndrome. Cardiovascular involvement in CKD is known as type-4 cardiorenal syndrome or chronic renocardiac syndrome.

4. Exercise has a multi-beneficial role in CKD. First, exercise is associated with significant improvements in aerobic capacity and muscle strength; this is important, given that CKD patients are characterized by low physical functioning, muscle weakness, and high risk of cachexia. Although evidence regarding the effect of exercise interventions on preventing renal failure is scarce, higher levels of physical activity have been associated with slower declines in kidney function in epidemiological studies, which provides some early proof of the potential preventive role of physical activity in CKD onset and progression. Finally, exercise has a beneficial effect on blood pressure, arterial stiffness, inflammation, oxidative stress, and reduced cardiovascular risk in the CKD population.

5. Exercise can be used as an adjunct treatment to help improve CKD-related morbidities, provided that potential risks are considered. The most important consideration for exercise in CKD is related to patients' cardiovascular health. Vigorous physical activity has been associated with a greater risk of sudden adverse cardiac events and should be undertaken with caution by CKD patients who are already at high cardiovascular risk. Other important considerations include the presence of hypertension (exercise is generally not recommended in uncontrolled hypertension), the risk of musculoskeletal injuries (exercise should be prescribed according to each patient's capabilities and fitness level), and whether the patient is on renal replacement therapy (exercise should best be avoided in the presence of severe fluid and electrolyte imbalances and weight should not be applied in the fistula arm). Potential risks from exercise can be minimized with appropriate patient education about abnormal symptoms, emphasis on low- and moderate-intensity exercise, which is generally safe, a gradual increase in exercise duration and intensity, and regular monitoring of responses to the exercise program.

6. CKD is accompanied by several complications that can affect nutritional status. For example, the accumulation of nitrogen-containing products from dietary and intrinsic protein catabolism in the body can distort taste and smell, which blunt patients' appetite and results in insufficient energy intake, while uremia can lead to abnormal gastrointestinal nutrient absorption. Therefore, as CKD progresses, nutritional status deteriorates, and the adoption of a balanced nutrition is crucial for preventing and/or managing protein-energy wasting. Besides malnutrition, CKD is characterized by serious metabolic complications, such as electrolyte imbalances, water and salt retention, and bone disorders, which can be managed, at least in part, through individualized dietary modifications.

7. True
8. False
9. False
10. True
11. False
12. <15 mL/min/1.73 m^2
13. positively; higher; inversely
14. the thickening of the arterial walls; the elasticity of arteries
15. 0.6–0.8 g/kg/d; 1.2–1.4 g/kg/d for CKD patients on dialysis or with malnutrition.
16. packaged products (e.g., salty snacks and pastries), processed foods (e.g., cold cuts) or pre-cooked meals; 1 teaspoon

CHAPTER 21:

1. There are several proposed mechanisms that explain the link between excess body weight and cancer development. At first, obesity is characterized by a chronic low-grade inflammatory state and abnormal levels of cytokines and adipokines, such as elevated levels of

leptin. Furthermore, it is well-established that insulin resistance, hyperinsulinemia, abnormalities in the IGF-1 axis, and increased levels of estrogen are common in obesity. These factors have been shown to promote carcinogenesis and increase the risk of developing cancer.

2. According to the PAGAC report, there is strong evidence that being physically active reduces the risk of breast, bladder, endometrial, colon, esophageal, adenocarcinoma, gastric cardia, and renal cancers. It is also reported that there is moderate evidence for lung cancer and limited evidence for hematologic, ovary, head and neck, pancreas, and prostate cancer.

3. According to Fearon et al., cancer cachexia is defined as a multifactorial syndrome characterized by the ongoing loss of muscle mass, with or without loss of fat mass, which cannot be completely reversed by conventional nutritional support and eventually leads to progressive functional impairments.

4. Given the absence of strong evidence regarding the association of lifestyle factors and the long-term survivorship after active treatments, current guidelines recommend individuals to follow cancer prevention guidelines. The main goals in this stage of survivorship are the reduction of cancer recurrence risk as well as the risk of other chronic diseases, like cardiovascular disease, diabetes mellitus, osteoporosis, and other primary types of cancer. Moreover, there is some evidence that following these recommendations is associated with a better quality of life and lower risk of morbidity and mortality.

5. False
6. False
7. True
8. False
9. True
10. False
11. False
12. False
13. smoking, curing, salting and fermentation as well as procedures used to preserve foods or enhance flavor
14. 25–30; 1; 1.5
15. any waking behavior characterized by an energy expenditure less than or equal to 1.5 METs while in a sitting or reclining posture
16. exercise, nutritional, and possible psychological

Abbreviations

%HRmax	Percentage of maximum heart rate	BWS	Beckwith-Wiedemann syndrome
1RM	1-repetition maximum	CAD	Coronary artery disease
5-mC	5-methylcytosine	CAMs	Cell-adhesion molecules
AA	Amino Acid	CASP-19	Control, autonomy, pleasure, and self-realization, quality of life scale 2019
AACC	American association of cereal chemists		
AASM	American Academy of Sleep Medicine	CB&M	Community balance and mobility scale
ABC	Atrial fibrillation better care	CD8+ T cells	Cytotoxic T cells expressing CD8 (cluster of differentiation 8) transmembrane glycoprotein
ACC	American College of Cardiology		
ACR	Albumin:creatinine ratio		
ACS	American Cancer Society	CDP	Computerized dynamic posturography
ACSM	American College of Sports Medicine	CEC	Circulating mature endothelial cells
ADA	American Dietetic Association	CES-D	Center for Epidemiological Studies depression scale
ADL	Activities of daily living		
ADMA	Asymmetric dimethylarginine	CETP	Cholesteryl-ester transfer protein
ADT	Androgen-deprivation therapy	CGMP	Cyclic guanosine monophosphate
AEE	Activity energy expenditure	CHD	Coronary heart disease
AFib	Atrial fibrillation	CHF	Chronic heart failure
AGE(s)	Advanced glycation end product(s)	CKD	Chronic kidney disease
AGS	American Geriatrics Society	CLA	Conjugated linoleic acid
AHA	American Heart Association	CNS	Central nervous system
AHF	acute heart failure	COPD	Chronic obstructive pulmonary disease
AHI	apnea-hypopnea index	COR	Class (strength) of recommendation
AI	apnea index	CPAP	Continuous positive airway pressure
AICR	American Institute for Cancer Research	CpG	Cytosine–phosphate–guanine
AKI	Acute kidney injury	CpGs	Cytosine–phosphate–guanine site
ANF	Atrial natriuretic factor	CR	Caloric restriction
ANS	Autonomic nervous system	CRF	Cardio-respiratory fitness
AP-1	Activator protein 1	CRP	C-reactive protein
Apo	Apolipoprotein	CTSIB	Clinical test of sensory integration in balance
APOE	Apolipoprotein E		
ART	Assisted reproductive technologies	CVD	Cardiovascular disease
ASCO	American Society of Clinical Oncology	DALYs	Disability-adjusted life-years
ASCVD	Atherosclerotic cardiovascular disease	DASH	Dietary approaches to stop hypertension
ATPIII	National Cholesterol Education Program Adult Treatment Panel III	DBP	Diastolic blood pressure
		DGA	Dietary Guidelines for Americans
BBS	Berg balance scale	DHA	Docosahexaenoic acid
BEST	Balance evaluation systems test	DKD	Diabetic kidney disease
BIA	Bioimpedance analysis	DM	Diabetes mellitus
BMI	Body-mass index	DNAmAge	DNA methylation age
BMR	Basal metabolic rate	DNMT	DNA methyltransferase
BodPod	Air-displacement plethysmography	DPA	Docosapentanoic acid
BOS	Base of support	DPP	Diabetes prevention program
BP	Blood pressure	DRIs	Dietary reference intakes
BPIFB4	BPI-fold-containing-family-B member 4	DXA	Dual-energy X-ray absorptiometry

Prevention and Management of Cardiovascular and Metabolic Disease: Diet, Physical Activity and Healthy Aging,
First Edition. Christina N. Katsagoni, Peter Kokkinos, and Labros S. Sidossis.
© 2023 John Wiley & Sons Ltd. Published 2023 by John Wiley & Sons Ltd.

EAA	Essential amino acids	HEI	Healthy eating index
EAR	Estimated average requirement	HF	Heart failure
EEG	Electroencephalogram	HI	Hypopnea index
EFSA	European Food Safety Authority	HIIE	High-intensity interval exercise
eGFR	Estimated glomerular filtration rate	HIIT	High-intensity interval training
EGIR	European Group for Study of Insulin Resistance	HMOD	Hypertension-mediated organ damage
		HPA	Hypothalamic-pituitary-adrenal axis
EKG	Electrocardiogram	HR	Heart rate
EMG	Electromyogram	HRR	Heart-rate reserve
EMPs	Endothelial microparticles	HTN	Hypertension
eNOS	Endothelial nitric-oxide synthase	IADL(s)	Instrumental activity(ies) of daily living
EPA	Eicosapentanoic acid	IARC	International Agency for Research on Cancer
EPCR	Endothelial protein-C receptor		
EPCs	Endothelial progenitor cells	ICAM-1	Intercellular cell-adhesion molecule 1
EPO	Erythropoietin	IDF	International Diabetes Federation
ER	Endoplasmic reticulum	IDL	Intermediate-density lipoprotein
ERAS	Enhanced recovery after surgery	IFG	Impaired fasting glucose
ESC/ESH	European Society of Cardiology/ European Society of Hypertension	IFN-γ	Interferon gamma
		IGF-1	Insulin-like growth factor
ESCs	Embryonic stem cells	IGFBP1	Insulin growth factor-binding proteins 1
ESPEN	European Society of Enteral and Parenteral nutrition	IGT	Impaired glucose tolerance
		IH	Intermittent hypoxia
ESRD	End-stage renal disease	IL	Interleukin (e.g., IL-1)
EVOO	Extra-virgin olive oil	IL-1ra	Interleukin-1 receptor antagonist
EWGSOP2	European Working Group on Sarcopenia in Older People	IR	Insulin resistance
		ISH	International Society of Hypertension
ExEE	Exercise energy expenditure	IV	Intravenous
FAO	Joint Food and Agriculture Organization of the United Nations	KA	Ketoacids
		Kcal	Kilocalories
FASD	Fetal alcohol spectrum disorder	Kg	Kilogram
FDA	(United States) Food and Drug Administration	LCD	Low-carbohydrate diets
		LDL	Low-density lipoprotein
FEV_1	Forced expiratory volume	LFDs	Low-fat diets
FFA	Free fatty acid	LOE	Level (quality) of evidence
FFM	Fat-free mass	LPD	Low-protein diet
FIM	Functional independence measure	LPS	Bacterial lipopolysaccharides
FM	Fat mass	LV	Left ventricle
FMD	Flow-mediated vasodilation	MAPK	Mitogen-activated protein kinase
FOXO	Forkhead box transcription factors (e.g., FOXO3A)	MCP-1	Monocyte chemoattractant protein 1
		MD	Mediterranean diet
FPG	Fasting plasma glucose	MET(s)	Metabolic equivalent(s) of task
FPS	Fried phenotype score	MI	Myocardial infarction
FVC	Forced vital capacity	MICT	Moderate-intensity continuous training
GATOR1	Gap activity toward Rags 1	MMSE	Mini Mental State Examination
GBD	Global burden of disease	MODY	Maturity-onset diabetes of the young
GC	Guanylate cyclase	MPS	Muscle protein synthesis
GDP	Guanosine diphosphate	MRI	Magnetic resonance imaging
GFR	Glomerular filtration rate	mRNA	Messenger ribonucleic acid
GH/IGF-I	Growth hormone/insulin-like growth factor I	MRV	Maximal reference value
		MTHFR	Methylenetetrahydrofolate reductase
GLP-1	Glucagon-like peptide 1	mTOR	Mammalian target of rapamycin
GTP	Guanosine triphosphate	MUFA	Mono-unsaturated fatty acids
HAAs	Heterocyclic aromatic amines	MVPA	Moderate-to-vigorous physical activity
HbA1C	Glycated hemoglobin	NADH	Nicotinamide adenine dinucleotide
HBV	High biologic value	NADPH	Nicotinamide adenine dinucleotide phosphate
HDL	High-density lipoprotein		

NCDs	Non-communicable diseases	SaO$_2$	Oxygen saturation
ncRNA	Non-coding RNA	SBP	Systolic blood pressure
ND	Nordic diet	SCFA	Short-chain fatty acid
NEAT	Non-exercise activity thermogenesis	SD	Social determinants
NF-κB	Nuclear factor-kappa B	SDA	Specific dynamic action
NFAT	Nuclear factor of activated T cells	SDAp	Seventh-day Adventist population
NHANES	National Health and Nutrition Examination Survey	sdLDL	Small dense low-density lipoprotein
		SES	Socio-economic status
NHLBI	The National Heart, Lung, and Blood Institute	SFA	Saturated fatty acids
		SNA	Sympathetic nervous system activity
NIDDM	Non-insulin-dependent diabetes mellitus	SOC	Components of successful aging: selection, optimization, and compensation
NK	Natural killer (cells)		
NO	Nitric oxide	SOD	Superoxide dismutase
NOAC	Novel oral anticoagulants	SPPB	Short physical performance battery
NPV	Non-pulmonary vein	SRS	Silver–Russell syndrome
NREM	Non-rapid eye movement	SSBs	Sugar-sweetened beverages
ODI	Oxygen desaturation index	sTNFr	Soluble tumor necrosis-factor receptors
OGTT	Oral glucose tolerance test	SWLS	Satisfaction with life scale
OSA	Obstructive sleep apnea	TC	Total cholesterol
PA	Physical activity	TEE	Total energy expenditure
PAGAC	Physical Activity Guidelines Advisory Committee	TEF	Thermic effect of food
		TF	Tissue factor
PAHs	Polycyclic aromatic hydrocarbons	TFA	Trans-fatty acids
PAI-1	Plasminogen-activator inhibitor 1	TFPI	Tissue factor pathway inhibitor
PAL	Physical-activity level	TG	Triglycerides
PANAS	Positive and negative affect schedule	TGF-β	Transforming growth-factor beta
PAP	Positive airway pressure	THF	Tetrahydrofolate
PAR	Physical-activity ratio	TM	Thrombomodulin
PBMCs	Peripheral blood mononuclear cells	TNF-α	Tumor necrosis-factor alpha
PCO$_2$	Partial pressure of carbon dioxide	TONE	Nonpharmacologic interventions in the elderly
PECAM-1	Platelet endothelial cell-adhesion molecule 1		
PEW	Protein-energy wasting	TOS	The Obesity Society
PGC	Peroxisome proliferator-activated receptor gamma co-activator	tPA	Tissue-type plasminogen activator
		TLR	Toll-like receptor
PNA	Parasympathetic nervous system activity	TUG	Timed up-and-go (test)
PNMS	Prenatal maternal stress	T1D	Type 1 diabetes mellitus
PO$_2$	Partial pressure of oxygen	T2D	Type 2 diabetes mellitus
POMA	Performance-oriented mobility assessment	UNU	United Nations University
PREDIMED	Prevencion con Dieta Mediterranea	USDA	United States Department of Agriculture
PSG	Polysomnography	VCAM-1	Vascular cell-adhesion molecule 1
PUFA	Poly-unsaturated fatty acids	VEGF	Vascular endothelial growth factor
PV	Pulmonary vein	VLCD	Very low-calorie diet
QOL	Quality of life	VLDL	Very low-density lipoprotein
RCT	Randomized controlled trial	VO$_2$max	Peak oxygen consumption
RDA	Recommended dietary allowance	VO$_2$R	Oxygen uptake reserve
RDI	Respiratory disturbance index	WC	Waist circumference
REE	Resting energy expenditure	WCRF	World Cancer Research Fund
REM	Rapid eye movement	WEMWBS	Warwick–Edinburgh mental well-being scale
RMR	Resting metabolic rate		
ROCs	Reactive oxygen-carbons	WHEL study	Women's healthy eating and living study
RoM	Range of motion	WHO	World Health Organization
ROS	Reactive oxygen species	WHOQOL-BREF	WHO quality of life-BREF
RR	Relative Risk	WINS	Women's intervention nutrition study
SACN	UK's Scientific Advisory Committee on Nutrition		

Glossary

4E-BP1: Member of the translation-repressor protein family that works as substrate of the mechanistic target of rapamycin (mTOR) signaling pathway.

***A posteriori* dietary pattern:** A data-driven approach in which dietary patterns are created using factor analysis, principal components analysis, or cluster analysis.

***A priori* dietary pattern:** Defined as the estimation of a dietary index/score based on previous food and disease association.

ABC pathway: An integrated approach for atrial fibrillation management across all healthcare levels and among different specialties. In the ABC pathway, A stands for "anticoagulation/avoid stroke", B for "better symptom management", and C for "comorbidity optimization". Compared with usual care, implementation of the ABC pathway has been associated with a lower risk of all-cause mortality, lower risk of a composite outcome of stroke/major bleeding/cardiovascular death and hospitalization, lower rates of cardiovascular events, and lower health-related costs.

Activity energy expenditure: Represents all energy expended above the resting level and includes the exercise energy expenditure (ExEE) as well as non-exercise activity thermogenesis (NEAT).

Activity theory: Asserts that an individual's life satisfaction is directly related to his degree of social interaction or level of activity.

Acute kidney injury: The sudden loss of kidney function over a period of hours or days.

Added/free sugar: Defined as "monosaccharides and disaccharides added to foods and beverages by the manufacturer, cook, or consumer, and sugars naturally present in honey, syrups, fruit juices, and fruit juice concentrates."

Adrenergic receptor: A class of G protein-coupled receptors that are targets of many catecholamines like norepinephrine (noradrenaline) and epinephrine (adrenaline) produced by the body, but also many medications like beta blockers, beta-2 (β_2) agonists and alpha-2 (α_2) agonists, which are used to treat high blood pressure and asthma.

Aerobic fitness: The ability of the circulatory and the respiratory systems to supply the necessary oxygen for the muscle during prolonged work.

Advanced glycation end products: Proteins or lipids that become glycated following exposure to sugars. They are a biomarker implicated in aging and the development, or worsening, of many degenerative diseases.

Agility: The ability to change the direction of speed and mode of response to a stimulus.

Aging: A complex process that, beyond genetic variations and biological factors, is strongly associated with the physical and social environment (race/ethnicity, culture, religion, security, social inequities, and scientific/technological advances) as well as personal characteristics (sex, ethnicity, or socio-economic status).

Aging well-being paradox: Despite age-related changes or declines in circumstances, health or income, many older adults can maintain subjective well-being in later life.

Albuminuria: Abnormal leakage of albumin into urine.

Alcohol spectrum disorders: A group of conditions that can occur in a person who was exposed to alcohol before birth. The most profound effects of prenatal alcohol exposure are cognitive and behavioral.

Amyloid beta (Aβ or Abeta): Series of peptides formed following the cleavage of the amyloid precursor protein (APP) by β- and γ-secretases that are thought to be involved in the pathogenesis of Alzheimer's disease.

Androgens: Hormones that contribute to the development and maintenance of male sex characteristics.

Angiogenesis: The physiological process through which new blood vessels are created from pre-existing vessels, formed in the earlier stage of vasculo-genesis, i.e., the process of blood-vessel formation in the embryo through the de novo production of endothelial cells.

Aromatase: An enzyme responsible for the biosynthesis of estrogens.

Atrial fibrillation: One of the most common types of cardiac arrhythmias, i.e., irregular heartbeats, which increases the risk of stroke, heart failure, and other cardiovascular-related complications.

Baroreceptors: A type of mechanoreceptors that allow for relaying information derived from blood pressure within the autonomic nervous system.

Prevention and Management of Cardiovascular and Metabolic Disease: Diet, Physical Activity and Healthy Aging,
First Edition. Christina N. Katsagoni, Peter Kokkinos, and Labros S. Sidossis.
© 2023 John Wiley & Sons Ltd. Published 2023 by John Wiley & Sons Ltd.

Binge drinking: A detrimental pattern of alcohol drinking. It is usually defined as consuming 5 or more drinks on an occasion for men or 4 or more drinks on an occasion for women. Often manifested by events such as drunkenness, hangovers, and difficulties with work.

Blue zones: Places around the world where people live longer and probably share common behavioral and lifestyle characteristics like family coherence, avoidance of smoking, plant-based diets, moderate and daily physical activity, and social engagement.

Caloric restriction: The reduction of dietary intake below energy requirements while maintaining optimal nutrition. Caloric restriction represents a nutritional intervention with the potential to attenuate aging.

Cancer survivors: People who have completed active anticancer treatments.

Cardiac rehabilitation: A medically supervised program designed to help improve cardiovascular health.

Cardio-renal syndrome: A condition in which the heart and kidneys are closely linked; the disease of one organ causes dysfunction of the other and ultimately leads to the failure of both.

Cardio-respiratory fitness: The ability of the circulatory and respiratory systems to supply oxygen during sustained physical activity.

Cardiovascular disease risk: The likelihood of an individual to experience an acute coronary or stroke event within a specific time period.

Chronic heart failure: A gradual loss of cardiac function that develops gradually over years or decades and it is characterized by trouble pumping blood through the body.

Chronic kidney disease: The gradual loss of kidney function over years or even decades, usually caused by a long-term medical condition and aggravated by additional risk factors. In general, it is defined as decreased kidney function with a glomerular filtration rate <60 mL/min/1.73 m^2 or kidney damage with an albumin:creatinine ratio ≥30 mg/g for ≥3 months.

Compression of morbidity theory: Asserts that the age of chronic illness onset may be postponed more than the age of death, thus squeezing most morbidity in life into a shorter period with less lifetime disability.

Continuous positive airway pressure: A form of positive airway pressure ventilation in which a constant level of pressure greater than atmospheric is continuously applied to the upper respiratory tract of a patient during sleep to prevent upper airway collapsing and respiratory events. It was introduced as a therapeutic approach for obstructive sleep apnea in 1981 and has been recommended as the first-line treatment for the disease ever since.

Continuous training: Endurance training characterized by a low-mid intensity, steady exercise whose duration is more than 20 min without resting intervals and that must be completed in a considerable time (e.g., sauntering or jogging).

Coordination: The ability to use the senses, such as sight and hearing, in conjunction with other body parts to perform tasks efficiently and accurately.

DASH (Dietary Approaches to Stop Hypertension) diet: The DASH diet is a plant-based dietary pattern characterized by a high intake of vegetables, fruits, whole grains, nuts; the addition of some fish, poultry, and low-fat dairy products; and the minimization of processed/red meat, sugar, and processed foods.

Developmental plasticity: The property by which a genotype produces distinct phenotypes depending on the environmental conditions during development. It is part of the organism's adaptability to environmental factors for the best chances to survive and reproduce.

Diabetes mellitus: A group of metabolic disorders characterized by chronic hyperglycemia (i.e., high concentrations of blood glucose) resulting from defects in insulin production, insulin action, or both that is associated with disturbances in glucose, lipid, and protein metabolism.

Dietary pattern: A model of eating habits according to which somebody consumes specific quantities, proportions, variety, or combinations of food groups, foods, drinks, and nutrients in his/her usual diet.

Disengagement theory: Posits that successful aging involves a voluntary disengagement from the social roles of active adult life.

Dynamic aerobic exercise: Activities with enough intensity, duration, and frequency to improve stamina or muscle strength.

Dynamic equilibrium theory: Posits that the proportion of the life span with serious illness or disability stabilizes or decreases, whereas the proportion with moderate disability or less severe illness increases.

Dynamic resistance exercise: Exercises designed to move the muscles through a specific range of motion.

Dyslipidemia/hyperlipidemia: High levels of total cholesterol, LDL-cholesterol, and/or triglycerides as well as low levels of HDL-cholesterol.

Eicosanoids: oxidized derivatives of 20-carbon poly-unsaturated fatty acids (PUFAs) formed by the cyclooxygenase (COX), lipoxygenase (LOX) and cytochrome P450 (cytP450) pathways.

eI4F4: A translation initiation factor.

Endocrine-disrupting chemicals: Chemicals such as drugs, pesticides, plastic softeners, and flame retardants that mimic, block, or interfere with hormones in the body's endocrine system and are associated with various health issues.

Endothelial dysfunction: The loss of normal endothelial function. It is a hallmark of vascular diseases and is recognized as a key early event in the development of atherosclerosis.

Endothelium: A special type of epithelium that lines the blood and lymphatic vessels. Although traditionally considered an inert, static layer in the circulatory system, the endothelium is a complex organ with important autocrine and paracrine functions.

Environmentally induced epigenetic changes: Nutritional factors, drugs, pesticides, environmental compounds, and inorganic contaminants (i.e., arsenic) that can alter the epigenome and may contribute to the development of abnormalities.

Epigenetic changes: Changes that may be caused by behavioral and environmental factors that can affect gene function.

Epigenetic diet: A class of bioactive dietary compounds such as isothiocyanates in broccoli, genistein in soybean, resveratrol in red grapes, and other commonly consumed foods that modify the epigenome leading to beneficial health outcomes.

Epigenetic marks: Modifications to DNA that regulate whether genes are turned on or off, which influences gene expression and phenotypic outcome. The most common epigenetic changes are DNA methylation, histone modification, and non-coding RNA.

Epigenetic plasticity: The ability of an individual genome to produce different phenotypes when exposed to environmental cues.

Epigenetics of aging: Epigenetics can mark accurate chronological time versus biological time, and since epigenetic modifications are often reversible, they might be a promising target for aging-intervention strategies.

Epigenetics: The study of changes in gene function that are mitotically and/or meiotically heritable and do not entail a change in the DNA sequence.

Epithelium: A type of tissue made of densely packed cells that rest on a basement membrane.

Estrogens: Hormones that contribute to the development and maintenance of female sex characteristics.

Exercise training: The use of repetitive body movements to increase endurance, flexibility, and/or muscular strength.

Exercise volume: The outcome of exercise: i) intensity, ii) duration, and iii) frequency.

Expansion of morbidity theory: Suggests that an increase in the life expectancy causes an increase in the proportion of life spent with underlying illness or disability.

Fat-free mass: Includes the skeleton, muscles, and body water.

Fetal and infant origins of adult disease hypothesis: Fetal undernutrition in middle-to-late gestation leads to disproportionate fetal growth, which predisposes individuals to certain diseases in adulthood.

Fiber(s): The edible part(s) of plants that are resistant to digestion and absorption in the human small intestine. Good fiber sources are whole grains, vegetables, pulses, and some fruits.

Fibrinolysis: A highly regulated enzymatic process that prevents unnecessary accumulation of intravascular fibrin and enables the removal of thrombi.

Fibrosis: Pathological wound healing in which connective tissue replaces normal parenchymal tissue unchecked that leads to considerable tissue remodeling and the formation of permanent scar tissue.

Flow-mediated vasodilation: The most common diagnostic assay for endothelial function in clinical practice. It measures endothelial-mediated vasorelaxation of the brachial artery in response to the release of external compression.

Folate-mediated, one-carbon metabolism: A complex network of interconnected metabolic pathways that supplies methyl groups for DNA, RNA, or protein methylation.

Forced vital capacity: The maximum amount of air that can be forcibly exhaled from the lungs after fully inhaling.

Frailty: A clinical state that frequently presents in older adults and is characterized by an increased risk of falls, institutionalization, care needs, and disability/death.

GATOR1: A subcomplex of the GATOR (SEA) complex. GATOR1 possesses Rag GTPase activating protein activity and inhibits TORC1 activity in response to amino acid starvation.

Gestational diabetes mellitus: A type of diabetes first diagnosed in the second or third semester of pregnancy without any prior diagnosis of Type 1 Diabetes or Type 2 Diabetes.

Glomerular filtration rate: A measure of how much blood (in mL) is cleaned by the kidneys per minute. It is estimated indirectly from the clearance rate of exogenous markers, such as inulin, or endogenous markers, such as creatinine and cystatin C, using equations that account for body size, assuming an average adult body size of $1.73\ m^2$.

Health: According to the World Health Organization, a state of complete physical, mental, and social well-being, and not merely the absence of disease or infirmity.

Healthy aging: The process of developing and maintaining the functional ability that enables well-being in older age.

Healthy biological aging: The maintenance, post maturity, of optimal physical and cognitive functioning for as long as possible, delaying the onset and rate of functional decline, and clinical disorders.

Healthy life expectancy: The average number of years that an individual is expected to live in a state of self-assessed good or very good health, based on current mortality rates and prevalence of good or very good health.

Healthy waist circumference: Less than 94 cm for men and 80 cm for women.

Heart failure: The American College of Cardiology/American Heart Association guidelines define HF as a "complex clinical syndrome that can result from any structural or functional cardiac disorder that impairs the ability of the ventricle to fill or eject blood."

Heavy alcohol intake: About 31–40 g per day and >50 g per day.

Heterocyclic amines: Compounds produced during cooking red meat at high temperatures, such as grilling or barbecuing and are characterized as carcinogenic.

High-intensity interval exercise: High-intensity interval training (HIIT) in combination with sprint interval training.

High-intensity interval training: Aerobic exercise at high intensity combined with active or passive recovery periods of lower intensity.

His bundle: A collection of heart muscle cells specialized for electrical conduction.

Human peripheral blood mononuclear cells: Immune cells with a single, round nucleus that originate in bone marrow and are secreted into peripheral circulation.

Hypercapnia: A condition of abnormally elevated carbon dioxide (CO_2) levels in the blood.

Hypercholesterolemia: High LDL-cholesterol levels, cardiovascular disease (CVD), or self-reported use of medication to control cholesterol.

Hypernatremia: An electrolyte problem, defined as serum sodium concentration <135 mg/L.

Hypertension: Either i) office SBP values ≥ 140 mmHg and/or DBP ≥90 mmHg following repeated examination or ii) SBP >130 mmHg or DBP >80 mmHg.

Hypoxemia: A decrease in blood oxygen saturation.

Immunosenescence: The process of immune dysfunction that occurs with age and includes remodeling of lymphoid organs that leads to changes in the immune function of the elderly.

Impaired fasting glucose: A condition in which the fasting blood-glucose level is 100 to 125 milligrams per deciliter (mg/dL), after an overnight fast.

Impaired glucose tolerance: A condition in which the blood-glucose level is 140 to 199 mg/dL (7.8 to 11.0 mmol/L) after a 2-hour OGTT.

Inflamm-aging: Chronic, sterile, low-grade inflammation during aging.

Insulin-like growth factor I: A polypeptide hormone produced mainly by the liver in response to the endocrine growth hormone (GH) stimulus. Insulin-like growth factor I is partly responsible for systemic GH activities as well as anabolic, antioxidant, anti-inflammatory, and cytoprotective actions.

Interval training: Relatively high in intensity, it includes repetitions of physical activity with periods of rest between.

Intradialytic exercise: Exercise performed on dialysis days in a renal unit, using a specially designed cycle ergometer.

Intrinsic capacity: All mental and physical capacities that a person can draw on such as their ability to walk, think, see, hear, and remember.

Isoflavones: Substituted derivatives of isoflavone, a type of naturally occurring isoflavonoids, many of which act as phytoestrogens in mammals.

Isometric resistance exercise: Contractions of a specific muscle or group of muscles.

Life-course aging model: The attainment of peak capacity for a body system that starts in early development when plasticity permits changes in structure and function induced by a range of environmental stimuli, followed by a period of decline, the rate of which depends on the peak attained and later life conditions.

Light-intensity activities: Defined as activities performed at or under 3 METs, which require the least amount of effort compared to moderate and vigorous activities.

Lipofuscin: A pigmented, heterogenous byproduct of failed intracellular catabolism conventionally found within lysosomes or the cytosol of aging postmitotic cells.

Longevity: Reaching extreme age, a standard age threshold does not exist. The synergistic result of random events, chance, environmental factors, and genetic predisposition.

Malnutrition: A state of deficiencies or excesses in energy or nutrient intake, imbalance of essential nutrients, or impaired nutrient utilization.

Mediterranean diet: The traditional dietary pattern adopted in olive-growing areas of the Mediterranean region. It is characterized by high consumption of extra-virgin olive oil (as the main edible fat), vegetables, legumes, whole grains, fruits, nuts, and seeds; moderate consumption of poultry and fish-seafood (varying with proximity to the sea); low consumption of full-fat dairy products, red meat, processed meat (cold cuts) and sweets; and low-to-moderate consumption of wine as the main source of alcohol accompanying meals.

Mediterranean lifestyle: The lifestyle of people in the Mediterranean region. It incorporates the Mediterranean diet with other lifestyle habits, such as consumption of seasonal and eco-friendly food products, regular exercise as part of family and social activities, adequate rest during the day, and traditional culinary activities, which have been identified as beneficial for health.

Meningioma: A type of central nervous system (brain or spinal cord) tumor.

Metabolic dyslipidemia: Obesity-induced dyslipidemia driven by insulin resistance.

Metabolic equivalent of task (MET): The energy cost of a given activity divided by the resting energy expenditure. Represents the amount of oxygen used during resting conditions or sitting quietly, and it is assumed to be 3.5 mL of oxygen per kg of body weight per minute (3.5 mL O_2/kg/min).

Metabolic syndrome: A clustering of metabolic abnormalities, including central obesity, insulin resistance, dyslipidemia, and hypertension that significantly increases the risk of cardio-metabolic diseases.

Metabolically healthy obesity: Obesity in the absence of a clearly defined cardio-metabolic disorder, such as metabolic syndrome, insulin resistance, hypertension, diabetes, or dyslipidemia.

Metastasis: Malignant tumors that are derived from a primary tumor and located in another part of the body.

Methods to quantify physical-activity intensity: Energy expenditure as a result of physical activity, metabolic equivalents (METs), oxygen consumption (VO_2), heart rate (HR), heart rate reserve (HRR), and specifying a percentage of oxygen uptake reserve (VO_2R).

Moderate-intensity activities: Activities that require 3.0 to 5.9 METs.

Moderate-intensity continuous training: Medium-intensity aerobic training.

Monocyte chemoattractant protein-1: One of the key chemokines that regulate the migration and infiltration of monocytes/macrophages.

mTOR signaling pathway: The mTOR signaling pathway regulates gene transcription and protein synthesis for cell proliferation and immune cell differentiation. Also plays an important role in tumor metabolism.

Mucositis: Ulceration and inflammation of gastrointestinal-tract membranes.

Multidimensional concept of successful aging: Successful aging occurs when a person has a high well-being, quality of life, and personal fulfillment.

Multiple myeloma: A type of bone-marrow cancer.

Muscular endurance: Defined as the ability of the muscle or muscle groups to perform repetitive contractions over a period of time against resistance, such as lifting a weight several times.

Muscular strength: Defined as the ability of the muscle or muscle groups to exert force during a voluntary contraction.

Myokines: Cytokines synthesized and released by myocytes during muscular contractions. They are implicated in the autocrine regulation of metabolism in the muscle and the paracrine/endocrine regulation of other tissues and organs.

Myosteatosis: Skeletal muscle fat infiltration.

Negative biology: The pathology-oriented approach for prevention and treatment.

NF-κB pathway: A family of highly conserved transcription factors that regulate inflammatory responses, cellular growth, and apoptosis.

Non-communicable diseases: Chronic medical conditions linked with genetic, physiological, behavioral, and environmental factors among others.

Obesity paradox: A phenomenon in which patients with overweight and obesity and several chronic diseases such as heart failure, atrial fibrillation, etc. as well as older adults present lower all-cause mortality compared to normal-weight and underweight patients.

Obstructive sleep apnea: A chronic pathological condition characterized by recurrent pauses of breathing during sleep due to obstruction of the upper airways, which leads to sleep disruption.

Oxidative stress: A persistent imbalance between free radicals and antioxidants in favor of the former. It is a mediator of inflammation, vascular injury, and atherosclerosis that is an important risk factor for the pathogenesis of most cardiometabolic diseases.

Peroxisome proliferator-activated receptor agonists: Substances that act upon the peroxisome proliferator-activated receptor.

Pescatarian: An individual who incorporates seafood into an otherwise vegetarian diet. Pescatarians may or may not consume other animal products such as eggs and dairy products.

Physical activity: Defined as "any bodily movement produced by skeletal muscles that requires energy expenditure."

Physical-activity domains: Opportunities for activity that include: i) occupational (i.e., work), ii) domestic (i.e., household chores), iii) transportation/utilitarian, and iv) leisure time.

Physical-activity level: A way to describe a person's daily physical activity.

Physical inactivity: Defined by an individual's inability to follow the current age group recommendations regarding weekly levels of physical activity.

Pituitary-adrenal axis: A complex set of direct influences and feedback interactions that control reactions to stress and regulate many body processes, including digestion, the immune system, mood, and emotions as well as energy storage and expenditure.

Polycyclic aromatic hydrocarbons: Compounds produced during smoking and the curing of red meat that are characterized as carcinogenic.

Polysomnography: The gold-standard method for obstructive sleep apnea diagnosis. It is non-invasive and consists of a simultaneous recording of multiple physiologic parameters related to sleep and wakefulness during night sleep in a laboratory under the supervision of specialized medical personnel.

Positive biology: Strives to understand positive phenotypes, why some individuals live a longer and healthier life without suffering from chronic diseases that most people confront much earlier in their lives.

Prediabetes: A condition characterized by blood-glucose levels that are higher than normal but not high enough to be classified as diabetes.

Prehabilitation: A process of improving the nutritional state and the functional capability of a patient before a surgery to minimize postoperative complications and improve postoperative parameters.

Prudent/healthy dietary pattern: Represents all foods and beverages consumed, including foods and beverages across all food groups in nutrient-dense forms, in the recommended amounts and within calorie limits. It is characterized by high consumption of fruits, vegetables, nuts, legumes, fish, vegetable oils (especially olive oil), and whole grains as well as low/modest consumption of red and processed meats, foods rich in refined carbohydrates (sugars), salt, and industrialized processed foods high in trans-fatty acids.

RagA/B: A heterodimer that localizes on the lysosome surface and functions to relay amino acid signals to activate the product of TOR by recruiting it to the lysosome where TOR is activated by Rheb (regulation of cell growth).

Rag GTPases: Heterodimeric complexes on vacuolar/lysosomal membranes, as central elements of an amino acid signaling network upstream of TORC1.

Reactive oxygen species: A generic term that defines a wide variety of oxidant molecules with vastly different properties and biological functions that range from signaling to causing cell damage.

Renal replacement therapy: The treatment for end-stage renal disease, usually advised to start once the estimated glomerular filtration rate is <15 mL/min/1.73 m^2. It includes dialysis, i.e., the process of removing excess water, solutes, and toxins from the blood in the form of hemodialysis, peritoneal dialysis, hemofiltration, hemodiafiltration, or intestinal dialysis as well as renal transplantation.

Residual volume: The amount of air that remains in a person's lungs after fully exhaling.

Resilience and longevity: Psychosocial resources of resilience are linked to overall functioning and survivorship among centenarians. A "robust" personality, cognitive reserves, and social and economic resources are salient resilience factors necessary for survival, optimal functioning, and well-being.

Resistance training: A type of exercise that increases muscles contraction because of an external resistance that builds strength.

Respiratory event: A temporary and partial or complete cessation/pause of breathing during sleep.

Resting energy expenditure: Represents the energy expended at rest by an individual in fasting conditions and a thermo-neutral environment.

Resting metabolic rate: See REE above.

S6K1: A serine/threonine kinase that acts downstream of PIP3 and phosphoinositide-dependent kinase-1 in the PI3 kinase pathway.

Salt-sensitivity: An increase in blood pressure in response to high dietary salt intake.

Sarcopenia: A type of progressive and generalized skeletal muscle mass and strength (muscle atrophy) that occurs with aging and/or immobility.

Sarcopenic obesity: Characterized by the combination of high percentage of body fat and sarcopenia.

Sedentary behaviors: Defined as any waking behaviors characterized by an energy expenditure ≤1.5 METs in a sitting, reclining, or lying position.

Selectins: Special adhesion molecules expressed by endothelial cells that take part in the process of atherosclerosis by contributing to the migration of monocytes to the subendothelial.

Skill-related physical fitness: It consists of six components; agility, speed, power, balance, coordination, and reaction time.

SOC successful aging: Successful aging encompasses selection of functional domains on which to focus one's resources, optimizing developmental potential (maximization of gains), and compensating for losses, thus ensuring the maintenance of functioning and a minimization of losses.

Speed: The ability to achieve high movement velocity within a short period of time.

Successful aging (Rowe's and Kahn's model): Successful aging is multidimensional, encompassing the avoidance of disease and disability, the maintenance of high physical and cognitive function, and sustained engagement in social and productive activities.

Synaptic plasticity: The ability of synapses to strengthen or weaken over time in response to increases or decreases in their activity.

Tau protein: a microtubule-associated protein predominantly expressed in the neurons that are closely associated with proper functioning of the cytoskeletal network in terms of microtubule assembly.

Telomere: A region of repetitive nucleotide sequences associated with specialized proteins at the ends of linear chromosomes.

TGF-β: Transforming growth factor-β (TGF-β) superfamily signaling plays a critical role in the regulation of cell growth, differentiation, and development in a wide range of biological systems.

Thrifty phenotype hypothesis: The epidemiological associations between poor fetal and infant growth and the subsequent development of type 2 diabetes and the metabolic syndrome result from the effects of poor nutrition in early life, which produces permanent changes in glucose-insulin metabolism.

Total energy expenditure: Represents the total energy that a person expends in a day for processes essential for life (e.g., to digest, absorb, and convert food) as well as exercise.

Trans-fatty acids: Unsaturated fatty acids with one or more unconjugated double bonds in the trans configuration.

Trans-generational epigenetics: The result of epigenetic inheritance through several different pathways, including direct inheritance through the germ line or somatic parental effects on the epigenetic state of germ cells or somatic cells.

Tumor: A mass of abnormal cells. Tumors may be benign (not cancer) or malignant (cancer).

Type 1 diabetes: Referred to as insulin-dependent diabetes mellitus.

Type 2 diabetes: Referred to as non-insulin-dependent diabetes mellitus.

Ultra-processed foods: Food that are made mainly from fats, added sugars, hydrogenated fats, and starches.

Urinary system: Also known as the renal system or urinary tract, it consists of the kidneys, ureters, bladder, and the urethra; its main function in the human body is the production, storage, and eventual removal of urine, the fluid waste excreted by the kidneys.

Uvulopalatopharyngoplasty: A surgical procedure for the management of obstructive sleep apnea that includes the removal of the tonsils, the uvula, and part of the soft palate.

Vegan diet: A dietary pattern in which animal products (e.g., meat, poultry, fish, seafood, eggs, and dairy) are not consumed.

Vegetarian diet: A dietary pattern that may include eggs (ovo-vegetarian), dairy products (lacto-vegetarian), eggs and dairy products (lacto-ovo-vegetarian), or eggs, dairy products, and fish and/or shellfish (pescetarian).

Vigorous intensity activities: Defined as activities that require 6.0 or more METs.

VO$_2$max: The maximum amount of oxygen (or true maximum aerobic capacity) that the body can use during work, and the value does not change despite an increase in workload over time.

Well-being: Represents positive emotional health, participation in valued social roles, engaging with others, leading meaningful lives, maintaining autonomy, and independence.

Whole-grain foods: A food might be labeled as whole grain "if it contains at least 30% whole-grain ingredients in the overall product and more whole grain than refined grain ingredients, both on a dry-weight basis."

Williams evolutionary hypothesis: Low adult death rates should be associated with low rates of senescence and high adult death rates with high rates of senescence. It is usually interpreted as a prediction that higher extrinsic mortality promotes either an earlier onset or a faster rate of senescence.

Xenobiotic metabolism: The process of bio transforming less polar compounds into more polar compounds that can be excreted more easily.

Index

A

AACC. *See* American Association of Cereal Chemists (AACC)
ACSM. *See* American College of Sports Medicine (ACSM)
Active aging, 98
Activities of Daily Living (ADL), 97
   assessment tools, 124–129
     Barthel index (BI), 125
     functional independence measure (FIM), 125
     Katz index (KI), 125
     Lawton Instrumental ADL Scale, 125
Activity energy expenditure (AEE), 70
Activity theory, 97
Acute decompensated HF (ADHF), 179
Acute heart failure (AHF), 172–174
Acute kidney injury (AKI), 327
Added/free sugar, 8–9
ADHF. *See* Acute decompensated HF (ADHF)
ADL. *See* Activities of Daily Living (ADL)
ADL Profile Instrumental (IADL), 125
ADT. *See* Androgen-deprivation therapy (ADT)
Adults
   BMI and waist circumference, 276
   dyslipidemia in, 268–269
   fat intake in, 141–142
   heart failure (HF) in, 176
   physical activity in, 81
   respiratory event scoring, 301
   sleep staging and arousal scoring, 301
AEE. *See* Activity energy expenditure (AEE)
Aerobic endurance, muscular endurance *vs.*, 65
Aerobic exercise/fitness, 63–64, 162, 184, 235, 250, 267, 290
Age-related diseases, 43, 110, 111
Agility, 65–66
Aging process. *See also* Healthy aging
   biology, 93–95
   cognitive decline with, 120
   hallmarks, 94
   immune system, 119
   multiple organ systems. *See* Multiple organ systems
   overview, 93–98
   phytochemicals on, 111
   procedures, 117
AHF. *See* Acute heart failure (AHF)
AHRE duration, 192
AKI. *See* Acute kidney injury (AKI)
Alcohol, 247, 350
   consumption, 29
   intake, 243, 244
All-cause mortality, 277, 336
   and cardiovascular mortality, 330
   DASH diet, 45
   hazard ratio of, 279
   MD, 39–40
   Nordic diet (ND), 48
   physical activity (PA), 81
Alzheimer's disease, 81
American Association of Cereal Chemists (AACC), 351
American College of Sports Medicine (ACSM), 83, 360
American Heart Association/American College of Cardiology (AHA/ACC), 50, 264
American Institute for Cancer Research (AICR), 347
American Society of Clinical Oncology (ASCO), 358, 359
Amygdala epigenome, 29
Anabolic resistance, 134, 371
Anaerobic fitness, 63–64
Androgen-deprivation therapy (ADT), 357
Angiogenesis, 214
Anti-atherogenic effects, 264
Anticoagulation/avoid stroke, 195, 208
Anti-inflammatory effects, 138, 142
Antioxidants, 209
Antioxidative properties plant, 144
Anxiety disorders, 28
Arachidonic acid, 141
ART. *See* Assisted reproductive technologies (ART)
ASCVD. *See* Atherosclerotic cardiovascular disease (ASCVD)
Assisted reproductive technologies (ART), 21
Atherosclerosis, 119
Atherosclerotic cardiovascular disease (ASCVD), 259, 261, 262
Atherosclerotic plaque, 260
Atrial fibrillation (AFib), 191, 374
   in athletes, 199
   complications, 194–195
   definition and classification, 192
   etiology, 192–194
   exercise training, 200
   gender-specific considerations in, 194
   management, 195–196
   nutrition in, 197–199
   physical activity and risk, 199–200
   prevalence, 191–192
   recommendations, 201
ATTICA study, 11
Autoimmune thyroid disease, 225, 230
Autonomic nervous system, 194

B

Balance, 65–66
Balance assessment, 124
Baltic Sea diet pyramid, 47
Bariatric surgery, 286
Barker hypothesis, 22–23
Barthel index (BI), 125
Basal metabolic rate (BMR), 70, 71
Basic or physical ADLs, 124
Beckwith Weidemann syndrome (BWS), 21
β-glucans, 262
Bioactive compounds, 24, 27
Biophenols, 143
Bisphenol A (BPA), 29
Blood-lipid levels, 260, 264
   exercise training and, 264–268
     HDL-cholesterol, 266–267
     intensity of, 267–268
     LDL-cholesterol, 266
   physical activity, 264–268
Blood pressure/hypertension, 50
Blue zones, 108, 136
BMI. *See* Body-mass index (BMI)
BMR. *See* Basal metabolic rate (BMR)
Body composition, 64, 276
Body fat, direct assessment of, 276
Body-mass index (BMI), 177, 178, 244
   classification, 276
   drawback, 276
Borg scale, 72
Brain-derived neurotrophic factor, 163
BWS. *See* Beckwith Weidemann syndrome (BWS)

C

Caffeine, 247
Calcium and dairy products, 352
Caloric restriction, 177
CAMs. *See* Cell adhesion molecules (CAMs)

Cancer, 42, 347
  alcoholic beverages, 350
  body composition, 357–358
  body weight, 357–358
  cachexia syndrome, 357
  calcium and dairy products, 352
  DASH diet, 46
  development, 347
  dietary fiber, 351–352
  dietary patterns, 352–353
  dietary supplements, 353
  excess body fat, 348–350
  long-term survivorship, 359–360
  mortality, 46
  nutrition, 356–359
  physical activity and, 353–354
  prehabilitation for surgery, 358–359
  prevention, 25, 355
  protective against, 26
  red and processed meat, 350–351
  risk factors, 347–350
  vegetarian dietary patterns, 51
  whole grains, 351–352
Canola oil, 46
Carbohydrates, 137–138
Carbon metabolism, 24
Cardiac rehabilitation (CR), 183
Cardio-cerebral syndrome, 176
Cardio-metabolic diseases, 10, 279, 303
Cardio-protective effects, 16-0
Cardio-renal syndrome, 329
Cardiorespiratory fitness, 64, 369
Cardiovascular diseases (CVDs), 3, 40–41, 47–48, 175, 379
  in CKD, 329
  DASH diet, 45
  dietary sodium intake and, 6
  incidence and mortality, 86
  mortality, 9
  multiple organ systems, 119
  physical-activity recommendations, 265
  risk assessment, 261
  and type 2 diabetes mellitus, 10
  unhealthy dietary patterns with, 11
  vegetarian dietary patterns, 50
Cardiovascular fitness, 64
Carotenoids, 151
Case-control studies, 11
Celiac disease, 230
Cell adhesion molecules (CAMs), 214
Cell-based assays, 207
Centenarians, 106, 109, 370
Cerebral tissue atrophy, 120
Cholesterol, 260
Chronic diseases, 3
  cancer prevention and, 25
  and non-communicable diseases (NCDs), 36
  risk, 23, 47–48
Chronic hyperglycemia, 223
Chronic hypertension, 242
Chronic kidney disease (CKD), 327, 379
  cardiovascular disorders in, 329
  complications, 329–330
  DASH diet, 46
  definition, 328
  dietary guidelines for, 332
  etiology, 329
  exercise training and, 336–338
  management, 330, 332
  mortality risk in, 335–336
  nutritional therapy in, 330
  nutrition in, 330–333
  physical activity and fitness, 333–336
  prevalence, 328–329
  protein intake for, 332
  recommendations for, 338–340
Chronic left heart failure, 172
Chronic obstructive pulmonary disease (COPD), 244
Chronic reno-cardiac syndrome, 329
Chronic sleep deprivation, 306
Cigarette smoking, 28–29, 42
cis-MUFA, 7
Cognitive-FIM, 125
Cognitive function, 100, 162–163
Cognitive impairment, 176
Coma, 230
Community-based environments, 159
Compression of morbidity theory, 108, 109
Continuous positive airway pressure (CPAP), 307–309, 377
Coordination, 65–66
Coronary heart disease (CHD), 140, 171
Costa Rican Nicoyan diet, 108
CPAP. See Continuous positive airway pressure (CPAP)
CpGs. See Cytosine–guanine site (CpGs)
C-reactive protein (CRP), 46, 309
CRP. See C-reactive protein (CRP)
CVDs. See Cardiovascular diseases (CVDs)
Cytosine–guanine site (CpGs), 20

D

Dairy products, 352
DALYs. See Disability-adjusted life-years (DALYs)
Danish Diet Cancer and Health cohort study, 47
DASH diet. See Dietary approaches to stop hypertension (DASH) diet
DCCT assay. See Diabetes control and complications trial (DCCT) assay
Dental disease, 229–230
Depression, 112
Developmental plasticity, 110
Device-based interventions, 86
DEW-IT trial, 44
Diabetes control and complications trial (DCCT) assay, 226
Diabetes mellitus (DM), 173, 176, 304, 375
  chronic complications, 229
  complications, 228–230
    amputations, 229
    dental disease, 229–230
    diabetic retinopathy, 228
    heart disease and stroke, 228
    kidney disease, 228–229
    neuropathy, 229
    of pregnancy, 230
  definition, 223
  diagnosis, 226
  epidemiology, 223–225
  exercise guidelines for, 236
  non-pharmacological, 232–236
  obesity and mortality in, 232
  physical inactivity/sedentary behavior and, 230–232
  physiology and pathophysiology, 230
  prediabetes, 226–228
  prevention/delay of, 232
  types of, 225–227
Diabetic ketoacidosis, 230
Diabetic kidney disease (DKD), 329
Diastolic blood pressure (DBP), 242, 245
Diet
  metabolic syndrome, 289–290
  and physical activity, 354–356
Dietary approaches to stop hypertension (DASH) diet, 37, 40, 44, 52, 290
  all-cause and specific-cause mortality, 45
  cancer, 46
  cardiovascular diseases, 45
  characteristics, 44
  chronic kidney disease, 46
  components, 149
  dietary pattern, 44–46
  dyslipidemia, 264
  health effects, 44–45
  hyperglycemia, 46
  hyperlipidemia, 46
  hypertension, 247–249
  to manage HF, 180
  obesity/metabolic syndrome, 45
  plant-based diets, 149–150
  type 2 diabetes mellitus, 46
Dietary fiber, 5, 137–138, 351–352
  intake, 36
  physicochemical characteristics of, 5
Dietary intervention, 111
Dietary methyl donors, 24
Dietary patterns, 209–210
  cancer, 352–353
  DASH diets, 44–46, 247
  as epigenetic mark, 25–27
  as healthy/prudent, 36
  heart failure (HF), 179–181
  Mediterranean-type, 37–44
  Nordic diet (ND), 46–48
  obesity, 280
  US-style, 51–53
  vegetarian, 48–49
Dietary Patterns Methods Project, 52
Dietary potassium, 332
Dietary reference intake (DRI), 5, 52, 246
Dietary sodium restriction, 332
Dietary sugars, 9
Diet–health interactions, 11
Dioxin, 29
Direct calorimetry, 70
Disability-adjusted life-years (DALYs), 3, 4, 79

Disease epidemiology, 21–22
Disengagement theory, 97
DKD. See Diabetic kidney disease (DKD)
DNAm. See DNA methylation (DNAm)
DNA methylation (DNAm), 20, 24, 110, 112, 133
DNA methyltransferase (DNMT), 133
Docosahexaenoic acid (DHA), 140, 308
Docosapentaenoic acid (DPA), 140
DPA. See Docosapentaenoic acid (DPA)
DRI. See Dietary reference intake (DRI)
Dry beriberi, 181
Dutch famine, 23
Dynamic equilibrium, 108
Dyslipidemia, 42
    DASH diet, 264
    diet, 262–264
    epidemiology, 259–260
    exercise training, 264–268
    LDL-cholesterol, 266
    management, 262, 263
    in older adults, 268–269
    pathophysiology, 260
    physical activity, 264–268
    prevention, 261
    risk factors, 260–261
    total cholesterol, 265
    triglycerides, 265

E

Early pregnancy, 29
EDCs. See Endocrine-disrupting chemicals (EDCs)
Eicosapentaenoic acid (EPA), 140, 246
Embryonic stem cells (ESCs), 20
Embryos, epigenetics reprogramming in, 22
Endocrine disorders, 242
Endocrine-disrupting chemicals (EDCs), 29
Endometrial cancer, 349
Endothelial dysfunction, 206–208
    angiogenesis, 214
    assessment, 207
    description, 207
    exercise training and, 211–215
    inflammation, 214–215
    management, 208
    Mediterranean diet on, 210
    nutrition and, 208–210
    oxidative stress, 211–213
    physical activity and, 210–211
Endothelial function, 205
Endothelium, 205, 206, 374
End-stage renal disease (ESRD), 327, 336
Endurance training, 64, 163, 184
Environmental factors, 20, 28, 110
EPA. See Eicosapentaenoic acid (EPA)
Epigenesis, 19
Epigenetic diet, 368
Epigenetics
    barker hypothesis, 22–23
    definition, 19–20
    and disease epidemiology, 21–22
    errors, 21
    and genetic information, 20
    mark, dietary pattern as, 25–27
    mechanisms, 20–21
    mechanisms and longevity, 110
    modifications, 21
    physical activity and alterations, 29
    reprogramming in embryos, 22
    and stress, 27–29
    in in utero and maternal lifestyle, 23–25
Epigenome, 23
Epithelium, 205, 374
Erythropoietin, 327
ESCs. See Embryonic stem cells (ESCs)
e-selectin, 46
ESPEN. See European society of enteral and parenteral nutrition (ESPEN)
ESRD. See End-stage renal disease (ESRD)
Essential amino acids supplementation, 181
Ethanol, 29
European Food Safety Authority (EFSA), 247
European Society of Cardiology (ESC) Guidelines, 179
European society of enteral and parenteral nutrition (ESPEN), 357
European Working Group on Sarcopenia in Older People (EWGSOP2), 120
EWGSOP2. See European Working Group on Sarcopenia in Older People (EWGSOP2)
Exceptional longevity, 112
Excess body fat, 348–350
ExEE. See Exercise energy expenditure (ExEE)
Exercise energy expenditure (ExEE), 70
Exercise/Exercise training, 164, 200, 235
    and chronic kidney disease (CKD), 336–338
    definition, 69
    for diabetes mellitus patients, 236
    on different tissues, 215
    duration, 76
    dyslipidemia, 264–268
    and endothelial dysfunction, 211–215
    and fibrinolysis, 213–214
    frequency, 76
    for heart failure, 182–185
    metabolic syndrome, 290
    obesity, 285–286
    and obstructive sleep apnea (OSA), 312–314
    in patients with heart failure, 184
    volume, 76
EXERDIET-HTA study, 252
Exocrine pancreas, 226
"Expansion of morbidity," 108
Expert Panel, 359

F

Fad diets, 283
FASD. See Fetal alcohol spectrum disorder (FASD)
Fast and ultraprocessed foods, 352
Fasting plasma glucose (FPG), 226
Fat-free mass (FFM), 64
Fat-free mass index (FFMI), 276
Fat intake, 138–142
Fat mass (FM), 64
Fat-mass index (FMI), 276
Fetal alcohol spectrum disorder (FASD), 29
FFM. See Fat-free mass (FFM)
FFMI. See Fat-free mass index (FFMI)
Fibrinolysis, 213–214
FIM. See Functional Independence measure (FIM)
Fitness
    aerobic and anaerobic, 63–64
    body composition, 64
    cardiorespiratory, 64
    cardiovascular, 64
    chronic kidney disease (CKD), 333–336
    flexibility, 65
    muscular, 64–65
    physical, 63
5-methylcytosine (5-mC), 20
Flexibility, 65
Flexitarian/semi-vegetarian diet, 48
Flow-mediated vasodilation (FMD), 207, 210
Fluid restriction, 179
FMD. See Flow-mediated vasodilation (FMD)
Folic acid, 209
Food groups, 36
    Mediterranean diet, 41
Foods
    meat consumption, 10–11
    nutrition and, 209
    in saturated fatty acids, 9–10
Forced vital capacity (FVC), 119
Four-stage balance test, 124
FPG. See Fasting plasma glucose (FPG)
FPS. See Fried phenotype score (FPS)
Frailty, 121–122, 176, 371
    and microbiota, 138
    physical activity and, 163
Free sugars, 137
Fried phenotype score (FPS), 121
Frugality, 37
Fruits, 351–352
    bioactive properties, 143
    flavonoids in, 143
    low consumption of, 7
    phenolic compounds in, 143
Functional ability, 99
Functional independence measure (FIM), 125
Functionality assessment tools, 124–125

G

Gait speed, 122–123
Gastrointestinal neuropathies, 229
GATOR1, 135
GDM. See Gestational diabetes mellitus (GDM)
Genetics, 19
Genocide, 28
Genome-wide association studies (GWAS), 110
Gestational age, 21
Gestational diabetes mellitus (GDM), 225, 226
Glucocorticoid receptors, 27
Glycemic index, 9
Gut-brain axis, 138
Gut microbiome, 9
GWAS. See Genome-wide association studies (GWAS)

H

Habitual physical activity, 250
Hallmarks, of aging process, 94
"Hallmarks of cancer," 347, 348
Hand-grip strength, 122, 123
Havighurst's model, 98
HDL cholesterol. *See* High-density lipoprotein (HDL) cholesterol
Health reserve, 99
Healthy aging, 42–44, 101–102. *See also* Aging process
  biomedical model, 97
  definition, 98–99
  domains and sub-domains, 101
  early concepts of, 96–97
  life-course approach to, 99–101
  longevity and. *See* Longevity
  and long-life span, 111–112
  macronutrients in, 134–142
  nutrition and, 133
  phenotype, 100, 101
  physical activity as. *See* Physical activity (PA)
Healthy biological health theory, 100
Healthy Grain Forum (2017), 8
Healthy Nordic food index, 47
Healthy/prudent diet
  definition, 36–37
  dietary patterns. *See* Dietary patterns
  effectiveness, 52
Heart contracts, 242
Heart disease, 228
Heart failure (HF), 171, 373
  ACC/AHA guidelines, 179
  classification, 172–173, 373
  clinical conditions associated with, 175
  cognitive impairment, 176
  definition, 172
  diabetes and, 176
  dietary patterns, 179–181
  exercise training in, 183–184
  intensity of activity, 184
  lifestyle factors and, 177
  malnutrition and sarcopenia, 175
  Mediterranean diet, 180–181
  nutritional supplements, 181–182
  nutrition and dietary approaches, 177–179
  obesity, 175–176
  in older adults, 176
  physical activity and exercise for, 182–185
  physical inactivity and, 182–183
  prevalence, 173–175
  tailored exercise advice in, 185
  therapeutic management, 176–177
Heart rate, 65
Heart rate reserve (HRR) method, 75–76
Helsinki Birth Cohort study, 48
Herbal infusions, 37
HF-preserved ejection fraction (HFpEF), 172, 175, 176, 181
High BP, 41
High-density lipoprotein (HDL) cholesterol, 48, 259, 260, 264, 266–267, 282
High dietary sodium intake, 5–7
High-energy density diet, 277
High-fat DASH diet (HF-DASH), 44
High-protein diets, 283
High saturated fatty acid intake, 7
High sodium intake, 3
High trans fatty acids intake, 7
Hip-bone mineral density, 143
Histone modifications, 20
Home-based CR, 184
HRmax. *See* Maximum heart rate (HRmax)
HRR method. *See* Heart rate reserve (HRR) method
Human cell membrane phospholipids, 141
Human genome, 133
Hypercholesterolemia, 259, 261, 268
Hyperglycemia, 46
Hyperkalemia, 330
Hyperlipidemia. *See* Dyslipidemia
Hypernatremia, 179
Hyperphosphatemia, 333
Hypertension, 171, 175, 228, 241, 329, 377
  classification of, 242
  co-morbidities and complications, 244
  DASH diet, 247–248
  definition, 242
  dietary strategies, 244–249
    alcohol, 247
    caffeine, 247
    dietary patterns, 247–249
    magnesium intake, 246
    sodium restriction, 245–246
    weight loss, 244–245
  management, 244, 251
  Mediterranean diet, 248–249
  Nordic diet, 249
  nutrition, 251–252
  physical activity and exercise, 250
  physical activity guidelines for, 250–251
  prevalence, 242, 244
  prevention, 244
  risk factors, 242–244
    alcohol intake, 243
    BMI, 244
    obesity, 244
    physical inactivity, 244
    sodium intake, 243
    unhealthy/poor diets, 243
  treatment goals for, 244
  vegetarian diets, 249
Hypocaloric diet, 284
Hypothalamus, 24

I

ICQC. *See* International Carbohydrate Quality Consortium (ICQC)
IDDM. *See* Insulin-dependent diabetes mellitus (IDDM)
IDL. *See* Intermediate-density lipoprotein (IDL)
IGF-1. *See* Insulin growth factor-1 (IGF-1)
IGF2 gene. *See* Insulin-like growth factor 2 (IGF2) gene
Immune system
  aging, 119
  physical activity, 162
Impaired endothelial function, 206
Inadequate dietary fiber, 138
Incidental PA, 69
Inflamm-aging, 119
Inflammation, 214–215
Instrumental ADLs (IADLs), 124
Insulin-dependent diabetes mellitus (IDDM), 225
Insulin growth factor-1 (IGF-1), 349, 350
Insulin-like growth factor 2 (IGF2) gene, 23
Insulin sensitivity index, 149
Intensity of activity, 184
INTERHEART study, 11
Intermediate-density lipoprotein (IDL), 259, 260
International Carbohydrate Quality Consortium (ICQC), 8
Intrauterine obesogenic environment, 25
Intrinsic capacity, 99
Intrinsic heart rate, 119
In utero, 23–25
  stimuli-associated epigenetic, 28
Iron supplementation, 181
Islet autoimmunity, 230, 231

K

Kahn's biomedical model, 97
Karvonen method, 75–76
"Katz-cluster," 98
Katz index (KI), 125
Kidney disease, 228–229, 327

L

Lacto-ovo-vegetarian diet, 50
Lacto-vegetarian dietary pattern, 286
Lawton Instrumental ADL Scale, 125
LCD. *See* Low-calorie diet (LCD)
Left ventricular ejection fraction (LVEF), 172, 179, 373
Leucine, 136
Life-course functional trajectories, 99
Life expectancy, 105, 106
Lipoproteins, 259
  metabolism, 260
Long-chain fatty acids, 139
Longevity, 107–108, 370
  boom, 107
  clusters, 108
  epigenetic mechanisms and, 110
  factors in blue zones, 112
  as healthy aging model, 109
  heritability of, 109–110
  sex differences, 107
Long-life span, 111–112
Long-term survivorship, 359–360
Look AHEAD trial, 236
Low-calorie diet (LCD), 281, 308, 310
Low-density lipoprotein (LDL) cholesterol, 140, 259, 260, 264, 266, 282

Low dietary fiber intake, 5
LVEF. *See* Left ventricular ejection fraction (LVEF)
Lymphatic endothelial cells, 205
Lyon diet, 180

M

Macronutrients, in healthy aging, 134–142
   carbohydrates, 137–138
   fat intake, 138–142
   protein, 134–137
Magnesium intake, 246
Malnutrition, 175
Mammalian target of rapamycin (mTOR) signaling pathway, 135
Maternal
   lifestyle, 23–25
   nutrition, 23
   overnutrition, 24–25
   undernutrition, 23–24
Maximal oxygen uptake (VO$_2$max), 74
Maximum heart rate (HRmax), 75
MD. *See* Mediterranean diet (MD)
Meat consumption, 10–11
Mediterranean diet (MD), 27, 111, 146–148, 210, 233, 372, 374, 378
   all-cause and disease-specific mortality, 39–40
   beneficial effects of, 311
   concepts and healthy properties, 27
   dietary pattern, 37–44
      all-cause and disease-specific mortality, 39–40
      beneficial effects of, 40
      cardiovascular diseases, 40–41
      dyslipidemia, 42
      foods and food groups of, 41
      healthy aging, 42–44
      hypertension, 41
      type 2 diabetes mellitus, 41–42
   dyslipidemia, 264
   health effects of, 39
   heart failure, 180–181
   hypertension, 248–249
   obesity, 283
   obstructive sleep apnea (OSA), 310–311
   plant-based diets, 146–148
Mediterranean Diet Foundation, 37, 39
Mediterranean lifestyle (MedLife), 37, 311
MedLife. *See* Mediterranean lifestyle (MedLife)
MedWeight study, 287
MET. *See* Metabolic equivalents (MET)
Metabolic acidosis, 330
Metabolically healthy obesity, 279
Metabolic disorders, 23, 24, 29
Metabolic equivalents (MET), 72–74
Metabolic syndrome (MetS), 9, 11, 42, 81, 288, 376
   DASH diet, 45
   diagnosis, 288
   epidemiology, 288
   lifestyle and risk, 288–289
   management, 289–290
   physical activity, 289, 290
   prevalence, 288
   and type 2 diabetes mellitus, 11, 23
   vegetarian dietary patterns, 50–51
Metabolism, 63
Methylenetetrahydrofolate reductase (MTHFR), 24
5,10-Methylene THF, 24
Methyl groups, 20
MetS. *See* Metabolic syndrome (MetS)
Microbiota, 138
Mini Mental State Examination (MMSE), 100
Mini Nutritional Assessment and Short Nutritional Assessment Questionnaire, 233
Mitogen-activated protein kinase (MAPK), 137
MMSE. *See* Mini Mental State Examination (MMSE)
Moderate-intensity activity, 314
Moderate-to-severe OSA, 312
Moderate-to-vigorous physical activity (MVPA), 165
Monogenic diabetes syndromes, 226
Mono-unsaturated fatty acids (MUFA), 141, 260, 264
Morbidity, concepts of, 108–109
Mortality, concepts of, 108–109
Motor-FIM, 125
MTHFR. *See* Methylenetetrahydrofolate reductase (MTHFR)
MUFA. *See* Mono-unsaturated fatty acids (MUFA)
Multidimensional approach, 97
Multiple organ systems, 118
   cardiovascular disease (CVD), 119
   frailty, 121–122
   immune system, 119
   measurements, 122–129
      balance assessment, 124
      complex balance measures, 124
      four-stage balance test, 124
      functionality assessment tools, 124–125
      gait speed, 122–123
      hand-grip strength, 122, 123
      short physical performance battery (SPPB), 124
      30-s chair test is, 124
      TUG test, 124
   musculoskeletal system, 120
   neurologic function, 120
   pulmonary, 119
   sarcopenia, 120–121
Muscular endurance, 65
   vs. aerobic endurance, 65
Muscular fitness, 64–65
   muscular endurance, 65
   oxygen consumption and heart rate, 65
   specificity principle, 65
Muscular strength, 64–65
Musculoskeletal health, 163–164
Musculoskeletal system, 120
   multiple organ systems, 120
MVPA. *See* Moderate-to-vigorous physical activity (MVPA)
Myokines, 214

N

NADPH. *See* Nicotinamide adenine dinucleotide phosphate (NADPH)
National Diabetes Prevention Program (DPP), 232
Natural biophenols, 143
NCDs. *See* Non-communicable diseases (NCDs)
ncRNA. *See* Non-coding RNA (ncRNA)
NEAT. *See* Non-exercise activity thermogenesis (NEAT)
"Negative" biology, 106
Neuroendocrine factors, 24
Neurological disorders, 81
Neurologic function, 120
Neuropathy, 229
Nicotinamide adenine dinucleotide phosphate (NADPH), 212
NIDDM. *See* Non-insulin-dependent diabetes mellitus (NIDDM)
Nocturnal symptoms, 300
Non-alcoholic fatty liver disease, 149
Non-coding RNA (ncRNA), 20, 21
Non-communicable diseases (NCDs), 3, 11
   chronic diseases and, 36
   physical inactivity, 11–13, 80
   sub-optimal diet
      dietary patterns, 11
      foods and food groups, 7–11
      in nutrients, 5–7
Non-exercise activity thermogenesis (NEAT), 70–71
Non-insulin-dependent diabetes mellitus (NIDDM), 225
Non-modifiable risk factors, 3
Non-REM (NREM) sleep, 300, 305
Nordic diet (ND), 46–48
   all-cause and specific-cause mortality, 48
   anti-inflammatory effects, 48
   chronic disease risk, 47
   health effects of, 47
   hypertension, 249
   inflammation, 48
   in older adults, 48
   plant-based diets, 148–149
n-3 poly-unsaturated fatty acids (n-3 PUFA), 140
n-6 poly-unsaturated fatty acids (n-6 PUFA), 140–141
Nutrigenomics, 27
Nutritional supplements, 181–182
   essential amino acids, 181
   iron, 181
   omega-3 poly-unsaturated fatty acid, 181–182
   thiamine, 181
Nutritional therapy, in CKD, 330

Nutrition/Nutrients
    in atrial fibrillation, 197–199
    cancer, 356–359
    in chronic kidney disease (CKD), 330–333
    and dietary approaches, 177–179
    and endothelial dysfunction, 208–210
        dietary patterns, 209–210
        obesity and weight loss, 208–209
    and exercise, 236
    and foods, 209
    and healthy aging, 133
    hypertension, 251–252
    metabolic syndrome, 290
    obesity, 285–286
    in obstructive sleep apnea (OSA), 308–311
    physical activity, 356–358
    sub-optimal diet in, 5–7
        high dietary sodium intake, 5–7
        high saturated fatty acid intake, 7
        high trans fatty acids intake, 7
        low dietary fiber intake, 5

O

Obesity, 9, 26, 42, 65, 177, 244
    assessment, 275–276
    causes, 277
    classification, 275–276
    complications and co-morbidities, 277
    DASH diet, 45
    definition, 275–276
    dietary fat model of, 277
    endothelial function, 208–209
    epidemiology, 276
    heart failure (HF), 175–176
    metabolically healthy, 279
    multi-system complications, 277
    overweight and, 275, 348
    pathogenesis, 276
    physical activity, 281
    prevention, 279–281
        dietary patterns, 280
        dietary sugar, 280
        early strategies, 279–280
        healthy weight, 280
    treatment, 281–286
        dietary strategies, 281–284
        goals, 281
        nutrition and exercise, 285–286
        pharmacotherapy and bariatric surgery, 286
        physical activity and, 284–285
        weight loss, 281
Obesity paradox, 175, 197, 276, 278–279
Obstructive sleep apnea (OSA), 378
    clinical presentation, 299
    complications, 305–306
    diagnosis, 300–302
    dietary modifications for, 308–310
    exercise training and, 312–314
    fitness, 311–312
    management, 307–308, 313
    Mediterranean diet/lifestyle in, 310–311
    nutrition in, 308–311
    pathophysiology and risk factors, 303–305
    physical activity and, 311–313
    prevalence, 302–303
    treatment modalities, 307
ODI. *See* Oxygen desaturation index (ODI)
OGTT. *See* Oral glucose tolerance test (OGTT)
Okinawan dietary patterns, 372
    plant-based diets, 150–151
Oleic acid, 42
Olive-oil polyphenols, 42
Omega-6, 140–141
Omega-3 poly-unsaturated fatty acid, 140, 181–182, 246
OmniHeart trial, 264
1-repetition maximum (1-RM), 64–65, 369
1-RM. *See* 1-repetition maximum (1-RM)
Oral glucose tolerance test (OGTT), 226
Organ-specific changes, 129
Overweight
    burden, 349
        classification, 275
        and obesity, 348
Oxidative metabolism, 29
Oxidative stress, 211–213
Oxygen consumption, 65
Oxygen desaturation index (ODI), 301

P

PAL. *See* Physical-activity level (PAL)
Pancreatitis, 226
PASS. *See* Performance assessment of self-care skills (PASS)
Pathology-oriented approach, 105
PBMCs. *See* Peripheral-blood mononuclear cells (PBMCs)
PCSK9. *See* Proprotein convertase subtilisin/ kexin type 9 (PCSK9)
Peak oxygen consumption (VO_2max), 333–334
Perceived exertion, 72
Performance assessment of self-care skills (PASS), 125
Periodontal disease, 229–230
Peripheral-blood mononuclear cells (PBMCs), 162
Peripheral muscle training, 184
Pharmacotherapy surgery, 286
Pharynx, 303
Phase-dependent therapy, 286
Physical activity (PA), 36, 112
    aerobic, 86
    atrial fibrillation, 199–200
    and cancer, 353–354
    chronic kidney disease (CKD), 333–336
    concepts of, 36
    definition, 69
    and diabetes mellitus, 230–232
    dimensions, 70
    domains, 70
    dyslipidemia, 264–268
    and endothelial dysfunction, 210–211
    and exercise. *See* Exercise
    and frailty, 163
    guidelines, 83–86
    health benefits in adults, 82
    health impact, 81–83
    of healthy aging, 161–164
        cardiovascular health, 161–162
        cognitive function, 162–163
        immune system, 162
        musculoskeletal health, 163–164
        VIVIFRAIL exercise protocol, 163–164
    for heart failure, 182–185
    hypertension, 250
        guidelines for, 250–251
    and inactivity estimations worldwide, 79–80
    intensity of, 69–76
        heart rate reserve (HRR) method, 75–76
        maximal oxygen uptake (VO_2max), 74
        maximum heart rate, 75
        metabolic equivalents, 72–74
        perceived exertion, 72
        physical-activity level, 71–72
        total energy expenditure, 69–71
        VO_2 reserve method, 76
    interventions to increase, 86–87
    metabolic syndrome (MetS), 290
    nutrition, 356–359
    and obesity, 281, 284–285
    obstructive sleep apnea (OSA), 311–312
    for older adults, 164–165
    physical inactivity, 159–161
    premature all-cause mortality, 81
    recommendations, 201
    recommendations for prevention, 354–356
    and sarcopenia, 163
    and sedentary behavior, 80–81, 159
    WHO guidelines on, 84–85
Physical Activity Guidelines Advisory Committee, 159
Physical-activity level (PAL), 71–72
Physical fitness, 64
    ACSM guidelines, 63
    components, 64
    definition, 63
    skill-related, 65
Physical function, 336–337
Physical health, 162
Physical inactivity, 11–13, 79–80, 159–161, 244, 373
    and heart failure (HF), 182–183
Phytosterols, 262
Plan de vida, 108
Plant-based diets, 49, 142–151
    DASH diet, 149–150
    Mediterranean diet (MD), 146–148
    Nordic diet (ND), 148–149
    Okinawan diet, 150–151
    plant polyphenols, 143–145
Plant polyphenols, 143–145
Plant protein sources, 136
Plasma glucose (PG), 226
Polycyclic aromatic hydrocarbons, 11

Polysomnography (PSG), 300
Poly-unsaturated fatty acids (PUFAs), 46
"Positive" biology, 106
Potassium intake, 246
Power, 65–66
Prediabetes, 226–228
PREDIMED-plus trial, 264
PREDIMED trial, 42, 283
Premature all-cause mortality, 81
Premature death, 160
PREMIER clinical trial, 44, 252
Prenatal alcohol exposure, 29
Primary hypertension, 242
Processed meat, 350–351
Progressive cellular damage, 118
Project Ice Storm, 28
Proprotein convertase subtilisin/kexin type 9 (PCSK9), 262
Protein, 134–137
Psychological stressors, 27, 28, 112
Pulmonary disease, multiple organ systems, 119
Pulmonary veins, 194

Q

Quality of life (QOL), 358

R

Randomized controlled trials (RCTs), 7, 10, 48
Range of motion (RoM), 65
Rapid eye movement (REM) sleep, 300, 301
Raw vegan diet, 142
RCTs. See Randomized controlled trials (RCTs)
Reaction time, 65–66
Reactive oxygen species (ROS), 207
Red and processed meat, 350–351
REE. See Resting energy expenditure (REE)
Renal replacement therapy, 330
Renal system, 327
Renin-angiotensin-systems, 11
REPLACE action package, 7, 8
Resistance exercise, 250
Resistance training, 65, 184, 267
Respiratory disturbance index (RDI), 301
Resting energy expenditure (REE), 70–71
Resting metabolic rate (RMR), 70
Reverse cholesterol transport, 264
Riboflavin (vitamin B2), 24
RMR. See Resting metabolic rate (RMR)
RoM. See Range of motion (RoM)
Routine physical activity, 81, 369
Rowe's biomedical model, 97
Ryuku Islands, 150

S

SACN. See Scientific Advisory Committee on Nutrition (SACN); UK Scientific Committee on Nutrition (SACN)
Salt, 6
Sarcopenia, 120–121, 163, 357, 371
  heart failure (HF), 175
  obesity in prostate cancer, 357
Saturated fatty acids (SFAs), 7, 138–140, 260
  content foods, 10
  foods and food groups rich in, 9–10
SBP. See Systolic blood pressure (SBP)
Scientific Advisory Committee on Nutrition (SACN), 8
SDA. See Seventh-day Adventist (SDA)
Secondary dyslipidemia, 259
Secondary hypertension, 242
Secondary prevention, 261
Sedentary behavior, 80–81, 369
  and diabetes mellitus, 230–232
  physical activity and, 159
  WHO guidelines on, 84–85
Sedentary time, 69
Seventh-day Adventist (SDA), 50, 108
SFAs. See Saturated fatty acids (SFAs)
Shear stress, 211
Short physical performance battery (SPPB), 124
Silver–Russell syndrome (SRS), 21
Sirtuin-FOXO pathway, 151
Skeletal-muscle gene expression, 160
Skill-related physical fitness, 65
Sleep apnea, 378
SOC. See Successful aging (SOC)
Sodium intake, 243, 244
Sodium restriction, 177–179, 245–246
Spanish centenarians, 110
Specificity principle, 65
Speed, 65–66
SPPB. See Short physical performance battery (SPPB)
SRS. See Silver–Russell syndrome (SRS)
SSBs. See Sugar-sweetened beverages (SSBs)
Stochastic events, 110
Stress, 27–29
  psychological, 28
  regulatory system, 28
Stroke, 195, 228
Structured PA, 69
Sub-optimal diet
  dietary patterns, 11
  foods and food groups, 7–11
  in nutrients, 5–7
Subsequent hypertension, 208
Successful aging (SOC), 96–98
Sugar-sweetened beverages (SSBs), 8–9, 280
Sugar-sweetened drinks, 352
Systolic blood pressure (SBP), 242, 245

T

T1D. See Type 1 diabetes mellitus (T1D)
T2D. See Type 2 diabetes mellitus (T2D)
TEE. See Total energy expenditure (TEE)
TFAs. See Trans fatty acids (TFAs)
Therapeutic management, of heart failure, 176–177
Thiamine supplementation, 181
30-s chair test, 124
Timed Up-and-Go (TUG) test, 124, 371
T-lymphocyte, 338
Total energy expenditure (TEE), 69–71
  for population group, 71–72
Toxicant, 20
t-PA antigens, 213
Trans fatty acids (TFAs), 7, 141, 260, 367
Transgenerational epigenetic inheritance, 20
TUG Test. See Timed Up-and-Go (TUG) test
Tutsi genocide study, 28
Type-4 cardio-renal syndrome, 329, 331
Type 1 diabetes mellitus (T1D), 225, 236
Type 2 diabetes mellitus (T2D), 9–11, 23, 26, 223–225, 230–236, 231
  DASH diet, 46
  Mediterranean-type dietary pattern (MD), 41–42
  vegetarian dietary patterns, 50

U

UK Scientific Committee on Nutrition (SACN), 137
Unhealthy/poor diets, 177, 242, 243
Unsaturated fatty acids
  omega-3, 140
  omega-6, 140–141
Upper-airway muscle fatigue, 303
Urinary system, 327
Urinary tract, 327
U-shaped association, 6, 9
US-style dietary pattern, 51–53

V

Vasodilation, 211
Vegetables, 351–352
  bioactive properties, 143
  flavonoids in, 143
  low consumption of, 7
  phenolic compounds in, 143
Vegetarian dietary patterns, 48–49, 142, 143
  blood pressure/hypertension, 50
  cancer, 51
  CVD risk and mortality, 50
  health effects of, 50–51
  metabolic syndrome, 50–51
  type 2 diabetes mellitus, 50
VEGF functions, 214
Ventilation–perfusion mismatching, 119
Very low-calorie diet (VLCD), 281
Very low-density lipoprotein (VLDL), 259, 260
Vigorous-intensity activity, 13, 314
Visceral adiposity index, 149
Visceral obesity, 306
Vitamin B6, 24
Vitamin B12, 24, 51
Vitamin E, 150
Vitamin K, 198
VIVIFRAIL exercise protocol, 163–164
VLCD. See Very low-calorie diet (VLCD)
VLDL. See Very low-density lipoprotein (VLDL)
VO_2 reserve method, 76

W

WCRF/AIRC. *See* World Cancer Research Fund/American Institute for Cancer Research (WCRF/AIRC)
Weight-loss, 208–209, 244–245
    diets, 281
    lifestyle modifications during, 286–287
    maintenance, 286–287
    needs, 281
Wellness programs, 86
Western diet, 11, 25, 243
Wet beriberi, 181
WHO guidelines, 137
Whole-body movements, 299
Whole-fat dairy products, 9
Whole grains, 351–352
    food products, 8
Wisconsin sleep cohort study, 302
Wolff-Parkinson-White syndrome, 191
World Cancer Research Fund/American Institute for Cancer Research (WCRF/AIRC), 42, 347, 350, 354